QUINOLONE
ANTIMICROBIAL
AGENTS 3rd Edition

QUINOLONE ANTIMICROBIAL AGENTS

3rd Edition

Edited by

DAVID C. HOOPER
Massachusetts General Hospital
Harvard Medical School
Boston, Massachusetts

and

ETHAN RUBINSTEIN
Sheba Medical Center and
Tel Aviv University
Faculty of Medicine
Tel Hashomer, Israel

ASM
PRESS

Washington, D.C.

Address editorial correspondence to ASM Press, 1752 N St. NW, Washington, DC 20036-2904, USA

Send orders to ASM Press, P.O. Box 605, Herndon, VA 20172, USA
Phone: (800) 546-2416 or (703) 661-1593
Fax: (703) 661-1501
E-mail: books@asmusa.org
Online: www.asmpress.org

Library of Congress Cataloging-in-Publication Data

Quinolone antimicrobial agents / edited by David C. Hooper and Ethan Rubinstein.—3rd ed.
      p. ; cm.
   Includes bibliographical references and index.
   ISBN 1-55581-231-7 (alk. paper)
   1. Quinolone antibacterial agents—Testing. 2. Bacterial diseases—Chemotherapy—Evaluation. I. Hooper,
David C. II. Rubinstein, Ethan.
   [DNLM: 1. Anti-Infective Agents, Quinolone—therapeutic use. 2. Bacterial Infections—drug therapy. 3.
Quinolones—pharmacology. QV 250 Q66 2003]
RM666.Q55Q56 2003
616.9'2061—dc21
                                                                                    2003051813

10 9 8 7 6 5 4 3 2 1

Cover photo: Crystal structure of the 92-kDa fragment of yeast topoisomerase II, as determined by Berger et al. (*Nature* **379**:225–232, 1996). Figure courtesy of Jonathan Heddle and Anthony Maxwell, John Innes Centre, Norwich, United Kingdom.

CONTENTS

CONTRIBUTORS

David R. Andes
Infectious Diseases and Clinical Pharmacology Sections, Department of Medicine, University of Wisconsin, and the William S. Middleton Memorial Veterans Hospital, Madison, WI 53792

Peter Ball
School of Biomedical Sciences, University of St. Andrews, Fife, Scotland, United Kingdom

Arnold S. Bayer
Division of Adult Infectious Diseases, Harbor-UCLA Medical Center, 1000 West Carson Street, Building RB2/Room 225, Torrance, CA 90509

Michael L. Bennish
Africa Centre for Health and Population Studies, P.O. Box 198, Mtubatuba, 3935, South Africa

Louis Bernard
Infectious Diseases Division and Medical Clinic II, Department of Medicine, Geneva University Hospitals, 24 Rue Micheli-du-Crest, CH-1211 Geneva 14, Switzerland

A. John Camm
Department of Cardiological Sciences, St. George's Hospital Medical School, Cranmer Terrance, London SW17 0RE, United Kingdom

William A. Craig
Infectious Diseases and Clinical Pharmacology Sections, Department of Medicine, University of Wisconsin, and the William S. Middleton Memorial Veterans Hospital, Madison, WI 53792

John M. Domagala
Department of Medicinal Chemistry, Pfizer Global Research and Development, 2800 Plymouth Road, Ann Arbor, MI 48105

Karl Drlica
Public Health Research Institute, 225 Warren Street, Newark, NJ 07103

Michael N. Dudley
Pharmacology and Microbiology, Essential Therapeutics, Inc., 850 Maude Ave., Mountain View, CA 94034

G. M. Eliopoulos
Department of Medicine, Beth Israel Deaconess Medical Center, Boston, MA 02215, and Harvard Medical School, Boston, MA 02115

Jørgen Engberg
Department of Gastrointestinal and Parasitic Infections, Division of Diagnostics, Statens Serum Institut, Artillerivej 5, DK-2300 Copenhagen S, Denmark

James Ferguson
Photobiology Unit, Ninewells Hospital and Medical School, Dundee DD1 9SY, Scotland, United Kingdom

Faryal Ghaffar
Southwestern Medical School, 5323 Harry Hines Boulevard, Dallas, TX 75235-9063

Thomas D. Gootz
Pfizer Global Research and Development, Mail stop 8200-40, Eastern Point Road, Groton, CT 06340

Jennifer Rubin Grandis
Department of Otolaryngology, University of Pittsburgh, Pittsburgh, PA 15213

Kalpana Gupta
Department of Medicine, Division of Allergy & Infectious Diseases, University of Washington School of Medicine, 1959 NE Pacific Street, BB1221, Mailstop 356523, Seattle, WA 98195

Susan E. Hagen
Department of Medicinal Chemistry, Pfizer Global
Research and Development, 2800 Plymouth Road,
Ann Arbor, MI 48105

David C. Hooper
Division of Infectious Diseases, Massachusetts
General Hospital, Harvard Medical School, 55 Fruit
Street, Boston, MA 02114-2696

Adolf W. Karchmer
Division of Infectious Diseases, Beth Israel
Deaconess Medical Center , 330 Brookline Avenue,
Kennedy-6A, Boston, MA 02215-5399

Thuan P. Le
Division of Pediatric Infectious Diseases, Harbor-
UCLA Medical Center, 1124 West Carson Street,
E-6, Torrance, CA 90509

Daniel Lew
Infectious Diseases Division and Medical Clinic II,
Department of Medicine, Geneva University
Hospitals, 24 Rue Micheli-du-Crest, CH-1211
Geneva 14, Switzerland

Hartmut Lode
Department of Pulmonary Infectious Diseases, City
Hospital Zehlendorf/Heckeshorn, Freie Universität
Berlin, Zum Heckeshorn 33, D-14109 Berlin,
Germany

Donald E. Low
Department of Microbiology, Toronto Medical
Laboratories and Mount Sinai Hospital, and
University of Toronto, 600 University Ave., Rm.
1487, Toronto, Ontario M5G 1X5, Canada

Lionel Mandell
Division of Infectious Diseases, McMaster
University, Hamilton, Ontario L8V 1C3, Canada

Martin Mayers
Department of Ophthalmology, Bronx Lebanon
Medical Center, Albert Einstein College of
Medicine, Bronx, NY 10457

George H. McCracken, Jr.
Southwestern Medical School, 5323 Harry Hines
Blvd, Dallas, TX 75235-9063

Michael H. Miller
Center for Immunology and Microbial Disease,
Departments of Ophthalmology and Medicine,
Albany Medical College, Albany, NY 12208

Kurt G. Naber
Urologic Clinic, Hospital St. Elisabeth, D-94315
Straubing, Germany

S. Ragnar Norrby
Swedish Institute for Infectious Disease Control,
Nobel's Vg 18, SE17182 Solna, Sweden

Neil Osheroff
Department of Biochemistry, School of Medicine,
Vanderbilt University, Nashville, TN 37232-0146

Rosanna W. Peeling
Sexually Transmitted Diseases Diagnostics
Initiative, The World Health Organization, Geneva,
Switzerland

Ronald E. Polk
Department of Pharmacy, School of Pharmacy,
Virginia Commonwealth University, Smith Building
Room 454, 410 North 12th Street, Richmond, VA
23298-0533

Roula Qaqish
St. Louis College of Pharmacy, 4588 Parkview
Place, St. Louis, MO 63110-1088

Didier Raoult
Unité des Rickettsies CNRS UMR 6020, Faculté de
Médecine, Université de la Méditerranée, 27,
Boulevard Jean Moulin, 13385 Marseille Cedex 05,
France

Jean-Marc Rolain
Unité des Rickettsies CNRS UMR 6020, Faculté de
Médecine, Université de la Méditerranée, 27,
Boulevard Jean Moulin, 13385 Marseille Cedex 05,
France

Allan R. Ronald
Division of Infectious Diseases, St. Boniface
Hospital, 409 Tache Avenue, Winnipeg, Manitoba
R2H 2A6, Canada

Ethan Rubinstein
Unit of Infectious Diseases, Sheba Medical Center,
Tel Aviv University, Tel Hashomer 52621, Israel

W. Michael Scheld
Department of Medicine, University of Virginia
School of Medicine, P.O. Box 801342,
Charlottesville, VA 22908-1342

Joseph S. Solomkin
Division of Trauma and Critical Care, Department
of Surgery, University of Cincinnati, 231 Albert B.
Sabin Way, Cincinnati, OH 45267-0558

Ralf Stahlmann
Institute of Clinical Pharmacology and Toxicology, Freie Universität Berlin, Garystrasse 5, D-14195 Berlin, Germany

Walter Stamm
Department of Medicine, Division of Allergy & Infectious Diseases, University of Washington School of Medicine, 1959 NE Pacific Street, BB1221, Mailstop 356523, Seattle, WA 98195

C. Thauvin-Eliopoulos
Department of Medicine, Beth Israel Deaconess Medical Center, Boston, MA 02215, and Harvard Medical School, Boston, MA 02115

Allan R. Tunkel
Division of Infectious Diseases, Department of Medicine, Drexel University College of Medicine, 3300 Henry Avenue, Philadelphia, PA 19129

Francis Waldvogel
Infectious Diseases Division and Medical Clinic II, Department of Medicine, Geneva University Hospitals, 24 Rue Micheli-du-Crest, CH-1211 Geneva 14, Switzerland

Henrik C. Wegener
Danish Zoonosis Centre, Danish Veterinary Institute, Bülowsvej 27, DK-1790 Copenhagen V, Denmark

Yee Guan Yap
Department of Cardiological Sciences, St. George's Hospital Medical School, Cranmer Terrance, London SW17 0RE, United Kingdom

Michael R. Yeaman
Division of Adult Infectious Diseases, Harbor-UCLA Medical Center, 1000 West Carson Street, Building RB2, Torrance, CA 90509

Lowell S. Young
Kuzell Institute for Arthritis & Infectious Diseases, California Pacific Medical Center, 2200 Webster Street, Suite 305, San Francisco, CA 94115

Victor L. Yu
Infectious Disease Section, VA Medical Center, and University of Pittsburgh, Pittsburgh, PA 15240

PREFACE

The quinolone class of antimicrobial agents has emerged as one of the most widely used classes of antimicrobials in clinical medicine. For this reason, the first edition of *Quinolone Antimicrobial Agents* was organized to bring together in a single volume information about their chemistry, antimicrobial activity, pharmacology, and clinical uses. As their use and numbers increased, additional information was covered in the second edition. Now with the substantial amount of new information on these agents that has become available since the publication of the second edition of *Quinolone Antimicrobial Agents* in 1993, an expanded third edition has been organized in a single, convenient volume to include comprehensive coverage of current information on a larger number of compounds, their clinical applications, and the limitations to their use, including updates on the important and expanding data on bacterial resistance and profiles of adverse effects. Like the first and second editions, this edition is designed for use by clinicians, clinical microbiologists, pharmacologists, pharmacists, basic scientists, and others needing information about these drugs.

The third edition of *Quinolone Antimicrobial Agents* now includes 30 chapters organized into sections on mechanisms and spectrum of activity and resistance (5 chapters), pharmacology (3 chapters), clinical applications (16 chapters), and adverse and other effects (6 chapters). All chapters are either new or completely updated. The area of greatest expansion has been in the section on adverse and other effects because of the substantial body of new information in this area that has become available since the second edition.

We are grateful for all of the considerable efforts of the authors of the individual chapters and the assistance and patience of the editors at ofthe American Society for Microbiology ASM Press. Particular thanks are due to our families for their patience, support, and inspiration during this project.

David C. Hooper
Ethan Rubinstein
April 2003

INTRODUCTION

The quinolones (also called fluoroquinolones, 4-quinolones, and quinolone carboxylic acids) are analogs of the earlier developed agent nalidixic acid. Although nalidixic acid is a related naphthyridone, this chemical group is now generally included within the quinolone class. Nalidixic acid, the first member of the class, was originally isolated by Lesher and associates (1) from a distillate during chloroquine synthesis and thus was a by-product of antimalarial research (2). Additional older analogs include oxolinic acid, pipemidic acid, and cinoxacin. These older or first-generation analogs are not considered further in this book, except for purposes of comparison with the newer agents.

The second generation of quinolones, about which we have considerable information, includes norfloxacin, ciprofloxacin, ofloxacin, enoxacin, and pefloxacin. These agents are substantially more potent in vitro and have broader antibacterial spectra than nalidixic acid but maintain the favorable property of being absorbed after oral administration. Additional advantageous pharmacologic properties include relatively long half-lives due to slow of elimination that allow twice-daily dosing, excellent distribution into many tissues and body fluids, and penetration into human cells, resulting in antimicrobial activity in so called "sanctuaries" as well as against some intracellular pathogens. Although differences in spectra of activity exist, this generation of quinolones in general exhibits striking potency against enteric gram-negative bacilli;, additional lesser activity against nonenteric, gram-negative bacilli and some staphylococci;, and generally marginal activity against streptococci and anaerobes.

The third generation of quinolones that followed maintained many of the favorable properties of the second generation and added increases in potency against gram-positive bacteria and, in some cases, against anaerobes and mycobacteria and in many cases also added longer half-lives of elimination that supported once-daily dosing. A few compounds in the second generation (e.g., lomefloxacin and fleroxacin) also had long half-lives and once-daily dosing, and others (e.g., sparfloxacin, and tosufloxacin) had enhancements of activity against gram-positive and anaerobic bacteria, but none became widely used in the United States and in Europe. The earliest of the third third-generation compounds was temafloxacin, and later in succession levofloxacin, trovafloxacin, gatifloxacin, and moxifloxacin became members of this group.

In general, the tolerability of many of the marketed quinolones has been good and comparable to that of other commonly used classes of antimicrobials, and with many of the second-generation agents and some of the third-generation agents have been given to millions of patients. Some adverse effects related to particular structural properties were recognized among second-generation agents, e.g., the photosensitivity caused by lomefloxacin and sparfloxacin due to a halide substituent at position 8, were recognized. Other adverse effects were unexpected and incompletely recognized until after drug release, e.g., a hemolytic uremic syndrome with temafloxacin and severe hepatotoxicity with trovafloxacin, were unexpected and incompletely recognized until after drug release, resulting in part because of the rarity of their occurrence. The mechanisms of some of these rare reactions are still incompletely understood, and thus the tolerability of each member of the quinolone class must be considered individually.

The information provided in the third edition of *Quinolone Antimicrobial Agents* is organized into sections on mechanisms and spectrum of activity and resistance (5 chapters), pharmacology (3 chapters), clinical applications (16 chapters), and adverse and other effects (6 chapters). All chapters are either new or completely updated. The area of greatest expansion has been in the section on adverse and other effects because of the substantial body of new information in this area that has become available since the second edition.

REFERENCES

Lesher, G.Y., E. D. Forelich, M. D. Gruet, J. H. Bailey, and R. P. Brudage. 1962. 1,8-Naphythyridine derivatives. A new class of chemotherapeutic agent. *J. Med. Pharm. Chem.* 5:1063-1068.

Neu, H.C. 1987. Ciprofloxacin: an overview and prospective appraisal. *Am. J. Med.* 82(Suppl. 4A):395-404.

I. MECHANISMS AND SPECTRUM OF ANTIBACTERIAL ACTIVITY AND RESISTANCE

Chapter 1

Structure-Activity Relationships of the Quinolone Antibacterials in the New Millennium: Some Things Change and Some Do Not

JOHN M. DOMAGALA AND SUSAN E. HAGEN

No one disputes the enormous impact of the fluoro-quinolones on the modern antibacterial armamentarium. Indeed, their broad spectrum of activity and excellent pharmacokinetic properties make the quinolones almost ideal antimicrobial agents and have propelled such compounds as ciprofloxacin, ofloxacin, and moxifloxacin to therapeutic success. However, no drug class is without its undesirable side effects, and the quinolones are no exception; phototoxicity, theophylline interactions, central nervous system (CNS) effects, and clastogenicity have all been observed. Since the late 1960s scientists have probed each position of the quinolone molecule attempting to improve potency, broaden spectrum, and reduce the recognized side effects. Indeed, many recently developed quinolones result from attempts to ameliorate side effects rather than from efforts to improve antibacterial potency.

The complex interrelationships between structure, antibacterial activity, and side-effect profile have been detailed in recent review articles such as (but not limited to) those authored by Lietman (70), Kim et al. (57), and Applebaum and Hunter (4). The review by Domagala in 1994 (18) represented one of the first attempts to simultaneously delineate the structure-activity relationships (SARs) of both activity and side effects providing some insights as to where the future of the quinolones might reside. A significant conclusion of this work was that the side chain at C-7 in conjunction with that at C-8 would be the main focus of successful quinolone manipulation; all other positions were viewed as optimal. Many of these observations from 1994 have been proven correct, although some recent developments in this area were not predicted. The purpose of this particular review is to summarize developments in the SAR of the quinolones with respect to potency and side-effect potential, with particular emphasis on those studies conducted after 1994.

THE 1 POSITION

Because of the toxicities associated with temafloxacin (structure 1) and trovafloxacin (structure 2), a great deal of scrutiny has been focused on substitution at N-1. Although both molecules contain a 2,4-difluorophenyl at this position, only circumstantial evidence exists to suggest that this particular N-1 substituent is to blame for the idiosyncratic organ toxicities that have restricted the use of these two agents. However, it has been postulated that agents with this particular moiety may be associated with a higher incidence of CNS adverse effects (71).

(1) temafloxacin   (2) trovafloxacin

New substituents at the 1 position include the chiral fluorocyclopropyl exemplified by sitafloxacin (DU-6859A, structure 3) (59, 84). Addition of the fluorine to the cyclopropyl group does not measurably improve antibacterial potency, gyrase activity, or solubility, when compared with the unsubstituted cyclopropyl. The chiral form of the fluorocyclopropyl group slightly affects the overall antibacterial activity, with a two- to fourfold difference in potency between the most active stereoisomer and the least active; overall, the *cis* isomer was more efficacious than the *trans* isomer. However, the fluorinated analog does not induce micronuclei when assayed in mouse bone marrow cells, suggesting that it is less genotoxic than the nonfluorinated parent (59).

John M. Domagala and Susan E. Hagen • Department of Medicinal Chemistry, Pfizer Global Research and Development, 2800 Plymouth Road, Ann Arbor, MI 48105.

(3) sitafloxacin

Researchers at Wakunaga synthesized a series of *N*-(5-amino-2,4-difluorophenyl) derivatives in an obvious extension of the trovafloxacin/temafloxacin work (3, 40a). The resulting compounds (structures 4 and 5) contain either an aminoazetidine (structure 4) or an amino group (structure 5) at the 7 position. In general, these compounds possess good in vitro activity (especially against gram-positive organisms) but display limited oral bioavailability. No SAR studies on this series have been published; however, it does not appear that the addition of the amino group to the difluorophenyl parent affects antibacterial potency to an appreciable degree.

(4)   (5)

This work was further elaborated to include *N*-fluoropyridyl analogs such as DW-116 (fandofloxacin) (51, 52, 110) (structure 6) and WQ-3034 (structure 7) (106). A SAR study of fandofloxacin analogs reveals that the 2-pyridyl is more active than the 4-pyridyl isomer in the monofluorinated series, although this activity is still greatly inferior to ofloxacin in vitro (110). In vivo, the activity of DW-116 approaches that of ofloxacin, an apparent contradiction attributed to its excellent pharmacokinetic properties (51, 110). Again, no direct comparisons between the phenyl and pyridyl compounds exist in the literature; it appears, however, that difloxacin (structure 8, the phenyl analog of DW-116) is similar to ciprofloxacin and ofloxacin in vivo (14). This result suggests that the pyridyl substitution offers little if any advantage over the original phenyl compound. Indeed, published data indicate that the phenyl compound (structure 8) possesses the same excellent pharmacokinetic properties attributed to the pyridyl derivative (DW-116) in single-dose human studies (35, 52). For example, after administration of a single 200-mg dose, the measured half-life ($t_{1/2}$) of the pyridyl analog 6 is reported to be 20.6 h, virtually identical to the half-life reported for the phenyl analog 8 (21.6 h [35])

(6) DW-116   (7) WQ-3034   (8) difloxacin

A formal quantitative structure-activity relationship (QSAR) study of the N-1 phenyls reveals that the presence of a hydroxyl group increases gyrase potency but decreases whole-cell activity. Smaller substituents at N-1 and lower lipophilicities also boost gyrase activity (53). It has been reported that a benzyl moiety at N-1 decreases activity, with these analogs displaying activity inferior to that of norfloxacin (95). *t*-Butyl groups continue to appear at the 1 position, especially in the design of mycobacterial agents, and in some cases appear as active as the cyclopropyl group, at least in vitro (62).

In summary, then, the new N-1 substituents offer no sustained significant advantages over previous benchmarks. Toxicity issues surrounding the 2,4-difluorophenyl moiety, although unexplained, have virtually eliminated these particular derivatives as potential antibacterial agents. Thus, the cyclopropyl group, with or without a fluorine substituent, remains the N-1 substituent of choice.

THE 2 PYRIDONES

The 2 pyridones, which were introduced in 1994, represent a new structural class of "quinolone-type" antibacterials. This new class was derived by moving the N-1 group of the quinolone core (structure 9) to the bridgehead position to form the 2-pyridone core 10. While no longer a quinolone by name or by numbering convention, molecular modeling calculations (30) and X-ray crystallography reveal close similarities to the prototypical quinolone structure.

(9)   (10)

At first glance the SAR of the 2 pyridones also appears to follow that of the quinolones: a C-1 cyclopropyl, the 7-fluoro (6-fluoro in structure 9) positioned next to a basic heterocyclic side chain at C-8, and the retention of the 3-carboxyl and the 4-carbonyl groups. But on closer inspection, the SAR differs from the quinolones by being more restrictive with less positional variation allowed (68). For example, the classical naphthyridines (X = N in the quinolone nucleus 9) represent a very robust group of agents including trovafloxacin, tosufloxacin, and gemifloxacin. However, in the 2-pyridone series, setting X to N reduces both in vitro and in vivo efficacy (69). In fact, for the quinolones X may be CH, CF, CC1, CBr, CCH$_3$, C–CH$_2$CH$_3$, C–OCH$_3$, and C–OCH$_2$CH$_3$, while for the 2 pyridones C–CH$_3$ is most preferred and the halogens actually diminish activity. It appears that the C-7 fluorine cannot be removed (68).

While the SAR is narrower, the 2-pyridone nucleus is often as active or more active than the closest quinolone comparator (69), as exemplified by comparing structures 11 and 12. The animal pharmacokinetics and in vivo efficacy are also superior for 11 (versus 12) and for the 2-pyridone isostere of ciprofloxacin versus ciprofloxacin. In addition, the 2 pyridones were always more active against ciprofloxacin-resistant organisms than the corresponding quinolone (Table 1; see row 2).

(11) ABT 719 2 Pyridone   (12) 4 Quinolone

After extensive side-chain optimization, two analogs were chosen for additional study. ABT 719 (structure 11) was selected initially because of its excellent activity in vitro and in vivo and because of its simpler side-chain structure. Unfortunately, the selectivity for gyrase over mammalian topoisomerase was poor, leading to clastogenicity (92). Following the published clastogenicity SAR, bulk was added to the side chain to produce A 170568 (structure 13, reference 5). Compound 13 was less toxic in general than ABT 719 and it showed no activity against mammalian topoisomerase II (Top II) at >100 µg/ml. For the most definitive review of the 2-pyridone area the article by Li et al. is highly recommended (69).

Table 1. MICs of structures 11 and 12

Organism	MIC (µg/ml)	
	11	12
Staphylococcus aureus	0.01	0.05
S. aureus (ciprofloxacin resistant)	0.78	12.5
Enterococcus faecium	0.02	0.1
Streptococcus pyogenes	0.02	0.1
Escherichia coli	0.002	0.01

(13) A 170568

POSITIONS 2, 3, AND 4

Conventional wisdom in the quinolone area dictates that the 3-carboxylic acid and the 4-carbonyl moieties are required for binding to the gyrase complex and are thereby essential for antibacterial activity. A broad series of quinolones containing various acid replacements at the 3 position was reported in which several such analogs did show activity in a limited in vitro screen (80). In particular, the nitroacetyl derivative 14 showed excellent activity against *Staphylococcus aureus* (0.025 µg/ml) and *Escherichia coli* (0.013 µg/ml). The authors concluded that antibacterial activity parallels the acidity of the functionality at C-3; in the nitroacetyl group, it was estimated that the pK$_a$ of the hydrogen at C-3 was just as acidic as the carboxyl proton in the standard quinolone.

(14)

Successful substitution in the 2 position remains limited to sulfur-bearing rings, such as NM394 (structure 15). As might be expected, the chirality of the methyl group in the N-1–C-2 ring is important, with the (*S*) form being favored by a factor of two- to fivefold. It has been shown previously that the (*S*) forms of chiral C-8–N-1 tricyclic quinolones (such as ofloxacin and T-3761) are much more potent than the corresponding (*R*) isomers (93). Attempts to substitute an oxygen atom at C-2 as part of a heterocyclic ring provide the expected results: the oxygen-containing analogs (structure 16) show no antibacterial activity (15).

(15) NM394   (16)

Extending the tricycle work into tetracycle analogs has been reported (structure 17). These derivatives contain no nitrogen at the 1 position but do have the requisite sulfur atom at the 2 position and a variety of heteroatoms at the 8 position. A slight preference for a nitrogen atom at C-8 versus oxygen was noted. The resulting derivatives possess good in vitro activity (MICs ranging from 0.0125 to 0.4 μg/ml against gram-positive organisms and 0.05 to 1.56 μg/ml for gram-negative organisms) but little in vivo efficacy (48). For this reason, these compounds remain more curiosity than true developmental candidates.

(17) X = NR, O, S

THE 5 POSITION

At the time of the 1994 review, only three substituents at position 5 had ever been shown to increase in vitro potency over hydrogen: NH_2 (19, 111), CH_3 (39), and OH (19). The former two have been exemplified in several advanced compounds (structures 18–21). Other small substituents such as F (77) and Cl (111) were neutral or caused decreased activity. All larger substituents, CH_2CH_3 (39), $NHCH_3$ (20, 111), $N(CH_3)_2$ (20, 111), and NHAc (20), were significantly less active. This SAR seems to hold true over all types of quinolones and 2 pyridones regardless of the other substitutions.

In general, the 5 substituent did not have a major impact on pharmacokinetics because its primary advantage was potency and improved spectrum. Sparfloxacin (structure 18) and grepafloxacin (structure 19) both displayed excellent in vitro potency and good pharmacokinetics in humans, but are less attractive because of side effects (6). Sparfloxacin showed a high incidence of phototoxicity (due to the 8-fluorine and a particularly high skin penetration). Interestingly, the 5-NH_2 group generally reduces phototoxicity (111). Both agents displayed QT prolongation (6), which is not related uniquely to the 5 substituent. In certain series, the 5-NH_2 and 5-CH_3 groups have been reported to enhance genetic toxicity risk (97).

(18) sparfloxacin

(19) grepafloxacin

(20) D61-1113 (86, 98)

(21) BMY 43748 (9)

THE 6 POSITION

The fluoroquinolones derived their name from the dogma that the 6-fluoro group was an essential feature of the broad-spectrum quinolones that first appeared in the late 1970s (11). The 6-fluorine was shown to improve gyrase inhibition of enoxacin and norfloxacin by 15- to 18-fold and cell penetration by another three- to fourfold, leading to MIC decreases of 10- to 100-fold over the respective 6-hydrogen derivatives (22). Nearly all medicinal chemists kept the 6-fluorine constant for the next 30 years with great success. In 1992, however, Ledoussal (66) reported that certain highly potent 6-fluoroquinolones (structure 22) could, in fact, retain their in vitro activity even when the 6-fluoro group was removed (structure 23). When the 6-fluoro group from the less potent derivative 24 was removed (producing structure 25), the loss in activity was substantial. Perhaps the strong inhibitory contributions of the N-1 cyclopropyl group, the C-8–F and the pyrolidine side chain found in structure 23 were more than enough to compensate for the loss of the C-6–F. Armed with these new data several groups reevaluated the fluoroquinolone SAR without the 6-fluorine.

	R-6	R-8
(22)	F	F
(23)	H	F
(24)	F	H
(25)	H	H

In the first approach, Cecchetti et al. examined a series of 6-aminoquinolones (12, 13). Simple replacement of the 6-fluoro of ciprofloxacin with NH_2 (structure 26) reduced the activity by 28- to 300-fold (12). The literature cited above suggested the need for a substituent at C-8 that was absent in ciprofloxacin. Leaving the 6-amino group constant, positions 5, 7, and 8 were optimized to produce the tetrahydroisoquinolone 27 (MF 5137) (13).

(26)   (27) MF 1537

This agent (MF 1537, structure 27) was 8 to 62 times more active than ciprofloxacin against gram-positive clinical isolates, although its gram-negative activity was less interesting (108). More importantly, MF 1537 maintained its potency versus ciprofloxacin-resistant isolates (13). The 6-amino group did not appear to enhance pharmacokinetic parameters in animals, as structure 27 was less active in mouse chemotherapy experiments than would have been predicted by its MIC (13). The 6-amino group did appear to reduce CNS liability when compared with a 6-H (17).

Other workers explored replacing the 6-fluorine with a methyl group (structure 28a,b) (44, 58). When compared with ciprofloxacin, structure 28a was four to eight times less active versus all organisms except for ciprofloxacin-resistant *Staphylococcus*, where the MIC of structure 28a was 2 µg/ml relative to >128 µg/ml for ciprofloxacin (58). The addition of a 5-amino group (structure 28b) (44) increased potency by two- to fourfold, making structure 28b quite similar to ciprofloxacin in vitro. The best compound from this research was LB 20226 (structure 29) (58), which was more active than ciprofloxacin against gram-positive organisms, but which also contains the aminomethyl pyrolidinyl side chain associated with genotoxicity (16, 97).

(28a) X = H   (29) LB 20226
(28b) X = NH$_2$

In a very systematic study, Gray and coworkers (36) compared a C-6 fluorine with a 6-NH$_2$, NO$_2$, H, Me, and Br in compound 30. The results (shown in Table 2) reveal that the 6-fluorine is superior to the amino substituent by 16- to 200-fold with superiority over Me and Br ranging from 4- to 100-fold. The analysis also reveals that, as suggested by Ledoussal, the 6 hydrogen is equivalent to the 6-fluoro substituent in conferring activity to structure 30, even at the enzyme level. Researchers at Procter and Gamble further examined the 7 and 8 positions holding R-6 = H. They found that for any side chain, a F, C1, OMe, or Me at C-8 were equally effective substituents in vitro but the 8-OMe showed the best selectivity for bacterial gyrase over mammalian topoisomerase (66). They also showed that the traditional fluorine at C-6 was a contributor to genotoxicity as shown in Table 3.

Table 2. MICs and gyrase inhibition of compound 30

Organism	MIC and gyrase inhibition (µg/ml) with the following at position 6:					
	F	H	NH$_2$	NO$_2$	Me	Br
S. aureus	0.03	0.008	8	4	0.25	0.25
S. pneumoniae	0.06	0.25	1	4	8.0	1
E. coli	0.016	0.008	0.25	0.5	0.03	0.06
Gyrase IC$_{50}$	0.2	0.5	3.2	1.6	1.6	3.2

(30)   (30a)

From this work three compounds (structures 31a to 31c) warranted further evaluation. These agents were highly active against *S. aureus*, methicillin-resistant *S. aureus* (MRSA), and *Streptococcus pneumoniae* while maintaining relevant gram-negative potency (7, 10). As with the previous desfluoro examples, compounds 31a to 31c display potent activity [MIC at which 90% of the isolates tested are inhibited (MIC$_{90}$) ″ 2.0 µg/ml] against quinolone-resistant isolates (88). The lack of the 6-fluoro did not reduce the spectrum since these quinolones were also very potent against *Mycoplasma*, *Chlamydia*, and *Legionella* (24). The pharmacokinetics in animals were also unaffected by the removal of the 6-fluorine (74), leading to excellent animal efficacy (8). With regard to side effects, these desfluoro quinolones showed less clastogenicity (40)

Table 3. Effect of a fluorine at position 6 on genotoxicity

Group at position 8	Group at position 6	% of micronucleated/binucleated cells at 64 µg/ml
F	F	50
	H	NS[a]
OMe	F	7.5
	H	NS[a]

[a]NS, no significant percent.

and less CNS activity (78) than their 6-fluoro quinolone comparators.

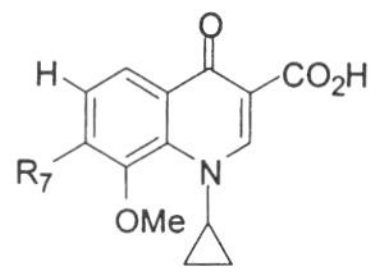

(31a) R-7 = 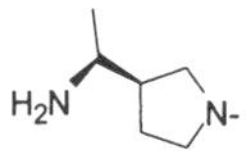   PGE 9262932

(31b) R-7 = 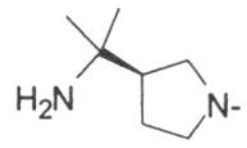   PGE 4175997

(31c) R-7 = 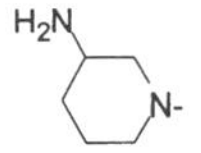   PGE 9509924

Another approach to removing the 6-fluorine involved the replacement of the carbon and the fluorine with nitrogen to give structure 32. This substitution was not favorable because structure 32a was much less active than the corresponding C-6–H analog (36); when R-8 was changed to methyl for several R-7 side chains, the loss in activity was consistently 2- to 10-fold (87).

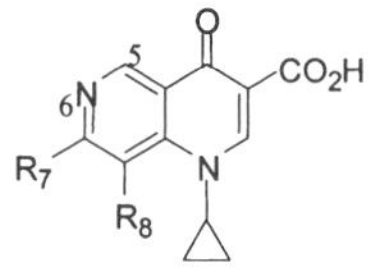

(32)

(32a) R-7 = 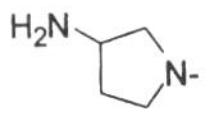   R-8 = Cl

In 1995, Reuman and coworkers (85) reported that aryl groups could be connected to the quinolone nucleus to give compounds such as structure 33 which were extremely potent against gram-positive organisms. It was observed that the potency of structure 33a was not diminished when the 6-fluorine was shifted to the 8 position to yield the 6-desfluoro derivative 33b.

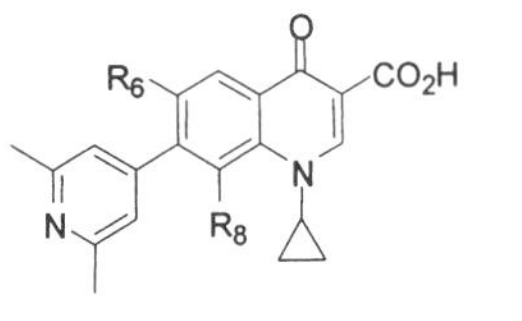

(33)
(33a) R-6 = F, R-8 = H
(33b) R-6 = H, R-8 = F

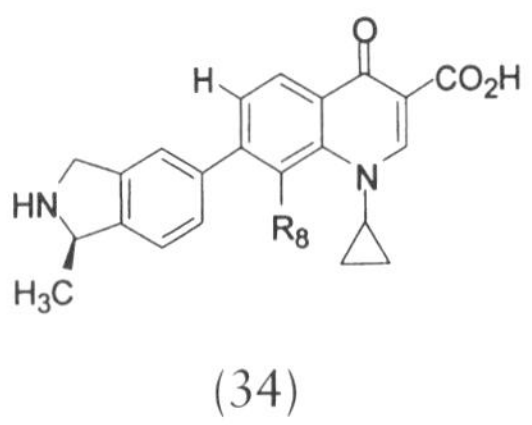

(34)
(34a) R-8 = OCHF$_2$
T-3811
BMS 284756

Consistent with this finding, the Toyama group chose a basic aryl side chain for their clinical candidate T-3811 (BMS 284756, garenoxacin, structure 34a) (102). Because the 2,3-dihydroisoindoyl side chain was optimized with the H at C-6, reintroducing the fluorine at that position had no effect on antibacterial potency (64). When R-8 in structure 34 was varied between H, CH$_3$, OCH$_3$, and OCHF$_2$, the methyl group provided the better potency, but the OCHF$_2$ (structure 34a) group gave the better pharmacokinetic properties in animals (42). The OCHF$_2$ substituent (structure 34a) also showed less CNS liability than OCH$_3$ and significantly less acute toxicity (42). The OCHF$_2$ groups of structure 34a also provided two to eight times more selectivity against mammalian Top II when compared with the other substituents (64). This selectivity advantage of garenoxacin (T-3811, BMS 284756) was also apparent when compared with several other quinolones (109). This finding is important because aromatic side chains had been observed to increase the risk of clastogenicity (107).

In vitro garenoxacin displayed MIC$_{90}$s versus MRSA 32 times superior to ciprofloxacin and was generally two times superior to trovafloxacin against the other gram-positive organisms. Against the gram-negative organisms, ciprofloxacin was generally more active by 4- to 16-fold (102). The pharmacokinetics of garenoxacin (structure 34a) in dogs were excellent ($t_{1/2}$, 4.3 h; 81% bioavailability) (101). As expected from any O-alkyl substituent at R-8, structure 34a showed no phototoxicity (79). Garenoxacin also displayed decreased CNS liability in animals (31, 33) with a low potential for drug interaction (33). Significantly, in vitro (32) and in vivo (54, 79) studies suggest that garenoxacin induces less articular toxicity than other quinolones. It will be interesting to see if the desfluoroquinolones as a class display less arthropathy than their 6-F counterparts.

The discussion in this section clearly shows that the 6-F can be replaced, especially if the C-7 and C-8 positions are reoptimized. The removal of the 6-F does not dramatically reduce potency or pharmacokinetics, and activity against quinolone-resistant organisms is retained. For the first time, we now are able to define the contribution of the C-6 fluorine to the overall side-effect profile of the fluoroquinolones. It seems clear that the C-6 fluorine is a significant contributor to genotoxicity and CNS liabilities as tested in animals. Final results of clinical trials with garenoxacin will prove if the reduced CNS liabilities are mirrored in humans.

THE 7 POSITION

As mentioned in the introduction, prior experience in the quinolone area dictates that the manipulation of the side chain at the 7 position holds great promise in improving potency and pharmacokinetics. For this reason, the substituent at C-7 continues to attract considerable synthetic attention. The favored groups at this position have traditionally been five- and six-membered nitrogen heterocycles substituted with a basic nitrogen moiety. Nothing in the past seven years has disproven this observation, despite extensive substitution and modification of the piperazine and pyrrolidine rings. Other ring sizes have been studied as well as carbocyclic derivatives that are attached to the quinolone nucleus via a carbon atom but which still contain a basic nitrogen.

Extensive SAR work on 7-(3-amino)-azetidinyl quinolones such as E-4695 (structure 35) (37) has been reported (27, 28, 34). Initial success with the 3-amino derivatives led to further exploration of 2-alkyl-3-amino analogs (structure 36) with particular emphasis on the effects of stereochemistry on antibacterial activity. Not unexpectedly, the *trans* isomer was the most active in vitro and was similar to ciprofloxacin against both gram-positive and gram-negative organisms (27). As in the 7-pyrrolidinyl quinolones, addition of a methyl group to the ring did affect physiochemical properties of the molecule (increased lipophilicity and basicity), and the in vivo potency was also improved two- to fourfold by the addition of this methyl group. Exposure levels in mice were also 2 to 15 times higher for the aminoazetidinyl analogs, as measured by the area under the curve.

(35) E-4695   (36)

Gemifloxacin (SB-265805, structure 37) is an excellent example of the ongoing modifications of the pyrrolidine ring at C-7 (73, 43). Addition of the oxime to the pyrrolidine ring imparts a slight to moderate boost (two- to eightfold) in in vitro potency over the simple aminomethyl comparator; however, the presence of the oxime dramatically affects pharmacokinetic parameters such as the area under the curve and the maximum concentration of drug in serum (43). Indeed, gemifloxacin exhibits a bioavailability of 95%, compared with 10% for the analogous desoximino parent (45). Gemifloxacin also appears less clastogenic when compared with other marketed quinolones (73). It is interesting to note that removal of the aminomethyl moiety from the pyrrolidine ring (giving the oxime analog 38) does not destroy antibacterial activity, because structure

38 is more active than ciprofloxacin against gram-positive organisms (and still equipotent against gram-negative organisms). Also interesting is the SAR of the alkyl substituents on the oximino group; increasing alkyl chain length resulted in increased gram-positive activity but decreased gram-negative potency (46). In this series, the napthyridine ring system proved superior to the C-8 fluoro- and chloroquinolones, an obvious reversal in the SAR previously seen for other C-7 substituents (43).

(37) gemifloxacin   (38)

Other modifications of the aminomethyl moiety on the C-7 pyrrolidine were also effective. Substitution of the methylene portion with a single methyl (structure 39 [21]), two methyls (structure 40 [38]), and a cyclopropyl (structure 41 [60]) have all been reported; this particular series of (aminoethyl) pyrrolidines was also important in the 6-desfluoroquinolones discussed earlier. In general, addition of the alkyl group(s) confers excellent in vitro gram-positive activity when compared with the simple aminomethyl parent, with an average two- to fourfold increase. Significant enhancement (5- to 10-fold) of oral efficacy is also observed. For the monomethyl derivatives such as structure 39, examination of all possible stereoisomers of the pyrrolidine reveals that dramatic differences in MIC and oral activity exist between isomers, with the (3R, 1S) isomer being most active on the order of 6- to 30-fold. This result contrasts sharply with a similar examination of the two isomers of 3-(aminomethyl) pyrrolidine, where there was little difference in activity between stereoisomers (21). Similarly, when the methylene is substituted with two methyls (structure 40)—thereby removing one center of chirality—the most active isomer is the R. A slight decrease in potency (approximately two- to fourfold) is observed for the dimethyl analog when compared with the more active monomethyl derivative, although good in vivo activity is retained. Excellent pharmacokinetic data have been reported for both the dimethyl and monomethyl compounds (94). Replacement of the two methyls with the cyclopropyl group (structure 41) further diminished activity, in particular against gram-negative bacteria. Apparently, the introduction of too much bulk to the methylene spacer is unfavorable for gram-negative potency (60).

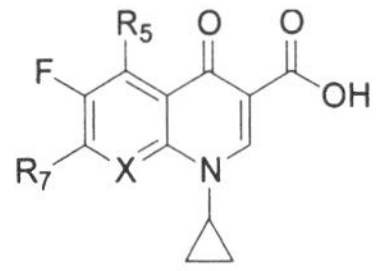

No.	R-5	X	R-7
39	Varies	Varies	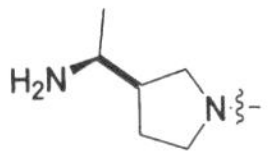
40	Varies	Varies	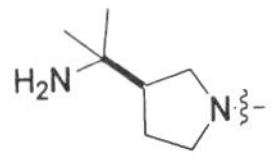
41	Varies	Varies	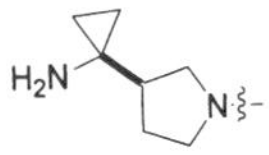

Adding a cyclopropyl group to the (3-amino) pyrrolidine ring gives both olamufloxacin (HSR-903, structure 42) (50) and sitafloxacin (structure 3). Little of the SAR of olamufloxacin analogs has been published. Nevertheless, when compared with the currently marketed quinolones, structure 42 appears to be at least equipotent with sparfloxacin against gram-negative organisms and superior in activity against gram-positive organisms in vitro (100). In head-to-head comparisons, the sitafloxacin side chain offers no advantage over the simple (3-amino)pyrrolidine either in antibacterial activity or pharmacokinetics (59). It was noted, though, that the cyclopropyl derivatives were less soluble than the parent compounds; previous SAR examinations also indicate that the bulk of the cyclopropyl group could reduce genetic toxicity (97).

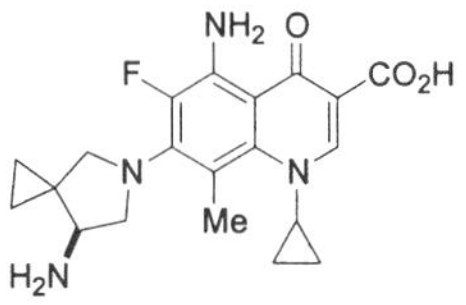

(42) olamufloxacin

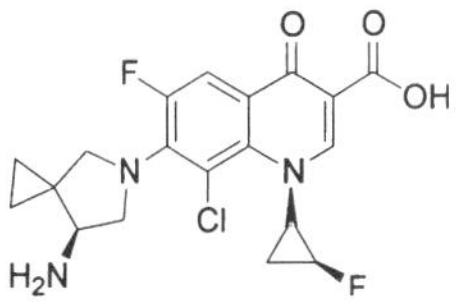

(3) sitafloxacin

Researchers at Daiichi substituted a fluoromethyl moiety on the 3-aminopyrrolidine to produce another series of C-7 pyrrolidines, exemplified by DC-756 (structure 43) (99). Although direct comparisons are few, it appears that the presence of the fluoromethyl does not greatly affect in vitro activity. Addition of two amino groups to the pyrrolidine ring (structure 44) did not improve in vitro potency (72). In a brief report, a small series of triazolyl pyrrolidines at C-7 (for example, SYN987, structure 45) were synthesized and tested against gram-positive

organisms only. In vitro activities were comparable with ciprofloxacin (61).

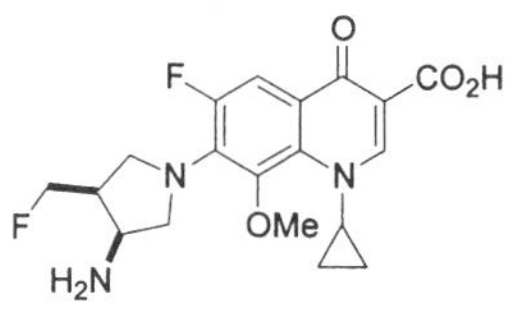

(43) DC-756

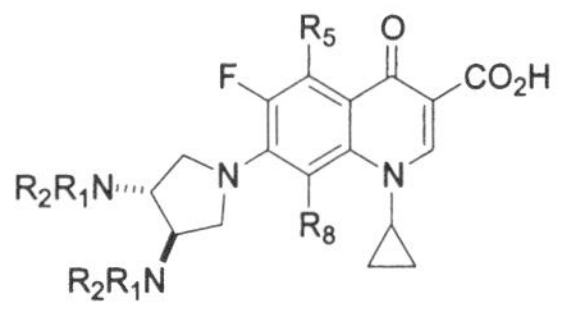

(44)

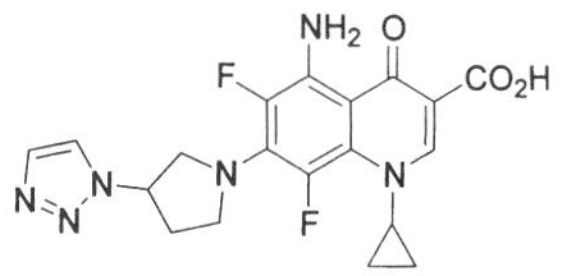

(45) SYN987

Work in the C-7 piperazine derivatives has also focused on several areas. Substitution of the distal piperazine nitrogen with a variety of oximino moieties gives the derivatives represented by phenyl (structure 46) (25), furan (structure 47) (26), and thiophene (structure 48) (76). In general, the oximino phenyl analogs were two- to eight-fold less active in vitro than the unsubstituted piperazine parent, especially against gram-negative organisms. A similar trend was noted when the phenyl group was replaced with a furan (structure 47), although the furan analogs (MICs of 0.13 to 1 μg/ml) were more potent than the phenyl comparators (MICs of 0.25 to 32 μg/ml). However, thiophene analogs such as structure 48 appear to be roughly equipotent with their unsubstituted counterparts, and structure 48 was actually 10 times more active than ciprofloxacin against gram-negative strains (76). In all cases, no in vivo results were reported.

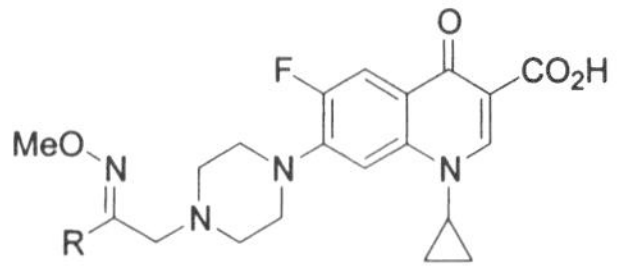

(46) R = phenyl
(47) R = 2-furyl
(48) R = 2-thienyl

This strategy of modifying the piperazine moiety via substitution of the distal nitrogen was further investigated to give a series of benzenesulfonamides represented by structure 49 (1, 81). When compared with the parent compound (ciprofloxacin) in vitro, the 4-aminophenyl analog showed an increase in antibacterial activity against both *S. aureus* (twofold improvement in MIC) (81) and MRSA (a 16-fold improvement) (1). QSAR analysis of these series reveals that electronic and steric effects on the benzenesulfonyl group are most important for improved activity (81). Further study in *S. pneumoniae* confirmed that the substituents on the benzenesulfonyl group affected not only the gram-positive activity but also altered the target preference of the quinolone from Top IV to gyrase (2).

(49)

Other recent modifications of the 7-piperazine moiety have been less successful. Addition of an extra nitrogen between the piperazine ring and the quinolone nucleus to give a "hydrazine bridge" (structure 50) resulted in derivatives with diminished antibacterial potency (96). Homologation of the six-membered ring piperazine to the seven-membered ring perhydrodiazepinone (structure 51) appears to boost gram-positive activity by two- to sixfold, but is detrimental to gram-negative potency by the same amount, at least in sparfloxacin analogs (47).

(50)   (51)

As previously stated, the preferred C-7 substituent has historically been either a piperazine or an aminopyrrolidine. Attempts to incorporate other ring systems have not produced superior replacements. In a limited series of aminopiperidines, the most potent analog (balofloxacin, Q-35, structure 52) offered a slight advantage over ciprofloxacin in vitro and maintained comparable activity against DNA gyrase (49). Several aminomethyl morpholine derivatives such as Y-26611 (structure 53) (90) and Y-34867 (structure 54) (89) have been studied for anti-*Helicobacter pylori* eradication. Overall, Y-34867 is reported to have excellent gram-positive activity (superior to levofloxacin and amoxicillin) but decreased gram-negative potency. The (*S*) stereoisomer appears to be the more active (89).

(52) Q-35   (53) R-1 = R-2 = H, R-8 = F
                   (54) R-1 = R-2 = Me, R-8 = OMe

Several bicyclic amines have been appended to the 7 position; of these, the most promising agents appear to be CFC-222 (structure 55) (56, 82) and moxifloxacin (structure 56) (75). Both have been compared with commercially available quinolones but few published SAR studies exist, especially comparisons of these pyrrolidine-type bicycles with pyrrolidine comparators. In general, CFC-222 possesses good activity against gram-positive organisms (2- to 16-fold more active than ciprofloxacin) but diminished gram-negative efficacy (two to four times). Compound 55 demonstrated excellent pharmacokinetics in mice with a serum half-life of 6 h, compared with 1.5 h for ciprofloxacin (82). Similarly, moxifloxacin was reported to have activity 4- to 16-fold better than ciprofloxacin against the gram-positive organisms and one to two times better against the gram-negative organisms. Pharmacokinetics also appear to be excellent, since it has been noted that moxifloxacin will have once-daily dosing in humans (75).

(55) CFC-222   (56) moxifloxacin

As expected, the stereochemistry of the bicyclic amines at C-7 is critical to activity. In an examination of derivatives such as structure 57, the (*R*) isomer was consistently more potent than the *S*, and the most active analogs were at least equipotent to sparfloxacin (83). According to a formal QSAR study, molecular surface area of the C-7 moiety as well as the net charge of the C-7 atom are the most predictive factors for gram-positive activity (67). A series of bridged 4-aminopiperidine analogs (structure 58) showed a preference for the endo isomer over the exo, although neither isomer proved more potent than the piperazine moiety they were designed to replace (55).

(57)   (58)

It has long been known that the C-7 substituent need not be attached through a nitrogen atom; indeed, attachment through a carbon atom can produce compounds with good in vitro and in vivo potency (63). The size of the ring and the hybridization of the linking carbon atom are both critical parameters for activity. It has been postulated that the success of a carbocyclic substituent at C-7 depends on the ease with which its conformation can approximate the piperazine or aminopyrrolidine structure in space; however, even simple alkyl substituents at C-7 (see structure 59) do show good activity in vitro (104). Indeed, the simple 7-vinyl analog was essentially equipotent to ciprofloxacin against gram-negative organisms.

Researchers at Dainippon synthesized a series of 7-alkynyl-amino-8-fluoroquinolones (structure 60) in an attempt to position a nitrogen atom in the region typically occupied by the piperazine (29). These prototypical acyclic carbon isosteres appear to be slightly less active (four- to eightfold) than the piperazines they were designed to replace. The compounds predicted by modeling to be the most active (i.e., structures 60, 61, and 62) were slightly less active than the alkene 63, which modeling predicted would be the least potent. In all cases, though, the most active compounds were still much less active than the reference standard, ciprofloxacin. Obviously, the correlation between activity and spatial orientation of the nitrogen is intriguing but not yet well defined.

(59) R-7 = cyclopropyl or vinyl   (60)

(61) R-7 = C–CHCH$_2$NH$_2$ (E)
(62) R-7 = CH$_2$CH$_2$CH$_2$NH$_2$
(63) R-7 = C=CHCH$_2$NH$_2$ (Z)

The most promising of these carbon-attached derivatives is pazufloxacin (structure 64), an ofloxacin-type compound that contains an aminocyclopropyl group at the 7 position (103). (In the 6-desfluoro quinolones reviewed earlier, garenoxacin also possesses a carbocylic side chain with excellent antibacterial activity and a good side-effect profile.) In an extensive SAR analysis, the 7-(1-aminocyclopropyl) group was held constant while varying the 1, 8, and 5 positions. The best all-around derivative was still structure 64, which displays good gram-negative activity in vitro. When compared with ofloxacin

(which contains the *N*-methylpiperazine at C-7), pazufloxacin appears to have comparable in vitro activity with a better side-effect profile; a lower induction of convulsion activity in mice and lower cell cytotoxicity are observed (103). In vivo activity of pazufloxacin is at least equivalent to ofloxacin. However, replacement of the piperazine in ofloxacin with the 1-aminocyclopropyl does reduce the half-life of the derivative by 50% (105). Nevertheless, the discovery of pazufloxacin exemplifies an important addition to the SAR of 7-carbocyclic analogs.

(64) pazufloxacin

In summary, then, what has the experience of the past six or seven years taught us about the effect of the substituent at C-7 on activity? Primarily, it appears that no new heterocycles have dethroned the piperazines and aminopyrrolidines as the side chains of choice. In fact, almost all of the "new" C-7 substituents are simple substitutions or modifications of the "old" five- and six-membered rings: addition of alkyl groups, introduction of new functional groups (such as oximes or benzenesulfonamides), and elaboration of the ring into a bicyclic structure. The old dogma remains valid: a piperazine core gives higher gram-negative activity and amino/aminomethylpyrrolidines confer higher gram-positive activity. However, it does appear that judicious substitution of the piperazine/pyrrolidine can subtly affect the overall activity and side-effect profile as well as pharmacokinetic properties.

THE 8 POSITION

It has been shown in an earlier section that the substituent at C-6 (for example, the 6-H versus the 6-F) greatly influences the SAR at C-8; therefore, this section will focus on those more traditional quinolones containing a fluorine at C-6. For this series, it has long been known that the substituent at C-8 controls in vivo efficacy and also affects the antibacterial spectrum. Historically, a fluorine or chlorine at this position conferred excellent potency but undesirable phototoxicity and in vitro genetic toxicity (18). Most recent work at this position has focused on the 8-methoxy substituent, since this moiety has proven to impart good antibacterial activity without concomitant phototoxicity. These attributes led to the development of Q-35 (49) and moxifloxacin (75). It has recently been suggested that the

8-OMe group might also limit the selection of quinolone-resistant bacterial mutants (23).

Extension of the 8-methoxy to the 8-ethoxy group produced analogs (structure 65) that were even less clastogenic in vitro but were also less active (two- to four-fold) against bacterial pathogens (91). Removal of the methyl ether to give the 8-OH (structure 66) essentially eliminated antibacterial activity, especially against clinical isolates; it was postulated that the acidic nature of the hydroxyl group was detrimental to potency. Other modifications, such as the OCH_2F analog 67 (fourfold less active than OCH_3) and the OCF_3 analog 68 (twofold less active), were also detrimental to in vitro activity, although to a lesser degree. Interesting to note is the $OCHF_2$ (structure 69) derivative, which was equipotent to the original 8-OMe parent (112). Replacement of the 8-OMe with 8-SMe to give structure 70 did not appreciably affect the antibacterial potency. None of the 8-alkoxy or 8-SMe analogs displayed any phototoxicity or clastogenicity. Unfortunately, no in vivo data were reported, which is especially important given the degree to which the C-8 substituent controls in vivo efficacy (112).

(65) R-8 = OEt
(66) R-8 = OH
(67) R-8 = OCH_2F
(68) R-8 = OCF_3
(69) R-8 = $OCHF_2$
(70) R-8 = SMe

(71)

Previous investigators have removed the C-8 substituent entirely and created another ring bridging the N-1 and C-8 positions; obviously, the most well-known examples of this strategy are ofloxacin and flumequin. A recent addition to this class is the tricyclic quinolone WQ-0835 (structure 71), which contains a hydrazine moiety at the N-1 position (41). Although few published SARs exist, it appears that these derivatives are essentially equipotent with levofloxacin (and reported to be two to four times more active against gram-positive organisms.) Good in vitro activity and pharmacokinetics in rats were also revealed.

SUMMARY

Since the early 1990s, the SAR of the 6-fluoroquinolones has remained relatively constant. At N-1,

efforts to find aryl replacements for the cyclopropyl group continue, but no substituent to date imparts activity superior to the cyclopropyl. Moreover, the uncertainty of the toxicity potentially induced by aryl N-1 substituents may thwart research in this area of the molecule. Positions 2, 3, 4, and 5 have seen no meaningful improvements; in fact, most groups now seem to leave the 5 position unsubstituted. The removal of the 6-fluorine provided new a SAR by demonstrating that the fluorine could be replaced, but the only replacement of value seemed to be hydrogen. The 6-desfluoroquinolones were never more potent than their fluorinated counterparts, but they did show less CNS and clastogenic risk, demonstrating for the first time which side effects are associated with the 6-fluoro group. Also important was that the desfluoro compounds maintained activity against quinolone-resistant clinical isolates. At C-7, countless new side chains appeared, yet only one extended the SAR beyond the piperazine and pyrrolidine theme. That one side chain was the 2,3-dihydroisoindole group on garenoxacin (structure 34), which is novel because of the aryl-carbon attachment to the quinolone nucleus rather than the usual nitrogen attachment. Such carbon-attached side chains may push the C-7 SAR in new directions with new properties and side-effect profiles. At the 8 position, the old groups of Me and OMe (and small modifications of them) still predominate as researchers have moved away from C-8 halogen. There is also nearly complete agreement that a C-8–H is no longer of value. As to the novel 2-pyridone template, it remains to be seen if this modification provides any added benefit to the quinolone area other than novelty. The SAR of the 2 pyridones closely follows that of the quinolones, and quinolone side effects have been reported as well.

The reality of the quinolone SAR efforts is that all the potency ever required was already in hand in the early 1990s. The continuous battle has been to reduce the side effects of the class and to retain activity versus the growing number of quinolone-resistant strains. In this battle, single atom replacements and simple modifications have proven effective at shifting the benefit/risk profile to the benefit side (sitafloxacin, gemifloxacin, and the desfluoro compounds, for example). Thus, challenges to the traditional SAR will continue, and the success or failure of these efforts will be the focus of intense scrutiny during the next several years.

REFERENCES

1. Allemandi, D. A., F. L. Alovero, and R. Manzo. 1994. In-vitro activity of new sulphanilil fluoroquinolones against *Staphylococcus aureus. J. Antimicrob. Chemother.* 34:261–265.

2. Alovero, F. L., X.-S. Pan, J. E. Morris, R. H. Manzo, and L. M. Fisher. 2000. Engineering the specificity of antibacterial fluoroquinolones: benzenesulfonamide modifications at C-7 of ciprofloxacin change its primary target in *Streptococcus pneumonia* from topoisomerase IV to gyrase. *Antimicrob. Agents Chemother.* 44:320–325.

3. Amano, H., N. Hayashi, Y. Ohshita, Y. Niino, and A. Yazaki. 1997. WQ-2724 and WQ-2743, Novel fluoroquinolones: in vitro and in vivo activities, pharmacokinetics and toxicity, Abstr. F-163. *In Proceedings of the 37th Interscience Conference on Antimicrobial Agents and Chemotherapy,* Toronto, Canada.

4. Applebaum, P. C., and P. A. Hunter. 2000. The fluoroquinolone antibacterials: past, present, and future perspectives. *Int. J. Antibacter. Agents* 5–15.

5. Armiger, Y. L., D. T. W. Chu, A. K. L. Fung, Q. Li, W. Wang, A. Nilius, J. Alder, P. Ewing, G. Stone, J. Meulbroek, M. Bui, L. L. Shen, L. Paige, Y. S. Or, and J. J. Plattner. 1998. The discovery of A-165753 and 170568, two potent broad spectrum antimicrobial agents, abstr. F-86. *In Proceedings of the 38th Interscience Conference on Antimicrobial Agents and Chemotherapy.* American Society for Microbiology, Washington, D.C.

6. Ball, P., A. Fernald, and G. Tillotson. 1998. Therapeutic advances of new fluoroquinolones. *Exp. Opin. Investig. Drugs* 7:761–783.

7. Barry, A. L., P. C. Fuchs, and S. D. Brown. 2001. In vitro activities of three nonfluorinated quinolones against representative bacterial isolates. *Antimicrob. Agents Chemother.* 45:1923–1927.

8. Bierman, J., D. Reichart, J. Emig, H. McKeever, B. Kuzmak, M. Gazda, and B. Ledoussal. 1999. In vivo efficacy of a series of non-fluoroquinolones (NFQ's) in mice, Abstr. F-551. *In Proceedings of the 39th Interscience Conference on Antimicrobial Agents and Chemotherapy.* American Society for Microbiology, Washington, D.C.

9. Bouzard, D., P. Di. Cesare, M. Essiz, J. P. Jacquet, B. Ledoussal, P. Remuzon, R. E. Kessler, and J. Fung-Tomc. 1992. Fluoronaphthyridines as antibacterial agents. 4. Synthesis and structure-activity relationships of 5-substituted 6-fluoro-7-(cycloalkylamino)-1,4-dihydro-4-oxo-1,8-naphthyri dine-3-carboxylic acids. *J. Med. Chem.* 35:518–525.

10. Brown, S. D., A. L. Barry, and P. C. Fuchs. 1999. In vitro antibacterial activity of a series of novel non-fluoroquinolones (NFQ's) against bacterial pathogens, abstr. F-549. *In Proceedings of the 39th Interscience Conference on Antimicrobial Agents and Chemotherapy.* American Society for Microbiology, Washington, D.C.

11. Bryskier, A., and J.-F. Chantot. 1995. Classification and structure-activity relationships of fluoroquinolones. *Drugs* 49(Suppl. 2):16–28.

12. Cecchetti, V., S. Clementi, G. Cruciani, A. Fravolini, P. G. Pagella, A. Savino, and O. Tabarrini. 1995. 6-Aminoquinolones: a new class of quinolone antibacterials? *J. Med. Chem.* 38:973–982.

13. Cecchetti, V., A. Fravolini, M. C. Lorenzini, O. T., P. Terni, and T. Xin. 1996. Studies on 6-aminoquinolones: synthesis and antibacterial evaluation of 6-amino-8-methylquinolones. *J. Med. Chem.* 39:436–445.

14. Chu, D. T. W., P. B. Fernandes, A. K. Claiborne, E. Pihuleac, C. W. Nordeen, R. E. Maleczka, Jr., and A. G. Pernet. 1985. Synthesis and structure-activity relationships of novel arylfluoroquinolone antibacterial agents. *J. Med. Chem.* 28:1558–1564.

15. Chung, S. J., and D. H. Kim. 1997. Synthesis and evaluation of 3-fluoro-2-piperazinyl-5,6,13-trihydro-5-oxoquino[1,2-a][3,1]benzox azine-6-carboxylic acids as potential antibacterial agents. *Arch. Pharm. Med. Chem.* 330:63–66.

16. Ciaravino, V., M. J. Suto, and J.C. Theiss. 1993. High capacity in vitro micronucleus assay for assessment of chromosome damage: Results with quinolone /napthyridone antibacterials. *Mutat. Res.* 298:227–236.

17. De Sarro, A., V. Cecchetti, V. Fravolini, F. Naccari, O. Tabarrini, and G. De Sarro. 1999. Effects of novel 6-desfluoroquinolones and classic quinolones on pentylenetetrazole-induced seizures in mice. *Antimicrob. Agents Chemother.* 43:1729–1736.

18. Domagala, J. M. 1994. Review: structure-activity and structure-side-effect relationships for the quinolone antibacterials. *J. Antimicrob. Chemother.* 33:685–706.

19. Domagala, J. M., A. J. Bridges, T. P. Culbertson, L. Gambino, S. E. Hagen, G. Karrick, K. Porter, J. P. Sanchez, J. A. Sesnie, F. G. Spense, D. D. Szotek, and J. Wemple. 1991. Synthesis and biological activity of 5-amino- and 5-hydroxyquinolones, and the overwhelming influence of the remote N_1- substituent in determining the structure-activity relationship. *J. Med. Chem.* 34:1142–1154.

20. Domagala, J. M., S. E. Hagen, M. P. Hutt, J. P. Sanchez, J. Sesnie, and A. K. Trehan. 1988. 5-Amino-7-(3-amino-1-pyrrolidinyl)-1-cyclopropyl-6,8-difluoro-1,4-dihydro-4 -oxo-3-quinolinecarboxylic acid (PD 124,816). Synthesis and biological evaluation of a new class of quinolone antibacterials. *Drugs Exp. Clin. Res.* 14:453–460.

21. Domagala, J. M., S. E. Hagen, T. Joannides, J. S. Kiely, E. Laborde, M. C. Schroeder, J. A. Sesnie, M. A. Shapiro, M. J. Suto, and S. Vanderroest. 1993. Quinolone antibacterials containing the new 7-[3-(1-aminoethyl)-1-pyrroldinyl] side chain: the effects of the 1-aminoethyl moiety and its stereochemical configurations on potency and in vivo efficacy. *J. Med. Chem.* 36:871–882.

22. Domagala, J. M., L. D. Hanna, C. L. Heifetz, M. P. Hutt, T. F. Mich, J. P. Sanchez, and M. Solomon. 1986. New structure-activity relationships of the quinolone antibacterials using the target enzyme. The development and application of a DNA gyrase assay. *J. Med. Chem.* 29:394–404.

23. Dougherty, T. J., D. Beulieu, and J. F. Barrett. 2001. New quinolones and the impact on resistance. *Drug Disc. Today* 6:529–536.

24. Felmingham D., M. J. Robbins, C. Dencer, I. Mathias, H. Salman, and G. L. Ridgway. 2000. Abstr. F-1511. In vitro activity of non-fluorinated quinolones (PGE-926932, -4175997, -9509924) against *Mycoplasma pneumoniae*, *Chlamydia pneumoniae* and *Legionella* spp., Abstr. F-1511. *In Proceedings of the 40th Interscience Conference on Antimicrobial Agents and Chemotherapy.* American Society for Microbiology, Washington, D.C.

25. Foroumadi, A., S. Emami, A. Davood, H. Moshafi, A. Sharifian, M. Tabatabaie, H. Farimanni, S. G. Tarhimi, and A. Shafiee. 1997. Synthesis and in-vitro antibacterial activities of N-substituted piperazinyl quinolones. *Pharm. Sci.* 3:559–563.

26. Foroumadi, A., S. Emami, P. Haghighat, and M. H. Moshafi. 1999. Synthesis and in-vitro antibacterial activity of new N-substituted piperazinyl quinolones. *Pharm. Pharmacol. Commun.* 5:591–594.

27. Frigola, J., A. Torrens, J.A. Castrillo, J. Mas, D. Vano, J. M. Berrocal, C. Calvet, L. Salgado, J. Redondo, S. Garcia-Granda, E. Valenti, and J. R. Quintana. 1994. 7-Azetidinylquinolones as antibacterial agents. 2. Synthesis and biological activity of 7-(2,3-disubstituted-1-azetidinyl)-4-oxoquinoline- and-1,8-naphthyridine-3-carboxylic acids. Properties and structure-activity relationships of quinolones with an azetidine moiety. *J. Med. Chem.* 37:4195–4210.

28. Frigola, J., D. Vano, A. Torrens, A. Gomez-Gomar, E. Ortega, and S. Garcia-Granda. 1995. 7-Azetidinyl-quinolones as antibacterial agents. 3. Synthesis, properties, and structure-activity relationships of the stereoisomers containing a 7-(3-amino-2-methyl-1-azetidinyl) moiety. *J. Med Chem.* **38:**1203–1215.

29. Fujita, M., K. Chiba, J. Nakano, Y. Tominaga, and J.-I. Matsumoto. 1998. Synthesis and structure-antibacterial activity relationships of 7-(3-amino-1-propynyl and 3-amino-1-propenyl)quinolones. *Chem. Pharm. Bull.* **46:**631–638.

30. Fung, A. K. L., and L. L. Shen. 1999. The 2-pyridone antibacterial agents: 8-position modifications. *Curr. Pharm. Design* **5:**515–543.

31. Furuhata, K., H. Fukuda, T. Nakamura, Y, Morita, H. Arai, Y. Todo, Y. Watanabe, and H. Narita. 1999. Pharmacological evaluation of T-3811ME (BMS-284756): toxicity to the central nervous system, abstr. F-551. *In Proceedings of the 39th Interscience Conference on Antimicrobial Agents and Chemotherapy.* American Society for Microbiology, Washington, D. C.

32. Furuhata, K., H. Fukuda, A. Shimamoto, H. Arai, Y. Todo, Y. Watanabe, and H. Narita. 1998. Pharmacological evaluation of T-3811ME: toxicity on articular chondrocytes in vitro, abstr. F-77. *In Proceedings of the 38th Interscience Conference on Antimicrobial Agents and Chemotherapy.* American Society for Microbiology, Washington, D.C.

33. Furuhata, K., K. Soumi, J. Matsumoto, A. Horikawa, N. Nojima, H. Arai, Y. Todo, Y. Watanabe, and H. Narita. 1997. T-3811, a novel des-F(6)-quinolone: comparative studies of the adverse reactions associated with quinolones, abstr. F-161. *In Proceedings of the 37th Interscience Conference on Antimicrobial Agents and Chemotherapy.* American Society for Microbiology, Washington, D.C.

34. Garcia-Rodriguez, J. A., J. E. Garcia Sanchez, M. I. Garcia Garcia, M. J. Fresnadillo, I. Trujiliano, and E. Garcia Sanchez. 1994. In-vitro activity of four new fluoroquinolones. *J. Antimicrob. Chemother.* **34:**53–64.

35. Granneman, G.R., K. M. Snyder, and V. S. Shu. 1986. Difloxacin metabolism and pharmacokinetics in humans after single oral dose. *Antimicrob. Agents and Chemother.* **30:**689–693.

36. Gray, J. L., J. K. Almstead, S. M. Flaim, C. P. Gallagher, X. E. Hu, N. K. Kim, H. D. McKeever, C. J. Miley, T. L. Twinem, S. X. Zheng, and B. Ledoussal. 2000. Synthesis and testing of non-fluorinated quinolones (NFQ's). A study on the influence of the C-6 position, abstr. F-1506. *In Proceedings of the 40th Interscience Conference on Antimicrobial Agents and Chemotherapy.* American Society for Microbiology, Washington, D.C.

37. Guinea, J., D. Gargallo-Viola, M. Robert, E. Tudela, M. A. Xicota, J. Garcia, M. Esteve, R. Coll, M. Pares, and R. Roser. 1995. E-4695, a new C-7 azetidinyl fluoronaphthyridine with enhanced activity against gram-positive and anaerobic pathogens. *Antimicrob. Agents Chemother.* **39:**413–421.

38. Hagen, S. E., J. M. Domagala, S. J. Gracheck, J. A. Sesnie, M. A. Stier, and M. J. Suto. 1994. Synthesis and antibacterial activity of new quinolones containing a 7-[3-(1-amino-1-methylethyl)-1-pyrrolidinyl] moiety. Gram-positive agents with excellent oral activity and low side-effect profile. *J. Med. Chem.* **37:**733–738.

39. Hagen, S., J. M. Domagala, C. L. Heifetz, and J. Johnson. 1991. Synthesis and biological activity of 5-alkyl-1,7,8-trisubstituted—6-fluoroquinoline-3-carboxylic acids. *J. Med. Chem.* **34:**1155–1161.

40. Hannon-Hardy, J., V. Murphy, B. Kuzmak, H. Murli, P. Curry, B. Ledoussal, J. Gray, S. Flaim, N. Kim, P. Young, E. Swing, N. Nikolaides, S. Mundla, M. Reilly, and T. Schunk. 1999. Acute IV toxicity and clastogenicity of novel, 8-methoxy-non-fluoroquinolones compared to 8-methoxy-fluoroquinolones, abstr. F-553. *In Proceedings of the 39th Interscience Conference on Antimicrobial Agents and Chemotherapy.* American Society for Microbiology, Washington, D.C.

40a. Hayashi, N., H. Amano, Y. Ohshita, Y. Niino, J. Yoshida, and A. Yazaki. 1996. In vitro and in vivo activities, pharmacokinetics and toxicity of WQ-2724 and WQ-2743, two novel fluoroquinolones, abstr. F-51. *In Proceedings of the 36th Interscience Conference on Antimicrobial Agents and Chemotherapy.* American Society for Microbiology, Washington, D.C.

41. Hayashi, N., Y Hirao, H. Amano, Y. Oshita, M. Yokomoto, S. Inoue, and A. Yazaki. 1995. WQ-0835, A prototypical tricyclic quinolone: in vitro and in vivo antibacterial activity and pharmacokinetics, abstr. F192. *In Proceedings of the 35th Interscience Conference on Antimicrobial Agents and Chemotherapy.* American Society for Microbiology, Washington, D.C.

41a. Hayashi, N., Y. Oshita, H. Amano, Y. Hirao, Y. Niino, and A. Yazaki. 1999. WQ-3330 and WQ-2942, structure-activity relationships of novel 8-methyl quinolones containing an aminophenyl group at the N-1 position, abstr. 557. *In Proceedings of the 39th Interscience Conference on Antimicrobial Agents and Chemotherapy.* American Society for Microbiology, Washington, D.C.

42. Hayashi, K., Y. Todo, S. Hamamoto, K. Ojima, M. Yamada, T. Kito, M. Takahata, Y. Watanabe, and H. Narita. 1997. T-3811, a novel des-F(6)-quinolone: synthesis and in vitro activity of 7-(isoindolin-5-yl) derivatives, abstr. F-158. *In Proceedings of the 37th Interscience Conference on Antimicrobial Agents and Chemotherapy.* American Society for Microbiology, Washington, D.C.

43. Hong, C. Y., Y. K. Kim, J. H. Chang, S. H. Kim, H. Choi, D. H. Nam, Y. Z. Kim, and J. H. Kwak. 1997. Novel fluoroquinolone antibacterial agents containing oxime-substituted (aminomethyl)pyrrolidines: synthesis and antibacterial activity of 7-(4-(aminomethyl)-3-(methoxyimino)pyrrolidin-1-yl)-1-cyclopropyl-6-fluoro- 4-oxo-1,4-dihydro[1,8]naphthyridine-3-carboxylic acids (LB 20304). *J. Med. Chem.* **40:**3584–1593.

44. Hong, C. Y., S. H. Kim, and Y. K. Kim. 1997. Novel 5-amino-6-methylquinolone antibacterials: a new class of non-fluoroquinolones. *Bioorg. Med. Chem. Lett.* **7:**1875–1878.

45. Hong, C. Y., Y. K. Kim, J. H. Jang, and M. Y. Kim. 1998. SB-265805 (LB20304a): Discovery of SB-265805, the synergistic effect of the methoxyloxime and aminomethyl groups of the C7-pyrrolidine on in vitro antibacterial activity, abstr. F-96. *In Proceedings of the 38th Interscience Conference on Antimicrobial Agents and Chemotherapy.* American Society for Microbiology, Washington, D.C.

46. Hong, C. Y., Y. K. Kim, D. H. Nam, H. Choi, J. H. Jang, K. S. Paek, and M. Y. Kim. 1998. SB-265805 (LB20304a): SAR of the oxime-derivatized pyrrolidine. The importance of the oximinoalkyl group on the in vitro antibacterial activity and pharmacokinetics, Abstr. F-95. *In Proceedings of the 38th Interscience Conference on Antimicrobial Agents and Chemotherapy.* American Society for Microbiology, Washington, D.C.

47. Imamori, K. 1995. In vitro antibacterial activity of FA103, a new quinolone derivative of C-7 position with 7-perhydrodiazepinone. *Jpn. J. Antibiot.* **48:**1891–1898.

48. Inoue, Y., H. Kondo, M. Taguchi, T. Jinbo, F. Sakamoto, and G. Tsukamoto. 1994. Synthesis and antibacterial activity

of thiazolopyrazine-incorporated tetracyclic quinolone antibacterials. *J. Med. Chem.* **37**:586–592.

49. Ito, T., K. Kojima, K. Koizuma, H. Nagano, and T. Nishino. 1994. Inhibitory activity on DNA gyrase and intracellular accumulation of quinolones: structure-activity relationship of Q-35 analogs. *Biol. Pharm. Bull.* **17**:927–930.

50. Jiraskova, N. 2000. Olamufloxacin. *Curr. Opin. Investig. Drugs* **1**:31–34.

51. Johnson, A. P. 1999. DW-116. *Curr. Opin. Anti-Infect. Investig. Drugs* **1**:488–492.

52. Jung, B. H., M. H. Choi, and B. C. Chung. 2000. Pharmacokinetics and urinary excretion of DW116, a new fluoroquinolone antibacterial agent, in humans as a Phase I study. *Drug Dev. Ind. Pharm.* **26**:103–106.

53. Jurgens, J., H. Schedletzky, P. Heisig, J. K. Seydel, B. Wiedemann, and U. Holzgrabe. 1996. Syntheses and biological activities of new N_1-aryl substituted quinolone antibacterials. *Arch. Pharm. Pharm. Med. Chem.* **329**:179–190.

54. Kawamura, Y., A. Nagai, M. Miyazaki, T. Sanzen, H. Fukumoto, H. Hayakawa, Y. Todo, N. Terashima, Y. Watanabe, and H. Narita. 2000. Articular toxicity of BMS-284756 (T-3811ME) administered orally to juvenile dogs, abstr. A-277. *In Proceedings of the 37th Interscience Conference on Antimicrobial Agents and Chemotherapy.* American Society for Microbiology, Washington, D.C.

55. Kim, J., Y. H. Yoon, I. H. Cho, J. M. Lee, K. Lee, J. H. Kim, and K. H. Hong. 1996. Synthesis and antibacterial activity of a new series of quinolones with 7-substituent of [3.1.1] bicyclic amines. *Kor. J. Med. Chem.* **6**:183–189.

56. Kim, J. H., J. A. Kang, Y. G. Kim, J. W. Kim, J. H. Lee, E. C. Choi, and B. K. Kim. 1997. In vitro and in vivo antibacterial efficacies of CFC-222, a new fluoroquinolone. *Antimicrob. Agents Chemother.* **41**:2209–2213.

57. Kim, O. K., J. F. Barrett, and K. Ohemeng. 2001. Advances in DNA gyrase inhibitors. *Exp. Opin. Investig. Drugs* **10**:199–212.

58. Kim, S. H., Y. K. Kim, H.-J. Kang, and C. Y. Hong. 1997. Novel 6-methylquinolone antibacterials: a new class of non-6-fluoroquinolones. *J. Med. Chem.* **7**:19–22.

59. Kimura, Y., S. Atarashi, K. Kawakami, K. Sato, and I. Hayakawa. 1994. (Fluorocyclopropyl)quinolones. 2. Synthesis and stereochemical structure-activity relationships of chiral 7-(-amino-5-azaspiro[2,4]heptan-5-yl-)-1-(2-fluorocyclopropyl)quinolone antibacterial agents. *J. Med. Chem.* **37**:3344–3352.

60. Kimura, Y., S. Atarashi, M. Takahashi, and I. Hayakawa. 1994. Synthesis and structure-activity relationships of 7-{3-(1-aminoalkyl)pyrrolidinyl]- and 7-[3-(1-aminocycloalkyl) pyrrolidinyl]-quinolone antibacterials. *Chem. Pharm. Bull.* **42**:1442–1454.

61. Kitzis, M. D., F. W. Goldstein, N. Ishida, and J. F. Acar. 1995. SYN987, SYN1193, and SYN1253, new quinolones highly active against gram-positive cocci. *J. Antimicrob. Chemother.* **36**:209–213.

62. Klopman, G., D. Fercu, T. E. Renau, M. R. Jacobs. 1996. N-1-tert-butyl-substituted quinolones: in vitro anti-*Mycobacterium avium* activities and structure-activity relationship studies. *Antimicrob. Agents Chemother.* **40**:2637–2643.

63. Laborde, E. , J. S. Kiely, T. P. Culbertson, and L. E. Lesheski. 1993. Quinolone antibacterials: synthesis and biological activity of carbon isosteres of the 1-piperazinyl and 3-amino-1-pyrrolidinyl side chains. *J. Med. Chem.* **36**:1964–1970.

64. Lawrence, L. E., P. G. Wu, L. Fan, K. Gouveia, A. Card, K. Denbleyker, and J. F. Barrett. 2000. The structure-activity

relationship of BMS-284756, a novel des-F(6)-quinolone, abstr. C-751. *40th Interscience Conference on Antimicrobial Agents and Chemotherapy.* American Society for Microbiology, Washington, D.C.

65. Ledoussal, B., J. K. Almstead, S. M. Flaim, C. P. Gallagher, J. L. Gray, X. E. Hu, N. K. Kim, H. D. MeKeever, C. J. Miley, T. L. Twinem, and S. X. Zheng. 1999. Novel non-fluoroquinolones (NFQ's), structure-activity, and design of new, potent and safe agents, abstr. F-544. *In Proceedings of the 39th Interscience Conference on Antimicrobial Agents and Chemotherapy.* American Society for Microbiology, Washington, D.C.

66. Ledoussal, B., D. Bouzard, and E. Coroneos. 1992. Potent non-6-fluoro-substituted quinolone antibacterials: synthesis and biological activity. *J. Med. Chem.* **35**:198–200.

67. Lee, K. W., S. Y. Kwon, S. Hwang, J.-U. Lee, and H. Kim. 1996. Quantitative structure-activity relationships (QSAR) study on C-7 substituted quinolone. *Bull. Kor. Chem. Soc.* **17**:147–152.

68. Li, Q., D. T. W. Chu, A. Claiborne, C. S. Cooper, C. M. Lee, K. Raye, K. B. Berst, P. Donner, W. Wang, L. Hasvold, A. Fung, Z. Ma, M. Tufano, R. Flamm, L. L. Shen, J. Baranowski, A. Nilius, J. Alder, J. Meulbroek, K. Marsh, D. Crowell, Y. Hui, L. Seif, L. M. Melcher, R. Henry, S. Spanton, R. Faghih, L. L. Klein, S. Ken Tanaka, and J. J. Plattner. 1996. Synthesis and structure-activity relationships of 2-pyridones: a novel series of potent DNA gyrase inhibitors as antibacterial agents. *J. Med. Chem.* **39**:3070–3088.

69. Li, Q., L. A. Mitscher, and L. L. Shen. 2000. The 2-pyridone antibacterial agents: bacterial topoisomerase inhibitors. *Med. Res. Rev.* **20**:231–293.

70. Lietman, P. S. 1995. Fluoroquinolone toxicities: An update. *Drugs* **49**(Suppl. 2):159–163.

71. Lode, H. 1999. Potential interactions of the extended-spectrum fluoroquinolones with the CNS. *Drug Safety* **21**:123–135.

72. Lohray, B. B., S. Baskaran, B. S. Rao, B. Mallesham, K. S. N. Bharath, B. Y. Reddy, S. Venkateswarlu, A. K. Sadhukhan, M. S. Kumar, and H. M. Sarnaik. 1998. Novel quinolone derivatives as potent antibacterials. *Bioorg. Med. Chem. Lett.* **8**:525–528.

73. Lowe, M. N., and H. M. Lamb. May 2000. Gemifloxacin. *Drugs* **59**:1137–1147.

74. Mallalieu, N. L., D. H. Ellis, P. H. Zoutendam, M. Gavin, M. K. Dirr, M. Martin, and B. Ledoussal. 1999. Preclinical pharmacokinetics of non-fluoroquinolone antibacterials, abstr. F-550. *In Proceedings of the 39th Interscience Conference on Antimicrobial Agents and Chemotherapy.* American Society for Microbiology, Washington, D.C.

75. Martel, A. M., P. A. Leeson, and J. Castaner. 1997. Moxifloxacin. *Drugs Future* **22**:109–113.

76. Mirzaei, M., and A. Foroumadi. 2000. Synthesis and in-vitro antibacterial activity of N-piperazinyl quinolone derivatives with a 2-thienyl group. *Pharm. Pharmacol. Commun.* **6**:351–354.

77. Moran, D. B., C. B. Ziegler, Jr., T. S. Dunne, N. A. Kuck, and Y. I. Lin. 1989. Synthesis of novel 5-fluoro analogues of norfloxacin and ciprofloxacin. *J. Med. Chem.* **32**:1313–1318.

78. Murphy, V., J. Hannah-Hardy, H. Murli, H. Raabe, G. Douds, K. Sealover, P. Young, E. Swing, N. Nikolaides, S. Mundla, M. Reilly, and T. Schunk. 1999. Preliminary toxicity of a series of non-fluoroquinolones (NFQ's), abstr. F-554. *In Proceedings of the 39th Interscience Conference on Antimicrobial Agents and Chemotherapy.* American Society for Microbiology, Washington, D.C.

79. Nagai, A., M. Takahata, M. Miyazaki, Y. Kawamura, T. Kodama, Y. Todo, Y. Watanabe, and H. Narita. 1997. T-3811, a novel des-F(6)-quinolone: toxicological evaluation, abstr. F-162. *In Proceedings of the 37th Interscience Conference on Antimicrobial Agents and Chemotherapy.* American Society for Microbiology, Washington, D.C.

80. Nam, K.-S., B.-J. Kim, T.-S. Lee, and W.-J. Kin. 1996. New quinolone antibacterial agents introducing new functional groups at C-3 position. *Kor. J. Med. Chem.* 6:203–238.

81. Nieto, M. J., F. Alovero, R. H. Manzo, and M. R. Mazzieri. 1999. A new class of fluoroquinolones: benzenesulfonamidefluoroquinolones (BSFQs), antibacterial activity and SAR studies. *Eur. J. Med. Chem.* 34:209–214.

82. Park, K. H., I. H. Cho, J. M. Lee, J. A. Kang, Y. G. Kim, K. H. Hong, J. H. Kim, and T. Nishino. 1995. In vitro and in vivo antibacterial activities of CFC-222, a novel broad spectrum fluoroquinolone. *Drugs* 49(Suppl. 2):240–242.

83. Park, T.-H., K.-S. Nam, Y.-H. Ha, Y.-J. Choi, J.-D. Ha, J.-Y. King, and Y.-H. Kim. 1997. Synthesis and antibacterial activity of KRQ-10018 and its analogues: potent DNA gyrase inhibitors, abstr. F-173. *In Proceedings of the 37th Interscience Conference on Antimicrobial Agents and Chemotherapy.* American Society for Microbiology, Washington, D.C.

84. Pavan, B., and F. Vesce. 1999. Sitafloxacin. *Curr. Opin. Anti-Infect. Investig. Drugs* 1:478–487.

85. Reuman, M., S. J. Daum, B. Singh, M. P. Wentland, R. B. Perni, P. Pennock, P. M. Carabateas, M. D. Gruett, M. T. Saindane, P. H. Dorff, S. A. Coughlin, D. M. Sedlock, J. B. Rake, and G. Y. Lesher. 1995. Synthesis and antibacterial activity of some novel 1-substituted 1,4 dihydro-4-oxo-7-pyridinyl-3-quinolinecarboxylic acids. Potent antistaphylococcal agents. *J. Med. Chem.* 38:2531–2540.

86. Ryan, B., H.-T. Ho, P. Wu, M.-B. Frosco, T. Dougherty, and J. F. Barrett. 2000. 40th Interscience Conference on antimicrobial agents and chemotherapy (ICAAC). *Exp. Opin. Investig. Drugs* 9:2945–2972.

87. Sabatini, S., V. Cecchetti, O. Tabarrini, and A. Fravolini. 1999. 8-Methyl-7-substituted-1, 6-napthyridine-3-carboxylic acids as new 6-desfluoroquinolone antibacterials [1]. *J. Heterocycl. Chem.* 36:953–957.

88. Sahm, D. F., A. M. Staples, I. A. Critchley, C. Thornsberry, K. S. Murfitt, J. A. Karlowsky, and D. C. Mayfield. 2000. Activities of non-fluorinated quinolones against recent clinical isolates of gram-positive cocci, including those resistant to currently available fluoroquinolones, abstr. 1509. *40th Interscience Conference on Antimicrobial Agents and Chemotherapy.* American Society for Microbiology, Washington, D.C.

89. Sakurai, N., F. Hirayama, M. Sano, S. Uemori, A. Moriguchi, Y. Yokoyama, K. Yamamoto, M. Miyoshi, Y. Ikeda, and T. Kawakita. 1998. Synthesis and anti-*Helicobacter pylori* activity of Y-34867, a new 7-morpholinoquinolone, abstr. F-085. *38th Interscience Conference on Antimicrobial Agents and Chemotherapy.* American Society for Microbiology, Washington, D.C.

90. Sakurai, N., M. Sano, F. Hirayama, T. Kuroda, S. Uemori, A. Moriguchi, K. Yamamoto, Y. Ikeda, and T. Kawakita. 1998. Synthesis and structure-activity relationships of 7-(2-aminoalkyl)morpholinoquinolones as anti-*Helicobacter pylori* agents. *Bioorg. Med. Chem. Lett.* 8:2185–2190.

91. Sanchez, J. P., R. D. Gogliotti, J. M. Domagala, S. J. Gracheck, M. D. Huband, J. A. Sesnie, M. A. Cohen, and M. A. Shapiro. 1995. The synthesis, structure-activity, and structure-side effect relationships of a series of 8-alkoxy- and 5-amino-8-alkoxyquinolone antibacterial agents. *J. Med. Chem.* 38:4478–4487.

92. Schultz, C. C., Y. Nan, T. Marron, A. Nilius, M. Bui, P. Raney, G. Stone, L. Shen, J. Baranowski, R. Snyder, and Y. S. Or. 1999. Synthesis and antibacterial activity of C-8 carbon linked 2-pyridones, Abstr. F-560. *In Proceedings of the 39th Interscience Conference on Antimicrobial Agents and Chemotherapy.* American Society for Microbiology, Washington, D.C.

93. Segawa, J., K. Kazuno, M. Matsuoka, I. Amimoto, M. Ozaki, M. Matsuda, Y. Tomii, M. Kitano, and M. Kise. 1995. Studies of pyridonecarboxylic acids. IV. Synthesis and antibacterial activity evaluation of S-(2)- and R-(1)-6-fluoro-1-methyl-4-oxo-7-(1-piperazinyl)-4H-[1,3]thiazeto[3, 2-a]quinoline-3-carboxylic acids. *Chem. Pharm. Bull.* 43:1238–1240.

94. Shapiro, M. A., J. A. Dever, T. Joannides, J. A. Sesnie, and S. Vanderroest. 1995. In vivo therapeutic efficacies of PD 138312 and PD 140248, two novel fluoronaphthyridines with outstanding gram-positive potency. *Antimicrob. Agents Chemother.* 39:2183–2186.

95. Sheu, J. Y., Y. L.Chen, K. C. Fang, T. C. Wang, C. H. Peng, and C. C. Tzeng. 1998. Synthesis and antibacterial activity of 1-(substituted-benzyl)-6-fluoro-1,4-dihydro-4-oxoquinoline-3-carboxylic acids and their 6,8-difluoro analogs. *J. Heterocycl. Chem.* 35:955–964.

96. Singh, R., R. Fathi-Afshar, G. Thomas, M. P.Singh, F. Higashitani, A. Hyodo, N. Unemi, and R. G. Micetich. 1998. Synthesis and antibacterial activity of 7-hydrazinoquinolones. *Eur. J. Med. Chem.* 33:697–703.

97. Suto, M. J., J. M. Domagala, G. E. Roland, G. B. Mailloux, and M. A. Cohen. 1992. Fluoroquinolones: relationships between structural variations, mammalian cell cytotoxicity, and antimicrobial activity. *J. Med. Chem.* 35:4745–4750.

98. Takahashi, H., K. Kawakami, K. Sugita, H. Ohki, K. Kimura, S. Miyauchi, H. Inagaki, R. Miyauchi, M. Tanaka, M. Chiba, E. Yamazaki, K. Sato, Y. Kurosaka, S. Nishida, Y. Murakami, T. Otani, K. Yabe, N. Haga, T. Jindo, K. Takasuna, F. Yamaguchi, M. Sekiguchi, I. Hayakawa, and M. Takemura. 2000. Synthesis and biological evaluation of D61–1113, a novel fluoroquinolone having potent activity against gram-positive bacteria including MRSA, PRSP, and VRE, abstr. F-1505. *In Proceedings of the 40th Interscience Conference on Antimicrobial Agents and Chemotherapy.* American Society for Microbiology, Washington, D.C.

99. Takahashi, H., K. Kawakami, K. Sugita, H. Ohki, K. Kimura, R. Miyauchi, K. Sato, and M. Takemura. 1998. DC-756: A new methoxyquinolone: synthesis and in vitro activity of 7-[(3-amino-4-substituted)pyrroldin-1-yl] derivatives, abstr. F-73. In *Proceedings of the 38th Interscience Conference on Antimicrobial Agents and Chemotherapy.* American Society for Microbiology, Washington, D.C.

100. Takahashi, Y., N. Masuda, M. Otsuki, M. Miki, and T. Nishino. 1997. In vitro activity of HSR-903, a new quinolone. *Antimicrob. Agents Chemother.* 41:1326–1330.

101. Takahata, M., J. Mitsuyama, Y. Yamashiro, H. Araki, H. Yamada, H. Hayakawa, Y. Todo, S. Minami, Y. Watanabe, and H. Narita. 1997. T-3811, a novel des-F(6)-quinolone: study of pharmacokinetics in animals, abstr. F-160. *In Proceedings of the 37th Interscience Conference on Antimicrobial Agents and Chemotherapy.* American Society for Microbiology, Washington, D.C.

102. Takahata, M., J. Mitsuyama, Y. Yamashiro, M. Yonezawa, H. Araki, Y. Todo, S. Minami, Y. Watanabe, and N. Hirokazu. 1999. In vitro and in vivo antimicrobial activities of T-3811ME, a novel des-F(6)-quinolone. *Antimicrob. Agents Chemother.* 43:1077–1084.

103. Todo, Y., J. Nitta, M. Miyajima, Y. Fukuoka, Y. Yamashiro, N. Nishida, I. Saikawa, and H. Narita. 1994. Pyridonecarboxylic acids as antibacterial agents. VIII. Synthesis and structure-activity relationship of 7-(1-aminocyclopropyl)-4-oxo-1,8-naphthyridine-3-carboxylic acids and 7-(1-aminocyclopropyl)-4-oxoquinolone-3-carboxylic acids. *Chem. Pharm. Bull.* 42:2063–2070.

104. Todo, Y., H. Takagi, F. Iino, Y. Fukuoka, Y. Ikeda, K. Tanaka, I. Saikawa, and H. Narita. 1994. Pyridonecarboxylic acids as antibacterial agents. VI. Synthesis and structure-activity relationship of 7-(alkyl, cycloalkyl, and vinyl)-1-cyclopropyl-6-fluoro-4-quinolone-3-carboxylic acids. *Chem. Pharm. Bull.* 42:2049–2054.

105. Todo, Y., H. Takagi, F. Iino, Y. Fukuoka, M. Takahata, S. Okamoto, I. Saikawa, and H. Narita. 1994. Pyridonecarboxylic acids as antibacterial agents. IX. Synthesis and structure-activity relationship of 3-substituted 10-(1-aminocyclopropyl)-9-fluoro-7-oxo-2,3-dihydro-7H-pyrido[1,2,3-*d/e*]-1,4-benzoxazine-6-carboxylic acids and their 1-thio and 1-aza analogues. *Chem. Pharm. Bull.* 42:2569–2574.

106. Tomioka, H., K. Sato, H. Kajitani, T. Akaki, and S. Shishido. 2000. Comparative antimicrobial activities of the newly synthesized quinolone WQ-3034, levofloxacin, sparfloxacin, and ciprofloxacin against *Mycobacterium tuberculosis* and *Mycobacterium avium* complex. *Antimicrob. Agents Chemother.* 44:283–286.

107. Wentland, M. P., G. Y. Lesher, M. Reuman, M. D. Gruett, B. Singh, S. C. Aldous, P. H. Dorff, J. B. Rake, and S. A. Coughlin. 1993. Mammalian topoisomerase II inhibitory activity of 1-cyclopropyl-6,8-difluoro-1,4-dihydro-7-(2,6-dimethyl-1-4-pyridinyl)-4-ox o-3-quinolinecarboxylic acid and related derivatives. *J. Med. Chem.* 36:2801–2809.

108. Wise, R., P. G. Pagella, V. Cecchetti, A. Fravolini, and O. Tabarrini. 1995. In vitro activity of MF 5137, a new potent 6-aminoqionolone. *Drugs.* 49(Suppl. 2):272–273.

109. Yamada, H., H. Hisada, J. Mitsuyama, M. Takahata, Y. Todo, S. Minami, N. Terashima, Y. Wantanabe, and H. Narita. 2000. BMS-284756 (T-3811ME), a des-fluoro(6)-quinolone. Selectivity between bacterial and human type II DNA topoisomerases, abstr. C-753. *In Proceedings of the 37th Interscience Conference on Antimicrobial Agents and Chemotherapy.* American Society for Microbiology, Washington, D.C.

110. Yoon, S. J., Y. H. Chung, C. H. Lee, Y. S. Oh, D. R. Choi, N. D. Kim, J. K. Lim, Y. H. Jin, D. K. Lee, and W. Y. Lee. 1997. Synthesis, pharmacokinetics, and biological activity of a series of new pyridonecarboxylic acid antibacterial agents bearing a 5-fluoro-2-pyridyl group or a 3-fluoro-4-pyridyl group at N-1. *J. Heterocycl. Chem.* 34:1021–1026.

111. Yoshida, T., Y. Yamamoto, H. Orita, M. Kakiuchi, Y. Takahashi, M. Itakura, N. Kado, K. Mitani, S. Yasuda, H. Kato, and Y. Itoh. 1996. Structure-activity relationships of antibacterial activity and side effects for 5- or 8- substituted and 5,8-disubstituted-7-(3-amino-1-pyrrolidinyl)-1-cyclopropyl-1, 4-dihydro-4-oxoquinoline-3-carboxylic acids. *Chem. Pharm. Bull.* 44:1074–1085.

112. Yoshido, T., Y. Yamamoto, H. Orita, M. Kakiuchi, Y. Takahashi, M. Itakura, N. Kado, K. Mitani, S. Yasuda, H. Kato, and Y. Itoh. 1996. Studies on quinolone anibacterials. IV. Structure-activity relationships of antibacterial activity and side effects for 5- or 8-substituted and 5,8-disubstituted-7-(3-amino-1-pyrroldinyl)-1-cyclopropyl-1,4-dihydro-4-oxo quinoline-3-carboxylic acids. *Chem. Pharm. Bull.* 44: 1074–1085.

Chapter 2

Mechanisms of Quinolone Action

KARL DRLICA AND DAVID C. HOOPER

The fluoroquinolones have as their targets two essential bacterial enzymes, DNA gyrase (topoisomerase II) (65) and DNA topoisomerase IV (99). These two topoisomerases act by passing one region of duplex DNA through another; during that process the quinolones trap a reaction intermediate containing drug, enzyme, and broken DNA. The resulting ternary complexes block DNA replication and lead to cell death. Because the topoisomerases are conserved enzymes, the quinolones exhibit activity against a broad spectrum of bacterial species.

The two topoisomerases share many mechanistic properties; consequently, conclusions about one can often be extrapolated from work with the other. Quinolone-topoisomerase-DNA complexes also share features with ternary complexes formed by antitumor drugs, eukaryotic topoisomerase II, and DNA. Thus, inferences about the bacterial enzymes can sometimes be drawn from studies of their eukaryotic counterpart. Since differences between the two bacterial enyzmes may reflect different chromosomal functions or locations, complexes with one target may be more cytotoxic than with another. Such information potentially contributes to a rationale for choosing one compound over another for treatment of a particular pathogen.

In this chapter the quinolones are introduced through a brief consideration of DNA topoisomerases and quinolone target preference. The discussion then turns to the question of how the agents block bacterial growth. Lethal action is a distinct process, and so it is described separately. Throughout the discussion attention is given to fluoroquinolone structure. Of particular interest are substituents at the C-8 position, since they affect target preference and render fluoroquinolones especially effective at killing cells. Also of interest are moieties attached to the C-7 position, since they, too, affect target preference. Both structural variations influence the attack of particular topoisomerase mutants in a way that contributes to

our understanding of intracellular quinolone action. Readers interested in earlier reviews are referred to references 22, 49, 83, and 104.

DNA TOPOISOMERASES

Many DNA molecules are very long, some are circular, and all require separation of the two duplex strands for most, if not all of their activities. These three general features of DNA lead to physical problems solved by the topoisomerases. For example, long DNA molecules are likely to become entangled, making them difficult to pull apart when cells divide. The double-stranded passage activity of the type II topoisomerases allows snarls to be resolved and interlinked circles (catenanes) to be unlinked (decatenated). Long DNA molecules are also likely to require condensation, not only to fit inside bacterial cells but also to properly segregate after replication. The negative supercoils introduced by gyrase contribute to chromosome condensation (35, 87).

Even short DNA molecules are faced with the problem of separating their complementary strands. The most obvious strand separation problem arises from the unwinding of DNA that must occur during DNA replication. Since the two strands are intertwined, the unreplicated portion of the chromosome would have to rotate rapidly (4,500 rpm to accomodate the known replication rate of the *Escherichia coli* chromosome [101]). Rapid strand separation, plus barriers to rotation such as chromosome circularity, is expected to cause positive superhelical stress to build up ahead of replication forks. That stress is relieved by topoisomerase action, as is the more local stress caused by translocation of transcription complexes through DNA.

Processes such as initiation of replication and transcription also require separation of DNA strands. For these activities local strand separation

Karl Drlica • Public Health Research Institute, 225 Warren Street, Newark, NJ 07103. **David C. Hooper** • Division of Infectious Diseases, Massachusetts General Hospital, 55 Fruit Street, Boston, MA 02114-2696.

occurs preferentially at particular sites and at particular times. Negative supercoiling participates in these processes through its energetic activation of DNA (local strand separation occurs more readily with negatively supercoiled DNA than with relaxed DNA). Control of topoisomerase action allows supercoiling to change in an orderly way that responds to the environment, thereby contributing to local control of DNA activity. Recently discovered examples include the relaxation of supercoils associated with infection of cultured macrophages by *Salmonella enterica* serovar Typhimurium (115) and with hydrogen peroxide treatment of *E. coli* (168). Clearly a knowledge of DNA topology and topoisomerases is of central importance to our understanding bacterial chromosome structure and function.

DNA topoisomerases act by altering the number of times one strand of a DNA duplex winds around its complementary strand; that is, topoisomerases selectively change the linking number of double-stranded DNA molecules. The bacterial topoisomerases are divided into three groups: type I (topoisomerases I and III), type II (gyrase and topoisomerase IV), and specialized topoisomerases (enzymes that catalyze transposition or integration/excision of bacteriophage DNA from the bacterial chromosome). The latter group is outside the scope of the present chapter and is not discussed further. The type I and type II enzymes differ in their mechanisms of action. Type I topoisomerases transiently cleave one strand of a double helix, altering the DNA-linking number in steps of one. Type II enzymes transiently break both strands of a duplex and pass another double-helical segment through the break. These enzymes act in steps of two with respect to linking number. Next we briefly describe the four major bacterial topoisomerases.

Topoisomerase I

James Wang reported the isolation of the first DNA topoisomerase in 1971 (166). The enzyme, now called topoisomerase I, is a monomeric, 110-kDa protein when extracted from *E. coli*. Crystallographic studies indicate that the enzyme is composed of four domains linked by putative hinge regions. Together these domains form a toroidal structure having a central hole large enough to accommodate double-stranded DNA (108). It has been proposed that a large conformational change exposes the active site and allows DNA to enter and leave the central cavity. Topoisomerase I from both prokaryotic and eukaryotic sources catalyzes the removal of negative supercoils from DNA in the absence of ATP; eukaryotic topoisomerase I has the additional ability to remove positive supercoils. The DNA-relaxing activity of *E. coli* topoisomerase I is inhibited by quinolones, but only at very high concentrations (123, 160).

Topoisomerase I is encoded by the *topA* gene. Since *topA* defects elevate chromosomal supercoiling (145) while compensatory gyrase mutations lower it (41, 145), topoisomerase I was proposed to have a safety-valve function that prevents excessive supercoiling from accumulating (45). The discovery that transcription could itself cause high levels of supercoiling in *topA* mutants (143) led to the idea that topoisomerase I removes negative supercoils behind transcription complexes, while gyrase removes positive supercoils ahead of them (109, 177). R-loop formation associated with transcription was subsequently identified as the source of a growth defect attributed to *topA* mutations. In an R loop, mRNA hybridizes to the template strand of DNA, leaving the complementary DNA strand unpaired; such strand separation in a topologically closed DNA molecule generates negative superhelical tension that is normally relaxed by topoisomerase I. Presumably the absence of topoisomerase I allows a buildup of negative supercoils and the accumulation of R loops. Overproduction of ribonuclease H, which digests hybridized RNA, partially relieves the growth defect of *topA* mutations (50). Overproduction of topoisomerase III also relieves the growth defect (19). Topoisomerase III, which is discussed below, is a poor relaxing enzyme unless negative supercoiling is very high. Thus, its ability to suppress *topA* mutations supports the idea that hypernegative supercoiling (46, 144) can actually accumulate in living cells. We conclude that one function of topoisomerase I is the topological destabilization of transcription-mediated R loops. Another is likely to be control of global supercoiling, since a *topA* defect that raises supercoiling also suppresses a *mukB* mutation, a defect that has a global effect on chromosome condensation (148).

Some forms of environmental stress, such as treatment with hydrogen peroxide, increase the expression of *topA* at about the same time that supercoiling drops (168). Such changes appear to be physiologically important, since *topA* mutants are hypersensitive to hydrogen peroxide (162). Increased expression of topoisomerase I would facilitate removal of R loops from highly expressed stress response genes, and the lower supercoiling might optimize the activity of particular promoters through changes in DNA twist (165). Heat shock may represent a similar situation, but in that case a net increase in topoisomerase I is not obvious (164).

Topoisomerase III

The second type I topoisomerase, topoisomerase III, is a monomeric, 83-kDa protein encoded by *topB*. This enzyme, first described in 1983 by Dean et al. (36), has a toroidal structure similar to that of topoisomerase I (24, 121). Although topoisomerase III is able to remove negative superhelical twists (156), its relaxing activity is much less efficient than its ability to decatenate nicked daughter DNA circles following a cycle of DNA replication (38). The decatenase activity is unaffected by quinolones (38, 79). Topoisomerase III binds to both RNA and DNA, and it can induce cleavage of both nucleic acids at identical nucleotide sequences, albeit with different site preference (40).

The physiological role of topoisomerase III is unclear. Survival of mutants with chromosomal deletions encompassing *topB* indicates that the enzyme is not essential (39). Topoisomerase III may have a role in DNA recombination, perhaps in conjunction with the RecQ helicase (79, 178). RecQ-topoisomerase III complexes (79) may normally suppress homologous recombination, since a *mutR* mutation, which increases the frequency of spontaneous DNA deletions (149, 170), is a *topB* allele (149). That finding would help explain how a deletion of *recA* suppresses the extensive cell filamentation observed when *topB* expression is restricted in the absence of topoisomerase I (190). This topoisomerase III-mediated cell filamentation is not mediated by the SOS response, nor is it eliminated by overexpression of topoisomerase IV (190), an activity that relaxes and decatenates DNA (discussed below). Whether topoisomerase III participates in resolving replicated chromosomes through its potent decatenating activity is unknown.

Gyrase

DNA gyrase was discovered by Gellert and associates (65) as an activity that introduces negative supercoils into DNA. This multisubunit enzyme is composed of two A subunits (GyrA, 97 kDa) and two B subunits (GyrB, 90 kDa) encoded by the *gyrA* and *gyrB* genes, respectively. The two subunit types are each divided into two domains (reviewed in reference 147). As discussed in more detail in a subsequent section, GyrA mediates DNA-strand breakage and reunion. A 59-kDa N-terminal tryptic fragment of GyrA, when complexed with GyrB, is sufficient to support weak DNA-supercoiling activity. Addition of the C-terminal 33-kDa GyrA fragment improves enzyme efficiency and is thought to stabilize the complex. GyrB mediates the ATPase activity of the enzyme. Its N-terminal domain contains the ATP-binding site; a 47-kDa C-terminal fragment, when complexed with GyrA, supports DNA relaxation but neither supercoiling nor ATP hydrolysis.

Gyrase is the only purified enzyme that can introduce negative supercoils into DNA. It can also catenate and decatenate covalently closed circular DNA molecules, and it ties and unties knots in double-stranded DNA molecules. These reactions require ATP, which the enzyme hydrolyzes to ADP and inorganic phosphate. DNA gyrase also has the ability to relax positive and negative DNA supercoils.

The ATPase activity of DNA gyrase is competitively inhibited by novobiocin and other coumarin antibacterials. These agents, which are structurally unrelated to quinolones, bind to the N-terminal portion of the *E. coli* GyrB protein. The availability of coumarins and temperature-sensitive gyrase mutations made it possible to study the intracellular action of the enzyme. The ability of the drugs and mutations to block the introduction of supercoils into phage DNA (64) and to cause a loss of chromosomal DNA supercoiling (48, 159) indicate that gyrase participates in the maintenance of supercoiling. The supercoiling activity of DNA gyrase is opposed by the relaxing activities of topoisomerase I and topoisomerase IV. Because transcription of the genes encoding DNA gyrase and topoisomerase I respond to the superhelicity of DNA in opposite ways (decreasing negative supercoiling stimulates transcription of the *gyrA* and *gyrB* genes and suppresses transcription of the *topA* gene [119, 163]), supercoiling is thought to be homeostatically regulated.

Gyrase probably plays two roles in DNA replication. One involves the introduction of negative supercoils needed for binding of initiation proteins to replication origins. The other involves the relaxation of positive supercoils arising from DNA strand unwinding during replication fork propagation. As pointed out below, topoisomerase IV also facilitates DNA unwinding (141). Whether gyrase participates in the decatenation of interlocked daughter DNA molecules may depend on the bacterial species. In *E. coli*, topoisomerase IV is a much more active decatenase than gyrase, and so the accumulation of partially segregated nucleoids in gyrase mutants (158) is generally attributed to the loss of supercoils preventing topoisomerase IV activity (84). However, some human pathogens lack topoisomerase IV (27, 60). In such organisms gyrase may assume responsibility for chromosome decatenation.

Transcription is also influenced by gyrase since negative supercoiling of DNA affects promoter activity and binding of regulatory proteins to DNA. Thus, it is likely that promoters of environment-sensitive genes have evolved to take advantage of the sensitivity of gyrase and supercoiling to environmental factors such as oxygen tension (44, 89), salt concentration (86, 90), and temperature (68, 120). Gyrase also facilitates RNA polymerase movement by removing positive supercoils expected to accumulate ahead of transcription complexes (177). Recent evidence for the generation of positive supercoils by transcription comes from the observation that they can be sensed by promoters more than 5 kb from the source (78).

DNA gyrase is also involved in aspects of DNA recombination and DNA repair, largely by virtue of its supercoiling activity (strand invasion and DNA bending occur more readily with a supercoiled substrate). Integrative recombination of bacteriophage lambda and transposition of transposon Tn5 are among the examples affected by a reduction in gyrase activity.

Topoisomerase IV

DNA topoisomerase IV was purified first by Kato et al. (99). The *E. coli* enzyme, which displays almost 40% homology with gyrase at the amino acid level, is composed of two ParC subunits (75 kDa, homologous to GyrA) and two ParE subunitis (70 kDa, homologous to GyrB). ParC is associated with the bacterial cell membrane, perhaps in a DNA-dependent manner. (Membrane association is enhanced by the presence of magnesium and reduced by treatment with DNase I.) Purified topoisomerase IV relaxes both negative and positive supercoils in an ATP-dependent reaction that is inhibited by the coumarins and by the quinolones.

While the ability of topoisomerase IV to relax negative supercoils is weak, it is sufficient to suppress a *topA* deficiency if the two subunits of the enzyme are overproduced (99, 118). Even at normal levels, topoisomerase IV may contribute to the control of supercoiling by opposing the activity of gyrase (186). An important feature of the enzyme is its preferential ability to relax positive supercoils. This occurs roughly 20 times faster than relaxation of negative supercoils, apparently because processivity is greater with a positively supercoiled substrate (30). This preference would allow topoisomerase IV to relieve positive torsional tension arising ahead of replication forks without competing strongly with the supercoiling activity of gyrase (101).

Topoisomerase IV also exhibits a potent decatenating activity. As pointed out above, one function of decatenation is the unlinking of daughter chromosomes at the end of a round of replication. A second function is the elimination of precatenanes arising from replication fork movement. (Some of the positive supercoils generated ahead of the replication fork can be manifested behind the fork as precatenanes.) Thus, topoisomerase IV is likely to facilitate replication-fork movement through a direct relaxation activity and through removal of precatenanes.

FLUOROQUINOLONE TARGETS

Bacteria fall into three general classes with respect to fluoroquinolone targets. One group, composed of the human pathogens *Mycobacterium tuberculosis*, *Helicobacter pylori*, and *Treponema pallidum*, appears to have only gyrase as a target, because the genomes of this group lack a close homologue of topoisomerase IV (27, 60, 161). In these bacteria gyrase probably assumes the function of topoisomerase IV. Many mycobacterial species, including *M. tuberculosis*, are also unusual in having an alanine at the position equivalent to amino acid 83 in the gyrase A (GyrA) protein of *E. coli* (75). In most organisms this position is occupied by serine or threonine. Since an alanine substitution at GyrA position 83 has no effect on the DNA-supercoiling activity of gyrase (12, 77), the change is expected to have little effect on growth. However, gyrases with a hydrophobic amino acid at this position are inherently less sensitive to quinolone attack (76). In the case of an Ala-83 substitution, the effect is about threefold with the purified *E. coli* protein (12). *T. pallidum* also carries the alanine seen with *M. tuberculosis*, while *H. pylori* has an asparagine substitution at the 83 position. Whether these changes are related to the absence of topoisomerase IV is not known. The net result, however, is that wild-type strains of *M. tuberculosis*, *M. avium*, *M. bovis*, *T. pallidum*, and probably *H. pylori* are equivalent in susceptibility to moderately susceptible, first-step gyrase mutants of other organisms.

The second and third groups of bacteria contain both gyrase and topoisomerase IV. In gram-negative organisms, such as *E. coli*, gyrase is more sensitive than topoisomerase IV to fluoroquinolone-mediated attack (Table 1). Consequently, in these bacteria first-step resistance mutations map in the genes encoding gyrase, generally in *gyrA*. (*gyrB* mutations, which can also reduce susceptibility [184], tend to be selected less often.) Resistance alleles mapping in *parC* or *parE*, two genes encoding topoisomerase IV, have little or no protective effect unless accompanied by a gyrase mutation (16, 18, 25, 102). In gram-positive bacteria, such as *Staphylococcus aureus*, gyrase is much less sensitive to fluoroquinolones than in

Table 1. Inhibition of purified topoisomerase activity by fluoroquinolones

Source of proteins	Fluoroquinolone	Inhibitory concentration (IC$_{50}$)^a		
		Topoisomerase IV	Gyrase	Topoisomerase IV/gyrase
E. coli	Ciprofloxacin	5	0.42	12
	Trovafloxacin	8	0.52	15
	Sparfloxacin	9.3	0.57	16
S. aureus	Ciprofloxacin	13.7	25	0.5
	Trovafloxacin	8.7	18.8	0.5
	Sparfloxacin	40	22	2^b

^{a} Drug concentration (μM) for half-maximal inhibition of catalytic activity. Topoisomerase IV was assayed for decatenation of kinetoplast DNA; gyrase activity was supercoiling of relaxed pBR322 plasmid DNA. Adapted from reference 70.
^{b} Gyrase may be the primary target for sparfloxacin.

gram-negative bacteria; topoisomerase IV tends to have about the same sensitivity in both types of organism (Table 1; exceptions are discussed below). This loss of sensitivity by gyrase causes first-step, ciprofloxacin-resistant mutations in gram-positive bacteria to map in *parC* rather than in *gyrA* (54, 55, 128).

In some gram-positive bacteria, fluoroquinolone structure can have a strong influence on target preference when defined genetically. For example, when compounds are compared for the identity of first-step mutations in *Streptococcus pneumoniae*, addition of a bulky benzenesulfonamide modification to the C-7 position shifts preference from topoisomerase IV to gyrase (3), probably by increasing the relative activity of the compound against gyrase (3). The substituent at the C-8 position is also important for target selection: fluoroquinolones with a C-8 halogen or methoxy group tend to prefer gyrase as a target, while many of the other compounds prefer topoisomerase IV (Table 2; Fig. 1, structures). Although many of the agents listed in Table 2 have too many structural differences to

attribute the target shift solely to a particular substituent, the C-8–H compound AM1121 has been compared with its C-8-methoxy derivative gatifloxacin and its C-5-methyl derivative grepafloxacin for the identity of first-step mutants. AM1121 selects a *parC* allele, and gatifloxacin and grepafloxacin both select a *gyrA* mutation (Table 2).

Sometimes genetic and biochemical data fail to agree on the identity of the primary target. Three laboratories reported that topoisomerase IV, when purified from *S. pneumoniae*, is much more sensitive than gyrase to sparfloxacin (126, 130, 135). However, genetic studies show that gyrase is the primary target of the drug (62, 132, 136, 139). Arguments have been provided against two trivial explanations. First, the genes encoding topoisomerase IV lack mutations that would account for the effect (136). Second, the relative amounts of the two proteins do not account for the difference between in vitro and in vivo observations (136). Thus, the difference in target preference probably reflects a greater cytotoxicity of quinolone complexes formed with gyrase than with topoisomerase

Table 2. Primary fluoroquinolone targets defined genetically in *S. pneumoniae*

Fluoroquinolone	C-8 substituent^a	Location of first-step resistance mutation	Reference(s)
Sparfloxacin	F	*gyrA*	62, 132, 139
Clinafloxacin	Cl	*gyrA, parC*	133
Moxifloxacin	OMe	*gyrA*	139
Gatifloxacin	OMe	*gyrA*	62
Garenoxacin^b	OF$_2$	*gyrA*	42
Gemifloxacin	na^c	*gyrA*	80
NSFQ-105	H	*gyrA*	3
Grepafloxacin^d	H	*gyrA*	124
AM1121	H	*parC*	63
Ciprofloxacin	H	*parC*	62, 132, 134, 138
Norfloxacin	H	*parC*	62
Trovafloxacin	na^c	*parC*	62, 138
Levofloxacin	na^c	*parC*	62, 138

^{a} Abbreviations: OMe, methoxy; F, fluorine; Cl, chlorine; H, hydrogen.
^{b} Lacks C-6 fluorine.
^{c} Not applicable.
^{d} Same structure as AM1121 but with C-5 methyl group.

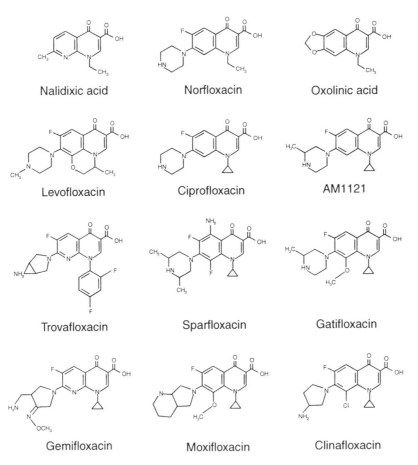

Figure 1. Structures of commonly studied fluoroquinolones.

IV. For example, gyrase-containing complexes block replication more rapidly than those containing topoisomerase IV (58, 100), which may make the repair of gyrase-containing lesions more difficult.

BACTERIOSTATIC ACTION

Overview of Type II Topoisomerase Structure and Action

As pointed out in the introduction, the hallmark of quinolone action is the trapping of gyrase and topoisomerase IV on DNA as drug-enzyme-DNA complexes. Some relaxation of chromosomal DNA supercoiling also occurs (153), but it is not enough to account for inhibition of growth (*gyrB* mutants grow well with substantially lower levels of supercoiling [145]). The ternary structures are called cleaved, cleavage, or cleavable complexes because the trapped DNA is broken. To provide a context for understanding how fluoroquinolones block bacterial growth, it is necessary to consider topoisomerase structure and activity, quinolone binding, and complex formation.

Crystal structures are available for portions of eukaryotic topoisomerase II (15, 53), bacterial GyrA (122), and bacterial GyrB (171). If we assume that the eukaryotic structure is representative, the two GyrA subunits are seen as forming dimers through two contact regions, one called the DNA gate and the other, the exit gate. Each GyrA subunit also interacts with a GyrB subunit. Although the order of events is not rigorously established, a general scheme for DNA-strand passage can be envisioned (Fig. 2) (167). First, one region of duplex DNA, the gate or G segment, binds to the surface of a GyrA dimer that is stabilized by binding to GyrB subunits. The gyrase subunits may assemble on the DNA, or perhaps more often, the DNA passes through the GyrB clamp (discussed below) to reach the GyrA surface (Fig. 2c) (172). Gyrase cleaves both strands of the G segment while the protein portion of the DNA gate is closed (Fig. 2d). (Cleavage occurs even when the gate is locked by protein cross-linking [173].) ATP binding to GyrB promotes dimerization and formation of a protein clamp that captures a second region of DNA, the transport or T segment (Fig. 2e) (172). The DNA gate opens, and the T segment passes through it (Fig. 2f).

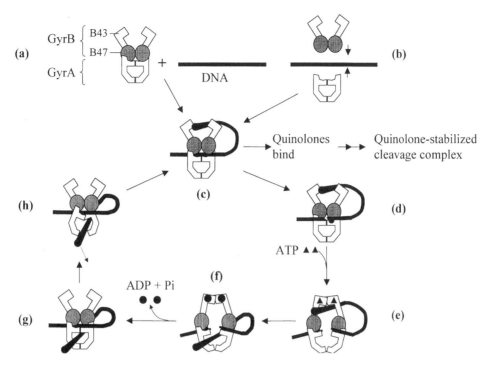

Figure 2. Model of supercoiling and relaxation by DNA gyrase. (a) The 43-kDa and 47-kDa regions of GyrB, along with the 64-kDa region of GyrA are shown as a tetramer. The 33-kDa C-terminal domains of GyrA are omitted for clarity, as is the DNA wrap around gyrase. Supercoiling occurs when gyrase either binds a G segment of DNA (a) or assembles onto the G segment (b). The resulting complex (c) is a substrate for quinolone binding. The ternary complex (c) cleaves DNA to form a cleavage complex (d). ATP binds to the 43-kDa domains of GyrB, causing them to close and capture the T segment of DNA (e). The T segment is transported through the break in the G segment and into the bottom cavity of gyrase (f). The break in the G segment is religated (g), and the T segment is then released from the bottom cavity through the exit gate in the enzyme (h). The exit gate closes, resetting the enzyme for a new round of supercoiling. Between capture of the T segment and resetting of the enzyme, ATP is hydrolyzed and released. The figure was provided by Dr. J. G. Heddle (John Innes Centre, Norwich, United Kingdom). Reprinted from reference 83 by courtesy of Marcel Dekker, Inc.

The G segment of DNA is then rejoined (Fig. 2g), and the T segment passes through the exit gate of the GyrA protein (Fig. 2h). The ATP-operated clamp of the GyrB protein reopens on ATP hydrolysis. Gyrase can act processively by remaining attached to the G segment and drawing T segments repeatedly into the GyrB clamp after each round of ATP hydrolysis.

Two ATPs are hydrolyzed per catalytic cycle (97, 167). With eukaryotic topoisomerase II, the two hydrolysis steps appear to be temporally distinct (11), with the faster one occurring before strand passage through the DNA gate and the second after it. Apparently ATP hydrolysis accelerates strand passage even though hydrolysis is not required for passage (11). Distinct hydrolysis steps have yet to be demonstrated with the bacterial enzymes.

Quinolone-Topoisomerase-DNA Complexes

A key advance in the dissection of complex formation was the identification of a gyrase mutation that prevents quinolone-dependent DNA cleavage (31). Quinolone binding to these mutant gyrase-DNA complexes induces a conformational change that can be detected in the GyrB subunit by limited proteolysis (95). The trapped complex is able to hydrolyze ATP, but at a slower rate than seen in the absence of quinolone (96). The effect on ATP hydrolysis may be related to the conformational changes, since ATP hydrolysis is a function of the GyrB subunit (1, 2). With wild-type gyrase, conversion to the quinolone-distinctive rate of ATP hydrolysis happens quickly after drug is added to gyrase and DNA. DNA cleavage, however, is a slower, subsequent process (96). Thus quinolone binding and trapping of cleaved DNA are distinct.

The DNA cleavage reaction consists of a pair of single-stranded scissions occurring on opposite strands of the duplex (57, 125). These nicks, which are staggered by 4 bp, allow the G segment to be pulled apart for passage of the T segment during topoisomerase action. Although both DNA strands must be broken in a coordinated way for the gate to open, trapping each single-stranded break by a quinolone appears to be an independent event (153). Thus, there are probably two drug binding sites, an idea that is supported by a stoichiometry of two quinolone molecules per gyrase (31, 95). When the protein portion of the DNA gate is cross-linked so that it cannot open wide enough to allow the passage of a DNA segment, quinolones are still able to bind and trap broken DNA (173). This observation is best explained by the drug-blocking religation.

Complexes formed with topoisomerase IV are probably similar to those with gyrase, although DNA does not wrap around topoisomerase IV as it does around gyrase (57, 98). As with gyrase, a topoisomerase IV mutation can block DNA cleavage while still allowing quinolone binding to complexes (114), and quinolones reduce the ATPase activity of topoisomerase IV (4). Even in the absence of cleavage, quinolones enhance both binding of topoisomerase IV to DNA and formation of a distortion in the DNA of the complex (114). Moreover, a conformational change may occur in the ParE protein, the topoisomerase IV homologue of GyrB; *parE* mutations have been obtained that render the enzyme defective at forming a cleaved complex with norfloxacin without interfering significantly with hydrolysis of ATP, dimerization of ParE, or DNA binding (10). As with gyrase, inhibition of religation is likely to be a major factor in complex formation, since inhibition correlates with yield of cleavage (5).

Anderson et al. (6) have suggested that the quinolones distort topoisomerase-bound DNA by placing the 3′ ends of the DNA out of the proper alignment needed for rejoining. In contrast, some antitumor drugs acting on eukaryotic topoisomerase II are thought to distort the bound DNA in a way that exerts more effect on the forward reaction (6).

Quinolone Binding Sites

Each subunit of the GyrA dimer contains on its presumed DNA binding surface a short recognition helix (α-helix 4; Fig. 3). The major quinolone-resistance mutations map on the exposed surface of this helix at amino acids numbered 83 and 87 in the *E. coli* protein (34, 122, 131, 155). Studies with purified gyrase indicate that mutations at these positions reduce drug binding (12, 175, 185). Since two recognition helices occur per GyrA dimer (122) and since biochemical studies indicate a stoichiometry of two quinolones per complex (31), it is likely that one quinolone binds to each recognition helix. Other resistance alleles are found in the same general region of GyrA (Fig. 3), but they confer less protection than those at positions 83 and 87 (111). The portion of GyrA shown in Fig. 3B is termed the quinolone-resistance-determining region (QRDR) (amino acids 51 to 106 [61, 183]).

The nature of the quinolone binding site can be studied by covariation of quinolone and gyrase structure, the latter via resistance mutations. For intracellular experiments it has been assumed that drug-topoisomerase-DNA complex formation can be measured by the ability of a compound to prevent colony formation on drug-containing agar plates. When the C-8-methoxyfluoroquinolone gatifloxacin was compared with its C-8–H derivative, AM1121, ten *gyrA* mutants of *E. coli* fell into two classes (111). Those alleles encoding changes in the recognition helix showed greater susceptibility to compounds with a C-8-methoxy group when compared with mutant alleles encoding changes located outside the helix (111). These data suggest that the C-8-methoxy moiety partially overcomes the protective effect of the helix mutations, a conclusion that is consistent with the recognition helix being part of the binding site.

Substitution of a proline into the helix (position 84) between the two major resistance mutation sites constitutes an exception to the general distinction between the allele classes, since the susceptibility of the Pro-84 mutant is unaffected by the C-8-methoxy group (111). Proline is known to disrupt α-helices; perhaps this proline alters the alignment between amino acids 83 and 87, thereby preventing proper positioning of the drug independent of the presence of a C-8-methoxy group.

Halogen substituents at the C-8 position also increase quinolone attack against mutants altered at GyrA positions 83 and 87 (43, 150). Inspection of the amino acid changes conferring resistance at those positions reveals that the electronegative character of serine (position 83) and aspartic acid (position 87) is lost, mainly by mutation to hydrophobic residues. Electron-rich methoxy or halogen substituents on the quinolone may restore an electron-dense microenvironment and thereby enhance attack of these mutants. In general, methoxy, chlorine, and bromine groups are more effective than fluorine substituents, as indicated by experiments with several *gyrA* mutants of *Mycobacterium smegmatis* (150). Work with gyrase purified from *E. coli* supports conclusions derived from cell growth studies (12). For example, addition of chlorine or bromine to fluoroquinolone C-8 increases the inhibitory activity against gyrase containing two alanine substitutions (GyrA positions 83 and 87). Addition of a fluorine has a smaller effect.

Quinolone orientation on gyrase has been deduced from the identity of the most resistant mutant selected by different compounds. With *M. smegmatis*, a C-8-methoxy fluoroquinolone having a C-7-ring ethyl at the N position selects for a GyrA

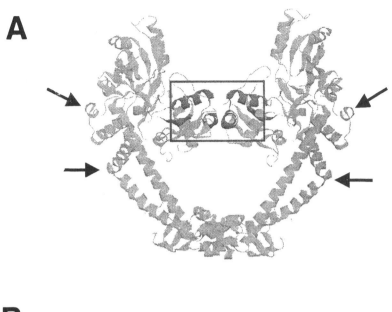

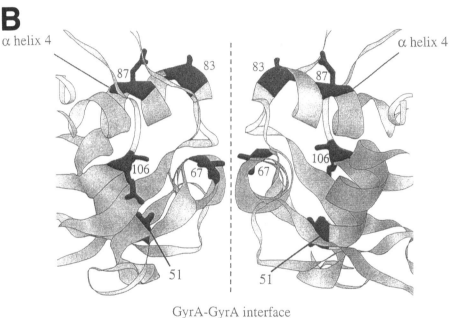

GyrA-GyrA interface

Figure 3. Structure of DNA gyrase GyrA59 dimer. The figure shows a ribbon representation (generated in RasMol) of the GyrA59 fragment (122), courtesy of J.G. Heddle (John Innes Centre). The upper panel shows the entire GyrA59 dimer while the lower panel is an enlargement of the boxed region in the upper panel. Amino acids that change to confer quinolone resistance are indicated in black and by the amino acid numbers. Amino acid 51 is in helix 2, amino acid 67 is in helix 3, and amino acids 83 and 87 are in helix 4. The figure was adapted from reference 61. Arrows in the upper panel indicate the location of changes that increase illegitimate recombination and spontaneous induction of lambda prophage as described in reference 7.

mutant whose alteration (Gly to Cys) is near the N-terminal end of the recognition helix (position 81 in the *E. coli* numbering system) (Fig. 4). That mutant exhibits the highest MIC at which 99% of the isolates tested are inhibited (MIC$_{99}$) of those tested (Fig. 5). In contrast, locating the C-7-ring ethyl at a carbon adjacent to the ring nitrogen is less discriminating (Fig. 5). Apparently Cys-81 interferes more with fluoroquinolone binding when an ethyl group is

attached to the C-7 piperazinyl ring nitrogen than when the ethyl is bound to a ring carbon. These data are consistent with the C-7 fluoroquinolone ring binding near the N terminus of the helix, while the remainder of the quinolone attaches more toward the C terminus (Fig. 4). Such an orientation would explain why in *E. coli* a mutation at position 81 confers resistance to fluoroquinolones but not to nalidixic acid (21), a compound that lacks a C-7 ring. For

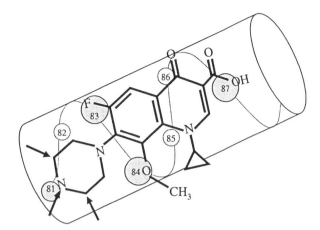

Figure 4. Proposed quinolone binding site. Orientation of fluoroquinolones and GyrA α-helix-4. α-Helix-4, adapted from the crystal structure of the breakage-reunion domain of the GyrA protein of *E. coli* (122), is drawn parallel to the long axis of the fluoroquinolone. For clarity, amino acid numbers represent positions in the *E. coli* GyrA protein. (The experiments were performed with *M. smegmatis*; position 81 in the figure corresponds to 89 in *M. smegmatis*.) Arrows indicate positions of an ethyl group that changes the identity of the most resistant mutant (see text). The figure was adapted from reference 150.

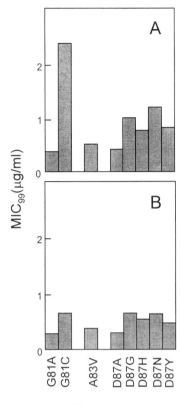

Figure 5. Effect of GyrA variation on susceptibility to fluoroquinolones. MIC_{99} was determined for two structurally similar fluoroquinolones with the indicated fluoroquinolone-resistant mutants of *M. smegmatis*. (The changes in the GyrA variants are indicated by standard amino acid abbreviations with the letter preceeding the number indicating the wild-type amino acid and the letter following the number representing the variant; the numbers used correspond to those shown in Fig. 4 and represent positions numbered according to the *E. coli* GyrA protein.) Panel A utilized fluoroquinolone PD161144, which has an ethyl group attached to the C-7 ring nitrogen as indicated by an arrow in Fig. 4. Panel B utilized fluoroquinolone PD161148, which has its ethyl group attached to a C-7 ring carbon adjacent to the nitrogen indicated in Fig. 4. The figure was adapted from data presented in reference 150.

reasons that are not yet understood, the effect of ethyl positioning is more pronounced when a methoxy group is at position C-8 (150), further supporting the idea that the presence of the methoxy group alters quinolone positioning on gyrase.

Work with purified topoisomerase IV has focused on compounds having commercial potential, and those compounds differ by too many moieties to draw structural conclusions. Nevertheless, two changes in the recognition helix of the *S. aureus* ParC (GrlA) protein (Phe-80 and Lys-84) interfere with the ability of ciprofloxacin and trovafloxacin to stimulate topoisomerase IV-mediated DNA cleavage (5). When drug concentrations are saturating, the mutation at position 84 allows about half as much cleavage as that at position 80 (5). As expected, mutants with changes at position 84 exhibit lower susceptibility than those with changes at position 80 (107). A comparable situation occurs in *S. pneumoniae* (136, 179).

Intracellular work directed at topoisomerase IV has also lacked structural variants that would allow conclusions to be drawn about particular fluoroquinolone structures. Nevertheless, a consistent story can be pieced together. For example, premafloxacin, a C-8-methoxy compound, preferentially attacks *S. aureus* topoisomerase IV (93). Standard ParC (GrlA) variants, which are equivalent to GyrA83 and 87 variants of *E. coli*, are only one-fourth as susceptible to ciprofloxacin as to premafloxacin (93). This is the result expected from a gyrase study (111) in which the C-8-methoxy group was shown to preferentially

enhance activity against mutants containing alterations in the recognition helix. Consequently, it is more difficult to select first-step mutants with premafloxacin than with ciprofloxacin (93). Indeed, the first-step, premafloxacin-resistant mutants that have been isolated map outside the recognition helix (93). It has been suggested that these mutations confer premafloxacin resistance because they make topoisomerase IV less likely to form stable complexes with DNA and therefore less likely to be converted to toxic complexes by quinolone action (93).

Chromosomal Distribution of Complexes

The location of the quinolone-gyrase-DNA complexes on the bacterial chromosome is likely to influence the potential damage that quinolones can cause. Complex distribution can be estimated by treating cells with quinolone, gently extracting the DNA with an ionic detergent to denature the topoisomerase, and then measuring the size of the resulting DNA fragments generated by the release of double-stranded DNA breaks. By this method two size classes of fragment have been detected with *E. coli* DNA when gyrase is the target: pulse-labeled (newly replicated) DNA is about 15 kbp (47), while fragments released from the chromosome as a whole average about 100 kbp (153). These data indicate that gyrase is associated with replication forks and also scattered around the chromosome.

Topoisomerase IV is estimated to be distributed over the *E. coli* chromosome at about 200-kbp intervals when ciprofloxacin is used as a probe and a *gyrA* resistance allele is present to reduce attack of gyrase (25). The spacing of topoisomerase IV has also been examined in *S. aureus* using norfloxacin as a probe and a *gyrA* mutation to minimize attack of gyrase. In this bacterium cleavage occurred every 30 kbp (58). Although understanding the quantitative difference between *E. coli* and *S. aureus* requires additional work, it is clear that the complexes are spaced closely enough in both organisms to readily interfere with DNA activities that involve translocating enzymes.

The rules determining the distribution of complexes are presently undefined. Strong interaction sites with DNA can be found (85, 114, 137), but topoisomerase IV and gyrase generally exhibit a low preference for specific sites (for examples, see references 56, 57, 59, 110, 129). Low sequence specificity would allow these enzymes to respond virtually anywhere on the chromosome to activities that require topological changes. Among the stronger interaction sites for gyrase are those present in *rep* (bacterial interspersed mosaic element, or BIME) sequences (8, 9, 17, 28, 52, 181, 182). These sequences, which are sometimes associated with binding sites for the small DNA-bending protein called integration host factor, are located at about 200 places around the chromosome near the 3′ ends of active genes, usually in nontranslated regions. At these sites gyrase is expected to relieve the positive supercoiling arising from active transcription (109, 177). Thus, the enzymes probably recognize DNA on the basis of both nucleotide sequence and local topology.

One of the topological problems handled by the topoisomerases may be the resolution of DNA entanglements. Moving pictures of ethidium-stained chromosomal DNA released from cells treated with proteinase and detergents show that most of the DNA molecules exist in the form of rosettes in which DNA loops emanate from one or more nodes (13). The number and size of the rosettes are reduced by mutation of *recA*, treatment with ribonuclease, or treatment with topoisomerase IV. When all three perturbations are combined, few nodes remain. Hecht and Pettijohn had previously shown that the RNA component responsible for constraining DNA of isolated chromosomes is nascent RNA (81). Thus it appears that transcription- and recombination-dependent DNA entanglements are present. Such entanglements may be responsible for the topological barriers (151) detected in vivo using site-specific recombination of γδ (157). In this assay the synapsis of two distant γδ *res* sites is blocked by barriers that prevent DNA branch migration and a slithering movement of two regions of interwound duplex DNA. Resolution of *res* sites occurs less often in topoisomerase IV and gyrase mutants, as if alterations in these enzymes result in defects in removing topological barriers on the chromosome.

Cytological assays, carried out with *Bacillus subtilis*, suggest that topoisomerase IV is localized at the cell poles (91). If the enzyme is also widely distributed on the *B. subtilis* chromosome, as seen with *E. coli* and *S. aureus* using the quinolone-mediated DNA cleavage assay, polar localization might reflect the restraint of DNA loops. Loop constraint fits well with the behavior of eukaryotic topoisomerase II, which can be seen at the base of loops in metaphase chromosomes (51). An interesting feature of *Drosophila* topoisomerase II is that it shows a cleavage preference for a sequence containing alternating AT dinucleotides (20). This preferred sequence is present at about 10^4 copies per genome, which corresponds in frequency to the number of DNA loops observed by microscopy.

Inhibition of DNA Synthesis

One of the consequences of quinolone-gyrase-DNA complex formation is the reversible interruption of DNA replication (72). Inhibition of DNA synthesis is rapid (within minutes) even when inhibition is only partial (58, 153). This result is consistent with gyrase being located immediately in front of replication forks where complex formation would block fork movement (47, 84, 100). Complexes formed on DNA with purified gyrase and ciprofloxacin block replication by bacteriophage T7 DNA polymerase at a location 10 to 14 nucleotides upstream from the gyrase cleavage site (169). Since almost 130 bp of DNA are wrapped around gyrase, DNA polymerase must be able to penetrate much of the wrapped portion of the complex. Replication is not blocked when gyrase is obtained from an active-site mutant that fails to allow cleavage. Thus DNA cleavage, not binding of the drug by the enzyme, is required to halt DNA replication. Collision of the replication apparatus with a drug-gyrase-DNA complex fails to stimulate the release of DNA breaks in vitro (169), a finding that is consistent with the reversible nature of inhibition of DNA replication in vivo (release of breaks is expected to be irreversible [103]).

The quinolone concentration required to block DNA synthesis correlates well with the MIC (26), and the MICs of different quinolones correlate with their ability to block the activity of purified gyrase, although higher drug concentrations are required in vitro than in vivo (69). These correlations make it reasonable to take inhibition of DNA synthesis and MIC as indicators of intracellular complex formation. Since DNA synthesis is blocked by complexes containing only one single-stranded break (153), inhibition of growth is expected to occur at lower concentrations than required to saturate all gyrase interactions.

Biochemical studies with topoisomerase IV have led to statements that are similar to those with gyrase. For example, complexes formed with quinolone and purified topoisomerase IV block passage of the replication apparatus, but only when DNA in the complex has been cleaved (a mutation that blocks cleavage prevents stoppage of replication fork movement) (85). Moreover, collision of the replication fork with the complex fails to release DNA breaks. However, the resulting complexes are irreversible, unlike the situation with gyrase (169). Other differences between the gyrase and topoisomerase IV become apparent when the fate of replication-generated torsional tension is considered. Replication fork movement creates positive supercoils that can either accumulate ahead of the fork or diffuse back across it to become precatenanes (right-handed, catenane-like windings [23, 84]). While positive supercoils can be removed by both gyrase and topoisomerase IV, precatenanes are removed only by topoisomerase IV (84).

The intracellular action of quinolones suggests that the two enzymes may normally occupy different compartments on the chromosome. For example, gyrase-containing complexes inhibit DNA replication rapidly (within minutes), while those with topoisomerase IV act more slowly (58, 102); under conditions in which inhibition is partial, norfloxacin directed at S. aureus topoisomerase IV inhibits DNA synthesis at a rate less than 10% of that seen when nalidixic acid, a less potent compound, attacks gyrase (58). Slow inhibition of replication by topoisomerase IV-containing complexes is consistent with this enzyme acting behind replication forks or at the end of a round of replication. Indeed, topoisomerase IV-dependent inhibition of synthesis is delayed by 40 min when E. coli cells are released from amino acid starvation (100). (Starvation prevents initiation of replication; after release about 40 min are required to complete a round of replication.) The delay is eliminated by mutations in gyrB or seqA (100). Thus topoisomerase IV-mediated complexes can act as barriers to fork movement that rapidly inhibit DNA replication (85) when gyrase is defective or inhibited (101) or when DNA synthesis initiates from multiple sites. But this direct relaxation of positive supercoils by topoisomerase IV appears to supplement gyrase activity and may not always be used.

The data sketched above lead to the general view that gyrase functions ahead of forks and that topoisomerase IV normally functions behind them. This idea explains how norfloxacin can trap topoisomerase IV in complexes on plasmid DNA without inhibiting DNA synthesis (100). One of the consequences of this enzyme dichotomy is that the preference for gyrase shown by some fluoroquinolones when attacking S. pneumoniae (Table 2) would allow these agents to block DNA synthesis more rapidly than fluoroquinolones that target topoisomerase IV. Still not understood is how quinolone-topoisomerase IV-DNA complexes can be distributed throughout the chromosome (58) and yet display delayed inhibition of DNA synthesis. (Less than a minute should be required for a replication fork to reach one of these complexes in S. aureus.)

Inhibition of RNA Synthesis

Early experiments with nalidixic acid showed that RNA synthesis is blocked by the drug, but more slowly than DNA synthesis (72). Thus, when culture turbidity is measured after drug treatment, it continues to increase for more than 30 min (71). Since little loss of supercoils occurs at concentrations that inhibit RNA synthesis (112), inhibition of RNA synthesis is not explained by DNA relaxation. It is more likely that drug-enzyme-DNA complexes block transcription, much as they block replication. Indeed, purified gyrase trapped on DNA by ciprofloxacin blocks transcription by purified RNA polymerase (174). Termination of transcription occurs upstream from the gyrase complex, consistent with steric hindrance. For bacteriophage T7 RNA polymerase, transcription termination occurs 10 bp from the center of the gyrase-mediated cleavage site (the distance is 20 bp for E. coli RNA polymerase [174]). Gyrase bound to DNA in the absence of quinolone allows transcription complexes to pass; thus, the broken DNA with its covalently bound protein appears to be the interfering lesion. As with replication, transcription fails to stimulate the release of DNA breaks from ternary drug-enzyme-DNA complexes (174). Thus, quinolone-mediated inhibition of transcription may be largely bacteriostatic.

LETHAL ACTION

Distinction between Blocking Growth and Killing Cells

Formation of quinolone-gyrase-DNA complexes cannot by itself be a lethal event because complex formation, as monitored by inhibition of DNA synthesis, is reversible (72). Moreover, comparison of closely related fluoroquinolones shows that one compound can be more effective than another at preventing colony formation but less effective at killing cells (189). In addition, compounds can have similar MICs for two strains but can kill one much more effectively than the other (67, 127). Thus, blocking growth, i.e., blocking DNA and RNA synthesis, must be distinct from killing cells even though complex formation and cell death are clearly connected (resistance alleles in the target genes reduce both effects [111, 174, 175]). The most straightforward model is that drug-gyrase-DNA complexes block cell growth while release of DNA breaks from those complexes is lethal (25). Double-stranded DNA breaks are indeed lethal (103), and the release of breaks from chromosomal drug-gyrase-DNA complexes correlates with cell death, not with inhibition of growth (25).

Since single-stranded DNA breaks are probably more easily repaired than double-stranded ones, lethal activity is expected to correlate better with the latter. About 5 to 10 times more quinolone (oxolinic acid) is required to trap double-stranded breaks, i.e., pairs of closely spaced single-stranded breaks, than solitary, single-stranded breaks (153). Lethal action during short incubation times also requires 5 to 10 times more quinolone than inhibition of DNA synthesis, a surrogate measure for the trapping of single-stranded lesions (25, 153). Thus, compounds that more easily trap both members of a pair of single-stranded breaks, or more readily cause release of double-stranded breaks, are expected to be more lethal.

Differences between bacteriostatic and lethal effects are sometimes obscured by the practice of measuring killing after long incubation periods. Lethal action can be detected after as little as an hour of incubation, but measurement of minimal bactericidal concentration (MBC) typically involves overnight incubation. When incubation periods are long, many secondary events, such as lethal filamentation, can occur (71, 140), and that may cause MBC and MIC to be quantitatively similar (26). Secondary events could be important for clinical efficacy, particularly when quinolone administration occurs only once per day and concentrations drop close to the MIC.

Proteins Affecting Release and Repair of DNA Breaks

Inhibitors of RNA or protein synthesis interfere with the lethal action of the quinolones without blocking quinolone-mediated inhibition of DNA replication (25, 37, 72). Thus quinolone lethality may depend on the expression of a suicide protein induced by quinolone treatment. The protein, which has not been identified, probably turns over rapidly, because addition of chloramphenicol, even after 120 min of nalidixic acid treatment, rapidly eliminates lethal activity (32, 33). Since *lexA* Ind– mutants fail to affect killing by nalidixic acid (105), the suicide gene(s) is not part of the SOS response. Many other proteins in addition to those in the SOS regulon are induced by quinolones (66). Some of those might be involved in lethal action. Spontaneous mutants have been obtained whose growth is blocked by nalidixic acid or other quinolones in the absence of cell death, but the presence of multiple mutations has made it difficult to identify the responsible genes (176; Zhao et al., unpublished observations).

Studies with eukaryotic systems establish the existence of proteins that repair topoisomerase-containing complexes. For example, a tyrosine-DNA phosphodiesterase has been purified from yeast that cleaves the DNA-topoisomerase I linkage formed in complexes trapped by camptothecin (180). Since mutants that lack the activity are hypersensitive to camptothecin, at least when a RAD9-repair pathway is absent (142), the diesterase is functional. Another factor in this system may be the tagging of complexes by conjugation to small proteins (SUMO-1) (113). SUMO-1 tagging could help mark the complexes for repair. Such a system would be applicable to quinolone action in bacteria if it were to conduct only a partial repair that releases DNA breaks.

Once breaks are released, recombination proteins are likely to be involved in their repair. RecA is one of these proteins, since defects in *recA* increase the rate and extent of killing by quinolones (74, 105, 116). High-level, induced expression of RecA, however, is not required for protection from the lethal action of nalidixic acid (*lexA* mutants that prevent induction of *recA* are not hypersusceptible to the drug [105]). Moreover, chloramphenicol, which would block induction of RecA expression, protects from quinolone-induced death. Protection by chloramphenicol occurs even with a *recA* mutant (140), consistent with RecA repairing breaks after their release from the complexes by some other protein.

Cells that are defective in *recBCD* are also hypersusceptible to killing by quinolones (140). RecBCD repairs interstrand cross-links (14); perhaps it also repairs double-stranded breaks. Participation of RecBCD in the SOS response, both in the induction process and as a product of the regulon, may be irrelevant to quinolone lethality since *lexA* Ind− mutants are not hypersusceptible to nalidixic acid (105).

Cell Death in the Absence of Protein Synthesis

Inhibition of protein synthesis only partially blocks the lethal action of fluoroquinolones such as ciprofloxacin (25, 152); consequently, these compounds kill bacteria even in the absence of the suicide protein, although not as extensively as in its presence. One possible mechanism is suggested by observations of Ikeda (92) in which quinolone-promoted illegitimate DNA recombination has been attributed to gyrase subunit dissociation. Subunit dissociation might account for chloramphenicol-insensitive death, since dissociation might release the equivalent of double-stranded breaks (25). Chloramphenicol-insensitive killing can be considered as a distinct mode of lethality because it requires higher drug concentrations than the chloramphenicol-sensitive mode (40-fold with *E. coli* [111, 189], and 7- to 10-fold with *Mycobacterium bovis* BCG [43] and *S. aureus* [188]).

From symmetry considerations we expect subunit dissociation to occur along the GyrA-GyrA and GyrB-GyrB axis (Fig. 3), since each GyrA monomer is expected to hold an end of the broken DNA. Currently no data directly address this idea. However, the change of Ser-67 to Ala, which occurs on the GyrA-GyrA dimer interface (Fig. 3), decreases survival in the presence of quinolones when chloramphenicol is present (normalization is made to MIC$_{99}$ to correct for complex formation differences with wild-type cells [111]). Most other resistance mutations in the *gyrA* QRDR do not exhibit this phenomenon (111).

Work with the *gyrB-225* mutation argues against dissociation of subunits occurring along the GyrA-GyrB dimer axis (82). This mutation, which compensates for a deficiency of topoisomerase I (41, 117, 145), facilitates the killing of *E. coli* cells by quinolones when chloramphenicol is present. Purified GyrB-225, when mixed with GyrA, is slightly

defective at introducing supercoils; however, the two gyrase subunits bind DNA and quinolone as well as wild-type gyrase. Moreover, the mutant GyrA-GyrB interaction is stronger than the wild-type interaction. Thus, dissociation along the GyrA-GyrA and GyrB-GyrB axis remains as the most likely explanation for enhanced lethality with the mutant when chloramphenicol is present.

The protein-synthesis-independent mode of killing is likely to exist in most bacteria, since gyrase and topoisomerase IV are conserved enzymes. Among the organisms that exhibit the pathway are *E. coli* (152, 189), *S. aureus* (152, 188), *M. bovis* BCG (43), and *Entercococcus faecalis* (73). The pathway is particulary prominent in *E. faecalis*.

The Concentration Paradox

One of the intriguing phenomena associated with quinolone lethality is the decline in bactericidal activity when drug concentrations are very high (33). This phenomenon has typically been explained by the need for the suicide protein, since the expression of this protein is expected to be blocked when high concentrations of quinolone block RNA synthesis (112, 174). However, the paradoxical concentration effect can be seen even when protein synthesis is blocked (140, 188, 189). Thus, the absence of a suicide protein cannot by itself account for the effect. The effect remains unexplained.

Topoisomerase IV as a Lethal Target

Little is known about topoisomerase IV as a lethal target. It is likely that many of the general statements for it will be similar to those developed with gyrase. For example, when topoisomerase IV is the lethal target, the paradoxical concentration effect occurs: treatment of *S. aureus* with increasing concentrations of ciprofloxacin is associated with a distinct minimum in lethal activity (188). As with gyrase, lethal action involving topoisomerase IV occurs at roughly five times the MIC$_{99}$ (188), the situation needed to accumulate pairs of double-stranded breaks from single-stranded ones (153). Moreover, chloramphenicol protects from ciprofloxacin-mediated killing of *S. aureus* (152), suggesting that an induced suicide protein is involved in topoisomerase IV-mediated cell death.

Involvement of DNA Replication in Cell Death

Inhibition of DNA synthesis by quinolones is reversible, but cell death is not; thus, blocking replication fork movement cannot be sufficient for the loss of viability that occurs shortly after treatment of cells with quinolones. Likewise, events that stem from rapid inhibition of replication also fail to kill cells. For example, the rapid degradation of DNA that accompanies inhibition of DNA synthesis (29) also occurs when cells are treated with quinolone (nalidixic acid) plus chloramphenicol, but the cells do not die (106). The irreversible complexes seen when replication forks collide with purified topoisomerase IV (85) must somehow be repaired in vivo. Repair also appears to occur when replication forks collide with bacteriophage T4 type II topoisomerase trapped on DNA by the antitumor drug amsacrine, since DNA cleavage is not detected (88).

Whether cells must be replicating for the quinolones to be lethal is a separate question. One can imagine two scenarios that would require replication for bactericidal action. First, there might be little gyrase or topoisomerase IV on nonreplicating chromosomes. If so, few DNA breaks could be released because few complexes would be created. Second, the release of DNA breaks might require the interaction of a replication fork with a complex before the putative suicide protein would act. Neither possibility has been addressed experimentally.

Effect of Fluoroquinolone Structure on Lethal Action

The influence of fluoroquinolone structure on lethality is still poorly defined, but one can envision several types of effect. For example, structure could affect drug uptake, efflux, and binding to topoisomerase-DNA complexes. Together these factors would influence the formation of complexes required for subsequent lethal steps. Once the complexes form, drug structure could also influence the release of DNA breaks. For example, it could affect the ability of the complex to serve as a substrate for the putative suicide protein. Experimentally, this effect would be observed as differences among compounds when lethal activity is normalized to complex formation, i.e., to bacteriostatic activity (50% infective dose or MIC). Structure could also influence the ability of the compounds to promote subunit dissociation. This phenomenon would be reflected as lethal activity when chloramphenicol or rifampin is present to block the expression of the putative suicide protein (25, 146).

Interpretation of intracellular experiments can be complicated by uncertainties with respect to which enzyme is trapped on the DNA. Many species have two targets, and drug structure can change target preference (Table 2). Mycobacteria have been particularly useful for attributing effects to gyrase

because that enzyme appears to be the only target, at least with *M. tuberculosis*. Gyrase is also the likely target with gram-negative bacteria since topoisomerase IV is generally less sensitive. Work with gram-positive organisms is more problematic because quinolone sensitivity can vary for the two targets. The following paragraphs piece together scattered statements that concern the effects of two aspects of fluoroquinolone structure.

The N-1 cyclopropyl group

Ciprofloxacin differs structurally from norfloxacin by the presence of a cyclopropyl rather than a methyl group at the N-1 position (Fig. 1); consequently, comparisons of these widely studied compounds can be used to attribute activity to the moiety. A striking feature of ciprofloxacin is its ability to kill *E. coli* in the presence of rifampin and chloramphenicol. Norfloxacin lacks the activity (152). According to the ideas developed in previous sections, these data indicate that the N-1 cyclopropyl group contributes to the lethal action of the quinolones, possibly by enhancing the dissociation of gyrase subunits. Other compounds that contain an N-1 cyclopropyl group are moxifloxacin, gatifloxacin, sparfloxacin, sitafloxacin, clinafloxacin, and gemifloxacin.

The cyclopropyl group does not seem to be sufficient for dissociation with topoisomerase IV, since chloramphenicol blocks the lethal activity of ciprofloxacin with *S. aureus* (152). (Topoisomerase IV is the primary target for ciprofloxacin in *S. aureus*.) Nor is the cyclopropyl group required, since with *S. aureus* the lethal activity of ofloxacin, a compound that lacks a cyclopropyl moiety, is only partially inhibited by chloramphenicol (152).

C-8-halogen/methoxy substituents

Substituents attached to the C-8 position are common to many of the newer fluoroquinolones (Fig. 1). When lethal activity is compared without correction for complex formation (i.e., MIC), C-8 halogen and methoxy substituents increase the activity of N-1 cyclopropyl fluoroquinolones. For example, a methoxy group improves lethal action (90% and 99% lethal dose) by about threefold with *M. bovis* BCG (43). With *E. coli* the C-8 methoxy group has little effect unless gyrase is resistant; with a GyrA S83L variant, the methoxy increases lethality (99.9% lethal dose) eightfold (189). In this situation topoisomerase IV may be the target. With *S. aureus*, the methoxy group improves lethality with cells that have mutations in both *parC* and *gyrA* (94, 188), and in some (188) but not all (94) cases it also improves lethality beyond its improvement of bacteriostatic activity. Collectively these data indicate that the methoxy group can increase lethal action with either gyrase or topoisomerase IV. A C-8 bromine also increases activity, but generally less than a methoxy group; a C-8 ethoxy group has no enhancing effect (188). In general, these effects parallel bacteriostatic action, which, as pointed out above, is probably influenced by a variety of factors.

When resistant gyrase is the target, the C-8 moiety affects lethal activity, in part because complex formation occurs more readily (discussed in previous sections). Examples have been observed with a variety of mycobacterial mutants and several different C-8 groups (43, 111, 187). *gyrA* mutants exhibit striking differences in susceptibility when lethal action is measured and then normalized to bacteriostatic activity to correct for differences in drug uptake and complex formation. With *E. coli*, for example, A51V and D82A GyrA variants exhibit low susceptibility, and a C-8 methoxy group has little or no enhancing effect (111). But susceptibility of other GyrA variants is generally increased by the presence of a C-8 methoxy group. These differences might reflect the suitability of the complexes for removal by the suicide protein. Surprisingly, introduction of a *parC* resistance allele sharply increases the susceptibility of the GyrA A51V and D82A variants and decreases susceptibility of some other mutants. This apparent involvement of topoisomerase IV is not understood. The interesting possibility has been raised that subunit exchange might occur between gyrase and topoisomerase IV (18, 154).

The methoxy group increases lethality for most GyrA variants of *E. coli* when chloramphenicol is present to block the presumed expression of the suicide protein (111). Under these conditions the A51V and A67S variants are unusual in their high degree of susceptibility, as if these perturbations facilitate subunit dissociation. (Amino acid 67 is located on the GyrA-GyrA dimer interface.) Complex effects are also seen in this assay when topoisomerase IV is altered; addition of a *parC* resistance allele to the strains eliminates the hypersensitivity of the A51V and A67S variants (111).

CONCLUDING REMARKS

The bacteriostatic effects of the quinolones are now understood at a level sufficient to allow structure-function interpretations. The recognition helices of the GyrA and ParC proteins (122) are

probably part of a site where drug binds shortly after DNA. Once gyrase has cleaved the DNA, the quinolone prevents religation. That leaves the topoisomerase covalently, but reversibly, bound to DNA. Neither the replication nor the transcription apparatus can pass through the drug-topoisomerase-cleaved DNA complexes, accounting for inhibition of growth. Future progress in this area may come from understanding how *gyrB* and *parE* mutations contribute to resistance.

Explanations for lethal action are currently based on indirect arguments because we do not have an in vitro assay for cell death. Since complex formation is reversible while death is not, events beyond complex formation must be involved. The most straightforward idea is that the release of double-stranded DNA breaks causes cell death. A major advance would be to isolate and characterize the putative break-releasing protein, since then we could begin to think about ways to stimulate its activity. Equally important would be to understand how some quinolones kill cells in the absence of protein synthesis. Then it might be possible to optimize drug structure to accentuate this activity. Methods for blocking the release of DNA breaks would then allow the study of other lethal events, such as cell filamentation, that are likely to stem from interruption of DNA replication.

From a clinical perspective we need to identify safe compounds that rapidly kill bacteria, especially resistant mutants. Some progress has been made by the development of the C-8-methoxy derivatives. However, further refinement could become an academic exercise if ways are not developed to slow the emergence of fluoroquinolone-resistant pathogens.

Acknowledgments. We thank the following for critical comments on the manuscript: Jonathan Heddle, Hiroshi Hiasa, Anthony Maxwell, Glenn Tillotson, and Xilin Zhao. We also thank Jonathan Heddle for supplying Fig. 2 and Tao Lu for assistance in preparation of the figures. The authors' work was supported by grants from Bayer Corp., Bristol-Myers Squibb, and Mylan Pharmaceutical Co., and by National Institutes of Health grants AI35257 (to K.D.) and AI23988 (to D.C.H).

REFERENCES

1. Ali, J., A. Jackson, A. Howells, and A. Maxwell. 1993. The 43-kDa N-terminal fragment of the gyrase B protein hydrolyses ATP and binds coumarin drugs. *Biochemistry* **32**: 2717–2724.
2. Ali, J. A., G. Orphanides, and A. Maxwell. 1995. Nucleotide binding to the 43-kilodalton N-terminal fragment of the DNA gyrase. *Biochemistry* **34**:9801–9808.
3. Alovero, F., X.-S. Pan, J. Morris, R. Manzo, and L. Fisher. 1999. Engineering the specificity of antibacterial fluoroquinolones: benzenesulfonamide modifications at C-7 of ciprofloxacin change its primary target in *Streptococcus*

pneumoniae from topoisomerase IV to gyrase. *Antimicrob. Agents Chemother.* **44**:320–325.

4. Anderson, V., T. Gootz, and N. Osheroff. 1998. Topoisomerase IV catalysis and the mechanism of quinolone action. *J. Biol. Chem.* **274**:17879–17885.

5. Anderson, V., R. Zaniewski, F. Raczmarek, T. Gootz, and N. Osheroff. 2000. Action of quinolones against *Staphylococcus aureus* topoisomerase IV; basis for DNA cleavage enhancement. *Biochemistry* **39**:2726–2732.

6. Anderson, V. E., R. P. Zaniewski, F. S. Kaczmarek, T. D. Gootz, and N. Osheroff. 1999. Quinolones inhibit DNA religation mediated by *Staphylococcus aureus* topoisomerase IV. *J. Biol. Chem.* **274**:35927–35932.

7. Ashizawa, Y., T. Yokochi, Y. Ogata, Y. Shobuike, J. Kato, and H. Ikeda. 1999. Mechanism of DNA gyrase-mediated illegitimate recombination: characterization of *Escherichia coli gyrA* mutants that confer hyper-recombination phenotype. *J. Mol. Biol.* **289**:447–458.

8. Bachellier, S., D. Perrin, M. Hoffnung, and E. Gilson. 1993. Bacterial interspersed mosaic elements (BIMEs) are present in the genome of *Klebsiella*. *Mol. Microbiol.* **7**:537–544.

9. Bachellier, S., W. Saurin, D. Perrin, M. Hofnung, and E. Gilson. 1994. Structural and functional diversity among bacterial interspersed mosaic elements (BIMEs). *Mol. Microbiol.* **12**:61–70.

10. Bahng, S., E. Mossessova, P. Nurse, and K. Marians. 2000. Mutational analysis of *Eshcerichia coli* topoisomerase IV. *J. Biol. Chem.* **275**:4112–4117.

11. Baird, C. L., T. T. Harkins, S. K. Morris, and J. E. Lindsley. 1999. Topoisomerase II drives DNA transport by hydrolyzing one ATP. *Proc. Natl. Acad. Sci. USA* **96**:13685–13690.

12. Barnard, F., and A. Maxwell. 2001. Interaction between DNA gyrase and quinolones: the effect of alanine mutations at A subunit residues Ser-83 and Asp-87. *Antimicrob. Agents Chemother.* **45**:1994–2000.

13. Bendich, A. 2001. The form of DNA molecules in bacterial cells. *Biochimie* **83**:177–186.

14. Berardini, M., P. L. Foster, and E. L. Loechler. 1999. DNA polymerase II (polB) is involved in a new DNA repair pathway for DNA interstrand cross-links in *Escherichia coli*. *J. Bacteriol.* **181**:2878–2882.

15. Berger, J. M., S. J. Gamblin, S. C. Harrison, and J. C. Wang. 1996. Structure and mechanism of DNA topoisomerase II. *Nature* **379**:225–232.

16. Blanche, F., B. Cameron, F.-X. Bernard, L. Maton, B. Manse, L. Ferrero, N. Ratet, C. Lecoq, A. Goniot, D. Bisch, and J. Crouzet. 1996. Differential behaviors of *Staphylococcus aureus* and *Escherichia coli* type II DNA topoisomerases. *Antimicrob. Agents Chemother.* **40**:2714–2720.

17. Boccard, F., and P. Prentki. 1993. Specific interaction of IHF with RIBs, a class of bacterial repetitive DNA elements located at the 39 end of transcription units. *EMBO J.* **12**:5019–5027.

18. Breines, D. M., S. Ouabdesselam, E. Y. Ng, J. Tankovic, S. Shah, C. J. Soussy, and D. C. Hooper. 1997. Quinolone resistance locus *nfxD* of *Escherichia coli* is a mutant allele of the *parE* gene encoding a subunit of topoisomerase IV. *Antimicrob. Agents Chemother.* **41**:175–179.

19. Broccoli, S., P. Phoenix, and M. Drolet. 2000. Isolation of the *topB* gene encoding DNA topoisomerase III as a multi-copy suppressor of *topA* null mutations in *Escherichia coli*. *Mol. Microbiol.* **35**:58–68.

20. Burden, D. A., and N. Osheroff. 1999. In vitro evolution of preferred topoisomerase II DNA cleavage sites. *J. Biol. Chem.* **274**:5227–5235.

21. Cambau, E., F. Borden, E. Collatz, and L. Gutmann. 1993. Novel *gyrA* point mutation in a strain of *Escherichia coli* resistant to fluoroquinolones but not to nalidixic acid. *Antimicrob. Agents Chemother.* **37**:1247–1252.

22. Champoux, J. J. 2001. DNA topoisomerases: structure, function, and mechanism. *Annu. Rev. Biochem.* **70**:369–413.

23. Champoux, J. J., and M. D. Been. 1980. Topoisomerases and the swivel problem, p. 809–815. *In* B. Alberts (ed.), *Mechanistic Studies of DNA Replication and Genetic Recombination: ICN-UCLA Symposia on Molecular and Cellular Biology*. Academic Press, New York, N.Y.

24. Changela, A., R. DiGate, and A. Mondragon. 2001. Crystal structure of a complex of a type 1A DNA topoisomerase with a single-stranded DNA molecule. *Nature* **411**:1077–1081.

25. Chen, C.-R., M. Malik, M. Snyder, and K. Drlica. 1996. DNA gyrase and topoisomerase IV on the bacterial chromosome: quinolone-induced DNA cleavage. *J. Mol. Biol.* **258**:627–637.

26. Chow, R., T. Dougherty, H. Fraimow, E. Bellin, and M. Miller. 1988. Association between early inhibition of DNA synthesis and the MICs and MBCs of carboxyquinolone antimicrobial agents for wild-type and mutant [*gyrA nfxB(ompF) acrA*] *Escherichia coli* K-12. *Antimicrob. Agents Chemother.* **32**:1113–1118.

27. Cole, S. T., R. Brosch, J. Parkhill, T. Garnier, C. Churcher, D. Harris, S. Gordon, K. Eiglmeier, S. Gas, C. E. Barry, F. Tekaia, K. Babcock, D. Basham, D. Brown, T. Chillingworth, R. Connor, R. Davies, K. Devlin, T. Feltwell, S. Gentles, N. Hamlin, S. Holroyd, T. Hornsby, K. Jagels, and B. Barrell. 1998. Deciphering the biology of *Mycobacterium tuberculosis* from the complete genome sequence. *Nature* **393**:537–544.

28. Condemine, G., and C. Smith. 1990. Transcription regulates oxolinic acid-induced DNA gyrase cleavage at specific sites on the *E. coli* chromosome. *Nucleic Acids Res.* **18**:7389–7395.

29. Cook, T. M., W. Deitz, and W. Goss. 1966. Mechanism of action of nalidixic acid on *Escherichia coli*. *J. Bacteriol.* **91**:774–779.

30. Crisona, N., T. Strick, D. Bensimon, V. Croquette, and N. Cozzarelli. 2000. Preferential relaxation of positively supercoiled DNA by *E. coli* topoisomerase IV in single-molecule and ensemble measurements. *Genes Dev.* **14**:2881–2892.

31. Critchlow, S. E., and A. Maxwell. 1996. DNA cleavage is not required for the binding of quinolone drugs to the DNA gyrase-DNA complex. *Biochemistry* **35**:7387–7393.

32. Crumplin, G., M. Kenwright, and T. Hirst. 1984. Investigations into the mechanism of action of the antibacterial agent norfloxacin. *J. Antimicrob. Chemother.* **13**:9–23.

33. Crumplin, G. C., and J. T. Smith. 1975. Nalidixic acid: an antibacterial paradox. *Antimicrob. Agents Chemother.* **8**:251–261.

34. Cullen, M., A. Wyke, R. Kuroda, and L. Fisher. 1989. Cloning and characterization of a DNA gyrase A gene from *Escherichia coli* that confers clinical resistance to 4-quinolones. *Antimicrob. Agents Chemother.* **33**:886–894.

35. Dasgupta, S., S. Maisnier-Patin, and K. Nordstrom. 2000. New genes with old *modus operandi*. *EMBO Rep.* **1**:323–327.

36. Dean, F., M. Krasnow, R. Otter, M. Matzuk, S. Spengler, and N. Cozzarelli. 1983. *Escherichia coli* type I topoisomerases: identification, mechanism and role in recombination. *Cold Spring Harbor Symp. Quant. Biol.* **47**:769–777.

37. Deitz, W. H., T. M. Cook, and W. A. Goss. 1966. Mechanism of action of nalidixic acid on *Escherichia coli*. III. Conditions required for lethality. *J. Bacteriol.* **91**:768– 773.

38. DiGate, R., and K. Marians. 1988. Identification of a potent decatenating enzyme from *Escherichia coli*. *J. Biol. Chem.* **263**:13366–13373.

39. DiGate, R., and K. Marians. 1989. Molecular cloning and DNA sequence analysis of *Escherichia coli topB*, the gene encoding topoisomerase III. *J. Biol. Chem.* **264**:17924–17930.

40. DiGate, R., and K. Marians. 1992. *Escherichia coli* topoisomerase III-catalyzed cleavage of RNA. *J. Biol. Chem.* **267**:20532–20535.

41. DiNardo, S., K. Voelkel, R. Sternglanz, A. Reynolds, and A. Wright. 1982. *Esherichia coli* DNA topoisomerase I mutants have compensatory mutations in DNA gyrase genes. *Cell* **31**:43–51.

42. Discotto, L. F., L. Lawrence, K. Denbleyker, and J. F. Barrett. 2001. *Staphylococcus aureus* mutants selected by BMS-284756. *Antimicrob. Agents Chemther.* **45**:3273–3275.

43. Dong, Y., C. Xu, X. Zhao, J. Domagala, and K. Drlica. 1998. Fluoroquinolone action against mycobacteria: effects of C8 substituents on bacterial growth, survival, and resistance. *Antimicrob. Agents Chemother.* **42**:2978–2984.

44. Dorman, C., G. Barr, N. NiBhriain, and C. Higgins. 1988. DNA supercoiling and the anaerobic growth phase regulation of *tonB* gene expression. *J. Bacteriol.* **170**:2816–2826.

45. Drlica, K. 1992. Control of bacterial DNA supercoiling. *Mol. Microbiol.* **6**:425–433.

46. Drlica, K., R. Franco, and T. Steck. 1988. Rifampicin and *rpoB* mutations can alter DNA supercoiling in *Escherichia coli*. *J. Bacteriol.* **170**:4983–4985.

47. Drlica, K., S. H. Manes, and E. C. Engle. 1980. DNA gyrase on the bacterial chromosome: possibility of two levels of action. *Proc. Natl. Acad. Sci. USA* **77**:6879–6883.

48. Drlica, K., and M. Snyder. 1978. Superhelical *Escherichia coli* DNA: relaxation by coumermycin. *J. Mol. Biol.* **120**:145–154.

49. Drlica, K., and X. Zhao. 1997. DNA gyrase, topoisomerase IV, and the 4-quinolones. *Microbiol. Mol. Biol. Rev.* **61**:377–392.

50. Drolet, M., P. Phoenix, R. Menzel, E. Masse, L. F. Liu, and R. J. Crouch. 1995. Overexpression of RNase H partially complements the growth defect of an *Escherichia coli* Δ*topA* mutant: R-loop formation is a major problem in the absence of DNA topoisomerase I. *Proc. Natl. Acad. Sci. USA* **92**:3526–3530.

51. Earnshaw, W. C., B. Halligan, C. A. Cooke, M. M. S. Heck, and L. F. Liu. 1985. Topoisomerase II is a structural component of mitotic chromosome scaffolds. *J. Cell Biol.* **100**:1706–1715.

52. Espeli, O., and F. Boccard. 1997. In vivo cleavage of *Escherichia coli* BIME-2 repeats by DNA gyrase: genetic characterization of the target and identification of the cut site. *Mol. Microbiol.* **26**:767–777.

53. Fass, D., C. E. Bogden, and J. M. Berger. 1999. Quaternary changes in topoisomerase II may direct orthogonal movement of two DNA strands. *Nat. Struct. Biol.* **6**:322–326.

54. Ferrero, L., B. Cameron, and J. Crouzet. 1995. Analysis of *gyrA* and *grlA* mutations in stepwise-selected ciprofloxacin-resistant mutants of *Staphylococcus aureus*. *Antimicrob. Agents Chemother.* **39**:1554–1558.

55. Ferrero, L., B. Cameron, B. Manse, D. Lagneaux, J. Crouzet, A. Famechon, and F. Blanche. 1994. Cloning and primary structure of *Staphylococcus aureus* DNA topoisomerase IV: a primary target of fluoroquinolones. *Mol. Microbiol.* **13**:641–653.

56. Fisher, L. M., H. A. Barot, and M. E. Cullen. 1986. DNA gyrase complex with DNA: determinants for site-specific DNA breakage. *EMBO J.* **5**:1411–1418.

57. Fisher, L. M., K. Mizuuchi, M. H. O'Dea, H. Ohmori, and M. Gellert. 1981. Site-specific interaction of DNA gyrase with DNA. *Proc. Natl. Acad. Sci. USA* **78**:4165–4169.

58. Fournier, B., X. Zhao, T. Lu, K. Drlica, and D. Hooper. 2000. Selective targeting of topoisomerase IV and DNA gyrase in *Staphylococcus aureus*: different patterns of quinolone-induced inhibition of DNA synthesis. *Antimicrob. Agents Chemother.* **44**:2160–2165.

59. Franco, R., and K. Drlica. 1988. DNA gyrase on the bacterial chromosome: oxolinic acid-induced DNA cleavage in the *dnaA-gyrB* region. *J. Mol. Biol.* **201**:229–233.

60. Fraser, C., S. Norris, G. Weinstock, O. White, G. Sutton, R. Dodson, M. Gwinn, E. Hickey, R. Clayton, K. Ketchum, E. Sodergren, J. Hardham, M. McLeod, S. Alzberg, J. Peterson, H. Khalak, D. Richardson, J. Howell, M. Chidambaram, T. Utterback, L. McDonald, P. Artiach, C. Bowman, M. Cotton, C. Fujii, S. Garland, B. Hatch, D. Horst, K. Roberts, M. Sandusky, J. Weidman, H. Smith, and J. Venter. 1998. Complete genome sequence of *Treponema pallidum*, the syphilis spirochete. *Science* **281**:375–388.

61. Friedman, S. M., T. Lu, and K. Drlica. 2001. A mutation in the DNA gyrase A gene of *Escherichia coli* that expands the quinolone-resistance-determining region. *Antimicrob. Agents Chemother.* **45**:2378–2380.

62. Fukuda, H., and K. Hiramatsu. 1999. Primary targets of fluoroquinolones in *Streptococcus pneumoniae*. *Antimicrob. Agents Chemother.* **43**:410–412.

63. Fukuda, H., R. Kishi, M. Takei, and M. Hosaka. 2001. Contributions of the 8-methoxy group of gatifloxacin to resistance selectivity, target preference, and antibacterial activity against *Streptococcus pneumoniae*. *Antimicrob. Agents Chemother.* **45**:1649–1653.

64. Gellert, M., M. H. O'Dea, T. Itoh, and J.-I. Tomizawa. 1976. Novobiocin and coumermycin inhibit DNA supercoiling catalyzed by DNA gyrase. *Proc. Natl. Acad. Sci. USA* **73**:4474–4478.

65. Gellert, M., M. H. O'Dea, K. Mizuuchi, and H. Nash. 1976. DNA gyrase: an enzyme that introduces superhelical turns into DNA. *Proc. Natl. Acad. Sci. USA* **73**:3872–3876.

66. Gmuender, H., K. Kuratli, K. DiPadova, C. P. Gray, W. Keck, and S. Evers. 2001. Gene expression changes triggered by exposure of *Haemophilus influenzae* to novobiocin or ciprofloxacin: combined transcription and translation analysis. *Genome Res.* **11**:28–42.

67. Goldman, J. D., D. G. White, and S. V. Levy. 1996. Multiple antibiotic resistance (*mar*) locus protects *Escherichia coli* from rapid cell killing by fluoroquinolones. *Antimicrob. Agents Chemother.* **40**:1266–1269.

68. Goldstein, E., and K. Drlica. 1984. Regulation of bacterial DNA supercoiling: plasmid linking number varies with growth temperature. *Proc. Natl. Acad. Sci. USA* **81**:4046–4050.

69. Gootz, T. D. 2001. Bactericidal assays for fluoroquinolones. *Methods Mol. Biol.* **95**:185–194.

70. Gootz, T. D., R. P. Zaniewski, S. L. Haskell, F. S. Kaczmarek, and A. E. Maurice. 1999. Activities of trovafloxacin compared with those of other fluoroquinolones against purified topoisomerases and gyrA and grlA mutants of *Staphylococcus aureus*. *Antimicrob. Agents Chemother.* **43**:1845–1855.

71. Goss, W., W. Deitz, and T. Cook. 1964. Mechanism of action of nalidixic acid on *Escherichia coli*. *J. Bacteriol.* **88**:1112–1118.

72. Goss, W., W. Deitz, and T. Cook. 1965. Mechanism of action of nalidixic acid on *Escherichia coli*. II. Inhibition of deoxyribonucleic acid synthesis. *J. Bacteriol.* **89**:068–1074.

73. Gradelski, E., B. Kolek, D. Bonner, L. Valera, B. Minassian, and J. Fung-Tomc. 2001. Activity of gatifloxacin and ciprofloxacin in combination with other antimicrobial agents. *Int. J. Antimicrob. Agents* **17**:103–107.

74. Green, M., J. Donch, and J. Greenburg. 1970. Effect of inhibitors of DNA synthesis on UV-sensitive derivatives of *Escherichia coli* strain K-12. *Mutat. Res.* **9**:149–154.

75. Guillemin, I., V. Jarlier, and E. Cambau. 1998. Correlation between quinolone sensitivity patterns and sequences in the A and B subunits of DNA gyrase in mycobacteria. *Antimicrob. Agents Chemother.* **42**:2084–2088.

76. Guillemin, I., W. Sougakoff, E. Cambau, V. Revel-Viravau, N. Moreau, and V. Jarlier. 1999. Purification and inhibition by quinolones of DNA gyrases from *Mycobacterium avium*, *Mycobacterium smegmatis* and *Mycobacterium fortuitum* bv. peregrinum. *Microbiology* **145**:2527–2532.

77. Hallett, P., and A. Maxwell. 1991. Novel quinolone resistance mutations of the *Escherichia coli* DNA gyrase A protein; enzymatic analysis of the mutant proteins. *Antimicrob. Agents Chemother.* **35**:335–340.

78. Hanafi, D., and L. Bossi. 2000. Activation and silencing of *leu-500* promter by transcription-induced DNA supercoiling in the *Salmonella* chromosome. *Mol. Microbiol.* **37**:583–594.

79. Harmon, F., R. DiGate, and S. Kowalczykowski. 1999. RecQ helicases adn topoisomerase III comprise a novel DNA strand passage function: a conserved mechanism for control of DNA recombination. *Mol. Cell* **3**:611–620.

80. Heaton, V. J., J. E. Ambler, and L. M. Fisher. 2000. Potent antipneumococcal activity of gemifloxacin is associated with dual targeting of gyrase and topoisomerase IV, an in vivo target preference for gyrase, and enhanced stabilization of cleavable complexes in vitro. *Antimicrob. Agents Chemother.* **44**:3112–3117.

81. Hecht, R. M., and D. E. Pettijohn. 1976. Studies of DNA bound RNA molecules isolated from nucleoids of *Escherichia coli*. *Nucleic Acids Res.* **3**:767–788.

82. Heddle, J., T. Lu, X. Zhao, K. Drlica, and A. Maxwell. 2001. *gyrB-225*, a mutation of DNA gyrase that compensates for topoisomerase I deficiency: investigation of its low activity and quinolone hypersensitivity. *J. Mol. Biol.* **309**:1219–1231.

83. Heddle, J. G., F. Barnard, L. Wentzell, and A. Maxwell. 2000. The interaction of drugs with DNA gyrase: a model for the molecular basis of quinolone action. *Nucleosides Nucleotides Nucleic Acids* **19**:1249–1264.

84. Hiasa, H., and K. J. Marians. 1996. Two distinct modes of strand unlinking during theta-type DNA replication. *J. Biol. Chem.* **271**:21529–21535.

85. Hiasa, H., D. Yousef, and K. Marians. 1996. DNA strand cleavage is required for replication fork arrest by a frozen topoisomerase-quinolone-DNA ternary complex. *J. Biol. Chem.* **271**:26424–26429.

86. Higgins, C. F., C. J. Dorman, D. A. Stirling, L. Waddell, I. R. Booth, G. May, and E. Bremer. 1988. A physiological role for DNA supercoiling in the osmotic regulation of gene expression in *S. typhimurium* and *E. coli*. *Cell* **52**:569–584.

87. Holmes, V., and N. Cozzarelli. 2000. Closing the ring: links between SMC proteins and chromosome partitioning, condensation, and supercoiling. *Proc. Natl. Acad. Sci. USA* **97**:1322–1324.

88. Hong, G., and K. Kreuzer. 2000. An antitumor drug-induced topoisomerase cleavage complex blocks a bacteriophage T4 replication fork in vivo. *Mol. Cell. Biol.* **20**:594–603.

89. Hsieh, L.-S., R. M. Burger, and K. Drlica. 1991. Bacterial DNA supercoiling and [ATP]/[ADP]: Changes associated with a transition to anaerobic growth. *J. Mol. Biol.* **219**:443–450.

90. Hsieh, L.-S., J. Rouviere-Yaniv, and K. Drlica. 1991. Bacterial DNA supercoiling and [ATP]/[ADP]: Changes associated with salt shock. *J. Bacteriol.* **173**:3914–3917.

91. Huang, W. M., J. Libbey, P. VanderHoeven, and S. X. Yu. 1998. Bipolar localization of *Bacillus subtilis* topoisomerase IV, an enzyme required for chromosome segregation. *Proc. Natl. Acad. Sci. USA* **95**:4652–4657.

92. Ikeda, H. 1994. DNA topoisomerase-mediated illegitimate recombination. *Adv. Pharmacol.* **29A**:147–165.

93. Ince, D., and D. Hooper. 2000. Mechanisms and frequency of resistance to premafloxacin in *Staphylococcus aureus*: Novel mutations suggest novel drug-target interactions. *Antimicrob. Agents Chemother.* **44**:3344–3350.

94. Ince, D., and D. C. Hooper. 2001. Mechanisms and frequency of resistance to gatifloxacin in comparison to AM-1121 and ciprofloxacin in *Staphylococcus aureus*. *Antimicrob. Agents Chemother.* **45**:2755–2764.

95. Kampranis, S., and A. Maxwell. 1998. Conformational changes in DNA gyrase revealed by limited proteolysis. *J. Biol. Chem.* **273**:22606–22614.

96. Kampranis, S., and A. Maxwell. 1998. The DNA gyrase-quinolone complex, ATP hydrolysis and the mechanism of DNA cleavage. *J. Biol. Chem.* **273**:22615–22626.

97. Kampranis, S., and A. Maxwell. 1998. Hydrolysis of ATP at only one GyrB subunit is sufficient to promote supercoiling by DNA gyrase. *J. Biol. Chem.* **273**:26305–25309.

98. Kampranis, S. C., and A. Maxwell. 1996. Conversion of DNA gyrase into a conventional type II topoisomerase. *Proc. Natl. Acad. Sci. USA* **93**:14416–14421.

99. Kato, J.-I., Y. Nishimura, R. Imamura, H. Niki, S. Hiraga, and H. Suzuki. 1990. New topoisomerase essential for chromosome segregation in *E. coli*. *Cell* **63**:393–404.

100. Khodursky, A., and N. Cozzarelli. 1998. The mechanism of inhibition of topoisomerase IV by quinolone antibacterials. *J. Biol. Chem.* **273**:27668–27677.

101. Khodursky, A., B. Peter, M. Schmid, J. DeRisi, D. Botstein, P. Brown, and N. Cozzarelli. 2000. Analysis of topoisomerase function in bacterial replication fork movement: use of DNA microarrays. *Proc. Natl. Acad. Sci. USA* **97**:9419–9424.

102. Khodursky, A. B., E. L. Zechiedrich, and N. R. Cozzarelli. 1995. Topoisomerase IV is a target of quinolones in *Escherichia coli*. *Proc. Natl. Acad. Sci. USA* **92**:11801–11805.

103. Krasin, F., and F. Hutchinson. 1977. Repair of DNA double-strand breaks in *Escherichia coli*, which requires *recA* function and the presence of a duplicate genome. *J. Mol. Biol.* **116**:81–98.

104. Levine, C., H. Hiasa, and K. Marians. 1998. DNA gyrase and topoisomerase IV: Biochemical activities, physiological roles during chromosome replication, and drug sensitivities. *Biochim. Biophys. Acta* **1400**:29–43.

105. Lewin, C., B. Howard, N. Ratcliffe, and J. Smith. 1989. 4-Quinolones and the SOS response. *J. Med. Microbiol.* **29**:139–144.

106. Lewin, C., and J. Smith. 1990. DNA breakdown by the 4-quinolones and its significance. *J. Med. Microbiol.* **31**:65–70.

107. Li, X., X. Zhao, and K. Drlica. 2002. Selection of *Streptococcus pneumoniae* mutants having reduced susceptibility to levofloxacin and moxifloxacin. *Antimicrob. Agents Chemother.* **46**:522–524.

108. Lima, C., J. C. Wang, and A. Mondragon. 1994. Three-dimensional structure of the 67K N-terminal fragment of *E. coli* DNA topoisomerase I. *Nature* **367**:138–146.

109. Liu, L., and J. Wang. 1987. Supercoiling of the DNA template during transcription. *Proc. Natl. Acad. Sci. USA* **84**: 7024–7027.

110. Lockshon, D., and D. R. Morris. 1985. Sites of reaction of *Escherichia coli* DNA gyrase on pBR322 *in vivo* as revealed by oxolinic acid-induced plasmid linearization. *J. Mol. Biol.* **181**:63–74.

111. Lu, T., X. Zhao, and K. Drlica. 1999. Gatifloxacin activity against quinolone-resistant gyrase: allele-specific enhancement of bacteriostatic and bactericidal activity by the C-8-methoxy group. *Antimicrob. Agents Chemother.* **43**:2969–2974.

112. Manes, S. H., G. J. Pruss, and K. Drlica. 1983. Inhibition of RNA synthesis by oxolinic acid is unrelated to average DNA supercoiling. *J. Bacteriol.* **155**:420–423.

113. Mao, Y., M. Sun, S. Desai, and L. Liu. 2000. SUMO-1 conjugation to topoisomerase I: a possible repair response to topoisomerase-mediated DNA damage. *Proc. Natl. Acad. Sci. USA* **97**:4046–4051.

114. Marians, K., and H. Hiasa. 1997. Mechanism of quinolone action: a drug-induced structural perturbation of the DNA precedes strand cleavage by topoisomerase IV. *J. Biol. Chem.* **272**:9401–9409.

115. Marshall, D., F. Bowe, C. Hale, G. Dougan, and C. Dorman. 2000. DNA topology and adaptation of *Salmonella typhimurium* to an intracellular environment. *Philos. Trans. R. Soc. Lond.* **355**:565–574.

116. McDaniel, L. S., L. H. Rogers, and W. E. Hill. 1978. Survival of recombination-deficient mutants of *Escherichia coli* during incubation with nalidixic acid. *J. Bacteriol.* **134**:1195–1198.

117. McEachern, F., and L. M. Fisher. 1989. Regulation of DNA supercoiling in *Escherichia coli*: genetic basis of a compensatory mutation in DNA gyrase. *FEBS Lett.* **253**:67–70.

118. McNairn, E., N. N. Bhriain, and C. Dorman. 1995. Overexpression of the *Shigella flexneri* genes coding for DNA topoisomerase IV compensates for loss of DNA topoisomerase I: effect on virulence gene expression. *Mol. Microbiol.* **15**:507–517.

119. Menzel, R., and M. Gellert. 1983. Regulation of the genes for *E. coli* DNA gyrase: homeostatic control of DNA supercoiling. *Cell* **34**:105–113.

120. Mizushima, T., Y. Ohtsuka, T. Miki, and K. Sekimizu. 1994. Temperature shift-up leads to simultaneous and continuous plasmid DNA relaxation and induction of DnaK and GroEL proteins in anaerobically growing *Escherichia coli* cells. *FEMS Microbiol. Lett.* **121**:333–336.

121. Mondragon, A., and R. DiGate. 1999. The structure of the *Escherichia coli* DNA topoisomerase III. *Structure (Lond.)* **7**:1373–1383.

122. MoraisCabral, J. H., A. P. Jackson, C. V. Smith, N. Shikotra, A. Maxwell, and R. C. Liddington. 1997. Crystal structure of the breakage-reunion domain of DNA gyrase. *Nature* **388**:903–906.

123. Moreau, N. J., H. Robaux, L. Baron, and X. Tabary. 1990. Inhibitory effects of quinolones on pro- and eucaryotic DNA topoisomerases I and II. *Antimicrob. Agents Chemother.* **34**:1955–1960.

124. Morris, J., X.-S. Pan, and L. M. Fisher. 2002. Grepafloxacin, a dimethyl derivative of ciprofloxacin, acts preferentially through gyrase in *Streptococcus pneumoniae*: role of the C-5 group in target specificity. *Antimicrob. Agents Chemother.* **46**:582–585.

125. Morrison, A., and N. R. Cozzarelli. 1979. Site-specific cleavage of DNA by *E. coli* DNA gyrase. *Cell* **17**:175–184.

126. Morrissey, I., and J. George. 1999. Activities of fluoroquinolones against *Streptococcus pneumoniae* type II topoi-

somerases purified as recombinant proteins. *Antimicrob. Agents Chemother.* **43**:2570–2585.

127. Morrissey, I., and J. George. 2000. Bactericial activity of gemifloxacin and other quinolones against *Streptococcus pneumoniae*. *J. Antimicrob. Chemother.* **45**(Suppl. S1): 107–110.

128. Ng, E. Y., M. Trucksis, and D. C. Hooper. 1996. Quinolone resistance mutations in topoisomerase IV: relationship to the *flqA* locus and genetic evidence that topoisomerase IV is the primary target and DNA gyrase is the secondary target of fluoroquinolones in *Staphylococcus aureus*. *Antimicrob. Agents Chemother.* **40**:1881–1888.

129. O'Connor, M. B., and M. H. Malamy. 1985. Mapping of DNA gyrase cleavage sites *in vivo*. Oxolinic acid induced cleavages in plasmid pBR322. *J. Mol. Biol.* **181**:545–550.

130. Onodera, Y., Y. Uchida, M. Tanaka, and K. Sato. 1999. Dual inhibitory activity of sitafloxacin (DU-6859a) against DNA gyrase and topoisomerase IV of *Streptococcus pneumoniae*. *J. Antimicrob. Chemother.* **44**:533–536.

131. Oram, M., and M. Fisher. 1991. 4-quinolone resistance mutations in the DNA gyrase of *Escherichia coli* clinical isolates identified by using the polymerase chain reaction. *Antimicrob. Agents Chemother.* **35**:387–389.

132. Pan, X., and L. M. Fisher. 1997. Targeting of DNA gyrase in *Streptococcus pneumoniae* by sparfloxacin: selective targeting of gyrase or topoisomerase IV by quinolones. *Antimicrob. Agents Chemother.* **41**:471–474.

133. Pan, X., and L. M. Fisher. 1998. DNA gyrase and topoisomerase IV are dual targets of clinafloxacin action in *Streptococcus pneumoniae*. *Antimicrob. Agents Chemother.* **42**:2810–2816.

134. Pan, X.-S., J. Ambler, S. Mehtar, and L. M. Fisher. 1996. Involvement of topoisomerase IV and DNA gyrase as ciprofloxacin targets in *Streptococcus pneumoniae*. *Antimicrob. Agents Chemother.* **40**:2321–2326.

135. Pan, X.-S., and L. M. Fisher. 1999. *Streptococcus pneumoniae* DNA gyrase and topoisomerase IV: overexpression, purification, and differential inhibition by fluoroquinolones. *Antimicrob. Agents Chemother.* **43**:1129–1136.

136. Pan, X.-S., G. Yague, and L. M. Fisher. 2001. Quinolone resistance mutations in *Streptococcus pneumoniae* GyrA and ParC proteins: mechanistic insights into quinolone action from enzymatic analysis, intracellular levels, and phenotypes of wild-type and mutant proteins. *Antimicrob. Agents Chemother.* **45**:3140–3147.

137. Pato, M. L., M. Karlock, C. Wall, and N. P. Higgins. 1995. Characterization of Mu prophage lacking the central strong gyrase binding site: localization of the block in replication. *J. Bacteriol.* **177**:5937–5942.

138. Pestova, E., R. Beyer, N. P. Cianciotto, G. A. Noskin, and L. R. Peterson. 1999. Contribution of topoisomerase IV and DNA gyrase mutations in *Streptococcus pneumoniae* to resistance to novel fluoroquinolones. *Antimicrob. Agents Chemother.* **43**:2000–2004.

139. Pestova, E., J. Millichap, G. Noskin, and L. Peterson. 2000. Intracellular targets of moxifloxacin: a comparison with other fluoroquinolones. *J. Antimicrob. Chemother.* **45**:583–590.

140. Piddock, L., and R. Walters. 1992. Bactericidal activities of five quinolones for *Escherichia coli* strains with mutations in genes encoding the SOS response or cell division. *Antimicrob. Agents Chemother.* **36**:819–825.

141. Postow, L., N. Crisona, B. Peter, C. Hardy, and N. Cozzarelli. 2001. Topological challenges to DNA replication: conformations at the fork. *Proc. Natl Acad. Sci. USA* **98**:8219–8226.

142. Pouliot, J., K. Yao, C. Robertson, and H. Nash. 1999. Yeast gene for a Tyr-DNA phosphodiesterase that repairs topoisomerase I complexes. *Science* **286:**552–555.

143. Pruss, G., and K. Drlica. 1986. Topoisomerase I mutants: the gene on pBR322 that encodes resistance to tetracycline affects plasmid DNA supercoiling. *Proc. Natl. Acad. Sci. USA* **83:**8952–8956.

144. Pruss, G. J. 1985. DNA Topoisomerase I mutants: increased heterogeneity in linking number and other replicon-dependent changes in DNA supercoiling. *J. Mol. Biol.* **185:**51–63.

145. Pruss, G. J., S. H. Manes, and K. Drlica. 1982. *Escherichia coli* DNA topoisomerase I mutants: increased supercoiling is corrected by mutations near gyrase genes. *Cell* **31:**35–42.

146. Ratcliffe, N. T., and J. T. Smith. 1984. Ciprofloxacin and ofloxacin exhibit a rifampicin-resistant bactericidal mechanism not detectable in other 4-quinolone antibacterial agents. *J. Pharm. Pharmacol.* **36:**59P.

147. Reece, R., and A. Maxwell. 1991. DNA gyrase: structure and function. *Crit. Rev. Biochem. Mol. Biol.* **26:**335–375.

148. Sawitzke, J. A., and S. Austin. 2000. Suppression of chromosome segregation defects of Escherichia coli muk mutants by mutations in topoisomerase I. *Proc. Natl. Acad. Sci. USA* **97:**1671–1676.

149. Schofield, M. A., R. Agbunag, M. Michaels, and J. Miller. 1992. Cloning and sequencing of *Escherichia coli mutR* shows its identity to *topB*, encoding topoisomerase III. *J. Bacteriol.* **1774:**5168–5170.

150. Sindelar, G., X. Zhao, A. Liew, Y. Dong, J. Zhou, J. Domagala, and K. Drlica. 2000. Mutant prevention concentration as a measure of fluoroquinolone potency against mycobacteria. *Antimicrob. Agents Chemother.* **44:**3337–3343.

151. Sinden, R. R., J. O. Carlson, and D. E. Pettijohn. 1980. Torsional tension in the DNA double helix measured with trimethylpsoralen in living *E. coli* cells. *Cell* **21:**773–783.

152. Smith, J. T., and C. S. Lewin. 1988. Chemistry and mechanisms of action of the quinolone antibacterials, p. 23–82. *In* V. T. Andriole (ed.), *The Quinolones*. Academic Press, San Diego, Calif.

153. Snyder, M., and K. Drlica. 1979. DNA gyrase on the bacterial chromosome: DNA cleavage induced by oxolinic acid. *J. Mol. Biol.* **131:**287–302.

154. Soussy, C., J. Wolfson, E. Ng, and D. Hooper. 1993. Limitations of plasmid complementation test for determination of quinolone resistance due to changes in gyrase A protein and identification of conditional quinolone resistance locus. *Antimicrob. Agents Chemother.* **37:**2588–2592.

155. Sreedharan, S., M. Oram, B. Jensen, L. Peterson, and L. Fisher. 1990. DNA gyrase *gyrA* mutations in ciprofloxacin-resistant strains of *Staphylococcus aureus*: close similarity with quinolone resistance mutations in *Escherichia coli*. *J. Bacteriol.* **172:**7260–7262.

156. Srivenugopal, K., D. Lockshon, and D. Morris. 1984. *Escherichia coli* DNA topoisomerase III: purification and characterization of a new type I enzyme. *Biochemistry* **23:**1899–1906.

157. Staczek, P., and N. P. Higgins. 1998. Gyrase and topo IV modulate chromosome domain size *in vivo*. *Mol. Microbiol.* **29:**1435–1448.

158. Steck, T. R., and K. Drlica. 1984. Bacterial chromosome segregation: evidence for DNA gyrase involvement in decatenation. *Cell* **36:**1081–1088.

159. Steck, T. R., G. J. Pruss, S. H. Manes, L. Burg, and K. Drlica. 1984. DNA supercoiling in gyrase mutants. *J. Bacteriol.* **158:**397–403.

160. Tabary, X., N. Moreau, C. Dureuil, and F. LeGoffic. 1987. Effect of DNA gyrase inhibitors pefloxacin, five other quinolones, novobiocin, and chlorobiocin on *Escherichia coli* topoisomerase I. *Antimicrob. Agents Chemother.* **31:**1925–1928.

161. Tomb, J., O. White, A. Kerlavage, R. Clayton, G. Sutton, R. Fleischmann, K. Ketchum, H. Klenk, S. Gill, B. Dougherty, K. Nelson, J. Quackenbush, L. Zhou, E. Kirkness, S. Peterson, B. Loftus, D. Richardson, R. Dodson, H. Khalak, A. Glodek, K. McKenney, L. Fitzegerald, N. Lee, M. Adams, and J. Venter. 1997. The complete genome sequence of the gastric pathogen *Helicobacter pylori*. *Nature* **388:**539–547.

162. Tse-Dinh, Y. 2000. Increased sensitivity to oxidative challenges associated with *topA* deletion in *Escherichia coli*. *J. Bacteriol.* **182:**829–832.

163. Tse-Dinh, Y.-C. 1985. Regulation of the *Escherichia coli* DNA topoisomerase I gene by DNA supercoiling. *Nucleic Acids Res.* **13:**4751–4763.

164. Tse-Dinh, Y.-C., H. Qi, and R. Menzel. 1997. DNA supercoiling and bacterial adaptation: thermotolerance and thermoresistance. *Trends Microbiol.* **5:**323–326.

165. Wang, J.-Y., and M. Syvanen. 1992. DNA twist as a transcriptional sensor for environmental changes. *Mol. Microbiol.* **6:**1861–1866.

166. Wang, J. C. 1971. Interaction between DNA and an *Escherichia coli* protein. *J. Mol. Biol.* **55:**523–533.

167. Wang, J. C. 1998. Moving one DNA double helix through another by a type II DNA topoisomerase: the story of a simple molecular machine. *Q. Rev. Biophys.* **31:**107–144.

168. Weinstein-Fischer, D., M. Elgrably-Weiss, and S. Altuvia. 2000. *Escherichia coli* response to hydrogen peroxide: a role for DNA supercoiling, topoisomerase I, and Fis. *Mol. Microbiol.* **35:**1413–1420.

169. Wentzell, L., and A. Maxwell. 2000. The complex of DNA gyrase and quinolone drugs on DNA forms a barrier to the T7 DNA polymerase replication complex. *J. Mol. Biol.* **304:**779–791.

170. Whoriskey, S., M. Scholfield, and J. Miller. 1991. Isolation and characterization of *Escherichia coli* mutants with altered rates of deletion formation. *Genetics* **127:**21–30.

171. Wigley, D. B., G. J. Davies, E. J. Dodson, A. Maxwell, and D. Dodson. 1991. Crystal structure of an N-terminal fragment of the DNA gyrase B protein. *Nature* **351:**624–629.

172. Williams, N., A. Howells, and A. Maxwell. 2001. Locking the ATP-operated clamp of DNA gyrase: probing the mechanism of strand passage. *J. Mol. Biol.* **306:**969–984.

173. Williams, N. L., and A. Maxwell. 1999. Locking the DNA gate of DNA gyrase: investigating the effects on DNA cleavage and ATP hydrolysis. *Biochemistry* **38:**14157–14164.

174. Willmott, C. J. R., S. E. Critchlow, I. C. Eperon, and A. Maxwell. 1994. The complex of DNA gyrase and quinolone drugs with DNA forms a barrier to transcription by RNA polymerase. *J. Mol. Biol.* **242:**351–363.

175. Willmott, C. J. R., and A. Maxwell. 1993. A single point mutation in the DNA gyrase A protein greatly reduces binding of fluoroquinolones to the gyrase-DNA complex. *Antimicrob. Agents Chemother.* **37:**126–127.

176. Wolfson, J. S., D. C. Hooper, D. J. Shih, G. L. McHugh, and M. N. Swartz. 1989. Isolation and characterization of an *Escherichia coli* strain exhibiting partial tolerance to quinolones. *Antimicrob. Agents Chemother.* **33:**705–709.

177. Wu, H.-Y., S.-H. Shyy, J. C. Wang, and L. F. Liu. 1988. Transcription generates positively and negatively supercoiled domains in the template. *Cell* **53:**433–440.

178. Wu, L., and I. Hickson. 2001. RecQ helicases and topoisomerases: components of a conserved complex for the regulation of genetic recombination. *CMLS Cell. Mol. Life Sci.* **58:**894–901.

179. Yague, G., J. Morris, X.-S. Pan, K. Gould, and L. M. Fisher. 2002. Cleavable-complex formation by wild-type and quinolone-resistant *Streptococcus pneumoniae* type II topoisomerases mediated by gemifloxacin and other fluoroquinolones. *Antimicrob. Agents Chemother.* **46:**413–419.

180. Yang, S.-W., A. B. Burgin, B. N. Huizenga, C. A. Robertson, K. C. Yao, and H. A. Nash. 1996. A eukaryotic enzyme that can disjoin dead-end covalent complexes between DNA and type I topoisomerases. *Proc. Natl. Acad. Sci. USA* **93:**11534–11539.

181. Yang, Y., and G. Ames. 1988. DNA gyrase binds to the family of prokaryotic repetitive extragenic palindromic sequences. *Proc. Natl. Acad. Sci. USA* **85:**8850–8854.

182. Yang, Y., and G. Ames. 1990. The family of repetitive extragenic palindromic sequences: interaction with DNA gyrase and histonelike protein HU, p. 211–225. *In* K. Drlica and M. Riley (ed.), *The Bacterial Chromosome.* American Society for Microbiology, Washington, D.C.

183. Yoshida, H., M. Bogaki, M. Nakamura, and S. Nakamura. 1990. Quinolone resistance-determining region in the DNA gyrase *gyrA* gene of *Escherichia coli. Antimicrob. Agents Chemother.* **34:**1271–1272.

184. Yoshida, H., M. Bogaki, M. Nakamura, L. Yamanaka, and S. Nakamura. 1991. Quinolone resistance-determining region in the DNA gyrase *gyrB* gene of *Escherichia coli. Antimicrob. Agents Chemother.* **35:**1647–1650.

185. Yoshida, H., M. Nakamura, M. Bogaki, H. Ito, T. Kojima, H. Hattori, and S. Nakamura. 1993. Mechanism of action of quinolones against *Escherichia coli* DNA gyrase. *Antimicrob. Agents Chemother.* **37:**839–845.

186. Zechiedrich, E. L., A. Khodursky, S. Bachellier, R. Schneider, D. Chen, D. Lilley, and N. Cozzarelli. 2000. Roles of topoisomerases in maintaining steady-state DNA supercoiling in *Escherichia coli. J. Biol. Chem.* **275:**8103–8113.

187. Zhao, B.-Y., R. Pine, J. Domagala, and K. Drlica. 1999. Fluoroquinolone action against clinical isolates of *Mycobacterium tuberculosis*: effects of a C8-methoxyl group on survival in liquid media and in human macrophages. *Antimicrob. Agents Chemother.* **43:**661–666.

188. Zhao, X., J.-Y. Wang, C. Xu, Y. Dong, J. Zhou, J. Domagala, and K. Drlica. 1998. Killing of *Staphylococcus aureus* by C-8-methoxy fluoroquinolones. *Antimicrob. Agents Chemother.* **42:**956–958.

189. Zhao, X., C. Xu, J. Domagala, and K. Drlica. 1997. DNA topoisomerase targets of the fluoroquinolones: a strategy for avoiding bacterial resistance. *Proc. Natl. Acad. Sci. USA* **94:**13991–13996.

190. Zhu, Q., P. Pongpech, and R. DiGate. 2001. Type I topoisomerase activity is required for proper chromosomal segregation in *Escherichia coli. Proc. Natl. Acad. Sci. USA* **98:**9766–9771.

Quinolone Antimicrobial Agents, 3rd ed.
Edited by David C. Hooper and Ethan Rubinstein
© 2003 ASM Press, Washington, D.C.

Chapter 3

Mechanisms of Quinolone Resistance

DAVID C. HOOPER

The fluoroquinolones are antibacterial agents that have been used widely in clinical medicine. With the continuing development of new congeners with expanded clinical indications reflecting an expanding antibacterial spectrum for some members of the class, an understanding of the limitations posed by the occurrence of bacterial resistance to fluoroquinolones is of increasing importance. Quinolone action and resistance are closely linked phenomena, and resistance related to alterations in drug targets informs understanding of the molecular details of quinolone action. Mechanisms of quinolone action are covered in detail in chapter 2, and the epidemiology of quinolone resistance in clinical settings is covered in chapter 23. In this chapter the mechanisms of quinolone resistance will be reviewed. This topic was recently reviewed and will be further updated here (89). Specifically, resistance due to alterations in drug targets and due to altered drug permeation, both resulting from chromosomal mutations, are covered in detail. Also covered is the recently described novel mechanism of plasmid-mediated resistance. No specific mechanisms of quinolone degradation effect resistance, although certain environmental fungi can degrade quinolones by metabolic pathways (232).

RESISTANCE DUE TO ALTERED DRUG TARGET ENZYMES

Differences in Enzyme Targets of Fluoroquinolones and First-Step Resistance in Gram-Negative and Gram-Positive Bacteria

Detailed information about the enzymes, DNA gyrase and topoisomerase IV, which are the targets of quinolone action, is covered in chapter 2. Because both of the known targets of quinolone drugs are essential bacterial enzymes and because ternary com-

plexes of either enzyme with DNA and quinolone can block DNA replication (51, 63, 85), drug interaction with either target can produce a block in cell growth and trigger the events leading to cell death (see chapter 2). The relative sensitivities of the two enzymes thereby affect MICs for both wild-type and mutant bacteria, with the more sensitive enzyme as the principal determinant of the MIC of the quinolone for the bacterium. Thus, the resistance phenotype of mutations in the genes encoding the subunits of one target enzyme, the primary or most sensitive target enzyme, will be affected by the level of drug sensitivity of the other or secondary target enzyme coexisting in the bacterial cell. In other terms, the level of sensitivity of the other target enzyme may set a ceiling on the increment in resistance of the cell conferred by a given mutation in the primary target enzyme. This concept is most easily understood in the setting in which the quinolone sensitivity of both enzymes within a cell is highly similar. In this circumstance, the levels of resistance conferred by single, first-step target mutations is small because the interaction of the quinolone with the highly sensitive second target sustains drug activity (83, 168). Thus, the magnitude of the resistance phenotype for the cell that is conferred by a given mutation is determined not only by the magnitude in reduction of sensitivity of the mutant target enzyme but also by the level of sensitivity of the other target enzyme. At each point in a series of mutational steps in target enzymes leading to increasing resistance, the level of susceptibility of the cell to a quinolone is predicted to be determined in part by the more sensitive of the two target enzymes.

DNA gyrase, which is a heterotetramer composed of two GyrA and two GyrB subunits, was shown to be a primary quinolone target in *Escherichia coli* on the basis of genetic studies in which single mutations in either the GyrA or GyrB subunit of this

David C. Hooper • Division of Infectious Diseases, Massachusetts General Hospital, Harvard Medical School, Boston, MA 02114-2696.

enzyme conferred increments in drug resistance (51, 83). Later work demonstrated that topoisomerase IV, which has a heterotetrameric structure similar to that of DNA gyrase and is composed of two ParC and two ParE subunits, which are similar to GyrA and GyrB, repectively, is a secondary drug target in *E. coli*. Mutations in ParC (104) or ParE (29) alone have no resistance phenotype but can contribute to an increase in the resistance phenotype when GyrA or GyrB mutations are also present.

In contrast, for *Staphylococcus aureus*, initial genetic studies showed that common first-step drug-resistance mutations were not in the subunits of DNA gyrase but in a distinct genetic locus *flqA* (83). *flqA* mutants were shown subsequently to have mutations in either the ParC (154) or ParE (60) subunits of topoisomerase IV. Whereas first-step resistant mutants have mutations in topoisomerase IV, second-step mutants have mutations in DNA gyrase (55, 91). In addition, mutations in the DNA gyrase subunits of *S. aureus* when present in the absence of mutations in a subunit of topoisomerase IV cause no change in susceptibility to most quinolones, except nalidixic acid (60). Thus, topoisomerase IV in *S. aureus* is a primary target of action of most quinolones (211). Recent studies, however, suggest that sparfloxacin, nadifloxacin, and garenoxacin, a novel desfluoroquinolone with potent gram-positive activity, have DNA gyrase as their primary target in *S. aureus* (50, 211), but this property is not consistent for all desfluoroquinolones (194).

These differences between *S. aureus* and *E. coli* have been shown to correlate with the differences in the relative quinolone sensitivities of DNA gyrase and topoisomerase IV in the two species (27). For many quinolones, *E. coli* DNA gyrase is more sensitive than *E. coli* topoisomerase IV (92). In contrast, for at least some of this same group of quinolones, *S. aureus* topoisomerase IV is more sensitive than *S. aureus* DNA gyrase (27, 211).

Although data are less complete for other species, there appears to be a pattern for many quinolones in which DNA gyrase is the primary quinolone target (and most sensitive target enzyme) in gram-negative bacteria and topoisomerase IV is the primary drug target (and most sensitive target enzyme) in gram-positive bacteria, thus affecting the nature of first-step resistance mutations relating to target alteration. For several gram-negative species in addition to *E. coli*, first-step resistant mutants selected with various quinolones have mutations in GyrA or GyrB; these include *Salmonella enterica* serovar Typhimurium (192), *Shigella dysenteriae* (188), *Campylobacter jejuni* (228), *Campylobacter fetus* (221), *Citrobacter freundii* (220), *Haemophilus*

influenzae (75), *Helicobacter pylori* (which lacks genes for topoisomerase IV) (142), and *Vibrio parahaemolyticus* (162). As discussed below, for many other gram-negative species, mutations in GyrA have been identified in quinolone-resistant clinical isolates, but it was not possible to determine whether the mutations were first or later step and in some cases the possible presence of mutations in ParC or ParE was not evaluated.

In two other gram-positive species studied in addition to *S. aureus*, topoisomerase IV also appears to be the principal target for some quinolones. Ciprofloxacin-selected first-step mutants of *Streptococcus pneumoniae* have mutations in the ParC or ParE subunits of topoisomerase IV similar to those reported in *S. aureus* (166, 173). In addition in *Enterococcus faecalis*, second- but not first-step resistant mutants selected with ciprofloxacin have mutations in GyrA (110). Furthermore, in resistant clinical isolates of *E. faecalis*, ParC mutations were found in low-level resistant isolates without a mutation in GyrA, and high-level resistant isolates had mutations in both ParC and GyrA, suggesting that first-step mutants may have mutations in topoisomerase IV (32, 53, 102). Thus, ciprofloxacin and other quinolones may have as their primary target topoisomerase IV rather than DNA gyrase in *S. pneumoniae* and *E. faecium* as well as in *S. aureus*. This pattern, however, can vary depending on quinolone structure in some species. Sparfloxacin- and clinafloxacin-selected, first-step mutants of *S. pneumoniae* have mutations in DNA gyrase. Furthermore, the mutations in topoisomerase IV that affected ciprofloxacin activity have no effect on the activity of sparfloxacin and clinafloxacin in the absence of mutations in DNA gyrase subunits (167, 168). Similar data in which first-step resistant mutants of *S. pneumoniae* have mutations in *gyrA* or *gyrB* have been reported for gatifloxacin (67) and moxifloxacin (147). These data vary with species as well, because first-step resistant mutants of *S. aureus* selected with gatifloxacin or moxifloxacin have mutations in *parC* but not *gyrA* (93, 95). Furthermore, in *S. pneumoniae*, removal of the 8-methoxy group of gatifloxacin results in a compound, AM-1121, which selects for first-step *parC* mutants (69). Structural modifications at position 7 of the quinolone molecule can also affect primary targeting of DNA gyrase or topoisomerase IV in *E. coli* as well (10).

For anaerobic bacteria, resistant mutants of the gram-negative anaerobe *Bacteroides fragilis* selected with levofloxacin, ciprofloxacin, or trovafloxacin were found to have mutations in *gyrA*, although in each case the *gyrA* mutations were only identified in second-step mutants, and the genes for topoisomerase IV were not identified and evaluated (13, 164). Similarly, although moxifloxacin-resistant clinical isolates of *Clostridium difficile*, a gram-positive anaerobe, had mutations in GyrA, first-step mutants selected directly with moxifloxacin in the laboratory did not, and mutations in ParC or ParE were not evaluated (1). Thus, definitive data on target preference patterns in anaerobes are not yet available.

For *Mycoplasma hominis*, which is more closely related to *S. pneumoniae* than to *E. coli* (20), first-step mutants selected with ofloxacin, pefloxacin, or ciprofloxacin had mutations in ParE or ParC, whereas first-step mutants selected with sparfloxacin had mutations in GyrA (21), providing a second example in addition to that in *S. pneumoniae* in which sparfloxacin differed from other quinolones in its primary target. For resistant mutants of *Chlamydia trachomatis* selected by four passages of cells in the presence of either ofloxacin or sparfloxacin, mutations in GyrA were found in the absence of mutations in GyrB, ParC, and ParE, suggesting that DNA gyrase is the primary quinolone target in this organism (49). First-step quinolone-resistant mutants of *Mycobacterium tuberculosis* (6, 214) and *Mycobacterium smegmatis* (191) have been found to have mutations in GyrA, and thus DNA gyrase appears to be the primary quinolone target. Total genome sequencing of *M. tuberculosis* indicates that this organism lacks genes for topoisomerase IV (43), and thus DNA gyrase is likely the only quinolone target. In addition to *M. tuberculosis* and *H. pylori*, *Treponema pallidum* also lacks genes for topoisomerase IV (65).

Athough the model in which the principal target of quinolones is determined by the more sensitive of the two target enzymes is conceptually appealing for quinolones, which act as DNA poisons to block progression of the DNA replication complex (see chapter 2), there are problems with this model that have not been fully explained. In particular, for *S. pneumoniae* in many cases with quinolones that target DNA gyrase in vivo (based on selection of first-step resistant mutants), purified DNA gyrase is substantially less sensitive than topoisomerase IV to these same quinolones (83, 144, 168). The approximately threefold excess of cellular levels of the subunits of DNA gyrase relative to those of topoisomerase IV were thought insufficient to compensate for the 20- to 40-fold differences in drug sensitivity found with the purified enzymes (169). Furthermore, in some cases first-step selections with the same quinolone may generate diverse resistant mutants, some with alterations in topoisomerase IV and others with alterations in DNA gyrase (224). Thus, differences between results in vitro and in vivo and primary and secondary target interactions suggest that other factors, as yet unidentified, may contribute to the interactions of quinolones with their target enzymes and to the phenotypic effects of resistance mutations in these targets in vivo.

DNA Gyrase

Gyrase A subunit changes

Alterations in DNA gyrase occur commonly in quinolone-resistant, gram-negative bacteria and for many species have been shown to contribute to the resistance phenotype in the absence of other mutations (Table 1). Alterations in GyrA are reported more often than alterations in GyrB, possibly reflecting the lower level of resistance conferred by single GyrB mutations relative to single GyrA mutations. In *E. coli*, one of the most extensively studied organisms, resistance mutations cluster in the amino terminus of GyrA between amino acid positions 67 and 106, termed the quinolone-resistance-determining region (QRDR), which is near to Tyr122, which is covalently bound to DNA phosphate groups during the enzyme's DNA strand-passing reactions (239). Resistance mutations, such as Ala51Val, have also been found outside this region, but substantially less often (66). Two amino acids, Ser83 and Asp87, are most commonly mutated in resistant isolates. The Ser83Trp mutation has been shown to cause reduced binding of norfloxacin to enzyme-DNA complexes (234). A dually mutant Ser83Ala Asp87Ala enzyme complexed with DNA was also recently shown to have approximately 10-fold reduction in affinity for ciprofloxacin (17). The pattern of binding of enoxacin to DNA complexes with wild-type gyrase holoenzyme and enzyme reconstituted with GyrA(Ser83Leu), however, was complex with little overall reduction in drug binding for the mutant enzyme-DNA complex but with the loss of an apparent high-affinity drug binding site suggested by analysis of Scatchard plots (242).

In the published crystal structure of a fragment of GyrA, the positions of amino acids involved in the QRDR were localized to a positively charged surface along which DNA is thought to bind (36). Thus, a common model envisions that amino acid changes in the QRDR of GyrA alter the structure of the site of quinolone binding near the interface of the enzyme and DNA and that resistance is then caused by reduced drug affinity for the modified enzyme-DNA complex. Direct structural information on the site of quinolone binding within the complex is not yet available.

Table 1. Mutations in the GyrA subunit of DNA gyrase and the ParC subunit of topoisomerase IV associated with quinolone resistance

Species	GyrA			ParC		
	Amino acid position[a]	Wild-type amino acid	Mutant amino acid	Amino acid position	Wild-type amino acid	Mutant amino acid
Gram-negative bacteria						
E. coli	51	Ala	Val[b]			
	67	Ala	Ser[b]			
	81	Gly	Cys[b], Asp[b]	78	Gly	Asp[b]
	82	Asp	Gly			
	83	Ser	Leu[b], Trp[b], Ala[b]	80	Ser	Leu[b], Ile[b], Arg
	84	Ala	Pro[b]			
	87	Asp	Asn[b], Val[b], Gly[b], Tyr[b], Ala[b], His	84	Glu	Lys[b], Gly, Val
	106	Gln	His[b], Arg[b]			
Salmonella spp.	67	Ala	Pro			
	83	Ser	Phe[b], Tyr[b], Ala			
	87	Asp	Asn[b], Tyr[b], Gly			
	119	Ala	Val, Glu			
Shigella spp.	83	Ser	Leu[b]			
	87	Asp	Gly			
Aeromonas spp.	83	Ser	Ile[b]			
V. parahaemolyticus	83	Ser	Leu[b]	85	Ser	Phe[b]
C. jejuni	70	Ala	Thr[b]			
	86	Thr[c]	Ile[b]			
	90	Asp[d]	Asn[b], Tyr[b]			
K. pneumoniae	83	Ser	Phe[b], Tyr[b]	80	Ser	Ile, Arg
	87	Asp	Gly[b], Asn, Ala	84	Glu	Gly, Lys
K. oxytoca	83	Thr[c]	Ile			
C. freundii	83	Thr[c]	Ile	80	Ser	Ile
	87	Asp	Tyr, Val, Gly	84	Glu	Lys
E. cloacae	83	Ser	Phe, Tyr, Thr, Ile			
	87	Asp	Asn			
E. aerogenes	83	Ser	Ile			
S. marcescens	81	Gly	Cys			
	83	Ser	Arg, Ile			
	87	Asp	Tyr, Asn			
P. stuartii	83	Ser	Arg, Ile			
H. influenzae	84	Ser	Tyr[b], Leu	84	Ser	Ile[b]
	88	Asp	Asn[b], Tyr	88	Glu	Lys[b]
N. gonorrhoeae	67	Ala	Ser			
	75	Ala	Ser			
	84	Ala	Pro			
				85	Gly	Cys
				86	Asp	Asn
	91	Ser	Phe, Tyr	87	Ser	Ile
				88	Ser	Phe, Pro
	95	Asp	Asn, Gly	91	Glu	Lys, Gly
				116	Arg	Leu
H. pylori	87	Asn	Lys[b]			
	88	Ala	Val[b]			
	91	Asp	Asn[b]			
	97	Ala	Val			
P. aeruginosa	83	Thr[c]	Ile[b,d], Ala	80	Ser	Leu[b,d], Trp
	84	Ala	Pro			
	87	Asp	Asn, Tyr, Gly, His	84	Glu	Lys
	106	Gln	Leu			
A. baumannii	81	Gly	Val			
	83	Ser	Leu			
B. fragilis	82	Asp	Asn[b]			
	83	Ser	Phe[b]			
Bacteroides spp.	83	Ser	Leu			

Continued on following page

Table 1. *Continued*

Species	GyrA			ParC		
	Amino acid position[a]	Wild-type amino acid	Mutant amino acid	Amino acid position	Wild-type amino acid	Mutant amino acid
Gram-positive bacteria						
S. aureus				23	Lys	Asn[b]
				41	Val	Gly
				43	Arg	Cys[b]
				45	Ile	Met
				48	Ala	Thr
				52	Ser	Arg
				69	Asp	Tyr[b]
				78	Gly	Cys[b]
	84	Ser	Leu[b], Ala, Val, Lys	80	Ser	Phe[b], Tyr[b]
	85	Ser	Pro[b]	81	Ser	Pro
	86	Glu	Lys[b], Gly	84	Glu	Lys[b], Leu[b], Val, Ala, Gly, Tyr
	88	Glu	Val, Lys			
	106	Gly	Asp	103	His	Tyr
				116	Ala	Glu[b], Pro[b]
				157	Pro	Leu[b]
				176	Ala	Thr[b], Gly
Coagulase-negative staphylococci	84	Ser	Leu, Phe, Ala	80	Ser	Leu, Phe, Tyr
				84	Asp	Tyr, Gly, Asn
S. pneumoniae				63	Ala	Tyr[b]
				78	Asp	Asn
	81	Ser	Phe[b], Tyr[b], Cys	79	Ser	Phe[b], Tyr[b], Ala
	84	Ser	Phe[b], Tyr[b]			
	85	Glu	Lys[b], Gln[b], Gly	83	Asp	Asn[b], Gly[b], Val
				85	Asp	Gly
				93	Lys	Glu[b]
				95	Arg	Cys
				102	His	Tyr
				115	Ala	Pro, Val
				129	Tyr	Ser
				137	Lys	Asn
S. oralis, S. mitis, S. sanguis, S. anginosus	81	Ser	Phe[b], Tyr[b]	79	Ser	Phe[b], Ile[b], Leu[b], Tyr, Arg
	85	Glu	Gln[b], Lys[b], Gly	83	Asp	Asn, His, Tyr
S. pyogenes	81	Ser	Phe	79	Ser	Tyr
	99	Met	Leu			
E. faecalis	83	Ser	Arg, Ile, Asn	80	Ser	Arg, Ile
	87	Glu	Lys, Gly	84	Glu	Ala
E. faecium	83	Ser	Arg, Leu, Ile, Tyr	80	Ser	Ile, Arg
	87	Glu	Leu, Gly, Lys	84	Glu	Lys, Thr
				97	Ser	Asn
C. difficile	83	Thr	Val, Ile			
Mycobacteria						
M. tuberculosis	88	Gly	Cys[b]			
	90	Ala	Val[b]			
	91	Ser[c]	Pro			
	94	Asp[d]	Asn[b], Ala, His, Tyr, Gly			
	95	Ser	Thr			
M. smegmatis	75	Ala	Ser[b]			
	89	Gly	Cys[b]			
	91	Ala[c]	Val[b]			
	92	Ser	Pro[b]			
	95	Asp	Gly[b], Ala[b], Asn[b], His[b]			

Continued on following page

Table 1. *Continued*

Species	GyrA			ParC		
	Amino acid position[a]	Wild-type amino acid	Mutant amino acid	Amino acid position	Wild-type amino acid	Mutant amino acid
Other bacteria						
M. hominis				69	Asp	Tyr
				73	Arg	His
	83	Ser	Leu[b], Trp[b]	80	Ser	Ile[b]
	84	Ser	Trp[b]	81	Ser	Pro
	87	Glu	Lys[b]	84	Glu	Lys[b], Gln[b], Gly
	119	Ala	Gln[b], Val			
C. trachomatis	83	Ser	Ile[b]			
C. burnetii	87	Gly	Lys[b]			

[a] Rows reflect alignments of homologous amino acids.
[b] Amino acids for which genetic data support a role for the mutation in causing resistance. Other mutant amino acids have been associated with resistance in clinical isolates.
[c] Homolog of GyrA Ser83 of *E. coli*.
[d] Homolog of GyrA Asp87 of *E. coli*.

Substitutions of amino acids in positions equivalent to Ser83 and Asp87 in many other gram-negative bacteria, mycobacteria, and *C. trachomatis* have been shown either to cause quinolone resistance by genetic studies or to be associated with resistance in clinical isolates (Table 1). In the case of clinical isolates of gram-negative bacteria, GyrA mutations were often seen in strains with lower levels of resistance and dual mutations in GyrA and ParC were seen in strains with higher levels of resistance without the finding of ParC mutations alone, suggesting that GyrA mutations likely preceded ParC mutations as levels of resistance progressed upward (5, 33, 204). Thus, models of quinolone resistance from alterations in DNA gyrase developed from studies of *E. coli* will likely be applicable to a broad range of gram-negative and other bacteria as well.

For many gram-positive bacteria, DNA gyrase serves as a secondary quinolone target, and, thus, resistance mutations in GyrA are only demonstrable when there are also resistance mutations in ParC or ParE. Changes in GyrA that cause incremental resistance when present together with ParC or ParE mutations in high-level resistant isolates of *S. aureus*, *S. pneumoniae*, *E. faecalis*, and *M. hominis* are similar to those causing resistance in gram-negative bacteria. Initial studies of resistant clinical isolates of *S. aureus* prior to the recognition of the role of topoisomerase IV in resistance commonly had GyrA mutations (97, 205), but when ParC and ParE were also evaluated, GyrA quinolone resistance mutations were not found in the absence of mutations in topoisomerase IV (56, 202). *gyrA* single mutants of *S. aureus* constructed in the laboratory exhibit little or no resistance to fluoroquinolones, but interestingly

exhibit a fourfold increase in resistance to nalidixic acid, the early nonfluorinated quinolone with low potency against gram-positive bacteria (59), suggesting that nalidixic acid has little or no activity against *S. aureus* topoisomerase IV.

Mutations in GyrA of gram-positive bacteria most often occur at positions 83 and 84, with Ser84Leu or Tyr in *S. aureus* and Ser83Phe or Tyr in *S. pneumoniae* being most common. Glu86Lys in *S. aureus* and Glu87Lys or Gln in *S. pneumoniae* are also common. Each of these GyrA mutations and the less common Ser85Pro mutation of *S. aureus* have been shown to contribute to ciprofloxacin resistance in the presence of mutant topoisomerase IV. The Ser83Phe or Tyr mutation of *S. pneumoniae* also confers resistance to sparfloxacin in the absence of mutant topoisomerase IV (167). Recently, data on mutations in GyrA (as well as GyrB, ParC, and ParE) were reported for resistant clinical isolates of viridans streptococci (78). Correlations of sequence differences with resistance were more difficult because of greater sequence heterogeneity among these streptococcal strains than was seen in *S. pneumoniae*. Ser81Tyr/ Phe mutations were found but only in the presence of ParC mutations. Other mutations, as listed in Table 1, have been associated with resistance in clinical isolates but have not yet been shown to contribute to resistance directly. Noteworthy is the similarity of the mutations in GyrA found in resistant clinical isolates of *E. faecalis* (Ser83Arg or Ile or Asn and Glu87Lys or Gly) to those found in *S. aureus* and *S. pneumoniae* (102, 110, 218). In the one study that evaluated both ParC and GyrA, no GyrA mutations were found in the absence of a ParC mutation (102). A GyrA subunit purified from another highly resistant but genetically uncharacterized clinical strain of *E. faecalis* when combined with a wild-type GyrB subunit was also shown to have quinolone-resistant enzymatic activity (149). Thus, it is likely that resistance caused by GyrA mutation in *E. faecalis* is highly similar to that in *S. pneumoniae* and *S. aureus*.

Gyrase B subunit changes

In general, resistance mutations in GyrB have been found less often than those in GyrA and have been reported in *E. coli*, *Salmonella*, *M. tuberculosis*, *S. aureus*, and *S. pneumoniae* (Table 2). Most is known about the two mutations studied in *E. coli* GyrB, Asp426Asn and Lys447Glu. Both mutations cause resistance to nalidixic acid, but they differ in their effects on susceptibility to fluoroquinolones with a piperazinyl substituent at position 7 of the quinolone ring (e.g., norfloxacin, enoxacin, ciprofloxacin, and others), causing either low-level resistance (four- to eightfold increase in MIC, Asp426Asn) or increased susceptibility (fourfold decrease in MIC, Lys447Glu) to ciprofloxacin. These differences in phenotype have been proposed to be caused by differences in direct electrostatic interactions between the affected amino acids in the wild-type and mutant GyrB subunits and drugs with and without the positively charged piperazinyl moiety (240). Thus, the positive charge of the piperazinyl substituent of enoxacin (or other piperazinylated quinolones) would have increased affinity for the Lys447Glu mutant enzyme because of the negative charge of the substituted glutamic acid, but decreased affinity for the Asp426Asn mutant enzyme because of the positive charge of the substituted asparagine. Relative to wild-type holoenzyme, gyrase reconstituted with GyrB(Asp426Asn) in complex with DNA bound substantially less enoxacin (242). Although DNA complexes with the GyrB(Lys447Glu) mutant enzyme and the wild-type enzyme bound similar amounts of enoxacin overall, increased binding to this mutant enzyme-DNA complex was demonstrable at low concentrations of enoxacin in analyses of Scatchard plots.

The location and structure of the domain that contains these amino acids (referred to as the QRDR domain of GyrB) are distant from the QRDR domain of GyrA in the enzyme conformation indicated by the original crystal structure of yeast topoisomerase II, which has homology to both GyrB (amino terminus) and GyrA (carboxy terminus) (25). Subsequent analysis of the crystal structures of other conformations of yeast topoisomerase II, however, revealed substantial domain shifts that bring the

yeast homolog of the QRDR domain of GyrB into proximity with that of GyrA (26), suggesting that these two domains may form a quinolone-binding pocket during one stage of the enzyme's catalytic cycle. Definitive information on the nature of the site and enzyme conformation to which quinolones bind must await further crystallographic studies on complexes of gyrase, DNA, and quinolone.

GyrB resistance mutations, in addition to the two mutations studied most extensively as discussed above, also include in the same domain the Ser463Tyr mutation found in a resistant mutant of *S. enterica* serovar Typhimurium (71) and the Asp495Arg or His mutations found in second-step resistant mutants of *M. tuberculosis* (105). Likewise, resistance mutations in GyrB of *S. aureus* and *S. pneumoniae* are in regions similar to those involved in resistance in *E. coli* GyrB (Table 2) and include Asp437Asn in *S. aureus* (97) and the equivalent Asp435Asn in *S. pneumoniae* (165) as well as Arg458Glu in *S. aureus* (97). A single GyrB Glu474Lys mutation of *S. pneumoniae* found in a first-step mutant selected on clinafloxacin (and without mutations in GyrA, ParC, and ParE) conferred low-level resistance to sparfloxacin and clinafloxacin, but not ciprofloxacin (168). Thus, the patterns of resistance for specific quinolones demonstrating first-step resistance mutations in GyrA also appear to be reflected in first-step mutations in GyrB as well, reflecting the holoenzyme as the unit that ultimately mediates resistance in vivo. The contribution of the GyrB mutations Glu474Lys and Asp435Glu found in clinical isolates to incremental resistance in combination with mutations in topoisomerase IV in *S. pneumoniae* has also been demonstrated by transformation experiments (230).

Topoisomerase IV

ParC subunit changes

The ParC subunit of topoisomerase IV is homologous to GyrA, and the ParE subunit is homologous to GyrB. Particularly highly conserved in the topoisomerase IV subunit homologs are the QRDR domains of GyrA and GyrB, a conservation that predicts similarity of drug interaction and resistance mutations for the two enzymes. The strongest genetic data for the secondary role of topoisomerase IV in quinolone resistance is from *E. coli*, in which mutations in ParC or ParE were shown to contribute to resistance only in the presence of mutant GyrA (29, 104). In gram-negative bacteria, ParC mutations have been found in high-level resistant clinical isolates, usually in combination with mutations in *gyrA*

Table 2. Mutations in the GyrB subunit of DNA gyrase and the ParE subunit of topoisomerase IV associated with quinolone resistance

Species	GyrB Amino acid position[a]	GyrB Wild-type amino acid	GyrB Mutant amino acid	ParE Amino acid position	ParE Wild-type amino acid	ParE Mutant amino acid
Gram-negative bacteria						
E. coli	426	Asp	Asn[b]			
				445	Leu	His[b]
	447	Lys	Glu[b]			
Salmonella sp.	463	Ser	Tyr[b]			
P. aeruginosa	464	Ser	Phe			
	466	Glu	Asp			
				473	Ala	Val
Gram-positive bacteria						
S. aureus				25	Pro	His[b]
				410	Ser	Pro
				422	Glu	Asp
	437	Asp	Asn[b]	432	Asp	Asn[b], Gly, Val
				451	Pro	Gln[b], Ser
	458	Arg	Gln[b]	470	Asn	Asp[b]
	477	Glu	Ala	472	Glu	Val, Lys
				478	His	Tyr
S. pneumoniae				103	His	Tyr[b]
	406	Gly	Ser, Asp			
				431	Leu	Ile
	435	Asp	Asn[b], Glu[b], Val	435	Asp	Asn[b], Val
	440	Ser	Tyr			
	445	Arg	Ser			
				447	Arg	Cys, Ser
	454	Pro	Ser	454	Pro	Ser[b]
				473	Asn	Ile
	474	Glu	Lys[b]	474	Glu	Lys
	475	Glu	Val			
				476	Ile	Phe
S. mitis, S. oralis				424	Pro	Gln
				474	Glu	Lys
	494	Ser	Thr			
Mycobacteria						
M. tuberculosis	495	Asp	Arg[b], His[b]			
Other bacteria						
M. hominis				426	Asp	Asn[b]
				440	Leu	Phe
				460	Gly	Lys[b]

[a] Rows reflect alignments of homologous amino acids
[b] Amino acids for which genetic data support a role for the mutation in causing resistance. Other mutant amino acids have been associated with resistance in clinical isolates.

in *E. coli* (84, 225), *Klebsiella pneumoniae* (33, 46, 47), *Klebsiella oxytoca* (33), *Enterobacter cloacae* (33), *Enterobacter aerogenes* (33), *C. freundii* (156), *Pseudomonas aeruginosa* (5, 150), *H. influenzae* (75), and *Neisseria gonorrhoeae* (23, 48, 204, 222), and directly selected mutants of *V. parahaemolyticus* (162). These mutations tended to occur in the positions equivalent to Ser80 and Glu84 of *E. coli* ParC

(Table 1). Unusual mutations were also found and include those in directly selected mutants, Gly78Asp in *E. coli* (84), and those associated with resistance in clinical isolates, Gly85Cys (222), Asp86Asn (48), Glu91Lys/Gly (23, 48), and Arg116Leu (222) in *N. gonorrhoeae*.

The largest body of information concerning the role of topoisomerase IV in quinolone resistance in gram-positive bacteria comes from studies of *S. aureus* and *S. pneumoniae*. Mutations encoding single amino acid changes in either the ParC (GrlA) or ParE (GrlB) subunits of *S. aureus* topoisomerase IV cause four- to eightfold increments in resistance to ciprofloxacin and many other quinolones (55, 154). ParC mutations appear more common than ParE mutations among clinical resistant strains and have clustered in the amino terminus, with Ser80Phe/Tyr mutations being most common (Table 1) (55, 57, 154, 201, 210, 212, 227, 237). Also common are Glu84Lys/Leu mutations. Both the purified Ser80Phe and Glu84Lys mutant ParC subunits contribute resistance in the enzymatic activity of topoisomerase IV, and a ParC subunit with both mutations contributes an even higher level of resistance (215). Ala116Glu/Pro mutations are less common but also cause quinolone resistance similar to that due to mutations at positions 80 or 84. In addition, Ala116Glu/Pro mutations confer slight increases in susceptibility to novobiocin and coumermycin (59), coumarins which act as competitive inhibitors of the ATPase activity of topoisomerase IV and DNA gyrase. Mutations at position 116 are in proximity to the active site Tyr122. In *S. pneumoniae* similar ParC mutations have been reported, including Ser79Tyr/Phe and Asp83Asn/Gly/Ala in resistant mutants selected in the laboratory and found in resistant clinical isolates (Table 1) (79, 100, 145, 165–168, 219). Resistant clinical isolates of *E. faecalis* have also been shown recently to have similar mutations in ParC (Ser80Arg/Ile and Glu84Ala). In one strain with low-level resistance, a mutation in ParC without a mutation in GyrA was found, and no GyrA mutants were found in the absence of a ParC mutation (102). A similar pattern was seen in resistant clinical isolates of viridans streptococci in which a Ser79Phe was found in a low-level resistant isolate in the absence of mutations in ParE, GyrA, and GyrB, and isolates with high-level resistance had an additional mutation in GyrA or GyrB (78). Resistant isolates with Ser79Ile and Ser79Tyr ParC mutations in addition to GyrA mutations were also found, and DNA from a Ser79Tyr mutant was able to transform low-level resistance to a susceptible recipient. Although genetic studies in *E. faecalis* have not yet proved the role of ParC mutations in resistance in this organism, the analogy to the patterns found in *S. aureus*, *S. pneumoniae*, and viridans streptococci for which genetic data are available strongly suggests that these ParC mutations contribute to resistance. High-level quinolone-resistant strains of *Enterococcus faecium* have been shown to contain mutations in both ParC and GyrA (53). In *M. hominis*, Ser80Ile and Arg73His ParC mutations were found

in separate multiresistant isolates, and Glu84Lys and Asp69Tyr mutations have been selected with sparfloxacin (second step) and ofloxacin (fourth step), respectively (21).

Although QRDR mutations in ParC have been most commonly identified, in vitro selections for resistance by plating on agar containing quinolones with enhanced potency against gram-positive bacteria have expanded the range of mutations shown to cause resistance, many of which are outside the canonical QRDR (Table 3) (94, 95).

ParE subunit changes

Mutations in ParE appear to be uncommon in laboratory and clinical resistant isolates, but *parE* has been evaluated less often than *parC* and *gyrA* in studies of resistant isolates. For gram-negative bacteria, a single example exists of a ParE mutation contributing to resistance in conjunction with a mutation in GyrA for a laboratory strain of *E. coli* (Leu445His) (29). Most reported ParE mutations have been in gram-positive bacteria. Mutations in ParE have been found to cause resistance in *S. aureus* (Asn470Asp) (60) and *S. pneumoniae* (Asp435Asn) (173, 175). Mutations His103Tyr, Pro454Ser, Arg447Cys, and Glu474Lys, usually in combination with ParC and GyrA mutations, have been found in the second or later steps of serial selections of *S. pneumoniae* with clinafloxacin, trovafloxacin, ciprofloxacin, and moxifloxacin (99, 148, 168), and Glu474Lys has been shown by transformational experiments to cause a twofold increase in the MIC of levofloxacin without effect on the MICs of newer fluoroquinolones (230). A Glu472Lys mutation has been reported to have arisen in a fifth-step mutant selected with the desfluoroquinolone garenoxacin (50). Other mutations, Glu422Asp, Asp432Gly, Asp432Asn, and Pro451Ser, have been reported in resistant clinical isolates of *S. aureus* but have not yet been shown to contribute to the resistance phenotype in vivo (Table 2) (216). Purified mutant *S. aureus* ParE subunits (Asp432Asn and Asn470Asp) have also been shown to cause quinolone-resistant topoisomerase IV activity when combined with the wild-type ParC subunit (215). The Asn470Asp mutation of *S. aureus* ParE, like the *S. aureus* ParC Ala116Glu mutation, causes hypersusceptibility to coumarins (60), and the purified Asn470Asp ParE subunit also contributes to hypersusceptibility to novobiocin in enzymatic activity (215). A Pro424Gln ParE mutation has been found in a resistant clinical isolate of *Streptococcus mitis* in the absence of mutations in GyrA, GyrB, and ParC (78). A first-step mutant of *M. hominis* selected on ofloxacin was found to have

Table 3. Efflux systems associated with quinolone resistance

Species	Mutant class	Pump components	Pump class	Additional resistance phenotype
Gram-negative bacteria				
E. coli	marR, soxS, robA	AcrAB-TolC	RND	Tetracycline, chloramphenicol
	emrR	EmrAB	MFS	CCCP, organomercurials, nalidixic acid
	?	MdfA	MFS	Chloramphenicol, tetracycline, erythromycin, neomycin
P. aeruginosa	mexR (nalB, cfxB)	MexAB-OprM	RND	Tetracycline, chloramphenicol, trimethoprim
	nfxB	MexCD-OprJ	RND	Erythromycin, trimethoprim, triclosan
	mexT (nfxC)	MexEF-OprN	RND	Chloramphenicol, trimethoprim, imipenem, triclosan
	?	MexXY-OprM	RND	Erythromycin, aminoglycosides, ethidium bromide, acriflavine
S. maltophilia	?	SmeDEF	RND	Erythromycin, chloramphenicol, tetracycline, nalidixic acid
V. parahaemolyticus	?	NorM	MATE	Streptomycin, ethidium bromide
V. cholerae	?	VceAB	MFS	Erythromycin, deoxycholate, CCCP, nalidixic acid
B. thetaiotaomicron	?	BexA	MATE	
Gram-positive bacteria				
S. aureus	flqB (promoter), arlRS, norR	NorA	MFS	Ethidium, acriflavine, rhodamine 6G, puromycin
B. subtilis	bmrR	Bmr	MFS	Ethidium, acriflavine, rhodamine 6G, TPP
	bltR	Blt (-BltD)	MFS	Ethidium, acriflavine, rhodamine 6G, TPP
	?	Bmr3	MFS	Puromycin
S. pneumoniae	?	PmrA	MFS	Ethidium bromide
L. lactis	?	LmrA	ABC	Aminoglycosides, macrolides, lincosamides, chloramphenicol, tetracycline
Mycobacteria				
M. smegmatis	?	LfrA	MFS	Ethidium, acriflavine, quarternary ammoniums

a Asp426Asn ParE mutation (21, 22). No ParE resistance mutations have yet been reported in E. faecalis.

Models for How Altered Drug Targets Cause Resistance

Direct data on quinolone interactions with topoisomerases come from studies of E. coli DNA gyrase for which it has been shown that quinolones bind to a complex of DNA and DNA gyrase rather than DNA gyrase alone (203). The Ser83Trp mutation in GyrA, the dual Ser83Ala Asp87Ala mutation in GyrA, and the Asp426Asn mutation in GyrB were also associated with reduced binding of norfloxacin, ciprofloxacin, or enoxacin to the gyrase-DNA complex, respectively (17, 233, 242). The GyrA Ser83Leu mutation, however, had a more complex pattern of binding of enoxacin (242). Thus, overall, it appears that reductions in the affinity of drug for the enzyme-DNA target may mediate resistance for some classes of mutants, in particular, those with

mutations in and around position 83 (84 for S. aureus GyrA and 80 for S. aureus ParC) in the QRDR. The recently published X-ray crystallographic structure of a fragment of E. coli GyrA localizes the QRDR to a positively charged surface along which DNA has been modeled to bind (36). This region is adjacent to the two tyrosines (Tyr 122, one from each GyrA subunit) that are linked to DNA during strand breakage and might be considered as a candidate for the site of quinolone binding (see chapter 2). Thus, in one model, amino acid changes in the QRDR of GyrA (and by homology ParC) alter the structure of a quinolone binding site near the interface of the enzyme and DNA, and resistance is effected by reduced drug affinity for the modified enzyme-DNA complex. As yet no topoisomerase crystal structures that include a quinolone molecule and DNA have been reported to enable direct proof of this model.

Resistance mediated by mutations in ParE or GyrB might act by a similar mechanism in some cases, in particular, for the GyrB Asp426Asn muta-

tion, as noted above. The original crystal structure of a fragment of topoisomerase II of yeast, which has homology with both GyrA (carboxy terminus) and GyrB (amino terminus), suggested that the regions of quinolone resistance mutations in GyrB or ParE were distant from the region involved to the QRDR of GyrA or ParC (25). In subsequent crystal structures of other conformations of the yeast enzyme, however, the domains homologous to the QRDR regions of GyrB and ParE are in greater proximity to the region homologous to the QRDR of GyrA and ParC (24), suggesting that there may be enzyme conformations in which the QRDRs of GyrA and GyrB (or ParC and ParE) together form a quinolone binding site in a region also involved in DNA binding, as originally proposed by Yoshida, Nakamura, and their associates (240).

Although the GyrA Ser83Ala mutation in the QRDR produced no measureable defect in catalytic function or intracellular DNA supercoiling, GyrA Asp87Ala caused reduced DNA-supercoiling activity of reconstituted holoenzyme (17), and the GyrA Asp87Gly subunit was associated with reduced intracellular DNA supercoiling (14). The coumarin hypersusceptibility of some ParE mutants suggests the possibility that impairment of catalytic function may contribute to quinolone resistance in these mutants (60). Because ParC116 mutants also exhibit a coumarin hypersusceptibility phenotype, and these mutations are in proximity to the Tyr122 active site, they too might be postulated to have such a mechanism (59). A similar phenotype was found in yeast mutants selected for amsacrine resistance that had mutations in the domain of topoisomerase II homologous to that of ParE and were shown to be catalytically impaired (229). In addition, other mutations in yeast topoisomerase II (in the GyrB domain) that conferred cellular resistance to CP-115,953, a quinolone congener with activity against this enzyme, were associated with decreased enzyme levels within the yeast cell, decreased enzyme stability, and no increase in drug resistance of the purified enzyme (195). Furthermore, some uncommon mutations outside the QRDR regions of ParC and ParE that were shown to cause quinolone resistance in *S. aureus* (94, 95) exhibited poor growth and had topoisomerase IV with reduced DNA decatenation specific activity (Hooper et al., unpublished observations). Thus, in an additional model of the mechanism of drug resistance by target mutation, some mutations that impair enzyme function and stability may result in reduced formation of competent enzyme-DNA complexes that constitute the target of quinolone binding, rather than directly affecting the affinity of the quinolone for the complex. Thus, for some mutations the presence of fewer competent enzyme-DNA complexes itself may result in fewer drug targets on the chromosome and thereby effect resistance. That such non-QRDR mutations have been found more often in the subunits of topoisomerase IV than in the subunits of DNA gyrase suggests that cells may tolerate a broader set of mutations that affect enzyme function and stability in topoisomerase IV than in DNA gyrase.

RESISTANCE DUE TO ALTERED ACCESS OF DRUG TO TARGET ENZYMES

Quinolones must traverse the cell wall and cytoplasmic membrane of gram-positive bacteria and additionally the outer membrane in gram-negative bacteria to reach DNA gyrase and topoisomerase IV present in the cytoplasm. The cell wall is thought to provide little or no barrier to diffusion of small molecules such as quinolones, which have molecular weights around 300 to 400 Da. Accumulation of quinolones by whole cells of *S. aureus* is nonsaturable under usual experimental conditions and likely occurs by simple diffusion across the cytoplasmic membrane. All active quinolones have a negatively charged carboxyl group at position 3, and most current quinolones have an additional positively charged group at position 7 (piperazinyl or pyrrolidinyl ring derivatives) and thus are zwitterionic. The proportions of positively charged, negatively charged, dually charged, and uncharged species of a given quinolone vary with pH, and it is presumed that it is the uncharged species that diffuses freely across the membrane and reaches equilibrium with the cytoplasm (155). Differences in the pH between the medium and the cytoplasm may thus affect partitioning of drug by altering the proportions of charged species which are "trapped" in the cytoplasmic compartment. These factors are likely reponsible for the reductions in activity of zwitterionic quinolone congeners that occur below pH 7. Little is known about nonspecific binding of quinolones to bacterial cytoplasmic proteins or any compartmentalization of quinolones within the bacterial cell.

Altered Permeation Mechanisms in Gram-Negative Bacteria

Some quinolone-resistant clinical isolates of many species of gram-negative bacteria were found in early reports to have alterations in the amounts of outer membrane proteins, some of which were reduced amounts of general diffusion porins (86, 87, 176). Subsequent studies have identified the necessary

additional role of energy-dependent efflux systems that pump drug out of the cell and act in concert with reduced diffusion due to reduced porin channels. These efflux pumps are generally multidrug pumps native to most if not all bacteria, and the reader is referred to recent reviews on this topic (171, 179, 180, 187). No quinolone-specific efflux pumps have yet been identified, as might be expected for a class of synthetic compounds. The best studied organisms have been *E. coli* and *P. aeruginosa*, but examples have also been found in a number of other gram-negative bacteria that have been studied.

Mar, Sox, and Rob regulons and the AcrAB-TolC pump of *E. coli* and *S. enterica* serovar Typhimurium

In one of the best-studied systems in *E. coli* multiply antibiotic-resistant (Mar) mutants (7), which could be selected with tetracycline, chloramphenicol (73, 74), or fluoroquinolones (41, 103), were found to have mutations in the *marRAB* regulon (12). *marR* mutants resulting in a defective MarR repressor exhibited increased expression of MarA, a transcriptional activator that led to increased expression of *micF* and other loci and to quinolone resistance (42, 117). *micF* encodes an antisense RNA species that is complementary to the 5′ end of *ompF* transcripts, which encode OmpF, one of the two major porins of *E. coli* (11). Expression of the *mar* regulon can be induced by salicylates, acetaminophen, dinitrophenol, clofibric acid, and ethacrynic acid but not by quinolones (15, 40). Thus, increased expression of MarA leads to increased *micF*, which in turn leads to reduced translation of *ompF* mRNA by formation of a double-stranded RNA that may bind poorly to the ribosome. Reduced amounts of OmpF in the *E. coli* outer membrane appear to slow diffusion of norfloxacin and other fluoroquinolones, leading to slower rates of accumulation, but reductions in OmpF alone found in *ompF* mutants resulted in less resistance and lesser reductions in norfloxacin accumulation than *marR* mutants (41). Furthermore, reduced norfloxacin accumulation in *marR* mutants was abolished by inhibitors of proton motive force (90), indicating that additional energy-dependent factors contribute to reduced steady-state levels of accumulation. An additional factor necessary for resistance in *marR* mutants is the endogenous AcrAB membrane efflux pump (157, 163). AcrB is a member of the restriction-nodulation-division (RND) family of multidrug resistance (MDR) efflux pumps, which have 12 membrane-spanning domains and broad substrate profiles and are driven by the energy of the proton gradient across the cell membrane

(Table 3) (171). AcrA is a member of the membrane fusion protein (MFP) family, members of which appear to link inner and outer membrane proteins (245). The resistance phenotype of Mar mutants is abolished in *acrAB* mutants, indicating the necessity of an intact AcrAB pump for *marRAB*-mediated resistance (157, 163). The importance of the AcrAB-TolC system for quinolone resistance was further highlighted by the observation that inactivation of the *acrAB* locus reduced the quinolone resistance of strains with mutations in *marR* that also had *gyrA* single and double mutations sufficiently to bring them below clinical breakpoints for susceptibility (157). Thus, reduced porin channels appear to act in concert with endogenous MDR pumps to reduce steady-state cellular levels of quinolones, with reduced inward diffusion through porins serving to enhance the efflux capabilities of AcrAB, the efficiency of which may be low for unnatural substrates such as quinolones. In gram-negative bacteria AcrAB and other MDR pump-MFP combinations appear to be functionally linked to outer-membrane proteins that complete a pathway from cytoplasm or inner membrane to the exterior of the cell. In AcrAB, the TolC outer membrane protein appears to serve such a function (64), in addition to other roles, including secretion of hemolysin (198, 226). The importance of the AcrAB-TolC system in affecting efflux-mediated drug susceptibility in *E. coli* was highlighted by the systematic disruption of a series of MDR pumps identified on the basis of genome sequences (208). Deletions of *acrAB* or *tolC* produced increases in susceptibility for the broadest number of compounds as well as the largest effect on quinolone susceptibilities (fourfold for norfloxacin and ciprofloxacin and twofold for nalidixic acid), suggesting that this pump system is the most important in determining drug susceptibility levels in wild-type cells. No deletion mutants in other pumps produced any changes in quinolone MICs, but it remains possible that under other conditions overexpression of others of the pumps studied could affect resistance to quinolones or other antibiotics, as can occur with overexpression of the EmrAB pump system, deletion of which did not affect quinolone susceptibility in wild-type cells (see below).

E. coli strains with mutations in the *soxRS* locus, which is involved in the cellular responses to oxidative stress, have an overlapping resistance phenotype with *marR* mutants including low-level resistance to quinolones (138). SoxS is a homolog of MarA and appears to affect the expression of an overlapping set of genes, including reductions of OmpF due to increases in *micF* RNA (38). The *E. coli* RobA protein also belongs to the same family of transcriptional

activators as MarA. Overexpression of RobA, like overexpression of MarA, causes reductions of OmpF by increasing *micF* expression and multidrug resistance including fluoroquinolones. Resistance from RobA overexpression is also dependent on intact AcrAB (217). Thus, there are several regulatory systems in *E. coli* that may be altered to effect pleiotropic resistance that includes quinolones.

Quinolone-resistant clinical isolates of *E. coli* have been shown to have overexpression of *marA* and *soxS* as well as AcrA protein, in addition to mutations in *gyrA* and *parC* (137, 158). Because Mar mutants can be selected with tetracycline or chloramphenicol, in addition to fluoroquinolones, there may be an additional risk of selection of these mutants in clinical settings as a result of exposure of patients to these other classes of antibiotics.

Genes homologous to *marRAB*, *soxRS*, *acrAB*, and *tolC* of *E. coli* not surprisingly also exist in *S. enterica* serovar Typhimurium (111, 177, 207). Increased expression of *acrB* and reduced accumulation of ciprofloxacin has been found in ciprofloxacin-resistant clinical isolates (177). Other resistant clinical strains have also been found to have constitutive expression of *soxRS* that contributed to the resistance phenotype (111). Mutants selected with enrofloxacin, a fluoroquinolone used in animals, have also been shown to have increased levels of AcrA protein, altered outer-membrane profiles, altered lipopolysaccharide profiles, and reduced ciprofloxacin accumulation (77). Thus, it seems likely that the role of the Mar and Sox regulons and the AcrAB efflux pump in quinolone resistance in *S. enterica* serovar Typhimurium will be similar to that in *E. coli*.

EmrAB and MdfA pumps of *E. coli*

EmrB is a member of the major facilitator superfamily (MFS) of MDR pumps with 14 membrane-spanning domains. EmrA belongs to the MFP family, and EmrR is a negative transcriptional regulator (122, 236). Expression of *emrAB* results in resistance to carbonyl cyanide-*m*-chlorophenylhydrazone (CCCP), organomercurials, and nalidixic acid but not to fluoroquinolones (70, 121). EmrB is induced by both CCCP and nalidixic acid (171).

Overexpression of another *E. coli* MFS pump, MdfA, which was originally termed Cmr and CmlA for its ability to confer resistance to chloramphenicol, also confers resistance to fluoroquinolones, erythromycin, neomycin, tetracycline, and many other compounds as well as reduced accumulation of chloramphenicol (52). The contribution of MdfA to intrinsic levels of susceptibility to fluoroquinolones

and the nature of possible interacting membrane fusion and outer-membrane proteins are not yet defined.

Mex-Opr efflux systems of *P. aeruginosa*

In *P. aeruginosa*, multidrug resistance that includes quinolones has been shown to involve four different efflux pump systems, MexAB-OprM, MexCD-OprJ, MexEF-OprN, and MexXY-OprM, each of which includes a set of three proteins, an inner-membrane MDR pump, an MFP periplasmic linking protein, and an outer-membrane protein (Table 3) (178, 179). Additional homologs of these genes exist on the *P. aeruginosa* chromosome, but only these four have been shown thus far to be involved in multidrug resistance (135). Genetic knockout and reconstitution experiments in which only one of MexAB-OprM, MexCD-OprJ, and MexXY-OprM was expressed have been used to define the levels of expression in wild-type bacteria and the broad but incompletely overlapping substrate profiles for each of these pumps (120, 136). MexAB-OprM is normally expressed in wild-type bacteria, and outer membrane impermeability and the MexAB-OprM pump act in concert (as was true for OmpF and AcrAB in *E. coli*) to determine the level of susceptibility to quinolones and other antibiotics (116). *P. aeruginosa* strains with dual resistance mutations in *gyrA* and *parC* become susceptible to levofloxacin by clinical breakpoint criteria when OprM is inactivated, highlighting the contribution of this pump to the reduced susceptibility of wild-type and mutant strains (120).

Overexpression of MexAB-OprM causes increased resistance to ciprofloxacin, nalidixic acid, tetracycline, and chloramphenicol (182), a phenotype seen in *nalB* (*cfxB*) mutants of *P. aeruginosa*, which showed overexpression of an outer-membrane protein consistent with OprM (133, 189, 193). MexAB-OprM expression also contributes to reduced susceptibility to the β-lactams carbenicillin, ceftazidime, and aztreonam but not imipenem (136). MexB is a protein predicted to have 12 membrane-spanning domains that belongs to the RND family of exporters. *mexA* (null) and *oprM* (null) mutants exhibit increased accumulation of norfloxacin and increased susceptibility to fluoroquinolones (115), and, as noted above, wild-type strains of *P. aeruginosa* have sufficient expression of MexAB-OprM to contribute to the intrinsic level of resistance of *P. aeruginosa* to norfloxacin, tetracycline, chloramphenicol, and trimethoprim (106, 114, 120). The *nalB* (*cfxB*) locus has been shown to be a mutant allele of *mexR*, which is upstream of the *mexAB-*

oprM operon and regulates its expression (183). Expression of *mexR* itself appears to be negatively autoregulated, and MexR protein may have both repressor and activator functions, with the *nalB* mutation promoting activator function.

Mutants overexpressing MexAB-OprM produce less pyocyanin, casein protease, and elastase, virulence factors that are regulated by quorum-sensing systems that involve homoserine lactones and quinolone-derivative signaling molecules (54, 174). It has been suggested that MexAB-OprM is involved in active efflux of the $3OC_{12}$-homoserine lactone and 2-heptyl-3-hydroxyl-4-quinolone signaling molecules (172, 174), suggesting a link between resistance and virulence mechanisms that awaits further delineation. The increased antibiotic resistance that occurs in *P. aeruginosa* growing in biofilms appears not to be due to overexpression of MexAB-OprM or other pumps (34, 45). Resistance emerging after therapy with quinolones, however, has been documented to occur due to selection of *mexR* mutations and has been associated with increased expression of OprM (250).

nfxB mutants of *P. aeruginosa* also exhibit increased resistance to fluoroquinolones, erythromycin, trimethoprim, and triclosan and hypersusceptibility to some β-lactams and aminoglycosides (39, 87, 108). The *nfxB* gene, which is upstream of *mexCD-oprJ* and transcribed in the opposite direction, appears to be a repressor, and mutations in it result in increased expression of the *mexCD-oprJ* operon (161, 181). NfxB also appears to be a repressor of its own expression. *nfxB*(null) mutations result in the highest level of expression of MexCD-OprJ and are associated with additional resistance to tetracycline and chloramphenicol not seen in the original missense *nfxB* mutants (181). In contrast to MexAB-OprM, little or no expression of MexCD-OprJ occurs in wild-type cells under usual laboratory conditions, but MexCD-OprJ expression increases with decreases in expression of MexAB-OprM (116), suggesting coordinate cellular regulation of different efflux systems. The mechanism of hypersusceptibility to β-lactams and aminoglycosides is not fully understood, but reduced induction of chromosomal AmpC β-lactamase was found in an *nfxB* mutant that also lacked *mexAB-oprM* (134).

The differences in the resistance profiles of *mexR* and *nfxB* mutants appear, however, not to be determined by the outer-membrane components of MexAB-OprM and MexCD-OprJ pumps, since MexAB-OprJ and MexCD-OprM hybrid pumps retain the resistance profiles of the respective MexAB-OprM and MexCD-OprJ native pumps (206). Hybrid systems produced by exchange of the inner membrane components MexB and MexD, however, appear to be inactive (238). The resistance phenotype of *nfxB* mutants correlates with reduced accumulation of norfloxacin and chloramphenicol in these mutants (181). Reduced accumulation in *nfxB* mutants is reversed by the protonphore, CCCP, consistent with energy dependence of a pump. *nfxB* mutations in combination with mutations in *gyrA* have been identified among resistant clinical isolates of *P. aeruginosa* from cystic fibrosis and other patients (98, 243).

nfxC mutants of *P. aeruginosa* are resistant to fluoroquinolones, chloramphenicol, trimethoprim, imipenem, and triclosan and overexpress MexEF-OprN (39, 107, 108, 132). MexEF-OprN has variable levels of expression in different strains of wild-type bacteria that also express MexAB-OprM (116, 184). In these strains there was an inverse relationship between levels of MexAB-OprM and MexEF-OprN (116). Aparently, MexEF can function together with OprM, but MexAB cannot function together with OprN (132). Upstream of *mexEF-oprN* is the *mexT* gene, which is predicted to encode a member of the LysR family of transcriptional activators. A DNA fragment containing *mexT* when cloned on a plasmid causes increased expression of MexEF-OprN, a finding consistent with positive activation. Some wild-type strains have mutations in *mexT*, which are apparently responsible for their lack of expression of MexEF-OprN, and *nfxC* mutants contain an intact *mexT* gene (109, 131). One *nfxC* mutant has been reported in a resistant clinical isolate of *P. aeruginosa* (68). *nfxC* mutants also exhibited decreased transcription of *rhlI*, the gene encoding the synthase gene for C4-homoserine lactone, another signaling molecule involved in regulation of expression of virulence factors (109). This reduction was reversed by addition of synthetic C4-homoserine lactone and the *Pseudomonas* quinolone-derivative signaling molecule, suggesting that MexEF-OprN may affect cellular levels of *Pseudomonas* quinolone-derivative signaling molecule.

The most recently identified efflux system in *P. aeruginosa* that affects quinolones is MexXY-OprM (139). Expression of *mexXY* genes in *E. coli* or *P. aeruginosa* requires either *E. coli* TolC or *P. aeruginosa* OprM, respectively, to cause a resistance, which includes fluoroquinolones, erythromycin, ethidium bromide, and acriflavine (135, 139). This system is distinctive because it also confers resistance to aminoglycosides and appears to be necessary for the antagonism of aminoglycoside action by divalent cations (124, 135, 136) and because its expression is inducible by growth in the presence of tetracycline, erythromycin, gentamicin, or ofloxacin in wild-type strains (135). The genetic determinants that affect expression of *mexXY* and underlie the induction phenotype have yet to be identified.

Although all four known efflux systems in *P. aeruginosa* cause increases in resistance to quinolones when overexpressed, quinolone congeners differ in the extent to which they are affected by each system, and use of different quinolones in resistance selections results in differential selection of mutants overexpressing these systems (108). Quinolones with a fluorine at position 6 and a positively charged substituent at the 7 position tend to select *nfxB*-type mutants, whereas quinolones lacking a positively charged substituent at position 7 tend to select *nalB*- and *nfxC*-type mutants. These differences presumably reflect the extent to which a particular quinolone is a substrate for a given efflux system. Quinolones, which are synthetic compounds, are not natural substrates for these or other efflux pumps. The natural substrates of MDR pumps remain to be defined clearly, but as noted above, expression of some pumps can affect expression of virulence factors, and it has been suggested that signaling molecules may be natural substrates of some pumps.

Broad-spectrum inhibitors of the MDR pumps of *P. aeruginosa* have recently been identified and shown to cause increased susceptibility to a number of antimicrobials that are pump substrates, including fluoroquinolones (123, 190). The inhibitors also blocked resistance acquired by overexpression of these pumps and reduced the frequency with which resistance could be selected with levofloxacin. Because of the multiplicity of pumps, inhibition of all of them appears to be necessary to reduce the frequency of selection of resistance (120). Surprisingly, the same inhibitor affected the substrates of MexXY differentially in overproducer strains, reducing fluoroquinolone resistance but increasing aminoglycoside resistance, suggesting that the inhibitor might act competitively with some drug substrates but in complex ways with others (124).

Efflux systems in other gram-negative bacteria

Considerably less is known about altered permeation and efflux contributing to quinolone resistance in other gram-negative bacteria. MarA homologs have been found in *K. pneumoniae* (RamA) (72), *Proteus vulgaris* (PqrA) (96), and several other bacterial species (7), suggesting that similar regulatory mechanisms may underlie some forms of multidrug resistance in these organisms as well.

A mutant with a pleiotropic resistance phenotype selected by passage of *C. jejuni* on pefloxacin

was found to have, in addition to a *gyrA* mutation, reduced accumulation of ciprofloxacin that was reversed with CCCP and expression of two new outer-membrane proteins (37), a pattern similar to that seen in other efflux mutants. Quinolone-resistant clinical isolates of *K. pneumoniae* have been shown to have, in addition to alterations in *gyrA*, slight reductions in accumulation of norfloxacin that are reversed with CCCP, and variable loss of outer membrane proteins (129). Resistant mutants of *C. freundii* selected in vitro also appeared to accumulate less norfloxacin than their parent strain (220). The *robA* homolog of *E. cloacae* when cloned on a plasmid in *E. coli* caused reduced OmpF by activation of *micF* and pleiotropic resistance to quinolones, chloramphenicol, tetracycline, and β-lactams (112).

Stenotrophomonas maltophilia, which is commonly resistant to multiple antibiotics, has been shown to have proteins that cross-react with antibodies to OprM and MexB of *P. aeruginosa* (246), and a new pump, SmeDEF, has recently been identified in this organism; SmeD is a member of the membrane fusion family, SmeE a member of the RND family of pumps, and SmeF similar to other outer-membrane proteins (8). Cloning of *smeDEF* in an *E. coli* ΔacrAB strain conferred multidrug resistance, including resistance to norfloxacin, ofloxacin, nalidixic acid, erythromycin, chloramphenicol, and tetracycline as well as reduced accumulation of norfloxacin. A multidrug-resistant laboratory mutant of *S. maltophilia* also exhibited increased levels of *smeDEF* mRNA relative to low levels of expression in the parent strain (8). For both mutant and wild-type strains, there was growth-phase-dependent regulation of levels of *smeDEF* RNA, with the highest levels in early exponential phase followed by a gradual decline. Deletion of *smeE* and *smeF* in wild-type strains caused two- to fourfold reductions in MICs of a number of quinolones and other antibiotics, suggesting that expression of SmeDEF also contributes to the intrinsic reduced susceptibility of *S. maltophilia* (247). In addition, 33 to 47% of clinical isolates also appear to overexpress *smeD* or SmeF, a finding that correlates with higher MICs of quinolones (9).

Accumulation of norfloxacin in cells of *V. parahaemolyticus* is increased by addition of CCCP, and the *norM* gene cloned from *V. parahaemolyticus* caused resistance to norfloxacin, ciprofloxacin, ethidium, and streptomycin in *E. coli* (143). NorM exhibited homology to the *E. coli* YdhE protein, which is predicted to be a membrane protein but lacks sequence similarity to other MDR pumps. NorM is now recognized to be a member of a new family of multidrug and toxic compound extrusion (MATE) pumps (187). Cloned *ydhE* also caused quinolone resistance but differed from *norM* in other aspects of the pleiotropic resistance phenotype. Thus, additional mechanisms of resistance associated with reduced drug accumulation appear to exist. *Vibrio cholerae* also encodes an MDR pump, VceAB, a homolog of EmrAB of *E. coli* that when inactivated causes increased susceptibility to nalidixic acid, erythromycin, deoxycholate, and CCCP (44).

Efflux of norfloxacin has been suggested previously in *Bacteroides fragilis* (140), and a new MATE family transporter, BexA, was recently identified in *Bacteroides thetaiotaomicron* and shown to cause increased resistance to norfloxacin and ciprofloxacin when overexpressed in *E. coli* and increased susceptibility to these quinolones when inactivated in its native host (141). Energy-dependent norfloxacin efflux from overexpression of *bexA* was observed in *E. coli*, and the norfloxacin MICs for these strains were reduced by known efflux inhibitors, including MC 207,110, the broad-spectrum inhibitor of the Mex-Opr pumps of *P. aeruginosa*.

Other MDR pumps such as that encoded by the *mtrCDE* operon of *N. gonorrhoeae* are homologous to the pumps encoded by *mexAB-oprM* in *P. aeruginosa* and *acrAB* in *E. coli* but are not known to be involved in quinolone resistance (82).

Altered Permeation Mechanisms in Gram-Positive Bacteria

In gram-positive bacteria the permeability barrier of the outer membrane does not exist, and alterations in expression of efflux pumps appear to mediate drug resistance due to altered permeation in these organisms. The two best-studied systems that effect quinolone resistance are NorA of *S. aureus* and Bmr and Blt of *Bacillus subtilis*, but additional examples are being identified and studied in other gram-positive bacteria.

NorA of *S. aureus*

Acquired quinolone resistance due to altered permeation in gram-positive bacteria has been identified in *S. aureus* and *B. subtilis* due to active efflux of drug across the cytoplasmic membrane. In *S. aureus*, resistance of this type has been shown to be due to increased levels of expression of *norA*, a chromosomal gene that encodes a protein with 12 predicted membrane-spanning domains that is a member of the MFS class of transporters (153, 241). Like other MDR transporters, NorA has a broad substrate profile mediating pleiotropic resistance, which in NorA includes ethidium bromide, rhodamine 6G, tetraphenylphosphonium

(TPP), chloramphenicol, and hydrophilic quinolones such a norfloxacin, ciprofloxacin, and ofloxacin (152, 241). The activity of hydrophobic quinolones such as sparfloxacin and trovafloxacin is less affected by NorA. Cloned *norA* mediates a similar resistance phenotype in *E. coli*. In everted membrane vesicles prepared from *E. coli* cells containing cloned *norA* but not cells containing the vector plasmid alone, uptake of labeled norfloxacin (which represents drug efflux because of the reversed membrane orientation in everted vesicles) is saturable and depends on the energy generated by the proton gradient across the membrane (153). Norfloxacin uptake in everted vesicles and the resistance phenotype associated with *norA* expression is inhibited by reserpine and verapamil (128, 153), which also inhibit other MDR transporters. NorA, like another MFS transporter, LmrP of *Lactococcus lactis* (186), also transports Hoechst 33342, a dye that exhibits strong fluorescence when in the membrane, but little fluorescence in an aqueous environment (244). Purified NorA reconstituted into proteoliposomes was also sufficient to mediate transport of Hoechst 33342, indicating the NorA pump can act alone to transport substrates. The inhibitor verapamil and the hydrophilic quinolone substrates norfloxacin and ciprofloxacin are competitive inhibitors of Hoechst 33342 transport by NorA in everted membrane vesicles, but interestingly, sparfloxacin behaves as a noncompetitive inhibitor, suggesting that drug binding sites differ for those quinolones that are good substrates and those that are not (244).

The level of expression of *norA* varies and is regulated. Increased steady-state levels of *norA* mRNA and pleiotropic resistance are associated with single-nucleotide changes upstream of *norA* in the 5' untranslated region of the *norA* promoter (101, 153). The increased levels of *norA* transcripts in one such mutant appear to be caused by the increased half-life and stability of the mutant *norA* mRNA (62). *norA* expression also varies with growth phase, being greatest during exponential phase, but this regulation appears to be independent of the *agr* or *sar* genes, which mediate growth-phase-dependent global regulation of excreted virulence factors and some surface proteins (58). *norA* expression is affected by a newly described two-component regulatory system *arlRS*, which also affects cellular adhesion, autolysis, and extracellular proteolytic activity (58, 61). An 18-kDa protein binding upstream of *norA*, named NorR, belongs to the MarR and SarR family of regulators (222a). *norR* overexpression on a plasmid results in increased levels of *norA* mRNA and increased resistance to quinolones and other NorA substrates. Thus, regulation of *norA* expression appears to be multifactorial. The environmental signals and the full extent of the genetic pathways that regulate its expression in different environments remain to be determined. Salicylate, which induces expression of the *marRAB* regulon of *E. coli* (40), also appeared to increase ciprofloxacin resistance in *S. aureus*, but the involvement of NorA or other staphylococcal transporters in this phenomenon was not studied (81). One mutant of *S. aureus* in which *norA* expression was induced by norfloxacin has also been described, but the genetic basis of the effect remains to be defined (101). Resistance has also been associated with a single mutation in the *norA* structural gene (160), but little is known about structure-activity relationships of NorA. Also undefined are the normal functions of NorA in the cell.

Although the *norA* gene appears to be nonessential on the basis of the isolation of knockout mutants (92a), it is widely present on the chromosomes of clinical isolates of *S. aureus* and coagulase-negative staphylococci (101). Blocking of NorA function with reserpine increases quinolone susceptibility (153) and reduces the frequency of selection of resistant mutants with norfloxacin (128), suggesting a role for NorA in determining quinolone susceptibility even in wild-type staphylococci. Apparent contributions of efflux to the quinolone resistance of clinical isolates of *S. aureus* has also been found in subsets of clinical isolates for which quinolone resistance was reduced in the presence of reserpine (146, 199). Most of these isolates had no mutations in promoter region or structural gene of *norA* (146, 200), suggesting the presence of extragenic mutations affecting *norA* expression or the involvement of other reserpine-inhibitable pumps in the resistance phenotype. Some but not all strains exhibited increased levels of *norA* mRNA (199). In addition to reserpine, other drugs in clinical use, including the widely used proton pump inhibitors omeprazole and lansoprazole, inhibit the resistance phenotype of strains overexpressing NorA, suggesting that combinations of antimicrobials with pump inhibitors may be feasible (2).

Bmr, Blt, and Bmr3 of *B. subtilis*

The Bmr protein of *B. subtilis* has 44% amino acid identity with NorA of *S. aureus* and also belongs to the MFS class (151, 152). The expression of the chromosomal *bmr* gene results in a resistance phenotype similar to that due to expression of *norA*. Expression of *bmr* is induced by rhodamine 6G and TPP, two Bmr substrates, and *bmrR*, which is upstream of *bmr*, has homology to other transcriptional activator proteins (3). BmrR has been shown to bind the *bmr* promoter with increased affinity in the presence of these inducers, and the purified carboxy-terminal half of the Bmr protein has also been

shown to bind rhodamine and TPP (127). The crystal structure of BmrR bound with TPP alone (249) and together with the *bmr* promoter (248), as well as targeted structural modifications of many pumps (187), has suggested the structural basis for the binding of multiple structurally diverse molecules to BmrR that may be relevant to the mechanism by which the pump itself recognizes such a wide variety of structural substrates, many of which are either amphiphilic with a positive or neutral charge or hydrophobic. This general model includes a pocket with hydrophobic and nonpolar residues and a buried negatively charged amino acid, such a Glu, which is exposed on drug binding, stabilizing the drug-protein interaction. Glu residues located in a hydrophobic domain have been found in many secondary transporters and are often essential for function. Kinetic experiments also suggest, however, that transporters can have different functional sites of binding for different substrates (185, 187, 244).

Blt, another transporter in *B. subtilis* related to Bmr, has an apparently identical substrate profile but is not expressed in wild-type cells (4). Its expression is regulated by the product of the upstream gene, *bltR*, which is not induced by rhodamine. There is also an additional downstream gene, *bltD*, which is cotranscribed with *blt* and appears to encode a specific polyamine acetyltransferase (235). The role of this acetyltransferase within the cell is as yet unknown, but these findings suggest that *bltD* and *blt* may have related, specific physiologic functions in the cell.

The most recently identified MDR transporter of *B. subtilis*, Bmr3, has 14 membrane-spanning segments and, when overexpressed, confers resistance to puromycin and to the quinolones norfloxacin and tosufloxacin, but not levofloxacin (159). Disruption of *bmr3* does not affect intrinsic susceptibility, indicating that the gene is not essential and is poorly expressed. *bmr3* transcripts appear to be lower in late log phase of growth in relation to early log phase. Thus, as in gram-negative bacteria, multiple pumps with overlapping substrate profiles occur in gram-positive bacteria as well.

Quinolones, which are synthetic compounds, appear to be incidental substrates for NorA, Bmr, Blt, and Bmr3. Specific mutations or the physiologic conditions that promote their expression will reduce quinolone activity and contribute to low-level resistance.

PmrA of *S. pneumoniae*

Quinolone-resistant clinical and laboratory strains of *S. pneumoniae* have been shown to have reduced accumulation of quinolones that is reversible with reserpine, suggesting the involvement of an efflux system(s) in quinolone resistance in this organism as well (16, 30). In addition, a *norA* homolog, *pmrA*, has been identified in *S. pneumoniae*, and its inactivation by introduction of a *norA::cat* insertion in the chromosome caused increased quinolone susceptibility and decreased whole-cell efflux of ethidium bromide (76). Reserpine was also able to reduce the selection of ciprofloxacin-resistant mutants of *S. pneumoniae* (126), as it was in *S. aureus* (128). Although clinical isolates of quinolone-resistant *S. pneumoniae* are relatively infrequent at present, it is noteworthy that as many as one third of resistant isolates studied appear to have an at least partially reserpine-reversible resistance phenotype, suggesting a common but not exclusive role for drug efflux, since target enzyme mutations were usually present as well (19, 31, 35). Also noteworthy is that a reserpine-induced reduction in MICs of quinolones of two- to fourfold can also be seen in susceptible *S. pneumoniae*, suggesting that for some resistant strains with a similar magnitude of reduction in MIC by reserpine, there may not necessarily be increased expression of PmrA or other pumps over that in wild-type cells. The nature of mutations in *S. pneumoniae* that can lead to increased expression of PmrA or other efflux pumps is unknown.

Quinolone-resistant clinical isolates of viridans streptococci have also been shown to have an efflux phenotype defined as lower MICs of quinolones in the presence of reserpine. DNA from such strains of *S. mitis* and *Streptococcus oralis* was able to transform *S. pneumoniae* to this phenotype in the laboratory. Transformation of resistance determinants from viridans streptococci to pneumococci, however, appears to be uncommon among ciprofloxacin-resistant clinical isolates of *S. pneumoniae* (18).

Efflux transporters in other gram-positive bacteria

Other MDR transporters reported in gram-positive bacteria, such as QacA/B and Smr of *S. aureus* and Ptr of *Streptomyces pristinaespiralis*, do not appear to include quinolones in their broad substrate profiles (113, 171). LmrA of *L. lactis*, however, confers resistance to quinolones and multiple other compounds (187) and is distinctive because it is a member of the ABC transporter family, which utilizes ATP hydrolysis, rather than the membrane proton gradient, as a source of energy (125, 223).

Some highly quinolone-resistant clinical isolates of *E. faecalis* also appear to accumulate lesser amounts of norfloxacin than susceptible strains, suggesting a possible role for efflux in resistance in this organism as well. The genes responsible for this phe-

nomenon and their role in resistance in *E. faecalis*, however, have not been defined (149).

Altered Permeation Mechanisms in Mycobacteria

The *lfrA* gene of *M. smegmatis* is predicted to encode an efflux pump of the MFS class with 14 membrane-spanning domains. LfrA is similar to QacA but not NorA of *S. aureus* (213). Expression of cloned *lfrA* in *E. coli* causes low-level resistance to hydrophilic quinolones such as ciprofloxacin and ofloxacin and to ethidium bromide, acriflavine, and some quarternary ammonium compounds. The activity of a more hydrophobic quinolone such as sparfloxacin was unaffected by *lfrA* expression, a pattern also seen with *norA* of *S. aureus*. Overexpression of cloned *lfrA* from a plasmid in *M. smegmatis* also causes resistance and reduced drug accumulation that is reversible with CCCP (118). Overexpression of chromosomal *lfrA*, however, has not yet been associated with resistance in *M. smegmatis*. Homologs of *lfrA* appear to be present in *M. tuberculosis* and *Mycobacterium avium* (213). A resistant mutant of *M. tuberculosis* strain H37Ra selected with ofloxacin was found to have no mutation in the QRDR of *gyrA* and exhibited reduced accumulation of norfloxacin that was abolished with CCCP, suggesting possible resistance due to efflux (105). The increments of resistance to ciprofloxacin were somewhat greater (fourfold) than those for ofloxacin and sparfloxacin (twofold). LfrA also appears to contribute to the innate reduced susceptibility of mycobacteria to quinolones (197).

OTHER MECHANISMS OF RESISTANCE

No specific quinolone-degrading enzymes have been identified as a mechanism of resistance, but fungi that are capable of degrading quinolones through metabolic pathways have been reported (231).

Recently, plasmid-mediated resistance to quinolones was identified and validated for the first time in clinical strains of *K. pneumoniae* (130). Resistance was transferable to *E. coli* by conjugation. The gene responsible for this resistance, *qnr*, has been cloned and sequenced and is related to the *mcbG* gene, which is in involved in immunity to microcin B17, an inhibitor of DNA gyrase (196). Overexpression of *mcbG* also confers low-level quinolone resistance as well (Yu and Hooper, unpublished observations) (119). Purified Qnr also protects purified *E. coli* DNA gyrase from ciprofloxacin (221a). *qnr* has been found in quinolone-resistant clinical isolates of both *K. pneu-*

moniae and *E. coli* within complex integrons on plasmids (226a).

No such plasmid-mediated quinolone resistance has been reported in natural isolates of gram-positive bacteria. One possible form of plasmid-mediated quinolone resistance in gram-positive bacteria, however, is due to MDR pumps. The QacA/B (170) and Smr (80) MDR pumps, which can cause resistance to other antimicrobials but not quinolones, are encoded on plasmids in *S. aureus*, and the *norA* gene cloned on a shuttle plasmid confers quinolone resistance in *S. aureus* (241). In addition, mutant resistant alleles of *grlA* and *grlB* of topoisomerase IV present on shuttle plasmids also confer resistance when introduced into wild-type *S. aureus* (59, 60). Overexpression of *norA* and genes for topoisomerases from plasmids are known, however, to have toxic effects on the cell that may limit the fitness of resistant bacteria containing them (209).

FUTURE PROSPECTS

With the continuing development of newer fluoroquinolones as well as some new nonfluorinated derivatives with increasing potency, some mutant bacteria that are resistant to earlier fluoroquinolones may by clinical-breakpoint criteria remain susceptible to the new, more potent agents, although in most cases the MICs of the newer agents for such mutant bacteria are increased relative to those for wild-type bacteria. The low frequency of resistance selection in vitro for drugs that appear to have similar activities against both DNA gyrase and topoisomerase IV is promising (168) (see chapter 2), but to be broadly applicable, this property of matched activity would need to be accomplished for many different species.

Other approaches to expanding and preserving the utility of fluoroquinolones include development of inhibitors of MDR efflux pumps, which might be used in conjunction with fluoroquinolones (or other antimicrobials that are substrates for these pumps) to enhance intrinsic activity as well as to circumvent efflux-type resistance mechanisms. Other classes of inhibitors of DNA gyrase and topoisomerase IV have also been explored (88), but no class has yet been as successful as the quinolones and related agents. Because of bacterial ingenuity, we, however, must also approach the problem of quinolone resistance from an epidemiologic perspective with efforts to focus quinolone use to limit the selection and to promote infection control practices to limit spread of resistance organisms once selected.

REFERENCES

1. Ackermann, G., Y. J. Tang, R. Kueper, P. Heisig, A. C. Rodloff, J. Silva, Jr., and S. H. Cohen. 2001. Resistance to moxifloxacin in toxigenic *Clostridium difficile* isolates is associated with mutations in *gyrA*. *Antimicrob. Agents Chemother.* **45:**2348–2353.

2. Aeschlimann, J. R., L. D. Dresser, G. W. Kaatz, and M. J. Rybak. 1999. Effects of NorA inhibitors on in vitro antibacterial activities and postantibiotic effects of levofloxacin, ciprofloxacin, and norfloxacin in genetically related strains of *Staphylococcus aureus*. *Antimicrob. Agents Chemother.* **43:**335–340.

3. Ahmed, M., C. M. Borsch, S. S. Taylor, N. Vazquez-Laslop, and A. A. Neyfakh. 1994. A protein that activates expression of a multidrug efflux transporter upon binding the transporter substrates. *J. Biol. Chem.* **269:**28506–28513.

4. Ahmed, M., L. Lyass, P. N. Markham, S. S. Taylor, N. Vazquez-Laslop, and A. A. Neyfakh. 1995. Two highly similar multidrug transporters of *Bacillus subtilis* whose expression is differentially regulated. *J. Bacteriol.* **177:**3904–3910.

5. Akasaka, T., M. Tanaka, A. Yamaguchi, and K. Sato. 2001. Type II topoisomerase mutations in fluoroquinolone-resistant clinical strains of *Pseudomonas aeruginosa* isolated in 1998 and 1999: role of target enzyme in mechanism of fluoroquinolone resistance. *Antimicrob. Agents Chemother.* **45:**2263–2268.

6. Alangaden, G. J., E. K. Manavathu, S. B. Vakulenko, N. M. Zvonok, and S. A. Lerner. 1995. Characterization of fluoroquinolone-resistant mutant strains of *Mycobacterium tuberculosis* selected in the laboratory and isolated from patients. *Antimicrob. Agents Chemother.* **39:**1700–1703.

7. Alekshun, M. N., and S. B. Levy. 1997. Regulation of chromosomally mediated multiple antibiotic resistance: the *mar* regulon. *Antimicrob. Agents Chemother.* **41:**2067–2075.

8. Alonso, A., and J. L. Martínez. 2000. Cloning and characterization of SmeDEF, a novel multidrug efflux pump from *Stenotrophomonas maltophilia*. *Antimicrob. Agents Chemother.* **44:**3079–3086.

9. Alonso, A., and J. L. Martinez. 2001. Expression of multidrug efflux pump SmeDEF by clinical isolates of *Stenotrophomonas maltophilia*. *Antimicrob. Agents Chemother.* **45:**1879–1881.

10. Alovero, F. L., X. S. Pan, J. E. Morris, R. H. Manzo, and L. M. Fisher. 2000. Engineering the specificity of antibacterial fluoroquinolones: benzenesulfonamide modifications at C-7 of ciprofloxacin change its primary target in *Streptococcus pneumoniae* from topoisomerase IV to gyrase. *Antimicrob. Agents Chemother.* **44:**320–325.

11. Andersen, J., N. Delihas, K. Ikenaka, P. J. Green, O. Pines, O. Ilercil, and M. Inouye. 1987. The isolation and characterization of RNA coded by the *micF* gene in *Escherichia coli*. *Nucleic Acids Res.* **15:**2089–2101.

12. Ariza, R. R., S. P. Cohen, N. Bachhawat, S. B. Levy, and B. Demple. 1994. Repressor mutations in the *marRAB* operon that activate oxidative stress genes and multiple antibiotic resistance in *Escherichia coli*. *J. Bacteriol.* **176:**143–148.

13. Bachoual, R., L. Dubreuil, C. J. Soussy, and J. Tankovic. 2000. Roles of *gyrA* mutations in resistance of clinical isolates and in vitro mutants of *Bacteroides fragilis* to the new fluoroquinolone trovafloxacin. *Antimicrob. Agents Chemother.* **44:**1842–1845.

14. Bagel, S., V. Hüllen, B. Wiedemann, and P. Heisig. 1999. Impact of *gyrA* and *parC* mutations on quinolone resistance, doubling time, and supercoiling degree of *Escherichia coli*. *Antimicrob. Agents Chemother.* **43:**868–875.

15. Balagué, C., and E. G. Véscovi. 2001. Activation of multiple antibiotic resistance in uropathogenic *Escherichia coli* strains by aryloxoalcanoic acid compounds. *Antimicrob. Agents Chemother.* 45:1815–1822.

16. Baranova, N. N., and A. A. Neyfakh. 1997. Apparent involvement of a multidrug transporter in the fluoroquinolone resistance of *Streptococcus pneumoniae*. *Antimicrob. Agents Chemother.* 41:1396–1398.

17. Barnard, F. M., and A. Maxwell. 2001. Interaction between DNA gyrase and quinolones: effects of alanine mutations at GyrA subunit residues Ser[83] and Asp[87]. *Antimicrob. Agents Chemother.* 45:1994–2000.

18. Bast, D. J., J. C. S. De Azavedo, T. Y. Tam, L. Kilburn, C. Duncan, L. A. Mandell, R. J. Davidson, and D. E. Low. 2001. Interspecies recombination contributes minimally to fluoroquinolone resistance in *Streptococcus pneumoniae*. *Antimicrob. Agents Chemother.* 45:2631–2634.

19. Bast, D. J., D. E. Low, C. L. Duncan, L. Kilburn, L. A. Mandell, R. J. Davidson, and J. C. S. De Azavedo. 2000. Fluoroquinolone resistance in clinical isolates of *Streptococcus pneumoniae*: contributions of type II topoisomerase mutations and efflux to levels of resistance. *Antimicrob. Agents Chemother.* 44:3049–3054.

20. Bébéar, C. M., A. Charron, J. M. Bové, C. Bébéar, and J. Renaudin. 1998. Cloning and nucleotide sequences of the topoisomerase IV *parC* and *parE* genes of *Mycoplasma hominis*. *Antimicrob. Agents Chemother.* 42:2024–2031.

21. Bébéar, C. M., H. Renaudin, A. Charron, J. M. Bové, C. Bébéar, and J. Renaudin. 1998. Alterations in topoisomerase IV and DNA gyrase in quinolone-resistant mutants of *Mycoplasma hominis* obtained in vitro. *Antimicrob. Agents Chemother.* 42:2304–2311.

22. Bebear, C. M., J. Renaudin, A. Charron, H. Renaudin, B. de Barbeyrac, T. Schaeverbeke, and C. Bebear. 1999. Mutations in the *gyrA*, *parC*, and *parE* genes associated with fluoroquinolone resistance in clinical isolates of *Mycoplasma hominis*. *Antimicrob. Agents Chemother.* 43:954–956.

23. Belland, R. J., S. G. Morrison, C. Ison, and W. M. Huang. 1994. *Neisseria gonorrhoeae* acquires mutations in analogous regions of *gyrA* and *parC* in fluoroquinolone-resistant isolates. *Mol. Microbiol.* 14:371–380.

24. Berger, J. M. 1998. Type II DNA topoisomerases. *Curr. Opin. Struct. Biol.* 8:26–32.

25. Berger, J. M., S. J. Gamblin, S. C. Harrison, and J. C. Wang. 1996. Structure and mechanism of DNA topoisomerase II. *Nature* 379:225–232.

26. Berger, J. M., and J. C. Wang. 1996. Recent developments in DNA topoisomerase II structure and mechanism. *Curr. Opin. Struct. Biol.* 6:84–90.

27. Blanche, F., B. Cameron, F. X. Bernard, L. Maton, B. Manse, L. Ferrero, N. Ratet, C. Lecoq, A. Goniot, D. Bisch, and J. Crouzet. 1996. Differential behaviors of *Staphylococcus aureus* and *Escherichia coli* type II DNA topoisomerases. *Antimicrob. Agents Chemother.* 40:2714–2720.

28. Reference deleted.

29. Breines, D. M., S. Ouabdesselam, E. Y. Ng, J. Tankovic, S. Shah, C. J. Soussy, and D. C. Hooper. 1997. Quinolone resistance locus *nfxD* of *Escherichia coli* is a mutant allele of *parE* gene encoding a subunit of topoisomerase IV. *Antimicrob. Agents Chemother.* 41:175–179.

30. Brenwald, N. P., M. J. Gill, and R. Wise. 1997. The effect of reserpine, an inhibitor of multidrug efflux pumps, on the in-vitro susceptibilities of fluoroquinolone-resistant strains of *Streptococcus pneumoniae* to norfloxacin. *J. Antimicrob. Chemother.* 40:458–460.

31. Brenwald, N. P., M. J. Gill, and R. Wise. 1998. Prevalence of a putative efflux mechanism among fluoroquinolone-resistant clinical isolates of *Streptococcus pneumoniae*. *Antimicrob. Agents Chemother.* 42:2032–2035.

32. Brisse, S., A. C. Fluit, U. Wagner, P. Heisig, D. Milatovic, J. Verhoef, S. Scheuring, K. Köhrer, and F. J. Schmitz. 1999. Association of alterations in ParC and GyrA proteins with resistance of clinical isolates of *Enterococcus faecium* to nine different fluoroquinolones. *Antimicrob. Agents Chemother.* 43:2513–2516.

33. Brisse, S., D. Milatovic, A. C. Fluit, J. Verhoef, N. Martin, S. Scheuring, K. Köhrer, and F. J. Schmitz. 1999. Comparative in vitro activities of ciprofloxacin, clinafloxacin, gatifloxacin, levofloxacin, moxifloxacin, and trovafloxacin against *Klebsiella pneumoniae*, *Klebsiella oxytoca*, *Enterobacter cloacae*, and *Enterobacter aerogenes* clinical isolates with alterations in GyrA and ParC proteins. *Antimicrob. Agents Chemother.* 43:2051–2055.

34. Brooun, A., S. Liu, and K. Lewis. 2000. A dose-response study of antibiotic resistance in *Pseudomonas aeruginosa* biofilms. *Antimicrob. Agents Chemother.* 44:640–646.

35. Broskey, J., K. Coleman, M. N. Gwynn, L. McCloskey, C. Traini, L. Voelker, and R. Warren. 2000. Efflux and target mutations as quinolone resistance mechanisms in clinical isolates of *Streptococcus pneumoniae*. *J. Antimicrob. Chemother.* 45:95–99.

36. Cabral, J. H., A. P. Jackson, C. V. Smith, N. Shikotra, A. Maxwell, and R. C. Liddington. 1997. Crystal structure of the breakage-reunion domain of DNA gyrase. *Nature* 388:903–906.

37. Charvalos, E., Y. Tselentis, M. M. Hamzehpour, T. Köhler, and J. C. Pechère. 1995. Evidence for an efflux pump in multidrug-resistant *Campylobacter jejuni*. *Antimicrob. Agents Chemother.* 39:2019–2022.

38. Chou, J. H., J. T. Greenberg, and B. Demple. 1998. Postranscriptional repression of *Escherichia coli* OmpF protein in response to redox stress: positive control of the *micF* antisense RNA by the *soxRS* locus. *J. Bacteriol.* 175:1026–1031.

39. Chuanchuen, R., K. Beinlich, T. T. Hoang, A. Becher, R. R. Karkhoff-Schweizer, and H. P. Schweizer. 2001. Cross-resistance between triclosan and antibiotics in *Pseudomonas aeruginosa* is mediated by multidrug efflux pumps: exposure of a susceptible mutant strain to triclosan selects *nfxB* mutants overexpressing MexCD-OprJ. *Antimicrob. Agents Chemother.* 45:428–432.

40. Cohen, S. P., S. B. Levy, J. Foulds, and J. L. Rosner. 1993. Salicylate induction of antibiotic resistance in *Escherichia coli*: activation of the *mar* operon and a *mar*-independent pathway. *J. Bacteriol.* 175:7856–7862.

41. Cohen, S. P., L. M. McMurry, D. C. Hooper, J. S. Wolfson, and S. B. Levy. 1989. Cross-resistance to fluoroquinolones in multiple-antibiotic-resistant (Mar) *Escherichia coli* selected by tetracycline or chloramphenicol: decreased drug accumulation associated with membrane changes in addition to OmpF reduction. *Antimicrob. Agents Chemother.* 33:1318–1325.

42. Cohen, S. P., L. M. McMurry, and S. B. Levy. 1988. *marA* locus causes decreased expression of OmpF porin in multiple-antibiotic-resistant (Mar) mutants of *Escherichia coli*. *J. Bacteriol.* 170:5416–5422.

43. Cole, S. T., R. Brosch, J. Parkhill, T. Garnier, C. Churcher, D. Harris, S. V. Gordon, K. Eiglmeier, S. Gas, C. E. Barry, F. Tekaia, K. Badcock, D. Basham, D. Brown, T. Chillingworth, R. Connor, R. Davies, K. Devlin, T. Feltwell, S. Gentles, N. Hamlin, S. Holroyd, T. Hornsby, K. Jagels, and B. G. Barrell. 1998. Deciphering the biology of

Mycobacterium tuberculosis from the complete genome sequence. *Nature* **393**:537–544.

44. Colmer, J. A., J. A. Fralick, and A. N. Hamood. 1998. Isolation and characterization of a putative multidrug resistance pump from *Vibrio cholerae*. *Mol. Microbiol.* **27**:63–72.

45. De Kievit, T. R., M. D. Parkins, R. J. Gillis, R. Srikumar, H. Ceri, K. Poole, B. H. Iglewski, and D. G. Storey. 2001. Multidrug efflux pumps: expression patterns and contribution to antibiotic resistance in *Pseudomonas aeruginosa* biofilms. *Antimicrob. Agents Chemother.* **45**:1761–1770.

46. Deguchi, T., A. Fukuoka, M. Yasuda, M. Nakano, S. Ozeki, E. Kanematsu, Y. Nishino, S. Ishihara, Y. Ban, and Y. Kawada. 1997. Alterations in the GyrA subunit of DNA gyrase and the ParC subunit of topoisomerase IV in quinolone-resistant clinical isolates of *Klebsiella pneumoniae*. *Antimicrob. Agents Chemother.* **41**:699–701.

47. Deguchi, T., T. Kawamura, M. Yasuda, M. Nakano, H. Fukuda, H. Kato, N. Kato, Y. Okano, and Y. Kawada. 1997. In vivo selection of *Klebsiella pneumoniae* strains with enhanced quinolone resistance during fluoroquinolone treatment of urinary tract infections. *Antimicrob. Agents Chemother.* **41**:1609–1611.

48. Deguchi, T., M. Yasuda, M. Nakano, S. Ozeki, T. Ezaki, I. Saito, and Y. Kawada. 1996. Quinolone-resistant *Neisseria gonorrhoeae*: correlation of alterations in the GyrA subunit of DNA gyrase and the ParC subunit of topoisomerase IV with antimicrobial susceptibility profiles. *Antimicrob. Agents Chemother.* **40**:1020–1023.

49. Dessus-Babus, S., C. M. Bébéar, A. Charron, C. Bébéar, and B. de Barbeyrac. 1998. Sequencing of gyrase and topoisomerase IV quinolone-resistance-determining regions of *Chlamydia trachomatis* and characterization of quinolone-resistant mutants obtained in vitro. *Antimicrob. Agents Chemother.* **42**:2474–2481.

50. Discotto, L. F., L. E. Lawrence, K. L. Denbleyker, and J. F. Barrett. 2001. *Staphylococcus aureus* mutants selected by BMS-284756. *Antimicrob. Agents Chemother.* **45**:3273–3275.

51. Drlica, K., E. C. Engle, and S. H. Manes. 1980. DNA gyrase on the bacterial chromosome: possibility of two levels of action. *Proc. Natl. Acad. Sci. USA* **77**:6879–6883.

52. Edgar, R., and E. Bibi. 1997. MdfA, an *Escherichia coli* multidrug resistance protein with an extraordinarily broad spectrum of drug recognition. *J. Bacteriol.* **179**:2274–2280.

53. El Amin, N., S. Jalal, and B. Wretlind. 1999. Alterations in GyrA and ParC associated with fluoroquinolone resistance in *Enterococcus faecium*. *Antimicrob. Agents Chemother.* **43**:947–949.

54. Evans, K., K. Passador, R. Srikumar, E. Tsang, J. Nezezon, and K. Poole. 1998. Influence of the MexAB-OprM multidrug efflux system on quorum sensing in *Pseudomonas aeruginosa*. *J. Bacteriol.* **180**:5443–5447.

55. Ferrero, L., B. Cameron, and J. Crouzet. 1995. Analysis of *gyrA* and *grlA* mutations in stepwise-selected ciprofloxacin-resistant mutants of *Staphylococcus aureus*. *Antimicrob. Agents Chemother.* **39**:1554–1558.

56. Ferrero, L., B. Cameron, B. Manse, D. Lagneaux, J. Crouzet, A. Famechon, and F. Blanche. 1994. Cloning and primary structure of *Staphylococcus aureus* DNA topoisomerase IV: a primary target of fluoroquinolones. *Mol. Microbiol.* **13**:641–653.

57. Fitzgibbon, J. E., J. F. John, J. L. Delucia, and D. T. Dubin. 1998. Topoisomerase mutations in trovafloxacin-resistant *Staphylococcus aureus*. *Antimicrob. Agents Chemother.* **42**:2122–2124.

58. Fournier, B., R. Aras, and D. C. Hooper. 2000. Expression of the multidrug resistance transporter NorA from *Staphylococcus aureus* is modified by a two-component regulatory system. *J. Bacteriol.* **182**:664–671.

59. Fournier, B., and D. C. Hooper. 1998. Effects of mutations in GrlA of topoisomerase IV from *Staphylococcus aureus* on quinolone and coumarin activity. *Antimicrob. Agents Chemother.* **42**:2109–2112.

60. Fournier, B., and D. C. Hooper. 1998. Mutations in topoisomerase IV and DNA gyrase of *Staphylococcus aureus*: novel pleiotropic effects on quinolone and coumarin activity. *Antimicrob. Agents Chemother.* **42**:121–128.

61. Fournier, B., and D. C. Hooper. 2000. A new two-component regulatory system involved in adhesion autolysis, and extracellular proteolytic activity of *Staphylococcus aureus*. *J. Bacteriol.* **182**:3955–3964.

62. Fournier, B., Q. C. Truong-Bolduc, X. Zhang, and D. C. Hooper. 2001. A mutation in the 5′ untranslated region increases stability of *norA* mRNA, encoding a multidrug resistance transporter of *Staphylococcus aureus*. *J. Bacteriol.* **183**:2367–2371.

63. Fournier, B., X. Zhao, T. Lu, K. Drlica, and D. C. Hooper. 2000. Selective targeting of topoisomerase IV and DNA gyrase in *Staphylococcus aureus*: different patterns of quinolone-induced inhibition of DNA synthesis. *Antimicrob. Agents Chemother.* **44**:2160–2165.

64. Fralick, J. A. 1996. Evidence that TolC is required for functioning of the Mar/AcrAB efflux pump of *Escherichia coli*. *J. Bacteriol.* **178**:5803–5805.

65. Fraser, C. M., S. J. Norris, G. M. Weinstock, O. White, G. G. Sutton, R. Dodson, M. Gwinn, E. K. Hickey, R. Clayton, K. A. Ketchum, E. Sodergren, J. M. Hardham, M. P. McLeod, S. Salzberg, J. Peterson, H. Khalak, D. Richardson, J. K. Howell, M. Chidambaram, T. Utterback, L. McDonald, P. Artiach, C. Bowman, M. D. Cotton, and J. C. Venter. 1998. Complete genome sequence of *Treponema pallidum*, the syphilis spirochete. *Science* **281**:375–388.

66. Friedman, S. M., T. Lu, and K. Drlica. 2001. Mutation in the DNA gyrase A gene of *Escherichia coli* that expands the quinolone resistance-determining region. *Antimicrob. Agents Chemother.* **45**:2378–2380.

67. Fukuda, H., and K. Hiramatsu. 1999. Primary targets of fluoroquinolones in *Streptococcus pneumoniae*. *Antimicrob. Agents Chemother.* **43**:410–412.

68. Fukuda, H., M. Hosaka, S. Iyobe, N. Gotoh, T. Nishino, and K. Hirai. 1995. *nfxC*-type quinolone resistance in a clinical isolate of *Pseudomonas aeruginosa*. *Antimicrob. Agents Chemother.* **39**:790–792.

69. Fukuda, H., R. Kishii, M. Takei, and M. Hosaka. 2001. Contributions of the 8-methoxy group of gatifloxacin to resistance selectivity, target preference, and antibacterial activity against *Streptococcus pneumoniae*. *Antimicrob. Agents Chemother.* **45**:1649–1653.

70. Furukawa, H., J. T. Tsay, S. Jackowski, Y. Takamura, and C. O. Rock. 1993. Thiolactomycin resistance in *Escherichia coli* is associated with the multidrug resistance efflux pump encoded by *emrAB*. *J. Bacteriol.* **175**:3723–3729.

71. Gensberg, K., Y. F. Jin, and L. J. Piddock. 1995. A novel *gyrB* mutation in a fluoroquinolone-resistant clinical isolate of *Salmonella typhimurium*. *FEMS Microbiol. Lett.* **132**:57–60.

72. George, A. M., R. M. Hall, and H. W. Stokes. 1995. Multidrug resistance in *Klebsiella pneumoniae*: a novel gene, *ramA*, confers a multidrug resistance phenotype in *Escherichia coli*. *Microbiology* **141**:1909–1920.

73. George, A. M., and S. B. Levy. 1983. Amplifiable resistance to tetracycline, chloramphenicol, and other antibiotics in *Escherichia coli*: involvement of a non-plasmid-determined efflux of tetracycline. *J. Bacteriol.* **155**:531–540.

74. George, A. M., and S. B. Levy. 1983. Gene in the major cotransduction gap of the *Escherichia coli* K- 12 linkage map required for the expression of chromosomal resistance to tetracycline and other antibiotics. *J. Bacteriol.* **155**:541–548.

75. Georgiou, M., R. Muñoz, F. Román, R. Cantón, R. Gómez-Lus, J. Campos, and A. G. de la Campa. 1996. Ciprofloxacin-resistant *Haemophilus influenzae* strains possess mutations in analogous positions of GyrA and ParC. *Antimicrob. Agents Chemother.* **40**:1741–1744.

76. Gill, M. J., N. P. Brenwald, and R. Wise. 1999. Identification of an efflux pump gene, *pmrA*, associated with fluoroquinolone resistance in *Streptococcus pneumoniae*. *Antimicrob. Agents Chemother.* **43**:187–189.

77. Giraud, E., A. Cloeckaert, D. Kerboeuf, and E. Chaslus-Dancla. 2000. Evidence for active efflux as the primary mechanism of resistance to ciprofloxacin in *Salmonella enterica* serovar Typhimurium. *Antimicrob. Agents Chemother.* **44**:1223–1228.

78. González, I., M. Georgiou, F. Alcaide, D. Balas, and A. G. de la Campa. 1998. Fluoroquinolone resistance mutations in the *parC*, *parE*, and *gyrA* genes of clinical isolates of viridans group streptococci. *Antimicrob. Agents Chemother.* **42**:2792–2798.

79. Gootz, T. D., R. Zaniewski, S. Haskell, B. Schmieder, J. Tankovic, D. Girard, P. Courvalin, and R. J. Polzer. 1996. Activity of the new fluoroquinolone trovafloxacin (CP-99,219) against DNA gyrase and topoisomerase IV mutants of *Streptococcus pneumoniae* selected in vitro. *Antimicrob. Agents Chemother.* **40**:2691–2697.

80. Grinius, L. L., and E. B. Goldberg. 1994. Bacterial multidrug resistance is due to a single membrane protein which functions as a drug pump. *J. Biol. Chem.* **269**:29998–30004.

81. Gustafson, J. E., P. V. Candelaria, S. A. Fisher, J. P. Goodridge, T. M. Lichocik, T. M. McWilliams, C. T. Price, F. G. O'Brien, and W. B. Grubb. 1999. Growth in the presence of salicylate increases fluoroquinolone resistance in *Staphylococcus aureus*. *Antimicrob. Agents Chemother.* **43**:990–992.

82. Hagman, K. E., W. Pan, B. G. Spratt, J. T. Balthazar, R. C. Judd, and W. M. Shafer. 1995. Resistance of *Neisseria gonorrhoeae* to antimicrobial hydrophobic agents is modulated by the *mtrRCDE* efflux system. *Microbiology* **141**:611–622.

83. Heaton, V. J., J. E. Ambler, and L. M. Fisher. 2000. Potent antipneumococcal activity of gemifloxacin is associated with dual targeting of gyrase and topoisomerase IV, an in vivo target preference for gyrase, and enhanced stabilization of cleavable complexes in vitro. *Antimicrob. Agents Chemother.* **44**:3112–3117.

84. Heisig, P. 1996. Genetic evidence for a role of *parC* mutations in development of high-level fluoroquinolone resistance in *Escherichia coli*. *Antimicrob. Agents Chemother.* **40**:879–885.

85. Hiasa, H., D. O. Yousef, and K. J. Marians. 1996. DNA strand cleavage is required for replication fork arrest by a frozen topoisomerase-quinolone-DNA ternary complex. *J. Biol. Chem.* **271**:26424–26429.

86. Hirai, K., H. Aoyama, T. Irikura, S. Iyobe, and S. Mitsuhashi. 1986. Differences in susceptibility to quinolones of outer membrane mutants of *Salmonella typhimurium* and *Escherichia coli*. *Antimicrob. Agents Chemother.* **29**:535–538.

87. Hirai, K., S. Suzue, T. Irikura, S. Iyobe, and S. Mitsuhashi. 1987. Mutations producing resistance to norfloxacin in *Pseudomonas aeruginosa*. *Antimicrob. Agents Chemother.* **31**:582–586.

88. Hooper, D. C. 1998. Bacterial topoisomerases, anti-topoisomerases, and anti-topoisomerase resistance. *Clin. Infect. Dis.* **27**:S54–S63.

89. Hooper, D. C. 1999. Mechanisms of quinolone resistance. *Drug Resist. Updates* **2**:38–55.

90. Hooper, D. C., J. S. Wolfson, K. S. Souza, E. Y. Ng, G. L. McHugh, and M. N. Swartz. 1989. Mechanisms of quinolone resistance in *Escherichia coli*: characterization of *nfxB* and *cfxB*, two mutant resistance loci decreasing norfloxacin accumulation. *Antimicrob. Agents Chemother.* **33**:283–290.

91. Hori, S., Y. Ohshita, Y. Utsui, and K. Hiramatsu. 1993. Sequential acquisition of norfloxacin and ofloxacin resistance by methicillin-resistant and -susceptible *Staphylococcus aureus*. *Antimicrob. Agents Chemother.* **37**:2278–2284.

92. Hoshino, K., A. Kitamura, I. Morrissey, K. Sato, J. Kato, and H. Ikeda. 1994. Comparison of inhibition of *Escherichia coli* topoisomerase IV by quinolones with DNA gyrase inhibition. *Antimicrob. Agents Chemother.* **38**:2623–2627.

92a. Hsieh, P. C., S. A. Siegel, B. Rogers, D. Davis, and K. Lewis. 1998. Bacteria lacking a multidrug efflux pump: a sensitive tool for drug discovery. *Proc. Natl. Acad. Sci. USA* **95**:6602–6606.

93. Ince, D., R. Aras, and D. C. Hooper. 1999. Mechanisms and frequency of resistance to moxifloxacin in comparison with ciprofloxacin in *Staphylococcus aureus*. *Drugs* **58**:132–133.

94. Ince, D., and D. C. Hooper. 2000. Mechanisms and frequency of resistance to premafloxacin in *Staphylococcus aureus*: novel mutations suggest novel drug-target interactions. *Antimicrob. Agents Chemother.* **44**:3344–3350.

95. Ince, D., and D. C. Hooper. 2001. Mechanisms and frequency of resistance to gatifloxacin in comparison to AM-1121 and ciprofloxacin in *Staphylococcus aureus*. *Antimicrob. Agents Chemother.* **45**:2755–2764.

96. Ishida, H., H. Fuziwara, Y. Kaibori, T. Horiuchi, K. Sato, and Y. Osada. 1995. Cloning of multidrug resistance gene *pqrA* from *Proteus vulgaris*. *Antimicrob. Agents Chemother.* **39**:453–457.

97. Ito, H., H. Yoshida, M. Bogaki-Shonai, T. Niga, H. Hattori, and S. Nakamura. 1994. Quinolone resistance mutations in the DNA gyrase *gyrA* and *gyrB* genes of *Staphylococcus aureus*. *Antimicrob. Agents Chemother.* **38**:2014–2023.

98. Jalal, S., O. Ciofu, N. Hoiby, N. Gotoh, and B. Wretlind. 2000. Molecular mechanisms of fluoroquinolone resistance in *Pseudomonas aeruginosa* isolates from cystic fibrosis patients. *Antimicrob. Agents Chemother.* **44**:710–712.

99. Janoir, C., E. Varon, M. D. Kitzis, and L. Gutmann. 2001. New mutation in ParE in a pneumococcal in vitro mutant resistant to fluoroquinolones. *Antimicrob. Agents Chemother.* **45**:952–955.

100. Janoir, C., V. Zeller, M. D. Kitzis, N. J. Moreau, and L. Gutmann. 1996. High-level fluoroquinolone resistance in *Streptococcus pneumoniae* requires mutations in *parC* and *gyrA*. *Antimicrob. Agents Chemother.* **40**:2760–2764.

101. Kaatz, G. W., and S. M. Seo. 1995. Inducible NorA-mediated multidrug resistance in *Staphylococcus aureus*. *Antimicrob. Agents Chemother.* **39**:2650–2655.

102. Kanematsu, E., T. Deguchi, M. Yasuda, T. Kawamura, Y. Nishino, and Y. Kawada. 1998. Alterations in the GyrA subunit of DNA gyrase and the ParC subunit of DNA topoisomerase IV associated with quinolone resistance in *Enterococcus faecalis*. *Antimicrob. Agents Chemother.* **42**:433–435.

103. Kern, W. V., M. Oethinger, A. S. Jellen-Ritter, and S. B. Levy. 2000. Non-target gene mutations in the development of fluoroquinolone resistance in *Escherichia coli*. *Antimicrob. Agents Chemother.* **44**:814–820.

104. Khodursky, A. B., E. L. Zechiedrich, and N. R. Cozzarelli. 1995. Topoisomerase IV is a target of quinolones in *Escherichia coli. Proc. Natl. Acad. Sci. USA* **92**:11801–11805.

105. Kocagöz, T., C. J. Hackbarth, I. Ünsal, E. Y. Rosenberg, H. Nikaido, and H. F. Chambers. 1996. Gyrase mutations in laboratory-selected, fluoroquinolone- resistant mutants of *Mycobacterium tuberculosis* H37Ra. *Antimicrob. Agents Chemother.* **40**:1768–1774.

106. Köhler, T., M. Kok, M. Michea-Hamzehpour, P. Plesiat, N. Gotoh, T. Nishino, L. K. Curty, and J. C. Pechère. 1996. Multidrug efflux in intrinsic resistance to trimethoprim and sulfamethoxazole in *Pseudomonas aeruginosa. Antimicrob. Agents Chemother.* **40**:2288–2290.

107. Köhler, T., M. Michea-Hamzehpour, U. Henze, N. Gotoh, L. Curty, and J. C. Pechère. 1997. Characterization of MexE-MexF-OprN, a positively regulated multidrug efflux system of *Pseudomonas aeruginosa. Mol. Microbiol.* **23**:345–354.

108. Köhler, T., M. Michea-Hamzehpour, P. Plesiat, A. L. Kahr, and J. C. Pechère. 1997. Differential selection of multidrug efflux systems by quinolones in *Pseudomonas aeruginosa. Antimicrob. Agents Chemother.* **41**:2540–2543.

109. Köhler, T., C. Van Delden, L. K. Curty, M. M. Hamzehpour, and J. C. Pechere. 2001. Overexpression of the MexEF-OprN multidrug efflux system affects cell-to-cell signaling in *Pseudomonas aeruginosa. J. Bacteriol.* **183**:5213–5222.

110. Korten, V., W. M. Huang, and B. E. Murray. 1994. Analysis by PCR and direct DNA sequencing of *gyrA* mutations associated with fluoroquinolone resistance in *Enterococcus faecalis. Antimicrob. Agents Chemother.* **38**:2091–2094.

111. Koutsolioutsou, A., E. A. Martins, D. G. White, S. B. Levy, and B. Demple. 2001. A *soxRS*-constitutive mutation contributing to antibiotic resistance in a clinical isolate of *Salmonella enterica* (serovar Typhimurium). *Antimicrob. Agents Chemother.* **45**:38–43.

112. Lee, E. H., E. Collatz, I. Podglajen, and L. Gutmann. 1996. A *rob*-like gene of *Enterobacter cloacae* affecting porin synthesis and susceptibility to multiple antibiotics. *Antimicrob. Agents Chemother.* **40**:2029–2033.

113. Lewis, K., D. C. Hooper, and M. Ouellette. 1997. Multidrug resistance pumps provide broad defense. *ASM News* **63**:605–610.

114. Li, X. Z., D. M. Livermore, and H. Nikaido. 1994. Role of efflux pump(s) in intrinsic resistance of *Pseudomonas aeruginosa*: resistance to tetracycline, chloramphenicol, and norfloxacin. *Antimicrob. Agents Chemother.* **38**:1732–1741.

115. Li, X. Z., H. Nikaido, and K. Poole. 1995. Role of *mexA-mexB-oprM* in antibiotic efflux in *Pseudomonas aeruginosa. Antimicrob. Agents Chemother.* **39**:1948–1953.

116. Li, X. Z., L. Zhang, and K. Poole. 2000. Interplay between the MexA-MexB-OprM multidrug efflux system and the outer membrane barrier in the multiple antibiotic resistance of *Pseudomonas aeruginosa. J. Antimicrob. Chemother.* **45**:433–436.

117. Linde, H. J., F. Notka, M. Metz, B. Kochanowski, P. Heisig, and N. Lehn. 2000. In vivo increase in resistance to ciprofloxacin in *Escherichia coli* associated with deletion of the C-terminal part of MarR. *Antimicrob. Agents Chemother.* **44**:1865–1868.

118. Liu, J., H. E. Takiff, and H. Nikaido. 1996. Active efflux of fluoroquinolones in *Mycobacterium smegmatis* mediated by LfrA, a multidrug efflux pump. *J. Bacteriol.* **178**:3791–3795.

119. Lomovskaya, O., F. Kawai, and A. Matin. 1996. Differential regulation of the *mcb* and *emr* operons of *Escherichia coli*: role of *mcb* in multidrug resistance. *Antimicrob. Agents Chemother.* **40**:1050–1052.

120. Lomovskaya, O., A. Lee, K. Hoshino, H. Ishida, A. Mistry, M. S. Warren, E. Boyer, S. Chamberland, and V. J. Lee. 1999. Use of a genetic approach to evaluate the consequences of inhibition of efflux pumps in *Pseudomonas aeruginosa. Antimicrob. Agents Chemother.* **43**:1340–1346.

121. Lomovskaya, O., and K. Lewis. 1992. *emr*, an *Escherichia coli* locus for multidrug resistance. *Proc. Natl. Acad. Sci. USA* **89**:8938–8942.

122. Lomovskaya, O., K. Lewis, and A. Matin. 1995. EmrR is a negative regulator of the *Escherichia coli* multidrug resistance pump EmrAB. *J. Bacteriol.* **177**:2328–2334.

123. Lomovskaya, O., M. S. Warren, A. Lee, J. Galazzo, R. Fronko, M. Lee, J. Blais, D. Cho, S. Chamberland, T. Renau, R. Leger, S. Hecker, W. Watkins, K. Hoshino, H. Ishida, and V. J. Lee. 2001. Identification and characterization of inhibitors of multidrug resistance efflux pumps in *Pseudomonas aeruginosa*: novel agents for combination therapy. *Antimicrob. Agents Chemother.* **45**:105–116.

124. Mao, W. M., M. S. Warren, A. Lee, A. Mistry, and O. Lomovskaya. 2001. MexXY-OprM efflux pump is required for antagonism of aminoglycosides by divalent cations in *Pseudomonas aeruginosa. Antimicrob. Agents Chemother.* **45**:2001–2007.

125. Margolles, A., M. Putman, H. W. Van Veen, and W. N. Konings. 1999. The purified and functionally reconstituted multidrug transporter LmrA of *Lactococcus lactis* mediates the transbilayer movement of specific fluorescent phospholipids. *Biochemistry* **38**:16298–16306.

126. Markham, P. N. 1999. Inhibition of the emergence of ciprofloxacin resistance in *Streptococcus pneumoniae* by the multidrug efflux inhibitor reserpine. *Antimicrob. Agents Chemother.* **43**:988–989.

127. Markham, P. N., M. Ahmed, and A. A. Neyfakh. 1996. The drug-binding activity of the multidrug-responding transcriptional regulator BmrR resides in its C-terminal domain. *J. Bacteriol.* **178**:1473–1475.

128. Markham, P. N., and A. A. Neyfakh. 1996. Inhibition of the multidrug transporter NorA prevents emergence of norfloxacin resistance in *Staphylococcus aureus. Antimicrob. Agents Chemother.* **40**:2673–2674.

129. Martínez-Martínez, L., I. García, S. Ballesta, V. J. Benedí, S. Hernández-Allés, and A. Pascual. 1998. Energy-dependent accumulation of fluoroquinolones in quinolone-resistant *Klebsiella pneumoniae* strains. *Antimicrob. Agents Chemother.* **42**:1850–1852.

130. Martínez-Martínez, L., A. Pascual, and G. A. Jacoby. 1998. Quinolone resistance from a transferable plasmid. *Lancet* **351**:797–799.

131. Maseda, H., K. Saito, A. Nakajima, and T. Nakae. 2000. Variation of the *mexT* gene, a regulator of the MexEF-OprN efflux pump expression in wild-type strains of *Pseudomonas aeruginosa. FEMS Microbiol. Lett.* **192**:107–112.

132. Maseda, H., H. Yoneyama, and T. Nakae. 2000. Assignment of the substrate-selective subunits of the MexEF-OprN multidrug efflux pump of *Pseudomonas aeruginosa. Antimicrob. Agents Chemother.* **44**:658–664.

133. Masuda, N., and S. Ohya. 1992. Cross-resistance to meropenem, cephems, and quinolones in *Pseudomonas aeruginosa. Antimicrob. Agents Chemother.* **36**:1847–1851.

134. Masuda, N., E. Sakagawa, S. Ohya, N. Gotoh, and T. Nishino. 2001. Hypersusceptibility of the *Pseudomonas aeruginosa* nfxB mutant to β-lactams due to reduced expression of the AmpC β-lactamase. *Antimicrob. Agents Chemother.* **45**:1284–1286.

135. Masuda, N., E. Sakagawa, S. Ohya, N. Gotoh, H. Tsujimoto, and T. Nishino. 2000. Contribution of the

MexX-MexY-OprM efflux system to intrinsic resistance in *Pseudomonas aeruginosa. Antimicrob. Agents Chemother.* **44:**2242–2246.

136. **Masuda, N., E. Sakagawa, S. Ohya, N. Gotoh, H. Tsujimoto, and T. Nishino.** 2000. Substrate specificities of MexAB-OprM, MexCD-OprJ, and MexXY-OprM efflux pumps in *Pseudomonas aeruginosa. Antimicrob. Agents Chemother.* **44:**3322–3327.

137. **Mazzariol, A., Y. Tokue, T. M. Kanegawa, G. Cornaglia, and H. Nikaido.** 2000. High-level fluoroquinolone-resistant clinical isolates of *Escherichia coli* overproduce multidrug efflux protein AcrA. *Antimicrob. Agents Chemother.* **44:** 3441–3443.

138. **Miller, P. F., L. Gambino, M. C. Sulavik, and S. J. Gracheck.** 1994. Genetic relationship between *soxRS* and *mar* loci in promoting multiple antibiotic resistance in *Escherichia coli. Antimicrob. Agents Chemother.* **38:**1773–1779.

139. **Mine, T., Y. Morita, A. Kataoka, T. Mizushima, and T. Tsuchiya.** 1999. Expression in *Escherichia coli* of a new multidrug efflux pump, MexXY, from *Pseudomonas aeruginosa. Antimicrob. Agents Chemother.* **43:**415–417.

140. **Miyamae, S., H. Nikaido, Y. Tanaka, and F. Yoshimura.** 1998. Active efflux of norfloxacin by *Bacteroides fragilis. Antimicrob. Agents Chemother.* **42:**2119–2121.

141. **Miyamae, S., O. Ueda, F. Yoshimura, J. Hwang, Y. Tanaka, and H. Nikaido.** 2001. A MATE family multidrug efflux transporter pumps out fluoroquinolones in *Bacteroides thetaiotaomicron. Antimicrob. Agents Chemother.* **45:** 3341–3346.

142. **Moore, R. A., B. Beckthold, S. Wong, A. Kureishi, and L. E. Bryan.** 1995. Nucleotide sequence of the *gyrA* gene and characterization of ciprofloxacin-resistant mutants of *Helicobacter pylori. Antimicrob. Agents Chemother.* **39:**107–111.

143. **Morita, Y., K. Kodama, S. Shiota, T. Mine, A. Kataoka, T. Mizushima, and T. Tsuchiya.** 1998. NorM, a putative multidrug efflux protein, of *Vibrio parahaemolyticus* and its homolog in *Escherichia coli. Antimicrob. Agents Chemother.* **42:**1778–1782.

144. **Morrissey, I., and J. T. George.** 2000. Purification of pneumococcal type II topoisomerases and inhibition by gemifloxacin and other quinolones. *J. Antimicrob. Chemother.* **45:**101–106.

145. **Munoz, R., and A. G. de la Campa.** 1996. ParC subunit of DNA topoisomerase IV of *Streptococcus pneumoniae* is a primary target of fluoroquinolones and cooperates with DNA gyrase A subunit in forming resistance phenotype. *Antimicrob. Agents Chemother.* **40:**2252–2257.

146. **Muñoz-Bellido, J. L., M. A. Manzanares, J. A. Andrés, M. N. Zufiaurre, G. Ortiz, M. S. Hernández, and J. A. García-Rodríguez.** 1999. Efflux pump-mediated quinolone resistance in *Staphylococcus aureus* strains wild type for *gyrA, gyrB, grlA,* and *norA. Antimicrob. Agents Chemother.* **43:**354–356.

147. **Nagai, K., T. A. Davies, B. E. Dewasse, M. R. Jacobs, and P. C. Appelbaum.** 2001. Single- and multi-step resistance selection study of gemifloxacin compared with trovafloxacin, ciprofloxacin, gatifloxacin and moxifloxacin in *Streptococcus pneumoniae. J. Antimicrob. Chemother.* **48:**365–374.

148. **Nagai, K., T. A. Davies, G. A. Pankuch, B. E. Dewasse, M. R. Jacobs, and P. C. Appelbaum.** 2000. In vitro selection of resistance to clinafloxacin, ciprofloxacin, and trovafloxacin in *Streptococcus pneumoniae. Antimicrob. Agents Chemother.* **44:**2740–2746.

149. **Nakanishi, N., S. Yoshida, H. Wakebe, M. Inoue, and S. Mitsuhashi.** 1991. Mechanisms of clinical resistance to fluoroquinolones in *Enterococcus faecalis. Antimicrob. Agents Chemother.* **35:**1053–1059.

150. **Nakano, M., T. Deguchi, T. Kawamura, M. Yasuda, M. Kimura, Y. Okano, and Y. Kawada.** 1997. Mutations in *gyrA* and *parC* genes in fluoroquinolone-resistant clinical isolates of *Pseudomonas aeruginosa. Antimicrob. Agents Chemother.* **41:**2289–2291.

151. **Neyfakh, A. A.** 1992. The multidrug efflux transporter of *Bacillus subtilis* is a structural and functional homolog of the *Staphylococcus* NorA protein. *Antimicrob. Agents Chemother.* **36:**484–485.

152. **Neyfakh, A. A., C. M. Borsch, and G. W. Kaatz.** 1993. Fluoroquinolone resistance protein NorA of *Staphylococcus aureus* is a multidrug efflux transporter. *Antimicrob. Agents Chemother.* **37:**128–129.

153. **Ng, E. Y., M. Trucksis, and D. C. Hooper.** 1994. Quinolone resistance mediated by *norA*: physiologic characterization and relationship to *flqB*, a quinolone resistance locus on the *Staphylococcus aureus* chromosome. *Antimicrob. Agents Chemother.* **38:**1345–1355.

154. **Ng, E. Y., M. Trucksis, and D. C. Hooper.** 1996. Quinolone resistance mutations in topoisomerase IV: relationship of the *flqA* locus and genetic evidence that topoisomerase IV is the primary target and DNA gyrase the secondary target of fluoroquinolones in *Staphylococcus aureus. Antimicrob. Agents Chemother.* **40:**1881–1888.

155. **Nikaido, H., and D. G. Thanassi.** 1993. Penetration of lipophilic agents with multiple protonation sites into bacterial cells: tetracyclines and fluoroquinolones as examples. *Antimicrob. Agents Chemother.* **37:**1393–1399.

156. **Nishino, Y., T. Deguchi, M. Yasuda, T. Kawamura, M. Nakano, E. Kanematsu, S. Ozeki, and Y. Kawada.** 1997. Mutations in the *gyrA* and *parC* genes associated with fluoroquinolone resistance in clinical isolates of *Citrobacter freundii. FEMS Microbiol. Lett.* **154:**409–414.

157. **Oethinger, M., W. V. Kern, A. S. Jellen-Ritter, L. M. McMurry, and S. B. Levy.** 2000. Ineffectiveness of topoisomerase mutations in mediating clinically significant fluoroquinolone resistance in *Escherichia coli* in the absence of the AcrAB efflux pump. *Antimicrob. Agents Chemother.* **44:**10–13.

158. **Oethinger, M., I. Podglajen, W. V. Kern, and S. B. Levy.** 1998. Overexpression of the *marA* or *soxS* regulatory gene in clinical topoisomerase mutants of *Escherichia coli. Antimicrob. Agents Chemother.* **42:**2089–2094.

159. **Ohki, R., and M. Murata.** 1997. *bmr3*, a third multidrug transporter gene of *Bacillus subtilis. J. Bacteriol.* **179:**1423–1427.

160. **Ohshita, Y., K. Hiramatsu, and T. Yokota.** 1990. A point mutation in *norA* gene is responsible for quinolone resistance in *Staphylococcus aureus. Biochem. Biophys. Res. Commun.* **172:**1028–1034.

161. **Okazaki, T., and K. Hirai.** 1992. Cloning and nucleotide sequence of the *Pseudomonas aeruginosa nfxB* gene, conferring resistance to new quinolones. *FEMS Microbiol. Lett.* **76:**197–202.

162. **Okuda, J., E. Hayakawa, M. Nishibuchi, and T. Nishino.** 1999. Sequence analysis of the *gyrA* and *parC* homologues of a wild-type strain of *Vibrio parahaemolyticus* and its fluoroquinolone-resistant mutants. *Antimicrob. Agents Chemother.* **43:**1156–1162.

163. **Okusu, H., D. Ma, and H. Nikaido.** 1996. AcrAB efflux pump plays a major role in the antibiotic resistance phenotype of *Escherichia coli* multiple-antibiotic-resistance (Mar) mutants. *J. Bacteriol.* **178:**306–308.

164. **Onodera, Y., and K. Sato.** 1999. Molecular cloning of the *gyrA* and *gyrB* genes of *Bacteroides fragilis* encoding DNA gyrase. *Antimicrob. Agents Chemother.* **43:**2423–2429.

165. **Pan, X. S., J. Ambler, S. Mehtar, and L. M. Fisher.** 1996. Involvement of topoisomerase IV and DNA gyrase as

ciprofloxacin targets in *Streptococcus pneumoniae*. *Antimicrob. Agents Chemother.* **40**:2321–2326.

166. **Pan, X. S., and L. M. Fisher.** 1996. Cloning and characterization of the *parC* and *parE* genes of *Streptococcus pneumoniae* encoding DNA topoisomerase IV: role in fluoroquinolone resistance. *J. Bacteriol.* **178**:4060–4069.

167. **Pan, X. S., and L. M. Fisher.** 1997. Targeting of DNA gyrase in *Streptococcus pneumoniae* by sparfloxacin: selective targeting of gyrase or topoisomerase IV by quinolones. *Antimicrob. Agents Chemother.* **41**:471–474.

168. **Pan, X. S., and L. M. Fisher.** 1998. DNA gyrase and topoisomerase IV are dual targets of clinafloxacin action in *Streptococcus pneumoniae*. *Antimicrob. Agents Chemother.* **42**:2810–2816.

169. **Pan, X. S., G. Yague, and L. M. Fisher.** 2001. Quinolone resistance mutations in *Streptococcus pneumoniae* GyrA and ParC proteins: mechanistic insights into quinolone action from enzymatic analysis, intracellular levels, and phenotypes of wild-type and mutant proteins. *Antimicrob. Agents Chemother.* **45**:3140–3147.

170. **Paulsen, I. T., M. H. Brown, T. G. Littlejohn, B. A. Mitchell, and R. A. Skurray.** 1996. Multidrug resistance proteins QacA and QacB from *Staphylococcus aureus*: membrane topology and identification of residues involved in substrate specificity. *Proc. Natl. Acad. Sci. USA* **93**: 3630–3635.

171. **Paulsen, I. T., M. H. Brown, and R. A. Skurray.** 1996. Proton-dependent multidrug efflux systems. *Microbiol. Rev.* **60**:575–608.

172. **Pearson, J. P., C. Van Delden, and B. H. Iglewski.** 1999. Active efflux and diffusion are involved in transport of *Pseudomonas aeruginosa* cell-to-cell signals. *J. Bacteriol.* **181**:1203–1210.

173. **Perichon, B., J. Tankovic, and P. Courvalin.** 1997. Characterization of a mutation in the *parE* gene that confers fluoroquinolone resistance in *Streptococcus pneumoniae*. *Antimicrob. Agents Chemother.* **41**:1166–1167.

174. **Pesci, E. C., J. B. Milbank, J. P. Pearson, S. McKnight, A. S. Kende, E. P. Greenberg, and B. H. Iglewski.** 1999. Quinolone signaling in the cell-to-cell communication system of *Pseudomonas aeruginosa*. *Proc. Natl. Acad. Sci. USA* **96**:11229–11234.

175. **Pestova, E., R. Beyer, N. P. Cianciotto, G. A. Noskin, and L. R. Peterson.** 1999. Contribution of topoisomerase IV and DNA gyrase mutations in *Streptococcus pneumoniae* to resistance to novel fluoroquinolones. *Antimicrob. Agents Chemother.* **43**:2000–2004.

176. **Piddock, L. J., and R. Wise.** 1986. The effect of altered porin expression in *Escherichia coli* upon susceptibility to 4-quinolones. *J. Antimicrob. Chemother.* **18**:547–549.

177. **Piddock, L. J. V., D. G. White, K. Gensberg, L. Pumbwe, and D. J. Griggs.** 2000. Evidence for an efflux pump mediating multiple antibiotic resistance in *Salmonella enterica* serovar Typhimurium. *Antimicrob. Agents Chemother.* **44**:3118–3121.

178. **Poole, K.** 1994. Bacterial multidrug resistance—emphasis on efflux mechanisms and *Pseudomonas aeruginosa*. *J. Antimicrob. Chemother.* **34**:453–456.

179. **Poole, K.** 2000. Efflux-mediated resistance to fluoroquinolones in gram-negative bacteria. *Antimicrob. Agents Chemother.* **44**:2233–2241.

180. **Poole, K.** 2000. Efflux-mediated resistance to fluoroquinolones in gram-positive bacteria and the mycobacteria. *Antimicrob. Agents Chemother.* **44**:2595–2599.

181. **Poole, K., N. Gotoh, H. Tsujimoto, Q. X. Zhao, A. Wada, T. Yamasaki, S. Neshat, J. I. Yamagishi, X. Z. Li, and T.** Nishino. 1996. Overexpression of the *mexC-mexD-oprJ* efflux operon in *nfxB*-type multidrug-resistant strains of *Pseudomonas aeruginosa*. *Mol. Microbiol.* **21**:713–724.

182. **Poole, K., K. Krebes, C. McNally, and S. Neshat.** 1993. Multiple antibiotic resistance in *Pseudomonas aeruginosa*: evidence for involvement of an efflux operon. *J. Bacteriol.* **175**:7363–7372.

183. **Poole, K., K. Tetro, Q. X. Zhao, S. Neshat, D. E. Heinrichs, and N. Bianco.** 1996. Expression of the multidrug resistance operon *mexA-mexB-oprM* in *Pseudomonas aeruginosa*: *mexR* encodes a regulator of operon expression. *Antimicrob. Agents Chemother.* **40**:2021–2028.

184. **Pumbwe, L., and L. J. V. Piddock.** 2000. Two efflux systems expressed simultaneously in multidrug-resistant *Pseudomonas aeruginosa*. *Antimicrob. Agents Chemother.* **44**:2861–2864.

185. **Putman, M., L. A. Koole, H. W. Van Veen, and W. N. Konings.** 1999. The secondary multidrug transporter LmrP contains multiple drug interaction sites. *Biochemistry* **38**:13900–13905.

186. **Putman, M., H. W. Van Veen, J. E. Degener, and W. N. Konings.** 2001. The lactococcal secondary multidrug transporter LmrP confers resistance to lincosamides, macrolides, streptogramins and tetracyclines. *Microbiology* **147**:2873–2880.

187. **Putman, M., H. W. Van Veen, and W. N. Konings.** 2000. Molecular properties of bacterial multidrug transporters. *Microbiol. Mol. Biol. Rev.* **64**:672–693.

188. **Rahman, M., G. Mauff, J. Levy, M. Couturier, G. Pulverer, N. Glasdorff, and J. P. Butzler.** 1994. Detection of 4-quinolone resistance mutation in *gyrA* gene of *Shigella dysenteriae* type 1 by PCR. *Antimicrob. Agents Chemother.* **38**:2488–2491.

189. **Rella, M., and D. Haas.** 1982. Resistance of *Pseudomonas aeruginosa* PAO to nalidixic acid and low levels of beta-lactam antibiotics: mapping of chromosomal genes. *Antimicrob. Agents Chemother.* **22**:242–249.

190. **Renau, T. E., R. Léger, E. M. Flamme, J. Sangalang, M. W. She, R. Yen, C. L. Gannon, D. Griffith, S. Chamberland, O. Lomovskaya, S. J. Hecker, V. J. Lee, T. Ohta, and K. Nakayama.** 1999. Inhibitors of efflux pumps in *Pseudomonas aeruginosa* potentiate the activity of the fluoroquinolone antibacterial levofloxacin. *J. Med. Chem.* **42**:4928–4931.

191. **Revel, V., E. Cambau, V. Jarlier, and W. Sougakoff.** 1994. Characterization of mutations in *Mycobacterium smegmatis* involved in resistance to fluoroquinolones. *Antimicrob. Agents Chemother.* **38**:1991–1996.

192. **Reyna, F., M. Huesca, V. Gonzalez, and L. Y. Fuchs.** 1995. *Salmonella typhimurium gyrA* mutations associated with fluoroquinolone resistance. *Antimicrob. Agents Chemother.* **39**:1621–1623.

193. **Robillard, N. J., and A. L. Scarpa.** 1988. Genetic and physiological characterization of ciprofloxacin resistance in *Pseudomonas aeruginosa* PAO. *Antimicrob. Agents Chemother.* **32**:535–539.

194. **Roychoudhury, S., C. E. Catrenich, E. J. McIntosh, H. D. McKeever, K. M. Makin, P. M. Koenigs, and B. Ledoussal.** 2001. Quinolone resistance in staphylococci: activities of new nonfluorinated quinolones against molecular targets in whole cells and clinical isolates. *Antimicrob. Agents Chemother.* **45**:1115–1120.

195. **Sabourin, M., J. A. Byl, S. E. Hannah, J. L. Nitiss, and N. Osheroff.** 1998. A mutant yeast topoisomerase II (top2G437S) with differential sensitivity to anticancer drugs in the presence and absence of ATP. *J. Biol. Chem.* **273**:29086–29092.

196. **San, M. J., C. Hernandez-Chico, P. Pereda, and F. Moreno.** 1985. Cloning and mapping of the genetic determinants for

microcin B17 production and immunity. *J. Bacteriol.* **163:**275–281.

197. **Sander, P., E. De Rossi, B. Böddinghaus, R. Cantoni, M. Branzoni, E. C. Böttger, H. Takiff, R. Rodriguez, G. Lopez, and G. Riccardi.** 2000. Contribution of the multidrug efflux pump LfrA to innate mycobacterial drug resistance. *FEMS Microbiol. Lett.* **193:**19–23.

198. **Schlor, S., A. Schmidt, E. Maier, R. Benz, W. Goebel, and I. Gentschev.** 1997. In vivo and in vitro studies on interactions between the components of the hemolysin (HlyA) secretion machinery of *Escherichia coli. Mol. Gen. Genet.* **256:**306–319.

199. **Schmitz, F. J., A. C. Fluit, M. Lückefahr, B. Engler, B. Hofmann, J. Verhoef, H. P. Heinz, U. Hadding, and M. E. Jones.** 1998. The effect of reserpine, an inhibitor of multidrug efflux pumps, on the in-vitro activities of ciprofloxacin, sparfloxacin and moxifloxacin against clinical isolates of *Staphylococcus aureus. J. Antimicrob. Chemother.* **42:**807–810.

200. **Schmitz, F. J., B. Hertel, S. Scheuring, J. Verhoef, and A. C. Fluit.** 1998. Correlation of norfloxacin MIC-values with mutations with the coding and promoter region of the *norA* gene in 42 unrelated clinical isolates of *Staphylococcus aureus. J. Antimicrob. Chemother.* **42:**561–563.

201. **Schmitz, F. J., B. Hofmann, B. Hansen, S. Scheuring, M. Lückefahr, M. Klootwijk, J. Verhoef, A. Fluit, H. P. Heinz, K. Köhrer, and M. E. Jones.** 1998. Relationship between ciprofloxacin, ofloxacin, levofloxacin, sparfloxacin and moxifloxacin (BAY 12-8039) MICs and mutations in *grlA, grlB, gyrA* and *gyrB* in 116 unrelated clinical isolates of *Staphylococcus aureus. J. Antimicrob. Chemother.* **41:**481–484.

202. **Schmitz, F. J., M. E. Jones, B. Hofmann, B. Hansen, S. Scheuring, M. F. A. Lückefahr, J. Verhoef, U. Hadding, H. P. Heinz, and K. Köhrer.** 1998. Characterization of *grlA, grlB, gyrA,* and *gyrB* mutations in 116 unrelated isolates of *Staphylococcus aureus* and effects of mutations on ciprofloxacin MIC. *Antimicrob. Agents Chemother.* **42:**1249–1252.

203. **Shen, L. L., W. E. Kohlbrenner, D. Weigl, and J. Baranowski.** 1989. Mechanism of quinolone inhibition of DNA gyrase. Appearance of unique norfloxacin binding sites in enzyme-DNA complexes. *J. Biol. Chem.* **264:**2973–2978.

204. **Shultz, T. R., J. W. Tapsall, and P. A. White.** 2001. Correlation of in vitro susceptibilities to newer quinolones of naturally occurring quinolone-resistant *Neisseria gonorrhoeae* strains with changes in GyrA and ParC. *Antimicrob. Agents Chemother.* **45:**734–738.

205. **Sreedharan, S., M. Oram, B. Jensen, L. R. Peterson, and L. M. Fisher.** 1990. DNA gyrase *gyrA* mutations in ciprofloxacin-resistant strains of *Staphylococcus aureus:* close similarity with quinolone resistance mutations in *Escherichia coli. J. Bacteriol.* **172:**7260–7262.

206. **Srikumar, R., X. Z. Li, and K. Poole.** 1997. Inner membrane efflux components are responsible for β-lactam specificity of multidrug efflux pumps in *Pseudomonas aeruginosa. J. Bacteriol.* **179:**7875–7881.

207. **Sulavik, M. C., M. Dazer, and P. F. Miller.** 1997. The *Salmonella typhimurium mar* locus: molecular and genetic analyses and assessment of the requirement for virulence. *J. Bacteriol.* **179:**1857–1866.

208. **Sulavik, M. C., C. Houseweart, C. Cramer, N. Jiwani, N. Murgolo, J. Greene, B. DiDomenico, K. J. Shaw, G. H. Miller, R. Hare, and G. Shimer.** 2001. Antibiotic susceptibility profiles of *Escherichia coli* strains lacking multidrug efflux pump genes. *Antimicrob. Agents Chemother.* **45:**1126–1136.

209. **Sun, L., S. Sreedharan, K. Plummer, and L. M. Fisher.** 1996. NorA plasmid resistance to fluoroquinolones: role of copy number and *norA* frameshift mutations. *Antimicrob. Agents Chemother.* **40:**1665–1669.

210. **Takahata, M., M. Yonezawa, S. Kurose, N. Futakuchi, N. Matsubara, Y. Watanabe, and H. Narita.** 1996. Mutations in the *gyrA* and *grlA* genes of quinolone-resistant clinical isolates of methicillin-resistant *Staphylococcus aureus. J. Antimicrob. Chemother.* **38:**543–546.

211. **Takei, M., H. Fukuda, R. Kishii, and M. Hosaka.** 2001. Target preference of 15 quinolones against *Staphylococcus aureus,* based on antibacterial activities and target inhibition. *Antimicrob. Agents Chemother.* **45:**3544–3547.

212. **Takenouchi, T., C. Ishii, M. Sugawara, Y. Tokue, and S. Ohya.** 1995. Incidence of various *gyrA* mutants in 451 *Staphylococcus aureus* strains isolated in Japan and their susceptibilities to 10 fluoroquinolones. *Antimicrob. Agents Chemother.* **39:**1414–1418.

213. **Takiff, H. E., M. Cimino, M. C. Musso, T. Weisbrod, R. Martinez, M. B. Delgado, L. Salazar, B. R. Bloom, and W. R. Jacobs, Jr.** 1996. Efflux pump of the proton antiporter family confers low-level fluoroquinolone resistance in *Mycobacterium smegmatis. Proc. Natl. Acad. Sci. USA* **93:**362–366.

214. **Takiff, H. E., L. Salazar, C. Guerrero, W. Philipp, W. M. Huang, B. Kreiswirth, S. T. Cole, W. R. Jacobs, Jr., and A. Telenti.** 1994. Cloning and nucleotide sequence of *Mycobacterium tuberculosis gyrA* and *gyrB* genes and detection of quinolone resistance mutations. *Antimicrob. Agents Chemother.* **38:**773–780.

215. **Tanaka, M., Y. Onodera, Y. Uchida, and K. Sato.** 1998. Quinolone resistance mutations in the GrlB protein of *Staphylococcus aureus. Antimicrob. Agents Chemother.* **42:**3044–3046.

216. **Tanaka, M., Y. Onodera, Y. Uchida, K. Sato, and I. Hayakawa.** 1997. Inhibitory activities of quinolones against DNA gyrase and topoisomerase IV purified from *Staphylococcus aureus. Antimicrob. Agents Chemother.* **41:**2362–2366.

217. **Tanaka, T., T. Horii, K. Shibayama, K. Sato, S. Ohsuka, Y. Arakawa, K. Yamaki, K. Takagi, and M. Ohta.** 1997. RobA-induced multiple antibiotic resistance largely depends on the activation of the AcrAB efflux. *Microbiol. Immunol.* **41:**697–702.

218. **Tankovic, J., F. Mahjoubi, P. Courvalin, J. Duval, and R. Leclercq.** 1996. Development of fluoroquinolone resistance in *Enterococcus faecalis* and role of mutations in the DNA gyrase *gyrA* gene. *Antimicrob. Agents Chemother.* **40:**2558–2561.

219. **Tankovic, J., B. Perichon, J. Duval, and P. Courvalin.** 1996. Contribution of mutations in *gyrA* and *parC* genes to fluoroquinolone resistance of mutants of *Streptococcus pneumoniae* obtained in vivo and in vitro. *Antimicrob. Agents Chemother.* **40:**2505–2510.

220. **Tavío, M. D., J. Vila, J. Ruiz, G. Amicosante, N. Franceschini, A. M. Martín-Sánchez, and M. T. J. De Anta.** 2000. *In vitro* selected fluoroquinolone-resistant mutants of *Citrobacter freundii:* analysis of the quinolone resistance acquisition. *J. Antimicrob. Chemother.* **45:**521–524.

221. **Taylor, D. E., and A. S. S. Chau.** 1997. Cloning and nucleotide sequence of the *gyrA* gene from *Campylobacter fetus* subsp *fetus* ATCC 27374 and characterization of ciprofloxacin-resistant laboratory and clinical isolates. *Antimicrob. Agents Chemother.* **41:**665–671.

221a. **Tran, J. H., and G. A. Jacoby.** 2002. Mechanism of plasmid-mediated quinolone resistance. *Proc. Natl. Acad. Sci. USA* **99:**5638–5642.

222. Trees, D. L., A. L. Sandul, W. L. Whittington, and J. S. Knapp. 1998. Identification of novel mutation patterns in the *parC* gene of ciprofloxacin-resistant isolates of *Neisseria gonorrhoeae*. *Antimicrob. Agents Chemother.* **42:**2103–2105.

222a. Truong-Bolduc, Q. C., X. Zhang, and D. C. Hooper. 2003. Characterization of NorR protein, a multifunctional regulator of *norA* expression in *Staphylococcus aureus*. *J. Bacteriol.* **185:**3127–3138.

223. Van Veen, H. W., K. Venema, H. Bolhuis, I. Oussenko, J. Kok, B. Poolman, A. J. M. Driessen, and W. N. Konings. 1996. Multidrug resistance mediated by a bacterial homolog of the human multidrug transporter MDR1. *Proc. Natl. Acad. Sci. USA* **93:**10668–10672.

224. Varon, E., C. Janoir, M. D. Kitzis, and L. Gutmann. 1999. ParC and GyrA may be interchangeable initial targets of some fluoroquinolones in *Streptococcus pneumoniae*. *Antimicrob. Agents Chemother.* **43:**302–306.

225. Vila, J., J. Ruiz, P. Goni, and M. T. Jimenez de Anta. 1996. Detection of mutations in *parC* in quinolone-resistant clinical isolates of *Escherichia coli*. *Antimicrob. Agents Chemother.* **40:**491–493.

226. Wandersman, C., and P. Delepelaire. 1990. TolC, an *Escherichia coli* outer membrane protein required for hemolysin secretion. *Proc. Natl. Acad. Sci. USA* **87:**4776–4780.

226a. Wang, M., J. H. Tran, G. A. Jacoby, Y. Zhang, F. Wang, and D. C. Hooper. Plasmid-mediated quinolone resistance in clinical isolates of *Escherichia coli* from Shanghai. *Antimicrob. Agents Chemother.*, in press.

227. Wang, T., M. Tanaka, and K. Sato. 1998. Detection of *grlA* and *gyrA* mutations in 344 *Staphylococcus aureus* strains. *Antimicrob. Agents Chemother.* **42:**236–240.

228. Wang, Y., W. M. Huang, and D. E. Taylor. 1993. Cloning and nucleotide sequence of the *Campylobacter jejuni gyrA* gene and characterization of quinolone resistance mutations. *Antimicrob. Agents Chemother.* **37:**457–463.

229. Wasserman, R. A., and J. C. Wang. 1994. Mechanistic studies of amsacrine-resistant derivatives of DNA topoisomerase II. Implications in resistance to multiple antitumor drugs targeting the enzyme. *J. Biol. Chem.* **269:**20943–20951.

230. Weigel, L. M., G. J. Anderson, R. R. Facklam, and F. Tenover. 2001. Genetic analyses of mutations contributing to fluoroquinolone resistance in clinical isolates of *Streptococcus pneumoniae*. *Antimicrob. Agents Chemother.* **45:**3517–3523.

231. Wetzstein, H. G., N. Schmeer, and W. Karl. 1997. Degradation of the fluoroquinolone enrofloxacin by the brown rot fungus *Gloeophyllum striatum*: identification of metabolites. *Appl. Environ. Microbiol.* **63:**4272–4281.

232. Wetzstein, H. G., M. Stadler, H. V. Tichy, A. Dalhoff, and W. Karl. 1999. Degradation of ciprofloxacin by basidiomycetes and identification of metabolites generated by the brown rot fungus *Gloeophyllum striatum*. *Appl. Environ. Microbiol.* **65:**1556–1563.

233. Willmott, C. J., S. E. Critchlow, I. C. Eperon, and A. Maxwell. 1994. The complex of DNA gyrase and quinolone drugs with DNA forms a barrier to transcription by RNA polymerase. *J. Mol. Biol.* **242:**351–363.

234. Willmott, C. J., and A. Maxwell. 1993. A single point mutation in the DNA gyrase A protein greatly reduces binding of fluoroquinolones to the gyrase-DNA complex. *Antimicrob. Agents Chemother.* **37:**126–127.

235. Woolridge, D. P., N. Vazquez-Laslop, P. N. Markham, M. S. Chevalier, E. W. Gerner, and A. A. Neyfakh. 1997. Efflux of the natural polyamine spermidine facilitated by the *Bacillus subtilis* multidrug transporter Blt. *J. Biol. Chem.* **272:**8864–8866.

236. Xiong, A., A. Gottman, C. Park, M. Baetens, S. Pandza, and A. Matin. 2000. The EmrR protein represses the *Escherichia coli emrRAB* multidrug resistance operon by directly binding to its promoter region. *Antimicrob. Agents Chemother.* **44:**2905–2907.

237. Yamagishi, J. I., T. Kojima, Y. Oyamada, K. Fujimoto, H. Hattori, S. Nakamura, and M. Inoue. 1996. Alterations in the DNA topoisomerase IV *grlA* gene responsible for quinolone resistance in *Staphylococcus aureus*. *Antimicrob. Agents Chemother.* **40:**1157–1163.

238. Yoneyama, H., A. Ocaktan, N. Gotoh, T. Nishino, and T. Nakae. 1998. Subunit swapping in the Mex-extrusion pumps in *Pseudomonas aeruginosa*. *Biochem. Biophys. Res. Commun.* **244:**898–902.

239. Yoshida, H., M. Bogaki, M. Nakamura, and S. Nakamura. 1990. Quinolone resistance-determining region in the DNA gyrase *gyrA* gene of *Escherichia coli*. *Antimicrob. Agents Chemother.* **34:**1271–1272.

240. Yoshida, H., M. Bogaki, M. Nakamura, L. M. Yamanaka, and S. Nakamura. 1991. Quinolone resistance-determining region in the DNA gyrase *gyrB* gene of *Escherichia coli*. *Antimicrob. Agents Chemother.* **35:**1647–1650.

241. Yoshida, H., M. Bogaki, S. Nakamura, K. Ubukata, and M. Konno. 1990. Nucleotide sequence and characterization of the *Staphylococcus aureus norA* gene, which confers resistance to quinolones. *J. Bacteriol.* **172:**6942–6949.

242. Yoshida, H., M. Nakamura, M. Bogaki, H. Ito, T. Kojima, H. Hattori, and S. Nakamura. 1993. Mechanism of action of quinolones against *Escherichia coli* DNA gyrase. *Antimicrob. Agents Chemother.* **37:**839–845.

243. Yoshida, T., T. Muratani, S. Iyobe, and S. Mitsuhashi. 1994. Mechanisms of high-level resistance to quinolones in urinary tract isolates of *Pseudomonas aeruginosa*. *Antimicrob. Agents Chemother.* **38:**1466–1469.

244. Yu, J.-L., L. L. Grinius, and D. C. Hooper. 2002. NorA functions as a multidrug transporter in everted membrane vesicles and proteoliposomes. *J. Bacteriol.* **184:**1370–1377.

245. Zgurskaya, H. I., and H. Nikaido. 2000. Cross-linked complex between oligomeric periplasmic lipoprotein AcrA and the inner-membrane-associated multidrug efflux pump AcrB from *Escherichia coli*. *J. Bacteriol.* **182:**4264–4267.

246. Zhang, L., X. Z. Li, and K. Poole. 2000. Multiple antibiotic resistance in *Stenotrophomonas maltophilia*: involvement of a multidrug efflux system. *Antimicrob. Agents Chemother.* **44:**287–293.

247. Zhang, L., X.-Z. Li, and K. Poole. 2001. SmeDEF multidrug efflux pump contributes to intrinsic multidrug resistance in *Stenotrophomonas maltophilia*. *Antimicrob. Agents Chemother.* **45:**3497–3503.

248. Zheleznova, E. E., and R. G. Brennan. 2000. Crystal structure of the transcription activator BmrR bound to DNA and a drug. *Nature* **409:**378–382.

249. Zheleznova, E. E., P. N. Markham, A. A. Neyfakh, and R. G. Brennan. 1999. Structural basis of multidrug recognition by BmrR, a transcription activator of a multidrug transporter. *Cell* **96:**353–362.

250. Ziha-Zarifi, I., C. Llanes, T. Köhler, J. C. Pechere, and P. Plesiat. 1999. In vivo emergence of multidrug-resistant mutants of *Pseudomonas aeruginosa* overexpressing the active efflux system MexA-MexB-OprM. *Antimicrob. Agents Chemother.* **43:**287–291.

Quinolone Antimicrobial Agents, 3rd ed.
Edited by David C. Hooper and Ethan Rubinstein
© 2003 ASM Press, Washington, D.C.

Chapter 4

Quinolones and Eukaryotic Topoisomerases

THOMAS D. GOOTZ AND NEIL OSHEROFF

An extensive body of evidence indicates that the prokaryotic type II topoisomerases, DNA gyrase and topoisomerase IV, are the primary targets through which quinolones exert their antibacterial activities. However, relatively little work has been done to examine the effects of quinolones on other types of topoisomerases in bacteria or eukaryotes (see also chapter 2). Topoisomerases fall into two general categories (types I and II) based on the biochemical mechanism responsible for DNA strand passage. Type I enzymes characteristically catalyze single-stranded DNA cleavage and strand passage in the absence of ATP, while type II topoisomerases mediate double-stranded breakage with passage of another helix through the transient break by a process requiring energy from the hydrolysis of ATP (135, 168, 181). The DNA strand passage reactions mediated by topoisomerases are essential for maintaining the appropriate state of DNA supercoiling in the cell, for efficient replication of DNA, and for separation of daughter DNA molecules during cell division (9, 52, 81, 168). Type I and II topoisomerases are found in all cells and act in concert to maintain the optimal DNA conformation in the cell.

Eukaryotic type II topoisomerases can decatenate, relax, and unknot DNA by a duplex-strand passage mechanism that is analogous to that conducted by bacterial DNA gyrase (168). In addition to their similar biochemical mechanisms, bacterial DNA gyrase and eukaryotic type II topoisomerases (referred to simply as topoisomerase II) also share significant homology at the amino acid level (69, 73, 119, 172, 174). Studies have shown that regions in the N terminus and the middle portion of the eukaryotic type II monomer share significant homology with the B and A subunits, respectively, of DNA gyrase (119). This conservation of sequence homology suggests that a gene fusion event between the prokaryotic A and B subunits occurred during the course of evolution to produce the single gene encoding the eukaryotic type II monomer (119). This high degree of homology, which appears to be common among the type II topoisomerases, is not found with the type I enzymes (43, 173).

Given the similarities in biochemical mechanisms and amino acid sequences between bacterial DNA gyrase and topoisomerase II, it is reasonable to question whether quinolone antibacterial agents demonstrate activity against topoisomerase II from higher organisms. It has been generally accepted that at concentrations routinely achieved in vivo, antibacterial quinolones do not affect the latter enzyme (15, 83, 96). The high selectivity of nalidixic acid and the newer fluoroquinolones for DNA gyrase or topoisomerase IV compared with that of the eukaryotic enzyme has been cited in numerous reports (83, 96, 123). However, several recent studies have described new quinolones that appear to have lost this selectivity for the bacterial type II enzymes and show significant effects against eukaryotic topoisomerase II in vitro at concentrations that are clinically relevant. These quinolones come from several different structural series, and classical structure-activity relationships characterizing their interaction with topoisomerase II are beginning to emerge. In addition, several studies have investigated the effects of fluoroquinolones on cultured eukaryotic cells. Some results have correlated the genotoxic or cytotoxic effects obtained with these newer quinolones to their effects on topoisomerase II in vitro. In addition, recent studies also have examined the mechanisms responsible for the photogenotoxic activity of some fluoroquinolones. It has been suggested (11) that such studies are relevant in assessing the potential toxicity of new quinolone antibacterial agents to advance only those agents with potent activity against DNA gyrase/topoisomerase IV and no effect on mammalian topoisomerase II.

This chapter reviews the literature with respect to the reported effects of quinolones on topoisomerase II

Thomas D. Gootz • Pfizer Global Research and Development, Mail Stop 8118W-211, Eastern Point Road, Groton, CT 06340.
Neil Osheroff • Department of Biochemistry, School of Medicine, Vanderbilt University, Nashville, TN 37232-0146.

in vitro and considers those reports relevant to the effects of quinolones on whole cells. The initial part of the chapter describes in more detail some of the enzymatic properties of topoisomerase II and the consequences to the cell of the actions of drugs that are known to target this important enzyme.

EUKARYOTIC DNA TOPOISOMERASE II

Physiological Roles and Regulation

The survival of eukaryotic cells depends on the presence of type II topoisomerases. These enzymes are highly conserved, are required for the unlinking (i.e., segregation) of daughter chromosomes during mitosis (47, 81, 152, 177) and meiosis (153), chromosome condensation (1, 130, 175, 188), and the maintenance of proper chromosome structure (16, 47, 53, 67, 68, 176). In addition, considerable evidence points to important functions for type II enzymes in DNA replication, transcription, and recombination (9, 34, 46, 105, 135, 139, 148, 168, 181).

Although some eukaryotes such as yeast and *Drosophila* contain only a single form of topoisomerase II, most other species (including humans) contain two isoforms, α and β (7, 25, 49, 50, 61, 182). These two isoforms share ~70% amino acid sequence identity (10, 100, 109), but are encoded by separate genes (8, 26, 27, 184) and have different protomer molecular masses (~170 kDa and ~180 kDa, respectively). Relationships between topoisomerase II isoforms are not well defined. Enzymological differences between topoisomerase IIα and β are subtle, and a clear definition of the physiological roles of the α and β isoforms has yet to be determined. However, recent evidence indicates that these isoforms cannot functionally compensate for each other, and both appear to be required for the development of mammalian species.

The cellular functions of topoisomerase IIα and β probably reflect their physiological regulation more than their enzymological characteristics (25, 61). Topoisomerase IIα is regulated over both cell and growth cycles (126, 184). Enzyme levels increase throughout the S phase and peak at the G_2/M boundary. Furthermore, this isoform is found almost exclusively in rapid-proliferation tissues. Taken together, these characteristics suggest that topoisomerase IIα has the major responsibility for events associated with DNA replication and chromosome segregation. In contrast, the concentration of topoisomerase IIβ is generally independent of cell and growth cycles (7). Moreover, this isoform appears to be present in most cell types regardless of their pro-

liferation status. Thus, topoisomerase IIβ probably functions in ongoing nuclear processes.

Topoisomerase IIα is the isoform originally described in vertebrate species and to a large extent represents the enzyme that was characterized as "topoisomerase II" in early studies. However, because the enzymological characteristics of all eukaryotic type II topoisomerases appear to be similar and distinctions between isoforms are not always apparent, unless specifically stated otherwise, the term topoisomerase II will be used to refer to either member of this enzyme family.

Catalytic Cycle

All of the cellular activities of topoisomerase II stem directly from the mechanism by which it alters DNA topology (135, 139). Thus, before the physiological functions of the enzyme can be effectively dissected or its drug interactions fully exploited, it is imperative to understand the pathway by which topoisomerase II carries out its catalytic cycle.

Topoisomerase II alters the topological state of nucleic acids by passing an intact helix of DNA through a transient break that it generates in a separate helix. As a consequence of its double-stranded DNA passage reaction, the enzyme can relax (i.e., remove superhelical twists) from supercoiled DNA as well as knot-unknot or catenate-decatenate double-stranded nucleic acids (135, 139, 155, 168, 181). Unlike the prokaryotic type II enzyme, DNA gyrase (168, 181), eukaryotic topoisomerase II has no intrinsic ability to introduce superhelical twists into DNA. The double-stranded DNA passage reaction of topoisomerase II takes place at the expense of ATP hydrolysis and requires the presence of magnesium (139, 181). Although the mechanism of the enzyme appears to be concerted and quite complex in nature, it can be broken down into a series of discrete and straightforward steps (139). The reaction steps that make up the catalytic cycle of topoisomerase II are shown in Fig. 1, which depicts one round of enzyme-mediated DNA relaxation. Two points should be mentioned before the catalytic cycle is discussed. First, as a result of its double-stranded DNA passage mechanism, topoisomerase II removes two superhelical twists per reaction cycle. Second, only the topological state of DNA is altered by the actions of the enzyme; both the nucleic acid sequence and the chemical structure of the relaxed DNA product are identical to those of the original supercoiled substrate.

The catalytic cycle of topoisomerase II comprises at least six steps. A brief description follows. (i) Topoisomerase II binds to DNA at points of helix-

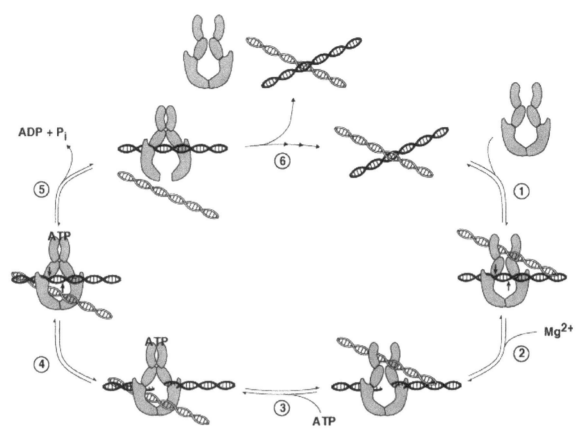

Figure 1. The six steps in the catalytic cycle of topoisomerase II. (i) The homodimer binds to DNA at points of helix-helix juxtaposition; (ii) in the presence of magnesium, topoisomerase II transiently cuts and religates the cleavage helix; (iii) on binding of two ATP molecules the enzyme-DNA complex undergoes a structural reorientation; (iv) following DNA strand passage topoisomerase II reestablishes a DNA cleavage-religation equilibrium; (v) topoisomerase II hydrolyzes the second bound ATP to ADP and P_i; (vi) the enzyme is recycled following hydrolysis of ATP.

helix juxtaposition (88, 193). Presumably, one of these helices is the DNA segment that the enzyme cleaves (i.e., cleavage helix) and the other is the segment that it passes through the break (i.e., passage helix). Neither DNA recognition nor enzyme DNA binding requires cofactors of any kind (134, 193). (ii) In the presence of a divalent cation (magnesium is used in vivo) (134, 138, 156), topoisomerase II transiently cuts and religates the cleavage helix (135, 139). This DNA cleavage-religation equilibrium can be readily reversed by the removal of the divalent cation (134), the addition of salt (116, 138) or a shift to suboptimal temperatures (90, 91, 116, 151). Cleavage takes place at preferred sequences within the nucleic acid backbone (3, 116, 125, 138, 156). Each cleaved DNA strand is complexed with a separate subunit of the homodimeric type II enzyme (192). This covalent topoisomerase II-DNA complex is referred to as the *cleavage complex* (66). (iii) On binding of two ATP molecules (75), the enzyme-DNA complex undergoes a structural reorientation (135, 139). During this reorientation, the

passage helix is translocated through the transient double-stranded break made in the cleavage helix. Although topoisomerase II does not require hydrolysis of the ATP to undergo DNA translocation, recent evidence suggests that this event takes place more rapidly if it is preceded by the hydrolysis of one of the bound ATP molecules (10). (iv) After DNA strand passage, topoisomerase II once again establishes a DNA cleavage-religation equilibrium (139). Hence, the enzyme generates cleavage complexes both prior to and following strand passage. Although the properties of these complexes are similar, the poststrand passage cleavage complex appears to be intrinsically more stable than its prestrand passage counterpart (133, 151). (v) Topoisomerase II hydrolyzes the second bound ATP to ADP and P_i (135, 139), which in turn triggers (vi) enzyme turnover (i.e., recycling). As described in the next section, the ability to analyze the individual steps of the catalytic cycle of the enzyme has contributed greatly to our understanding of the actions of topoisomerase II-targeted drugs.

TOPOISOMERASE II-TARGETED ANTINEOPLASTIC DRUGS

Beyond its critical physiological functions, topoisomerase II is the target for some of the most potent antineoplastic drugs currently used for the treatment of human cancers. Among the topoisomerase II-targeted drugs in clinical use are the epipodophyllotoxins (etoposide and teniposide), 4'-(9-acridinylamino)methane-sulfon-*m*-anisidide (*m*-AMSA), adriamycin, and mitoxantrone (114, 117, 158, 196).

Although all of these compounds inhibit the overall catalytic activity of the enzyme, their clinical efficacies correlate with their ability to stabilize covalent topoisomerase II-DNA cleavage complexes (114, 117). (In other words, they shift the DNA cleavage-religation equilibria of the enzyme toward the cleavage event.) At least in vitro, both the prestrand passage (29, 136, 143, 150) and poststrand passage (151) DNA cleavage complexes of topoisomerase II are targets for these drugs. For several years, the tight coupling of the DNA cleavage and religation reactions of topoisomerase II proved to be a formidable stumbling block to describing the detailed mechanism of drug action. Although, in general, it was assumed that antineoplastic agents enhanced enzyme-mediated breakage by inhibiting DNA religation (114, 158), it was impossible to confirm this assumption until assays that uncoupled religation from the forward DNA cleavage reaction were developed. Recently, three different assays specific for religation have been established. The first takes advantage of the fact that topoisomerase II-DNA cleavage complexes established in the presence of calcium (rather than magnesium) can be trapped in a kinetically competent form following chelation of the divalent cation (138, 192). The other two take advantage of the finding that the religation reaction of the enzyme is less sensitive to extremes of temperature (either high or low) than is its DNA cleavage reaction (90, 91, 116, 138, 151). By determining the effects of etoposide and *m*-AMSA on the apparent first-order rate constant for topoisomerase II-mediated DNA cleavage, it was demonstrated experimentally that these two structurally disparate antineoplastic drugs stabilize enzyme-DNA cleavage complexes primarily by impairing the ability of topoisomerase II to religate cleaved nucleic acids (136, 150, 151).

Despite the fact that structure-activity relationships have been established within individual drug series (13, 118), the common features that link these structurally disparate agents are not yet known. Even the site of drug action has yet to be characterized. All of the topoisomerase II-targeted antineo-plastic drugs discussed above interact with DNA, but there is no common mode of binding (the first two are nonintercalative, while the last three are intercalative) (32, 154, 183, 187). Moreover, there is no correlation between drug potency and either drug-DNA-binding affinity (32, 187) or -binding thermodynamics (179). These findings may be explained by recent kinetic and binding studies with etoposide and other anticancer drugs that suggest that these agents enter the topoisomerase II-DNA complex primarily through interactions with the enzyme (24, 63–65, 106, 197). These findings stand in contrast with those of gyrase-targeted antibacterial quinolones (160) or topoisomerase I-targeted anticancer camptothecins (77), which indicate that these latter agents bind primarily to the enzyme-DNA complex, as opposed to either the enzyme or the DNA. Because of the mechanism of drug action, cells that are treated with topoisomerase II-targeted agents accumulate high levels of protein-associated breaks in their genetic material (114, 117, 158, 194). The pathway that leads from increased concentrations of cleavage complexes to cell death has not been fully elucidated. However, topoisomerase II-mediated recombination (4, 52, 113, 142, 144, 158) and cellular events resembling apoptosis (101) both have been implicated. In addition, the lethal processing of these cleavage complexes appears to require ATP (111), calcium (17), and protein synthesis (31, 33, 159), and it is exacerbated by DNA transcription (80, 139, 158) and replication (139, 158). Supporting a role for DNA replication in drug-induced cell death, topoisomerase II-targeted agents appear to be considerably more lethal in S phase (during which DNA synthesis takes place) than in any other phase of the cell cycle (58, 121, 158). Treated cells generally progress until G_2 phase, dying prior to mitosis (58, 158).

Since topoisomerase II-targeted drugs act primarily by converting the type II enzyme into a cellular poison (109), the higher the physiological content of topoisomerase II, the more sensitive the cell is toward these agents (19, 42, 121, 165, 166, 196). Enzyme levels usually are elevated in rapidly proliferating or neoplastic cells (19, 40, 51, 76, 79, 92, 110, 126). Thus, clinically aggressive tumors appear to be most sensitive to these drugs (19, 166). Hypersensitivity to topoisomerase II-targeted agents has been associated with an overexpression of the enzyme or mutations in genes that encode DNA recombination/repair systems (44, 99, 109, 131, 166). Drug resistance has been correlated with decreased drug accumulation (14), decreased expression of topoisomerase II (28, 45, 62, 145), or mutations in topoisomerase II that decrease its sensitivity toward these agents (114, 117, 158, 196).

REPORTED EFFECTS OF QUINOLONES ON THE CATALYTIC ACTIVITY OF EUKARYOTIC TOPOISOMERASE II IN VITRO

As in the classical antineoplastic agents, the effects of quinolones on topoisomerase II have been assessed by using assays that measure either catalytic activity or the potential of the drugs to stimulate enzyme-mediated DNA cleavage. In general, it is believed that drug potency correlates best with formation of a drug-enzyme cleavage complex; however, many early studies measured inhibition of catalytic activity. The methods employed for measuring catalytic relaxation, catenation, or unknotting activity with purified topoisomerase II and various DNA substrates have been reviewed elsewhere (12). Such assays are most useful when performed in a manner that allows quantitation of the effects of a test agent (11).

Several investigators have assessed the effects of quinolones on the various catalytic activities of topoisomerase II. As reviewed previously (72), most of these studies have found that the quinolones developed for clinical use are not potent inhibitors of these activities in vitro. Miller et al. found that nalidixic and oxolinic acids had 50% inhibitory concentrations (IC_{50}s) of 500 and 100 μg/ml, respectively, for decatenation mediated by topoisomerase II isolated from HeLa cell nuclei (123). A similar degree of activity was found by Hussy et al., who used topoisomerase II isolated from calf thymus nuclei (96). These investigators determined the following IC_{50}s of ciprofloxacin, norfloxacin, ofloxacin, and nalidixic acid by using a catenation reaction: 150, 300, 1,300, and 1,000 μg/ml, respectively. Such studies also suggested that no correlation existed between the potencies of quinolones against bacterial DNA gyrase and their relative levels of inhibition of topoisomerase II (96). Using an assay for measuring the relaxation activity of topoisomerase II isolated from *Drosophila melanogaster* nuclei, Osheroff et al. found K_i values for nalidixic and oxolinic acids of 625 and 340 μg/ml, respectively (137). These relatively high drug levels required for inhibition may explain the failure of earlier studies to demonstrate any inhibition of *D. melanogaster* and rat liver topoisomerase II by low levels of nalidixic acid analogues (96, 115, 137, 141). In contrast, coumermycin A1 and novobiocin, two DNA gyrase B subunit inhibitors, are 10- to 100-fold more potent at inhibiting topoisomerase II relaxation activity in vitro than are quinolones (137).

Several investigators have characterized the inhibitory effects of quinolones on topoisomerase II relative to the drugs' inhibition of DNA gyrase and expressed results in terms of a selectivity ratio.

Hoshino et al. (86) studied the inhibition of *Escherichia coli* DNA gyrase supercoiling activity compared with the DNA relaxation activity of calf thymus topoisomerase II by nalidixic acid and fluoroquinolones. The data obtained indicate that IC_{50}s of ofloxacin, ciprofloxacin, lomefloxacin, enoxacin, CI-934, and nalidixic acid against gyrase ranged between 0.13 and 23.0 μg/ml (Table 1). The IC_{50}s against topoisomerase II-mediated relaxation varied considerably, with ofloxacin being the least inhibitory and CI-934 having the lowest IC_{50}. These results confirmed earlier studies indicating that no direct correlation exists between inhibitory potencies against bacterial and mammalian enzymes for the quinolones studied. Those authors also expressed their results in terms of a selectivity ratio by dividing the IC_{50}s obtained for topoisomerase II by the IC_{50}s generated against DNA gyrase. By means of this exercise, ofloxacin and ciprofloxacin demonstrated a high selectivity for DNA gyrase, while enoxacin, CI-934, and nalidixic acid possessed poor selectivity (86). Such calculations may prove misleading when the relative inhibitory potencies of quinolones against these enzymes are compared, and it should be remembered that the absolute inhibitory levels against topoisomerase II are also important. For example, while nalidixic acid had the lowest selectivity ratio of the quinolones in this study (Table 1), it also had one of the highest IC_{50}s against topoisomerase II.

This type of selectivity analysis has been reported for various quinolones in other studies (96), which in general agree that relatively high concentrations of compound are required to inhibit the catalytic activity of topoisomerase II in vitro. Although it has been established that some quinolones are more active than others at inhibiting the catalytic activity of topoisomerase II, very few studies have attempted to probe the structure-activity relationship of quinolones that may account for these differences.

Table 1. Relative DNA gyrase selectivities of some quinolones

Compound	IC_{50} (μg/ml)[a]		Selectivity ratio[d]
	DNA gyrase from *E. coli* KL-16[b]	Topoisomerase II from calf thymus[c]	
Ofloxacin	0.76	1,870	2,461
Ciprofloxacin	0.13	155	1,192
Lomefloxacin	0.78	280	359
Enoxacin	1.72	93	54
CI-934	3.55	64	18
Nalidixic acid	23	385	17

[a] Data from Hoshino et al. (86).
[b] Measured by DNA supercoiling assay.
[c] Measured by DNA relaxation assay.
[d] Determined by dividing IC_{50} for topoisomerase II by IC_{50} for DNA gyrase.

Hoshino et al. (85) studied several structurally related analogs of ofloxacin for their inhibitory effects on DNA gyrase supercoiling and calf thymus topoisomerase II relaxation activities. Their study presents some of the most direct evidence that the structural features of quinolones that confer potency against DNA gyrase do not necessarily impart increased inhibition of topoisomerase II. As illustrated in Table 2, the stereochemistry at the 3 position of the oxazine ring significantly influenced the relative potency against each enzyme (85). The pure S isomer of ofloxacin, DR-3355, was twofold more potent than ofloxacin against DNA gyrase, and it was severalfold more inhibitory than either the corresponding pure R isomer (DR-3354), or the desmethyl derivative (DL-8165) in this regard. The desmethyl derivative was 10 times more active at inhibiting topoisomerase II than the corresponding methylated analogs. The exomethylene derivative (DN-9494) was the most potent analog against calf thymus topoisomerase II relaxation activity (IC$_{50}$ of 64 µg/ml), yet it was twofold less potent than the S isomer against gyrase. This divergence in potency with regard to stereochemistry and substitution on the oxazine ring for these ofloxacin derivatives implies that the active sites for DNA gyrase and topoisomerase II recognize different spatial characteristics of quinolones.

Given the relatively weak inhibition of the catalytic activity of topoisomerase II exhibited by quinolones in vitro, the relevance of this activity for the eukaryotic cell remains uncertain. Very few studies have attempted to establish whether there is a relationship between the topoisomerase II inhibition observed in vitro and cell viability. Oomori et al.

(132), however, studied the cytotoxicities of several fluoroquinolones for HeLa cells in relation to their relative potencies against the relaxation activity of topoisomerase II purified from the same cell line. These investigators found the K_i values for cell growth after 48 h of exposure to the drugs to be 253, 204, 140, 113, and 230 µg/ml for fleroxacin, ofloxacin, norfloxacin, ciprofloxacin, and nalidixic acid, respectively (132). IC$_{50}$s for relaxation inhibition were 193, 169, 132, 87.3, and 34.4 µg/ml for fleroxacin, nalidixic acid, ofloxacin, norfloxacin, and ciprofloxacin, respectively (132). The relationship between the inhibitory potencies of these agents against the enzyme and their cytotoxicities was linear. Ciprofloxacin was also the most inhibitory quinolone against DNA, RNA, and protein synthesis as measured in this HeLa cell line (132). Those authors pointed out, however, that the inhibitory potencies observed with these quinolones were 2 orders of magnitude above the levels required for antibacterial activity.

IN VITRO EFFECTS OF QUINOLONES ON TOPOISOMERASE I

A limited number of studies that evaluate the interactions of quinolones with eukaryotic topoisomerase I are available. Quinolones have been shown to be less inhibitory for *E. coli* topoisomerase I than for DNA gyrase. Tabary et al. (169) found that the IC$_{50}$s of pefloxacin, ciprofloxacin, norfloxacin, and ofloxacin against bacterial topoisomerase I ranged between 35 and 50 µg/ml in the relaxation assay. This level of relaxation inhibition was approximately

Table 2. Influence of stereochemistry on the inhibitory activities of ofloxacin derivatives for DNA gyrase and topoisomerase II[a]

Quinolone	Substituent at position:		IC$_{50}$[b] (µg/ml)	
	R-1	R-2	DNA gyrase	Topoisomerase II
Ofloxacin	CH$_3$	H	0.76	1,870
DR-3355	CH$_3$	H	0.38	1,380
DR-3354	H	CH$_3$	4.7	2,550
DL-8165	H	H	3.1	178
DN-9494	CH$_2$	CH$_2$	0.70	64

[a] Data are from Hoshino et al. (85).
[b] Concentration of drug that inhibits 50% of *E. coli* KL-16 DNA gyrase supercoiling activity or calf thymus topoisomerase II relaxation activity.

10-fold lower than what was observed against DNA gyrase supercoiling activity. It is not surprising, therefore, that little inhibition of eukaryotic topoisomerase I has been observed with quinolones (169). In one study (96), nalidixic acid and ofloxacin at concentrations of up to 1,000 μg/ml showed no inhibitory activity against calf thymus nuclear topoisomerase I relaxation activity. Norfloxacin and ciprofloxacin exhibited limited inhibition in these tests, with IC$_{50}$s between 300 and 400 μg/ml (96).

ENHANCEMENT OF TOPOISOMERASE II-MEDIATED DNA CLEAVAGE BY QUINOLONES

The majority of studies in the literature that have investigated the effects of quinolones on eukaryotic topoisomerase II have studied inhibition of catalytic activity. While this is a valid approach that has also been used with the antitumor topoisomerase II inhibitors, it is not necessarily the most relevant parameter with which to correlate the cytotoxic potentials of these agents. As pointed out above, topoisomerase II-targeted drugs such as the epipodophyllotoxins stabilize a cleavage intermediate formed between double-stranded DNA and topoisomerase II in vitro. Formation of this cleavage complex also has been observed in DNA breakage assays using whole cells cultured in the presence of topoisomerase II inhibitors. A direct correlation between cell toxicity and cleavage complex stabilization by drug has been established for many topoisomerase II inhibitors and is a central theme of the "poison hypothesis" accounting for the cytotoxic effects of these drugs (109).

Given the relevance of cleavage complex formation to the mechanism of action of known topoisomerase II inhibitors, some studies have evaluated quinolones for their ability to stimulate topoisomerase II-mediated DNA cleavage in vitro. As described above, the generation of linear DNA in the presence of topoisomerase II and drug is a stoichiometric process: the amount of linear DNA formed is dependent on the concentrations of enzyme, DNA, and drug (66, 113, 150, 151). These double-stranded DNA breaks can be observed following treatment of the complexes with denaturing agents and protease, with subsequent electrophoresis of the DNA in agarose gels (6, 66). By quantitating the linear DNA cleavage products, the relative potency of topoisomerase II inhibitors can be assessed.

Nelson et al. (127) were the first to report that oxolinic acid stimulated DNA cleavage in vitro in the presence of T4 phage topoisomerase II (which has many characteristics in common with the eukaryotic enzyme). Barrett et al. (11) studied more thoroughly the effects of some newer quinolones on topoisomerase II purified from calf thymus. They found that ciprofloxacin, norfloxacin, oxolinic acid, and nalidixic acid were weak inhibitors of the catalytic unknotting and catenation activities of this enzyme. These quinolones also were not very active at inducing topoisomerase II-mediated DNA cleavage compared with the antitumor agents. Barrett et al. used two types of cleavage assays: one utilizing a nonradiolabeled DNA substrate and a second, which was more sensitive, using a linearized DNA substrate end labeled with ^{32}P. In the assay with radiolabeled substrate, ciprofloxacin stimulated enzyme-mediated DNA cleavage (concentration of drug that produces half-maximal DNA cleavage [CC$_{50}$s] of 120 μg/ml) but was 27-fold less potent than etoposide in this regard. That study, however, identified a novel 6,8-difluoro-7-pyridyl quinolone, CP-67,015 (Fig. 2), that was significantly more potent than other quinolones in stimulating DNA cleavage. In the radiolabeled and nonradiolabeled DNA cleavage assays, CP-67,015 demonstrated CC$_{50}$s of 33 and 73 μg/ml, respectively (11). The linear DNA cleavage patterns generated in the presence of CP-67,015 in the assay with radiolabeled DNA showed qualitative and quantitative differences from those generated with etoposide (11). These results are consistent with previously published results, which indicate that different structural families of topoisomerase II inhibitors generate unique cleavage patterns with enzyme in vitro and therefore likely recognize different DNA cleavage sites in the presence of the enzyme (29, 127, 170, 190).

An important aspect of the study with CP-67,015 was that both catalytic (unknotting and catenation) and cleavage activities obtained with calf thymus topoisomerase II were compared. As with etoposide, the CC$_{50}$s for the cleavage assays run with CP-67,015 were usually lower than the corresponding IC$_{50}$ obtained for inhibition of catalytic activity (11). This was particularly true for the cleavage assay using ^{32}P-radiolabeled DNA as substrate. This suggests that cleavage assays may be more sensitive for detecting the effects of quinolones on topoisomerase II. It is interesting that a similar observation has been made by Domagala and colleagues (48) with DNA gyrase; for a number of quinolones, they observed a better correlation between the generation of gyrase-mediated DNA cleavage and the MIC than between the MIC and the IC$_{50}$s for gyrase supercoiling. While CP-67,015 was shown to be a potent antibacterial agent and highly inhibitory for DNA gyrase (11), its increase in potency against topoisomerase II was an

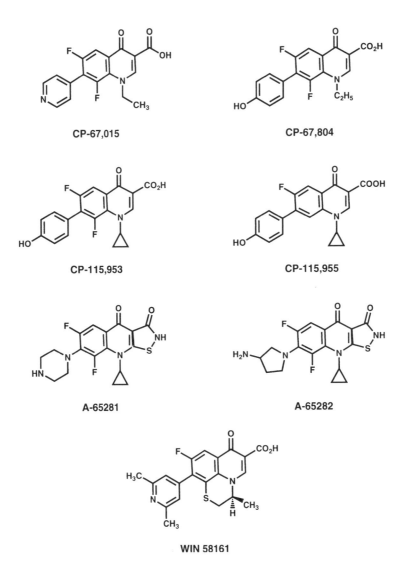

Figure 2. Structures of novel fluoroquinolones that act against topoisomerase II.

important finding, distinguishing this compound from other quinolones. This activity was also a critical consideration in determining the overall safety of CP-67,015, as will be discussed in the section describing the genotoxic effects of this quinolone.

Although CP-67,015 was one of the first quinolones shown to have potent activity against topoisomerase II, other quinolone analogs have recently been shown to enhance enzyme-mediated DNA cleavage. Kohlbrenner et al. (108) examined the activities of novel isothiazoloquinolones for stimulating calf thymus topoisomerase II-mediated DNA breakage in vitro. Two of these quinolones, A-65281 and A-65282 (Fig. 2), had IC$_{50}$s in the DNA-unknotting assay of 8 μg/ml and showed strong DNA cleavage activities, i.e., down to 4 μg/ml in the presence of the enzyme (108). The structure-activity relationship in these studies revealed that both the 6,8-difluoro substitution and an N-1 cyclopropyl

group were important in determining potency for enhancing topoisomerase II-mediated DNA cleavage (108). Both A-65281 and A-65282 were nearly as potent as the antitumor agent etoposide with respect to this activity. Thus, studies with the isothiazoloquinolone derivatives add to the information generated with CP-67,015, indicating that specific substitutions on the quinolone nucleus can lead to compounds that have significant activities against both DNA gyrase and eukaryotic topoisomerase II in vitro.

Another series of studies described the topoisomerase II inhibitory activity of several 10-(3′,5′-dimethyl-4′-pyridinyl)-6-pyridobenzothiazinyl (oxazine) carboxylic acids (39, 186). The most potent of these quinolones, WIN 58161 (Fig. 2), formed covalent complexes between purified HeLa cell topoisomerase II and DNA with a 50% effective concentration (EC$_{50}$) of 9.4 μM (4 μg/ml). WIN

58161 was about 12-fold less potent than etoposide in these in vitro cleavage assays. Additional in vitro studies indicated that the compound did not intercalate into DNA and established that protein-associated DNA strand breaks were produced when P388 cells were exposed to WIN 58161 (39). Enantiomeric specificity was again demonstrated to influence potency against topoisomerase II, since the pure 3-*S*-methyl enantiomer was over 2 orders of magnitude more active at inducing cleavage than the *R*-methyl enantiomer.

Evidence that quinolones and antitumor inhibitors of topoisomerase II show both a common inhibitor-binding site and a common mechanism of action (i.e., increase in levels of enzyme-DNA cleavage complexes) comes from studies using mutants of the T4 phage enzyme. While the mammalian enzyme is a homodimer, T4 phage topoisomerase II contains three subunits, designated by their sizes as 39-kDa (catalyzes ATP hydrolysis), 52-kDa (conducts DNA breakage and resealing), and 60-kDa (confers structural stability) (94, 95). T4 topoisomerase II is involved in phage DNA replication and has many properties in common with the mammalian enzyme; it is normally inhibited by *m*-AMSA, ellipticine, teniposide, and etoposide, but is insensitive to oxolinic acid (94). Mutant T4 phage were isolated under selection with *m*-AMSA, and one drug-resistant mutant was found to contain topoisomerase II with an alteration in the 39-kDa subunit (94). The enzyme from this mutant demonstrated *m*-AMSA-resistant DNA relaxation activity and was insensitive to *m*-AMSA-enhanced DNA cleavage. This mutation conferred a DNA gyrase-like sensitivity to oxolinic acid, as measured in a cleavage assay. The mutant enzyme was also ultrasensitive to the epipodophyllotoxins etoposide and teniposide (94). Those authors hypothesized that the mutant topoisomerase II had an altered binding site that decreased the binding of some antitumor agents while favoring binding of other compounds, including the quinolone antibiotic oxolinic acid. These results suggest that the binding sites on T4 topoisomerase II for some antitumor drugs and oxolinic acid are either the same or overlapping. If the sites for these two classes of drugs are similar, it might be expected that minor structural modifications on the quinolone nucleus could significantly increase their affinities for topoisomerase II. This conclusion is consistent with the observations reported above for some quinolones discussed in this review.

These corroborating observations cause us to reconsider the previously held doctrine that all quinolones are highly selective for bacterial type II topoisomersases. Studies using purified topoisomerase II have also led to important new observations addressing the biochemical mechanism by which these novel quinolones interact with the eukaryotic type II enzyme.

MECHANISTIC STUDIES OF C-7-HYDROXYPHENYL-SUBSTITUTED QUINOLONES: THE CP-115,953 SERIES

As already described, most quinolone antimicrobial agents are poor effectors of eukaryotic topoisomerase II (72, 84, 195). While all antibacterial quinolones in clinical use contain an aliphatic group at the C-7 position (35, 185), compounds with aromatic C-7 groups (pyridine, 2,6-dimethylpyridine, and quinoline) also have been reported (11, 98, 186). These latter compounds are distinguished from quinolone antimicrobial agents by their increased activity toward the eukaryotic enzyme (11, 98, 186). However, in all cases, potency was still considerably lower than that of a topoisomerase II-targeted antineoplastic drug such as etoposide. To further assess the influence of aromatic C-7 substituents on the activities of quinolones, the effects of quinolone derivative CP-115,953 and analogous compounds (all of which contain a hydroxyphenyl ring at C-7) on eukaryotic topoisomerase II were examined (148, 149). Structures of these quinolones are shown in Fig. 2. All members of the CP-115,953 series are nonintercalative with respect to DNA (149). Furthermore, in addition to their activities against eukaryotic topoisomerase II, all are extremely effective against bacterial DNA gyrase (148, 149). In fact, CP-115,953 is approximately fourfold more effective than ciprofloxacin at inducing gyrase-mediated DNA cleavage (148). Because CP-115,953 is the most potent of these compounds in all respects, it will be the primary focus of this section.

Initial studies used topoisomerase II from *D. melanogaster* (148, 149). As shown in Fig. 3A, CP-115,953 is a potent enhancer of enzyme-mediated DNA breakage. Similar results were found for the effects of the quinolone on both the prestrand passage and poststrand passage DNA cleavage-religation equilibria (148). In addition, CP-115,953 was considerably more potent (relative to etoposide) against the mammalian type II enzyme (148). Thus, CP-115,953 is the first quinolone reported to have greater activity against eukaryotic topoisomerase II than does an antineoplastic drug in clinical use. Substitution of an ethyl group for the cyclopropyl at N-1 (CP-67,804) or removal, of the fluorine at C-8 (CP-115,955) reduced quinolone activity to ~40%

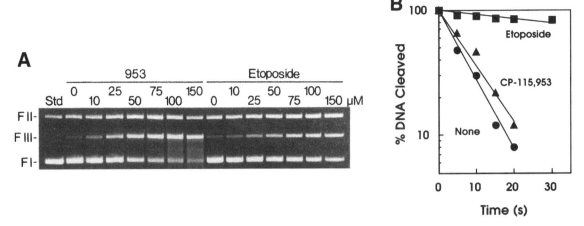

Figure 3. Effects of CP-115,953 on the DNA cleavage (A) and religation (B) reactions of *Drosophila* topoisomerase II. (A) Comparative cleavage titration of CP-115,953 and etoposide tested at the concentrations shown on the top of the gel photograph. CP-115,953 is more potent at enhancing topoisomerase II-mediated DNA cleavage product (form III DNA) from supercoiled DNA (form I) than is etoposide at comparable concentrations. (B) Religation of cleavage product was initiated by shifting assay mixtures from 30 to 55°C. Results obtained with 50 µM CP-115,953 are compared with those obtained in the absence of drug or in the presence of 100 µM etoposide. The drug concentrations used generated similar levels of enzyme-mediated DNA breakage. Data are plotted in a semilogarithmic fashion as the loss of linear DNA versus time. The percent linear DNA for each assay was set arbitrarily to 100% at time zero. Plots represent the averages of three independent experiments (average standard error, ≤5%). Panel B is reproduced from reference 148 with permission.

that of CP-115,953 (148, 149). It should be noted, however, that despite their decreased activities, CP-67,804 and CP-115,955 still were considerably more potent against the *Drosophila* type II enzyme than any other quinolone previously reported (except CP-115,953). Previously proposed models for quinolone action suggest that the C-7 substituent is important for drug-gyrase interactions (161, 191). In this regard, CP-115,955 differs from ciprofloxacin only at its C-7 position, yet is ~20-fold more potent at enhancing *Drosophila* topoisomerase II-mediated DNA cleavage (149). Thus, the presence of the hydroxyphenyl ring at position C-7 appears to be critical to the dramatic activities of quinolones in the CP-115,953 series.

As previously mentioned, two different topoisomerase II-targeted antineoplastic drugs enhanced enzyme-mediated DNA breakage primarily by inhibiting DNA religation (136, 150, 151). This was not the case for CP-115,953. As seen in the heat-induced DNA religation assay of Fig. 3B, the quinolone displayed little ability to inhibit DNA religation (148). These findings, which are in marked contrast to those with etoposide, were confirmed by using the other two religation assays described earlier (148). Furthermore, comparable results were obtained when religation was carried out in the presence of either CP-67,804 or CP-115,953 (148, 149). Since these quinolones have little effect on DNA religation, it is likely that they enhance topoisomerase

II-mediated DNA breakage primarily by stimulating the forward rate of nucleic acid cleavage. Therefore, quinolones in the CP-115,953 series appear to represent a novel mechanistic class of potent topoisomerase II-targeted drugs.

The mechanistic basis for quinolone action does not appear to have been conserved across divergent species. In contrast to results with eukaryotic topoisomerase II, CP-115,953 significantly inhibits the DNA religation reaction of *S. aureus* topoisomerase IV (4). Furthermore, there is a strong correlation between the potency of enhancement of topoisomerase IV-mediated DNA cleavage by the antibacterial quinolones ciprofloxacin, trovafloxacin, levofloxacin, and sparfloxacin and the ability of these drugs to inhibit the DNA religation reaction of the enzyme ($R = 0.96$) (5).

EVOLUTIONARY CONSERVATION OF THE QUINOLONE INTERACTION DOMAIN ON TYPE II TOPOISOMERASES

The fact that specific members of the quinolone family display high activity against both prokaryotic and eukaryotic type II topoisomerases suggests that the drug-interaction domain on these enzymes has been conserved over the course of evolution. Several lines of evidence indicate that this is most likely the case. First, at high concentrations, the antibacterial quinolone ciprofloxacin is a modest enhancer of DNA cleavage mediated by eukaryotic topoisomerase II (6, 57) and the anticancer drug etoposide is a modest enhancer of bacterial topoisomerase IV (5).

Second, etoposide competes with ciprofloxacin for the stimulation of DNA cleavage mediated by topoisomerase IV (6, 57). Even at DNA sites unique to the quinolone, cleavage is diminished in the presence of etoposide (5). In comparable competition studies conducted with the eukaryotic type II enzyme, ciprofloxacin is a competitive inhibitor of etoposide and CP-115,953 (57). Although not analyzed by a similar kinetic approach, ciprofloxacin also competes for DNA-cleavage enhancement with the anticancer drugs amsacrine and genistein 953 (57).

Third, mutations at serine 80 and glutamic acid 84 in *S. aureus* topoisomerase IV, which result in clinical resistance to quinolones, also confer resistance to etoposide in vitro (5). Furthermore, mutations at serine 740 in yeast topoisomerase II or serine 763 in human topoisomerase IIα decrease the sensitivity of these enzymes to CP-115,953 (89) (V. E. Anderson, J. L. Nitiss, and N. Osheroff, unpublished results). These residues are equivalent to serine 83 of GyrA and serine 80 of ParC/GrlA, respectively, and are believed to be at the center of the quinolone-resistance-determining region in bacterial type II topoisomerases (18, 22, 82, 93, 112).

Taken together, the evidence above strongly supports the concept that the drug-interaction domain on type II topoisomerases has been conserved over widely divergent species. This finding suggests that differences in quinolone mechanism between the bacterial and eukaryotic enzymes are probably due to minor differences in the geometry of the enzyme-drug-DNA ternary complex, rather than a gross change in the site of drug binding.

REPORTED EFFECTS OF FLUOROQUINOLONES ON EUKARYOTIC CELLS

Numerous studies have reported a wide range of effects of fluoroquinolones on eukaryotic cells. Major effects include direct breakage of chromosomal DNA by free radical-mediated phototoxicity or by topoisomerase II-mediated mechanisms. Several recent publications describe fluoroquinolone-induced DNA breakage by each of these mechanisms (71, 107, 162).

In the direct mechanism, UV light waves interact with fluoroquinolone acting as a sensitizing agent allowing passage of energy to DNA. The efficiency of this energy-transfer process is structure-related and a number of fluoroquinolones are known to be fairly potent photosensitizing agents for the skin. While wavelengths of light below 320 nm can directly cause DNA damage, longer wavelengths require the presence of light-absorbing chemical sensitizers that can directly transfer their chemical energy-producing damage to DNA. Alternatively, sensitizers can use secondary carriers such as free oxygen radicals to transfer energy to DNA. By this mechanism, which does not require the participation of topoisomerase II, fluoroquinolones or their metabolites can produce photochemical genotoxic events in eukaryotic cells (71). Irradiation of whole-cell systems or animal models with UV light in the presence of fluoroquinolones can result in DNA breakage, mutagenicity, and tumorigenicity. The observation that clastogenic events induced by ultraviolet light and fluoroquinolones can be modified by antioxidants suggests that reactive oxygen species are involved in the phototoxic mechanism (30). In addition, the UVA photoirradiation of fluoroquinolones has led to production of reactive oxygen species, including $-OH$, $-O_2^-$, H_2O_2, and singlet oxygen ($^1O_2$) (162, 180); however, no correlation between the level of these free oxygen radicals and phototoxicity has been established (178). The presence of a halogen in the 8 position of the fluoroquinolone molecule has also been correlated with a predilection for enhanced phototoxicity in vivo. Since photocarcinogenicity studies have shown that some fluoroquinolones possess the ability to enhance UVA-induced skin tumor formation (107), requirements for long-term photocarcinogenicity studies to assess the safety of new fluoroquinolones, were initiated by the Food and Drug Administration in the United States in the 1990s.

Such tests are difficult to perform, and many investigators have attempted to better understand the mechanism(s) of photochemical genotoxic events observed with fluoroquinolones at the cellular level. One study tested the ability of the Chinese hamster V79 lung cell micronucleus assay to predict both the phototoxic and photogenotoxic potential of a number of modern fluoroquinolones (162). In these studies, V79 cells were cultured and irradiated (290 to 400 nm) at a dose between 1,250 and 30,000 J/m^2 with or without fluoroquinolone (162). After irradiation, cell medium was removed and replaced with fresh medium followed by incubation for another 16 h. Cells were removed by trypsin-EDTA treatment and fixed for microscopic examination. Of the fluoroquinolones tested, clinafloxacin was the most potent for inducing micronucleated binucleate cells (IC$_{50}$ of 30 µg/ml) without UV irradiation (162). When irradiation effects were tested (UV source of

3,000 J/m^2) in the presence of drug defining the IC$_{50}$ for inhibition of cell proliferation, clinafloxacin was the most phototoxic compound, while lomefloxacin, nalidixic acid, and sparfloxacin were somewhat less phototoxic. Ciprofloxacin, ofloxacin and trovafloxacin were least phototoxic, requiring between 12,000 and 30,000 J/m^2 at the IC$_{50}$. Results indicated that the antiproliferative phototoxic and photoclastogenic activities of these fluoroquinolones were correlated in a parallel fashion (162). These in vitro results also correlate well with in vivo observations indicating that lomefloxacin and some other fluoroquinolones are more commonly phototoxic (92). These results also implicate C-6 and C-8 dihalogen substitution with heightened phototoxicity. Addition of 10 to 20 mM sodium azide to the cell culture for as little as 1 min prior to irradiation prevented the phototoxic damage. Since this effect has also been observed with etoposide and other inhibitors of mammalian topoisomerase II during cell proliferation, it was suggested that fluoroquinolone-induced phototoxicity may result from drug interaction with topoisomerase (162).

Other studies have examined the photogenotoxic activity of fluoroquinolones with UV light. In the Ames mutagenicity test fleroxacin, lomefloxacin, and ciprofloxacin induced weak increases in the number of revertants observed with *Salmonella enterica* serovar Typhimurium TA104 and TA100 (30). All three fluoroquinolones failed to show photomutagenic activity against *Saccharomyces cerevisiae* D7. In the Comet assay the fluoroquinolones caused DNA damage with UV irradiation using mouse lymphoma cells. Lomefloxacin was the most active of the agents tested with 50% of cells producing DNA damage with 3 µg/ml drug and exposure to UVA at 500 mJ/cm^2 (30). The three compounds also demonstrated clear concentration-dependent, UV-associated chromosomal aberrations in Chinese hamster V79 cells. The minimum concentrations at which more than one chromosomal aberration per cell was observed were 25 µg/ml for lomefloxacin, 100 µg/ml for fleroxacin, and 200 µg/ml for ciprofloxacin. Statistically significant increases in the frequency of aberrant cells were seen with lomefloxacin down to 6.5 µg/ml using a UVA source of 500 mJ/cm^2 (30).

The relative phototoxic potency of fluoroquinolones appears to be correlated with their individual instability to UV light. The unstable quinolones degrade on irradiation resulting in oxidative DNA damage that can be measured by the formation of 8-oxo-7,8-dihydro-2′-deoxyguanosine (8-oxodGuo) in the DNA (163). The amount of 8-oxodGuo formed in cultured cells or with cell-free

DNA samples due to fluoroquinolone and UVA (330 to 400 nm) or UVB (280 to 320 nm) light was correlated inversely with their relative photostability (163). The experimental fluoroquinolone BAY y3118 and lomefloxacin were found to be highly unstable to UV and, as a result, produced the highest amounts of 8-oxodGuo in vitro with purified calf thymus DNA. With a constant exposure to UVA irradiation of 1 J/cm^2, the relative potency for formation of 8-oxodGuo with calf thymus DNA was in the order BAY y3118 > lomefloxacin > ciprofloxacin > moxifloxacin (179). It is believed that such quantitative in vitro tests may be predictive of photocarcinogenicity as well, since lomefloxacin has been found to be highly active both in in vitro tests for phototoxicity and in animal models for photocarcinogenicity (30, 120, 140, 153, 163, 171). It is possible that the in vitro tests for photogenotoxicity, such as the Chinese hamster V79 model, may be helpful in identifying unacceptable toxic potential in new fluoroquinolone analogues at an early stage of development.

GENOTOXICITY IN THE ABSENCE OF UV IRRADIATION

The genotoxic potency of some antibacterial fluoroquinolones may correlate with their affinity to mammalian topoisomerase II protein rather than with either direct binding or transfer of energy to DNA. Several studies have reported on the genotoxic effects of fluoroquinolones in tests that do not depend on irradiation with UV light. Two reviews have described the reported genotoxic effects of quinolones in various in vitro cell systems (41, 72). Ciprofloxacin, norfloxacin, ofloxacin, and pefloxacin have been claimed to be mutagenic in the mouse lymphoma cell assay and to also produce a positive response in the rat hepatocyte unscheduled DNA synthesis (UDS) assay (157). These quinolones, however, did not show abnormal effects in either the Ames or the Chinese hamster V79 cell tests for gene mutagenicity or in the micronucleus or dominant lethal tests in mice (157, 164). The activity of ciprofloxacin in the UDS assay was confirmed in a separate study in which the compound produced a UDS response in human lymphocytes in vitro when tested at 5 µg/ml (4). A recent study indicates that ciprofloxacin induces double-stranded DNA breaks in human lymphoblastoid cells exposed to 80 µg of drug per ml (20). Tests with norfloxacin and fleroxacin (AM-833) indicated that these two drugs are not mutagenic, do not induce DNA strand breakage, and do not elicit a UDS response in either human or mouse skin fibroblasts (87).

A more recent study examined the structure-activity relationships of 17 quinolones with regard to their activity in various genotoxicity test systems (2). The purpose of the side-by-side comparison of these compounds was to establish a risk assessment for genotoxicity with respect to their activity in cell assays relative to known topoisomerase II inhibitors. All of the quinolones showed genotoxic activity in the *S. enterica* serovar Typhimurium TA102 and the SOS test, with newer, potent fluoroquinolones such as ciprofloxacin demonstrating lower mutagenic doses than nalidixic acid. Because all of these compounds are inhibitors of bacterial topoisomerase II (DNA gyrase) yet have well established safety profiles in humans, results of such positive Ames tests (bacterial mutagens) can be considered to have little predictive value in determining human safety. Only one fluoroquinolone that was shown to be active against mammalian topoisomerase II, CP-67,804, was also mutagenic in the Chinese hamster V79 cell assay at a clinically relevant concentration of 10 μg/ml (2). CP-67,804 also was mutagenic in the mouse lymphoma cell HPRT and TK loci at 5 and 15 μg/ml, respectively. It also caused chromosome aberrations in CHO cells at 10 μg/ml. As detailed elsewhere in this chapter, the heightened mutagenicity and clastogenic activity of CP-67,804 compared with those of other fluoroquinolones are likely a result of its potent cleavage complex formation with mammalian topoisomerase II. This highlights the importance of maintaining a high selectivity between the bacterial DNA gyrase target and its mammalian homologue for ensuring the safety of these agents.

While all of the in vitro effects described for marketed fluoroquinolones are of potential medical interest, no direct evidence indicates that they result from inhibition of topoisomerase II. In addition, the literature contains much debate concerning the relevance of positive in vitro genotoxicity results observed in a single test system, since the majority of quinolones appear not to induce the same responses in in vivo test systems (23, 122, 124, 164). This position is consistent with the good overall safety record that has been achieved for those fluoroquinolones in clinical use. From this experience, it has generally been accepted that the safety of new quinolone antibacterial agents in terms of their low-mutagenicity potential can be reliably determined by establishing their lack of genotoxic activities in a standard battery of in vitro and in vivo tests.

Much less is known, however, about the genotoxicity of other fluoroquinolones described in this chapter, which have demonstrated significantly increased potency toward topoisomerase II. One of the first quinolones described for its activity against topoisomerase II, the 6,8-difluoro-7-pyridyl-4-quinolone CP-67,015, has been characterized with regard to its genotoxic activity (78). CP-67,015 was not mutagenic in the Ames test but was a direct-acting mutagen in the mouse lymphoma cell assay, the Chinese hamster ovary cell hypoxanthine-guanine phosphoribosyl transferase gene (HGPRT) assay, and the V-79 cell-HGPRT forward mutation assay (78). This quinolone also induced chromosome aberrations in cultured human lymphocytes at concentrations of 250 μg/ml and produced genetically abnormal bone-marrow cells in mice given five daily parenteral doses of 500 mg/kg of body weight per day. Surprisingly, sister chromatid exchange was only marginally stimulated with CP-67,015 in human lymphocytes or CHO cells in vitro, even at levels that produced severe chromosome breakage (78). As described above, this quinolone was only 7- to 10-fold less potent than the antitumor agent etoposide for stimulating topoisomerase II-mediated DNA cleavage in vitro, thus establishing a probable link with topoisomerase II and its reported genotoxic activity in cells.

The cytotoxic activity of the potent topoisomerase II-acting quinolones CP-115,953 and CP-67,804 also have been investigated (148). Two tissue culture lines were used for this purpose: a wild-type CHO cell line and its VpmR-5 mutant, which was derived as a result of its resistance to epipodophyllotoxins (70, 74, 167). The mutant line is 10- to 20-fold more resistant than its wild type to etoposide and is cross-resistant to a number of other topoisomerase II-targeted antineoplastic drugs (70). Drug resistance in the VpmR-5 cell line results from a mutant, resistant form of topoisomerase II and not from reduced drug accumulation (167).

CP-115,953 and etoposide were equally cytotoxic to the wild-type CHO cells, with an EC_{50} of 9 μM (148). CP-67,804, which was less potent at enhancing topoisomerase II-mediated DNA cleavage than either CP-115,953 or etoposide, demonstrated an EC_{50} of 70 μM against wild-type CHO cells. While the VpmR-5 mutant cell line showed some degree of cross-resistance to CP-67,804 and CP-115,953 (3.7- and 1.3-fold increases in EC_{50}, respectively), resistance was not as pronounced as that observed with etoposide (12-fold increase in EC_{50} over that of wild type). Regardless of the magnitude of the increase in resistance against the VpmR-5 cell line, the cytotoxicity results obtained considered along with the activities of these quinolones against purified topoisomerase II (described above) strongly suggest that this enzyme is a target for these quinolones in mammalian cells.

Conclusive evidence for quinolone targeting in eukaryotic cells comes from two complementary genetic approaches in yeast. The first demonstrated that decreasing the cellular activity of topoisomerase II, which dramatically lowers the sensitivity of cultures to topoisomerase II-targeted anticancer drugs, also led to CP-115,953 resistance (56). The second showed that expression of mutated type II enzymes that displayed either resistance or hypersensitivity to quinolones in vitro conferred a corresponding phenotype to yeast in vivo (54, 89).

Further support for the conclusion that quinolones target topoisomerase II in cells came from two independent studies with mammalian tissue culture cells. In the first, the ability of CP-115,953 and several analogues to enhance topoisomerase II-mediated cleavage was compared with their ability to kill CHO cells in culture (55). A strong correlation ($R \approx 0.9$) between these two activities was observed. In the second, WIN 58161 was shown to induce protein-linked DNA strand breaks in P388 murine leukemia cells in a dose-dependent manner, and derivatives that displayed poor activity against mammalian topoisomerase II in vitro failed to induce these strand breaks in cultured cells (38). Furthermore, strand breaks were reversed on removal of drug, a hallmark of topoisomerase-targeted agents (38).

Antitumor Activity of Fluoroquinolones

Given the recent understanding of the enhanced ability of some fluoroquinolones to form stable cleavage complexes with mammalian topoisomerase II, it is not surprising that many of these unusual agents demonstrate antitumor activity in mouse models. One of the first published studies to evaluate a large number of structurally diverse fluoroquinolones for in vivo antitumor activity was from Yamashita et al. (189). These investigators tested 90 fluoroquinolones including the clinically available agents norfloxacin, ofloxacin, and ciprofloxacin for antitumor and topoisomerase II activity. Eighty of the compounds showed no stimulation of DNA cleavage with calf thymus topoisomerase II, nor did they demonstrate any antitumor activity against P388 leukemia in mice. It is clear, that as determined by numerous investigators, the majority of fluoroquinolone structural analogues are highly selective for bacterial DNA gyrase and possess no biologically meaningful activity against the mammalian homologue. As discussed more fully in this chapter, some structural moieties on the fluoroquinolone nucleus decrease gyrase selectivity and some of these agents have meaningful activity for stimulating topoisomerase II-mediated DNA cleavage. This subset of fluoroquinolones often contains common structural

features, including two halogens at C-6 and C-8 and an aromatic ring at C-7 (189). Ten such compounds in the study demonstrated stimulation of cleavage complex formation at test concentrations from 12.5 to 250 µM. However, all of these active experimental fluoroquinolones were significantly less potent in the cleavage assays than the control antitumor compound etoposide (189). Compared with recently published studies with other experimental fluoroquinolones such as CP-67,804 and CP-115,953, in which eukaryotic topoisomerase II cleavage studies were performed, the compounds examined by Yamashita et al. were relatively impotent in the cleavage assays. Despite this, all ten fluoroquinolones showed some degree of antitumor activity in the P388 leukemia model following a single intraperitoneal dose 24 h after tumor challenge. The most efficacious fluoroquinolone in these studies produced a 50% prolongation of life span compared with drug-free controls (189). In similar models, etoposide produced a 150% increase in life span, consistent with its greater activity in the in vitro cleavage assays with topoisomerase II. This early study, in general, is consistent with other antitumor model studies with topoisomerase II-active fluoroquinolones, indicating that they are not more active than conventional antitumor agents against topoisomerase II or with in vivo tumor models (37, 38, 97). As mentioned elsewhere in this chapter, CP-115,953 is the most potent fluoroquinolone examined to date in topoisomerase II-mediated DNA cleavage assays and it is more potent than etoposide against human tumor cell lines (148). So far, these antineoplastic fluoroquinolone leads have not advanced to a successful program of novel anticancer agents. The available data in the literature do highlight the fact that significant cross-species variability occurs with regard to the susceptibility of type II topoisomerases to different fluoroquinolones.

Antiparasitic Activity of Fluoroquinolones

Recent studies have also revealed the susceptibility of other eukaryotic cells to some fluoroquinolones, presumably mediated by a topoisomerase II mechanism (128). A number of structurally unrelated fluoroquinolones were shown to have modest killing activity against the bloodstream form of *Trypanosoma brucei brucei* (129). The most active compound was a tetracyclic experimental fluoroquinolone, KB-5246, with a 50% effective concentration for inhibiting trypanosome growth of 1.7 µM. While the other five quinolones tested were less potent in vitro than KB-5246, all prevented growth by a mechanism that was associated with formation of protein-DNA complexes. Unfortunately, as might be expected, cytotoxicity of these agents against L1210 cells paralleled their relative potencies against the parasite (129).

In studies with *Toxoplasma gondii*, trovafloxacin and some of its structural analogues demonstrated significant activity against this parasite, with IC_{50}s ranging from 0.53 to 14.09 μM (102–104). Trovafloxacin and a C-5 methylated derivative at the 1,8-naphthyridone ring had parasitic inhibition values of 98 and 99%, respectively, which was at least fivefold below their cytotoxic levels (102). Few additional studies have explored the direct anti-*Toxoplasma* activity of the fluoroquinolones.

Effects on Immune Cells

Effects of quinolones on mammalian immune cells have also been reported in the literature (20, 21, 41, 72, 87, 146; see also chapter 30). Quinolones have been shown to stimulate thymidine incorporation in phytohemagglutinin-stimulated lymphocytes and inhibit cell cycle progression, mitogen-induced mononuclear cell proliferation, and immunoglobulin secretion in vitro (21, 59, 60). The synthesis of interleukin-1 was reported to be inhibited at high concentrations of ciprofloxacin, while the production of interleukin-2 was up-regulated at the mRNA level (146, 147). Involvement of quinolone interactions with topoisomerase II in mediating these effects has not yet been demonstrated.

SUMMARY

In recent years, quinolones have been optimized for their activities against DNA gyrase and/or topoisomerase IV, leading to compounds with potent antibacterial activities. Although a homologous type II topoisomerase exists in eukaryotic cells, quinolones developed to date for medical use against bacterial infections have demonstrated effects on this enzyme only at concentrations that are 2 to 3 orders of magnitude above that required for antibacterial activity. However, the doctrine that all quinolones are poor antagonists of eukaryotic topoisomerase II needs to be changed in light of the recently reported effects of some quinolones from structurally diverse series. These quinolones induce significant topoisomerase II-mediated DNA cleavage in vitro and produce potent cytotoxic effects in cultured cells. In addition, WIN 58161 has demonstrated DNA-strand breakage in whole cells by alkaline elution. Evidence indicates that some of these quinolones demonstrate antitumor effects in experimental ani-

mal models. Mechanistic studies with CP-115,953 indicate that it is nonintercalating and, unlike the epipodophyllotoxins, fails to block DNA religation mediated by topoisomerase II. Quinolones such as CP-67,015, CP-115,953, A-65281, A-65282, and WIN 58161 are clearly different from quinolones developed so far for clinical use with respect to their potency against topoisomerase II. These observations underscore the importance of carefully testing new quinolones against eukaryotic topoisomerase II and in standard systems for genotoxicity to ensure their safety for future use as antibacterial agents.

REFERENCES

1. **Adachi, Y., M. Luke, and U. K. Laemmli.** 1991. Chromosome assembly in vitro: topoisomerase II is required for condensation. *Cell* **64:**137–148.
2. **Albertini, S., A.-A. Chetelat, B. Miller, W. Muster, E. Pujadas, R. Strobel, and E. Gocke.** 1995. Genotoxicity of 17 gyrase- and four mammalian topoisomerase II-poisons in prokaryotic and eukaryotic test systems. *Mutagenesis* **10:**343–351.
3. **Andersen, A. H., K. Christiansen, E. L. Zechiedrich, E. S. Jensen, N. Osheroff, and O. Westergaard.** 1989. Strand specificity of the topoisomerase II-mediated double-stranded DNA cleavage reaction. *Biochemistry* **28:**6237–6244.
4. **Anderson, V. E., R. P. Zaniewski, F. S. Kaczmarek, T. D. Gootz, and N. Osheroff.** 1999. Quinolones inhibit DNA religation mediated by *Staphylococcus aureus* topoisomerase IV; changes in drug mechanism across evolutionary boundaries. *J. Biol. Chem.* **274:**35927–35932.
5. **Anderson, V. E., R. P. Zaniewski, F. S. Kaczmarek, T. D. Gootz, and N. Osheroff.** 2000. Action of quinolones against *Staphylococcus aureus* topoisomerase IV: basis for DNA cleavage enhancement. *J. Biochem.* **39:**2726–2732.
6. **Andersson, H. C., and B. A. Kihlman.** 1989. The production of chromosomal alterations in human lymphocytes by drugs known to interfere with the activity of DNA topoisomerase II. I. m-AMSA. *Carcinogen* **10:**123–130.
7. **Austin, C. A., and K. L. Marsh.** 1998. Eukaryotic DNA topoisomerase II. *Bioessays* **20:**215–226.
8. **Austin, C. A., J. H. Sng, S. Patel,, and L. M. Fisher.** 1993. Novel HeLa topoisomerase II is the II beta isoform:complete coding sequence and homology with other type II topoisomerases. *Biochim. Biophys. Acta* **1172:**283–291.
9. **Bae, Y.-S., I. Kawasaki, H. Ikeda, and L. F. Liu.** 1988. Illegitimate recombination mediated by calf thymus DNA topoisomerase II in vitro. *Proc. Natl. Acad Sci. USA* **85:**2076–2080.
10. **Baird, C. L., T. T. Harkins, S. K. Morris, and J. E. Lindsley.** 1999. Topoisomerase II drives DNA transport by hydrolyzing one ATP. *Proc. Natl. Acad. Sci. USA* **96:**13685–13690.
11. **Barrett, J. F., T. D. Gootz, P. R. McGuirk, C. A. Farrell, and S. A. Sokolowski.** 1989. Use of in vitro topoisomerase II assays for studying quinolone antibacterial agents. *Antimicrob. Agents Chemother.* **33:**1697–1703.
12. **Barrett, J. F., J. A. Sutcliffe, and T. D. Gootz.** 1990. In vitro assays used to measure the activity of topoisomerases. *Antimicrob. Agents Chemother.* **34:**1–7.
13. **Baugley, B. C.** 1990. The possible role of electron-transfer complexes in the antitumor action of amsacrine analogues. *Biophys. Chem.* **35:**203–212.

14. **Beck, W. T., and M. K. Danks.** 1991. Characterization of multidrug resistance in human tumor cells, p. 3–55. *In* I. G. Robinson (ed.), *Molecular and Cellular Biology of Multidrug Resistance in Tumor Cells.* Plenum Publishing Corp., New York, N.Y.

15. **Bergan, T.** 1988. Pharmacokinetics of fluorinated quinolones, p. 119–154. *In* V. T. Andriole (ed.), *The Quinolones.* Academic Press, Inc., New York, N.Y.

16. **Berrios, M., N. Osheroff, and P. A. Fisher.** 1985. In situ localization of DNA topoisomerase II, a major polypeptide component of the *Drosophila* nuclear matrix fraction. *Proc. Natl. Acad. Sci. USA* **82:**4142–4146.

17. **Bertrand, R., D. Kerrigan, M. Sarang, and Y. Pommier.** 1991. Cell death induced by topoisomerase II inhibitors: role of calcium in mammalian cells. *Biochem. Pharmacol.* **42:**77–85.

18. **Blondeau, J. M.** 1999. Expanded activity and utility of the new fluoroquinolones: a review. *Clin. Ther.* **21:**3–40.

19. **Bodley, A. L., H.-Y. Wu, and L. F. Liu.** 1987. Regulation of DNA topoisomerases during cellular differentiation. *Natl. Cancer Inst. Monogr.* **4:**31–35.

20. **Bredberg, A., M Brant, and M. Jaszyk.** 1991. Ciprofloxacin-induced inhibition of topoisomerase II in human lymphoblastoid cells. *Antimicrob. Agents Chemother.* **35:**448–450.

21. **Bredberg, A., M. Brant, K. Riesbeck, Y. Azou, and A. Forsgren,** 1989. 4-Quinolone antibiotics: positive genotoxic screening tests despite an apparent lack of mutation induction. *Mutat. Res.* **211:**171–180.

22. **Brighty, K. E. and Gootz, T. D.** 2000. Chemistry and mechanism of action of the quinolone antibacterials, p. 34–82. *In* V. T. Andriole (ed.), *The Quinolones*, 3rd ed. Academic Press, New York, N.Y.

23. **Bugg, B. Y., M. K. Danks, W. T. Beck, and D. P. Suttle.** 1991. Expression of a mutant DNA topoisomerase II in CCRF-CEM human leukemic cells selected for resistance to teniposide. *Proc. Natl. Acad. Sci. USA* **88:**7654–7658.

24. **Burden, D. A., P. S. Kingma, S. J. Froelich-Ammon, M.-A. Bjornsti, M. W. Patchan, R. B. Thompson, and N. Oseroff.** 1996. Topoisomerase II-etoposide interactions direct the formation of drug-induced enzyme-DNA cleavage complexes. *J. Biol. Chem.* **271:**29238–29244.

25. **Burden, D. A., and N. Osheroff.** 1998. Mechanism of action of eukaryotic topoisomerase II and drugs targeted to the enzyme. *Biochim. Biophys. Acta* **1400:**139–154.

26. **Burden, D. A., and D. M. Sullivan.** 1994. Phosphorylation of the alpha- and beta-isoforms of DNA topoisomerase II is qualitatively different in terphase and mitosis in Chinese hamster ovary cells. *Biochemistry* **33:**14651–14655.

27. **Capranico, G., S. Tinelli, C. A. Austin, M. L. Fisher, and F. Zunio.** 1992. Different patterns of gene expression of topoisomerase II isoforms in differentiated tissues during murine development. *Biochim. Biophys. Acta* **1132:**43–48.

28. **Charcosset, J.-Y., J.-M. Saucier, and A. Jacquemin-Sablon.** 1988. Reduced DNA topoisomerase II activity and drug-stimulated DNA cleavage in 9-hydroxyellipticine-resistant cells. *Biochem. Pharmacol.* **37:**2145–2149.

29. **Chen, G. L., L. Yang, T. C. Rowe, B. D. Halligan, K. M. Tewey, and L. F. Liu.** 1984. Nonintercalative antitumor drugs interfere with the breakage-reunion reaction of mammalian DNA topoisomerase II. *J. Biol. Chem.* 1984 **259:**13560–13566.

30. **Chetelat, A. A., S. Albertini, and E. Gocke.** 1996. The photomutagenicity of fluoroquinolones in tests for gene mutation, chromosomal aberration, gene conversion and DNA breakage (comet assay). *Mutagenesis* **11:**497–504.

31. **Chow, K.-C., C. K, King, and W. E. Ross.** 1988. Abrogation of etoposide-mediated cytotoxicity by cycloheximide. *Biochem. Pharmacol.* **31:**1117–1122.

32. **Chow, K-C.,T. L. MacDonald, and W. E. Ross.** 1988. DNA binding by epipodophyllotoxins and N-acetyl anthracyclines: implications for mechanism of topoisomerase II inhibition. *Mol. Pharmacol.* **34:**467–473.

33. **Chow, K.-C., and W. E. Ross.** 1987. Topoisomerase-specific drug sensitivity in relation to cell cycle progression. *Mol. Cell. Biol.* **7:**3119–3123.

34. **Chistman, M. F., F. S. Dietrich, and G. R. Fink.** 1988. Mitotic recombination in the rDNA of *S. cerevisiae* is suppressed by the combined action of DNA topoisomerases I and II. *Cell* **55:**413–425.

35. **Chu, D. T. W., and P. B. Fernandes.** 1989. Structure-activity relationships of the fluoroquinolones. *Antimicrob. Agents Chemother.* **33:**131–135.

36. **Christ, W., T. Lehnert, and V. Ulbrich.** 1988. Specific toxicologic aspects of the quinolones. *Rev. Infect. Dis.* **10**(Suppl. 1):S141–S146.

37. **Clement, J. J., N. Burres, K. Jarvis, D. T. Chu, J. Swinlarski, and J. Alder.** 1995. Biological characterization of a novel antitumor quinolone. *Cancer Res.* **55:**830–835.

38. **Coughlin, S. A., D. W. Danz, R. G. Robinson, K. M. Klingbeill, M. P. Wentland, T. H. Corbett, W. R. Waud, L. A. Zwelling, E. Altschuler, E. Bales, and J. B. Rake.** 1995. Mechanism of action and antitumor activity of (S)-10-(2,6-dimethyl-4-pyridinyl)-9-fluoro-3-methyl-7-oxo-2,3-dihydro-7H-pyridol[1,2,3-de]-[1,4]benzothiazine-6-carboxylic acid (WIN 58161). *Biochem. Pharmacol.* **50:**111–122.

39. **Coughlin, S. A., D. W. Danz, R. G. Robinson, P. S. Moskwa, M. P. Wentland, G. Y. Lesher, and J. B. Rake.** 1991. Mechanism of action of WIN-58161. *Proc. Am. Assoc. Cancer Res.* **32:**337.

40. **Crespi, M. D., A. G. Mladovan, and A. Baldi.** 1988. Increment of DNA topoisomerases in chemically and virally transformed cells. *Exp. Cell Res.* **175:**206–215.

41. **Crumplin, G. C.** 1990. In vitro genotoxicity assessment and the effects of 4-quinolones upon human cells, p. 173–200. *In* G. C. Crumplin (ed.), *The 4-Quinolones: Antibacterial Agents In Vitro.* Springer-Verlag, London, United Kingdom.

42. **Danks, M. K., C. A. Schmidt, M. C. Cirtain, D.P. Suttle, and W. T. Beck.** 1988. Altered catalytic activity of and DNA cleavage by DNA topoisomerase II from human leukemic cells selected for resistance to VM-26. *Biochemistry* **27:**8861–8869.

43. **D'Arpa, P., P. S. Machlin, H. Ratrie, III, N. F.Rothfeld, D. W. Cleveland, and W. C. Earnshaw.** 1988. cDNA cloning of human DNA topoisomerase I: catalytic activity of a 67.7-kDa carboxyl-terminal fragment. *Proc. Natl. Acad. Sci. USA* **85:**2543–2547.

44. **Davies, S. M., C. N. Robson, S. L. Davies, and I. D. Hickson.** 1988. Nuclear topoisomerase II levels correlate with the sensitivity of mammalian cells to intercalating agents and epipodophyllotoxins. *J. Biol. Chem.* **263:**17724–17729.

45. **Deffie, A. M., J. K. Batra, and G. J. Goldenberg.** 1989. Direct correlation between DNA topoisomerase II activity and cytotoxicity in adriamycin-sensitive and -resistant P388 leukemia cell lines. *Cancer Res.* **48:**58–62.

46. **Dillehay, L. E., D. Jacobson-Kram, and J. R. Williams.** 1989. DNA topoisomerases and models of sister-chromatid exchange. *Mutat. Res.* **215:**15–23.

47. **DiNardo, S., K. Voelkel, and R. Sternglanz.** 1984. DNA topoisomerase II mutant *Saccharomyces cerevisiae*: topoisomerase II is required for segregation of daughter molecules at the termination of DNA replication. *Proc. Natl. Acad. Sci. USA* **81:**2616–2620.

48. Domagala, J. M., L. D. Hanna, C. L. Heifetz, M.P. Hutt, T. F. Mich, J. P. Sanchez, and M. Solomon. 1986. New structure-activity relationships of the quinolone antibacterials using the target enzyme. The development and application of a DNA gyrase assay. *J. Med. Chem.* **29**:394–404.

49. Drake, F. H., G. A. Hofmann, H. F. Bartus, M. R. Mattern, S. T. Crooke, and C. K. Mirabelli. 1989. Biochemical and pharmacological properties of p170 and p180 forms of topoisomerase II. *Biochemistry* **28**:8154–8160.

50. Drlica, K., and X. Zhao. 1997. DNA gyrase, topoisomerase IV, and the 4-quinolones. *Microbiol. Mol. Biol. Rev.* **61**:377–392.

51. Duget, M., C. Lavenot, F Harper, G. Mirambeau, and A. De Recondo. 1983. DNA topoisomerases from rat liver: physiological variations. *Nucleic Acids Res.* **11**:1059–1075.

52. Earnshaw, W. C., B. Halligan, C. A. Cooke, M. M. S. Heck, and L. F. Liu. 1985. Topoisomerase II is a structural component of mitotic chromosome scaffolds. *J. Cell Biol.* **100**:1706–1715.

53. Earnshaw, W. C., and M. M. S. Heck. 1985. Localization of topoisomerase II in mitotic chromosomes. *J. Cell Biol.* **100**:1716–1725.

54. Elsea, S. H., Y. Hsiung, J. L. Nitiss, and N. Osheroff. 1995. A yeast type II topoisomerase selected for resistance to quinolones. Mutation of histidine 1012 to tyrosine confers resistance to nonintercalative drugs but hypersensitivity to ellipticine. *J. Biol. Chem.* **270**:1913–1920.

55. Elsea, S. H., P. R. McGuirk, T. D. Gootz, M. Moynihan, and N. Osheroff. 1993. Drug features that contribute to the activity of quinolones against mammalian topoisomerase II and cultured cells: correlation between enhancement of enzyme-mediated DNA cleavage in vitro and cytotoxic potential. *Antimicrob. Agents Chemother.* **37**:2179–2186.

56. Elsea, S. H., N. Osheroff, and J. Nitiss. 1992. Cytotoxicity of quinolones toward eukaryotic cells. Identification of topoisomerase II as the primary cellular target for the quinolone CP-115,953 in yeast. *J. Biol. Chem.* **267**:13150–13153.

57. Elsea, S. H., M. Westergaard, D. A. Burden, J. P. Lomenick, and N. Osheroff. 1997. Quinolones share a common interaction domain on topoisomerase II with other DNA cleavage-enhancing antineoplastic drugs. *Biochemistry* **36**:2919–2924.

58. Estey, E., R. C. Adlakha, W. N. Hittelman, and L. A. Zwelling. 1987. Cell cycle dependent variations in drug-induced topoisomerase II-mediated DNA cleavage and cytotoxicity. *Biochemistry* **26**:4338–4344.

59. Forsgren, A., A. Bredberg, A. B. Pardee, S. F. Schlossman, and T. E Tedder. 1987. Effects of ciprofloxacin on eucaryotic pyrimidine nucleotide biosynthesis and cell growth. *Antimicrob. Agents Chemother.* **31**:774–779.

60. Forsgren, A., S. E Schlossman, and T. F. Tedder. 1987. 4-Quinolone drugs affect cell cycle progression and function of human lymphocytes in vitro. *Antimicrob. Agents Chemother.* **31**:768–773.

61. Fortune, J. M., and N. Osheroff. 2000. Topoisomerase II as a target for anticancer drugs: when enzymes stop being nice. *Progr. Nucleic Acids Res. Mol. Biol.* **64**:221–253.

62. Friche, E., M. K. Danks, C. A. Schmidt, and W. T. Beck. 1991. Decreased DNA topoisomerase II in daunorubicin-resistant Ehrlich ascites tumor cells. *Cancer Res.* **51**:4213–4218.

63. Froelich-Ammon, S. J., D. A. Burden, M. W. Patchan, S. H. Elsea, R. B. Thompson and N. Osheroff. 1995. Increased drug affinity as the mechanistic basis for drug hypersensitivity of a mutant type II topoisomerase. *J. Biol. Chem.* **270**:28018–28021.

64. Froelich-Ammon, S. J., and N. Osheroff. 1995. Topoisomerase poisons: harnessing the dark side of enzyme mechanism. *J. Biol. Chem.* **270**:21429–21432.

65. Froelich-Ammon, S. J., M. W. Patchan, N. Osheroff, and R. B. Thompson. 1995. Topoisomerase II binds to ellipticine in the absence or presence of DNA: characterization of enzyme-drug interactions by fluorescence spectroscopy. *J. Biol. Chem.* **270**:14998–15005.

66. Gale, K. C., and N. Osheroff. 1990. Uncoupling the DNA cleavage and religation activities of topoisomerase II with a single-stranded nucleic acid substrate: evidence for an active enzyme-cleaved DNA intermediate. *Biochemistry* **29**:9538–9545.

67. Gasser, S. M., and U. K. Laemmli. 1986. The organization of chromatin loops: characterization of a scaffold attachment site. *EMBO J.* **5**:511–518.

68. Gasser, S. M., T. Laroche, J. Falquet, E. Boy de la Tour, and U. K. Laemmli. 1986. Metaphase chromosome structure: involvement of topoisomerase II. *J. Mol. Biol.* **188**:613–629

69. Giaever, G., R. Lynn, T. Goto, and J. C.Wang. 1986. The complete nucleotide sequence of the structural gene *TOP2* of yeast DNA topoisomerase ll. *J. Biol. Chem.* **261**:12448–12454.

70. Glisson, B., R. Gupta, S. Smallwood-Kentro, and W. Ross. 1986. Characterization of acquired epipodophyllotoxin resistance in a Chinese hamster ovary cell line: loss of drug-stimulated DNA cleavage activity. *Cancer Res.* **46**:1934–1938.

71. Gocke, E., S. Albertini, A. A. Chetelat, S. Kirchner, and W. Muster. 1998. The photomutagenicity of fluoroquinolones and other drugs. *Toxicol. Lett.* **102–103**:375–381.

72. Gootz, T. D., J. F. Barrett, and J. A. Sutcliffe. 1990. Inhibitory effects of quinolone antibacterial agents on eucaryotic topoisomerases and related test systems. *Antimicrob. Agents Chemother.* **34**:8–12.

73. Goto, T., and J. C. Wang. 1984. Yeast DNA topoisomerase II is encoded by a single-copy, essential gene. *Cell* **36**: 1073–1080.

74. Harkins, T. T., T. J. Lewis, and J. E. Lindsley. 1998. Pre-steady-state analysis of ATP hydrolysis by *Saccharomyces cerevisiae* DNA topoisomerase II. 2. Kinetic mechanism for the sequential hydrolysis of two ATPs. *Biochemistry* **37**:7299–7312.

75. Harkins, T. T. and J. E. Lindsley. 1998. Pre-steady-state analysis of ATP hydrolysis by *Saccharomyces cerevisiae* DNA topoisomerase II. 1. A DNA-dependent burst in ATP hydrolysis. *Biochemistry* **37**:7292–7298.

76. Heck, M. M. S., and W. C. Earnshaw. 1986.Topoisomerase II: a specific marker for cell proliferation. *J. Cell Biol.* **103**:2569–2581.

77. Hertzberg, R. P., R. W. Busby, M. J. Caranfa, K. G. Holden, R. K. Johnson, S. M. Hecht, and W. D. Kingsbury. 1990. Irreversible trapping of the DNA-topoisomerase I covalent complex: affinity labeling of the camptothecin binding site. *J. Biol. Chem.* **265**:19287–19295.

78. Holden, H. E., J. F. Barrett, C. M. Huntington, P. A. Muehlbauer, and M. G. Wahrenburg. 1989. Genetic profile of a nalidixic acid analog: a model for the mechanism of sister chromatid exchange induction. *Environ. Mol. Mutagen.* **13**:238–252.

79. Holden, J. A., D.H. Rolfson, and C. T. Wittwer. 1990. Human DNA topoisomerase II: evaluation of enzyme activity in normal and neoplastic tissue. *Biochemistry* **29**:2127–2134.

80. Holm, C., J. M. Covey, D. Kerrigan, and Y. Pommier. 1989. Differential requirement of DNA replication for the cytotox-

icity of DNA topoisomerase I and II inhibitors in Chinese hamster DC3F cells. *Cancer Res.* **49**:6365–6368.

81. Holm, C., T. Goto, J. C. Wang, and D. Botstein. 1985. DNA topoisomerase II is required at the time of mitosis in yeast. *Cell* **41**:553–563.

82. Hooper, D. C. 1998. Bacterial topoisomerases, anti-topoisomerases, and anti-topoisomerase resistance. *Clin. Infect. Dis.* **27**:S54-S63.

83. Hooper, D. C., and J. S. Wolfson. 1989. Adverse effects of quinolone antimicrobial agents, p. 249–271. *In* J. S. Wolfson and D. C. Hooper (ed.), *Quinolone Antimicrobial Agents.* American Society for Microbiology, Washington, D.C.

84. Hooper, D. C., and J. S. Wolfson. 1991. Fluoroquinolone antimicrobial agents. *N. Engl. J. Med.* **324**:384–394.

85. Hoshino, K., K. Sato, K. Akahane, A. Yoshida, I. Hayakawa, M. Sato, T. Une, and Y. Osada. 1991. Significance of the methyl group on the oxazine ring of ofloxacin derivatives in the inhibition of bacterial and mammalian type II topoisomerases. *Antimicrob. Agents Chemother.* **35**:309–312.

86. Hoshino, K., K. Sato, T. Une, and Y. Osada. 1989. Inhibitory effects of quinolones on DNA gyrase of *Escherichia coli* and topoisomerase Il of fetal calf thymus. *Antimicrob. Agents Chemother.* **33**:1816–1818.

87. Hosomi, J., A. Maeda, Y. Oomori, T. Irikura, and T. Yokota. 1988. Mutagenicity of norfloxacin and AM-833 in bacteria and mammalian cells. *Rev. Infect. Dis.* **10**(Suppl. 1):S148–S149.

88. Howard, M. T., M. P. Lee, T.-S. Hsieh, and J. D. Griffith. 1990. *Drosophila* topoisomerase II-DNA interactions are affected by DNA structure. *J. Mol. Biol.* **217**:53–62.

89. Hsiung, Y., S.H. Elsea, N. Osheroff, and J. L. Nitiss. 1995. Identification of a eukaryotic topoisomerase II mutation conferring hypersensitivity to etoposide: the amino acid homologous to Ser83 of gyrA interacts with eukaryotic topoisomerase inhibitors. *J. Biol. Chem.* **270**:20359–20364.

90. Hsiang, Y.-H., J. B. Jiang, and L. F. Liu. 1989. Topoisomerase II-mediated DNA cleavage by amonafide and its structural analogs. *Mol. Pharmacol.* **36**:371–376.

91. Hsiang, Y.-H., and L. F. Liu. 1989. Evidence for the reversibility of cellular DNA lesions induced by mammalian topoisomerase II poisons. *J. Biol. Chem.* **264**:9713–9715.

92. Hsiang, Y.-H., H.-Y. Wu, and L. F. Liu. 1988. Proliferation-dependent regulation of DNA topoisomerase II in cultured cells. *Cancer Res.* **48**:3230–3235.

93. Huang, W. M. 1996. Bacterial diversity based on type II DNA topoisomerase II genes. *Annu. Rev. Genet.* **30**:79–107.

94. Huff, A. C., and K. N. Kreuzer. 1990. Evidence for a common mechanism of action for antitumor and antibacterial agents that inhibit type II DNA topoisomerases. *J. Biol. Chem.* **265**:20496–20505.

95. Huff, A. C., J. K. Leatherwood, and K. N. Kreuzer. 1989. Bacteriophage T4 DNA topoisomerase is the target of antitumor agent 4′-(9-acridinylamino) methane sulfon-*m*-anisidide (*m*-AMSA) in T4-infected *Escherichia coli. Proc. Natl. Acad. Sci. USA* **86**:1307–1311.

96. Hussy, P., G. Maass, B. Tummler, F. Grosse, and U. Schomburg. 1986. Effect of 4-quinolones and novobiocin on calf thymus DNA polymerase a primase complex, topoisomerase I and II, and growth of mammalian lymphoblasts. *Antimicrob. Agents Chemother.* **29**:1073–1078.

97. Jeffrey, A.M., L. Shao, S.Y. Brendler-Schwaab, G. Schlutter, and G. M. Williams. 2000. Photochemical mutagenicity of phototoxic and photochemically carcinogenic fluoro-

quinolones in comparison with the photostable moxifloxacin. *Arch. Toxicol.* **74**:555–559.

98. Jefson, M. R., P. R. McGuirk, A. E. Girard, T. D. Gootz, and J. F. Barrett. 1989. The synthesis and properties of optically pure C10-heteroaryl quinolones structurally related to ofloxacin, abstr. 1190. *In Program Abstracts 29th Interscience Conference on Antimicrobial Agents Chemotherapy.* American Society for Microbiology Washington, D.C.

99. Jeggo, P. A., K. Caldecott, S. Pidsley, and G.R. Banks. 1989. Sensitivity of Chinese hamster ovary mutants defective in DNA double-strand break repair to topoisomerase II inhibitors. *Cancer Res.* **49**:7057–7063.

100. Jenkins, J. R., P. Ayton, T. Jones, S. L. Davies, D. L. Simmons, A. L. Harris, D. Sheer, and I. D. Hickson. 1992. Isolation of cDNA clones encoding the beta isozyme of human DNA topoisomerase II and localization of the gene to chromosome 3p24. *Nucleic Acids Res.* **20**:5587–5592.

101. Kaufman, S. H. 1989. Induction of endonucleolytic DNA cleavage in human acute myelogenous leukemia cells by etoposide, camptothecin, and other cytotoxic anticancer drugs: a cautionary note. *Cancer Res.* **49**:5870–5878.

102. Khan, A. A., F. G. Araujo, K. E. Brighty, T. D. Gootz, and J. S. Remington. 1999. Anti-*Toxoplasma gondii* activities and structure-activity relationships of novel fluoroquinolones related to trovafloxacin. *Antimicrob. Agents Chemother.* **43**:1783–1787.

103. Khan, A. A., T. Slifer, F. G. Araujo, R. J. Polzer, and J. S. Remington. 1997. Activity of trovafloxacin in combination with other drugs for treatment of acute murine toxoplasmosis. *Antimicrob. Agents Chemother.* **41**:893–897.

104. Khan, A. A., T. Slifer, F. G. Araujo, and J. S. Remington. 1996. Trovafloxacin is active against *Toxoplasma gondii. Antimicrob. Agents Chemother.* **40**:1855–1859.

105. Kim, R. A., and J. C. Wang. 1989. A sub-threshold level of DNA topoisomerases leads to the excision of yeast rDNA as extrachromosomal rings. *Cell* **57**:975–985.

106. Kingma, P. S., D. A. Burden, and N. Osheroff. 1999. Binding of etoposide to topoisomerase II in the absence of DNA: decreased affinity as a mechanism of drug resistance. *Biochemistry* **38**:3457–3461.

107. Klecak, G., F. Urbach, and H. Urwyler. 1997. Fluoroquinolone antibacterials enhance UVA-induced skin tumors. *J. Photochem. Photobiol. B* **37**:174–181.

108. Kohlbrenner, W. E., N. Wideburg, D. Weigl, A. Saldivar, and D. T. W. Chu. 1992. Induction of calf thymus topoisomerase II-mediated DNA breakage by the antibacterial isothiazolo-quinolones A-65281 and A-65282. *Antimicrob. Agents Chemother.* **36**:81–86.

109. Kreuzer, K. N., and N. R. Cozzarelli. 1979. *Escherichia coli* mutants thermosensitive for deoxyribonucleic acid gyrase subunit A: effects on deoxyribonucleic acid replication, transcription and bacteriophage growth. *J. Bacteriol.* **140**:424–435.

110. Kroll, D. J., and T. C. Rowe. 1991. Phosphorylation of DNA topoisomerase II in a human tumor cell line. *J. Biol.Chem.* **266**:7957–7961.

111. Kupfer, F. A. , L. Bodley, and L. F. Liu. 1987. Involvement of intracellular ATP in cytotoxicity of topoisomerase II-targeting antitumor drugs. *Natl. Cancer Inst. Monogr.* **4**:37–40.

112. Levine, C., H. Hiasa, and K. J. Marians. 1998. DNA gyrase and topoisomerase IV: biochemical activities, physiological roles during chromosome replication and drug sensitivities. *Biochim. Biophys. Acta* **1400**:29–43.

113. Lin, M., L. F. Liu, D. Jacobson-Kram, and J. R. Williams. 1986. Induction of sister chromatid exchanges by inhibitors of topoisomerases. *Cell Biol. Toxicol.* **2**:485–494.

114. Liu, L. F. 1989. DNA topoisomerase poisons as antitumor drugs. *Annu. Rev. Biochem.* **58:**351–375.

115. Liu, L. F., J. L. Davis, and R. Calendar. 1981. Novel topologically knotted DNA from bacteriophage P4 capsids: studies with DNA topoisomerases. *Nucleic Acids Res.* **9:**3979–3989.

116. Liu, L. F., T. C. Rowe, L. Yang, K. M. Tewey, and G. L. Chen. 1983. Cleavage of DNA by mammalian DNA topoisomerase II. *J. Biol. Chem.* **258:**15365–15370.

117. Lock, R. B., and W. E. Ross. 1987. DNA topoisomerases in cancer therapy. *Anticancer Drug Design* **2:**151–154.

118. Long, B. H. 1987. Structure-activity relationships of podophyllin congeners that inhibit topoisomerase II. *Natl. Cancer Inst. Monogr.* **4:**123–127.

119. Lynn, R., G. Giaever, S. L. Swanberg, and J. C. Wang. 1986. Tandem regions of yeast DNA topoisomerase II share homology with different subunits of bacterial gyrase. *Science* **233:**647–649.

120. Makinen, M., P. D. Forbes, and F. Stenback. 1997. Quinolone antibacterials: a new class of photochemical carcinogens. *J. Photochem. Photobiol. B* **37:**182–187.

121. Markovits, J., Y. Pommier, D. Kerrigan, J. M. Covey, E. J. Tilden, and K. W. Kohn. 1987. Topoisomerase II-mediated DNA breaks and cytotoxicity in relation to cell proliferation and the cell cycle in NIH 3T3 fibroblasts and L1210 leukemia cells. *Cancer Res.* **47:**2050–2055.

122. McQueen, C. A,, and G. M. Williams. 1987. Effects of quinolone antibiotics in tests for genotoxicity. *Am. J. Med.* **82**(Suppl. 4A):94–96.

123. Miller, K. G., L.F. Liu, and R. T. Englund. 1981. A homogeneous type II DNA topoisomerase from HeLa cell nuclei. *J. Biol. Chem.* **256:**9334–9339.

124. Mitelman, F., A.-M. Kolnig, B. Strombeck, R. Norrby, B. Kromann-Andersen, P. Sommer, and J. Wadstein. 1988. No cytogenetic effects of quinolone treatment in humans. *Antimicrob. Agents Chemother.* **32:**936–937.

125. Muller, M. T., J. R. Spitzner, J. A. DiDonato, V. B. Mehta, and K. Tsutsui. 1988. Single-strand DNA cleavages by eukaryotic topoisomerase II. *Biochemistry* **27:**8369–8379.

126. Nelson, W., K. Cho, Y. Hsiang, L. F. Liu, and D. S. Coffey. 1987. Growth-related elevations of DNA topoisomerase II levels found in Dunning R3327 rat prostatic adenocarcinomas. *Cancer Res.* **47:**3246–3250.

127. Nelson, E. M., K. M. Tewey, and L. F Liu. 1984. Mechanism of antitumor drug action: poisoning of mammalian DNA topoisomerase II on DNA by 4'-(9-acridinylamino) methane-sulfon-*m*-anisidide. *Proc. Natl. Acad. Sci. USA* **81:**1361–1365.

128. Nenortas, E. C., A. L. Bodley, and T. A. Shapiro. 1998. DNA topoisomerases: a new twist for antiparasitic chemotherapy? *Biochim. Biophys. Acta* **1400:**349–354.

129. Nenortas, E. C., C. Burri, and T. A. Shapiro. 1999. Antitrypanosomal activity of fluoroquinolones. *Antimicrob. Agents Chemother.* **43:**2066–2068.

130. Newport, J., and T. Spann. 1987. Disassembly of the nucleus in mitotic extracts: membrane vesicularization, lamin disassembly, and chromosome condensation are independent processes. *Cell* **48:**219–230.

131. Nitiss, J., and J. C. Wang. 1988. DNA topoisomerase-targeting antitumor drugs can be studied in yeast. *Proc. Natl. Acad. Sci. USA* **85:**7501–7505.

132. Oomori, Y., T. Yasue, H. Aoyama, K. Hirai, S. Suzue, and T. Yokota. 1988. Effects of fleroxacin on HeLa cell functions and topoisomerase II. *J. Antimicrob. Chemother.* **22**(Suppl. D):91–97.

133. Osheroff, N. 1986. Eukaryotic topoisomerase II: characterization of enzyme turnover. *J. Biol. Chem.* **261:**9944–9950.

134. Osheroff, N. 1987. Role of the divalent cation in topoisomerase II-mediated reactions. *Biochemistry* **26:**6402–6406.

135. Osheroff, N. 1989. Biochemical basis for the interactions of type I and type II topoisomerases with DNA. *Pharmacol. Ther.* **41:**223–241.

136. Osheroff, N. 1989. Effect of antineoplastic agents on the DNA cleavage/religation equilibrium of eukaryotic topoisomerase II: inhibition of DNA religation by etoposide *Biochemistry* **28:**6157–6160.

137. Osheroff, N., E. R. Shelton, and D. L. Brutlag. 1983. DNA topoisomerase II from *Drosophila melanogaster:* relaxation of supercoiled DNA. *J. Biol. Chem.* **258:**9536–9543.

138. Osheroff, N., and E. L. Zechiedrlch. 1987. Calcium-promoted DNA cleavage by eukaryotic topoisomerase II: trapping the covalent enzyme-DNA complex in an active form. *Biochemistry* **26:**4303–4309.

139. Osheroff, N., E. L. Zechiedrich, and K. C. Gale. 1991. Catalytic function of DNA topoisomerase II. *Bioessays* **13:**269–275.

140. Ouedraogo, G., P. Morliere, R. Santus, M.A. Miranda, and J.V. Castell. 2000. Damage to mitochondria of cultured human skin fibroblasts photosensitized by fluoroquinolones. *J. Photochem. Photobiol. B.* **58:**20–25.

141. Phillips, I. 1987. Bacterial mutagenicity and the 4-quinolones. *J. Antimicrob. Chemother.* **20:**771–773.

142. Pommier, Y., D. Kerrigan, J. M. Covey, C.-S. Kao-Shan, and J. Whang-Peng. 1988. Sister chromatid exchanges, chromosomal aberrations, and cytotoxicity produced by antitumor topoisomerase II inhibitors in sensitive (DC3F) and resistant (DC3F/9-OHE) Chinese hamster cells. *Cancer Res.* **48:**512–516.

143. Pommier, Y., J. K. Minford, R. E. Schwartz, L. A. Zwelling, and K. W. Kohn. 1985. Effects of the intercalators 4'-(9-acridinylamino)-*m*-anisidide (*m*-AMSA, amsacrine) and 2-methyl-9-hydroxyellipticinium (2-Me-9-OH-E+) on topoisomerase II-mediated DNA strand cleavage and strand passage. *Biochemistry* **24:**6410–6416.

144. Pommier, Y., L. A. Zwelling, C.-S. Kao-Shan, J. Whang-Peng, and M. O. Bradley. 1985. Correlations between intercalator-induced DNA strand breaks and sister chromatid exchanges, mutations, and cytotoxicity in Chinese hamster ovary cells *Cancer Res.* **45:**3143–3149.

145. Potmesil, M., Y.-H. Hsiang, L. F. Liu, B. Bank, H. Grossberg, S. Kirschenbaum, T. J. Forlenzar, A. Penziner, D. Kanganis, D. Knowles, F. Tranganos, and R. Silber. 1988. Resistance of human leukemic and normal lymphocytes to drug-induced DNA cleavage and low levels of DNA topoisomerase II. *Cancer Res.* **48:**3537–3543.

146. Riesbeck, K., J. Andersson, M. Gullberg, and A. Forsgren. 1989. Fluorinated 4-quinolones induce hyperproduction of interleukin 2. *Proc. Natl. Acad. Sci. USA* **86:**2809–2813.

147. Riesbeck, K. and A. Forsgren. 1995. CP-115,953 stimulates cytokine production by lymphocytes. *Antimicrob. Agents Chemother.* **39:**476–483.

148. Robinson, M. J., B. A. Martin, T. D. Gootz, P. R. McGuirk, M. Moynihan, J. A. Sutcliffe, and N. Osheroff. 1991. Effects of quinolone derivatives on eukaryotic topoisomerase II: a novel mechanism for enhancement of enzyme-mediated DNA cleavage. *J. Biol. Chem.* **266:**14585–14592.

149. Robinson, M. J., B. A. Martin, T. D. Gootz, P. R. McGuirk, and N. Osheroff. 1992. Effects of novel fluoroquinolones on the catalytic activities of eukaryotic topoisomerase II: influence of the C-8 fluorine group. *Antimicrob. Agents Chemother.* **36:**751–756.

150. Robinson, M. J., and N. Osheroff. 1990. Stabilization of the topoisomerase II-DNA cleavage complex by antineoplastic

drugs: inhibition of enzyme-mediated DNA religation by 4'-(9-acridinyl-amino) methane sulfon-m-anisidide. *Biochemistry* **29:**2511–2515.

151. Robinson, M. J., and N. Osheroff. 1991. Effects of antineoplastic drugs on the post-strand passage DNA cleavage/religation equilibrium of topoisomerase II. *Biochemistry* **30:**1807–1813.

152. Rose, D., W. Thomas, and C. Holm. 1990. Segregation of recombined chromosomes in meiosis I required DNA topoisomerase II. *Cell* **60:**1009–1017.

153. Rosen, J. E., A. K. Prahalad, G. Schluter, D. Chen, and G. M. Williams. 1997. Quinolone antibiotic photodynamic production of 8-oxo-7,8-dihydro-2'-deoxyguanine in cultured liver epithelial cells. *Photochem. Photobiol.* **65:**990–996.

154. Ross, W. E., T. Rowe, B. Glisson, J. Yalowich, and L. Liu. 1984. Role of topoisomerase II in mediating epipodophyllotoxin-induced DNA cleavage. *Cancer Res.* **44:**5857–5860.

155. Sander, M. and T.-S. Hsieh. 1983. Double-strand DNA cleavage by type II DNA topoisomerase from *Drosophila melanogaster. J. Biol. Chem.* **258:**8421–8428.

156. Sander, M., and T.-S.Hsieh. 1985. *Drosophila* topoisomerase II double-strand DNA cleavage: analysis of DNA sequence homology at the cleavage site. *Nucleic Acids Res.* **13:**1057–1072.

157. Schluter, G. 1986. Toxicology of ciprofloxacin, p. 61–70. *In* H.C. Neu and H. Wenta (ed.), *Proceedings of the First International Ciprofloxacin Workshop.* Elsevier Science Publishing Inc., Amsterdam, The Netherlands.

158. Schneider, E., Y.-H. Hsiang, and L. F. Liu. 1990. DNA topoisomerases as anticancer drug targets. *Adv. Pharmacol.* **21:**149–183.

159. Schneider, E., P. A. Lawson, and R. K. Ralph. 1989. Inhibition of protein synthesis reduces the cytotoxicity of 4'-(9-acridinylamino)methane sulfon-*m*-anisidide without affecting DNA breakage and DNA topoisomerase II in murine mastocytoma cell line. *Biochem. Pharmacol.* **38:**263–269.

160. Shen, L. L., W. E. Kohlbrenner, D. Weigl, and J. Baranowski. 1989. Mechanism of quinolone inhibition of DNA gyrase: appearance of unique norfloxacin binding sites in enzyme-DNA complexes. *J. Biol. Chem.* **264:**2973–2978.

161. Shen, L. L., L. A. Mitscher, P. N. Sharma, T. J. O'Donnell, D. W. T. Chu, C. S. Cooper, T. Rosen, and A. G. Pernet. 1989. Mechanism of inhibition of DNA gyrase by antibacterials: a cooperative drug-DNA binding model. *Biochemistry* **28:**3886–3894.

162. Snyder, R. D., and C. S. Cooper. 1999. Photogenotoxicity of fluoroquinolones in Chinese hamster V79 cells:dependency on active topoisomerae II. *Photochem. Photobiol.* **69:**288–293.

163. Spratt, T. E., S. S. Schultz, D. E. Levy, D. Chen, G. Schluter, and G. M. Williams. 1999. Different mechanisms for the photoinduced production of oxidative DNA damage by fluoroquinolones differing in photostability. *Chem. Res. Toxicol.* **12:**809–815.

164. Stahlmann, R., and H. Lode. 1988. Safety overview: toxicity adverse effects and drug interactions, p. 201–233. *In* V. T. Andriole (ed.), *The Quinolones,* 3rd ed. Academic Press, Inc., New York, N.Y.

165. Sullivan, D. M., K.-C. Chow, B. S. Glisson, and W. E. Ross. 1987. Role of proliferation in determining sensitivity to topoisomerase II-active chemotherapy agents. *Natl. Cancer Inst. Monogr.* **4:**73–78.

166. Sullivan, D. M., M. D. Latham, and W. E. Ross. 1987. Proliferation-dependent topoisomerase II content as a determinant of antineoplastic drug action in human, mouse, and Chinese hamster ovary cells. *Cancer Res.* **47:**3973–3979.

167. Sullivan, D. M., M. D. Latham, T. C. Rowe, and W. E. Ross. 1989. Purification and characterization of an altered topoisomerase II from a drug-resistant Chinese hamster ovary cell line. *Biochemistry* **28:**5680–5687.

168. Sutcliffe, J. A., T. D. Gootz, and J. F. Barrett. 1989. Biochemical characteristics and physiological significance of major DNA topoisomerases. *Antimicrob. Agents Chemother.* **33:**2027–2033.

169. Tabary, X., N. Moreau, C. Dureuil, and F. LeGoffic. 1987. Effect of DNA gyrase inhibitors pefloxacin, five other quinolones, novobiocin, and clorobiocin on *Escherichia coli* topoisomerase I. *Antimicrob. Agents Chemother.* **31:**1925–1928.

170. Tewey, K. M., G. L. Chen, E. M. Nelson, and L. F. Liu. 1984. Intercalative antitumor drugs interfere with the breakage-reunion reaction of mammalian topoisomerase II. *J. Biol. Chem.* **259:**9182–9187.

171. Traynor, N. J., and N. K. Gibbs. 1999. The phototumorigenic fluoroquinolone lomefloxacin photosensitizes pyrimidine dimer formation in human keratinocytes in vitro. *Photochem. Photobiol.* **70:**957–959.

172. Tsai-Pflugfelder, M., L. F. Liu, A. A. Liu, K. M. Tewey, J. Whang-Peng, T. Knutsen, K. Huebner, C. M. Croce, and J. C. Wang. 1988. Cloning and sequencing of cDNA encoding human DNA topoisomerase II and localization of the gene to chromosome region 17q21–22. *Proc. Natl. Acad. Sci. USA* **85:**7177–7181.

173. Tse-Ding, Y.-C., and J. C. Wang. 1986. Complete nucleotide sequence of the *topA* gene encoding *Escherichia coli* DNA topoisomerase I. *J. Mol. Biol.* **191:**321–331.

174. Uemura, T., K. Morikawa, and M. Yanagida. 1986. The nucleotide sequence of the fission yeast DNA topoisomerase II gene; structural and functional relationships to other DNA topoisomerases. *EMBO J.* **5:**2355–2361.

175. Uemura, T., H. Ohkuru, Y. Adachi, K. Morino, K. Shiozaki, and M. Yanagida. 1987. Topoisomerase II is required for condensation and separation of mitotic chromosomes in *S. pombe. Cell* **50:**917–925.

176. Uemura, T., and M. Yanagida. 1984. Isolation of type I and II DNA topoisomerase mutants from fission yeast; single and double mutants show different phenotypes in cell growth and chromatin organization. *EMBO J.* **3:**1737–1744.

177. Uemura, T., and M. Yanagida. 1986. Mitotic spindle pulls but fails to separate chromosomes in type II DNA topoisomerase mutants: uncoordinated mitosis. *EMBO J.* **5:**1003–1010.

178. Umezawa, N., K. Arakane, A. Ryu, S. Mashiko, M. Hirobe, and T. Nagano. 1997. Participation of reactive oxygen species in phototoxicity induced by quinolone antibacterial agents. *Arch. Biochem. Biophys.* **342:**275–281.

179. Wadkins, R. M., and D. E. Graves. 1991. Interactions of anilinoacridines with nucleic acids: effects of substituent modifications on DNA binding properties. *Biochemistry* **30:**4278–4283.

180. Wagi, N., and K. Tawara. 1992. Possible direct role of reactive oxygens in the cause of cutaneous phototoxicity induced by five quinolones in mice. *Arch. Toxicol.* **66:**392–397.

181. Wang, J. C. 1985. DNA topoisomerases. *Annu. Rev. Biochem.* **54:**665–697.

182. Wang, J. C. 1996. DNA topoisomerases. *Annu. Rev. Biochem.* **65:**635–692.

183. Waring, M. J. 1981. DNA modification and cancer. *Annu. Rev. Biochem.* **50:**159–192.

184. Watanabe, M., K. Tsutsui, K. Tsutsui, and Y. Inoue. 1994. Differential expressions of the topoisomerase II alpha and II beta mRNAs in developing rat brain. *Neurosci. Res.* **19:**51–57.

185. Wentland, M. P. 1990. Structure-activity relationships of fluorquinolones, p. 1–43. *In* C. Siporin, C. L. Heifetz, and J. M. Domagala (ed.), *The New Generation of Quinolones.* Marcel Dekker, Inc., New York, N.Y.

186. Wentland, M. P. G. Y. Lesher, M. Reuman, G. M. Pilling, M. T. Saindane, R. B. Perni, M. A. Eissenstat, J. D. Weaver III, J. B. Rake, and S. A. Coughlin. 1991. Mammalian topoisomerase II inhibitory activity of 1,8-bridged-7-(2,6 dimethy-4-pyridinyl)-3-quinolone carboxylic acids. *Proc. Am. Assoc. Cancer Res.* 32:336.

187. Wilson, W. R., B. C. Baugley, L. P. G. Wakelin, and M. J. Waring. 1981. Interaction of the antitumor drug 4′-(9-acridinylamino) methane sulfon-*m*-anisidide and related acridines with nucleic acids. *Mol. Pharmacol.* 20:404–414.

188. Wood, E. R., and W. C. Earnshaw. 1990. Mitotic chromatin condensation in vitro using somatic cell extracts and nuclei with variable levels of endogenous topoisomerase II. *J. Cell Biol.* 111:2839–2850.

189. Yamashita, Y., T. Ashizawa, M. Morimoto, J. Hosomi, and H. Nakano. 1992. Antitumor quinolones with mammalian topoisomerase II-mediated DNA cleavage activitiy. *Cancer Res.* 52:2818–2822.

190. Yang, L., T. C. Rowe, E. M. Nelson, and L. F. Liu. 1985. In vivo mapping of DNA topoisomerase II-specific cleavage sites on SV40 chromatin. *Cell* 41:127–132.

191. Yoshida, H., M. Bogaki, M. Nakamura, L. M. Yamanaka, and S. Nakamura. 1991. Quinolone resistance determining region in the DNA gyrase *gyrB* gene of *Escherichia coli. Antimicrob. Agents Chemother.* 35:1647–1650.

192. Zechiedrich, E. L., K. Christiansen, A. H. Andersen, O. Westergaard, and N. Osheroff. 1989. Double-stranded DNA cleavage religation reaction of eukaryotic topoisomerase II: evidence for a nicked DNA intermediate. *Biochemistry* 28:6229–6236.

193. Zechiedrich, E. L., and N. Osheroff. 1990. Eukaryotic topoisomerases recognize nucleic acid topology by preferentially interacting with DNA crossovers. *EMBO J.* 9:4555–4562.

194. Zhang, H., P. D'Arpa, and L. F. Liu. 1990. A model for tumor cell killing by topoisomerase poisons. *Cancer Cells* 2:23–27.

195. Zimmer, C., K. Storl, and J. Storl. 1990. Microbial DNA topoisomerases and their inhibition by antibiotics. *J. Basic Microbiol.* 30:209–224.

196. Zwelling, L. A. 1989. Topoisomerase II as a target of antileukemia drugs: a review of controversial areas. *Hematol. Pathol.* 3:101–112.

197. Zwelling, L. A., M. Hinds, D. Chan, J. Mayes, K. L. Sie, E. Parker, L. Silberman, A. Radcliffe, M. Beran, and M. Blick. 1989. Characterization of an amsacrine-resistant line of human leukemia cells. *J. Biol. Chem.* 264:16411–16420.

Quinolone Antimicrobial Agents, 3rd ed.
Edited by David C. Hooper and Ethan Rubinstein
© 2003 ASM Press, Washington, D.C.

Chapter 5

Activity In Vitro of the Quinolones

C. THAUVIN-ELIOPOULOS AND G. M. ELIOPOULOS

In the decade since our previous review of this topic (45), the fluoroquinolones have become established as an indispensable class of antimicrobials in the hospital setting as well as in the community. At the same time, resistance has become an increasing concern. Resistance to fluoroquinolones emerged rapidly among staphylococci, particularly among methicillin-resistant strains of *Staphylococcus aureus*. Much of this can be attributed to clonal spread (133). Rates of resistance among *Pseudomonas aeruginosa* have also risen. In the United States, more than 23% of nosocomial intensive care unit isolates of this species recovered in 1999 were resistant to fluoroquinolones (www.cdc.gov/ncidod/hip/NNIS/ar_surv99.pdf). During treatment of *P. aeruginosa* infections in the hospital setting, resistance to ciprofloxacin emerged in 11% of patients treated with this fluoroquinolone (24). With the widespread use of fluoroquinolones for treatment of community-acquired pneumonia following the introduction of treatment guidelines, there is concern that rates of resistance to the class will climb among strains of *Streptococcus pneumoniae* as well. Therefore, considerable effort has been devoted to the development of new fluoroquinolones with enhanced activity against gram-positive bacteria.

This chapter will review the in vitro activities of the currently available and several investigational fluoroquinolones on the basis of data from published literature. Our primary purpose is to explore the potential antimicrobial spectrum of the class rather than to highlight specific agents. Therefore, neither inclusion nor omission of individual agents should be interpreted as reflecting a judgment on our part of their current or likely future roles in clinical therapy. The in vitro activity of these compounds is only one of several factors that ultimately define the potential contribution of these or any other antimicrobial agents. Clearly, the pharmacokinetic attributes of specific agents (chapter 6), as well as their individual safety profiles (chapters 25–29), are also critical factors in determining their eventual

contributions. Because of the possible drifts in levels of susceptibility to the fluoroquinolones that might have occurred in organisms collected during several years, this chapter will focus primarily on data derived since the publication of the previous edition of this book.

ANTIMICROBIAL ACTIVITY

Gram-Negative Bacteria

Enterobacteriaceae

Against the *Enterobacteriaceae*, ciprofloxacin remains among the most potent of the fluoroquinolones developed to date. In one large study reported in 1995 that included >11,000 strains of this family, ciprofloxacin inhibited 90% of isolates at a concentration of 0.25 μg/ml or less (124). Approximately 95% of recent isolates of *Escherichia coli* remain susceptible to ciprofloxacin and levofloxacin (128). In some regions, fluoroquinolone resistance among *E. coli* has risen to high levels. Only 67% of *E. coli* isolates collected in 1998 from 44 medical centers in Taiwan were susceptible to ciprofloxacin; 11.3% were fully resistant (102). High rates of resistance were seen among isolates from adult outpatients (11.9%) as well as from hospital inpatients (17.5%). Although some agents such as clinafloxacin or sitafloxacin may appear more active than ciprofloxacin against ciprofloxacin-resistant isolates (10, 20, 112), activities of the former drugs are substantially reduced also, compared with their activities against fluoroquinolone-susceptible isolates (Tables 1 and 2). Approximately 94% of recent *Klebsiella pneumoniae* isolates were susceptible to ciprofloxacin or levofloxacin (86, 128), and most studies report MICs at which 90% of the isolates tested are inhibited (MIC$_{90}$s) of these agents of ≤0.25 μg/ml (Tables 1 and 2). Most strains of *Klebsiella oxytoca* remain susceptible as well (10, 16, 53, 112, 124, 146).

C. Thauvin-Eliopoulos and G. M. Eliopoulous • Department of Medicine, Beth Israel Deaconess Medical Center, Boston, MA 02215, and Harvard Medical School, Boston, MA 02115.

Table 1. Susceptibility of *Enterobacteriaceae* to earlier fluoroquinolones[a]

Organism	Representative MIC$_{90}$ (range) (µg/ml) of:								
	CPX	OFX	LVX	SPX	LOM	CLX	TOS	SIT	TVX
Escherichia coli	0.25 (0.015->128)	0.25 (0.06-0.25)	0.5 (0.025-32)	0.5 (0.05-0.5)	0.25 (0.25-0.39)	0.06 (0.008-4)	0.06 (0.05-0.06)	1	0.5 (0.025-32)
Klebsiella pneumoniae	0.5 (0.05-0.5)	2 (0.25-2)	0.5 (0.05-1)	0.5 (0.1-1)	2	0.12 (0.03-0.12)	0.5 (0.1-0.5)	0.12	0.5 (0.1-1)
Klebsiella oxytoca	0.06 (0.015-0.12)	0.5 (0.12-0.5)	0.12 (0.06-0.13)	0.06 (0.05-0.06)	0.5	0.03 (0.03)	0.06 (0.025-0.06)	0.03	0.12 (0.12-0.13)
Klebsiella spp.	0.5 (0.25-8)	1 (1-8)	1 (1-8)	1 (0.5-8)					1 (0.5-4)
Serratia marcescens	2 (0.5-12.5)	4 (1-25)	2 (0.25-8)	12.5	4	0.25 (0.125-2)	6.25 (2-6.25)	0.5	4 (0.5-8)
Enterobacter cloacae	0.25 (0.025-2)	1 (0.12-1)	0.5 (0.05-2)	0.2	2 (2-3.13)	0.25 (0.016-0.25)	0.2 (0.2-1)	0.25	0.5 (0.05-2)
Enterobacter aerogenes	0.5 (0.03->16)	0.25 (0.1-1)	0.5 (0.06-16)		2 (0.39-2)	0.5 (0.06-2)		1	0.5 (0.12->16)
Enterobacter agglomerans	0.12 (0.015-1)	0.25 (0.06-0.5)			0.5	0.5			
Citrobacter freundii	0.25 (0.05-2)	1 (0.25-4)	0.5 (0.06-2)	1.56	8	0.12 (0.06-0.25)	0.78 (0.25-0.78)	0.5	1 (0.1-4)
Citrobacter diversus	0.06 (0.015-0.06)	0.25 (0.06-0.25)	0.13 (0.03-0.13)		0.25	0.13			0.25
Proteus mirabilis	0.12 (0.025-4)	0.25 (0.12-0.5)	0.12 (0.05-4)	0.5 (0.25-0.78)	0.5	0.12 (0.06-0.5)	0.25 (0.2-0.25)	0.5	0.5 (0.2-16)
Proteus vulgaris	0.06 (0.03-0.12)	0.5 (0.12-0.5)	0.12 (0.06-0.25)	0.5 (0.39-0.5)		0.06 (0.03-0.06)	0.39	0.12	0.5 (0.25-1)
Morganella morganii	0.06 (0.015-1)	0.25 (0.12-0.25)	0.12 (0.06-1)	0.5	0.39	0.12 (0.03-0.25)		0.25	0.5 (0.03-4)
Providencia rettgeri	0.5 (0.025-4)	2 (2-4)	1 (0.1-4)		2	0.06	1		0.5 (0.2-4)
Providencia stuartii	4-8 (0.12->16)	>8 (1->16)	4 (0.25->16)		>8	0.06	>4		1 (0.25->16)
Hafnia alvei	0.03 (≤ 0.06)	0.06 (0.03-0.25)	0.06 (0.03-0.25)		0.25	0.016			0.06 (0.03-0.06)

[a] Data were derived from the following references: for ciprofloxacin (CPX), 4, 7, 10, 16, 26, 34, 50, 53, 54, 86, 93, 112, 115, 123, 124, 128, 138, 146, 150, 151; ofloxacin (OFX), 4, 16, 50, 54, 86, 93, 115, 124, 146; levofloxacin (LVX), 7, 10, 16, 34, 50, 86, 112, 115, 128, 138, 150, ; sparfloxacin (SPX), 53, 86, 115, 146, 151; clinafloxacin (CLX), 10, 26, 34, 112; sitafloxacin (SIT), 112; tosulfoxacin (TOS), 54, 146; lomefloxacin (LMX), 93, 124; trovafloxacin (TVX), 7, 10, 26, 34, 50, 112, 115, 138, 150, 151. Data for fleroxacin can be found in references 54 and 124.

Table 2. Susceptibility of *Enterobacteriaceae* to more recent quinolone antimicrobials[a]

Organism	Representative MIC$_{90}$ (range) (μg/ml) of:							
	GAT	MOX	GEM	GARE	PGE-932	PGE-924	PGE-997	E-4767
Escherichia coli	0.25 (0.016–8)	0.25 (0.008–32)	0.016 (0.015–1)	0.1 (0.06–0.1)	0.12	0.12	0.5	0.007
Klebsiella pneumoniae	1 (0.1–1)	1 (0.13–1)	(0.12–0.25)	0.5 (0.1–0.5)	4	4	8	0.06
Klebsiella oxytoca	0.12 (0.06–0.12)	0.25 (0.12–0.25)	(0.03–0.25)	0.25	1	1	2	0.015
Klebsiella spp.	1 (0.5–1)	8	0.25					
Serratia marcescens	4 (2–12.5)	4 (0.5–8)	(0.25–1)	2	4	4	16	0.25
Enterobacter cloacae	0.5 (0.06–1)	1 (0.06–2)	(0.25–1)	0.25 (0.1–0.5)	1	1	2	0.06
Enterobacter aerogenes	1 (1–16)	2 (0.25–>16)	(0.12–0.25)	0.25	2	2	4	0.007
Enterobacter agglomerans	1	2	0.015					≤0.003
Citrobacter freundii	2 (1–4)	2 (1–4)	2	0.2 (0.2–0.25)	2	2	4	0.015
Citrobacter diversus	0.25	0.25						
Proteus mirabilis	0.25 (0.2–4)	0.5 (0.25–16)	0.12	1	1	2	2	0.03
Proteus vulgaris	0.39 (0.25–0.5)	1 (0.5–1)	0.12	(1.56–8)	1	1	2	
Morganella morganii	0.5 (0.25–2)	0.5 (0.13–4)	0.12 (0.06–0.12)	1	1	2	2	
Providencia rettgeri	0.5	1 (0.5–2)	8	2	2	4	2	0.25
Providencia stuartii	0.5	1 (0.5–2)	(0.25–>8)	2	>16	>16	>16	0.5
Hafnia alvei	0.06	0.13	0.03					

[a] Data were derived from the following references: for gatifloxacin (GAT), 10, 86, 112, 146, 151; moxifloxacin (MOX), 10, 50, 112, 115; gemifloxacin (GEM), 30, 47, 110a, 150; garenoxacin (GARE), 50, 138; PGE-932, PGE-924, PGE-997, 7; E-4767 and E-5065, 54. Data on additional compounds can be found as follows: CFC-222 (93); DV-7751a (16); AF-3013 (115).

The 7-azetidin, 8-chlorofluoroquinolone compounds E-4767 and E-5065 appear to be slightly more active than ciprofloxacin against *Klebsiella* spp., but the test panels did not include fluoroquinolone-resistant strains (54). Although fluoroquinolone MIC$_{90}$ against *Citrobacter freundii* are generally higher than those against *Citrobacter diversus*, resistant strains of both species are encountered (10, 16, 124).

Fluoroquinolones are an important option for the treatment of *Enterobacter* spp. infections because of high rates of resistance to β-lactams in this genus due to production of chromosomal enzymes (89). Results from a 1999 U.S. nationwide survey revealed that approximately 95% of *Enterobacter aerogenes* remained ciprofloxacin and levofloxacin susceptible; however, only 88% of *Enterobacter cloacae* were susceptible to ciprofloxacin (128). Again, certain investigational agents appeared more potent than ciprofloxacin against strains with reduced fluoroquinolone susceptibility, but with little evidence of useful levels of activity against the more highly ciprofloxacin-resistant organisms (10, 34, 112). In the aforementioned nationwide survey, ciprofloxacin susceptibility was reported for approximately 91% of *Proteus mirabilis*, but only 63% of *Providencia* spp. (128). Several studies show *Proteus stuartii* to be generally more resistant to fluoroquinolones than *Proteus rettgeri* (54, 124, 138, 150), while others show either the reverse, or little difference (10, 16, 146). Reduced susceptibility to ciprofloxacin and other fluoroquinolones is encountered more often among *Morganella morganii* than among *Proteus vulgaris* (10, 112, 138, 150, 151) (Tables 1 and 2).

Pseudomonas spp. and other gram-negative organisms

The activity demonstrated by ciprofloxacin against *P. aeruginosa* when this drug was first released, together with its availability in an oral formulation, represented a breakthrough in antimicrobial chemotherapy. Over time, the frequency of resistance has continued to rise, however. Only 76% of 380 *P. aeruginosa* isolates from 1997 and 71% of 464 isolates collected in 1999 were susceptible to ciprofloxacin (86, 128). Clinafloxacin and sitafloxacin are more potent than ciprofloxacin against some strains (Table 3), but none of the agents introduced into clinical practice in the United States or Western Europe since the approval of ciprofloxacin offers any obvious advantage compared with the earlier agent. The MIC$_{90}$ of ciprofloxacin was >1 μg/ml in 15 of 19 studies cited in Table 3. This stands in contrast to the situation that prevailed when this subject was reviewed in 1993, when only 6 of 44 studies reported MIC$_{90}$s exceeding 1 μg/ml (45).

The evaluation of antimicrobial susceptibilities of certain nonfermenting gram-negative organisms is limited by the lack of clearly defined standard testing methods for some members of this group. Only 6% of 66 strains of *Burkholderia cepacia* studied by Bonacorsi et al. (18) using Mueller-Hinton agar demonstrated susceptibility to ciprofloxacin (Table 3). In a study by Biedenbach et al. (15), 46% of 52 isolates of this species studied by broth microdilution were inhibited by gatifloxacin at ≤1 μg/ml. Examining 11 isolates of *Burkholderia mallei*, Heine

Table 3. Susceptibility of nonfermenting organisms to fluoroquinolones[a]

Organism	Range of MIC$_{90}$s (μg/ml) for:								
	CPX	OFX	LVX	TVX	GAT	MOX	GEM	SIT	CLX
P. aeruginosa	0.5–128	4–>128	2–128	2–>128	>4–32	8–>128	4	4	0.5–4
P. fluorescens	1–2	8	2–4	4–8	4	16			0.5
P. putida	1–8	>8	2	8	4				1
P. stutzeri	0.06–1	0.25–2	0.25–0.5	0.13–0.5	0.25	1			0.06
B. cepacia	>2–>256	4–25	4–256	4–>256	12.5–256	4–256		4	4–128
S. maltophilia	>2–32	8–64	2–32	1–64	2–32	1–128	4	0.25–8	0.5–8

[a] Data derived from the following references: for ciprofloxacin (CPX), 7, 10, 15, 16, 18, 26, 28, 34, 46, 50, 53, 54, 78, 86, 93, 112, 115, 123, 124, 128, 138, 146, 150, 151; ofloxacin (OFX), 15, 16, 46, 50, 54, 86, 115, 116, 124, 146; levofloxacin (LVX), 7, 10, 15, 16, 28, 34, 50, 78, 86, 112, 115, 123, 128, 138, 150; trovafloxacin (TVX), 7, 10, 15, 26, 34, 46, 50, 78, 112, 115, 116, 123, 138, 150, 151; gatifloxacin (GAT), 10, 15, 28, 86, 112, 116, 146, 151; moxifloxacin (MOX), 10, 50, 112, 115, 116; gemifloxacin (GEM), 150; sitafloxacin (SIT), 112, 116; and clinafloxacin (CLX), 10, 26, 34, 112. Additional data are available as follows: sparfloxacin (15, 53, 86, 115, 146, 151), tosufloxacin (54, 146), fleroxacin (124), grepafloxacin (116), lomefloxacin (124), T-3811 (123, 138), DV-7751a (16), CFC-222 (93), PGE-932, PGE-924. PGE-997 (7), E-4767, E-5065 (54), AF-3013 (115).

et al. (70) found lower fluoroquinolone MICs using an E-test method as compared with a microdilution method using cation-adjusted Mueller-Hinton broth. The MIC$_{90}$ of ciprofloxacin was 0.25 μg/ml by the former method and 1 μg/ml by the latter; results for ofloxacin were 1 μg/ml and 8 μg/ml, respectively. Isolates of *Stenotrophomonas maltophilia* are more likely to be susceptible to levofloxacin than to ciprofloxacin. In three studies, 53, 57, and 89% of strains were susceptible to levofloxacin, while 8, 29, and 34% were susceptible to ciprofloxacin in the corresponding collections (28, 34, 128). Against *S. maltophilia*, trovafloxacin is often ≥fourfold more active than ciprofloxacin based on MIC$_{90}$s (26, 34, 78, 112, 150). Moxifloxacin and gatifloxacin also appear to be more active than ciprofloxacin; clinafloxacin and sitafloxacin MIC$_{90}$s of ≤1 μg/ml have been reported (26, 34, 112). Additional data on fluoroquinolone activity against less commonly encountered isolates of nonfermenting bacteria are also available (10, 46).

Data presented on *Aeromonas* spp. suggest high degrees of susceptibility to a wide variety of fluoroquinolones (Table 4). The MIC$_{90}$s of ciprofloxacin and

ofloxacin against 10 isolates of *Flavobacterium meningosepticum* were >8 μg/ml (124). The susceptibilities to fluoroquinolones of *Acinetobacter* spp. vary. In the largest series of 428 isolates, >90% of which were *Acinetobacter baumannii*, MIC$_{90}$s were as follows: sitafloxacin, 2 μg/ml; clinafloxacin, 4 μg/ml; gatifloxacin, 8 μg/ml; moxifloxacin, trovafloxacin, levofloxacin, 16 μg/ml; ciprofloxacin, >16 μg/ml (112). Sahm et al. (128) reported that 51% of *Acinetobacter* spp. were susceptible to ciprofloxacin and 54% were susceptible to levofloxacin. Deshpande et al. (34) found 67 and 75% susceptible to these two agents, respectively. Fung-Tomc et al. (50) found the desfluoro(6) quinolone, garenoxacin (BMS-284756, T-3811ME), to be fourfold more active than levofloxacin or moxifloxacin and eightfold more active than ciprofloxacin against *A. baumannii*.

Gastrointestinal pathogens

The fluoroquinolones have been widely used to treat infectious diarrhea. Most bacterial pathogens are susceptible to this class (Table 5). Studying a collection

Table 4. Activities of fluoroquinolones against miscellaneous gram-negative bacteria[a]

Organism	Range of MIC$_{90}$s (μg/ml) of:							
	CPX	OFX	LVX	SPX	TVX	GAT	CLX	MOX
Acinetobacter spp.	0.06–>256	0.25–>8	0.05–32	0.1–16	0.025–32	0.03–8	0.13–8	>0.25–16
Aeromonas spp.	0.008–≤0.06	0.03–≤0.06	≤0.015–0.03	0.12	0.008–0.03	0.03	0.008	0.03
Alcaligenes spp.	4–32	4–32	2–32	32	8		8	2
Flavobacterium spp.	4–>8	4–>8	2–32	4–16	0.25–4		4	0.5
Eikenella corrodens	0.016	0.01	0.016–0.03	0.03–0.06	0.016	0.016		0.125
Pasteurella multocida	0.008–0.016	0.03	0.016–0.03	0.004–0.008	0.016	0.016		0.06

[a] Data derived from the following references: for ciprofloxacin (CPX), 7, 10, 16, 34, 47, 50, 53, 58, 59, 71, 93, 112, 120, 124, 128, 138, 145, 146, 150, 151; for ofloxacin (OFX), 16, 47, 50, 58, 93, 120, 124, 145, 146; for levofloxacin (LVX), 7, 10, 16, 34, 47, 50, 71, 112, 128, 138, 150; for sparfloxacin (SPX), 53, 58, 59, 120, 145, 146, 151; for trovafloxacin (TVX), 7, 10, 34, 47, 50, 59, 71, 112, 138, 145, 150, 151; for gatifloxacin (GAT), 10, 59, 71, 112, 146, 151; for clinafloxacin (CLX), 10, 34, 71, 112, 145; for moxifloxaxin (MOX), 10, 50, 60, 71, 112. Additional data are available for: fleroxacin (124), norfloxacin (47), sitafloxacin (112), lomefloxacin (124), grepafloxacin (47), T-3811 (138), CFC-222 (93), PGE-924, PGE-932, PGE-997 (7), DV-7751a (16), gemifloxacin (47, 71, 150).

Table 5. Susceptibilities of gastrointestinal tract pathogens to fluoroquinolone antimicrobials[a]

| Drug | Range of MIC$_{90}$s (μg/ml) against: | | | | | |
	Salmonella spp.	Shigella spp.	Campylobacter jejuni	Yersinia enterocolitica	Vibrio cholerae	Helicobacter pylori
Ciprofloxacin	0.01–0.25	0.008–≤0.06	0.12–64	0.016–0.06	0.004	0.06–0.5
Norfloxacin	0.5–1	0.06	>128	0.06		
Ofloxacin	0.12–0.5	0.06–0.12	0.25–32	0.12–0.25	0.016	0.12
Levofloxacin	0.03–0.25	0.016–0.03	0.12–32	0.03–0.06	0.008	0.25–0.5
Trovafloxacin	0.03–1	≤0.015–0.03	0.03–8	0.03–0.06	0.008	0.13–0.25
Gatifloxacin	0.06–0.25	0.016–0.03	0.25–4	0.06		0.25
Moxifloxacin	0.12–0.25	0.03–0.06	0.06–0.13	0.06–0.12	0.03	0.5
Gemifloxacin	0.015–0.12	≤0.015–0.25	128	0.015–0.03		
Garenoxacin	0.12	0.03	0.12	0.06	0.008	0.06

[a] Data derived from the followiing references: for ciprofloxacin, 10, 16, 47, 50, 53, 54, 67, 73, 75, 112, 124, 138, 150, 151; for norfloxacin, 47, 73; for ofloxacin, 16, 47, 50, 54, 73, 124; for levofloxacin, 10, 16, 47, 50, 73, 150; for trovafloxacin, 10, 47, 50, 112, 138, 150, 151; for gatifloxacin, 10, 67, 112, 151; for moxifloxacin, 10, 50, 112; for gemifloxacin, 47, 150; for garenoxacin, 50, 138. Additional data are available for other compounds: lomefloxacin (124), tosufloxacin (73), fleroxacin (124), sparfloxacin (53, 73, 151), grepafloxacin (47), sitafloxacin (112), clinafloxacin (10, 112), DV-7751a (16), E-4767 and E-5065 (54).

of 284 enteropathogens from Asia, Africa, and the Americas, Gomi et al. (61) found 90% of isolates susceptible to ciprofloxacin and levofloxacin at ≤0.25 μg/ml and ≤0.5 μg/ml, respectively. MIC$_{90}$s of ciprofloxacin against both enterotoxigenic and enteroaggregative *E. coli* were 0.25 μg/ml (61). Most strains of *Shigella* spp. are exquisitely susceptible to ciprofloxacin and other agents. However, strains of *S. sonnei* for which ciprofloxacin MICs are >8 μg/ml have been reported (124). In addition, failures of fluoroquinolone therapy of *S. sonnei* diarrhea have been noted in several patients with strains that demonstrated resistance to nalidixic acid (MIC > 100 μg/ml) and reduced susceptibility to ciprofloxacin and sparfloxacin (MICs, 0.19–0.39 μg/ml) and to ofloxacin (MICs, 0.78–1.56 μg/ml) (75). In our previous review (45), strains of *Salmonella* spp. studied were highly susceptible to ciprofloxacin (MIC$_{90}$s ≤ 0.06 μg/ml). In more recent articles, MIC$_{90}$s up to 0.25 μg/ml have been reported (53, 73, 151). A community outbreak of nalidixic acid-resistant *Salmonella enterica* serotype Typhimurium DT104 occurred in Denmark in 1998 (114). Although MICs of ciprofloxacin still fell within the susceptible range, the MICs of ciprofloxacin were 10-fold higher against these nalidixic acid-resistant strains than expected for fully susceptible isolates. In the United Kingdom, nalidixic acid resistance was seen in 21% of *S. enterica* serovar Typhi isolates collected in 1998 and in 23% of those recovered in 1999 (141, 142). Fluoroquinolone treatment failures have been described. MICs of the fluoroquinolones (ciprofloxacin, levofloxacin, tosufloxacin, sparfloxacin) against nalidixic acid-resistant strains of *S. enterica* serovar Typhi were 4 to 16 times higher than those against nalidixic acid-susceptible isolates (73).

Against ciprofloxacin-susceptible isolates of *Campylobacter jejuni*, Bauernfeind (10) found moxifloxacin and trovafloxacin (MIC$_{90}$s, 0.13 μg/ml) to be more active than levofloxacin (MIC$_{90}$, 0.5 μg/ml) or ciprofloxacin (MIC$_{90}$, 1 μg/ml). Unfortunately, fluoroquinolone resistance has increased significantly in this species as well (136). Only 32% of 91 strains of *C. jejuni* from patients with gastroenteritis reported in a study from Spain were susceptible to any of several fluoroquinolones (47). Gatifloxacin appears to be more active than ciprofloxacin against this species (10, 67). Ciprofloxacin inhibited all strains of two aerotolerant species, *Campylobacter cryaerophila* (12 isolates) and *Campylobacter butzleri* (64 isolates), at ≤0.25 μg/ml (92). Most strains of *Yersinia enterocolitica* are quite susceptible to various fluoroquinolones (Table 5). However, ciprofloxacin and trovafloxacin MICs up to 2 μg/ml have been documented (112). Several of the newer fluoroquinolones inhibit *Helicobacter pylori* at concentrations ≤0.5 μg/ml; however, the rank order of potencies differs between studies (10, 50).

Respiratory tract pathogens

The fluoroquinolones display potent activity against many gram-negative respiratory pathogens. MIC$_{90}$s of ciprofloxacin against *Haemophilus influenzae* are generally ≤0.03 μg/ml, irrespective of whether strains are β-lactamase producers (Table 6). The more recently introduced agents, such as levofloxacin, sparfloxacin, trovafloxacin, moxifloxacin, and gatifloxacin, share high levels of activity against these organisms. In a survey conducted in 1998 in the United States, 100% of >6,500 isolates were susceptible to ciprofloxacin at concentrations of 0.5

µg/ml or less (82). Occasionally, resistant strains are encountered, but these are uncommon (21, 124, 138). While rare strains of *Moraxella catarrhalis* with ciprofloxacin MICs of 1 to 4 µg/ml exist (52, 85, 112, 150), virtually all isolates are inhibited at ≤0.5 µg/ml. Against a recent collection of >3,600 strains, the MIC_{90} of ciprofloxacin was 0.06 µg/ml (82). Against the rare isolates with MICs of ciprofloxacin or levofloxacin >0.5 µg/ml, activities of gemifloxacin, trovafloxacin, gatifloxacin, or moxifloxacin may be substantially greater, with MICs of 0.25 µg/ml or less (52, 85, 112, 150).

Neisseria meningitidis remain exquisitely susceptible to various fluoroquinolones. MIC_{90}s as low as 0.001 µg/ml have been recorded for trovafloxacin (151). Eleven strains of *Bordetella pertussis* were inhibited by levofloxacin and clinafloxacin at a concentration of 0.03 µg/ml, by moxifloxacin at 0.015 µg/ml, and by ciprofloxacin, trovafloxacin, and gatifloxacin at 0.008 µg/ml (10). Against 45 isolates of *B. pertussis* recovered in northern California from December 1998 to August 1999, the MIC_{90}s of ciprofloxacin (range, ≤0.002 to 0.064 µg/ml), gatifloxacin, and trovafloxacin were 0.032, 0.06, and 0.032 µg/ml, respectively (62). Various agents, including ciprofloxacin, trovafloxacin, clinafloxacin, levofloxacin, moxifloxacin, gemifloxacin, and the desfluoro(6) quinolone, garenoxacin, are highly active against strains of *Legionella* spp., with MICs of 0.03 µg/ml or less (42, 81, 138). For several members of this class, activity against intracellular organisms has been validated using infected monocyte or pulmonary alveolar macrophage cultures, or in animal models, or both (42, 45, 81).

The role of atypical bacteria in community-acquired respiratory tract infections has been increasingly well appreciated. Activity against such organisms is a major reason why antimicrobials of this class (Table 6) have been widely adopted for the treatment of community-acquired pneumonia (8). Ciprofloxacin and levofloxacin MIC_{90}s against *Mycoplasma pneumoniae* typically range from 1 to 2 µg/ml (12, 13, 50, 90, 123). The fluoroquinolone, Q-35, inhibited 50 strains of this species at ≤0.78 µg/ml (56). MIC_{90}s of trovafloxacin and gatifloxacin of approximately 0.5 µg/ml have been reported (12, 90, 123), while potencies of moxifloxacin, sparfloxacin, and grepafloxacin (0.12 to 0.3 µg/ml) were greater still (11, 12, 13, 66, 90). In one study, garenoxacin proved 32-fold more potent than levofloxacin, inhibiting 10 strains of *M. pneumoniae* at 0.03 µg/ml (123). In another article, overall potencies or the two agents were comparable, but the desfluoro(6) quinolone inhibited all strains at 0.12 µg/ml, while levofloxacin did so only at 1 µg/ml (50).

Ciprofloxacin generally inhibits *Chlamydia pneumoniae* at approximately 2 µg/ml (113, 151). Several of the newer agents are more potent: gatifloxacin, sparfloxacin, sitafloxacin, and tosufloxacin MIC_{90}s are reported to be in the range of 0.06 to 0.12 µg/ml (113, 151). Garenoxacin inhibited 20 strains of *C. pneumoniae* at ≤0.03 µg/ml, while in the same study levofloxacin and moxifloxacin MIC_{90}s and MIC_{100}s were both 1 µg/ml (103). Sitafloxacin and sparfloxacin inhibited seven isolates of *Chlamydia psittaci* at concentrations of 0.063 µg/ml or less; ciprofloxacin inhibited these isolates at concentrations of 1 to 2 µg/ml (113). The in vitro activity of fluoroquinolones against *C. psittaci* predicted success in a mouse model of pneumonia. The 50% effective doses of sitafloxacin, sparfloxacin, tosufloxacin, ofloxacin, and ciprofloxacin were 1.1, 0.95, 1.56, 7.6, and 9.20 mg/kg, respectively (113). Chlamydiacidal activity within one dilution of the MICs has been reported (113). However, experiments utilizing long-term cell cultures suggest that viable *Chlamydia trachomatis* or *C. pneumoniae* may persist intracellularly for long periods even after treatment with potent fluoroquinolones (39, 100).

Gram-Positive Bacteria

Staphylococci

In recent years, efforts to develop new fluoroquinolones have led primarily to compounds with enhanced activity against gram-positive organisms (43). Activities of representative fluoroquinolones against staphylococci and other gram-positive bacteria are shown in Table 7. Several new series of agents that demonstrate enhanced activities against gram-positive bacteria have been explored. These include desfluoro(6) quinolones (50, 138), nonfluorinated quinolones (7, 50, 126), C-7 sulfonyl compounds (1, 3), C-7 bicyclic amines (93, 94), and C-7 azetidins (29, 53, 64). Although 90% or more of methicillin-susceptible strains of *Staphylococcus aureus* will be susceptible even to ciprofloxacin or ofloxacin (6, 37, 112, 124, 146), the great majority of methicillin-resistant *S. aureus* (MRSA) isolates are now resistant to these older agents. The newer agents, while substantially more potent than earlier compounds against both fluoroquinolone-susceptible and -resistant strains, nevertheless demonstrate reduced levels of activity against the latter. Reported MICs against MRSA sometimes vary over a substantial range, suggesting either heterogeneity in strain collections or methodological differences in testing. Against MRSA, representative MIC_{90}s from studies of the most active quinolones are: gemifloxacin, 8 µg/ml

Table 6. Susceptibility of gram-negative and atypical respiratory pathogens to quinolone antimicrobials[a]

Organism	Range of MIC90s (µg/ml) for:							
	CPX	OFX	LVX	TVX	GAT	MOX	GEM	GARE
Haemophilus influenzae	≤0.015-0.06	0.05-0.12	0.015-≤0.5	0.002-0.03	0.013-0.03	0.03-0.06	≤0.004-0.03	0.03
Moraxella catarrhalis	≤0.015-0.12	0.06-0.12	≤0.03-≤0.5	≤0.015-0.03	≤0.03-0.05	≤0.015-0.12	≤0.004-0.015	0.03
Neisseria meningitidis	0.004-0.008	0.03	≤0.008-0.016	0.001-≤0.008	≤0.008	≤0.008-0.016	0.002	0.008
Mycoplasma pneumoniae	1-5	1	0.5-2.5	0.25-1	0.13-0.5	0.12-0.3	0.25	0.03-0.06
Chlamydia pneumoniae	2	1	(0.5)-1	1	0.12	(0.06)-1	0.25	(0.008)
Legionella spp.	0.016-0.06	0.03-0.12	0.016-0.03	≤0.002-0.06	0.03	0.06	0.003-(0.008)	0.06

a Data from references as follows: ciprofloxacin (CPX), 6, 7, 10, 12, 13, 16, 21, 35, 40, 50, 52, 53, 62, 66, 81, 83, 85, 86, 93, 95, 112, 113, 115, 123, 124, 134, 138, 146, 149, 150, 151; ofloxacin (OFX), 6, 12, 13, 16, 50, 83, 113, 115, 124, 146; levofloxacin (LVX), 7, 10, 16, 21, 35, 42, 50, 52, 66, 81, 85, 86, 90, 95, 112, 115, 123, 134, 138, 150; trovafloxacin (TVX), 7, 10, 12, 21, 35, 50, 52, 62, 81, 85, 90, 112, 115, 123, 134, 138, 150; gatifloxacin (GAT), 10, 40, 62, 85, 86, 90, 112, 134, 146, 151; moxifloxacin (MOX), 10, 11, 21, 35, 50, 66, 81, 82, 90, 112, 115; gemifloxacin (GEM), 35, 42, 51, 52, 125, 150; garenoxacin (GARE), 123, 138, 139. Additional data are available for: Q-35 (56), lomefloxacin (93, 124), fleroxacin (124), sparfloxacin (6, 11, 12, 13, 21, 53, 66, 83, 85, 86, 90, 95, 113, 115, 146, 151), tosufloxacin (113, 146), clinafloxacin (10, 21, 35, 81, 112), grepafloxacin (13, 35, 52, 90, 149), sitafloxacin (35, 112, 113), AF-3013 (115), CFC-222 (93), DV-7751a (16), and norfloxacin (146).
b Parentheses indicate fewer than 10 strains tested.

Table 7. Susceptibility of gram-positive bacteria to U.S. approved fluoroquinolone antimicrobials[a]

Organism	Representative MIC90 (range) (µg/ml) of:						
	CPX	OFX	LVX	SPX	TVX	GAT	MOX
MSSA	0.5 (0.03-2)	0.5 (0.25-1)	0.25 (0.25-0.5)	0.12 (0.06-0.25)	0.03 (0.03-0.12)	0.12 (0.10-0.25)	0.12 (0.06-0.25)
MRSA	≥32 (25-128)	32 (6.25-50)	16 (8->32)	12.5 (8-16)	4 (0.05-32)	16 (4->32)	4 (2-16)
MSSE	2 (0.25-16)	0.5 (0.5)	1 (0.5-2)	0.12	0.13 (0.06-0.2)	(0.25-4)	0.13 (0.12-1)
MRSE	>16 (0.39-64)	32 (>8-32)	(0.39-16)	8	8 (0.1-8)	(0.25-8)	4 (0.13-8)
Streptococcus pneumoniae	2 (1-8)	2 (1-8)	1 (1-2)	0.5 (0.12-1)	0.12 (0.1-0.25)	0.5 (0.25-1)	0.25 (0.06-0.5)
Streptococcus pyogenes	2 (0.5-3.13)	2 (1-4)	1 (0.5-2)	1 (0.25-3.13)	0.25 (0.12-0.5)	0.5 (0.39-0.5)	0.25 (0.12-0.25)
Streptococcus agalactiae	2 (0.5-2)	4 (1-4)	1	(0.5-4)	0.5 (0.25-0.5)	0.5 (0.5)	0.5 (0.12-0.5)
Streptococci, other β-hemolytic	1 (1-8)	2 (2-4)	2 (1-2)	0.5 (0.5)	0.25 (0.12-1)	0.5 (0.25-0.5)	0.25 (0.13-1)
Streptococci, viridans group	4 (1-8)	4 (2-8)	2 (1-2)	0.5 (0.25-0.5)	0.25 (0.25-0.5)	0.5 (0.5-1)	0.25 (0.25-2)
Enterococcus faecalis	(1-128)	(2-32)	(2-50)	(0.78-32)	(0.25-32)	(1->4)	(0.5-16)
Enterococcus faecium	(2->128)	(4-100)	(2-64)	(4-50)	(2->32)	(3->32)	(4-≥32)
Listeria monocytogenes	1 (0.5-4)	4 (2-4)	1 (1-2)	2 (1-2)	0.5 (0.12-0.5)	0.5	0.5 (0.5)

a Abbreviations: MSSA, methicillin-susceptible *Staphylococcus aureus*; MRSA, methicillin-resistant *S. aureus*; MSSE, methicillin-susceptible *Staphylococcus epidermidis*; MRSE, methicillin-resistant *S. epidermidis*. Data were derived from the following references: ciprofloxacin (CPX), 4, 6, 7, 9, 10, 16, 21, 26, 27, 34, 35, 37, 38, 48, 50, 52, 53, 54, 66a, 74, 79, 83, 86, 91, 93, 94, 104, 105, 106, 112, 115, 122, 124, 126, 131, 134, 138, 140, 144, 146, 149, 150, 151; ofloxacin (OFX), 4, 6, 16, 21, 27, 38, 48, 50, 52, 54, 66a, 83, 87, 93, 94, 104, 106, 115, 122, 124, 144, 146, 151; levofloxacin (LVX), 7, 10, 16, 21, 34, 35, 37, 38, 48, 50, 52, 74, 82, 86, 91, 104, 106, 112, 115, 117, 122, 126, 131, 134, 137, 138, 140, 150; sparfloxacin (SPX), 6, 21, 48, 53, 66a, 74, 79, 82, 83, 84, 86, 87, 91, 94, 104, 106, 115, 122, 131, 144, 146, 151; trovafloxacin (TVX), 7, 10, 21, 26, 34, 35, 41, 50, 52, 66a, 74, 82, 84, 87, 91, 94, 104, 106, 115, 122, 126, 131, 134, 146, 151; gatifloxacin (GAT), 9, 10, 37, 38, 41, 84, 86, 87, 112, 126, 131, 134, 146, 151; moxifloxacin (MOX), 9, 10, 21, 26, 34, 35, 41, 50, 52, 66a, 74, 79, 82, 104, 112, 115, 122, 131; .Additional data are available for norfloxacin (106, 146), lomefloxacin (93, 124), and grepafloxacin (withdrawn) (35, 52, 66a, 79, 82, 104, 131, 149).

(66a, 150); garenoxacin, 2 to 6 μg/ml (50, 138); nonfluorinated quinolones PGE-932, PGE-924, PGE-997, 2 μg/ml (7, 126); clinafloxacin, 1 to 8 μg/ml (10, 26, 112); azetidins E-4767, 0.25 μg/ml, and E-5065, 2 μg/ml (54).

In most studies, methicillin-resistant strains of coagulase-negative staphylococci, like MRSA, are more resistant to fluoroquinolones (7, 37, 66a, 112, 115, 124, 150). Diekema et al. (37) found that 81% of 101 oxacillin-susceptible coagulase-negative staphylococci were susceptible to levofloxacin, whereas only 32% of 308 oxacillin-resistant strains were susceptible. In other studies, such a relationship is less obvious (10, 138). Data for *Staphylococcus epidermidis* are shown in Table 7. Ciprofloxacin MIC$_{90}$s against *Staphylococcus saprophyticus* are typically 0.5 to 1 μg/ml (10, 124, 150, 151). However, more resistant strains do occur. For 20 methicillin-resistant isolates of this species (ciprofloxacin MIC$_{90}$, 16 μg/ml), Bauernfeind (10) reported MIC$_{90}$ of newer agents as follows: levofloxacin and gatifloxacin, 8 μg/ml; trovafloxacin and moxifloxacin, 1 μg/ml; and clinafloxacin, 0.5 μg/ml. Fluoroquinolone susceptibilities of *Staphylococcus haemolyticus* vary over a broad range (66a, 84, 124); methicillin-resistant strains are usually more resistant to fluoroquinolones as well (112). Additional data for individual species or for nonspeciated collections of coagulase-negative staphylcocci have been presented: levofloxacin (7, 10, 16, 37, 50, 74, 112, 115, 138, 150), trovafloxacin (7, 10, 37, 50, 66a, 74, 84, 112, 115, 126, 138, 150, 151), gemifloxacin (66a, 150), gatifloxacin (10, 37, 84, 112, 126, 146, 151), moxifloxacin (10, 50, 66a, 74), garenoxacin (50, 138), PGE-932, PGE-924, and PGE-997 (7, 126), E-4767and E5065 (54), AF3013 (150), tosufloxacin (54, 146), DV7751a (16), clinafloxacin (10, 112, 126), and sitafloxacin (112).

Streptococci

The activities of new fluoroquinolones against *S. pneumoniae* (as well as against *H. influenzae* and agents of atypical pneumonia) have merited the inclusion of "respiratory quinolones" in treatment guidelines for community-acquired pneumonia (8). Surveys which have examined several thousand pneumococci collected in the United States since 1997 reveal resistance rates to levofloxacin, sparfloxacin, or moxifloxacin of <1% (38, 82, 130). Of concern, however, is that such large surveys have detected subtle trends toward increasing resistance to the class in the most recent years studied (130, 147). Geographic differences in resistance rates have

also been noted. Rates of resistance to levofloxacin from pneumococci collected in Asia (0.8 to 0.9%) were higher than those of >1,000 strains collected in Europe (0%) in one survey of isolates from 1997 to 1998 (129). Data from >6,000 *S. pneumoniae* isolated in the United States during 2000 to 2001 revealed 99.1% to be susceptible to levofloxacin (32). That study estimated that approximately 4.5% of levofloxacin-susceptible strains would have a single mutation in *parC* or *parE* of the quinolone resistance-determining region, and thus constitute a group from among which resistant strains might emerge in the future (32). Whereas MIC$_{90}$s of levofloxacin against *S. pneumoniae* range from 1 to 2 μg/ml, several compounds demonstrate greater potency, with MIC$_{90}$s as low as 0.03 to 0.06 μg/ml (e.g., gemifloxacin, sitafloxacin, PGE-924, PGE-997, E-4767) (Table 8).

A number of the newer agents inhibit *Streptococcus pyogenes* and other β-hemolytic streptococci at concentrations lower than those of ciprofloxacin or levofloxacin required to inhibit growth (Table 8). Strains of β-hemolytic streptococci with MICs of >4 μg/ml of one or both of the latter agents have been encountered (4, 122, 126). Against *Streptococcus agalactiae*, MIC$_{90}$s of 0.12 μg/ml have been recorded for moxifloxacin (74), garenoxacin (50), and gemifloxacin (91, 150). PGE-932 inhibited 77 strains of this species at 0.03 μg/ml or less (7). Fluoroquinolone resistance appears to be more common among viridans group streptococci, including *S. bovis*, than among β-hemolytic streptococci. In some cases (10, 74, 79, 112), but not others (122), newer agents such as moxifloxacin retain activity, with MICs of ≤0.5 μg/ml.

Enterococci and *Listeria monocytogenes*

Resistance to fluoroquinolones is now common among enterococci. MICs of ciprofloxacin against resistant strains may exceed 128 μg/ml. Although several of the newer agents are more potent than the early fluoroquinolones, activity is substantially reduced compared with that against susceptible isolates (Tables 7 and 8). For example, in one study that found 65% of 192 *Enterococcus faecalis* strains to be levofloxacin susceptible, clinafloxacin was only marginally superior, with only 69% of strains susceptible to this agent (34). That study also demonstrated the low rates of fluoroquinolone susceptibility among recent isolates of *Enterococcus faecium*. Only 15% of vancomycin-susceptible isolates and only 1% of vancomycin-resistant isolates were susceptible to levofloxacin; for clinafloxacin, one of the most active agents against enterococci, susceptibility rates for the two groups were 34% and 4%, respectively (34). MIC$_{90}$s of PGE-932 and garenoxacin against vancomycin-resistant enterococci were 8 µg/ml (7, 50).

Against *L. monocytogenes*, gemifloxacin MIC$_{90}$s of ≤0.25 µg/ml (104, 105) and moxifloxacin, trovafloxacin, or garenoxacin MIC$_{90}$s of ≤0. 5 µg/ml (50, 74, 104, 115) have been presented. Thus, these agents are more potent than ciprofloxacin or levofloxacin, for which MIC$_{90}$s typically range from 1 to 2 µg/ml (10, 50, 53, 104, 105, 106, 115).

Other gram-positive bacteria

Fluoroquinolone resistance is frequent among *Corynebacterium jeikeium*, and the newer agents do not appear to confer a consistent advantage against these organisms. For moxifloxacin and clinafloxacin, MIC$_{90}$s of 2 µg/ml against 26 strains of *C. jeikeium* have been reported (74). The MIC$_{90}$ of trovafloxacin against this collection was 16 µg/ml. Gatifloxacin with MICs of >4 µg/ml or >32 µg/ml against ciprofloxacin-resistant corynebacteria (84) and against *Corynebacterium* spp. (37), respectively, have been described elsewhere. Against 20 to 30 strains of other *Corynebacterium* spp., levofloxacin MIC$_{90}$s were 2 µg/ml for *C. striatum*, 4 µg/ml for *C. minutissimum*, and >16 µg/ml for *C. urealyticum* and *C. amycolatum* (106). Gemifloxacin was up to 32-fold more active than ciprofloxacin against several *Corynebacterium* spp. (105). Against 21 isolates of *Bacillus* spp., MIC$_{90}$s of ciprofloxacin, levofloxacin, and gatifloxacin were identical at 0.25 µg/ml (37). Ciprofloxacin inhibited 61 strains of *Bacillus anthracis*, including 12 clinical isolates from 2001, at concentrations ≤0.06 µg/ml (113a). Others reported a higher upper range of MICs against *B. anthracis*; ciprofloxacin and levofloxacin had comparable activities with MIC ranges from 0.06 to 2 µg/ml (69a). Little benefit of newer compounds is apparent against *Nocardia asteroides*. MIC$_{90}$s of trovafloxacin, sparfloxacin, and moxifloxacin were 16, 16, and 8 µg/ml, respectively (74). This study showed clinafloxacin to be more active (MIC$_{90}$, 2 µg/ml), but this compound is not presently under development.

Anaerobic Bacteria

Ciprofloxacin demonstrates weak activity against most gram-negative anaerobes (Table 9). Activities of levofloxacin are better but vary over a wide range. For example, published MIC$_{90}$s of this agent against *Bacteroides fragilis* range from 2 µg/ml to >16 µg/ml (10, 50, 88, 112, 138, 150). Newer

agents such as trovafloxacin, moxifloxacin, gatifloxacin, gemifloxacin, and garenoxacin are more active than older compounds against *B. fragilis* and other *Bacteroides* spp. (10, 50, 68, 88). Deshpande et al. (34) reported that 94% of gram-negative anaerobes studied were susceptible to trovafloxacin. *Fusobacterium* spp. may be somewhat more susceptible to older fluoroquinolones than are *Bacteroides* spp. (50, 68, 88, 119). MIC$_{90}$s of ciprofloxacin against *Clostridium perfringens* of 1 µg/ml or less have been reported (50, 57, 68, 88, 112, 119, 150). In contrast, *Clostridium difficile* are usually resistant to ciprofloxacin, MIC$_{90}$s of >6.25 µg/ml (10, 50, 88, 112, 119, 138, 148, 150). Newer agents with MICs of ≤1 µg/ml against *C. difficile* include trovafloxacin (10, 50, 112, 150), moxifloxacin (50), garenoxacin (50, 138), sitafloxacin (112, 119), and clinafloxacin (112); however, higher MIC$_{90}$s have been reported in other studies for several of these compounds. Against peptostreptococci, results are variable, but MIC$_{90}$s of ≤1 µg/ml have been reported for several of the newer compounds including moxifloxacin, trovafloxacin, gemifloxacin, garenoxacin, tosufloxacin, sitafloxacin, and clinafloxacin (26, 50, 68, 88, 97, 112, 138, 150). Kato et al. (88) reported MIC$_{90}$s of 0.78 µg/ml of ciprofloxacin and levofloxacin against *Mobiluncus* spp. and *Propionibacterium acnes*. For the latter organisms, others have reported results in a similar range (50, 57). Lower levels of activity of ciprofloxacin against these species have been reported previously (45). The activity of ciprofloxacin against *Actinomyces* spp. is variable, with MICs ranging from <0.06 µg/ml to 16 µg/ml (57).

Genital Pathogens

Bacterial pathogens

Most isolates of *Neisseria gonorrhoeae* are highly susceptible to fluoroquinolones (Table 10). Ciprofloxacin MICs are typically ≤0.1 µg/ml (7, 10, 33, 50, 112, 146, 150, 151) and often ≤0.016 µg/ml (10, 16, 33, 50, 112, 150, 151). However, strains with reduced susceptibility have emerged. MICs of ciprofloxacin may reach 8 µg/ml with multiple mutations, including dual *gyrA* plus *parC* mutations (33). Sitafloxacin (33, 112), PGE-932 (7), clinafloxacin (112), and garenoxacin (50) have greater activity than ciprofloxacin against isolates with reduced susceptibility to the older fluoroquinolone. Recently reported MIC$_{90}$s against *Gardnerella vaginalis* were: ciprofloxacin, 2 µg/ml; levofloxacin and trovafloxacin, 1 µg/ml; moxifloxacin and garenoxacin, 0.5 µg/ml (50).

Table 8. Susceptibility of gram-positive bacteria to investigational quinolone antimicrobials[a]

Organism	Representative MIC (range) (μg/ml) of:									
	CLX	GEM	SIT	TOS	GARE	PGE-932	PGE-924	PGE-997	E-4767	E-5065
MSSA	0.03 (0.03–0.06)	0.06 (0.03–0.06)	0.03	0.05 (0.05–0.12)	0.06 (0.03–0.06)	0.03	0.03	0.03	0.007	0.03
MRSA	2 (1–8)	8 (1–8)	0.5	6.25 (0.03–6.25)	(0.03–6.25)	2	2	2	0.25	2
MSSE	0.25	0.3 (0.015–0.3)			(0.1–2)					
MRSE	0.25	2 (0.25–2)			(0.1–4)					
Streptococcus pneumoniae	0.12 (0.06–0.5)	0.06 (0.015–0.06)	0.06	0.25 (0.25–1.56)	0.12 (0.05–0.12)	0.016	0.06	0.03	0.03	0.25
Streptococcus pyogenes		0.06 (0.015–0.06)		0.39	0.25 (0.1–0.25)	≤0.008	0.06	0.03		
Streptococcus agalactiae		0.12 (0.03–0.25)			0.25 (0.1–0.25)	0.016	0.06	0.06		
Streptococci, other β-hemolytic	0.12 (0.12–0.25)	0.06 (0.06)	0.03		0.12 (0.12–0.25)					
Streptococci, viridans group	0.12 (0.12)	0.12	0.12		0.25	0.03	0.12	0.06		
Enterococcus faecalis	(0.12–8)	2 (2–4)	2	(0.39–2)	(0.5–>4)	0.5	2	2		
Enterococcus faecium	(0.5–32)	8 (8)	(4–8)	25	32 (>4–32)	8	>16	16		
Listeria monocytogenes	0.25 (0.12–0.5)	0.25 (0.12–0.25)			0.5					

[a] Data derived from the following references: clinafloxacin (CLX), 10, 17, 21, 26, 27, 34, 35, 74, 104, 112, 124, 126, 131, 144; gemifloxacin (GEM), 30, 35, 38, 52, 66a, 79, 91, 104, 105, 120, 150; sitafloxacin (SIT), 35, 38, 112; tosufloxacin (TOS), 54, 146; garenoxacin (GARE), 9, 41, 134, 138; PGE-932, PGE-924 and PGE-997, 7, 126; E-4767 and E-5065, 54. Additional data are available for AF-3013 (115), CFC-222 (93, 94), and DV-7751a (16).

Table 9. Susceptibilities of anaerobic bacteria to fluoroquinolones[a]

Organism	Range of MIC₉₀s (μg/ml) of:									
	CPX	LVX	SPX	TVX	GAT	MOX	GEM	GARE	CLX	SIT
Bacteroides fragilis	4–64	2–>16	1–6.25	0.25–8	0.25–8	0.5–8	0.5–4	0.5–0.78	0.25–2	0.25–1
Bacteroides spp.	16–>64	4–16	3.13	1–8	2–8	8		0.5	1–2	0.39–1
Fusobacterium spp.	2–4	0.39	0.78–2	0.5		2	0.5	2		0.032–0.05
Prevotella spp.	>16	4–6.25	12.5	1–2	2	1–2	2		0.5	0.25–0.39
Clostridium perfringens	0.5–1.56	0.39	0.2–1.56	0.25	0.39–1	1	0.12	1	0.125	0.05–0.125
Clostridium difficile	6.25–12.5	6.25–128	4–32	1–16	1.56–2	2–16	2	0.78–1	0.25–4	0.12–0.25
Peptostreptococcus spp.	0.39–12.5	0.39–0.78	0.39–1	0.12–1.56	2	1–2	0.125–0.5	0.25	0.5	0.008–0.12

[a] Data derived from the following references (see previous tables for abbreviations): ciprofloxacin, 2, 7, 10, 16, 26, 50, 54, 57, 68, 69, 88, 93, 112, 119, 138, 146, 148, 150, 151; levofloxacin (LVX), 10, 50, 69, 88, 112, 138, 150; sparfloxacin (SPX), 57, 88, 119, 146, 151; trovafloxacin (TVX), 7, 10, 26, 34, 68, 112, 138, 150, 151; gatifloxacin (GAT), 10, 112, 146, 151; moxifloxacin (MOX), 10, 50, 97, 112; gemifloxacin (GEM), 97, 150; garenoxacin (GARE), 50, 138; clinafloxacin (CLX), 10, 26, 34, 57, 112; sitafloxacin (SIT), 88, 112, 119. Additional data are available for: ofloxacin (50, 57, 68, 69, 119, 146), tosufloxacin (88, 146), lomefloxacin (119), DV-7751a (16), CFC-222 (93), PGE-932, PGE-924, PGE-997 (7), and E-4767, E-5065 (54).

Table 10. Expected susceptibilities of genital pathogens to fluoroquinolones[a]

Agent	Range of MIC$_{90}$s (μg/ml) against:			
	Neisseria gonorrhoeae	Chlamydia trachomatis	Ureaplasma urealyticum	Mycoplasma hominis
Ciprofloxacin	0.001–2	0.5–2	2–8	0.5–4
Ofloxacin	0.03–2	1–2	1–4	0.5–8
Levofloxacin	≤0.008–2	0.25–0.5	1–4	0.5–2
Sparfloxacin	0.001–1	0.06	0.25–0.5	0.03–0.06
Trovafloxacin	<0.0005–0.5	0.06	0.12–0.5	0.03–0.06
Gatifloxacin	0.004–0.025	0.06	1	0.12
Moxifloxacin	0.015–1	0.06	0.25–1	0.06–0.12
Garenoxacin	0.008–0.25	0.008–0.016	0.25	0.03

[a] Data from references: ciprofloxacin (7, 10, 12, 13, 16, 33, 50, 90, 112, 113, 123, 143, 146, 150, 151), ofloxacin (12, 13, 50, 90, 113, 143, 146), levofloxacin (7, 10, 33, 50, 90, 112, 123, 143, 150), sparfloxacin (11, 12, 13, 33, 90, 113, 146, 151), trovafloxacin (7, 10, 12, 50, 90, 112, 123, 150, 151), gatifloxacin (10, 90, 112, 146, 151), moxifloxacin (10, 11, 50, 90, 112), and garenoxacin (50, 123). Additional data are available for: norfloxacin (146), fleroxacin (143), tosufloxacin (113, 146), sitafloxacin (33, 112, 113), grepafloxacin (13, 90), gemifloxacin (150), clinafloxacin (10, 112), and PGE-932, PGE-924, and PGE-997 (7).

Chlamydia trachomatis

Ciprofloxacin inhibits 90% of Chlamydia trachomatis strains at approximately 2 μg/ml (50, 113, 151). Ofloxacin and levofloxacin inhibit isolates at 1.0 and 0.5 μg/ml, respectively (50, 113). MIC$_{90}$s for other agents appear to be lower: tosufloxacin, 0.125 μg/ml (113); moxifloxacin, sparfloxacin, and sitafloxacin, 0.06 μg/ml; garenoxacin, 0.016 μg/ml (50, 113). Gatifloxacin inhibited three isolates at concentrations of 0.06 to 0.12 μg/ml (151) and trovafloxacin one strain at 0.063 μg/ml (123).

Mycoplasmas and ureaplasmas

In the largest series that examined 57 isolates of Mycoplasma hominis, MIC$_{90}$s of ciprofloxacin, fleroxacin, ofloxacin, and levofloxacin were 4, 4, 2, and 1 μg/ml, respectively (143). In other reports, MIC$_{90}$s of sparfloxacin and trovafloxacin were 0.03 to 0.06 μg/ml (11, 12, 13, 50, 90); those of moxifloxacin or gatifloxacin were 0.06 to 0.12 μg/ml (11, 50, 90). Garenoxacin inhibited 90% and 100% of isolates tested at 0.03 and 0.25 μg/ml (50). Eleven strains of Mycoplasma fermentans were inhibited by ciprofloxacin and ofloxacin at 0.25 μg/ml, and by sparfloxacin and trovafloxacin at 0.03 μg/ml (12).

MIC$_{90}$s of ciprofloxacin against Ureaplasma urealyticum range between 2 and 8 μg/ml, with a mode of 4 μg/ml (12, 13, 50, 143). Levofloxacin MIC$_{90}$s range from 1 μg/ml to 4 μg/ml (50, 90, 143). Reported MIC$_{90}$s of grepafloxacin and gatifloxacin were 1 μg/ml (13, 90). Several new agents are more potent (MIC$_{90}$s): moxifloxacin, 0.25 to 1 μg/ml; sparfloxacin, 0.25 to 0.5 μg/ml; trovafloxacin, 0.12 to 0.5 μg/ml; garenoxacin, 0.25 μg/ml (11, 12, 50, 90).

Other Organisms

Rickettsia and rickettsia-like organisms

Several older fluoroquinolones have demonstrated activity against Rickettsia rickettsii, Rickettssia conorii, and Coxiella burnetii (45). Levofloxacin inhibited isolates of the species and of the "Israeli spotted fever group rickettsia" at concentrations from 0.5 to 1 μg/ml (109). Three strains of C. burnetii were inhibited at concentrations of 0.5, 1, and 2 μg/ml but without bactericidal activity at concentrations up to 4 μg/ml (109).

Klein et al. (96) tested three strains of the agent of human granulocytic ehrlichiosis and found that ciprofloxacin and ofloxacin inhibited growth at 2 μg/ml, while trovafloxacin was inhibitory at ≤0.125 μg/ml. Horowitz et al. (76) examined six isolates of Ehrlichia phagocytophila from New York state, excluding one that was included in the study by Klein et al. (96). The MICs reported were: ofloxacin, ≤2 μg/ml; levofloxacin, ≤1 μg/ml; and trovafloxacin, ≤0.032 μg/ml. It has been suggested that the Ehrlichia canis group of organisms (which includes E. chaffeensis) is inherently more resistant to fluoroquinolones than the E. phagocytophila group because of sequence differences in the quinolone-resistance-determining regions (QRDR) (107). Comparison of sequences of the QRDR of the susceptible and resistant groups revealed that a serine in the gyrA gene of the former corresponding to position 83 in E. coli numbering was replaced by alanine in the fluoroquinolone-resistant organisms (107).

Mycobacteria

Against Mycobacterium tuberculosis, MIC$_{90}$s of ciprofloxacin or levofloxacin range from 0.12 to

1 μg/ml (50, 123, 127, 135, 151). Resistant strains, with MICs of 4 to 16 μg/ml for ciprofloxacin (50, 127) and 8 μg/ml for levofloxacin (127), have been detected in these series. Sparfloxacin, MIC_{90}, 0.125 μg/ml (135), moxifloxacin, MIC_{90}, 0.125 μg/ml (50) and gatifloxacin, MICs, 0.12 to 0.5 μg/ml (151) also demonstrate activity against *M. tuberculosis*. Activity of garenoxacin against *M. tuberculosis* appears to be method dependent (MIC_{90}s, 0.06 to 2 μg/ml), but comparable with that of ofloxacin (50, 123). Activities of trovafloxacin (MIC_{90}, 64 μg/ml) and gemifloxacin (MIC_{90}, 8 μg/ml) are poor against this organism, a property which has been attributed to the naphthyridone structural core (127). Various fluoroquinolones demonstrate activity against several other mycobacterial species (45). However, *Mycobacterium avium* complex strains are usually resistant to ciprofloxacin, and at best show variable susceptibilities to levofloxacin or garenoxacin (14, 45, 50). Evaluating growth inhibition through measurements of metabolic activity, clinafloxacin at 0.75 μg/ml and sparfloxacin at 1.5 μg/ml, were found to inhibit one strain of *Mycobacterium leprae* (36).

Borrelia burgdorferi

Against a collection of 11 strains of *Borrelia* spp. (which included nine *Borrelia burgdorferi*), MIC_{90}s of ciprofloxacin, ofloxacin, and levofloxacin were 2, 8, and 4 μg/ml, respectively (99). Similar estimates of activity were obtained in another study that examined six isolates of *B. burgdorferi*, with median MICs of 4 μg/ml for each of these agents (50). The highest MICs obtained in these studies were: moxifloxacin, 2 μg/ml (99) and 8 μg/ml (50); and trovafloxacin or gatifloxacin, 2 μg/ml (99, 50). The most active agents were gemifloxacin (MIC_{100}, 0.25 μg/ml [99]) and garenoxacin (MIC_{100}, 0.5 μg/ml [50]).

Bartonella spp.

Maurin and Roult (108) examined the activities of fluoroquinolones against one strain each of *Bartonella henselae*, *Bartonella quintana*, and *Bartonella vinsonii* tested at two inocula. At the higher inoculum, growth was inhibited by ciprofloxacin at 1 μg/ml, by ofloxacin at 1 (for *B. henselae*) to 2 μg/ml, and by sparfloxacin at 0.5 μg/ml. In another study, three strains of *Bartonella* spp. were inhibited by ciprofloxacin and levofloxacin at 1 to 2 μg/ml and by moxifloxacin, trovafloxacin, and garenoxacin at 0.5 to 1 μg/ml (50).

FACTORS INFLUENCING ASSESSMENT OF QUINOLONE ANTIMICROBIAL ACTIVITY

In the past, considerable attention has been devoted to the assessment of factors that modify the activities of fluoroquinolones as measured in vitro. From our previous review of the topic (45), several generalizations can be made. (i) Results obtained by microdilution broth and agar dilution methods are generally comparable. Data presented in the tables of this chapter are derived from studies using either method. (ii) Except for fluoroquinolones that are highly protein bound, the addition of serum to test medium usually influences results only to a minor degree. (iii) The activities of most compounds are reduced under conditions of low pH and high magnesium concentrations that prevail in urine. (iv) The inoculum size can influence fluoroquinolone activity, but usually to a lesser degree than that seen for other antimicrobials, such as β-lactam antibiotics.

There are, of course, exceptions to these generalizations. For example, susceptibility test results for anaerobic bacteria do appear to be influenced by the media chosen, and considerable attention has been devoted to this issue in the generation of NCCLS recommendations for susceptibility testing of anaerobes (69). Lower MICs of various agents, including ciprofloxacin, levofloxacin, and trovafloxacin, are obtained on brain heart infusion agar with supplements than on Brucella agar when testing members of the *B. fragilis* group (68, 69).

The sulfonyl fluoroquinolones designated NSFQ-104 and NSFQ-105 represent exceptions to the generalization about pH effects on activity. These compounds are more active at pH 5.5 than at pH 7.4 (1). For the C-7 azetidin compounds, E-4767 and E-5065, maximum activities are reached at pH 6.8; variations of pH in either direction result in reduced activity (54).

The influence of serum on activities of fluoroquinolones in vitro is usually of minimal consequence. However, the effects are not always predictable. For example, in one study MICs of fluoroquinolones against pneumococci were determined in broth alone and in the presence of 80% serum (5). For the strains that were most susceptible to ciprofloxacin, the MICs of gemifloxacin and trovafloxacin were fourfold and eightfold higher in serum, respectively, but all strains were susceptible to both fluoroquinolones under either condition. In contrast, for ciprofloxacin-resistant isolates, the MICs of gemifloxacin and trovafloxacin were only twofold higher in the presence of serum than in broth alone. Nevertheless, even this small further reduction in activity resulted in a substantial increase in the percent of isolates classified as resistant (5).

BACTERICIDAL ACTIVITY

MBCs of the various fluoroquinolone antimicrobials reviewed previously were almost always within two dilutions of the MIC (45). The newer agents seem to behave similarly. Clinafloxacin and gatifloxacin minimal bactericidal concentrations (MBCs) are generally within two dilutions of MICs (27, 146). The C-7 bicyclic amine fluoroquinolone, CFC-222, like ofloxacin and ciprofloxacin, killed several reference strains at concentrations within one to two dilutions of the MICs (93). Similar results were noted for the C-7 azetidin compounds (54), and for AF-3013 and six comparator agents (115). Minimal bactericidal concentrations at which 90% of strains tested are killed (MBC_{90}s) within one dilution of MIC_{90}s were noted when ciprofloxacin, levofloxacin, moxifloxacin, and sparfloxacin were tested against *M. pneumoniae* (66); for Q-35, the MBC_{90} was within two dilutions of MIC_{90} (56). It has been suggested that the C-8 methoxy substituent enhances the in vitro bactericidal activity of fluoroquinolones against *M. tuberculosis* and decreases survival of the organisms within macrophages (153). The C-8 methoxy group of gatifloxacin also appears to confer bactericidal activity of the compound against *S. aureus* with *grlA gyrA* dual mutations, a property that is lost by the fluoroquinolone AM-1121, which has an identical structure except for replacement of the $-OCH_3$ with $-H$ at C-8 (77).

When examined by time-kill curve techniques, the bactericidal activity of fluoroquinolones at concentrations of two to four times the MIC of susceptible gram-negative bacteria is usually rapid (45). Rapid killing of *E. coli*, *P. aeruginosa*, and *S. aureus* was seen when organisms were exposed to twice the respective MICs of gatifloxacin (146). Killing of *S. aureus* exposed to ciprofloxacin, ofloxacin, sparfloxacin, or temafloxacin was slower when measured under anaerobic conditions, as opposed to room air; nevertheless, the MBCs were not altered (152). Moxifloxacin, levofloxacin, and garenoxacin, each at a concentration of four times the MIC, exerted bactericidal activity (99.9% killing) by 24 h against 12 strains of *S. pneumoniae* (121). At these multiples of the MIC, killing was infrequently seen at 6 h of incubation. By 12 h, only five to eight of the strains were killed, depending on the antimicrobial used.

The bactericidal activities of fluoroquinolones have also been studied in vitro, in pharmacodynamic models that simulate serum antimicrobial concentrations following standard dosing in humans. Although much more complex to perform than traditional time-kill assays, these models address an important limitation of time-kill curves, which is that only a few concentrations of a drug are examined. When ciprofloxacin-susceptible *S. pneumoniae* were incorporated into fibrin clots and exposed to antimicrobials in such a dynamic system, the newer agents, trovafloxacin, gatifloxacin, clinafloxacin, sparfloxacin, and levofloxacin, exerted superior bactericidal activities during 48 h of incubation (72). When ciprofloxacin-resistant *S. pneumoniae* were studied in a dynamic model in which bacteria were suspended in broth, moxifloxacin, gatifloxacin, and grepafloxacin all exerted a sustained bactericidal effect over 48 h (31). When one isolate was exposed to levofloxacin (MIC, 2 μg/ml), regrowth occurred after 28 h of incubation, following an initial period of killing. When another isolate that was not susceptible to levofloxacin (MIC, 4 μg/ml) was examined, regrowth was evident after modest killing over the first 8 h of incubation (31).

RESISTANCE TO FLUOROQUINOLONES

The frequencies of isolation of single-step mutants resistant to fluoroquinolones, at four to eight times the MIC, from populations of fully susceptible organisms are low (45). Gilbert et al. (55) examined 13 to 20 isolates each of several bacterial species and found comparable frequencies of recovery of resistant mutants when strains of MRSA, *E. coli*, *K. pneumoniae*, or *P. aeruginosa* were exposed for 48 h to ciprofloxacin, levofloxacin, or trovafloxacin at concentrations of four times the MICs. In other cases, differences were seen. For example, for *E. cloacae*, the resistance frequency for ciprofloxacin (4.2×10^{-7}) was significantly greater than that for trovafloxacin or levofloxacin (2.0 or 2.9×10^{-8}, respectively); however, the reverse was true for *Serratia marcescens* (55).

In another study, single-step mutants from 10 strains of *S. pneumoniae* were detected at different frequencies, depending on the fluoroquinolone and MIC multiple used for selection. At four times the MIC, resistance was not detected for ciprofloxacin, trovafloxacin, or clinafloxacin (118). At two times the MIC, frequencies of resistance ranged from approximately 10^{-6} to $<10^{-11}$ for trovafloxacin or ciprofloxacin using the various strains, to $<2 \times 10^{-10}$ with all strains tested with clinafloxacin. Fukuda et al. (49) studied resistance selection in *S. pneumoniae* with gatifloxacin, AM-1121 (which is similar to gatifloxacin but with $-H$ instead of $-OCH_3$ at position C-8), ciprofloxacin and AM-1147 (similar to ciprofloxacin but with $-OCH_3$ instead of $-H$ at C-8). They found that none of the compounds examined selected mutants at four times the MIC or higher concentrations. However, at the MIC or twice the MIC, resistance frequencies were lower (approximately 10^{-9} or less) with the C-8 methoxyfluoroquinolones than with the corresponding C-8 –H analogs (approximately 10^{-6} or greater).

Ince and Hooper (77) found similar results for *S. aureus*. At low multiples of the MICs, the frequency of selecting single-step mutants was much lower with gatifloxacin than with AM-1121 (the C-8 –H analog) or with ciprofloxacin. At four times the respective MICs, the C-8 methoxy compound (gatifloxacin) also retained bactericidal activity against a *grlA gyrA* double mutant, while neither ciprofloxacin nor AM-1121 demonstrated any killing activity against this organism.

By repeated passage of initially susceptible bacterial colonies through incremental concentrations of various fluoroquinolones, colonies with stable resistance to the various agents can be obtained (45). With initially susceptible strains of *S. pneumoniae* subjected to up to 50 serial passages in fluoroquinolones, colonies were obtained with MICs as high as 128 µg/ml for ciprofloxacin, 8 µg/ml for trovafloxacin, and 2 µg/ml for clinafloxacin (33-fold increase) (118). Boos et al. (19) were able to select colonies of *S. pneumoniae*, *S. pyogenes,* and *S. aureus* with severalfold increases in MIC after passage through increasing concentrations of various fluoroquinolones. They did not note obvious differences between the agents in terms of likelihood to select resistant colonies. Later, however, this group examined a larger number of *S. pneumoniae* isolates (70 strains) and found that the estimated daily rate of MIC increase during serial passage was lowest for gatifloxacin and moxifloxacin, followed by levofloxacin, and highest for gemifloxacin and ciprofloxacin (132). Others have also found that the rapidity with which resistant colonies are detected during serial passage appears to depend on the organisms, on the selecting fluoroquinolone, and on the inoculum size. It was recently estimated that approximately 4.5% of 2000 to 2001 U.S. isolates of levofloxacin-susceptible *S. pneumoniae* already contain one mutation in the QRDR (32). It would be from among this subgroup of isolates that fully resistant strains might be expected to emerge over time, with the acquisition of a second mutation.

Resistance in *S. aureus* was detected after fewer passages in ciprofloxacin than in levofloxacin or trovafloxacin (55). In contrast, in the same study, the development of resistance in *P. aeruginosa* was significantly retarded when carried out under selection by ciprofloxacin as compared with the other agents.

Additional insights have been provided by studies of resistance in experimental animal models. Join-Lambert et al. (80) used a rat model of *P. aeruginosa* pneumonia to assess resistance emergent during treatment with ciprofloxacin or trovafloxacin, dosed to produce comparable antimicrobial exposures as measured by area under the curve/MIC ratios. Both treatments reduced the residual number of viable colonies to a comparable degree. Colonies overproducing efflux pumps were recovered almost 10-fold more frequently from animals treated with ciprofloxacin than from rats receiving trovafloxacin (80). Organisms recovered after ciprofloxacin treatment overproduced the MexEF-OprN efflux proteins; those recovered from rats receiving trovafloxacin overproduced the MexCD-OprJ efflux proteins. Although these in vivo results confirmed earlier in vitro observations by these investigators (98), an additional observation was that the frequency of efflux mutants recovered from *untreated* control rats was higher than that detected in the original bacterial inoculum. This finding implied that merely passage of a strain in vivo in such an infection model, even in the absence of antibiotic selective pressure, may contribute to the emergence of resistance.

ANTIMICROBIAL COMBINATIONS

In the treatment of infections due to gram-negative bacteria, it is not uncommon to witness the use of fluoroquinolones in combination with other antibiotics that display a similar antibacterial spectrum. In part, this use of combination antibiotics occurs in an effort to minimize the risk of providing inadequate coverage in the event of resistance to either agent. In other cases, it is hoped that using two antibiotics may enhance levels of inhibition or killing, or will prevent or delay the emergence of resistance.

Against 200 strains of *Enterobacteriaceae* collected more than 15 years ago, Haller (65) found little or no consistent evidence of either synergistic or antagonistic interactions between ciprofloxacin and any of five aminoglycosides. In that study, synergism between ciprofloxacin and several penicillins or cephalosporins was also uncommon (<5% of combinations). In one study, ciprofloxacin-imipenem combinations resulted in synergistic activity against approximately 20% of *Enterobacter* spp. (25), but this rate is higher than seen by other investigators (23). In an animal model of *Enterobacter* infection, dual therapy with ceftriaxone plus pefloxacin completely prevented the emergence of resistant colonies that was seen in 10 of 14 animals treated with the cephem alone, and in 6 of 11 treated with the fluoroquinolone alone (111). On the other hand, when *Serratia* infection was studied in the model, pefloxacin resistance was prevented by this combination, but more ceftriaxone resistance was encountered. Resistance was noted in none of 12 animals treated with ceftriaxone alone, but in 5 of 13 animals treated with the combination.

Favorable in vitro interactions between fluoroquinolones and either aminoglycosides or β-lactams has been noted more frequently against *P. aeruginosa* than against *Enterobacteriaceae*, but often at rates that vary widely (44, 45, 63). Mayer and Nagy (110) examined combinations of a fluoroquinolone (ciprofloxacin, ofloxacin, or pefloxacin) with a cephalosporin (ceftazidime, cefoperazone, ceftriaxone) against 18 strains of *Pseudomonas* spp. Using a microtiter broth system and a standard definition of synergism (fractional inhibitory concentration [FIC]$_{index}$ ≤ 0.5), these authors documented synergistic interaction between the various combinations against only 11 to 33% of the strains. Antagonism was not observed.

When antimicrobial combinations are studied against gram-negative bacteria by time-kill methods, it is often difficult to assess precisely the nature of interactions observed. One study examined combinations of piperacillin-tazobactam plus either ciprofloxacin or trovafloxacin, each drug at twice the MIC or one-fourth the MIC, against four clinical isolates of *P. aeruginosa* (22). Evidence of "synergistic" activity (combination resulting in 100-fold lower CFU/ml than the most active single agent at 24 h *and* at least 100-fold killing compared with inoculum density) was detected for 33% of the piperacillin-tazobactam plus trovafloxacin combinations and 8% of the piperacillin-tazobactam plus ciprofloxacin combinations. Other combinations were described as indifferent.

Using a dynamic in vitro model that simulated human serum concentrations achieved with administration of ciprofloxacin 200 mg every 12 h and azlocillin 4 g every 12 h, Dudley et al. (41) did provide evidence of an enhanced bactericidal effect, even against a strain resistant to both agents. In the aforementioned animal model (111), results were not clear-cut with *P. aeruginosa*. Even when pefloxacin was administered with ceftriaxone, resistance to the former remained high (12 or 15 animals) while resistance to the β-lactam increased from 3 of 15 animals treated with ceftriaxone alone to 6 of 15 receiving the combination (111). The question of whether combinations of a fluoroquinolone with a β-lactam would prevent the emergence of resistance to either or both antimicrobials in *P. aeruginosa* is complicated. *P. aeruginosa* strains that overexpress the various multidrug resistance efflux pumps found in this species may demonstrate cross-resistance to members of both classes (fluoroquinolones and β-lactams) and to other antimicrobials as well (101).

CONCLUSIONS

The fluoroquinolones continue to provide excellent in vitro activity against most commonly encountered gram-negative bacteria. However, in certain areas of the world or in specific institutional settings, significant numbers of *E. coli* or *Klebsiella* spp. are now resistant to available agents of this class. Rates of resistance among clinical isolates of *P. aeruginosa* are higher still. Nevertheless, the fluoroquinolones have revolutionized the treatment of many infections and still remain extremely valuable antimicrobials today. Resistance to fluoroquinolones is common among staphylococci, especially among methicillin-resistant strains of *S. aureus*. Several newer agents demonstrate increased potency against these organisms as compared with the activities of early fluoroquinolones; however, activities of even the newer agents are substantially reduced compared with their potency against fully susceptible strains. Several of the newer quinolones demonstrate potent in vitro activity against *S. pneumoniae*. High levels of activity against pneumococci, *H. influenzae*, and other respiratory gram-negative bacteria, and against the atypical pulmonary pathogens, have earned this class a major role in the treatment of community-acquired pneumonia. Thus, it is both the broad-spectrum antimicrobial activity of these drugs, and their high potency against many susceptible strains, that position the fluoroquinolone antimicrobials among our most valuable therapeutic classes.

REFERENCES

1. Allemandi, D. A., L. Fabiana, A. Manzo, and R. H. Manzo. 1994. In-vitro activity of new sulphanilil fluoroquinolones against *Staphylococcus aureus*. *J. Antimicrob. Chemother.* 34:261–265.
2. Alonso, R., T. Peláez, M. J. González-Abad, L. Alcalá, P. Muñoz, M. Rodríguez-Créixems, and E. Bouza. 2001. *In vitro* activity of new quinolones against *Clostridium difficile*. *J. Antimicrob. Chemother.* 47:195–197.
3. Alovero, F. L., X. S. Pan, J. E. Morris, R. H. Manzo, and L. M. Fisher. 2000. Engineering the specificity of antibacterial fluoroquinolones: benzenesulfonamide modifications at C-7 of ciprofloxacin change its primary target in *Streptococcus pneumoniae* from topoisomerase IV to gyrase. *Antimicrob. Agents Chemother.* 44:320–325.
4. Amyes, S. G. B., D. R. Baird, D. W. Crook, S. H. Gillespie, A. J. Howard, B. A. Oppenhiem, S. J. Pedler, A. Paull, D. S.

Tompkins, and S. A. Lawrie. 1994. A multicentre study of the in-vitro activity of cefotaxime, cefuroxime, ceftazidime, ofloxacin and ciprofloxacin against blood and urinary pathogens. *J. Antimicrob. Chemother.* 34:639–648.

5. Balcabao, I. P., L. Alou, L. Aguilar, M. L. Gomez-Lus, and J. Prieto. 2001. Influence of the decrease in ciprofloxacin susceptibility and the presence of human serum on the *in vitro* susceptibility of *Streptococcus pneumoniae* to five new quinolones. *J. Antimicrob. Chemother.* 48:907–909.

6. Ballow, C. H., R. N. Jones, D. M. Johnson, J. A. Deinhart, J. J. Schentag, and SPAR Study Group. 1997. Comparative in vitro assessment of sparfloxacin activity and spectrum using results from over 14,000 pathogens isolated at 190 medical centers in the USA. *Diagn. Microbiol. Infect. Dis.* 29:173–186.

7. Barry, A. L., P. C. Fuchs, and S. D. Brown. 2001. In vitro activities of three nonfluorinated quinolones against representative bacterial isolates. *Antimicrob. Agents Chemother.* 45:1923–1927.

8. Bartlett, J. G., R. F. Breiman, L. A. Mandell, and T. M. File, Jr. 1998. Community-acquired pneumonia in adults: guidelines for management. *Clin. Infect. Dis.* 26:811–838.

9. Bassetti, M., L. M. Dembry, P. A. Farrel, D. A. Callan, and V. T. Andriole. 2002. Antimicrobial activities of BMS-284756 compared with those of fluoroquinolones and β-lactams against gram-positive clinical isolates. *Antimicrob. Agents Chemother.* 46:234–238.

10. Bauernfeind, A. 1997. Comparison of the antibacterial activities of the quinolones Bay 12-8039, gatifloxacin (AM 1155), trovafloxacin, clinafloxacin, levofloxacin and ciprofloxacin. *J. Antimicrob. Chemother.* 40:639–651.

11. Bébéar, C. M., H. Renaudin, A. Boudjadja, and C. Bébéar. 1998. In vitro activity of BAY 12-8039, a new fluoroquinolone, against mycoplasmas. *Antimicrob. Agents Chemother.* 42:703–704.

12. Bébéar, C. M., H. Renaudin, A. Charron, D. Gruson, M. Lefrancois, and C. Bébéar. 2000. In vitro activity of trovafloxacin compared to those of five antimicrobials against mycoplasmas including mycoplasma hominis and *Urealplasma urealyticum* fluoroquinolone-resistant isolates that have been genetically characterized. *Antimicrob. Agents Chemother.* 44:2557–2560.

13. Bébéar, C. M., H. Renaudin, T. Schaeverbeke, F. Leblanc, and C. Bébéar. 1999. In-vitro activity of grepafloxacin, a new fluoroquinolone, against mycoplasmas. *J. Antimicrob. Chemother.* 43:711–714.

14. Bermudez, L. E., C. B. Inderlied, P. Kolonoski, M. Wu, L. Barbara-Burnham, and L. S. Young. 1996. Activities of Bay Y 3118, levofloxacin, and ofloxacin alone or in combination with ethambutol against *Mycobacterium avium* complex in vitro, in human macrophages, and in beige mice. *Antimicrob. Agents Chemother.* 40:546–551.

15. Biedenbach, D. J., M. A. T. Croco, T. J. Barrett, and R. N. Jones. 1999. Comparative in vitro activity of gatifloxacin against *Stenotrophomonas maltophilia* and *Burkholderia* species isolates including evaluation of disk diffusion and E test methods. *Eur. J. Clin. Microbiol. Infect. Dis.* 18:428–431.

16. Biedenbach, D. J., and R. N. Jones. 1995. In vitro evaluation of DV-7751a, a new fluoroquinolone with an enhanced spectrum of activity against gram-positive aerobic organisms and anaerobes. *Antimicrob. Agents Chemother.* 39:1636–1643.

17. Boisivon, A., N. Dhoyen, and C. Carbon. 1995. Activity of CI-960 alone and in combination with amoxycillin against *Listeria monocytogenes*, and comparison with other quinolones. *J. Antimicrob. Chemother.* 36:527–530.

18. Bonacorsi, S., F. Fitoussi, S. Lhopital, and E. Bingen. 1999. Comparative in vitro activities of meropenem, imipenem, temocillin, piperacillin, and ceftazidime in combination with tobramycin, rifampin, or ciprofloxacin against *Burkholderia cepacia* isolates from patients with cystic fibrosis. *Antimicrob. Agents Chemother.* 43:213–217.

19. Boos, M., S. Mayer, A. Fischer, K. Köhrer, S. Scheuring, P. Heisig, J. Verhoef, Ad. C. Fluit, and F.-J. Schmitz. 2001. In vitro development of resistance to six quinolones in *Streptococcus pneumoniae*, *Streptococcus pyogenes*, and *Staphylococcus aureus*. *Antimicrob. Agents Chemother.* 45:938–942.

20. Brisse, S., D. Milatovic, A. C. Fluit, J. Verhoef, N. Martin, S. Scheuring, K. Köhrer, and F.-J. Schmitz. 1999. Comparative in vitro activities of ciprofloxacin, clinafloxacin, gatifloxacin, levofloxacin, moxifloxacin, and trovafloxacin against *Klebsiella pneumoniae*, *Klebsiella oxytoca*, *Enterobacter cloacae*, and *Enterobacter aerogenes* clinical isolates with alterations in GyrA and ParC proteins. *Antimicrob. Agents Chemother.* 43:2051–2055.

21. Brueggemann, A. B., K. C. Kugler, and G. V. Doern. 1997. In vitro activity of BAY 12-8039, a novel 8-methoxyquinolone, compared to activities of six fluoroquinolones against *Streptococcus pneumoniae*, *Haemophilus influenzae*, and *Moraxella catarrhalis*. *Antimicrob. Agents Chemother.* 41:1594–1597.

22. Burgess, D. S., and R. W. Hastings. 2000. Activity of piperacillin/tazobactam in combination with amikacin, ciprofloxacin, and trovafloxacin against *Pseudomonas aeruginosa* by time-kill. *Diagn. Microbiol. Infect. Dis.* 38:37–41.

23. Bustamante, C. I., G. L. Drusano, R. C. Wharton, and J. C. Wade. 1987. Synergism of the combinations of imipenem plus ciprofloxacin and imipenem plus amikacin against *Pseudomonas aeruginosa* and other bacterial pathogens. *Antimicrob. Agents Chemother.* 31:632–634.

24. Carmeli, Y., N. Troillet, G. M. Eliopoulos, and M. N. Samore. 1999. Emergence of antibiotic-resistant *Pseudomonas aeruginosa*: comparison of risks associated with different antipseudomonal agents. *Antimicrob. Agents Chemother.* 43:1379–1382.

25. Chin, N.-X., and H. C. Neu. 1987. Synergy of imipenem—a novel carbapenem, and rifampin and ciprofloxacin against *Pseudomonas aeruginosa*, *Serratia marcescens*, and *Enterobacter* species. *Chemotherapy* 33:183–188.

26. Cohen, M. A., M. D. Huband, J. W. Gage, S. L. Yoder, G. E. Roland, and S. J. Gracheck. 1997. In-vitro activity of clinafloxacin, trovafloxacin, and ciprofloxacin. *J. Antimicrob. Chemother.* 40:205–211.

27. Cohen, M. A., S. L. Yoder, M. D. Huband, G. E. Roland, and C. L. Courtney. 1995. In vitro and in vivo activities of clinafloxacin, CI-990 (PD 131112), and PD 138312 versus enterococci. *Antimicrob. Agents Chemother.* 39:2123–2127.

28. Cohn, M. L., and K. B. Waites. 2001. Antimicrobial activities of gatifloxacin against nosocomial isolates of *Stenotrophomonas maltophilia* measured by MIC and time-kill studies. *Antimicrob. Agents Chemother.* 45:2126–2128.

29. Coll, R., D. Gargallo-Viola, E. Tudela, M. A. Xicota, S. Llovera, and J. Guinea. 1996. Antibacterial activity and pharmacokinetics of four new 7-azetidinyl fluoroquinolones. *Antimicrob. Agents Chemother.* 40:274–277.

30. Cormican, M. G., and R. N. Jones. 1997. Antimicrobial activity and spectrum of LB20304, a novel naphthyridone. *Antimicrob. Agents Chemother.* 41:204–211.

31. Coyle, E. A., G. W. Kaatz, and M. J. Rybak. 2001. Activities of newer fluoroquinolones against ciprofloxacin-resistant

Streptococcus pneumoniae. Antimicrob. Agents Chemother. 45:1654–1659.

32. Davies, T. A., A. Evangelista, S. Pfleger, K. Bush, D. F. Sahm, and R. Goldschmidt. 2002. Prevalence of single mutations in topoisomerase type II genes among levofloxacin-susceptible clinical strains of *Streptococcus pneumoniae* isolated in the United States in 1992 to 1996 and 1999 to 2000. *Antimicrob. Agents Chemother.* 46:119–124.

33. Deguchi, T., M. Yasuda, M. Nakano, E. Kanematsu, S. Ozeki, S. Ishihara, I. Saito, and Y. Kawada. 1997. Antimicrobial activity of a new fluoroquinolone, DU-6859a, against quinolone-resistant clinical isolates of *Neisseria gonorrhoeae* with genetic alterations in the GyrA subunit of DNA gyrase and the ParC subunit of topoisomerase IV. *J. Antimicrob. Chemother.* 39:247–249.

34. Deshpande, L. M., D. J. Diekema, and R. N. Jones. 1999. Comparative activity of clinafloxacin and nine other compounds tested against 2000 contemporary clinical isolates from patients in United States hospitals. *Diagn. Microbiol. Infect. Dis.* 35:81–88.

35. Deshpande, L. M., and R. N. Jones. 2000. Antimicrobial activity of advanced-spectrum fluoroquinolones tested against more than 2000 contemporary bacterial isolates of species causing community-acquired respiratory tract infections in the United States (1999). *Diagn. Microbiol. Infect. Dis.* 37:139–142.

36. Dhople, A. M., and M. A. Ibanez. 1993. In-vitro activity of three new fluoroquinolones and synergy with ansamycins against *Mycobacterium leprae. J. Antimicrob. Chemother.* 32:445–451.

37. Diekema, D. J., R. N. Jones, and K. V. I. Rolston. 1999. Antimicrobial activity of gatifloxacin compared to seven other compounds tested against gram-positive organisms isolated at 10 cancer-treatment centers. *Diagn. Microbiol. Infect. Dis.* 34:37–43.

38. Doern, G. V., K. P. Heilmann, H. K. Huynh, P. R. Rhomberg, S. L. Coffman, and A. B. Brueggemann. 2001. Antimicrobial resistance among clinical isolates of *Streptococcus pneumoniae* in the United States during 1999–2000, including a comparison of resistance rates since 1994–1995. *Antimicrob. Agents Chemother.* 45:1721–1729.

39. Dreses-Werringloer, U., I. Padubrin, B. Jürgens-Saathoff, A. P. Hudson, H. Zeidler, and L. Köhler. 2000. Persistence of *Chlamydia trachomatis* is induced by ciprofloxacin and ofloxacin in vitro. *Antimicrob. Agents Chemother.* 44:3288–3297.

40. Dubois, J., and C. St.-Pierre. 1999. In vitro activity of gatifloxacin compared with ciprofloxacin, clarithromycin, erythromycin, and rifampin, against Legionella species. *Diagn. Microbiol. Infect. Dis.* 33:261–265.

41. Dudley, M. N., J. Blaser, D. Gilbert, K. H. Mayer, and S. H. Zinner. 1991. Combination therapy with ciprofloxacin plus azlocillin against *Pseudomonas aeruginosa*: effect of simultaneous versus staggered administration in an in vitro model of infection. *J. Infect. Dis.* 164:499–506.

42. Edelstein, P. H., T. Shinzato, E. Doyle, and M. A. C. Edelstein. 2001. In vitro activity of gemifloxacin (SB-265805, LB20304a) against *Legionella pneumophila* and its pharmacokinetics in guinea pigs with *L. pneumophila* pneumonia. *Antimicrob. Agents Chemother.* 45:2204–2209.

43. Eliopoulos, G. 1999. Activity of newer fluoroquinolones *in vitro* against gram-positive bacteria. *Drugs* 58(Suppl. 2):23–28.

44. Eliopoulos, G. M., and C. T. Eliopoulos. 1989. Ciprofloxacin in combination with other antimicrobials. *Am. J. Med.* 87(Suppl. 5A):17S–22S.

45. Eliopoulos, G. M., and C. T. Eliopoulos. 1993. Activity in vitro of the quinolones, p. 161–193. *In* D. C. Hooper and J. S. Wolfson (ed.), *Quinolone Antimicrobial Agents*, 2nd ed. American Society for Microbiology, Washington, D.C.

46. Fass, R. J., J. Barnishan, M. C. Solomon, and L. W. Ayers. 1996. In vitro activities of quinolones, β-lactams, tobramycin, and trimethoprim-sulfamethoxazole against nonfermentative gram-negative bacilli. *Antimicrob. Agents Chemother.* 40:1412–1418.

47. Fernández-Roblas, R., F. Cabria, J. Esteban, J. C. López, I. Gadea, and F. Soriano. 2000. *In vitro* activity of gemifloxacin (SB-265805) compared with 14 other antimicrobials against intestinal pathogens. *J. Antimicrob. Chemother.* 46:1023–1027.

48. Frémaux, A., G. Sissia, and P. Geslin. 1999. In-vitro bacteriostatic activity of levofloxacin and three other fluoroquinolones against penicillin-susceptible and penicillin-resistant *Streptococcus pneumoniae. J. Antimicrob. Chemother.* 43(Suppl. C):9–14.

49. Fukuda, H., R. Kishii, M. Takei, and M. Hosaka. 2001. Contributions of the 8-methoxy group of gatifloxacin to resistance selectivity, target preference, and antibacterial activity against *Streptococcus pneumoniae. Antimicrob. Agents Chemother.* 45:1649–1653.

50. Fung-Tomc, J. C., B. Minassian, B. Kolek, E. Huczko, L. Aleskunes, T. Stickle, T. Washo, E. Gradelski, L. Valera, and D. P. Bonner. 2000. Antibacterial spectrum of a novel desfluoro(6) quinolone, BMS-284756. *Antimicrob. Agents Chemother.* 44:3351–3356.

51. Garcia, M. T., C. Pelaz, M. J. Gimenez, and L. Aguilar. 2000. In vitro activities of gemifloxacin versus five quinolones and two macrolides against 271 Spanish isolates of *Legionella pneumophila*: influence of charcoal on susceptibility test results. *Antimicrob. Agents Chemother.* 44:2176–2178.

52. García-Garrote, F., E. Cercenado, J. Martín-Pedroviejo, O. Cuevas, and E. Bouza. 2001. Comparative *in vitro* activity of the new quinolone gemifloxacin (SB-265805) with other fluoroquinolones against respiratory tract pathogens. *J. Antimicrob. Chemother.* 47:681–684.

53. García-Rodríguez, J. A., J. E. García Sánchez, M. I. García García, M. J. Fresnadillo, I. Trujillano, and E. García Sánchez. 1994. In-vitro activity of four new fluoroquinolones. *J. Antimicrob. Chemother.* 34:53–64.

54. Gargallo-Viola, D., S. Ferrer, E. Tudela, M. Robert, R. Coll, R. Roser, and J. Guinea. 2001. Antibacterial activities and pharmacokinetics of E-4767 and E-5065, two new 8-chloro-fluoroquinolones with a 7-azetidin ring substituent. *Antimicrob. Agents Chemother.* 45:3113–3121.

55. Gilbert, D. N., S. J. Kohlhepp, K. A. Slama, G. Grunkemeier, G. Lewis, R. J. Dworkin, S. E. Slaughter, and J. E. Leggett. 2001. Phenotypic resistance of Staphylococcus aureus, selected Enterobacteriaceae, and Pseudomonas aeruginosa after single and multiple in vitro exposures to ciprofloxacin, levofloxacin, and trovafloxacin. *Antimicrob. Agents Chemother.* 45:883–892.

56. Gohara, Y., S. Arai, A. Akashi, K. Kuwano, C-C. Tseng, S. Matsubara, M. Matumoto, and T. Furudera. 1993. In vitro and in vivo activities of Q-35, a new fluoroquinolone, against *Mycoplasma pneumoniae. Antimicrob. Agents Chemother.* 37:1826–1830.

57. Goldstein, E. J., and D. M. Citron. 1992. Comparative activity of ciprofloxacin, ofloxacin, sparfloxacin, temafloxacin, CI-960, CI-990, and WIN 57273 against anaerobic bacteria. *Antimicrob. Agents Chemother.* 36:1158–1162.

58. Goldstein E. J., D. M. Citron, S. Hunt Gerardo, M. Hudspeth, and C. V. Merriam. 1997. Comparative in vitro

activities of DU-6859a, levofloxacin, ofloxacin, sparfloxacin, and ciprofloxacin against 387 aerobic and anaerobic bite wound isolates. *Antimicrob. Agents Chemother.* 41:1193–1195.

59. Goldstein, E. J., D. M. Citron, C. V. Merriam, K. Tyrrell, and Y. Warren. 1999. Activity of gatifloxacin compared to those of five other quinolones versus aerobic and anaerobic isolates from skin and soft tissue samples of human and animal bite wound infections. *Antimicrob. Agents Chemother.* 43:1475–1479.

60. Goldstein, E. J., D. M. Citron, C. V. Merriam, Y. Warren, and K. Tyrrell. 2000. Comparative in vitro activities of GAR-936 against aerobic and anaerobic animal and human bite wound pathogens. *Antimicrob. Agents Chemother.* 44:2747–2751.

61. Gomi, H., Z.-D. Jiang, J. A. Adachi, D. Ashley, B. Lowe, M. P. Verenkar, R. Steffen, and H. L. Dupont. 2001. In vitro antimicrobial susceptibility testing of bacterial enteropathogens causing traveler's diarrhea in four geographic regions. *Antimicrob. Agents Chemother.* 45:212–216.

62. Gordon, K. A., J. Fusco, D. J. Biedenback, M. A. Pfaller, and R. N. Jones. 2001. Antimicrobial susceptibility testing of clinical isolates of Bordetella pertussis from Northern California: report from the SENTRY antimicrobial surveillance program. *Antimicrob. Agents Chemother.* 45:3599–3600.

63. Gradelski, E., L. Valera, D. Bonner, and J. Fung-Tomc. 2001. Synergistic activities of gatifloxacin in combination with other antimicrobial agents against *Pseudomonas aeruginosa* and related species. *Antimicrob. Agents Chemother.* 45:3220–3222.

64. Guinea, J., M. Robert, D. Gargallo-Viola, M. A. Xicota, J. Garcia, E. Tudela, M. Esteve, R. Coll, M. Pares, and R. Roser. 1993. In vitro and in vivo antibacterial activities of E-4868, a new fluoroquinolone with a 7-azetidin ring substituent. *Antimicrob. Agents Chemother.* 37:868–874.

65. Haller, I. 1985. Comprehensive evaluation of ciprofloxacin-aminoglycoside combinations against *Enterobacteriaceae* and *Pseudomonas aeruginosa* strains. *Antimicrob. Agents Chemother.* 28:663–666.

66. Hamamoto, K., T. Shimizu, N. Fujimoto, Y. Zhang, and S. Arai. 2001. In vitro activities of moxifloxacin and other fluoroquinolones against *Mycoplasma pneumoniae*. *Antimicrob. Agents Chemother.* 45:1908–1910.

66a. Hardy, D., D. Amsterdam, L. A. Mandell, and C. Rotstein. 2000. Comparative in vitro activities of ciprofloxacin, gemifloxacin, grepafloxacin, moxifloxacin, ofloxacin, sparfloxacin, trovafloxacin, and other antimicrobial agents against bloodstream isolates of gram-positive cocci. *Antimicrob. Agents Chemother.* 44:802–805.

67. Hayward, C. L., M. E. Erwin, M. S. Barrett, and R. N. Jones. 1999. Comparative antimicrobial activity of gatifloxacin tested against *Campylobacter jejuni* including fluoroquinolone-resistant clinical isolates. *Diagn. Microbiol. Infect. Dis.* 34:99–102.

68. Hecht, D. W., and J. R. Osmolski. 1996. Comparison of activities of trovafloxacin (CP-99,219) and five other agents against 585 anaerobes with use of three media. *Clin. Infect. Dis.* 23(Suppl. 1):S44–S50.

69. Hecht, D. W., and H. M. Wexler. 1996. In vitro susceptibility of anaerobes to quinolones in the United States. *Clin. Infect. Dis.* 23(Suppl. 1):S2–S8.

69a. Heine, H. S., R. Dicks, and G. Andrews. 2001. In vitro activity of oritavancin (LY 333328), levofloxacin, meropenem, GAR936 and linezolid against strains of *Bacillus anthracis*. abstr. E-524. *In Program and Abstracts of the 41st Interscience Conference on Antimicrobial Agents and Chemotherapy.* American Society for Microbiology, Washington, D.C.

70. Heine, H. S., M. J. England, D. M. Waag, and W. R. Byrne. 2001. In vitro antibiotic susceptibilities of *Burkholderia mallei* (causative agent of glanders) determined by broth microdilution and E-test. *Antimicrob. Agents Chemother.* 45:2119–2121.

71. Heinemann, B., H. Wisplinghoff, M. Edmond, and H. Seifert. 2000. Comparative activities of ciprofloxacin, clinafloxacin, gatifloxacin, gemifloxacin, levofloxacin, moxifloxacin, and trovafloxacin against epidemiologically defined *Acinetobacter baumannii* strains. *Antimicrob. Agents Chemother.* 44:2211–2213.

72. Hershberger, E., and M. J. Rybak. 2000. Activities of trovafloxacin, gatifloxacin, clinafloxacin, sparfloxacin, levofloxacin, and ciprofloxacin against penicillin-resistant *Streptococcus pneumoniae* in an in vitro infection model. *Antimicrob. Agents Chemother.* 44:598–601.

73. Hirose, K, K. Tamura, H. Sagara, and H. Watanabe. 2001. Antibiotic susceptibilities of *Salmonella enterica* Serovar Typhi and *S. enterica* Serovar Paratyphi A isolated from patients in Japan. *Antimicrob. Agents Chemother.* 45:956–958.

74. Hoogkamp-Korstanje, J. A. A., and J. Roelofs-Willemse. 2000. Comparative *in vitro* activity of moxifloxacin against gram-positive clinical isolates. *J. Antimicrob. Chemother.* 45:31–39.

75. Horiuchi, S., Y. Inagaki, N. Yamamoto, N. Okamura, Y. Imagawa, and R. Nakaya. 1993. Reduced susceptibilities of *Shigella sonnei* strains isolated from patients with dysentery to fluoroquinolones. *Antimicrob. Agents Chemother.* 37:2486–2489.

76. Horowitz, H. W., T.-C. Hsieh, M. E. Aguero-Rosenfeld, F. Kalantarpour, I. Chowdhury, G. P. Wormser, and J. M. Wu. 2001. Antimicrobial susceptibility of Ehrlichia phagocytophila. *Antimicrob. Agents Chemother.* 45:786–788.

77. Ince, D., and D. C. Hooper. 2001. Mechanisms and frequency of resistance to gatifloxacin in comparison to AM-1121 and ciprofloxacin in *Staphylococcus aureus*. *Antimicrob. Agents Chemother.* 45:2755–2764.

78. Isenberg, H. D., P. Alperstein, and K. France. 1999. In vitro activity of ciprofloxacin, levofloxacin, and trovafloxacin, alone and in combination with β-lactams, against clinical isolates of *Pseudomonas aeruginosa*, *Stenotrophomonas maltophilia*, and *Burkholderia cepacia*. *Diagn. Microbiol. Infect. Dis.* 33:81–86.

79. Johnson, D. M., R. N. Jones, M. E. Erwin, and the Quality Control Study Group. 1999. Antistreptococcal activity of SB-265805 (LB20304), a novel fluoronaphthyridone, compared with five other compounds, including quality control guidelines. *Diagn. Microbiol. Infect. Dis.* 33:87–91.

80. Join-Lambert, O. F., M. Michea-Hamzehpour, T. Kohler, F. Chau, F. Faurisson, S. Dautrey, C. Vissuzaine, C. Carbon, and J. Pechère. 2001. Differential selection of multidrug efflux mutants by trovafloxacin and ciprofloxacin in and experimental model of *Pseudomonas aeruginosa* acute pneumonia in rats. *Antimicrob. Agents Chemother.* 45:571–576.

81. Jonas, D., I. Engels, C. Friedhoff, B. Spitzmüller, F. D. Daschner, and U. Frank. 2001. Efficacy of moxifloxacin, trovafloxacin, clinafloxacin and levofloxacin against intracellular *Legionella pneumophila*. *J. Antimicrob. Chemother.* 47:147–152.

82. Jones, M. E., A. M. Staples, I. Critchley, C. Thornsberry, P. Heinze, H. D. Engler, and D. F. Sahm. 2000. Benchmarking the in vitro activities of moxifloxacin and comparator agents against recent respiratory isolates from 377 medical centers

throughout the United States. *Antimicrob. Agents Chemother.* **44:**2645–2652.

83. Jones, R. N., C. H. Ballow, J. J. Schentag, D. M. Johnson, J. A. Deinhart, and the SPAR Study Group. 1998. In vitro evaluation of sparfloxacin activity and spectrum against 24,940 pathogens isolated in the United States and Canada, the final analysis. *Diagn. Microbiol. Infect. Dis.* **31:**313–325.

84. Jones, R. N., M. L. Beach, M. A. Pfaller, and G. V. Doern. 1998. Antimicrobial activity of gatifloxacin tested against 1676 strains of ciprofloxacin-resistant gram-positive cocci isolated from patient infections in North and South America. *Diagn. Microbiol. Infect. Dis.* **32:**247–252.

85. Jones, R. N., D. J. Biedenbach, M. E. Erwin, M. L. Beach, M. A. Pfaller, and the Quality Control Study Group. 1999. Activity of gatifloxacin against *Haemophilius influenzae* and *Moraxella catarrhalis,* including susceptibility test development, E-test comparisons, and quality control guidelines for *H. influenzae. J. Clin. Microbiol.* **37:**1999–2002.

86. Jones, R. N., M. A. T. Croco, K. C. Kugler, M. A. Pfaller, M. L. Beach, and the SENTRY Participants Group (North America). 2000. Respiratory tract pathogens isolated from patients hospitalized with suspected pneumonia: frequency of occurrence and antimicrobial susceptibility patterns from the SENTRY Antimicrobial Surveillance Program (United States and Canada, 1997). *Diagn. Microbiol. Infect. Dis.* **37:**115–125.

87. Jones, R. N., D. M. Johnson, M. E. Erwin, M. L. Beach, D. J. Biedenbach, M. A. Pfaller, and the Quality Control Study Group 1999. Comparative antimicrobial activity of gatifloxacin tested against *Streptococcus* spp., including quality control guidelines and Etest method validation. *Diagn. Microbiol. Infect. Dis.* **34:**91–98.

88. Kato, N., H. Kato, K. Tanaka-Bando, K. Watanabe, and K. Ueno. 1996. Comparison of in vitro activities of DU-6859a and other fluoroquinolones against Japanese isolates of anaerobic bacteria. *Clin. Infect. Dis.* **23**(Suppl. 1):S31–S5.

89. Kaye, K. S., S. Cosgrove, A. Harris, G. M. Eliopoulos, and Y. Carmeli. 2001. Risk factors for emergence of resistance to broad-spectrum cephalosporins among *Enterobacter* spp. *Antimicrob. Agents Chemother.* **45:**2628–2630.

90. Kenny, G. E., and F. D. Cartwright. 2001. Susceptibilities of *Mycoplasma hominis, M. pneumoniae,* and *Ureaplasma urealyticum* to GAR-936, dalfopristin, dirithromycin, evernimicin, gatifloxacin, linezolid, moxifloxacin, quinupristin-dalfopristin, and telithromycin compared to their susceptibilities to reference macrolides, tetracyclines, and quinolones. *Antimicrob. Agents Chemother.* **45:**2604–2608.

91. Kerawala, M., J. E. Ambler, P. Y. C. Lee, and Y. J. Drabu. 2001. In vitro activity of gemifloxacin (SB-265805) compared to eleven other antimicrobial agents against streptococcal isolates, excluding *Streptococcus pneumoniae. Eur. J. Clin. Microbiol. Infect. Dis.* **20:**271–275.

92. Kiehlbauch, J. A., C. N. Baker, and I. K. Wachsmuth. 1992. In vitro susceptibilities of aerotolerant *Campylobacter* isolates to 22 antimicrobial agents. *Antimicrob. Agents Chemother.* **36:**717–722.

93. Kim, J. H., J. A. Kang, Y. G. Kim, J. W. Kim, J. H. Lee, E. C. Choi, and B. K. Kim. 1997. In vitro and in vivo antibacterial efficacies of CFC-222, a new fluoroquinolone. *Antimicrob. Agents Chemother.* **41:**2209–2213.

94. Kim, J. H., J. A. Kang, Y. Lee, K. H. Lee, J. H. Lee, E. C. Choi, and B. K. Kim. 1998. Susceptibility of penicillin-susceptible and -resistant pneumococci to CFC-222, a new fluoroquinolone. *J. Antimicrob. Chemother.* **42:**527–530.

95. Kitzis, M.-D., F. W. Goldstein, M. Miegi, and J.-F. Acar. 1999. In-vitro activity of levofloxacin, a new fluoro-

quinolone: evaluation against *Haemophilus influenzae* and *Moraxella catarrhalis. J. Antimicrob. Chemother.* **43**(Suppl. C):21–26.

96. Klein, M. B., C. M. Nelson, and J. L. Goodman. 1997. Antibiotic susceptibility of the newly cultivated agent of human granulocytic ehrlichiosis: promising activity of quinolones and rifamycins. *Antimicrob. Agents Chemother.* **41:**76–79.

97. Kleinkauf, N., G. Ackermann, R. Schaumann, and A. C. Rodloff. 2001. Comparative in vitro activities of gemifloxacin, other quinolones, and nonquinolone antimicrobials against obligately anaerobic bacteria. *Antimicrob. Agents Chemother.* **45:**1896–1899.

98. Köhler, T., M. Michea-Hamzehpour, P. Plesíat, A.-L. Kahr, and J.-C. Pechere. 1997. Differential selection of multidrug efflux systems by quinolones by *Pseudomonas aeruginosa. Antimicrob. Agents Chemother.* **41:**2540–2543.

99. Kraiczy, P., J. Weigand, T. A. Wichelhaus, P. Heisig, H. Backes, V. Schäfer, G. Acker, V. Brade, and K.-P. Hunfeld. 2001. In vitro activities of fluoroquinolones against the spirochete *Borrelia burgdorferi. Antimicrob. Agents Chemother.* **45:**2486–2494.

100. Kutlin, A., P. M. Roblin, and M. R. Hammerschlag. 2002. Effect of prolonged treatment with azithromycin, clarithromycin, or levofloxacin on *Chlamydia pneumoniae* in a continuous-infection model. *Antimicrob. Agents Chemother.* **46:**409–412.

101. Lee, A., W. Mao, M. S. Warren, A. Mistry, K. Hoshino, R. Okumura, H. Ishida, and O. Lomovskaya. 2000. Interplay between efflux pumps may provide either additive or multiplicative effects on drug resistance. *J. Bacteriol.* **182:**3142–3150.

102. McDonald, L. C., F.-J. Chen, H.-J. Lo, H.-C. Yin, P.-L. Lu, C.-H. Huang, P. Chen, T.-L. Lauderdale, and M. Ho. 2001. Emergence of reduced susceptibility and resistance to fluoroquinolones in *Escherichia coli* in Taiwan and contributions of distinct selective pressures. *Antimicrob. Agents Chemother.* **45:**3084–3091.

103. Malay, S., P. M. Roblin, T. Reznik, A. Kutlin, and M. R. Hammerschlag. 2002. In vitro activities of BMS-284756 against Chlamydia trachomatis and recent clinical isolates of *Chlamydia pneumoniae. Antimicrob. Agents Chemother.* **46:**517–518.

104. Marco, F., M. Almela, J. Nolla-Salas, P. Coll, I. Gasser, M. D. Ferrer, M. de Simon. 2000. In vitro activities of 22 antimicrobial agents against *Listeria monocytogenes* strains isolated in Barcelona, Spain. *Diagn. Microbiol. Infect. Dis.* **38:**259–261.

105. Martínez-Martínez, L., P. Joyanes, A. I. Suárez, and E. J. Perea. 2001. Activities of gemifloxacin and five other antimicrobial agents against *Listeria monocytogenes* and coryneform bacteria isolated from clinical samples. *Antimicrob. Agents Chemother.* **45:**2390–2392.

106. Martínez-Martínez, L., A. Pascual, A. I. Suárez, and E. J. Perea. 1999. In-vitro activity of levofloxacin, ofloxacin and D-ofloxacin against coryneform bacteria and *Listeria monocytogenes. J. Antimicrob. Chemother.* **43**(Suppl. C):27–32.

107. Maurin, M., C. Abergel, and D. Raoult. 2001. DNA gyrase-mediated natural resistance to fluoroquinolones in *Ehrlichia* spp. *Antimicrob. Agents Chemother.* **45:**2098–2105.

108. Maurin, M., and D. Raoult. 1993. Antimicrobial susceptibility of *Rochalimaea quintana, Rochalimaea vinsonii,* and the newly recognized *Rochalimaea henselae. J. Antimicrob. Chemother.* **32:**587–594.

109. Maurin, M., and D. Raoult. 1997. Bacteriostatic and bactericidal activity of levofloxacin against *Rickettsia rickettsii,*

Rickettsia conorii, 'Israeli spotted fever group rickettsia' and *Coxiella burnetii*. *J. Antimicrob. Chemother.* **39**:725–730.

110. Mayer, I., and E. Nagy. 1999. Investigation of the synergic effects of aminoglycoside-fluoroquinolone and third-generation cephalosporin combinations against clinical isolates of *Pseudomonas* spp. *J. Antimicrob. Chemother.* **43**:651–657.

110a. McClosky, L. M., T. Moore, N. Niconovich, B. Donald, J. Broskey, C. Jakielaszek, S. Rittenhouse, and K. Colman. 2000. In vitro activity of gemifloxacin against a broad range of recent clinical isolates from the USA. *J. Antimicrob. Chemother.* **45**(Suppl. 1):13–21.

111. Michea-Hamzehpour, M., J. C. Pechère, B. Marchou, and R. Auckenthaler. 1986. Combination therapy: a way to limit emergence of resistance? *Am. J. Med.* **80**(Suppl. 6B):138–142.

112. Milatovic, D., F.-J. Schmitz, S. Brisse, J. Verhoef, and A. C. Fluit. 2000. In vitro activities of sitafloxacin (DU-6859a) and six other fluoroquinolones against 8,796 clinical bacterial isolates. *Antimicrob. Agents Chemother.* **44**:1102–1107.

113. Miyashita, N., Y. Niki, and T. Matsushima. 2001. In vitro and in vivo activities of sitafloxacin against *Chlamydia* spp. *Antimicrob. Agents Chemother.* **45**:3270–3272.

113a. Mohammed, J., C. K. Marston, T. Popovic, R. S. Weyant, and F. C. Tenover. 2001. Antimicrobial susceptibility testing of *Bacillus anthracis*. abstr. UL-9. *In Program and Abstracts of the 41st Interscience Conference on Antimicrobial Agents and Chemotherapy*. American Society for Microbiology, Washington, D.C.

114. Mølbak, K., D. L. Baggesen, F. M. Aarestrup, J. M. Ebbesen, J. Engberg, K. Frydendahl, P. Gerner-Smidt, A. M. Petersen, and H. C. Wegener. 1999. An outbreak of multidrug-resistant, quinolone-resistant *Salmonella enterica* serotype Typhimurium DT104. *N. Engl. J. Med.* **341**:1420–1425.

115. Montanari, M. P., M. Mingoia, and P. E. Varaldo. 2001. In vitro antibacterial activities of AF 3013, the active metabolite of prulifloxacin, against nosocomial and community Italian Isolates. *Antimicrob. Agents Chemother.* **45**:3616–3622.

116. Muños Bellido, J. L., F. J. Sánchez Hernández, M. N. Gutiérrez Zufiaurre, and J. A. García-Rodríguez. 2000. In vitro activity of newer fluoroquinolones against *Stenotrophomonas maltophilia*. *J. Antimicrob. Chemother.* **46**:334–335.

117. Murdoch, D. R., and L. B. Reller. 2001. Antimicrobial susceptibilities of Group B streptococci isolated from patients with invasive disease: 10-year perspective. *Antimicrob. Agents Chemother.* **45**:3623–3624.

118. Nagai, K., T. A. Davies, G. A. Pankuch, B. E. Dewasse, M. R. Jacobs, and P. C. Appelbaum. 2000. In vitro selection of resistance to clinafloxacin, ciprofloxacin, and trovafloxacin in *Streptococcus pneumoniae*. *Antimicrob. Agents Chemother.* **44**:2740–2746.

119. Nord, C. E. 1996. In vitro activity of quinolones and other antimicrobial agents against anaerobic bacteria. *Clin. Infect Dis.* **23**(Suppl. 1):S15–S18.

120. Oh, J.-I., K.-S. Paek, M.-J. Ahn, M.-Y. Kim, C. Y. Hong, I.-C. Kim, and J.-H. Kwak. 1996. In vitro and in vivo evaluations of LB20304, a new fluoronaphthyridone. *Antimicrob. Agents Chemother.* **40**:1564–1568.

121. Pankuch, G. A., K. Nagai, T. A. Davies, M. R. Jacobs, and P. C. Appelbaum. 2002. Antipneumococcal activity of BMS-284756 compared with those of six other agents. *Antimicrob. Agents Chemother.* **46**:252–354.

122. Pfaller, M. A., and R. N. Jones. 1997. Comparative antistreptococcal activity of two newer fluoroquinolones, levofloxacin and sparfloxacin. *Diagn. Microbiol. Infect. Dis.* **29**:199–201.

123. Pfaller, M. A., and R. N. Jones. 2000. MYSTIC (Meropenem Yearly Susceptibility Test Information Collection) results from the Americas: resistance implications in the treatment of serious infections. *J. Antimicrob. Chemother.* **46**:25–37.

124. Prosser, B. L. T., and G. Beskid. 1995. Multicenter in vitro comparative study of fluoroquinolones against 25,129 gram-positive and gram-negative clinical isolates. *Diagn. Microbiol. Infect. Dis.* **21**:33–45.

125. Roblin, P. M., T. Reznik, A. Kutlin, and M. R. Hammerschlag. 1999. In vitro activities of gemifloxacin (SB 265805, LB20304) against recent isolates of *Chlamydia pneumoniae*. *Antimicrob. Agents Chemother.* **43**:2806–2807.

126. Roychoudhury, S., C. E. Catrenich, E. J. McIntosh, H. D. McKeever, K. M. Makin, P. M. Koenigs, and B. Ledoussal. 2001. Quinolone resistance in staphylococci: activities of new nonfluorinated quinolones against molecular targets in whole cells and clinical isolates. *Antimicrob. Agents Chemother.* **45**:1115–1120.

127. Ruiz-Serrano, M. J., L. Alcalá, L. Martínez, M. Díaz, M. Marín, M. J. González-Abad, and E. Bouza. 2000. In vitro activities of six fluoroquinolones against 250 clinical isolates of *Mycobacterium tuberculosis* susceptible or resistant to first-line antituberculosis drugs. *Antimicrob. Agents Chemother.* **44**:2567–2568.

128. Sahm, D. F., I. A. Critchley, L. J. Kelly, J. A. Karlowsky, D. C. Mayfield, C. Thornsberry, Y. R. Mauriz, and J. Kahn. 2001. Evaluation of current activities of fluoroquinolones against gram-negative bacilli using centralized in vitro testing and electronic surveillance. *Antimicrob. Agents Chemother.* **45**:267–274.

129. Sahm, D. F., M. E. Jones, M. L. Hickey, D. R. Diakun, S. V. Mani, and C. Thornsberry. 2000. Resistance surveillance of *Streptococcus pneumoniae*, *Haemophilus influenzae* and *Moraxella catarrhalis* isolated in Asia and Europe 1997–1998. *J. Antimicrob. Chemother.* **45**:457–466.

130. Sahm, D. F., J. A. Karlowsky, L. J. Kelly, I. A. Critchley, M. E. Jones, C. Thornsberry, Y. Mauriz, and J. Kahn. 2001. Need for annual surveillance of antimicrobial resistance in *Streptococcus pneumoniae* in the United States: 2-year longitudinal analysis. *Antimicrob. Agents Chemother.* **45**:1037–1042.

131. Saravolatz, L., O. Manzor, C. Check, J. Pawlak, and B. Belian. 2001. Antimicrobial activity of moxifloxacin, gatifloxacin and six fluoroquinolones against *Streptococcus pneumoniae*. *J. Antimicrob. Chemother.* **47**:875–877.

132. Schmitz, F.-J., M. Boos, S. Mayer, D. Hafner, H. Jagusch, J. Verhoef, and A. C. Fluit. 2001. Propensity of fluoroquinolones with different moieties at position 8 to cause resistance development in clinical isolates of *Streptococcus pneumoniae*. *Antimicrob. Agents Chemother.* **45**:2666–2667.

133. Schmitz, F. J., A. C. Fluit, D. Hafner, A. Beeck, A. M. Perdikouli, M. Boos, S. Scheuring, J. Verhoef, K. Kohrer, and C. von Eiff. 2000. Development of resistance to ciprofloxacin, rifampin, and mupirocin in methicillin-susceptible and -resistant *Staphylococcus aureus* isolates. *Antimicrob. Agents Chemother.* **44**:3229–3231.

134. SENTRY participants group (Latin America), A. Gales, and R. N. Jones. 2001. Activities of BMS 284756 (T-3811) against *Haemophilus influenzae*, *Moraxella catarrhalis*, and *Streptococcus pneumoniae* isolates from SENTRY Antimicrobial Surveillance Program Medical Centers in Latin America (1999). *Antimicrob. Agents Chemother.* **45**:1463–1466.

135. Skinner, P. S., S. K. Furney, D. A. Kleinert, and I. M. Orme. 1995. Comparison of activities of fluoroquinolones in murine macrophages infected with *Mycobacterium tuberculosis*. *Antimicrob. Agents Chemother.* **39**:750–753.

136. Smith, K. E., J. M. Besser, C. W. Hedberg, F. T. Leano, J. B. Bender, J. H. Wicklund, B. P. Johnson, K. A. Moore, M. T. Osterholm. 1999. Quinolone-resistant *Campylobacter jejuni* infections in Minnesota, 1992–1998. *N. Engl. J. Med.* 340:1525–1532.

137. Soussy, C.-J., M. Cluzel, M.-C. Ploy, M.-D. Kitzis, C. Morel, A. Bryskier, and P. Courvalin. 1999. In-vitro antibacterial activity of levofloxacin against hospital isolates: a multicenter study. *J. Antimicrob. Chemother.* 43(Suppl. C):43–50.

138. Takahata, M., J. Mitsuyama, Y. Yamashiro, M. Yonezawa, H. Araki, Y. Todo, S. Minami, Y. Watanabe, and H. Narita. 1999. In vitro and in vivo antimicrobial activities of T-3811ME, a novel Des-F (6)-quinolone. *Antimicrob. Agents Chemother.* 43:1077–1084.

139. Takahata, M., M. Shimakura, R. Hori, K. Kizawa, Y. Todo, S. Minami, Y. Watanabe, and H. Narita. 2001. In vitro and in vivo efficacies of T-3811ME (BMS-284756) against *Mycoplasma pneumoniae. Antimicrob. Agents Chemother.* 45:312–315.

140. Teng, L.-J., P.-R. Hsueh, S.-W. Ho, and K.-T Luh. 2001. High prevalence of inducible erythromycin resistance among *Streptococcus bovis* isolates in Taiwan. *Antimicrob. Agents Chemother.* 45:3362–3365.

141. Threlfall, E. J., and L. R. Ward. 2001. Decreased susceptibility to ciprofloxacin in *Salmonella enterica* serotype Typhi, United Kingdom. *Emerg. Infect. Dis.* 7:448–450.

142. Threlfall, E. J., L. R. Ward, J. A. Skinner, H. R. Smith, and S. Lacey. 1999. Ciprofloxacin-resistant *Salmonella typhi* and treatment failure. *Lancet* 353:1590–1591.

143. Ullmann, U., S. Schubert, and R. Krausse. 1999. Comparative in-vitro activity of levofloxacin, other fluoroquinolones, doxycycline and erythromycin against *Ureaplasma urealyticum* and *Mycoplasma hominis. J. Antimicrob. Chemother.* 43(Suppl. C):33–36.

144. Verhaegen, J., and L. Verbist. 1999. In-vitro activities of 16 non-β-lactam antibiotics against penicillin-susceptible and penicillin-resistant *Streptococcus pneumoniae. J. Antimicrob. Chemother.* 43:563–567.

145. Visalli, M. A., S. Bajaksouzian, M. R. Jacobs, and P. C. Appelbaum. 1997. Comparative activity of trovafloxacin, alone and in combination with other agents, against gram-negative nonfermentative rods. *Antimicrob. Agents Chemother.* 41:1475–1481.

146. Wakabayashi, E., and S. Mitsuhashi. 1994. In vitro antibacterial activity of AM-1155, a novel 6-fluoro-8-methoxy quinolone. *Antimicrob. Agents Chemother.* 38:594–601.

147. Whitney, C. G., M. M. Farley, J. Hadler, L. H. Harrison, C. Lexau, A. Reingold, L. Lefkowitz, P. R. Cieslak, M. Cetron, E. R. Zell, J. H. Jorgensen, and A. Schuchat. 2000. Increasing prevalence of multidrug-resistant *Streptococcus pneumoniae* in the United States. *N. Engl. J. Med.* 343:1917–1924.

148. Wilcox, M. H., W. Fawley, J. Freeman, and J. Brayson. 2000. *In vitro* activity of new generation fluoroquinolones against genotypically distinct and indistinguishable *Clostridium difficile* isolates. *J. Antimicrob. Chemother.* 46:551–555.

149. Wise, R., and J. M. Andrews. 1997. The activity of grepafloxacin against respiratory pathogens in the UK. *J. Antimicrob. Chemother.* 40(Suppl. A):27–30.

150. Wise, R., and J. M. Andrews. 1999. The in-vitro activity and tentative breakpoint of gemifloxacin, a new fluoroquinolone. *J. Antimicrob. Chemother.* 44:679–688.

151. Wise, R., N. P. Brenwald, J. M. Andrews, and F. Boswell. 1997. The activity of the methylpiperazinyl fluoroquinolone CG 5501: a comparison with other fluoroquinolones. *J. Antimicrob. Chemother.* 39:447–452.

152. Zabinski, R. A., K. J. Walker, A. J. Larsson, J. A. Moody, G. W. Kaatz, and J. C. Rotschafer. 1995. Effect of Aerobic and Anaerobic environments on antistaphylococcal activities of five fluoroquinolones. *Antimicrob. Agents Chemother.* 39:507–512.

153. Zhao, B. Y., R. Pine, J. Domagala, and K. Drlica. 1999. Fluoroquinolone action against clinical Isolates of *Mycobacterium tuberculosis*: Effects of a C-8 methoxyl group on survival in liquid media and in human macrophages. *Antimicrob. Agents Chemother.* 43:661–666.

II. PHARMACOLOGY

Chapter 6

Pharmacokinetics of Fluoroquinolones

MICHAEL N. DUDLEY

During the past two decades, fluoroquinolones have emerged as an important class of antimicrobials for treatment of a variety of infections. The success of this class in the clinic can largely be attributed to excellent pharmacokinetic properties of the class as a whole. The predictability of pharmacokinetic properties in patients enabled elucidation of pharmacokinetic-pharmacodynamic relationships in patients and application treatment of infections.

This chapter reviews important aspects of the pharmacokinetic properties of fluoroquinolones. Rather than provide an exhaustive tabular summary of published pharmacokinetic parameters, a topical discussion on important topics and principles is provided. Key fluoroquinolones discussed in this chapter are shown in Fig. 1.

ABSORPTION

Fluoroquinolones are generally well absorbed after oral administration. Table 1 summarizes the bioavailability of several fluoroquinolones in normal human healthy volunteers. The extent of bioavailability generally exceeds 75% for most agents. Fluoroquinolones have a low intrinsic hepatic clearance, and thus there is little first pass extraction.

Mechanisms of Drug Absorption

The precise mechanisms for absorption of fluoroquinolones are poorly understood. Studies in vitro (e.g., Caco-2 cells) and in vivo show that fluoroquinolones are largely absorbed by passive diffusion. Since many agents are zwitterionic, the pH-dependent solubility and permeability complicates assessment of bioavailability of agents, including determination of regional absorption.

Although most of the absorption of ofloxacin appears to be passive, a small proportion of ofloxacin absorption may be mediated by an active

transport system (63). Studies in rats show that ofloxacin absorption is saturable, suggesting the role of a transporter; this system appears to be different from the peptide transport system, that may be involved in sparfloxacin absorption (86).

In humans and in vitro Caco-2 cells, absorption of ciprofloxacin and enoxacin appears to have an active component that may be present in certain regions of the gastrointestinal (GI) tract. The absorption of ciprofloxacin was studied in healthy male volunteers by loading the ciprofloxacin dose in a device that releases drug upon remote control activation. Using this capsule, the drug can be released at various regions of the GI tract to determine absorption distal to the site of release. Bioavailability was reduced as the dose was "triggered" at more distal portions of the gut; for example, bioavailability was reduced to 37, 23, and 10% when the dose was delivered in the jejunum, ileum, and colon, respectively, suggesting that a major portion of ciprofloxacin absorption occurs in more proximal regions of the gut (31). However, it can not be deduced if these data reflect regional transport differences, or differences in pH-mediated changes in solubility with this zwitterionic compound.

A small but measurable amount of gastrointestinal secretion of drug has been shown in some preclinical and human systems. However, this does not appear to be a major route of elimination or obstacle for bioavailability. Studies in Caco-2 cells and in rats show that secretion could be inhibited by verapamil and other substrates for a common secretory mechanism, suggesting that these may be substrates for intestinal P-glycoprotein (P-gp) (63).

Factors Affecting Absorption

Dose

Dose proportionality in oral bioavailability is generally shown over the range of oral-dose studies (e.g.,

Michael N. Dudley • Essential Therapeutics, Inc., 850 Maude Ave., Mountain View, CA 94034.

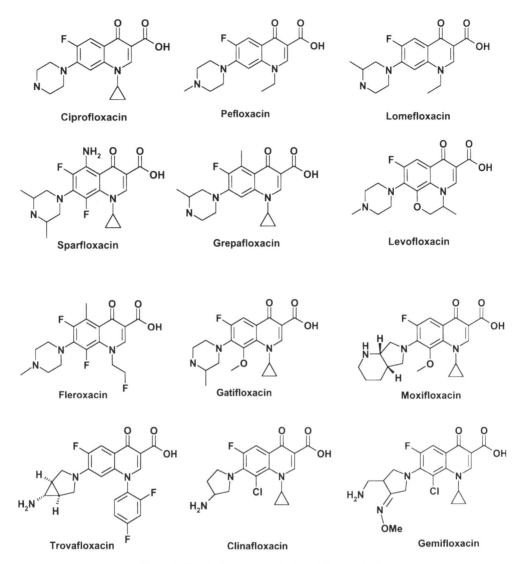

Figure 1. Chemical structures of selected fluoroquinolones.

25 to 1,000 mg). Levofloxacin has been studied as single and multiple intravenous (i.v.) or oral doses up to 750 and 1,000 mg, respectively, and showed maximum concentration of drug in serum (C_{max}) and area under the curve (AUC) values proportional to those observed with lower doses ($\leq$500 mg) (7, 8, 10).

Enantiomeric forms

Several fluoroquinolones have *R* and *S* enantiomers due to chiral centers located in heterocyclic rings fused or appended to the quinolone nucleus. In general, the pharmacokinetic properties of the enantiomeric forms are similar. Ofloxacin is available clinically as a racemic mixture of the *S*-(−) and *R*-(−) enantiomers, with the *S*-(−) form largely responsible for the antimicrobial activity. Studies in rats

with ofloxacin showed the *S*-(−) enantiomer of ofloxacin appeared to have slightly higher absorption than the *R*-(+) form (63). Assay of the separate enantiomers following administration of ofloxacin showed that the more active form [*S*-(−)] has a slight but statistically significant lower total and renal clearance, and a longer elimination half-life than the other enantiomer. The differences in serum AUCs were not due to protein binding (binding was the same for both enantiomers) (58). This difference served as one of the factors to further develop the *S*-(−) form (as levofloxacin) for clinical use. Studies with the *R* and *S* enantiomers of clinafloxacin in humans also showed no significant differences in oral bioavailability and pharmacokinetic disposition (33). Studies with gatifloxacin showed no difference in pharmacokinetic properties among the racemates.

Table 1. Summary of the pharmacokinetics of fluoroquinolones following a single dose in normal human volunteers[a]

Drug	Dose (mg/ml)	Route	Protein binding (%)	C_{max} (µg/ml)	V_{ss} (V_{area}) (liters/kg)	AUC (mg·h/liter)	Clearance (ml/min)[b]	Bioavailability (%)	CL_R (ml/min)	Fe (%)	$t_{1/2}$ (h)	Reference(s)
Ciprofloxacin	400	i.v.	30	3.4–6.7	1.9	8.1–14.2	417–568				3–4	14, 17, 26
	500	p.o.	30	1.5–2.9	2.1–5.0	9–11	700–902	55–70		25–35	3–5	
Clinafloxacin	400	i.v.	50–60	3.5	1.9	22.6	298		109.0	49–74	6.2	64
		p.o.	50–60	2.4	2.3	18.5	299	87		64	6.1	
Gatifloxacin	400	i.v.	20	4.5	1.5	35.1	180–206		124	62–82	7–9	23, 27
	400	p.o.	20	3.8	1.8	33.0	188–212	96	148–156	72–80	7–10	
Grepafloxacin	400	p.o.		0.93	8.1	11.4	480–800	72	0.67	8.5	11.7	18
Levofloxacin	500	i.v.	24–52	5.7	0.95	44–55	186–195		116.0	61	6.7	6, 7
	500	p.o.	24–52	4.8–5.7	1.3	45–61		95–100	100.0	63	6.4–7.4	
Moxifloxacin	400	i.v.	39–52	3.7–5.0	2.0	23–45	147–194		43.0	15–22	8.2–15.4	53, 69, 70, 74, 81
	400	p.o.	39–52	2.5–5.0	3.1(3.6)	20–45		86–100	23–50	15–20	8.3–15.6	
Sparfloxacin	400	p.o.	40	0.56–1.6	4.6	16.4–34.8		90	12.1–12.8	10	16–20	25
Trovafloxacin	300	p.o.	88	2.6		39.5		88	9	5	12.4	76
(alatrofloxacin)	300	i.v.		4.3	1.4	43.4	113		13	10	11	80

[a] Abbreviations: p.o., orally; V_{ss}, volume of distribution at steady state; V_{area}, volume of distribution in the area; CL_R, renal clearance.
[b] V/F and CL/F for oral doses.

Food and enteral feedings

Significant food-drug interactions are generally absent for fluoroquinolones. In general, food may delay the onset but not the extent of absorption of fluoroquinolones. Meals containing standard carbohydrate content or even high-fat breakfasts have been shown to delay absorption, but no major changes in the extent of oral bioavailability for ciprofloxacin, trovafloxacin, enoxacin, lomefloxacin, ofloxacin, and pefloxacin. Gemifloxacin oral bioavailability for a 320- or 640-mg oral dose was unaffected by a high-fat breakfast (1).

The early commercial unavailability of parenteral formulations (or their high cost) for use in critically ill patients has led to consideration of administration of suspensions of crushed tablets of some agents via a nasogastric tube. In studies with ciprofloxacin, ofloxacin, and trovafloxacin in normal volunteers as well as patients receiving enteral feedings through a nasogastric, gastrostomy, or jejunosotomy tubes, the bioavailability appears to be acceptable. Some studies have reported significant reductions in serum concentrations in patients administered ciprofloxacin as crushed tablets mixed with a variety of feeding solutions through enteral feeding tubes (16, 32, 48).

Several diseases or treatments are associated with alterations in the structure and function of the GI tract. Studies with i.v. and oral administration of ciprofloxacin in diabetic patients with gastroparesis showed the mean absolute bioavailability was 67% (range 43 to 82%), which is slightly lower than that reported in normal healthy volunteers (>80%) (46). Patients with human immunodeficiency virus infection and AIDS frequently have achlorhydria, and may be infected with opportunistic infections that produce chronic diarrhea and malabsorption syndromes. Cancer chemotherapy is associated with damage at the mucosal layer, and this may affect oral bioavailability and the efficacy of fluoroquinolone prophylaxis of infection in this patient group. Studies with ciprofloxacin showed that bioavailability was diminished slightly in patients after chemotherapy, but this reduction appeared to be more pronounced following recovery of cell division as measured by recovery in peripheral granulocyte counts (M. Dudley, unpublished observations).

DISTRIBUTION

Protein Binding

The serum protein binding of fluoroquinolones is generally low, owing to the charge and lipophilicity of the core molecule and its substituents. Protein binding generally fits in the low to moderate range (Table 1). Although low relative to other classes of drugs, correction for protein binding should be undertaken when comparing pharmacologic data for members of the class at the extreme ranges (e.g., trovafloxacin versus levofloxacin).

Methods for Describing the Extravascular Distribution of Fluoroquinolones

Tissue homogenates versus interstitial fluid

Studies of the tissue pharmacokinetic properties of antiinfectives and their importance in the outcome of infection continue to generate misunderstanding and controversy. Fluoroquinolones readily traverse cell membranes by passive and active processes (see below), and appear to distribute in a space exceeding total body water. This large volume of distribution occurs due to partitioning into cells, often where extracellular bacteria associated with clinical infections do not reside. Thus, high concentrations of drug in tissue homogenates signal drug sequestration at sites that may not be accessible to bacteria infecting an interstitial space, and hence are irrelevant. Situations in which intracellular penetration of drug can be relevant and should be considered include intracellular infections, such as those due to *Chlamydia* spp., *Mycoplasma* spp., *Legionella* spp., and for intracellular killing of phagocytized bacteria.

Sampling and reporting of results

Sampling of tissues from patients has several limitations. Given the invasiveness of the procedures, it is usually impossible to collect multiple samples from tissue biopsy or other sites. Thus, one has a "population" of single samples from a single patient. Most studies use tissues collected during surgical procedures deemed medically necessary for treatment of noninfectious ailments. The nature of the procedures may bias collection of tissues around a certain sampling time. Recently, population pharmacokinetic methods have been applied to analysis of tissue distribution data; studies with levofloxacin from patients undergoing prostate surgery demonstrated that high concentrations in prostate tissue could be expected, with modeling of data from more than 700 patients, showing levofloxacin AUC-tissue to AUC-plasma ratios exceeding 1 for most patients (16).

Blister fluid and microdialysis

Distribution of drug in experimentally induced blisters remains a standard method for comparison of the extravascular distribution of drugs. The blisters may be formed by application of an irritant (cantharides) or by suction through small holes in a plastic block applied to the skin of a volunteer. Wise and colleagues have studied the pharmacokinetics of several fluoroquinolones in serum and cantharides-induced blister fluid under relatively consistent conditions that provide a useful comparison among agents (Table 2). In general, the ratio of the AUC in blister fluid to serum is high and generally approaches 1. Other than for pefloxacin and possibly trovafloxacin, it would appear that all agents have similar distribution properties into interstitial fluids. It would appear that partitioning into blister fluid (as well as saliva) is based on serum pharmacokinetic properties and protein binding and not on physicochemical properties such as log D (38).

Although drug bound in tissues may be released over time, concentrations of drug in the interstitial fluid and other compartments (not influenced by active transport or efflux processes) tend change in parallel with the unbound (non-protein-bound) serum concentrations of drug. This relationship was recently demonstrated using microdialysis measurement of moxifloxacin in the interstitial fluid in vastus muscle and subcutaneous tissue in humans. Moxifloxacin concentrations in the dialysates paralleled those in plasma and were consistent with calculated unbound moxifloxacin concentrations in plasma (based on 52% protein binding). Measures of moxifloxacin concentrations in cantharides-induced skin blisters in the same subjects also agreed with concentrations measured using microdialysis probes (53).

Positron emission tomography

Positron emission tomography is an additional novel technique for tracing the distribution of drugs in animals and in humans. The fluorine atom common to fluoroquinolones enables ^{18}F labeling of compounds and detection using sensitive positron emission tomographic instruments. Trovafloxacin and fleroxacin pharmacokinetics were studied in healthy normal volunteers and confirmed the high distribution of these drugs into various tissues. As expected, concentrations of drug were highest in excretory organs (liver, kidney) (19, 20). Total concentrations and amounts of drug were also high in other tissues associated with infection due to susceptible organisms (e.g., lung); however, as with measures of tissue homogenates, the relevance to these concentrations to MICs for infecting pathogens requires careful consideration of the fraction of drug remaining unbound in the tissue.

Studies in Normal versus Infected Tissue

In view of the problems in estimating the amount of pharmacologically active fluoroquinolone in tissue homogenates, microdialysis has been used to compare drug distribution in normal versus infected tissues. Muller et al. (52) compared ciprofloxacin concentrations in inflamed foot lesions and normal tissues in diabetic patients following a single dose. Ciprofloxacin concentrations in serum, diabetic ulcers, and "normal" tissue in the contralateral limb were similar, indicating the agent was able to diffuse adequately to the site. A high degree of distribution

Table 2. Pharmacokinetics of fluoroquinolones in serum and cantharides-induced blister fluids in normal volunteers

Drug	Dose	Route	AUC (mg·h/liter)			C_{max} (mg/liter)			Reference(s)
			Serum	Blister	Blister:serum ratio	Serum	Blister	Blister:serum ratio	
Ciprofloxacin	100	i.v.	2.8	3.4	1.21		0.6		83
	400	i.v.	14.2	13.8	0.97	6.7	2.6	0.39	5
	500	p.o.	9.9	11.6	1.17	2.3	1.4	0.61	83
	750	p.o.	19.2	20.3	1.06	3.9	2.3	0.59	5
Clinafloxacin	200	p.o.	9.86	9.2	0.93	1.34	1.13	0.84	82
Enoxacin	400	i.v.	17.8	23.1	1.30	5.5	2.2	0.40	83
	600	p.o.	28.8	32.8	1.14	3.7	2.9	0.78	83
Grepafloxacin	400	p.o.	12.4	22.0	1.77	1.5	1.1	0.73	9
Lomefloxacin	400	p.o.	32.2	32.4	1.01	4.7	3.5	0.74	73
Moxifloxacin	400	i.v.	45.3	42.7	0.94	5.1	3.2	0.63	81
	400	p.o.	45.5	40.3	0.84	5	2.6	0.52	81
Norfloxacin	400	p.o.	5.4	5.7	1.06	1.45	1	0.69	83
Ofloxacin	600	p.o.	57.5	71.8	1.25	10.7	5.2	0.49	83
Pefloxacin	400	i.v.	56.1	38.8	0.69	NA[a]	3.3	NA	83
Sparfloxacin	400	p.o.	32.3	37.4	1.17	1.6	1.3	0.81	36
Trovafloxacin	200	p.o.	24.4	15.3	0.63	2.9	1.2	0.41	84

[a] NA, not available.

of levofloxacin into inflammatory skin-blister fluid has also been confirmed, with blister fluid:serum AUCs (both extrapolated to infinity) exceeding 100% (77).

Use of positron emission tomography has been extended to tracking the distribution of drugs to infected sites. Administration of [18F]fleroxacin to normal volunteers and patients with infections under treatment showed rapid accumulation in tissue sites. While accumulation was greater in kidneys or prostate when active urinary infection was present, there was no difference (or a slight reduction) in drug partitioning into lung tissue in patients with bronchitis (ca. 25% reduction in peak concentration). There was no change in drug distribution over time (20).

Distribution into Cerebrospinal Fluid

The high potency of several fluoroquinolones against pathogens associated with bacterial meningitis and resistance to other drug classes has prompted the investigation of fluoroquinolines in the treatment of bacterial meningitis. Studies using brain microdialysis in animals show that concentrations of drug in cerebrospinal fluid (CSF) are lower than those in serum, consistent with the role of a blood-brain barrier limiting the extent of distribution. Studies in mice have further shown that a multidrug resistance protein MRP1, P-glycoprotein, and an anion exchange transporter appear to be involved in efflux of grepafloxacin, levofloxacin, and sparfloxacin from CSF (75).

Although fluoroquinolones are removed from the CSF by active transport mechanisms, several agents appear to achieve concentrations in CSF that are associated with antimicrobial activity in vitro. Trovafloxacin was detected in the CSF from 13 adult healthy volunteers following a single 300-mg i.v. infusion (as the ala-ala prodrug ala-trovafloxacin). Trovafloxacin concentrations in CSF ranged between 0.14 and 0.91 up to 24 h after the dose. The CSF:serum trovafloxacin ratios ranged between 0.14 and 0.33 and increased over time, indicating that the terminal half-life in CSF was longer than that in serum. Since active transport mechanisms may mediate drug entry into CSF, it is likely that the terminal half-life is influenced by the input of drug into CSF (12).

Gatifloxacin distribution in the CSF has been noted in patients receiving 150–200 mg twice daily. Although absolute concentrations were not reported, the ratio of concentrations in CSF:serum ranged between 0.21 and 0.45 (60).

Distribution into Ocular Tissues

The pharmacokinetics of fluoroquinolones in the aqueous and vitreous in animals as well as humans have been described. Studies in a rabbit model clearly show that the partitioning of ciprofloxacin, fleroxacin, ofloxacin, and sparfloxacin into vitreous humor correlates with lipophilicity (measured by octanol-water partitioning). Removal from the vitreous appears to be mediated by both passive as well as active processes, with probenecid and heat-killed bacteria capable of slowing the removal of drug following direct intraocular injection (43).

Mean ciprofloxacin, levofloxacin, and moxifloxacin concentrations in human aqueous humor following single (moxifloxacin, levofloxacin) or two doses (12 h apart; ciprofloxacin) ranged from 0.5 to 2.3 µg/ml (24). However, it is only possible to obtain single samples from the chambers in both animals and humans; population pharmacokinetic approaches have proven to be valuable in characterizing drug movement into these compartments. Morlet and colleagues studied ciprofloxacin pharmacokinetics in the aqueous and vitreous chambers of human eyes in patients undergoing cataract/glaucoma surgery or retina repair. Data from these patients, as well as additional data in the literature, were used to construct a population pharmacokinetic model for ciprofloxacin pharmacokinetics in serum and the chambers of the eye. The mean ratios of concentrations in aqueous and vitreous humor to concentration in plasma were 0.23 and 0.17, respectively. The modeling and subsequent simulations led to development of a recommendation of a prophylactic regimen consisting of two 750-mg oral doses given 12 h apart, with surgery commencing within 12 h after administration of the second dose (51).

METABOLISM

Metabolism appears to be a significant mode for elimination of active drug for only a few fluoroquinolones. The piperazine ring at the C-7 appears to be the major site for biotransformation of most fluoroquinolones; the extent and rate of biotransformation can be modulated by substitutions on the ring. Some evidence exists that stereochemistry may play a role in altering metabolism on this substituent (4).

Pefloxacin

Pefloxacin is the most extensively metabolized fluoroquinolone in clinical use. The major metabolites in serum are the *N*-oxide, norfloxacin, and oxonorfloxacin and oxopefloxacin (49)

Gatifloxacin

Gatifloxacin is highly stable to metabolizing enzymes in vitro and in vivo. Only a small percentage of the dose is excreted as the ethylenediamine or methlethylenediamine metabolites of gatifloxacin. Although amino and glucuronide metabolites were observed in preclinical animal species, neither metabolite was observed in human urine (27).

Levofloxacin

Although urinary recovery of levofloxacin is among the highest of available fluoroquinolones, three minor metabolites have been identified in preclinical animal species and humans: β-D-glucuronide (M1, animals only), desmethyl-levofloxacin (M2), and an levofloxacin N-oxide (M3). Urinary excretion of M2 and M3 in humans accounts for less than 5% of a dose (56). These metabolites do not have significant antimicrobial activity.

Grepafloxacin

Metabolism of grepafloxacin in normal volunteers shows formation of five metabolites. These metabolites are reported to have minimal antibacterial activity. Phase 2 metabolites include the 4′-glucuronide, and 4′-sulfate conjugates of grepafloxacin. Oxidative metabolism occurs on the piperazinyl ring, including opening of the ring to the (2-aminopropyl)amino metabolite (18).

Moxifloxacin

Approximately 45 to 48% of a dose of moxifloxacin is recovered as unchanged drug in urine and feces. The remainder undergoes phase II metabolism in humans by glucuronidation on the 3 carboxy group (M2), and sulfation (M1) on the diazabicyclic ring of the 7 position of the quinolone nucleus. Both metabolites have a prolonged elimination half-life like moxifloxacin (half-life, 7 to 15 h) following oral or intravenous moxifloxacin. Most of the M1 metabolite is recovered in feces (ca. 35% of moxifloxacin), whereas ca. 13% of the dose of moxifloxacin was recovered as the M1 metabolite in urine. The M1 metabolite is 89.5% bound in human serum, whereas the M2 metabolite is only 4.8% bound (70).

EXCRETION

Dose Linearity

Levofloxacin has been studied at high doses (750 and 1,000 mg) in normal healthy volunteers. The pharmacokinetic parameter values observed in these subjects were proportional to those observed with 500-mg doses, and were not altered over several days of dosing (8). Grepafloxacin pharmacokinetics appeared to be nonlinear, with a disproportional increase in serum AUC at single oral doses of 600 to 1,200 mg. This increase could be due to saturation in hepatic uptake and clearance, resulting in an increase in oral bioavailability as well as a reduced systemic clearance. Studies with an i.v. formulation are not available to clarify the mechanism (18).

Renal Excretion

Most fluoroquinolones are excreted in moderate to high amounts as unchanged drug in the urine. Drugs with a high degree of renal excretion (e.g., ofloxacin-levofloxacin, gatifloxacin) show a correlation between total and renal clearance with creatinine clearance. Levofloxacin total clearance was highly correlated with creatinine clearance with single or multiple i.v. doses as high as 750 mg (10).

The zwitterionic nature of the fluoroquinolones makes them possible candidates for transport by both the anion- and cation-transport systems. Studies in vitro and in vivo with cimetidine and probenecid show that levofloxacin and grepafloxacin transport appears to be related to transport by both the organic cation transport system (OCT) and the organic anion transport system (OAT). P-gp did not appear to be involved in levofloxacin uptake and transport (34, 57, 87). However, these anion- and cation-antiport systems involved in transport of some fluoroquinolones do not appear to be limited to those inhibited by tetraethylammonium or probenecid (35). Tubular uptake from the apical membrane in a kidney epithelial cell line (LLC-PK$_1$) has also been demonstrated (47). Renal tubular secretion in humans is confirmed by comparison of measured renal clearance with creatinine clearance, and protein binding measurement, and a reduced renal clearance with concomitant administration of probenecid or cimetidine.

Urinary fluoroquinolone concentrations

Although the extent of urinary excretion of unchanged drug differs among fluoroquinones, drug concentrations in urine tend to be high and prolonged relative to the MIC of target urinary pathogens even with agents that have a relatively low degree of excretion in urine. For example, studies in normal volunteers with single doses of gemifloxacin (320 mg) or ofloxacin (400 mg) show that concentrations in urine produced detectable bactericidal activity against gram-negative pathogens for at least 24 h (55). Studies with levofloxacin show a single 250-mg dose produced mean urinary concentrations exceeding 60 µg/ml for 24 h, which is far in excess of the MICs for most urinary pathogens (56).

Hepatic Uptake and Biliary Excretion

Several fluoroquinolones are excreted to a significant extent as unchanged drug in the bile. In rats, the hepatic uptake can be rapid and approach that of hepatic blood flow. Studies with grepafloxacin in the rat show that uptake is due to an active transport system, which appears to be distinct from that involved in the transport of known organic anion or cationic transport (OAT and OCT, respectively), steroid, or bile acid systems (67). Further studies in rats with a hereditary defect in bile canalicular multispecific organic anion transport system showed that grepafloxacin transport into bile was primarily mediated by this transporter, and was much more efficient for grepafloxacin than levofloxacin (66, 69).

Intestinal Transport

Several fluoroquinolones appear to be substrates for transporters in the gut. Studies evaluating the extent and mechanisms for transport in rat and rabbit models demonstrated intestinal elimination (basolateral-to-apical transport) in the jejunal, ileal, and caecal segments. Lomefloxacin, sparfloxacin, moxifloxacin, and ciprofloxacin have been demonstrated to have a small but measurable fraction of their excretion through these segments (54). Secretion of grepafloxacin and levofloxacin has been demonstrated in human Caco-2 cell line, and was inhibited by cyclosporin, suggesting a role of P-gp. Additional studies suggested that other specific transport systems were involved in basolateral to apical efflux and were distinct from OAT, OCT, and multidrug resistance-related protein systems (85).

When ciprofloxacin was studied in vivo in rats cotreated with substrates/competitive inhibitors of P-gp (cyclosporin, verapamil, and quinidine), as well as β-lactams, ciprofloxacin biliary and intestinal elimination were decreased two- to eightfold; however, sparfloxacin, another known P-gp substrate, had no effect. It appears that ciprofloxacin may be a substrate for several transporters distinct from P-gp, including OAT or OCT (13). In the human Caco-2 system, it appears that several fluoroquinolones (e.g., ciprofloxacin, norfloxacin, pefloxacin) have a common carrier at the basal-lateral membrane, resulting in accumulation in the enterocye. Secretion is accomplished by facilitated exit across the apical membrane (29, 30)

COMPARISON OF THE PHARMACOKINETIC PROPERTIES OF FLUOROQUINOLONES IN NORMAL VOLUNTEERS

Table 1 summarizes data from pharmacokinetic studies in normal healthy volunteers who received a single oral or i.v. dose. One study has compared the pharmacokinetics of ciprofloxacin, gatifloxacin, grepafloxacin, levofloxacin, trovafloxacin, and moxifloxacin in 12 healthy volunteers; the results from this valuable comparative study are shown in Table 3, with serum drug levels shown in Fig. 2. All agents had a statistically significantly lower total clearance compared to ciprofloxacin, with moxifloxacin, levofloxacin, and trovafloxacin having the lowest values. Urinary recovery of unchanged drug was greatest for levofloxacin and gatifloxacin (>75% of a dose excreted unchanged), and was lowest for trovafloxacin, moxifloxacin, and grepafloxacin (<25% excreted unchanged). Ciprofloxacin remained the best example of an agent where excretion is balanced between renal and nonrenal routes (41% excreted unchanged) (44).

PHARMACOKINETICS IN SPECIAL PATIENT POPULATIONS

Race

Since most fluoroquinolones are metabolized to a small extent, differences in pharmacokinetics arising from pharmacogenetic differences are expectedly low. Pharmacokinetic properties of gatifloxacin were similar in Japanese and Caucasian male volunteers. In a population pharmacokinetic study in patients of African or Hispanic decent, there were no differences in pharmacokinetic parameters (27).

Gender

Most studies have not demonstrated major differences in pharmacokinetic properties between men and women. When differences have been noted, they often can be accounted for by differences in body

Table 3. Pharmacokinetic parameters for six fluoroquinolones tested in 12 volunteers[a]

Drug (mg dose)	C_{max} (μg/ml/70 kg)	C_{max} (μg/ml/70 kg), dose normalized	T_{max} (h)	T_{lag} (h)	Half-life (h)	MRT[b] (h)	AUC_{tot} (μg·h/ml/70 kg)	AUC_{tot} (μg·h/ml/70 kg), dose normalized	Total urinary recovery (% of dose)	Renal clearance (ml/min/1.73 m²)	V_{ss} (liters/70 kg)
Ciprofloxacin (250)	1.5 ± 0.43	1.2 ± 0.34	0.78 ± 0.33	0.27 ± 0.17	05.37 ± 0.82	5.8 ± 0.94	5.75 ± 1.25	4.6 ± 1.0	40.8 ± 7.48	266 ± 40.6	231 ± 61.8
Gatifloxacin (400)	3.42 ± 0.74*	1.71 ± 0.37	1.49 ± 0.65	0.21 ± 0.19	6.52 ± 0.87	9.28 ± 1.12*	30 ± 3.8*	15 ± 1.9*	76.9 ± 5.6	153 ± 21	110 ± 20
Grepafloxacin (600)	1.98 ± 0.52*	0.66 ± 0.17	2.77 ± 1.11	0.34 ± 0.06	12.12 ± 3.92*	14.15 ± 2.67*	23.5 ± 4.73*	7.85 ± 1.58*	9.36 ± 2.91	35.2 ± 6.9	306 ± 54.3
Levofloxacin (500)	6.21 ± 1.34*	2.48 ± 0.53*	0.8 ± 0.38	0.33 ± 0.15	6.95 ± 0.81	8.65 ± 0.8**	44.8 ± 4.4*	17.9 ± 1.76*	75.9 ± 11.6	124 ± 19.1	88 ± 9.92
Moxifloxacin (400)	4.34 ± 1.61*	2.17 ± 0.81*	1.02 ± 0.72	0.18 ± 0.16	9.51 ± 1.62	12.5 ± 2.03*	39.3 ± 5.35*	19.7 ± 2.67*	19.9 ± 4.55	30.5 ± 6.18	122 ± 19.6
Trovafloxacin (200)	2.09 ± 0.58	2.09 ± 0.58	0.95 ± 0.61	0.12 ± 0.16	10.3 ± 3.4	13.2 ± 5.37*	19.5 ± 3.1*	19.5 ± 3.1	9.27 ± 2.47	14.2 ± 3.5	129 ± 58

[a] Drugs were given orally. Data were determined by HPLC for original doses (200 mg) and for normalized doses compared to those for ciprofloxacin. Reprinted from reference 44 with permission. P values for results that were statistically significant compared to those for ciprofloxacin. Reprinted from reference 44 with permission.
[b] MRT, mean retention time.

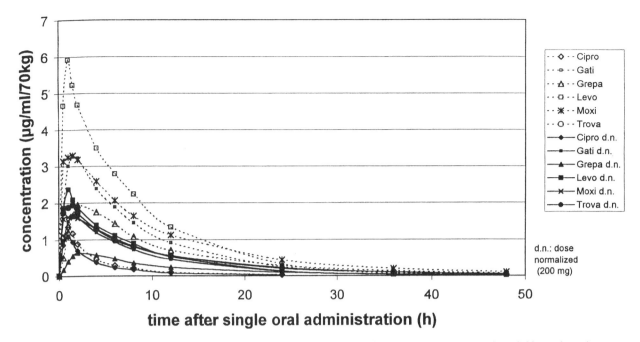

Figure 2. Comparison of fluoroquinolone concentrations in 12 healthy volunteers in a crossover study. Solid lines, dn = dose normalized values. Reprinted from reference 44 with permission.

weight. Chien et al. demonstrated that there was only a small difference (15% decrease) in volume of distribution for levofloxacin in women compared with that in men. Weight-adjusted values for oral and renal clearance showed no significant differences (6).

Fleroxacin pharmacokinetics in men and premenopausal women were compared to account for an apparent increase in side effects in women administered this drug. There was a slight reduction in steady-state volume of distribution in women compared with that in men; however, when adjusted for total body weight, the differences were not statistically significant. The weight-unadjusted value was smaller in women, thus resulting in higher concentrations in tissues and serum with a fixed dose that may underlie a higher frequency of adverse reactions in women (2).

Grepafloxacin pharmacokinetics varied slightly among men and women volunteers, but the differ-

ences were shown to be attributable to differences in lean or total body weight (18).

Cystic Fibrosis

In view of its potency against *Pseudomonas aeruginosa*, ciprofloxacin has been the most extensively studied agent in patients with cystic fibrosis. A summary of the major pharmacokinetic parameters is shown in Table 4.

In general, ciprofloxacin clearance and half-life are similar to those reported in normal healthy volunteers. In one recent study, the clearance and volume of distribution were significantly decreased compared with other patient groups and may have reflected study of an older population of patients with cystic fibrosis who had received multiple courses of aminoglycosides (50). In a study of young patients with cystic fibrosis (age, 6 to 16 years), the

Table 4. Comparison of pharmacokinetics of ciprofloxacin in cystic fibrosis patients[a]

Source or reference	No. of patients	V_1 (liters/kg)	V_{ss} (liters/kg)[b]	CL_R (liters/kg/h)	$t_{1/2}$ (h)
15	12	0.42 ± 0.38	2.21 ± 0.89	0.51 ± 0.11[c]	0.45 ± 1.9
72	9	NA[d]	NA	0.61 ± 0.17	2.8 ± 1.42
11	14	NA	2.71 ± 0.705	0.62 ± 0.10	NA
50	12	0.29 ± 0.20	1.1 ± 0.38	0.34 ± 0.12	2.9 ± 0.52

[a] Adapted from reference 50.
[b] V_{ss} was calculated as $V_1 + V_p$, where V_p = volume of the peripheral compartment.
[c] In this study, CL_T was expressed in liters per hour. For comparison purposes, the CL_T was divided by the mean weight of the CF patients.
[d] NA, not available.

population pharmacokinetics of ciprofloxacin was estimated using nonlinear mixed effects modeling. Ciprofloxacin pharmacokinetic parameters were related to total body weight. Dosage recommendations for younger children with cystic fibrosis were designed to produce exposures similar to those for efficacious regimens in adults. Ciprofloxacin 20 to 28 mg/kg orally twice daily for children 14 to 28 kg, and 15 to 20 mg/kg twice daily for older children (28 to 42 kg) were recommended (68).

Population Pharmacokinetic Studies

Population pharmacokinetic methods allow estimation of pharmacokinetic parameters in patients undergoing treatment in phase II or III clinical trials. These methods can require minimal sampling across one or several dosage intervals in treated patients, and can allow identification of patient or drug factors that influence pharmacokinetic properties. In addition, post hoc analyses using population model estimates can be used to generate individual patient parameters and exposure information. This information can subsequently be used to identify pharmacokinetic-pharmacodynamic relationships associated with clinical and microbiologic outcomes. Population pharmacokinetic analyses have been reported for several fluoroquinolones.

Levofloxacin

In a prospective trial of 272 patients with urinary tract, respiratory, or skin/skin structure infections, the population pharmacokinetics of levofloxacin was studied. The patient population was divided to form model "generation" and "validation" groups. This study demonstrated that for control of levofloxacin exposure (as AUC), models that included creatinine clearance (CL_{CR}), age, and race explained 40% of the variance in plasma drug concentrations; however, there was notable bias toward underprediction of levofloxacin clearance at higher measured values. The final regression equation for total levofloxacin clearance was:

$$CL = 5.9 + race + (age \times -0.032) + (CL_{CR} \times 0.70)$$

where race = −1.49 for Caucasian; −0.48 for black; −3.17 for Hispanic; and 5.14 for "others" (62).

Gatifloxacin

Gatifloxacin population pharmacokinetic parameters were estimated in a group of patients receiving treatment for ABECB. The model was able to identify the effects of body weight and creatinine clearance on key gatifloxacin pharmacokinetic properties, and estimated parameters comparable with those observed in normal healthy volunteers in controlled phase I studies. There was no effect of sex, age, or race on gatifloxacin pharmacokinetics (28).

Grepafloxacin

Grepafloxacin populations pharmacokinetics was studied in 76 patients with acute bacterial exacerbations of chronic bronchitis to assess factors associated with efficacy in these patients. Patients received daily doses of 200, 400, or 600 mg, and data were fit using an iterative two-stage analysis. Similar to what was shown in the healthy volunteer studies, there was evidence of nonlinear pharmacokinetic properties at the 600-mg dose, resulting in a disproportionate increase in exposure (by AUC). However, age, gender, and dose were not found to be significant predictors of grepafloxacin pharmacokinetics. Clearance in these patients was shown to be similar to that reported in young or healthy normal volunteers (22).

Patients with Severe Infections

Higher-dose ciprofloxacin (400 mg every 8 h) has been studied in patients with severe sepsis but normal renal function (assessed by calculated creatinine clearance). Systemic clearance averaged 0.4 liters/h/kg of body weight, with a 50% coefficient of variation. Average serum ciprofloxacin area under the curve from 0 to 8 h values ranged between 13.3 and 16.8 mg h/liter (42).

Ciprofloxacin (i.v.) was studied in 12 critically ill patients with major burn injury. Serum ciprofloxacin concentrations were comparable to those observed in normal volunteers. The pharmacokinetic properties were similar during the immediate postburn period and during clinical sepsis (79). In contrast, Lesne-Hulin et al. studied ciprofloxacin pharmacokinetics in patients with major burns and found that, while ciprofloxacin elimination was reduced, higher doses (e.g., 600 mg every 8 h) were required to achieve target exposures (AUC:MIC ≥ 125 liters/h) for organisms with an MIC of 0.5 mg/liter (41).

Elderly

Although changes in drug clearance in the elderly with drugs largely excreted unchanged in the urine are most often ascribed to age-related reduction in creatinine clearance, nonrenal mechanisms of clearance may be affected in this patient population. The best example can be shown for levofloxacin, a drug with high urinary recovery. When values for total and renal levofloxacin clearance were compared with creatinine clearance in two studies examining an age/gender effect on levofloxacin pharmacokinetics was combined with a study of pharmacokinetics in renal impairment, and excellent correlation ($r^2 >$ 0.8) between drug clearance and creatinine clearance was observed in both the elderly and younger patients with renal impairment (21).

Clinafloxacin pharmacokinetics were compared in elderly patients, and younger patients and healthy subjects with varying degrees of renal function. Clinafloxacin clearance was reduced in elderly subjects, but as with other fluoroquinolones, this reduction in excretion was explained by the decrement in renal function (65).

The combined effects of age and gender were studied for gatifloxacin. Elderly women had a higher peak plasma concentration and AUC (by 21 and 32%, respectively) compared with younger women; as in previous studies, most of the effect of age on clearance was explained by decrements in renal function in the elderly women. Gender effects were more pronounced in comparisons among the elderly patients; when adjusted for differences in body weight, the differences in C_{max} and AUC were 11 and 20% higher for elderly women and elderly men, respectively (39).

Changes in fluoroquinolone pharmacokinetics in the elderly may not be limited to just those associated with the established decline in creatinine clearance with advanced age. Grepafloxacin (an agent with urinary recovery of <15% in normal human volunteers) was shown to have an oral clearance in elderly subjects approximately 50% of that in normal healthy volunteers (37). No correlation between renal clearance and creatinine clearance was observed in elderly patients (18).

Advanced age is also associated with reduced lean body mass and can reduce the volume of distribution of drugs. Levofloxacin volume of distribution was observed to be reduced in elderly subjects (18% decrease) (56); the clinical significance of this change is low, as the effects of changes in renal function with age have a predominant effect on the disposition of the drug (6).

AIDS

Patients with AIDS have been reported to have altered GI function (e.g., achlorhydria) that can result in altered bioavailability of drugs. In view of the usefulness of several fluoroquinolones for opportunistic as well a traditional pathogens, the oral bioavailability and pharmacokinetics of several agents have been studied in this patient group.

Ciprofloxacin pharmacokinetics and oral bioavailability were studied in 12 patients with AIDS (according to 1993 Centers for Disease Control and Prevention criteria) with a median CD4 cell count of 45 cells/mm^3. Subjects had no symptomatic GI disease, and many were on several nucleoside antiretrovirals as well as prophylaxis for *Pneumocystis carinii*. Bioavailability averaged 82%, which was similar to those reported in normal healthy volunteers, with C_{max} and elimination half-lives similar to those reported in normal healthy volunteers (59).

Trovafloxacin pharmacokinetics were studied following a single oral or i.v. (as the double-alanine prodrug alatrovafloxacin) in 12 patients with AIDS. Despite receipt of several antiretroviral medications (no protease inhibitors), the pharmacokinetic properties were similar to those reported in normal healthy volunteers, with oral bioavailability ranging from 52 to 124% (40).

Levofloxacin pharmacokinetics in HIV-infected patients were also reported to be similar to those reported in normal healthy volunteers (56). Piscitelli et al. studied 750-mg doses given once daily for 14 days, followed by 750 or 1,000 mg given three times weekly for an additional 14 days. There was a trend toward a lower oral clearance in patients with CD4 cell numbers less than 250 cells/mm^3; a regression analysis did not show a correlation between cell number and clearance (61).

Pediatric Patients

Recent advances in the understanding of the pathogenesis and structure-activity relationships for fluoroquinolone-induced bone and cartilage toxicity has fostered the investigation of the pharmacokinetics of newer agents with improved activity against gram-positive bacteria in children. Trovafloxacin pharmacokinetics were studied in infants (age, 3 to 12 months) and children (2 to 12 years) following a single dose of the prodrug alatrofloxacin. Total drug clearance, volume of distribution, and elimination half-life averaged 151 mg/min/kg, 1.7 liters/kg, and 9.8 h, respectively, which are similar to values reported in healthy adults. No age-related differences in pharmacokinetic properties were detected, although the number of patients studied was relatively small (20 infants/children total) (3).

Single-dose oral ciprofloxacin was studied in infants (age, 5 to 14 months) and children up to 5 years of age. The average half-life ranged between

1.3 and 2.7 in the children and infants, respectively (14), values that were somewhat lower than those in adults.

Effect of Renal Dysfunction

Table 5 compares the pharmacokinetics and dosage adjustment for several fluoroquinolones in varying degrees of renal impairment.

Levofloxacin

The pharmacokinetics of levofloxacin are altered in patients with renal dysfunction; this change is expected because of the high degree of urinary excretion of unchanged drug observed in normal volunteers.

Gatifloxacin

Gatifloxacin pharmacokinetics are altered in patients with renal insufficiency. Total clearance of gatifloxacin correlates with creatinine clearance. Dosage reduction is recommended in patients with a creatinine clearance <40 ml/min.

Grepafloxacin

Grepafloxacin renal clearance was reduced in patients with varying degrees of renal impairment; however, total clearance remained unchanged due to the extensive degree of nonrenal clearance of this drug (18).

Hemodialysis and hemoperfusion

Although the drugs are readily permeable across dialysis and peritoneal membranes, hemodialysis and peritoneal dialysis have little effect of removing a significant amount of the fluoroquinolone from the body. This lack of effect is because of the high degree of intracellular distribution of these agents, as reflected in the volume of distribution. Therefore, replacement doses are not needed after dialysis other than doses scheduled on the basis of renal failure dosage regimens.

Continuous renal replacement therapy (CRRT)

Newer modes for temporary support of renal function in critically ill patients with renal dysfunction can have a marked effect on drug pharmacokinetics. Adjustment of dosage regimens on the basis of data derived in patients undergoing hemodialysis can be inappropriate. Levofloxacin and cipro-

floxacin have been studied in patients undergoing continuous venovenous hemofiltration or hemodiafiltration. Given that levofloxacin is largely excreted as unchanged drug in man, levofloxacin clearance (off continuous venovenous hemofiltration or hemodiafiltration) was substantially reduced in these patients. Levofloxacin clearance with CRRT with either technique ranged from 0.06 to 0.29 ml/min/kg, representing a significant component (16 to 70%) of the total serum clearance measured in these patients. However, since ciprofloxacin clearance was less affected in this patient group, clearance due to CRRT only represents 6 to 37% of drug clearance. From these data, levofloxacin doses of 250 mg/day (or 500 mg every 48 h) and ciprofloxacin doses of 400 to 600 mg/day would result in plasma drug concentrations consistent with those associated with efficacy in serious infections (45, 78).

Hepatic Disease

Hepatic metabolism and biliary excretion are a major route of excretion for several fluoroquinolones. Dosage adjustments in hepatic disease have been found to be required for only a few fluoroquinolones, likely because of the balance between this route and renal excretion, and that drug clearance is generally only altered in severe liver disease.

Ciprofloxacin

No adjustment was found to be necessary for ciprofloxacin in patients with cirrhosis documented by biopsy and Childs A and B level cirrhosis; however, adjustments in severe liver dysfunction (patients not examined in the two studies conducted to date) may be warranted.

Gatifloxacin

Gatifloxacin was studied in eight subjects with grade B or C hepatic dysfunction. Peak plasma drug concentrations and AUC were increased 32 and 22%, respectively, in these patients. This was associated with a statistically significant increase in oral clearance (about 20%); however, this difference was not considered to be clinically significant, and thus dose adjustment of gatifloxacin is not recommended in patients with moderate to severe hepatic impairment (28).

Grepafloxacin

Patients with hepatic impairment (as assessed by the Child-Pugh class A or B) had significantly differ-

Table 5. Pharmacokinetics and dosage adjustment of selected fluoroquinolones in renal impairment[a]

Drug	Normal renal function (CL_CR > 80) dosage rec.	Mild CL_CR (ml/min)	CL_{TOT} (ml/min)/ $t_{1/2}$ (h)	Dosage rec.	Moderate CL_CR (ml/min)	CL_{TOT} (ml/min)/$t_{1/2}$ (h)	Dosage rec.	Severe CL_CR (ml/min)	CL_{TOT} (ml/min)/ $t_{1/2}$ (h)	Dosage rec.	Very severe/dialysis dependent CL_CR (ml/min)	CL_{TOT} (ml/min)/ $t_{1/2}$ (h)	Dosage rec. (after dialysis)	Reference(s)
Ciprofloxacin[b]	250–750 mg twice daily	60–100	440/6.1	No. adj.	31–60	250/7.7	250–500, twice daily max.	<30		250–500 mg per day	<10	250/8.6	250–500 mg per day	14
Gatifloxacin	400 mg once daily	60–90	126/8.9	No. adj.	<40	81.1/16.5	200 mg once daily	10–30	34.9/29.6	200 mg once daily			200 mg once daily	60
Levofloxacin	500–750 mg once daily	50–80	NA/9.1	No. adj.	20–49	NA/26.6	500 × 1, then 250 mg daily[c]	<20	NA/34.8	500 mg × 1, then 250 q48h	<10	NA/50–76	500 mg × 1, then 250 q48h	21
Moxifloxacin[b]	400 mg once daily	60–90	167/15.2	No. adj.	30–60	187/16.2	No adj.	≤30	152/14.5	No. adj.			No. adj.	71

[a] Abbreviations: CL_CR, creatinine clearance; q48h, every 48 h; NA, not available.
[b] Values are oral clearance (CL/F) for ciprofloxacin, moxifloxacin.
[c] For infections outside the urinary tract.

128

ent values of oral clearance and volume of distribution relative to normal volunteers. Total oral clearance and volume of distribution were reduced by more than 50 and 30%, respectively, in patients with moderate (class B) impairment. The changes resulted in approximately a 50% increase in serum half-life compared with normal volunteers. In subjects with mild hepatic impairment, the dose of grepafloxacin should be reduced by ca. 1/3 (e.g., 600 mg per day reduced to 400 mg/day) (18).

Moxifloxacin

Patients with Childs-Pugh class A or B (mild to moderate) hepatic dysfunction had only minor increases in drug exposure (<25% increase in C_{max} or AUC) compared to normal subjects; thus dose adjustment in hepatic impairment is not recommended.

CONCLUSIONS

Fluoroquinolone antiinfectives are a remarkable class of drugs with potent activity against a variety of important human and animal pathogens. The pharmacokinetic properties, coupled with their potency, make them an extremely useful class of drug for oral and parenteral treatment of infection. The balanced renal and nonrenal routes of excretion tend to reduce the extent of interpatient variability in drug clearance, resulting in consistent exposure among patients. The ultimate challenges in this class remain in preserving their activity against key pathogens while using dosage regimens that produce exposures in vivo associated with good tolerability and safety.

REFERENCES

1. Allen, A., E. Bygate, D. Clark, A. Lewis, and V. Pay. 2000. The effect of food on the bioavailability of oral gemifloxacin in healthy volunteers. *Int. J. Antimicrob. Agents* 16:45–50.
2. Bertino, J. S., Jr., and A. N. Nafziger. 1996. Pharmacokinetics of oral fleroxacin in male and premenopausal female volunteers. *Antimicrob. Agents Chemother.* 40:789–791.
3. Bradley, J. S., G. L. Kearns, M. D. Reed, E. V. Capparelli, and J. Vincent. 2000. Pharmacokinetics of a fluoronaphthyridone, trovafloxacin (CP 99,219), in infants and children following administration of a single intravenous dose of alatrofloxacin. *Antimicrob. Agents Chemother.* 44:1195–1199.
4. Bryskier, A., and J. F. Chantot. 1995. Classification and structure-activity relationships of fluoroquinolones. *Drugs* 49(Suppl. 2):16–28.
5. Catchpole, C., J. M. Andrews, J. Woodcock, and R. Wise. 1994. The comparative pharmacokinetics and tissue penetration of single-dose ciprofloxacin 400 mg i.v. and 750 mg po. *J. Antimicrob. Chemother.* 33:103–110.
6. Chien, S. C., A. T. Chow, J. Natarajan, R. R. Williams, F. A. Wong, M. C. Rogge, and R. K. Nayak. 1997. Absence of age and gender effects on the pharmacokinetics of a single 500-milligram oral dose of levofloxacin in healthy subjects. *Antimicrob. Agents Chemother.* 41:1562–1565.
7. Chien, S. C., M. C. Rogge, L. G. Gisclon, C. Curtin, F. Wong, J. Natarajan, R. R. Williams, C. L. Fowler, W. K. Cheung, and A. T. Chow. 1997. Pharmacokinetic profile of levofloxacin following once-daily 500-milligram oral or intravenous doses. *Antimicrob. Agents Chemother.* 41:2256–2260.
8. Chien, S. C., F. A. Wong, C. L. Fowler, S. V. Callery-D'Amico, R. R. Williams, R. Nayak, and A. T. Chow. 1998. Double-blind evaluation of the safety and pharmacokinetics of multiple oral once-daily 750-milligram and 1-gram doses of levofloxacin in healthy volunteers. *Antimicrob. Agents Chemother.* 42:885–888.
9. Child, J., J. M. Andrews, and R. Wise. 1995. Pharmacokinetics and tissue penetration of the new fluoroquinolone grepafloxacin. *Antimicrob. Agents Chemother.* 39:513–515.
10. Chow, A. T., C. Fowler, R. R. Williams, N. Morgan, S. Kaminski, and J. Natarajan. 2001. Safety and pharmacokinetics of multiple 750-milligram doses of intravenous levofloxacin in healthy volunteers. *Antimicrob. Agents Chemother.* 45:2122–2125.
11. Christensson, B. A., I. Nilsson-Ehle, B. Ljungberg, A. Lindblad, A. S. Malmborg, L. Hjelte, and B. Strandvik. 1992. Increased oral bioavailability of ciprofloxacin in cystic fibrosis patients. *Antimicrob. Agents Chemother.* 36:2512–2517.
12. Cutler, N. R., J. Vincent, S. S. Jhee, R. Teng, T. Wardle, G. Lucas, L. C. Dogolo, and J. J. Sramek. 1997. Penetration of trovafloxacin into cerebrospinal fluid in humans following intravenous infusion of alatrofloxacin. *Antimicrob. Agents Chemother.* 41:1298–1300.
13. Dautrey, S., K. Felice, A. Petiet, B. Lacour, C. Carbon, and R. Farinotti. 1999. Active intestinal elimination of ciprofloxacin in rats: modulation by different substrates. *Br. J. Pharmacol.* 127:1728–1734.
14. Davis, R., A. Markham, and J. A. Balfour. 1996. Ciprofloxacin. An updated review of its pharmacology, therapeutic efficacy and tolerability. *Drugs* 51:1019–1074.
15. Davis, R. L., J. R. Koup, J. Williams-Warren, A. Weber, L. Heggen, D. Stempel, and A. L. Smith. 1987. Pharmacokinetics of ciprofloxacin in cystic fibrosis. *Antimicrob. Agents Chemother.* 31:915–919.
16. Drusano, G. L., S. L. Preston, M. Van Guilder, D. North, M. Gombert, M. Oefelein, L. Boccumini, B. Weisinger, M. Corrado, and J. Kahn. 2000. A population pharmacokinetic analysis of the penetration of the prostate by levofloxacin. *Antimicrob. Agents Chemother.* 44:2046–2051.
17. Dudley, M. N., J. Ericson, and S. H. Zinner. 1987. Effect of dose on serum pharmacokinetics of intravenous ciprofloxacin with identification and characterization of extravascular compartments using noncompartmental and compartmental pharmacokinetic models. *Antimicrob. Agents Chemother.* 31:1782–1786.
18. Efthymiopoulos, C. 1997. Pharmacokinetics of grepafloxacin. *J. Antimicrob. Chemother.* 40(Suppl. A):35–43.
19. Fischman, A. J., J. W. Babich, A. A. Bonab, N. M. Alpert, J. Vincent, R. J. Callahan, J. A. Correia, and R. H. Rubin. 1998. Pharmacokinetics of [18F]trovafloxacin in healthy human subjects studied with positron emission tomography. *Antimicrob. Agents Chemother.* 42:2048–2054.
20. Fischman, A. J., E. Livni, J. W. Babich, N. M. Alpert, A. Bonab, S. Chodosh, F. McGovern, P. Kamitsuka, Y. Y. Liu,

R. Cleeland, B. L. Prosser, J. A. Correia, and R. H. Rubin. 1996. Pharmacokinetics of [^{18}F]fleroxacin in patients with acute exacerbations of chronic bronchitis and complicated urinary tract infection studied by positron emission tomography. *Antimicrob. Agents Chemother.* 40:659–664.

21. Fish, D. N., and A. T. Chow. 1997. The clinical pharmacokinetics of levofloxacin. *Clin. Pharmacokinet.* 32:101–119.

22. Forrest, A., S. Chodosh, M. A. Amantea, D. A. Collins, and J. J. Schentag. 1997. Pharmacokinetics and pharmacodynamics of oral grepafloxacin in patients with acute bacterial exacerbations of chronic bronchitis. *J. Antimicrob. Chemother.* 40(Suppl. A):45–57.

23. Gajjar, D. A., F. P. LaCreta, H. D. Uderman, G. D. Kollia, G. Duncan, M. J. Birkhofer, and D. M. Grasela. 2000. A dose-escalation study of the safety, tolerability, and pharmacokinetics of intravenous gatifloxacin in healthy adult men. *Pharmacotherapy* 20:49S–58S.

24. Garcia-Saenz, M. C., A. Arias-Puente, M. J. Fresnadillo-Martinez, and C. Carrasco-Font. 2001. Human aqueous humor levels of oral ciprofloxacin, levofloxacin, and moxifloxacin. *J. Cataract. Refract. Surg.* 27:1969–1974.

25. Goa, K. L., H. M. Bryson, and A. Markham. 1997. Sparfloxacin. A review of its antibacterial activity, pharmacokinetic properties, clinical efficacy and tolerability in lower respiratory tract infections. *Drugs* 53:700–725.

26. Gonzalez, M. A., A. H. Moranchel, S. Duran, A. Pichardo, J. L. Magana, B. Painter, A. Forrest, and G. L. Drusano. 1985. Multiple-dose pharmacokinetics of ciprofloxacin administered intravenously to normal volunteers. *Antimicrob. Agents Chemother.* 28:235–239.

27. Grasela, D. M. 2000. Clinical pharmacology of gatifloxacin, a new fluoroquinolone. *Clin. Infect. Dis.* 31(Suppl. 2):S51–S58.

28. Grasela, D. M., B. Christofalo, G. D. Kollia, G. Duncan, R. Noveck, J. A. Manning, Jr., and F. P. LaCreta. 2000. Safety and pharmacokinetics of a single oral dose of gatifloxacin in patients with moderate to severe hepatic impairment. *Pharmacotherapy* 20:87S–94S.

29. Griffith, N., B. Hirst, and N. Simmons. 1994. Active intestinal secretion of the fluoroquinolone antibacterials ciprofloxacin, norfloxacin and pefloxacin; a common secretory pathway? *J. Pharmacol. Exp. Ther.* 269:496–502.

30. Griffith, N., B. Hirst, and N. Simmons. 1993. Active secretion of the fluoroquinolone ciprofloxacin by human intestinal epithelial Caco-2 cell layers. *Br. J. Pharmacol.* 108:575–576.

31. Harder, S., U. Fuhr, D. Beermann, and A. H. Staib. 1990. Ciprofloxacin absorption in different regions of the human gastrointestinal tract. Investigations with the hf-capsule. *Br. J. Clin. Pharmacol.* 30:35–39.

32. Healy, D. P., M. C. Brodbeck, and C. E. Clendening. 1996. Ciprofloxacin absorption is impaired in patients given enteral feedings orally and via gastrostomy and jejunostomy tubes. *Antimicrob. Agents Chemother.* 40:6–10.

33. Humphrey, G. H., M. A. Shapiro, E. J. Randinitis, R. J. Guttendorf, and J. I. Brodfuehrer. 1999. Pharmacokinetics of clinafloxacin enantiomers in humans. *J. Clin. Pharmacol.* 39:1143–1150.

34. Ito, T., I. Yano, Y. Hashimoto, and K. Inui. 2000. Transepithelial transport of levofloxacin in the isolated perfused rat kidney. *Pharm. Res.* 17:236–241.

35. Ito, T., I. Yano, S. Masuda, Y. Hashimoto, and K. Inui. 1999. Distribution characteristics of levofloxacin and grepafloxacin in rat kidney. *Pharm. Res.* 16:534–539.

36. Johnson, J. H., M. A. Cooper, J. M. Andrews, and R. Wise. 1992. Pharmacokinetics and inflammatory fluid penetration of sparfloxacin. *Antimicrob. Agents Chemother.* 36:2444–2446.

37. Kozawa, O., T. Uematsu, H. Matsuno, M. Niwa, S. Nagashima, and M. Kanamaru. 1996. Comparative study of pharmacokinetics of two new fluoroquinolones, balofloxacin and grepafloxacin, in elderly subjects. *Antimicrob. Agents Chemother.* 40:2824–2828.

38. Kozjek, F., L. J. Suturkova, G. Antolic, I. Grabnar, and A. Mrhar. 1999. Kinetics of 4-fluoroquinolones permeation into saliva. *Biopharm. Drug Dispos.* 20:183–191.

39. LaCreta, F. P., G. D. Kollia, G. Duncan, D. Behr, and D. M. Grasela. 2000. Age and gender effects on the pharmacokinetics of gatifloxacin. *Pharmacotherapy* 20:67S–75S.

40. Lacy, M. K., D. P. Nicolau, C. H. Nightingale, A. Geffken, R. Teng, J. Vincent, and R. Quintiliani. 1999. Oral bioavailability and pharmacokinetics of trovafloxacin in patients with AIDS. *Antimicrob. Agents Chemother.* 43:3005–3007.

41. Lesne-Hulin, A., P. Bourget, F. Ravat, C. Goudin, and J. Latarjet. 1999. Clinical pharmacokinetics of ciprofloxacin in patients with major burns. *Eur. J. Clin. Pharmacol.* 55:515–519.

42. Lipman, J., J. Scribante, A. G. Gous, H. Hon, and S. Tshukutsoane. 1998. Pharmacokinetic profiles of high-dose intravenous ciprofloxacin in severe sepsis. The Baragwanath Ciprofloxacin Study Group. *Antimicrob. Agents Chemother.* 42:2235–2239.

43. Liu, W., Q. F. Liu, R. Perkins, G. Drusano, A. Louie, A. Madu, U. Mian, M. Mayers, and M. H. Miller. 1998. Pharmacokinetics of sparfloxacin in the serum and vitreous humor of rabbits: physicochemical properties that regulate penetration of quinolone antimicrobials. *Antimicrob. Agents Chemother.* 42:1417–1423.

44. Lubasch, A., I. Keller, K. Borner, P. Koeppe, and H. Lode. 2000. Comparative pharmacokinetics of ciprofloxacin, gatifloxacin, grepafloxacin, levofloxacin, trovafloxacin, and moxifloxacin after single oral administration in healthy volunteers. *Antimicrob. Agents Chemother.* 44:2600–2603.

45. Malone, R. S., D. N. Fish, E. Abraham, and I. Teitelbaum. 2001. Pharmacokinetics of levofloxacin and ciprofloxacin during continuous renal replacement therapy in critically ill patients. *Antimicrob. Agents Chemother.* 45:2949–54.

46. Marangos, M. N., A. T. Skoutelis, C. H. Nightingale, Z. Zhu, A. G. Psyrogiannis, D. P. Nicolau, H. P. Bassaris, and R. Quintiliani. 1995. Absorption of ciprofloxacin in patients with diabetic gastroparesis. *Antimicrob. Agents Chemother.* 39:2161–2163.

47. Matsuo, Y., I. Yano, T. Ito, Y. Hashimoto, and K. Inui. 1998. Transport of quinolone antibacterial drugs in a kidney epithelial cell line, LLC-PK1. *J. Pharmacol. Exp. Ther.* 287:672–678.

48. Mimoz, O., V. Binter, A. Jacolot, A. Edouard, M. Tod, O. Petitjean, and K. Samii. 1998. Pharmacokinetics and absolute bioavailability of ciprofloxacin administered through a nasogastric tube with continuous enteral feeding to critically ill patients. *Intensive Care Med.* 24:1047–1051.

49. Montay, G., Y. Goueffon, and F. Roquet. 1984. Absorption, distribution, metabolic fate, and elimination of pefloxacin mesylate in mice, rats, dogs, monkeys, and humans. *Antimicrob. Agents Chemother.* 25:463–472.

50. Montgomery, M. J., P. M. Beringer, A. Aminimanizani, S. G. Louie, B. J. Shapiro, R. Jelliffe, and M. A. Gill. 2001. Population pharmacokinetics and use of Monte Carlo simulation to evaluate currently recommended dosing regimens of ciprofloxacin in adult patients with cystic fibrosis. *Antimicrob. Agents Chemother.* 45:3468–3473.

51. Morlet, N., G. G. Graham, B. Gatus, A. J. McLachlan, C. Salonikas, D. Naidoo, I. Goldberg, and C. M. Lam. 2000. Pharmacokinetics of ciprofloxacin in the human eye: a clinical study and population pharmacokinetic analysis. *Antimicrob. Agents Chemother.* 44:1674–1679.

52. Muller, M., M. Brunner, U. Hollenstein, C. Joukhadar, R. Schmid, E. Minar, H. Ehringer, and H. G. Eichler. 1999. Penetration of ciprofloxacin into the interstitial space of inflamed foot lesions in non-insulin-dependent diabetes mellitus patients. *Antimicrob. Agents Chemother.* 43:2056–2058.

53. Muller, M., H. Stass, M. Brunner, J. G. Moller, E. Lackner, and H. G. Eichler. 1999. Penetration of moxifloxacin into peripheral compartments in humans. *Antimicrob. Agents Chemother.* 43:2345–2349.

54. Musafija, A., J. Ramon, Y. Shtelman, G. Yoseph, B. Rubinovitz, S. Segev, and E. Rubinstein. 2000. Trans-epithelial intestinal elimination of moxifloxacin in rabbits. *J. Antimicrob. Chemother.* 45:803–5.

55. Naber, C. K., M. Hammer, M. Kinzig-Schippers, C. Sauber, F. Sorgel, E. A. Bygate, A. J. Fairless, K. Machka, and K. G. Naber. 2001. Urinary excretion and bactericidal activities of gemifloxacin and ofloxacin after a single oral dose in healthy volunteers. *Antimicrob. Agents Chemother.* 45:3524–3530.

56. North, D. S., D. N. Fish, and J. J. Redington. 1998. Levofloxacin, a second-generation fluoroquinolone. *Pharmacotherapy* 18:915–35.

57. Okano, T., H. Maegawa, K. Inui, and R. Hori. 1990. Interaction of ofloxacin with organic cation transport system in rat renal brush-border membranes. *J. Pharmacol. Exp. Ther.* 255:1033–1037.

58. Okazaki, O., C. Kojima, H. Hakusui, and M. Nakashima. 1991. Enantioselective disposition of ofloxacin in humans. *Antimicrob. Agents Chemother.* 35:2106–2109.

59. Owens, R. C., Jr., K. B. Patel, M. A. Banevicius, R. Quintiliani, C. H. Nightingale, and D. P. Nicolau. 1997. Oral bioavailability and pharmacokinetics of ciprofloxacin in patients with AIDS. *Antimicrob. Agents Chemother.* 41:1508–1511.

60. Perry, C. M., J. A. Barman Balfour, and H. M. Lamb. 1999. Gatifloxacin. *Drugs* 58:683–698.

61. Piscitelli, S. C., K. Spooner, B. Baird, A. T. Chow, C. L. Fowler, R. R. Williams, J. Natarajan, H. Masur, and R. E. Walker. 1999. Pharmacokinetics and safety of high-dose and extended-interval regimens of levofloxacin in human immunodeficiency virus-infected patients. *Antimicrob. Agents Chemother.* 43:2323–2327.

62. Preston, S. L., G. L. Drusano, A. L. Berman, C. L. Fowler, A. T. Chow, B. Dornseif, V. Reichl, J. Natarajan, F. A. Wong, and M. Corrado. 1998. Levofloxacin population pharmacokinetics and creation of a demographic model for prediction of individual drug clearance in patients with serious community-acquired infection. *Antimicrob. Agents Chemother.* 42:1098–1104.

63. Rabbaa, L., S. Dautrey, N. Colas-Linhart, C. Carbon, and R. Farinotti. 1997. Absorption of ofloxacin isomers in the rat small intestine. *Antimicrob. Agents Chemother.* 41:2274–2277.

64. Randinitis, E. J., J. I. Brodfuehrer, I. Eiseman, and A. B. Vassos. 2001. Pharmacokinetics of clinafloxacin after single and multiple doses. *Antimicrob. Agents Chemother.* 45:2529–3500.

65. Randinitis, E. J., J. R. Koup, G. Rausch, R. Abel, N. J. Bron, N. J. Hounslow, A. B. Vassos, and A. J. Sedman. 2001. Clinafloxacin pharmacokinetics in subjects with various degrees of renal function. *Antimicrob. Agents Chemother.* 45:2536–2542.

66. Sasabe, H., Y. Kato, T. Terasaki, A. Tsuji, and Y. Sugiyama. 1999. Differences in the hepatobiliary transport of two quinolone antibiotics, grepafloxacin and lomefloxacin, in the rat. *Biopharm. Drug Dispos.* 20:151–158.

67. Sasabe, H., T. Terasaki, A. Tsuji, and Y. Sugiyama. 1997. Carrier-mediated hepatic uptake of quinolone antibiotics in the rat. *J. Pharmacol. Exp. Ther.* 282:162–171.

68. Schaefer, H. G., H. Stass, J. Wedgwood, B. Hampel, C. Fischer, J. Kuhlmann, and U. B. Schaad. 1996. Pharmacokinetics of ciprofloxacin in pediatric cystic fibrosis patients. *Antimicrob. Agents Chemother.* 40:29–34.

69. Stass, H., A. Dalhoff, D. Kubitza, and U. Schuhly. 1998. Pharmacokinetics, safety, and tolerability of ascending single doses of moxifloxacin, a new 8-methoxy quinolone, administered to healthy subjects. *Antimicrob. Agents Chemother.* 42:2060–2065.

70. Stass, H., and D. Kubitza. 1999. Pharmacokinetics and elimination of moxifloxacin after oral and intravenous administration in man. *J. Antimicrob. Chemother.* 43(Suppl. B):83–90.

71. Stass, H., D. Kubitza, A. Halabi, and H. Delesen. 2002. Pharmacokinetics of moxifloxacin, a novel 8-methoxy-quinolone, in patients with renal dysfunction. *Br. J. Clin. Pharmacol.* 53:232–237.

72. Steen, H. J., E. M. Scott, M. I. Stevenson, A. E. Black, A. O. Redmond, and P. S. Collier. 1989. Clinical and pharmacokinetic aspects of ciprofloxacin in the treatment of acute exacerbations of pseudomonas infection in cystic fibrosis patients. *J. Antimicrob. Chemother.* 24:787–795.

73. Stone, J. W., J. M. Andrews, J. P. Ashby, D. Griggs, and R. Wise. 1988. Pharmacokinetics and tissue penetration of orally administered lomefloxacin. *Antimicrob. Agents Chemother.* 32:1508–1510.

74. Sullivan, J. T., M. Woodruff, J. Lettieri, V. Agarwal, G. J. Krol, P. T. Leese, S. Watson, and A. H. Heller. 1999. Pharmacokinetics of a once-daily oral dose of moxifloxacin (Bay 12–8039), a new enantiomerically pure 8-methoxy quinolone. *Antimicrob. Agents Chemother.* 43:2793–2797.

75. Tamai, I., J. Yamashita, Y. Kido, A. Ohnari, Y. Sai, Y. Shima, K. Naruhashi, S. Koizumi, and A. Tsuji. 2000. Limited distribution of new quinolone antibacterial agents into brain caused by multiple efflux transporters at the blood-brain barrier. *J. Pharmacol. Exp. Ther.* 295:146–152.

76. Teng, R., L. C. Dogolo, S. A. Willavize, H. L. Friedman, and J. Vincent. 1997. Oral bioavailability of trovafloxacin with and without food in healthy volunteers. *J. Antimicrob. Chemother.* 39(Suppl. B):87–92.

77. Trampuz, A., M. Wenk, Z. Rajacic, and W. Zimmerli. 2000. Pharmacokinetics and pharmacodynamics of levofloxacin against *Streptococcus pneumoniae* and *Staphylococcus aureus* in human skin blister fluid. *Antimicrob. Agents Chemother.* 44:1352–1355.

78. Traunmuller, F., R. Thalhammer-Scherrer, G. J. Locker, H. Losert, R. Schmid, T. Staudinger, and F. Thalhammer. 2001. Single-dose pharmacokinetics of levofloxacin during continuous veno-venous haemofiltration in critically ill patients. *J. Antimicrob. Chemother.* 47:229–231.

79. Varela, J. E., S. M. Cohn, M. Brown, C. G. Ward, N. Namias, and P. B. Spalding. 2000. Pharmacokinetics and burn eschar penetration of intravenous ciprofloxacin in patients with major thermal injuries. *J. Antimicrob. Chemother.* 45:337–342.

80. Vincent, J., J. Venitz, R. Teng, B. A. Baris, S. A. Willavize, R. J. Polzer, and H. L. Friedman. 1997. Pharmacokinetics and safety of trovafloxacin in healthy male volunteers following administration of single intravenous doses of the prodrug, alatrofloxacin. *J. Antimicrob. Chemother.* 39(Suppl. B):75–80.

81. Wise, R., J. M. Andrews, G. Marshall, and G. Hartman. 1999. Pharmacokinetics and inflammatory-fluid penetration of moxifloxacin following oral or intravenous administration. *Antimicrob. Agents Chemother.* 43:1508–1510.

82. **Wise, R., S. Jones, I. Das, and J. M. Andrews.** 1998. Pharmacokinetics and inflammatory fluid penetration of clinafloxacin. *Antimicrob. Agents Chemother.* **42:**428–430.

83. **Wise, R., D. Lister, C. A. McNulty, D. Griggs, and J. M. Andrews.** 1986. The comparative pharmacokinetics of five quinolones. *J. Antimicrob. Chemother.* **18**(Suppl. D):71–81.

84. **Wise, R., D. Mortiboy, J. Child, and J. M. Andrews.** 1996. Pharmacokinetics and penetration into inflammatory fluid of trovafloxacin (CP-99,219). *Antimicrob. Agents Chemother.* **40:**47–49.

85. **Yamaguchi, H., I. Yano, Y. Hashimoto, and K. I. Inui.** 2000. Secretory mechanisms of grepafloxacin and levofloxacin in the human intestinal cell line caco-2. *J. Pharmacol. Exp. Ther.* **295:**360–366.

86. **Yamaguchi, T., M. Yokogawa, M. Sekine, and Y. Hashimoto.** 1991. Intestinal absorption characteristics of sparfloxacin. *Drug Metab. Dispos.* **6:**53–59.

87. **Yano, I., T. Ito, M. Takano, and K. Inui.** 1997. Evaluation of renal tubular secretion and reabsorption of levofloxacin in rats. *Pharm. Res.* **14:**508–511.

Quinolone Antimicrobial Agents, 3rd ed.
Edited by David C. Hooper and Ethan Rubinstein
© 2003 ASM Press, Washington, D.C.

Chapter 7

Drug-Drug Interactions

ROULA QAQISH AND RONALD E. POLK

Pharmacokinetic drug-drug interactions occur when the absorption, metabolism, distribution, or elimination of one drug is altered by coadministration of another. Compared with many antimicrobial drugs, the fluoroquinolones cause relatively few pharmacokinetic drug-drug interactions. Absorption interactions are the most important, and the absorption of all fluoroquinolones is reduced when they are given with multivalent cations, including those frequently found in antacids such as aluminum, magnesium, and calcium. Nutritional cationic supplements including iron and zinc also reduce fluoroquinolone absorption. In addition, metabolic interactions are important for select fluoroquinolones that inhibit a relatively minor cytochrome P450 enzyme, CYP1A2. Inhibition of this enzyme's function by enoxacin, pefloxacin, ciprofloxacin and clinafloxacin can interfere with the metabolism of methylxanthines and a few additional drugs metabolized by this pathway (Table 1). In contrast to these pharmacokinetic interactions, pharmacodynamic drug-drug interactions occur when the pharmacologic response to one drug is altered by the coadministration of another, but without a change in drug pharmacokinetics. For example, coadministration of sparfloxacin with cisapride was found to not change the area under the concentration-time curve (AUC) of either drug (112), but since both drugs can independently increase the QTc interval, it is recommended that this combination be avoided (8). Adverse cardiovascular effects resulting from pharmacodynamic interactions are discussed in chapter 26.

The purpose of this chapter is to review fluoroquinolone pharmacokinetic drug-drug interactions, with an emphasis on newer agents, as well as to discuss some remaining controversial issues. The current prescribing information for each fluoroquinolone should be consulted for the most recent drug-drug interaction information.

PHARMACOKINETIC INTERACTIONS INVOLVING ABSORPTION

Antacids

One advantage of the fluoroquinolone class is high oral bioavailability. In 1985 Hoffken et al. reported that absorption of ciprofloxacin was dramatically impaired when it was coadministered with magnesium-aluminum antacid (Maalox) (34). The mean peak concentration of ciprofloxacin in serum following a 500-mg dose to normal volunteers was 1.8 μg/ml and was reduced to 0.13 μg/ml when the same dose was given with the antacid. Since this report, all drugs in this class have been investigated for cationic interactions. So dramatic is the effect that there is a suggestion that magnesium salts can be used to treat ciprofloxacin "poisoning" (67).

Early investigations

All fluoroquinolones are chelated by di- and trivalent cations, such as Mg^{2+}, Al^{3+}, and Ca^{2+} that are often present in antacids, and by iron supplements, sucralfate, and multivitamins (Table 2). The mechanism of this interaction is believed to be formation of an insoluble complex between the cation and the 4-keto and 3-carboxyl group common to the fluoroquinolone class (Fig. 1). Bismuth-based antacids such as bismuth subsalicylate have no significant effects on norfloxacin or ciprofloxacin absorption (7, 75). The magnitude of the effect depends on the specific fluoroquinolone, the specific cation and its dosage form (liquid or solid), and the timing of administration (Table 2). Thermodynamic investigations reveal that there are differences between quinolones and the strength of ligand binding with cations (97). These differences in binding affinity may be responsible for differences in absorp-

Roula Qaqish • St. Louis College of Pharmacy, 4588 Parkview Place, St. Louis, MO 63110-1088. Ronald E. Polk • Department of Pharmacy, School of Pharmacy, 410 N. 12th St., Smith Building Room 454, Richmond, VA 23298-0533.

Table 1. Substrates, inducers, and inhibitors of the CYP450 isoenzymes[a]

Agent	CYP1A2	CYP2C9	CYP2C19	CYP2D6	CYP3A4	CYP2E1
Substrates	Caffeine	Amitriptyline	Imipramine	Amitriptyline	Alprazolam	Dapsone
	Clozapine	Celecoxib	Diazepam	Amphetamine	Amiodarone	Chloroxazone
	Estradiol	Diclofenac	Omeprazole	Captopril	Amitriptyline	
	Grepafloxacin	Naproxen	Propranolol	Codeine	Atorvastatin	
	Haloperidol	Nelfinavir	(S) Mephenytoin	Debrisquine	Cisapride	
	Mirtazapine	Phenytoin	Voriconazole	Desipramine	Clarithromycin	
	Mexiletine	Piroxicam		Ecanide	Cyclosporine	
	(R) Warfarin	Pravastatin		Flecanide	Dapsone	
	Tacrine	Rosiglitazone		Fluoxetine	Docetaxel	
	Theophylline	(S) Warfarin		Haloperidol	Efavirenz	
	Zileuton	Tolbutamide		Imipramine	Erythromycin	
		Glyburide		Mirtazapine	Etoposide	
				Methoxyamphetamine	Fentanyl	
				Nortriptyline	Granisetron	
				Paroxetine	Itraconazole	
				Risperidone	Ketoconazole	
				Venlafaxine	Lidocaine	
					Loratadine	
					Lovastatin	
					Midazolam	
					Mirtazapine	
					Nefazadone	
					NNRTIs	
					Paclitaxel	
					Pioglitazone	
					Posaconazole	
					Prednisone	
					Protease inhibitors	
					Quinidine	
					Sertraline	
					Sildenafil	
					Sirolimus	
					Simvistatin	
					Tacrolimus	
					Telithromycin	
					Testosterone	
					Triazolam	
					Triazolam	
					Verapamil	
					Vinblastine	
					Ziprazidone	
Inhibitor	Cimetidine	Fluconazole	Fluoxetine	Cimetidine	Azole antifungals	Disulfiram
	Ciprofloxacin	Fluoxetine	Fluvoxamine	Fluoxetine	Clarithromycin	Isoniazid
	Clinafloxacin	Fluvoxamine		Omeprazole	Delavirdine	
	Fluvoxamine	Isoniazid		Paroxetine	Diltiazem	
	Paroxitine	Sertraline		Quinidine	Efavirenz	
		Sulfaphenozole			Erythromycin	
					Fluoxetine	
					Fluvoxamine	
					Grapefruit juice (GI only)	
					HIV-1 protease inhibitors	
					Nefazodone	
					Quinupristin/ Dalfopristin	
					Telithromycin	

Continued on following page

Table 1. *Continued*

Agent	CYP1A2	CYP2C9	CYP2C19	CYP2D6	CYP3A4	CYP2E1
Inducer	Carbamazepine Cigarette smoke Omeprazole Phenytoin Phenobarbital Rifampin Ritonavir	Rifampin		Carbamazepine Phenytoin Phenobarbital Rifampin	Carbamazepine Dexamethasone Efavirenz Nevirapine Phenytoin Phenobarbital Rifampin Rifabutin Ritonavir St. John's wort Troglitazone	Isoniazid

a CYP, cytochrome P450 enzymes; NNRTIs, nonnucleoside reverse transcriptase inhibitors; HIV, human immunodeficiency virus.

tion between quinolones when coadministered with the same cation.

Many investigations report that a reduction in absorption may persist even if administration times of magnesium and aluminum antacid (and sucralfate, an aluminum complex) are staggered for 2 h or more (Fig. 2; Table 2) (67, 68). Early studies with calcium-containing antacids were conflicting; some reported no significant interactions (18, 85) and others reported significant reduction in quinolone absorption (83). Additionally, the bioavailability of quinolones is decreased when they are administered with multivitamins that contain minerals such as zinc, copper, magnesium, or manganese, and iron supplements (41, 50, 71, 90). Dairy products (milk and yogurt) containing calcium also decrease absorption of ciprofloxacin by ~33%, whereas ofloxacin is less affected (62).

Recent investigations

The administration of oral levofloxacin (100 mg) simultaneously with aluminum hydroxide (1,000 mg), ferrous sulfate (160 mg elemental iron), and magnesium oxide (500 mg), resulted in a significant decrease in the mean AUC of levofloxacin by 44, 19, and 22%, respectively (85). In contrast, levofloxacin AUC was not altered by simultaneous administration of calcium carbonate (1,000 mg) or when sucralfate (1 g orally) was given one-half hour after oral levofloxacin (47, 85). The AUC of trovafloxacin was reduced by 66% when given one-half hour after a magnesium- and aluminum hydroxide-containing antacid (99), by 70% when given with 1 g of sucralfate, and by 48% when given with ferrous sulfate (120 mg elemental iron) (79a). A 20% decrease in the AUC of trovafloxacin was observed when given orally with 1,000 mg of calcium carbonate (79a).

Gatifloxacin (400 mg oral) AUC was significantly decreased when it was simultaneously given with ferrous sulfate (325 mg) or Maalox (44, 52). Calcium carbonate (500 mg) resulted in an 8% decrease in mean gatifloxacin AUC, a change that was not significant (44). The AUC of moxifloxacin (400 mg) was significantly reduced when simultaneously administered with oral ferrous sulfate (Eryfer 100, equivalent to 100 mg of Fe^{2+}), and sucralfate (1 g), but not by Ca^{2+} carbonate (500 mg) (90, 91, 92, 94). The impacts of Maalox administered at different times on the AUC of moxifloxacin are representative of these effects on all of the newer quinolones (Fig. 1).

Gemifloxacin AUC is reduced by a mean of 53% when it was given 3 h after a 2-g dose of sucralfate, and by 11% when given 3 h after 325 mg of ferrous sulfate (1). When given 2 h before sucralfate and iron, there was no significant effect on gemifloxacin absorption. Similar to that seen with other quinolones, gemifloxacin AUC is reduced by 85% when it is given 10 min before Maalox and by 15% when given 3 h after Maalox; there is no effect when it was given 2 h before Maalox (2).

Clinical importance

The clinical importance of an absorption interaction depends on the magnitude of reduction in absorption, the susceptibility (MIC) of the pathogen, and the site of infection. For example, a 50% reduction in absorption is not likely to have a clinically important effect in the treatment of an uncomplicated urinary tract infection caused by a susceptible strain of *Escherichia coli*. However, a 50% reduction in absorption when treating chronic osteomyelitis caused by a relatively resistant pathogen is more likely to result in clinical failure. There are few case reports of patients whose infection failed to respond to fluoroquinolone therapy most likely as a result of an absorption inter-

Table 2. Pharmacokinetic absorption interactions between cations and fluoroquinolones

Quinolone	Dose (mg)	Cation dose and dosage schedule[a]	Mean % reduction in AUC[b]	References
Ciprofloxacin	500	Ca carbonate (500 mg elemental calcium), simultaneous with ciprofloxacin	43*	83
	750	Didanosine-cation, three doses. Dose 3 given simultaneous with ciprofloxacin	98*	84
	500	Fe gluconate (600 mg) simultaneous with ciprofloxacin	67*	41
	500	$FeSO_4$ (325 mg t.i.d. for 7 days) simultaneous ciprofloxacin	63*	71
	500	Multivitamins with Zn for 7 days, simultaneous with ciprofloxacin	22*	71
	750	Sucralfate (1 g) simultaneous with ciprofloxacin	96*	103
	750	Mg/Al antacid single 30-ml dose, 2 h before 750 mg p.o. ciprofloxacin	85*	65
Enoxacin	400	Mg/Al antacid (30 ml) (MgO 1.85 g/AlOH 3.6 g) 0.5 h (before) enoxacin	73*	25
Gatifloxacin	400	Ca carbonate, (1 g) simultaneous with gatifloxacin	8	44
	400	$FeSO_4$ (325 mg) simultaneous with gatifloxacin	35*	44
	400	Mg/Al antacid (20 ml) simultaneous with gatifloxacin	64*	52
Gemifloxacin	320	Mg/Al antacid, 10 min after gemifloxacin	85*	2
	320	$FeSO_4$ (325 mg) 3 h before gemifloxacin	11	1
	320	Sucralfate 2 g, 3 h pre-gemifloxacin	60*	1
Lomefloxacin	400	Ca carbonate (500 mg) simultaneous with lomefloxacin	2	48
	400	$FeSO_4$ (100 mg elemental iron), simultaneous with lomefloxacin	14	48
	200	Mg/Al antacid (MgO 200 mg/AlOH 400 mg), simultaneous with lomefloxacin	41*	86
	400	Sucralfate (1 g) simultaneous with lomefloxacin	51*	48
Levofloxacin	100	AlOH (1 g) simultaneous with levofloxacin	44*	85
	100	Ca carbonate (1 g) simultaneous with levofloxacin	3	85
	100	$FeSO_4$ (160 mg) simultaneous with levofloxacin	19*	85
	100	MgOH (500 mg) simultaneous with levofloxacin	22*	85
	500	Sucralfate (1 g) 2 h after levofloxacin	5	47
Moxifloxacin	400	Ca carbonate (500 mg) simultaneous with 400 mg p.o. of moxifloxacin	2	91
	400	$FeSO_4$ (Eryfer 100 equivalent to 100 mg of Fe^{2+}) q.d. for 2 days, last dose simultaneous with moxifloxacin	39*	90
	400	Mg/Al antacid (10 ml) (900 mg/600 mg) simultaneous with moxifloxacin	60*	92
	400	Sucralfate (1 g) simultaneous with moxifloxacin	60*	94
Norfloxacin	400	AlOH (10 ml) (640 mg AlOH) simultaneous with norfloxacin	86*	7
	400	Ca carbonate (Titralac) (30 ml) 5 min after norfloxacin	62*	66
	400	$FeSO_4$ (300 mg) simultaneous with norfloxacin	55**	7
	400	Mg/Al antacid (Maalox) (30 ml) 5 min after norfloxacin	91*	66
	400	Sucralfate (1 g) simultaneous with norfloxacin	98*	69
	400	$ZnSO_4$ (200 mg) simultaneous with norfloxacin	56**	7
Ofloxacin	200	$AlPO_4$ (11 g) simultaneous with ofloxacin	7	54
	400	Ca carbonate (5 ml) 2 h before ofloxacin	4	18
	400	$FeSO_4$ (100 elemental Fe) simultaneous with ofloxacin	25	50
	400	Mg/Al antacid (15 ml) 2 h before ofloxacin	21*	18
	200	Sucralfate (1 g) simultaneous with ofloxacin	61*	42, 49
Pefloxacin	400	Mg/Al antacid (MgO 600 mg/AlOH 900 mg), 1 h after pefloxacin	54*	37
Rufloxacin	400	Mg/Al antacid (30 ml) 5 min after rufloxacin	38*	45
Sparfloxacin	400	Sucralfate (1 g) q.i.d. for 2 days, last dose given 0.5 h before sparfloxacin	47*	112
Temafloxacin	400	Mg/Al antacid (Maalox 70) (8 doses day prior to study and 5 doses day of study) temafloxacin	61*	22
Trovafloxacin	300	Mg/Al antacid (30 ml) 0.5 h before trovafloxacin	66*	99

[a] Abbreviations: t.i.d., three times a day; p.o., orally; q.d., once a day; q.i.d., four times a day.
[b] *, Statistically significant reduction in AUC (area under the plasma or serum concentration-versus-time curve); **, % reduction in urine excretion.

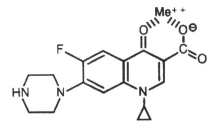

Figure 1. Proposed mechanism by which metal (Me^{++}) cations chelate fluoroquinolones.

action. One report described an elderly woman whose urinary tract infection caused by a norfloxacin-susceptible strain of *Pseudomonas aeruginosa* (MIC, <1 µg/ml) persisted during norfloxacin therapy and progressed to bacteremia (70). This unexpected finding was explained by the fact that the norfloxacin has been mashed up in Maalox before administering the dose into the patient's nasogastric tube.

Based on the preceding evidence of a substantial decrease in the bioavailability, concomitant use of

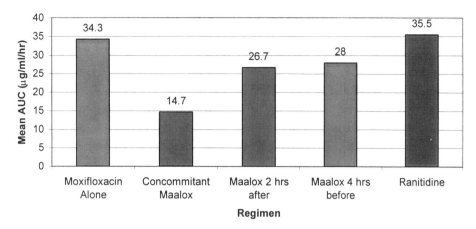

Figure 2. Effects of Maalox and ranitidine on absorption of moxifloxacin. Data from reference 92.

magnesium-, aluminum-, or calcium-containing antacids, sucralfate, or iron/vitamin-mineral preparations with all quinolones should be avoided. Because magnesium-aluminum antacids and sucralfate have the greatest effects, if they must be used, it is best to administer the quinolone at least 2 h before the antacid, or 4 h after, to allow for maximum absorption. It is equally important to remember that some drugs, such as didanosine chewable tablets, but not the enteric coated tablets, are formulated with an aluminum-magnesium buffer, and that the effect of coadministration with a fluoroquinolone is the same as with antacid (Fig. 3; 82).

Enteral Feedings and Absorption of Fluoroquinolones

A study in six normal volunteers found that the AUC following administration of a crushed ciprofloxacin 750-mg tablet given via a nasogastric tube with water or enteral feedings was the same as that following administration of an intact oral tablet (111). The same investigators reported that ciprofloxacin AUC given with enteral feeding solutions was significantly higher when administered via a nasoduodenal tube in comparison with a nasogastric tube (110). In 1992 it was reported that ciprofloxacin did not bind to gastric feeding tubes (15), and in 1994 Mueller et al. reported that the bioavailability of ciprofloxacin was significantly reduced, by a mean of 28%, when it was given to normal volunteers with Ensure in comparison with ciprofloxacin and water (61). Healy et al. reported in 1996 that when a ciprofloxacin 500-mg tablet was given orally to patients receiving Sustacal (240 ml given 8 h before, simultaneously with, and 4 h after ciprofloxacin), the mean AUC was significantly reduced, from 13.4 to 9.4 µg/ml/h (29). In the same investigation, when a ciprofloxacin 500-mg

tablet was crushed and given to patients with Jevity via gastrostomy or jejunostomy tubes, the mean AUC was further reduced to 7.4 and 5.8 µg/ml/h, respectively. Three subsequent investigations in seriously ill patients in the intensive care unit found that ciprofloxacin bioavailability was generally reduced when crushed and given through a nasogastric tube with enteral feedings (9, 12, 57). However the AUC following a 750-mg dose given in this manner was found to result in an AUC similar to that following a 400-mg intravenous dose. Finally, an in vitro study reported that when ciprofloxacin and levofloxacin were crushed and mixed with Ensure, there was an unexplained loss in fluoroqunolone, 82% and 61% for ciprofloxacin and levofloxacin, respectively, when measured by high-performance liquid chromatography (109). There was no loss in fluoroquinolone when ciprofloxacin was mixed with calcium and magnesium chloride.

Taken together, these data suggest that there is a reduction in ciprofloxacin absorption when mixed

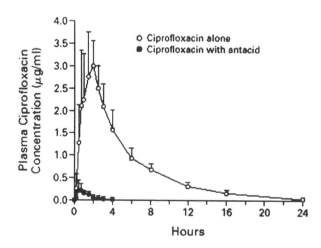

Figure 3. Effects of didanosine table formulation on absorption of ciprofloxacin. Reprinted from reference 82 with permission.

with enteral feeding solutions and given via a feeding tube. The presumed mechanism is chelation of ciprofloxacin by metal cations present in the enteral feeding solution, but there may be other mechanisms. Since bioavailability is certain when a fluoroquinolone is given intravenously, this route of administration is preferred in the seriously ill patient. If it is necessary to administer a crushed tablet via a feeding tube, it appears that a dose of 750 mg of ciprofloxacin will generally produce serum concentrations that are similar to those following an intravenous dose of 400 mg.

H₂ Blockers, Proton Pump Inhibitor Drugs, and Quinolones

Numerous investigations have found that non-antacid drugs that increase gastric pH, including proton pump inhibitors such as omeprazole (3, 99) and histamine (H₂)-receptor blockers such as ranitidine (65, 73, 85, 87, 92) have no appreciable effect on the bioavailability of quinolones (Table 2, Fig. 2). These drugs can be used as an alternative to antacids and sucralfate in the patient requiring protection from gastric acid.

Phosphate Binder

The relative bioavailability of ciprofloxacin was significantly reduced by 50% when coadministered with sevelamer hydrochloride (Renagel) (43). The mechanism of this interaction is unknown. It is prudent to avoid concomitant use of sevelamer with all fluoroquinolones until this interaction is investigated more fully.

PHARMACOKINETIC INTERACTIONS INVOLVING METABOLISM

Methylxanthine Interactions

Wijnands et al. were the first to report that quinolones could delay clearance of theophylline (107). Eight of ten patients with chronic bronchial disease treated with enoxacin (600 mg twice daily) and theophylline experienced severe nausea, vomiting, and occasionally convulsions. In another early report, ciprofloxacin was found to significantly decrease clearance of theophylline, occasionally leading to death from theophylline toxicity (35). Since theophylline is now less commonly used than in the past, this interaction is of less concern. Nevertheless, all new fluoroquinolones are investigated for their effects on theophylline metabolism (Table 3).

Unlike chelation interactions, which appear to be a class effect, metabolic interactions are quinolone specific. Enoxacin, ciprofloxacin, pefloxacin, grepafloxacin, and clinafloxacin are all inhibitors of methylxanthine metabolism (16, 30, 43, 53, 76, 108). The structure-activity relationships responsible for metabolic interactions have been investigated. Wijnands et al. initially hypothesized that the 4-oxo-metabolite of certain quinolones was responsible for inhibition of theophylline metabolism (108), but later work did not support this hypothesis (70). The sequence of N*—C—N–C–N—C (where N* is a nitrogen on the piperazine ring) was proposed to predict inhibition of xanthine metabolism (20, 27). A bulky substituent at position 8 is associated with less enzyme inhibition in rats, and the presence of 4'-nitrogen atom in the 7-piperazinyl group is reported to be essential for metabolic interactions to occur (58). Whatever the responsible structural elements, all available quinolones that inhibit metabolism of other drugs do so via a common mechanism: competitive inhibition of the cytochrome P450 hepatic enzyme, CYP1A2 (19, 20). During early clinical development, fluoroquinolones had a reputation for being "inhibitors of P450 enzymes," with no differentiation of specificity for different P450 isoforms. Currently, however, potential effects of a new fluoroquinolone on drug-metabolizing enzymes are routinely assessed during preclinical development. For example, the product information for moxifloxacin states: "In vitro studies with cytochrome P450 isoenzymes (CYP) indicates that moxifloxacin does not inhibit CYP3A4, CYP2D6, CYP2C9, 2C19, or CYP1A2, suggesting that moxifloxacin is unlikely to alter the pharmacokinetics of drugs metabolized by these enzymes (e.g., midazolam, cyclosporine, warfarin, theophylline) (3a).

Theophylline is 1,3-dimethylxanthine. CYP1A2 catalyzes N-demethylations to 1-methylxanthine and 3-methylxanthine, as well as an 8 oxidation reaction. Caffeine is 1,3,7-trimethylxanthine, and it is also N-demethylated via CYP1A2 (Table 3). All of the CYP1A2 inhibitory quinolones demonstrate dose-dependent enzyme inhibition and are considered by clinical pharmacologists to be prototype inhibitors of CYP1A2. The clinical investigations with clinafloxacin are used to illustrate the effects seen when an inhibitor of CYP1A2 is given with methylxanthines (76). As illustrated in Fig. 4A, administration of clinafloxacin twice daily for 5 days followed by theophylline increased the mean AUC for theophylline from a baseline value of 55 to 114 μg/ml/h (for a 200-mg dose of clinafloxacin) and to 145 μg/ml/h (for a 400-mg dose). Clinafloxacin also inhibits caffeine metabolism (Fig. 4B). The mean

Table 3. Summary of fluoroquinolone-methylxanthine interactions[a]

Fluoroquinolone and dose schedule	Interacting drug	Mean % change in C_{ss} or AUC[b]	Mean % change in CL	Reference
Clinafloxacin				
400 mg b.i.d. × 5 d	Caffeine		−84*	76
	Theophylline		−68*	76
200 mg b.i.d. × 5 d	Theophylline		−25.7*	76
Ciprofloxacin				
500 mg b.i.d. × 5 d	Theophylline	+66*	−30*	108
750 mg b.i.d. × 3 doses	Caffeine		−45*	30
750 mg b.i.d. × 5 d	Theophylline		−31*	84
Enoxacin				
400 mg b.i.d. × 5 d	Caffeine		−78*	89
400 mg b.i.d. × 5 d	Theophylline	+163*	−64*	108
Gatifloxacin				
400 mg b.i.d.	Theophylline		0	63
Gemifloxaicn				
320 mg q.d. × 7 d	Theophylline	+1.1		10
Grepafloxacin				
600 mg q.d. × 10 d	Theophylline		−52*	16
Levofloxacin				
500 mg b.i.d. × 9 doses	Theophylline		+3	21
Lomefloxacin				
400 mg q.d. × 3 d	Caffeine	−6	−3	31
400 mg b.i.d. × 7 d	Theophylline		−2	79
400 mg q.i.d. × 7 d	Theophylline		−7	64
Moxifloxacin				
200 mg b.i.d. × 3 d	Theophylline		−4	93
Ofloxacin				
200 mg b.i.d. × 5 d	Caffeine		+4	95
400 mg b.i.d. × 5 d	Theophylline	+2	−5	108
Norfloxacin				
400 mg b.i.d. × 4 d	Theophylline		−10*	4
400 mg b.i.d. × 5 d	Theophylline	+2	−5*	108
200 mg t.i.d. × 3 d	Theophylline		0	81
Pefloxacin				
400 mg b.i.d. × 5 d	Theophylline		−29*	108
Sparfloxacin				
200 mg q.d. × 8 d	Theophylline		−9	96
Temafloxacin				
600 mg b.i.d. × 7 d	Caffeine	+1.25		53
400 mg b.i.d. × 7 d	Theophylline	−55	−10	88
Trovafloxacin				
200 mg q.d.	Caffeine	+15	−17	46
200 mg q.d. × 7 d	Theophylline		−7	105
300 mg q.d. × 7 d	Theophylline	8		13

[a] Asterisk indicates statistical significance; % change, percent change from baseline or placebo control; CL, total body clearance; C_{ss}, steady-state concentration; q.d., once a day; t.i.d., three times a day; d, day.

AUC in healthy volunteers following a 200-mg dose of caffeine was 48 μg/ml/h, and this was increased to 250 μg/ml/h following pretreatment with clinafloxacin (400 mg). Since this increase in AUC represents the difference between one strong cup of coffee (200 mg of caffeine) and five strong cups of coffee, it is tempting to speculate that some of the adverse central nervous system (CNS) effects for fluoroquinolones are secondary to caffeine accumulation and toxicity (95). Many of the noninhibitory quinolones such as levofloxacin, however, also cause CNS adverse events and it has been difficult to sep-

arate drug-interaction effects from intrinsic adverse events (89). Norfloxacin, levofloxacin, lomafloxacin, sparfloxacin, gemifloxacin, torovafloxacin, gatifloxacin, and moxifloxacin do not significantly inhibit methylxanthine metabolism (4, 10, 13, 21, 31, 46, 64, 93, 96, 105).

In contrast to CYP1A2, the most important human hepatic P450 metabolic enzyme is CYP3A4. This enzyme is involved in the metabolism of a large number of drugs that have a narrow therapeutic index, including cyclosporine, terfenadine, cisapride, and ergotamine (Table 1). That certain quinolones

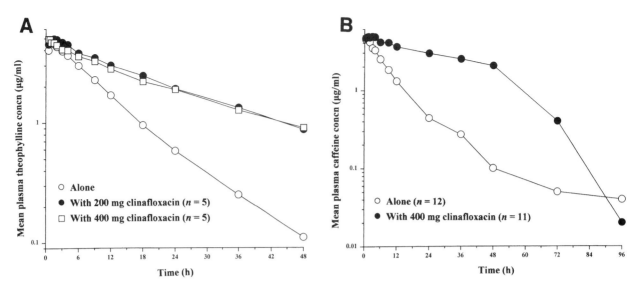

Figure 4. Effects of clinafloxacin on clearance of theophylline (a) and caffeine (b). Reprinted from reference 76 with permission.

(above) selectively inhibit a relatively unimportant human metabolic enzyme, CYP1A2, explains why there are relatively few important fluoroquinolone metabolic drug-drug interactions compared with potent inhibitors of CYP3A4 such as itraconazole, macrolides, the ketolide telithromycin, and the human immunodeficiency virus protease inhibitors (Table 1). The specificity of certain quinolones to inhibit only CYP1A2 is also important in understanding some of the other reported metabolic drug-drug interactions (below).

Warfarin

Many case reports have described bleeding in patients receiving warfarin when a quinolone was added (summarized by Ellis et al. [17]). They reported two additional patients taking warfarin in whom bleeding developed during ciprofloxacin therapy, and their review summarized an additional 64 reports submitted to the U.S. Food and Drug Administration. They concluded that, "clinicians should be aware of the potential bleeding complications that can occur with the ciprofloxacin-warfarin drug-drug interaction." In contrast to these case reports, all but one prospective trial in patients and normal volunteers have failed to document a statistically or clinically important effect on bleeding times (Table 4). How can these apparent disparities be reconciled?

Warfarin is a mixture of two enantiomers, (R) warfarin and (S) warfarin. The (S) enantiomer is responsible for most of the anticoagulant effect. At least 80% of (S) warfarin is metabolized by CYP2C9 (Table 1) and inhibitors of CYP2C9 increase bleed-

ing time in patients receiving warfarin (100). The relatively inactive (R) enantiomer of warfarin is metabolized in part by CYP1A2, and drug-interaction studies that have measured both enantiomer concentrations have found that enoxacin, ciprofloxacin, and clinafloxacin delay clearance of (R) warfarin but have no effect on (S) warfarin concentrations (36, 76, 102). For example, Israel et al. studied 36 adult patients who were attending a warfarin clinic (36). Ciprofloxacin (750 mg twice a day [b.i.d.]) or placebo was given for 2 weeks, followed by a washout period, and then followed by the alternate treatment. There was no change in (S) warfarin concentration and no patient had to discontinue treatment. There were small yet statistically significant decreases in concentrations of clotting factors II and VI, consistent with a modest increase in (R) warfarin concentrations. The magnitude of the (R) warfarin concentration, however, was not considered sufficient to cause a noticeable increase in prothrombin time (PT) or International Normalized Ratio (INR). There was no statistically significant change in mean PT, with the maximum estimated change in PT being ~1 s.

A single prospective study (out of 10 reviewed) did report a statistically significant change in coagulation. Randinitis et al. administered clinafloxacin (200 mg b.i.d.) for 14 days to 12 healthy males (age range, 21 to 31 years) who had been previously anticoagulated with warfarin (76). At the end of 2 weeks of clinafloxacin treatment, (R) warfarin plasma concentrations were significantly increased (32%) but there was no change in (S) warfarin concentrations. The magnitude of increase in (R), warfarin concentration was not considered sufficient to cause a noticeable increase in PT or the INR. There was also

Table 4. Summary of warfarin-fluoroquinolone interactions[a]

Quinolone	Dose/schedule/duration	Warfarin dosage	n	Effect on enantiomer	Effect on PT/INR	Reference
Enoxacin	400 mg b.i.d. × 14 d	25 mg day 1 and 8	6 HV	↑ R	↔	102
Clinafloxacin	200 mg b.i.d. × 14 d	Titrated over 14 days to INR between 1.5 and 2.0	12 HV	↑ R	↑ INR	76
Ciprofloxacin	750 mg b.i.d. × 12 d (2-wk washout)	Average dose 42 ± 13 mg (20–70 mg) weekly	36 P	↑ R	↔	36
Levofloxacin	500 mg b.i.d. × 9 d	30 mg single dose on day 4	16 HV	↔	↔	51
Moxifloxacin	400 mg q.d. × 8 d	25 mg single dose	24 HV	↔	↔	60
Norfloxacin	400 mg b.i.d. × 9 d	30 mg single dose on day 4	10 HV	NM	↔	77
Gemifloxacin	320 mg q.d. × 7 d (day 18–24)	Titrated over 14 days to INR between 1.3 and 1.8; day 14–24 fixed warfarin dose	35 HV	NM	↔	11
Grepafloxacin	600 mg q.d. × 14 d	Warfarin 10 mg × 2 days, then titrated on days 3–10 for INR 1.5–2.5	16 HV	NM	↔	16
Temafloxacin	600 mg b.i.d. on study days 13 and 15, and q.d. on day 16	Titrated over 16 days to INR between 1.3 and 1.7	10 HV	↔	↔	56
Trovafloxacin	200 mg q.d. × 7 d	Daily 21 days	NR	↔	↔	101

[a] ↑ Indicates significant increase; ↔ indicates no significant change; HV, healthy volunteers; P, patients; NM, not measured; NR, not reported; R, *R* enantiomer; q.d., once a day; d, days.

a significant increase in the mean INR values, from ~1.7 to 2.0 after 12 to 14 days of clinafloxacin administration, representing a 9 to 17% increase in individual values. The authors speculated that the change in INR might result from reduced vitamin K production by intestinal bacteria.

After reviewing these data it seems reasonable to conclude one of two things: case reports of bleeding in patients taking warfarin and a fluoroquinolone reflect a real, yet rare, interaction, or the case reports are confounded by an alternative mechanism. It is possible that quinolones reduce the numbers of gastrointestinal bacteria that produce vitamin K, resulting in exaggerated response to warfarin in a small subset of patients, but supporting data are few. It is also conceivable that a rare subset of patients has an unusual metabolic profile for warfarin, or unusual sensitivity to (*R*) warfarin, and fluoroquinolone therapy may somehow exaggerate the anticoagulant response. However, a more likely reason for reports of bleeding in patients receiving warfarin is "infection" itself. Infection is known to release numerous cytokines and many are known to down-regulate P450 metabolic enzyme activity (28). For example, viral infection is known to delay clearance of theophylline, and there are many reports of theophylline toxicity during viral infection (28). Likewise, the patient receiving warfarin who develops an infection will release cytokines, and it is a reasonable hypothesis that this results in inhibition of warfarin metabolism leading to bleeding. The quinolone, or any antimicrobial, may then be falsely blamed for "causing" bleeding. Additional research

is needed to determine the correct explanation. In the mean time, it is prudent to monitor the INR in every patient taking warfarin who develops an infection, and during antimicrobial treatment. On the basis of our current data, however, quinolones are not contraindicated in patients receiving warfarin.

Miscellaneous Interactions

Benzodiazepines

Benzodiazepines undergo extensive metabolism, usually by P450 enzymes and/or glucuronidation (26). None of the currently available benzodiazepines is known to be metabolized by CYP1A2; thus, a metabolic interaction with fluoroquinolones is not expected a priori.

Results of interaction studies between ciprofloxacin and diazepam are controversial. Diazepam is metabolized by CYP3A4 and CYP2C19 (26). The effects of pretreatment with a 7-day course of ciprofloxacin on an intravenous 5-mg dose of diazepam were investigated in 12 healthy volunteers in a double-blind placebo-controlled crossover study. In this study ciprofloxacin was found to impair the clearance of diazepam with a doubling of its half-life. However, no significant changes were detected in psychometric tests of digit symbol substitution, tapping rate, and short memory, as well as levels of concentration, vigilance, and tension measured by visual analogue scales (40). In a second investigation, the pharmacokinetics of a single intravenous dose of 10 mg of diazepam and the renal excretion of its metabolites were investigated in 10 healthy volunteers when diazepam was administered alone and on day 3 of ciprofloxacin (500 mg twice daily) (106). No significant changes in diazepam half-life, total body clearance, or renal clearance were observed. In addition, the renal excretion of the metabolites desmethyldiazepam, 3-hydroxydiazepam (temazepam), and 3-hydroxydesmethyldiazepam (oxazepam) were not altered by ciprofloxacin comedication. Although it is possible that excessive sedation could occur in patients receiving diazepam and a quinolone, there is no known mechanism to explain such an interaction, and this does not represent a contraindication to quinolone use.

Gatifloxacin was given in multiple doses to 14 patients (ages, 23 to 45 years) to assess its effect on the pharmacokinetics of midazolam, a model substrate of CYP3A4. Subjects received a 0.0145 mg/kg dose of intravenous midazolam on day 1, followed by 400 mg once-daily oral gatifloxacin on days 2 to 6. On day 6, midazolam was given 1 h before the last dose of gatifloxacin. As expected, no significant change occurred in the pharmacokinetics of midazolam or its metabolites (23).

Cyclosporine

Similar to the quinolone warfarin interaction, several early case reports suggested that quinolones may impair the metabolism of cyclosporine and promote nephrotoxicity (55). Multiple prospective investigations have failed to show any effect on cyclosporine metabolism by a fluoroquinolone (14, 33). This class of drugs is often recommended as a treatment of choice for infection caused by *Legionella pneumophila* in transplant patients receiving cyclosporine (see chapter 20), since macrolides and rifampin, the alternative agents for this infection, are well known inhibitors and inducers of cyclosporine metabolism, respectively. Cyclosporine is metabolized exclusively by CYP3A4 (Table 1), and the lack of a fluoroquinolone interaction is expected. The possible effect of infection on cyclosporine metabolism has not been investigated but may have been responsible for the appearance of an "interaction" in the early case reports.

Glyburide (glybenclamide)

Conflicting data exist regarding a quinolone-glyburide interaction. Glyburide is most likely metabolized by CYP2C9 (5) and a pharmacokinetic interaction with a quinolone is not anticipated (Table 1). Gatifloxacin was found not to alter glyburide pharmacokinetics or glucose tolerance in a

prospective investigation (24). There is, however, a case report of elevated serum glyburide levels and hypoglycemia in a patient receiving long-term glyburide after 1 week of ciprofloxacin therapy (78). It is possible that some quinolones have intrinsic insulin-like activity that may contribute to these reports (see chapter 25). It is also possible that infection may suppress glyburide metabolism, resulting in hypoglycemia in a susceptible individual.

Phenytoin

There have been case reports of a decrease in serum phenytoin concentrations when ciprofloxacin was initiated, followed by a return to therapeutic concentrations when ciprofloxacin was stopped (6, 72). A prospective investigation found that ciprofloxacin had no significant effect on phenytoin pharmacokinetics, although one subject showed a marked reduction in phenytoin AUC. Phenytoin is metabolized via CYP 2C9 and CYP 2C19 (Table 1). Although there is no mechanistic pathway to explain an interaction, a rare, idiosyncratic interaction is possible.

Like enoxacin, clinafloxacin is a potent inhibitor of CYP1A2. However, it can also inhibit other isoenzymes, including CYP2C9 and CYP2C19 in vitro, though it is considerably less potent for these isoforms (76). Randinitis et al. reported that clinafloxacin treatment (200 mg b.i.d.) resulted in a mean increase in phenytoin AUC of 20% in a group of healthy volunteers, consistent with a modest inhibition of CYP2C9 and CYP2C19 (76).

Rifampin

Though rifampin is one of the most potent inducers known of multiple P450 enzymes, there appears to be little effect on metabolism of most quinolones (98). One would expect rifampin to increase metabolism of quinolones that are metabolized by P450 enzymes that are induced by rifampin. For example, grepafloxacin is metabolized by CYP1A2 and rifampin induces this enzyme, so an interaction would be expected (Table 1). Because fluoroquinolones may have a role in treatment of infections caused by *Mycobacterium tuberculosis*, selection of a quinolone that does not undergo metabolism may be a preferred option.

Narcotics

There are rare reports that certain quinolones may interact adversely with some narcotics. Intravenous morphine may decrease the bioavailability of oral ciprofloxacin (59) and trovafloxacin (104) by ~50 and 38%, respectively, although the clinical significance is unclear. A prospective investigation found that morphine had no effect on pharmacokinetics of garenoxacin (BMS-284756) (80).

A convincing case report described that symptoms of methadone excess occurred in a patient receiving maintenance methadone during each of four courses of ciprofloxacin therapy for urosepsis (32). Since methadone is metabolized, in part, by CYP1A2, caution is advised when quinolones that inhibit this isoform are prescribed. Additional data are needed regarding this interaction.

Nonsteroidal anti-inflammatory drugs (NSAIDs)

An early report from the Ministry of Welfare in Japan found an alarmingly high number of patients with convulsions receiving fenbufen (NSAID) and enoxacin (38). Research has focused on the neuroinhibitory effects of quinolones, on gamma amino butyric acid receptors, CNS adverse effects of the fluoroquinolones, and a possible pharmacodynamic interaction with certain NSAIDs (see chapter 29). A prospective investigation, however, found that ciprofloxacin had no effects on the pharmacokinetics of fenbufen (39). Since thousands of patients have probably received quinolones and other NSAIDs through the years, with no reports of serious neurotoxicity, this interaction appears not to be a general phenomenon for all quinolones or NSAIDs and is of mostly historical interest.

Clozapine

The antipsychotic agent clozapine is metabolized by CYP1A2 (Table 1). A prospective investigation found that 250 mg of ciprofloxacin b.i.d. administered to seven schizophrenic patients resulted in a 29% mean increase in the serum concentrations of clozapine, and its N-desmethyl metabolite, 12 h after the clozapine dose (74) The increase in clozapine concentrations was proportional to ciprofloxacin concentrations. Larger doses of ciprofloxacin would be expected to have greater effects.

REFERENCES

1. Allen, A., E. Bygate, H. Faessel, L. Isaac, and A. Lewis. 2000. The effect of ferrous sulphate and sucralfate on the bioavailability of oral gemifloxacin in healthy volunteers. *Int. J. Antimicrob. Agents* 15:283–289.

2. Allen, A., M. Vousden, A. Porter, and A. Lewis. 1999. Effect of Maalox on the bioavailability of oral gemifloxacin in healthy volunteers. *Chemotherapy* 45:504–511.

3. Allen, A., M. Vousden, and A. Lewis. 1999. Effect of omeprazole on the pharmacokinetics of oral gemifloxacin in healthy volunteers. *Chemotherapy* 45:496–503.

3a. Bayer Corporation. 2001. Moxifloxacin (Avelox). Bayer Corp. Pharmaceutical Division, West Haven, Conn.

4. Bowels, S. K., Z. Popovski, M. J. Rybak, H. B. Beckman, and D. J. Edwards. 1988. Effect of norfloxacin on theophylline pharmacokinetics at steady state. *Antimicrob. Agents Chemother.* 32:510–512.

5. Brian W. R. 2000. Hypoglycemic agents, p. 529–543. *In* R. Levy, K. E. Thummel, W. F. Trager, P. D. Hansten, and M. Eichelbaum (ed.), *Metabolic Drug Interactions*. Lippincott, Williams and Wilkins, Philadelphia, Pa.

6. Brouwers, P. J., L. E. BeBoer, and H. J. Guchelaar. 1997. Ciprofloxacin-phenytoin interaction. *Ann. Pharmacother.* 31:498.

7. Campbell, N. R., M. Kara, B. Hasinoff, W. M. Haddara, and D. W. McKay. 1992. Norfloxacin interaction with antacids and minerals. *Br. J. Clin. Pharmacol.* 33:115,116.

8. Cisapride (Propulsid). 2000. *Revised Prescribing Information.* Janssen Pharmaceutica, Titusville, N.J.

9. Cohn, S. M., M. D. Sawyer, G. A. Burns, C. Tolomeo, and K. A. Milner. 1996. Enteric absorption of ciprofloxacin during tube feeding in the critically ill. *J. Antimicrob. Chemother.* 38:871–976.

10. Davy, M., N. Bird, K. L. Rost, and H. Fuder. 1999. Lack of effect of gemifloxacin on the steady-state pharmacodynamics of theophylline in healthy volunteers. *Chemotherapy* 45:478–484.

11. Davy, M., N. Bird, K. L. Rost, and H. Fuder. 1999. Lack of effect of gemifloxacin on the steady-state pharmacodynamics of warfarin in healthy volunteers. *Chemotherapy* 45:491–495.

12. de Marie, S. M. F. VandenBergh, S. L. Buijk, H. A. Bruining, A. van Vliet, J. A. Kluytmans, and J. W. Mouton. 1998. Bioavailability of ciprofloxacin after multiple enteral and intravenous doses in ICU patients with severe gram-negative intra-abdominal infections. *Intens. Care Med.* 24:343–346.

13. Dickens, G. R., D. Wermeling, and J. Vincent. 1997. Phase I pilot study of the effects of trovafloxacin (CP-99,219) on the pharmacokinetics of theophylline in healthy men. *J. Clin. Pharmacol.* 37:248–252.

14. Doose, D. R., S. A. Walker, S. C. Chien, R. R. Williams, and R. K. Nayak. 1998. Levofloxacin does not alter cyclosporine disposition. *J. Clin. Pharmacol.* 38:90–93.

15. Druckenbrod, R. W., and D. P. Healy. 1992. In vitro delivery of crushed ciprofloxacin through a feeding tube. *Ann. Pharmacother.* 26:494–495.

16. Efthymiopoulos, C., S. L. Bramer, A. Maroli, and B. Blum. 1997. Theophylline and warfarin interaction studies with grepafloxacin. *Clin. Pharmacokinet.* 33(Suppl. 1):39–46.

17. Ellis, R. J., M. S. Mayo, and D. M. Bodensteiner. 2000. Ciprofloxacin-warfarin coagulopathy: a case series. *Am. J. Hematol.* 63:28–31.

18. Flor, S., D. R. O. Guay, J. A. Opsahl, K. Tack, and G. R. Matzke. 1990. Effects of magnesium-aluminum hydroxide and calcium carbonate antacids on bioavailability of ofloxacin. *Antimicrob. Agents Chemother.* 34:2436–2438.

19. Fuhr, U., E-M. Anders, G. Mahr, F. Sörgel, A. H. Staib. 1992. Inhibitory potency of quinolone antibacterial agents against cytochrome P450IA2 activity in vivo and in vitro. *Antimicrob. Agents Chemother.* 36:942–948.

20. Fuhr, U., G. Strobl, F. Manaut, E. M. Anders, F. Sorgel, E. Lopez-de-Brinas, D. T. Chu, A. G. Pernet, G. Mahr, and F. Sanz. 1993. Quinolone antibacterial agents: relationship between structure and in vitro inhibition of the human cytochrome P-450 isoform CYP1A2. *Mol. Pharmacol.* 43:191–199.

21. Gisclon, L. G., C. R. Curtin, C. L. Fowler, R. R. Williams, B. Hafkin, and J. Natarajan. 1997. Absence of a pharmacokinetic interaction between intravenous theophylline and orally administered levofloxacin. *J. Clin. Pharmacol.* 37:744–750.

22. Granneman, G. R., U. Stephan, B. Birner, F. Sorgel, and D. Mukherjee D. 1992. Effect of antacid medication on the pharmacokinetics of temafloxacin. *Clin. Pharmacokinet.* 22(Suppl. 1):83–89.

23. Grasela, D. M., F. P. LaCreta, G. D. Kollia, D. M. Randall, and H. D. Uderman. 2000. Open-lable, nonrandomized study of the effect of gatifloxacin on the pharmacokinetics of midazolam in healthy male volunteers. *Pharmacotherapy.* 20:330–335.

24. Grasela, D., F. Lacreta, G. Kollia, D. Randall, R. Stoltz, and S. Berger. Lack of effect of multiple-dose gatifloxacin on oral glucose tolerance, glucose and insulin homeostasis, and glyburide pharmacokinetics in patients with Type II non-insulin-dependent diabetes mellitus, abstr. 196. *In Program and Abstracts of the 39th Interscience Conference on Antimicrobial Agents and Chemotherapy.* American Society for Microbiology, Washington, D.C.

25. Grasela, T. H., Jr., J. J. Schentag, A. T. Sedman, J. H. Wilton, D. J. Thomas, R. W. Schultz, M. E. Lebsack, and A. W. Kinkel. 1989. Inhibition of enoxacin absorption by antacids or ranitidine. *Antimicrob. Agents Chemother.* 33:615–617.

26. Greenblatt D. J., and L. L. von Moltke. 2000. Sedative-hypnotic and anxiolytic agents, p. 259–270. *In* R. Levy, K. E. Thummel, W. F. Trager, P. D. Hansten, and M. Eichelbaum (ed.), *Metabolic Drug Interactions.* Lippincott, Williams and Wilkins. Philadelphia, Pa.

27. Harder, S., A. H. Staib, C. Beer, A. Papenburg, W. Stille, and P. M. Shah. 1988. 4-Quinolones inhibit biotransformation of caffeine. *Eur. J. Clin. Pharmacol.* 35:651–656.

28. Hass, C. E. 2001. Drug-cytokine interactions, p. 287–310. *In* S. C. Piscatelli and K. A. Rodvold (ed.), *Drug Interactions in Infectious Diseases.* Humana Press, Totowa, N.J.

29. Healy, D. P. M. C. Brodbeck, and C. E. Clendening. 1996. Ciprofloxacin absorption is impaired in patients given enteral feedings orally and via gastrostomy and jejunostomy tubes. *Antimicrob. Agents Chemother.* 40:6–10.

30. Healy, D. P., R. E., Polk, L. Kanawati, D. T. Rock, and M. L. Mooney. 1989. Interaction between oral ciprofloxacin and caffeine in normal volunteers. *Antimicrob. Agents Chemother.* 33:474–478.

31. Healy, D. P., J. R. Schoenle, J. Stotka, and R. E. Polk. 1991. Lack of interaction between lomefloxacin and caffeine in normal volunteers. *Antimicrob. Agent Chemother.* 35:660–734.

32. Herrlin, K., M. Segerdahl, L. L. Gustafsson, and E. Kalso. 2000. Methadone, ciprofloxacin, and adverse drug reactions. *Lancet* 356:2069–2070.

33. Hoey, L. L., and K. D. Lake. 1994. Does ciprofloxacin interact with cyclosporine? *Ann. Pharmacother.* 28:93–96.

34. Hoffken, G., K. Borner, P. D. Glatzel, P. Koeppe, and H. Lode. 1985. Reduced enteral absorption of ciprofloxacin in the presence of antacids. *Eur. J. Clin. Microbiol.* 4:345.

35. Holden, R. Probable fatal interaction between ciprofloxacin and theophylline. 1988. *Br. Med. J.* 297:1339.

36. Israel, D. S., J. L. Stotka, W. Rock, C. D. Sintek, A. K. Kamada, C. Klein, W. R. Swaim, R. E. Pluhar, J. P. Toscano, J. T. Lettieri, A. H. Heller, and R. E. Polk. 1996. Effect of ciprofloxacin on the pharmacokinetics and pharmacodynamics of warfarin. *Clin. Infect. Dis.* 22:251–256.

37. Jaehde, U., F. Sorgel, U. Stephan, and W. Schunack. 1994. Effect of an antacid containing magnesium and aluminum on absorption, metabolism, and mechanism of renal elimination of pefloxacin in humans. *Antimicrob. Agents Chemother.* 38:1129–1133.

38. Janknegt, R. 1990. Drug interactions with quinolones. *J Antimicrob. Chemother.* 26(Suppl. D):7–29.

39. Kamali F., C. H. Ashton, V. R. Marsh, and J. Cox. 1998. Assessment of the effects of combination therapy with ciprofloxacin and fenbufen on the central nervous systems of healthy volunteers by quantitative electroencephalography. *Antimicrob. Agents Chemother.* 42:1256–1258.

40. Kamali, F., S. H. Thomas, and C. Edwards. 1993. The influence of steady-state ciprofloxacin on the pharmacokinetics and dose of diazepam in healthy volunteers. *Eur. J. Clin. Pharmacol.* 44:365–367.

41. Kara, M., B. B. Hasinoff, D. McKay, and N. R. C. Campbell. 1991. Clinical and chemical interactions between iron preparations and ciprofloxacin. *Br. J. Clin. Pharmacol.* 31:257–261.

42. Kawakami, J., T. Matsuse, H. Kotaki, T. Seino, Y. Fukuchi, H. Orimo, Y. Sawada, and T. Iga. 1994. The effect of food on the interaction of ofloxacin with sucralfate in healthy volunteers. *Eur. J. Clin. Pharmacol.* 47:67–69.

43. Kay, M. B., B. R. Overholser, B. A. Mueller, S. M. Moe, and K. M. Sowinski. 2002. Effect of sevelamer hydrochloride and calcium acetate on the relative oral bioavailability of ciprofloxacin, abstr. 174. *Proceedings of the American College of Clinical Pharmacy.* American College of Clinical Pharmacy, Kansas City, Mo.

44. Lacreta, F. P., S. Kaul, G. D. Kollia, G. Duncan, D. M. Randall, and D. M. Grasela DM. 1999. Pharmacokinetics (PK) and safety of gatifloxacin in combination with ferrous sulfate or calcium carbonate in healthy volunteers, abstr. 198. *In Proceedings of the 39th Interscience Conference on Antimicrobial Agents and Chemotherapy.* American Society for Microbiology, Washington, D.C.

45. Lazzaroni, M., B. P. Imbimbo, S. Bargiggia, O. Sangaletti, L. Dal Bo, G. Broccali, and G. B. Porro. 1993. Effects of magnesium-aluminum hydroxide antacid on absorption of rufloxacin. *Antimicrob. Agents Chemother.* 37:2212–2216.

46. LeBel, M., R. Teng, L. C. Dogolo, S. Willavize, H. L. Friedman, and J. Vincent. 1996. The effect of steady-state trovafloxacin on the steady-state pharmacokinetics of caffeine in healthy subjects, abstr A1. *In Proceedings of the 36th Interscience Conference on Antimicrobial Agents and Chemotherapy.* American Society for Microbilogy, Washington, D.C.

47. Lee, L-J., B. Hafkin, I-D. Lee, J. Hoh, and R. Dix. 1997. Effects of food and sucralfate on single oral dose of 500 mg of levofloxacin in healthy subjects. *Antimicrob. Agents Chemother.* 41:2196–2200.

48. Lehto, P., and K. T. Kivisto. 1994. Different effects of products containing metal ions on the absorption of lomefloxacin. *Clin. Pharmacol. Ther.* 56:477–482.

49. Lehto, P., and K. T. Kivisto. 1994. Effect of sucralfate on absorption of norfloxacin and ofloxacin. *Antimicrob. Agents Chemother.* 38:248–251.

50. Lehto, P., K. T. Kivisto, and P. J. Neuvonen. 1994. The effect of ferrous sulphate on the absorption of norfloxacin, ciprofloxcin, and ofloxacin. *Br. J. Clin. Pharmacol.* 37:82–85.

51. Liao, S., M. Palmer, C. Fowler, and R. K. Nayak. 1996. Absence of an effect of levofloxacin on warfarin pharmacokinetics and anticoagulantion in male volunteers. *J. Clin. Pharmacol.* 36:1072–1077.

52. Lober, S., S. Ziege, M. Rau, G. Schreiber, A. Mignot, P. Koeppe, and H. Lode. 1999. Pharmacokinetics of gati-

floxacin and interaction with an antacid containing aluminum and magnesium. *Antimicrob. Agents Chemother.* 43:1067–1071.

53. Mahr, G., F. Sorgel, R. Granneman, M. Kinzig, P. Muth, K. Patterson, U. Fuhr, P. Nickel, and U. Stephan. 1992. Effects of temafloxacin and ciprofloxacin on the pharmacokinetics of caffeine. *Clin. Pharmacokinet.* 22(Suppl. 1):90–97.

54. Martinez Cabarga, M., A. Sanchez Navarro, C. I. Colino Gandarillas, and A. Dominguez-Gil. 1991. Effects of two cations on gastrointestinal absorption of ofloxacin. *Antimicrob. Agents Chemother.* 35:2102–2105.

55. McLellan, R. A., R. K. Drobitch, H. McLellan, P. D. Acott, J. F. Crocker, and K. W. Renton. 1995. Norfloxacin interferes with cyclosporine disposition in pediatric patients undergoing renal transplantation. *Clin. Pharmacol. Ther.* 58:322–327.

56. Millar, E, S. Coles, P. Wyld, and W. Nimmo. 1992. Temafloxacin dose not potentiate the anticoagulant effect of warfarin in healthy subjects. *Clin. Pharmacokinet.* 22(Suppl. 1):102–106.

57. Mimoz, O., V. B. Binter, A. Jacolot, A. Edouard, M. Tod, O. Petitjean, and K. Samii. 1998. Pharmacokinetics and absolute bioavailability of ciprofloxacin administered through a nasogastric tube with continues enteral feeding to critically ill patients. *Intens. Care Med.* 24:1047–1051.

58. Mizuki, Y., I. Fujiwara, and T. Yamaguchi. 1996. Pharmacokinetic interactions related to the chemical structures of fluoroquinolones. *J. Antimicrob. Chemother.* 37(Suppl. A):41–55.

59. Morran, C., C. McArdle, L. Pettit, D. Sleigh, C. Gemmell, M. Hichens, D. Felmingham, and G. Tillotson. 1989. Brief report: pharmacokinetics of orally administered ciprofloxacin in abdominal surgery. *Am. J. Med.* 87(Suppl. 5A):86–88.

60. Reference deleted.

61. Mueller, B. A., D. G. Brieton, S. R. Abel, and L. Bowman. 1994. Effect of enteral feeding with ensure on oral bioavailabilities of ofloxacin and ciprofloxacin. *Antimicrob. Agents Chemother.* 38:2101–2105.

62. Neuvonen P. J., K. T. Kivisto, and P. Lehto. 1991. Interference of dairy products with the absorption of ciprofloxacin. *Clin. Pharmacol. Ther.* 50:498–502.

63. Niki, Y., K. Hashiguchi, N. Miyashita, M. Nakajima, T. Matsushima, and R. Soejima. 1996. Effects of AM-1155 on serum concentration of theophylline, abstr. F73. *In Proceedings of the 36th Interscience Conference on Antimicrobial Agents and Chemotherapy.* American Society for Microbiology, Washington, D.C.

64. Nix, D. E., A. Norman, and J. J. Schentag. 1989. Effect of lomefloxacin on theophylline pharmacokinetics. *Antimicrob. Agents Chemother.* 33:1006–1008.

65. Nix, D. E., W. A. Watson, M. E. Lener, R. W. Frost, G. Krol, H. Goldstein, J. Lettieri, and J. J. Schentag. 1989. Effects of aluminum and magnesium antacids and ranitidine on the absorption of ciprofloxacin. *Clin. Pharmacol. Ther.* 46:700–705.

66. Nix, D. E., J. H. Wilton, B. Ronald, R. W. Frost, G. Krol, H. Goldstein, J. Lettieri, and J. J. Schentag. 1989. Inhibition of norfloxacin absorption by antacids and sucralfate. *Rev. Infect. Dis.* 11(Suppl. 5):S1096.

67. Ofoefule S. I., and M. Okonta. 1999. Adsorption studies of ciprofloxacin: evaluation of magnesium trisilicate, kaolin and starch as alternatives for the management of ciprofloxacin poisoning. *Boll. Chim. Farm.* 138:239–242.

68. Okhamafe, A. O., J. O. Akerele, and C. S. Chukuka. 1991. Pharmacokinetic interactions of norfloxacin with some

metallic medicinal agents. *J. Antimicrob. Chemother.* 28:87–94.

69. Parpia, S. H., D. E. Nix, L. G. Hejmanowsk, H. R. Goldstein, J. H. Wilton, and J. J. Schentag. 1989. Sucralfate reduces the gastrointestinal absorption of norfloxacin. *Antimicrob. Agents Chemother.* 33:99–102.

70. Polk, R. E. 1989. Drug-drug interactions with ciprofloxacin and other fluoroquinolones *Am. J. Med.* 87(Suppl. 5A):76–81.

71. Polk, R. E., D. P. Healy, DP, J. Sahai, L. Drwal, and E. Racht. 1989. Effect of ferrous sulfate and multivitamins with zinc on absorption of ciprofloxacin in normal volunteers. *Antimicrob. Agents Chemother.* 33:1841–1844.

72. Pollak, P. T., and K. L. Slayter. 1997. Comment: ciprofloxacin-phenytoin interaction. *Ann. Pharmacother.* 31:1549–1550.

73. Purkins, L., S. D. Oliver, and S. A. Willavize. 1998. An open, controlled, crossover study on the effects of cimetidine on the steady-state pharmacokinetics of trovafloxacin. *Eur. J. Clin. Microbiol. Infect. Dis.* 17:431–433.

74. Raaska, K., and P. J. Neuvonen. 2000. Ciprofloxacin increases serum clozanine and N-desmethylclozapine: a study in patients with schizophrenia. *Eur. J. Clin. Pharmacol.* 56:585–589.

75. Rambout, L., J. Sahai, K. Gallicano, L. Oliveras, and G. Garber. 1994. Effect of bismuth subsalicylate on ciprofloxacin bioavailability. *Antimicrob. Agents Chemother.* 38:2187–2190.

76. Randinitis, E. J., C. W. Alvey, J. R. Koup, G. Rausch, R. Abel, N. J. Bron, N. J. Hounslow, A. B. Vassos, and A. J. Sedman. 2001. Drug interactions with clinafloxacin. *Antimicrob. Agents Chemother.* 45:2543–2552.

77. Rocci, M. L, Jr, P. H. Vlasses, L. M. Distlerath, M. H. Gregg, S. C. Wheeler, W. Zing, and T. D. Bjornsson. 1990. Norfloxacin does not alter warfarin's disposition or anticoagulant effect. *J. Clin. Pharmacol.* 30:728–732.

78. Roberge, R. J., R. Kaplan, R. Frank, and C. Fore. 2000. Glyburide-ciprofloxacin interaction with resistant hypoglycemia. *Ann. Emerg. Med.* 36:160–3

79. Roboson, R. A., E. J. Begg, H. C. Atkinson, C. A. Saunders, and C. M. Frampton. 1990. Comparative effects of ciprofloxacin and lomefloxacin on the oxidative metabolism of theophylline. *Br. J. Clin. Pharmacol.* 29:491–493.

79a. Roerig. 2000. Trovafloxacin (Trovan) Prescribing Information. Roerig, division of Pfizer, Inc., New York, N.Y.

80. Russo, R., A. Bello, L. Christopher, Z. Ge, and D. Gajjar. 2001. Lack of a pharmacokinetic interaction between intravenous morphine sulfate and oral BMS-284756 in healthy subjects, abstr. A-47. *In Program and Abstracts of the 41st Interscience Conference on Antimicrobial Agents and Chemotherapy.* American Society for Microbiology, Washington, D.C.

81. Sano, M., I. Yamamoto, J. Ueda, E. Yoshikawa, H. Yamashina, and M. Goto. 1987. Comparative pharmacokinetics of theophylline following two fluoroquinolones coadministration. *Eur. J. Clin. Pharmacol.* 32:431–432.

82. Sahai, J., K. Gallicano, L. Oliveros, S. Khaliq, N. Hawley-Foss, and G. Garber. 1993. Cations in the didanosie tablet reduce ciprofloxacin bioavailability. *Clin. Pharmacol. Ther.* 53:292–297.

83. Sahai, J., D. Healy, J. Stotka, and R. Polk. 1993. The influence of chronic administration of calcium carbonate on the bioavailability of oral ciprofloxacin. *Br. J. Clin. Pharmacol.* 35:302–304.

84. Schwartz, J., L. Jauregui, J. Lettieri, and K. Bachmann. 1988. Impact of ciprofloxacin on theophylline clearance and

steady-state concentrations in serum. *Antimicrob. Agents Chemother.* **32:**75–77.

85. Shiba, K., O. Sakai, J. Shimada, O. Okazaki, H. Aoki, and H. Hakusui. 1992. Effect of antacids, ferrous sulfate, and ranitidine on absorption of DR-3355 in humans. *Antimicrob. Agents Chemother.* **36:**2270–2274.

86. Shimada, J., K. Shiba, T. Oguma, H. Miwa, Y. Yoshimura, T. Nishikawa, Y. Okabayashi, T. Kitagawa, and S. Yamamoto. 1992. Effect of antacid on absorption of the quinolone lomefloxacin. *Antimicrob. Agents Chemother.* **36:**1219–1224.

87. Sorgel, F., G. R. Granneman, U. Stephan, and C, Locke. 1992. Effect of cimetidine on the pharmacokinetics of temafloxacin. *Clin. Pharmacokinet.* **22**(Suppl. 1):75–82.

88. Sorgel, F., G. Mahr, G. R. Granneman, and U. Stephan. 1992. Effects of two quinolone antibacterials, temafloxacin and enoxacin, on thephylline pharmacokinetics. *Clin Pharmacokinet.* **22**(Suppl. 1):65–74.

89. Staib, A. H., S. Harder, S. Mieke, C. Beer, W. Stille W, and P. Shah. 1987. Gyrase-inhibitors impair caffeine metabolism in man. *Methods Find. Exp. Clin. Pharmacol.* **9:**193–198.

90. Stass, H, and D. Kubitza. 2001. Effects of iron supplements on the oral bioavailability of moxifloxacin, a novel 8-methoxyfluoroquinolone, in humans. *Clin. Pharmacokinet.* **40**(Suppl. 1):57–62.

91. Stass, H., C. Wandel, H. Delesen, and J. G. Moller. 2001. Effect of calcium supplements on the oral bioavailability of moxifloxacin in healthy male volunteers. *Clin. Pharmacokinet.* **40**(Suppl. 1):27–32.

92. Stass, H., M. F. Bottcher, and K. Ochmann. 2001. Evaluation of the influence of antacids and H2 antagonists on the absorption of moxifloxacin after oral administration of a 400mg dose to healthy volunteers. *Clin. Pharmacokinet.* **40**(Suppl. 1):39–48.

93. Stass, H., and D. Kubitza. 2001. Lack of pharmacokinetic interaction between moxifloxacin, a novel 8-methoxyfluoroquinolone, and theophylline. *Clin. Pharmacokinet.* **40**(Suppl. 1):63–70.

94. Stass, H., U. Schuhly, J. G. Moller, and H. Delesen. 2001. Effects of sucralfate on the oral bioavailability of moxifloxacin, a novel 8-methoxyfluoroquinolone, in healthy volunteers. *Clin. Pharmacokinet.* **40**(Suppl. 1):49–55.

95. Stille, W., S. Harder, S. Mieke, C. Beer, P. M. Shah, K. Frech, and A. H. Staib. 1987. Decrease of caffeine elimination in man during co-administration of 4-quinolones. *J. Antimicrob. Chemother.* **20:**729–734.

96. Takagi, K., K. Yamaki, M. Nadai, T. Kuzuya, and T. Hasegawa. 1991. Effect of new quinolone, sparafloxacin, on the pharmacokinetics of theophylline in asthmatic patients. *Antimicrob. Agents Chemother.* **35:**1137–1141.

97. Teixeira, M. H., F. Teixeira, M. L. Leitao, and J. S. Redinha. 2000. A thermodynamic study of complexation of ciprofloxacin and lomefloxacin with aluminum ion. *J. Chemother.* **12:**499–502.

98. Temple M. E., M. C. Nahata. 1999. Interaction between ciprofloxacin and rifampin. *Ann. Pharmacother.* **33:**868–870.

99. Teng, R., L. C. Dogolo, S. A. Willavize, H. L. Friedman, and J. Vincent. 1997. Effect of Maalox and omeprazole on the bioavailability of trovafloxacin. *J. Antimicrob. Chemother.* **39**(Suppl. B):93–97.

100. Trager W. 2000. oral Anticoagulants, p. 403–413. *In* R., Levy, K. E. Thummel, W. F. Trager, P. D. Hansten, and M. Eichelbaum (ed.) *Metabolic Drug Interactions.* Lippincott, Williams and Wilkins, Philadelphia, Pa.

101. Reference deleted.

102. Toon, S., K. J. Hopkins, F. M. Garstang, L. Aarons, A. Sedman, and M. Rowland. 1987. Enoxacin-warfarin interaction: pharmacokinetic and stereochemical aspects. *Clin. Pharmacol. Ther.* **42:**33–41.

103. Van Slooten, A. D., D. E. Nix, H. L. Wilton, J. H. Love, J. M. Spivey, and H. R. Goldstein. 1991. Combined use of ciprofloxacin and sucralfate. *DICP Ann. Pharmacother.* **25:**578–582.

104. Vincent, J., T. Hunt, R. Teng, L. Robarge, S. A. Willavize, and H. L. Friedman. 1998. The pharmacokinetic effects of coadministration of morphine and trovafloxacin in healthy subjects. *J. Surg.* **176**(Suppl. 6A):32–38.

105. Vincent, J., R. Teng, L. C. Dogolo, S. A. Willavize, and H. L. Friedman. 1997. Effect of trovafloxacin, a new fluoroquinolone antibiotic, on the steady-state pharmacokinetics of theophyllline in healthy volunteers. *J. Antimicrob. Chemother.* **39**(Suppl. B):81–86.

106. Wijnands, W. J., J. F. Trooster, P. C. Teunissen, H. A. Cats, and T. B. Vree. 1990. Ciprofloxacin does not impair the elimination of diazepam in humans. *Drug Metab. Dispos.* **18:**954–957.

107. Wijnands, W. J. C. L. A. van Herwaarden, and T. B. Vree. 1984. Enoxacin raises plasma theophylline concentrations. *Lancet* **2:**108–109.

108. Wijnands, W. J., T. B. Vree, and C. L. A. van Herwaarden. 1986. The influence of quinolone derivatives on theophylline clearance. *Br. J. Clin. Pharmacol.* **22:**677–683.

109. Wright, D. H., S. L. Pietz, F. N. Konstantinides, and J. C. Rotschafer. 2000. Decreased in vitro fluoroquinolone concentration after admixture with an enteral feeding formulation. *J. Parenter. Enteral Nutr.* **24:**42–48.

110. Yuk, J. H., C. H. Nightingale, R. Quintiliani, N. S. Yeston, R. Orlando 3rd, E. D. Dobkin, J. C. Kambe, K. R. Sweeney, and E. A. Buonpane. 1990. Absorption of ciprofloxacin administered through a nasogastric or a nasoduodenal tube in volunteers and patients receiving enteral nutrition. *Diagn. Microbiol. Infect. Dis.* **13:**99–102.

111. Yuk, J. H., C. H. Nightingale, K. R., Sweeney, R. Quintiliani, J. T. Lettieri, and R. W. Frost. 1989. Relative bioavailability in healthy volunteers of ciprofloxacin administered through a nasogastric tube with and without enteral feeding. *Antimicrob. Agents Chemother.* **33:**1118–1120.

112. Zix, J. A., H. F. Geerdes-Fenge, M. Rau, J. Vockler, K. Borner, P. Koeppe, and H. Lode. 1997. Pharmacokinetics of sparafloxacin and interaction with cisapride and sucralfate. *Antimicrob. Agents Chemother.* **41:**1668–1672.

Quinolone Antimicrobial Agents, 3rd ed.
Edited by David C. Hooper and Ethan Rubinstein
© 2003 ASM Press, Washington, D.C.

Chapter 8

Pharmacodynamics of Quinolone Antimicrobial Agents

WILLIAM A. CRAIG AND DAVID R. ANDES

Pharmacodynamics describes the relationship between measures of drug levels in serum and tissue fluids and the antimicrobial and toxicologic effects of drugs (5, 10, 17, 49). While there have been numerous studies describing the pharmacokinetics of fluoroquinolones in serum and tissues, there has been much less emphasis on describing the time course of antimicrobial activity with these drugs. The MIC and minimal bactericidal concentration have been the major measures of the antimicrobial effect of the quinolones. Although these parameters are useful in defining the potency of the drug against a particular pathogen, they do not provide any information on the time course of antimicrobial activity. Other measures, such as the rate of bacterial killing with increasing concentrations of drug and persistent effects that last after antimicrobial exposure, provide a much better description of the time course of antimicrobial activity. This chapter focuses on the pharmacodynamic characteristics of the quinolone antimicrobials in in vitro models, in animal infection models, and in humans. We hope to demonstrate that there are many more similarities in results among the various models than there are differences.

TIME COURSE OF ANTIMICROBIAL ACTIVITY

Bacterial Killing

Numerous in vitro and in vivo studies have demonstrated that the quinolone antimicrobial agents exhibit concentration-dependent killing across a wide range of concentrations (2, 5, 8, 13, 18, 28, 31, 47). Thus, increases in the dose and concentration of the drug will result in faster and more extensive killing of bacterial organisms. Killing of some organisms such as *Streptococcus pneumoniae*

is exceedingly rapid, and some investigators have suggested that the quinolones do not produce concentration-dependent killing with these organisms. However, in vivo studies, where the growth and killing are somewhat slower, have still demonstrated concentration-dependent killing for the quinolones with *S. pneumoniae* (2, 4, 7, 13).

A variety of different parameters have been used to characterize the killing characteristics of the quinolone antimicrobials. Three major types of analysis have been used (20, 33). Some measures reflect the time to a certain magnitude of organism reduction (e.g., 2 log kill and 3 log kill), while others measure the magnitude of log reduction at specific times (e.g., 12 or 24 h). Others depend on changes in bacterial numbers over time and are referred to as integrated measures. These would include the slope of the kill curve, area above or under the kill curves, and the "intensity of effect." With all of these measurements, increasing concentrations of the fluoroquinolones have resulted in a greater antimicrobial effect.

Persistent Effects

There are a variety of in vitro and in vivo persistent effects that have been characterized for the quinolone antimicrobial agents (11, 37, 38, 39, 48). The in vitro postantibiotic effect determines the delay in organism regrowth after short periods of drug exposure. Multiple studies with the fluoroquinolones with both gram-positive cocci and gram-negative bacilli have demonstrated in vitro postantibiotic effects (PAEs) of short to moderate duration (1 to 3 h) (11, 39). Much longer PAEs have been observed for fluoroquinolones with some slowly growing organisms such as mycoplasmas and *Legionella pneumophila* (11).

Further exposure of organisms during the PAE phase to sub-MIC concentrations can greatly

William A. Craig and David R. Andes • University of Wisconsin, Department of Medicine, Infectious Diseases and Clinical Pharmacology Sections and the William S. Middleton Memorial Veterans Hospital, Madison, WI 53792.

enhance the duration of the PAE (37, 38). For example, several gram-positive cocci and gram-negative bacilli in the PAE phase following exposure to trovafloxacin and grepafloxacin for 2 h at 10 times the MIC were placed in drug-free broth or exposed to drug concentrations at 3/10 of the MIC. The in vitro MIC was increased 2- to 19-fold by the sub-MIC concentrations.

In vivo PAE studies combine the effects of supra-MIC and sub-MIC concentrations (2, 4, 7). Studies in the neutropenic murine thigh infection model with various fluoroquinolones have exhibited in vivo PAEs of 1.5 to 5 h with both gram-positive cocci and gram-negative bacilli. The in vivo PAE can be significantly enhanced by the presence of neutrophils. Studies with ciprofloxacin and a strain of *Klebsiella pneumoniae* showed that an in vivo PAE of 2.4 h in neutropenic mice was increased to 7.5 h in normal mice (11). Recent studies with several fluoroquinolones have demonstrated that the duration of the in vivo PAE with a strain of *S. pneumoniae* is even more enhanced by the presence of neutrophils (more than 10-fold) than observed with *K. pneumoniae* (27).

PK/PD PARAMETERS

By using the MIC as a measure of potency, specific pharmacokinetic/pharmacodynamic (PK/PD) parameters have been identified to correlate measures of drug exposure with antimicrobial activity (10). The duration that concentrations exceed the MIC and peak and area under the curve (AUC) to MIC ratios have been the primary PK/PD parameters evaluated. However, identifying the major PK/PD parameter correlating with efficacy is complicated by the high degree of interdependence among these parameters. Comparing the effects of dosing regimens using different dosing intervals or half-lives of the drug have been able to reduce much of the interdependence among PK/PD parameters.

In Vitro Models

Studies using a combination of dose escalation, dosage regimen fractionation, and strains with different MICs have suggested that the AUC/MIC ratio is the major PK/PD parameter determining efficacy of fluoroquinolones against *Pseudomonas aeruginosa* and *S. pneumoniae* (28, 35). However, there are some differences, depending on which measure of antibacterial activity is used in the in vitro model. With fluoroquinolones initial killing as measured by the time-to-a-3-log kill was best related to the peak/MIC ratio, whereas regrowth and the intensity

of effect were related more to the time above MIC (8, 20). When areas under and above the killing curve were used, the AUC/MIC ratio was the best parameter. Peak/MIC ratio has also been more important in dose-fractionation studies for organisms for which resistant subpopulations can readily emerge (8).

Animal Models

Dose-fractionation studies at several different total doses have been used to identify the primary PK/PD parameter determining in vivo activity (3). Studies in the neutropenic murine thigh infection and pneumonia models have consistently demonstrated that the 24-h AUC/MIC ratio best correlates with in vivo activity (2, 5, 10, 29, 30). The peak/MIC ratio also tends to show a reasonable correlation, while time of MIC does not. This is illustrated in Fig. 1 for temafloxacin against *S. pneumoniae* ATCC 10813.

Drusano et al. used survival as an indicator of efficacy in rats infected with *P. aeruginosa* (18). The efficacy of lomefloxacin was related to the peak level when the peak/MIC ratio was greater than 10 and related to the AUC when the peak/MIC ratio was less than 10. This is similar to that reported in in vitro models that use strains from which resistant subpopulations can emerge. Thus, high peak concentrations appear to be important in preventing the emergence of resistant subpopulations of bacteria.

Human Studies

Although pharmacodynamic studies have been performed in humans, none of these studies have used dose fractionation to reduce the interdependence among the various parameters. For example, in the study with levofloxacin by Preston et al., all three PK/PD parameters were highly correlated with outcome, with *P* values from <0.001 to 0.006 (41).

MAGNITUDE OF PK/PD PARAMETER REQUIRED FOR EFFICACY

In Vitro Studies

The magnitude of the AUC/MIC ratio required in in vitro models depends markedly on which measure of antibacterial activity is used. AUC/MIC ratios greater than 40 generally result in 3 to 4 log reductions, while values greater than 250 are required for the lowest areas under the kill curve (20, 28, 34, 50, 51). However, it is not yet known which in vitro measure of antibacterial activity best correlates with drug efficacy in animals or humans.

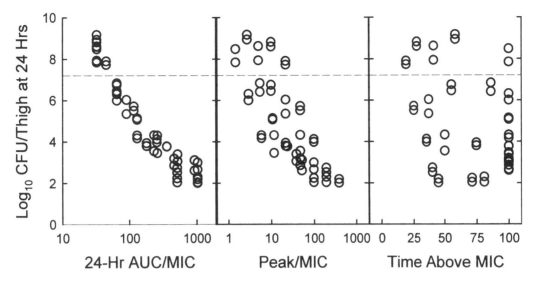

Figure 1. Relationship among PK/PD parameters for temafloxacin and $\log_{10}$ CFU per thigh of *S. pneumoniae* after 24 h of therapy in a murine thigh infection model. Reprinted from reference 5 with permission from Elsevier.

Animal Studies

Many of the animal infection models that use bacterial numbers as an indicator of efficacy have also not fully established a relationship between the reduction in organisms after short-treatment times with survival after more prolonged durations of therapy. Studies in our own laboratory using the neutropenic murine thigh infection and pneumonia models have demonstrated that the static dose (i.e., the dose producing no net change in bacterial numbers) after 24 h of therapy is very similar to the dose protecting 50% of the animals from death (i.e., PD_{50}) following 4 to 5 days of therapy (5, 14). However, the degree of bacterial reduction at 24 h required to produce 90 to 100% survival has not yet been established and appears to vary depending on the type of organism. Still the static dose after 24 h of therapy has been useful to identify differences in the magnitude of the PK/PD parameter for various quinolones, dosing intervals, organisms, and sites of infection.

Fantin et al. used the neutropenic murine infection model to demonstrate with pefloxacin a linear relationship between the static dose and the drug's MIC (19). Because the slope of this relationship was approximately 1, the 24-h AUC/MIC ratio for the static dose is a parameter that allows one to compare the activity of different quinolones against various bacterial pathogens. The 24-h AUC/MIC values for most organisms have varied from 10 to 70 (5, 7, 10). Initial analysis suggested that the mean values were approximately 25 for gram-negative bacilli and 50

for gram-positive cocci. However, more recent studies with the newer fluoroquinolones and desfluoroquinolones have exhibited relatively similar values for *Enterobacteriaceae*, *Staphylococcus aureus*, and *S. pneumoniae*.

The impact of drug resistance on the magnitude of the 24-h AUC/MIC ratio has been assessed primarily in *S. pneumoniae*. Studies with several of the newer fluoroquinolones have demonstrated that the static dose generally rises to the same degree as the MIC in ciprofloxacin-resistant strains (2, 4). Thus, the 24-h AUC/MIC does not change for these more resistant organisms. However, studies with gemifloxacin against three strains with higher MICs due to efflux did not show much of an increase in the static dose (4). These initial data suggest that the efflux mechanism of resistance in pneumococci may not be as active in vivo as it is in broth. Similar differences between in vivo and in vitro resistance have been observed in strains of *P. aeruginosa* expressing the MexEF pump (25).

Differences in the 24-h AUC/MIC values for the static doses among the various fluoroquinolones have been small unless there is significant protein binding. As shown in Fig. 2, the magnitude of the 24-h AUC for the static doses of the lowly bound sitafloxacin and gatifloxacin against six strains of *S. pneumoniae* were significantly lower than those for the highly bound gemifloxacin (2, 4, 7). However, similar values were observed when free drug levels of gemifloxacin were used to calculate the 24-h AUC/MIC ratios for the static doses. Similar differences have been observed between garenoxacin with

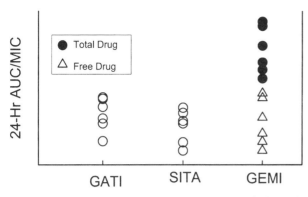

Figure 2. Relationship between the magnitude of the 24-h AUC/MIC for the static doses of the lowly protein-bound sitafloxacin and gatifloxacin and the highly protein-bound gemifloxacin against six strains of *S. pneumoniae* in a murine infection model.

about 80% binding in mice and another desfluoroquinolone (PGE-9509924) with low protein binding (6, 15). These studies strongly suggest that free drug concentrations should be used for calculating the magnitude of PK/PD parameters.

Since the AUC is the primary determinant of in vivo activity, one would not expect that the dosing regimen would be an important determinant of the antibacterial activity of quinolones. The static dose for 24-h dosing regimens tends to be higher that those observed at 1- to 12-h dosing intervals (2, 4, 7). Because of the rapid half-life of these drugs in small animals, the duration of persistent effects is rarely long enough to span the time that serum drug concentrations are below the MIC when these drugs are administered once daily. Similar effects have been observed with fluoroquinolones and desfluoroquinolones in animal models of meningitis (32, 42). Thus, dosing regimens of 12 h or less are necessary to accurately establish the magnitude of the 24-h AUC/MIC ratio in small animals.

We have also used the murine thigh infection and pneumonia models to compare the magnitude of the 24-h AUC/MIC for the static doses at different sites of infection and in the presence and absence of neutrophils (2, 4, 7). Very similar values have been observed in the thigh and lung models for multiple fluoroquinolones against a strain of *K. pneumoniae* that grows well in both tissues (2, 4, 7). The presence of neutrophils (i.e., values in normal mice compared with neutropenic mice) reduces the static dose about 25 to 50% when mice are infected with *K. pneumoniae*. However, marked reductions in the static dose (80 to 90%) are observed by the presence of neutrophils in mice infected with *S. pneumoniae*. These differences are largely due to differences in the enhancement of the in vivo PAE by the presence of

neutrophils, as discussed previously (27). The presence of neutrophils also slightly increases the extent of killing of the pneumococcus but not of *K. pneumoniae*.

Many other animal studies of fluoroquinolones have used survival rather than bacterial numbers as a measure of outcome. For those studies that also give the pharmacokinetics of the drug, one can calculate the 24-h AUC/MIC ratio for each dose studied. Fig. 3 examines the relationship between the 24-h AUC/MIC ratio and mortality in various experimental infections (5, 13). The great majority of these studies were in neutropenic or other immunocompromised animals. Many of the studies that use survival as an outcome follow mortality for prolonged periods of time after the end of therapy. This practice may allow organisms that have not been eradicated to regrow and produce mortality.

Mortality at 7 to 12 days after the end of therapy has proven to correlate poorly with the 24-h AUC/MIC values for the quinolone antimicrobial agents (5). Thus, only those studies that treated animals for at least 2 days, reported survival results within 24 h of the end of therapy, and observed at least 80% mortality by the end of therapy in untreated or saline-treated controls were used. This analysis included studies of pneumonia, peritonitis, sepsis, and soft tissue infections in mice, rats, and guinea pigs due to various organisms but primarily gramnegative bacilli. An excellent correlation between the 24-h AUC/MIC ratio and mortality was observed. In general, AUC/MIC ratios less than 30 were associated with greater than 50% mortality, whereas values of 100 or greater were associated with 90 to 100% survival.

Animal studies of endocarditis due to gram-negative bacilli or staphylococci have also been analyzed to determine the relationship between the 24-h

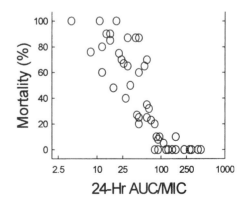

Figure 3. Relationship between mortality at the end of therapy and the 24-h AUC/MIC of fluoroquinolones with multiple pathogens in different animal models. Reprinted from reference 5 with permission from Elsevier.

AUC/MIC ratio and bacterial numbers in the vegetations (3). Dosing regimens with 24-h AUC/MIC ratios of 100 or greater produced bacterial numbers in vegetations after 3 to 6 days of therapy that were at least 2 logs lower than regimens with AUC/MIC ratios less than 100. Thus, the pharmacodynamic parameters predictive of efficacy of fluoroquinolones in the treatment of experimental endocarditis are similar to those for other infectious models.

Studies correlating mortality with the 24-h AUC/MIC ratios are also available for strains of *S. pneumoniae* in nonneutropenic animals (5, 12). Fig. 4 demonstrates the relationship between the 24-h AUC/MIC ratio and mortality for these infections. In some of these studies, specific genetic species of mice (e.g., CBA-J) were required to produce disease in the absence of neutropenia. In these studies the curve was shifted to the left and 90 to 100% survival could be observed as soon as the 24-h AUC/MIC value reached 25 to 35.

An earlier analysis, as shown in Fig. 5, examined the relationship between mortality and the 24-h AUC/MIC for intracellular and extracellular pathogens (13). The data for the extracellular pathogens are the same as many of the values shown in Fig. 3. The values for the intracellular pathogens were obtained from experimental studies in mice or guinea pigs infected with *Chlamydia psittaci*, *L. pneumophila*, *Mycobacterium tuberculosis*, and *Salmonella enterica* serovar Typhimurium. Although the intracellular concentrations of fluoroquinolones are higher than those in serum, this did not result in any difference in the relationship between the 24-h AUC/MIC and mortality for intracellular versus extracellular pathogens. Thus, concentrations of the quinolones in serum may also be good predictors of their in vivo activity against intracellular pathogens.

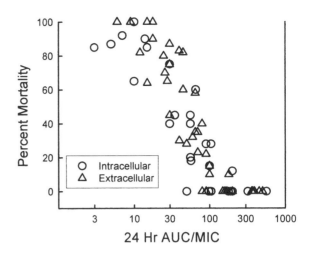

Figure 5. Relationship between the 24-h AUC/MIC ratio and mortality for extracellular (open triangles) and intracellular (open circles) pathogens in various experimental infection models in mice, rats, and guinea pigs. Reprinted from reference 13 with permission of Springer-Verlag.

Human Studies

The first study correlating PK/PD parameters of the fluoroquinolones with clinical response in humans was published by Peloquin et al. (40). In this study, which evaluated intravenous ciprofloxacin in seriously ill patients with lower respiratory tract infections, time above MIC was reported to be the important parameter for eradication of the organism from respiratory secretions. However, patients infected with *P. aeruginosa* failed because of the emergence of resistance. These patients not only had a low time above MIC, they also had low peak/MIC and low AUC/MIC ratios. The results of a subsequent analysis of the data with additional patients by Forrest et al. demonstrated that the 24-h AUC/MIC value was the best predictor of the clinical and microbiologic efficacy of ciprofloxacin (24). As shown in Fig. 6, a 24-h AUC/MIC value of 125 or higher was associated with much higher rates of clinical and bacteriologic cure than values less than 125. These investigators also demonstrated that 24-h AUC/MIC values of 250 or higher resulted in faster eradication (mean, 1.9 days) of the organisms from respiratory secretions than patients that had values of 125 to 250 (mean, 7 days) (36). This is what one would expect for drugs that exhibit concentration-dependent killing.

Preston et al. correlated PK/PD parameters for levofloxacin with both clinical and microbiologic efficacy in patients with urinary tract, pulmonary, skin, and soft tissue infections (41). Although significant covariations existed among the PK/PD parameters, these investigators demonstrated that patients

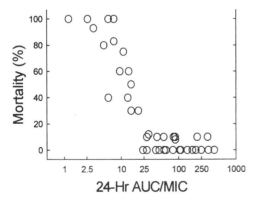

Figure 4. Relationship between mortality at the end of therapy and the 24-h AUC/MIC of fluoroquinolones against *S. pneumoniae* in nonneutropenic mice. Reprinted from reference 5 with permission from Elsevier.

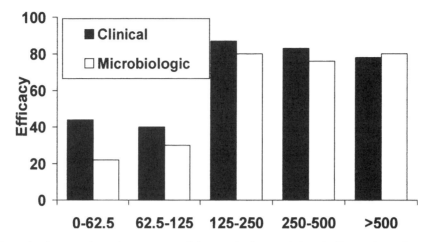

Figure 6. Relationship between the 24-h AUC/MIC and the microbiologic and clinical efficacy of ciprofloxacin in 64 patients with serious bacterial infections. Reprinted from reference 10 with permission of The University of Chicago Press.

who had a peak/MIC ratio of 12.2 or higher eradicated the infecting pathogen 100% of the time compared with 80.8% for those with peak/MIC ratios less than 12.2. The breakpoint for bacterial eradication using the peak/MIC ratio was similar to a 24-h AUC/MIC value of 100. Thus, the 24-h AUC/MIC ratios associated with microbiologic eradication in humans and high survival in animal infection models are very similar at values of 100 to 125.

One-third of the 21 patients infected with *S. pneumoniae* and treated with levofloxacin had 24-h AUC/MIC values from 30 to 100, and none of these patients failed therapy. This suggests that the 24-h AUC/MIC value for bacterial eradication of *S. pneumoniae* is lower than that for gram-negative bacilli. More recently, Ambrose and Grasela reported the relationship between the free drug 24-h AUC/MIC ratio and the eradication of *S. pneumoniae* from the blood or respiratory secretions of patients with community-acquired pneumonia and acute exacerbations of chronic bronchitis following treatment with levofloxacin or gatifloxacin (1). As shown in Fig. 7, bacterial eradication was less than 100% when the AUC/MIC ratio fell to the 30 to 40 range. More specifically, the rate of eradication was 100% when the AUC/MIC ratio was greater than 33.7 and only 64% when the ratio was less than 33.7. This breakpoint value is very similar to the 25 to 35 values observed for high survival in the animal models infected with *S. pneumoniae*.

There are also a few cases of clinical and bacteriologic failure with levofloxacin in patients infected with strains of *S. pneumoniae* that have MICs of 8 mg/liter (22, 23). The estimated 24-h AUC/MIC ratios in these patients would be less than 10. Failures in patients with pneumococcal pneumonia have also been reported for ciprofloxacin where the

24-h AUC/MIC ratio has been estimated to be about 10 to 20. These studies also support a 24-h AUC/MIC breakpoint of 25 to 35 for clinical and bacteriologic success with quinolones in patients infected with pneumococci.

PK/PD PARAMETERS AND THE EMERGENCE OF RESISTANCE

A variety of in vitro and in vivo studies have examined the relationship between PK/PD parameters and the eradication or emergence of resistant organisms. Several animal and in vitro studies have suggested that peak concentrations of fluoroquinolones that are 8 to 10 times higher than the MIC of the starting inoculum can significantly

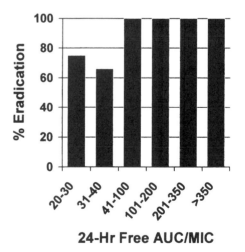

Figure 7. Relationship between fluoroquinolone free drug 24-h AUC/MIC and microbiologic eradication of *S. pneumoniae* in community-acquired respiratory tract infections. Adapted from reference 1.

reduce the emergence of resistant subpopulations (18, 26). More recent studies with in vitro models have determined the 24-h AUC/MIC ratios associated with enhancing and reducing the emergence of resistance (21, 33, 34, 44, 45). With *P. aeruginosa*, *K. pneumoniae*, and *S. aureus* the 24-h AUC/MIC values often range from 90 to 200 for preventing the selection of resistant organisms. On the other hand, the emergence of resistance in *S. pneumoniae* has been difficult to select in in vitro models.

Thomas et al. studied the emergence of resistance in patients treated with ciprofloxacin as combination or monotherapy (46). As shown in Table 1, 86% of patients receiving ciprofloxacin monotherapy that had 24-h AUC/MIC ratios less than 100 developed resistance. This was 100% for strains of *P. aeruginosa* and 50% for other gram-negative bacilli. Ciprofloxacin monotherapy resulting in 24-h AUC/MIC ratios of 100 or higher developed resistance in only 10% of the patients. The value was 25% for *P. aeruginosa* and only 7% for other gram-negative bacilli. All the patients receiving combination therapy had 24-h AUC/MIC ratios greater than 100, and none of these patients developed resistance. Although the peak/MIC ratio was not evaluated in this report, the earlier publication by Peloquin et al. showed that a peak/MIC ratio of 8 or higher was similarly predictive as a 24-h AUC/MIC greater than 100 in reducing the selection of resistant organisms during therapy (40). It should also be pointed out that the 24-h AUC/MIC value of 100 is also incorrectly applied to infections caused by gram-positive organisms. The study by Thomas et al. had only a few of these organisms treated with ciprofloxacin, and none of the patients developed resistance.

The mutation prevention concentration (MPC) is another measurement that has been receiving increasing interest among many investigators (9, 16, 33, 43). It is defined as the lowest drug concentration in agar that prevents the growth of any colonies from very large inocula of susceptible organisms. Several studies have demonstrated that the MPC can vary for different organisms and for different fluoroquinolones. For *S. pneumoniae*, the MPC values have varied from four to eight times the MIC. The difference between the MIC and MPC has been called the selection window for resistance. Some investigators have suggested that concentrations of quinolones in serum should exceed the MPC for the entire dosing interval (9). A recent study with levofloxacin, gatifloxacin, and moxifloxacin in an in vitro model using *S. aureus* was designed to produce peak concentrations that were equal to the MIC, between the MIC and MPC, and above the MPC (21). Resistant subpopulations were primarily selected when peak concentrations were within the selection window. Much more data including animal and human studies are needed on the significance of the MPC and the relationship of PK/PD parameters to the emergence of resistance.

APPLICATIONS OF QUINOLONE PHARMACODYNAMICS

Knowledge of the major PK/PD parameter determining efficacy and the magnitude of that target required for efficacy of specific pathogens has proven to be helpful for developing new quinolone agents, predicting the activity of new quinolone formulations, developing guideline recommendations, and establishing susceptibility and resistance breakpoints for susceptibility testing. Because the magnitudes of the PK/PD parameters appear to be relatively similar in animals and humans, animal studies can be useful for predicting clinical activity especially in situations where it is difficult to obtain sufficient clinical data (e.g., new emerging resistance). Initial studies suggest that pharmacodynamics can also be important in preventing the emergence of resistance. More in vitro, animal and human studies are necessary to fully document the usefulness of pharmacodynamic evaluation in optimizing therapy with the quinolone antimicrobial agents.

Table 1. Relationship of the 24-h AUC/MIC ratio and monotherapy and combination therapy to the emergence of resistant organisms during therapy with ciprofloxacin

Therapy	24-h AUC/MIC	No. of patients with resistant organisms/total no. of patients (%)[a]		
		All patients	*Pseudomonas*	Other GNB
Monotherapy	<100	12/14 (86)	10/10 (100)	2/4 (50)
Monotherapy	≥100	4/40 (10)	2/8 (25)	2/28 (7)
Combination	≥100	0/16 (0)	0/7 (0)	0/8 (0)

[a] GNB, gram-negative bacilli.

REFERENCES

1. Ambrose, P. G., D. M. Grasela, T. H. Grasela, J. Passarell, H. B. Mayer, and P. F. Pierce. 2001. Pharmacodynamics of fluoroquinolones against *Streptococcus pneumoniae* in patients with community-acquired respiratory tract infections. *Antimicrob. Agents Chemother.* 45:2793–2797.

2. Andes D., and W. A. Craig. 2002. Pharmacodynamics of the new fluoroquinolone gatifloxacin in murine thigh and lung infection models. *Antimicrob. Agents Chemother.* 46:1665–1670.

3. Andes, D. R., and W. A. Craig. 1998. Pharmacodynamics of fluoroquinolones in experimental models of endocarditis. *Clin. Infect. Dis.* 27:47–50.

4. Andes, D. R., and W. A. Craig. 1999. Pharmacodynamics of gemifloxacin against quinolone-resistant strains of *S. pneumoniae* with known resistance mechanisms, abstr. 27. *In Abstracts of the 39th Interscience Conference on Antimicrobial Agents and Chemotherapy.* American Society for Microbiology, Washington, D.C.

5. Andes, D., and W. A. Craig. 2002. Animal model pharmacokinetics and pharmacodynamics: a critical review. *Int. J. Antimicrob. Agents* 19:261–268.

6. Andes, D. 2001. Pharmacokinetics and pharmacodynamics of the non-fluorinated quinolones. *In Abstracts from the 7th International Symposium on New Quinolones*, Edinburgh, Scotland.

7. Andes, D. R., and W. A. Craig. 1999. In vivo pharmacodynamic activity of sitafloxacin against multiple bacterial pathogens, abstr. 28. *In Abstracts of the 39th Interscience Conference on Antimicrobial Agents and Chemotherapy.* American Society for Microbiology, Washington, D.C.

8. Blaser J., B. B. Stone, M. C. Groner, and S. H. Zinner. 1987. Comparative study with enoxacin and netilmicin in a pharmacodynamic model to determine importance of ratio of antibiotic peak concentration to MIC for bactericidal activity and emergence of resistance. *Antimicrob. Agents Chemother.* 31:1054–1060.

9. Blondeau, J. M., X. Zhao, G. Hansen, and K. Drlica. 2001. Mutant prevention concentrations of fluoroquinolones for clinical isolates of *Streptococcus pneumoniae*. *Antimicrob. Agents Chemother.* 45:433–438.

10. Craig, W. A. 1998. Pharmacokinetic/pharmacodynamic parameters: rationale for antibacterial dosing of mice and men. *Clin. Infect. Dis.* 26:1–12.

11. Craig, W. A., and S. Gudmundsson. 1996. Postantibiotic effect, p. 296–329. *In* V. Lorian (ed.), *Antibiotics in Laboratory Medicine*, 4th ed. The Williams and Wilkins Co., Baltimore, Md.

12. Craig, W. A. 2001. Does the dose matter? *Clin. Infect. Dis.* 33(Suppl. 3):233–237.

13. Craig, W. A., and A. Dalhoff. 1998. Pharmacodynamics of fluoroquinolones in experimental animal models, p. 207–232. *In* J. Kulman, A. Dalhoff, and H. J. Zeiler (eds.), *Quinolone Antibacterials.* Springer-Verlag, Heidelberg, Germany.

14. Craig, W. A., and D. R. Andes. 2000. Correlation of the magnitude of the AUC/MIC for 6 fluoroquinolones against *Streptococcus pneumoniae* with survival and bactericidal activity in an animal model, abstr. 289. *In Abstracts of the 40th Interscience Conference on Antimicrobial Agents and Chemotherapy.* American Society for Microbiology, Washington, D.C.

15. Craig, W. A., and D. R. Andes. 2001. In vivo pharmacodynamics of PGE-9509924, a new non-fluorinated quinolone, abstr. F-561. *In Abstracts of the 41st Interscience Conference on Antimicrobial Agents and Chemotherapy.* American Society for Microbiology, Washington, D.C.

16. Dong, Y., X. Zhao, J. Domagala, and K. Drlica. 1999. Effect of fluoroquinolone concentration on selection of resistant mutants of *Mycobacterium bovis* BCG and *Staphylococcus aureus*. *Antimicrob. Agents Chemother.* 43:1756–1758.

17. Drusano, G. L., S. L. Preston, R. C. Owens, and P. G. Ambrose. 2001. Fluoroquinolone pharmacodynamics. *Clin. Infect. Dis.* 33:2091–2096.

18. Drusano, G. L., D. E. Johnson, M. Rosen, and H. C. Standiford. 1993. Pharmacodynamics of a fluoroquinolone antimicrobial agent in a neutropenic rat model of *Pseudomonas* sepsis. *Antimicrob. Agents Chemother.* 37: 483–490.

19. Fantin, B., J. Leggett, S. Ebert, and W. A. Craig. 1991. Correlation between in vitro and in vivo activity of antimicrobial agents against gram-negative bacilli in a murine infection model. *Antimicrob. Agents Chemother.* 35:1413–1422.

20. Firsov, A. A., S. N. Vostrov, A. A. Shevchenko, Y. A. Protnoy, and S. H. Zinner. 1998. A new approach to in vitro comparisons of antibiotics in dynamic models: equivalent area under the curve/MIC breakpoints and equiefficient doses of trovafloxacin and ciprofloxacin against bacteria of similar susceptibilities. *Antimicrob. Agents Chemother.* 42:2841–2847.

21. Firsov, A. A., S. N. Vostrov, L. Y. Lubenko, S. H. Zinner, and Y. A. Portnoy. 2002. Concept of "mutant selection window" examined with quinolones: preventing the production of resistant mutants of *Staphylococcus aureus* in an in vitro dynamic model simulating normal and impaired elimination, abstr. A-1210. *In Abstracts of the 42th Interscience Conference on Antimicrobial Agents and Chemotherapy.* American Society for Microbiology, Washington, D.C.

22. Fish, D. N., S. C. Piscitelli, and L. H. Danziger. 1995. Development of resistance during antimicrobial therapy: a review of antibiotic class and patient characteristics in 173 studies. *Pharmacotherapy* 15:279–291.

23. Fishman, N. O., B. Suh, W. M. Weigel, B. Lorver, S. Gelone, A. L. Truant, T. D. Gootz, J. D. Christie, and P. H. Edelstein. 1999. Three levofloxacin treatment failures of pneumococcal respiratory tract infections. *In Abstracts of the 39th Interscience Conference on Antimicrobial Agents and Chemotherapy.* American Society for Microbiology, Washington, D.C.

24. Forrest, A., D. Nix, C. H. Ballow, T. F. Goss, M. C. Birmingham, and J. J. Schentag. 1993. Pharmacodynamics of intravenous ciprofloxacin in seriously ill patients. *Antimicrob. Agents Chemother.* 37:1073–1081.

25. Griffith, D. C., E. Corcoran, D. Cho, O. Lomovskaya, and M. N. Dudley. 2001. Pharmacodynamics of levofloxacin against *P. aeruginosa* with reduced susceptibility from different Mex efflux pump systems: do elevated MICs always predict reduced in vivo efficacy? *In Abstracts of the 41st Interscience Conference on Antimicrobial Agents and Chemotherapy.* American Society for Microbiology, Washington, D.C.

26. Join-Lambert, O. F., M. Michéa-Hamzehpour, T. Köhler, F. Chau, F. Faurisson, S. Dautney, C. Vissuzaine, C. Carbon, and J.-C. Pechère. 2001. Differential selection of multidrug efflux mutants by trovafloxacin and ciprofloxacin in an experimental model of Pseudomonas aeruginosa acute pneumonia in rats. *Antimicrob. Agents Chemother.* 45:571–576.

27. Kiem, S., and W. A. Craig. 2002. Why do neutrophils markedly reduce the 24-h AUC/MIC required for efficacy of fluoroquinolones against *Streptococcus pneumoniae*, abstr. A-492. *In Abstracts of the 42th Interscience Conference on Antimicrobial Agents and Chemotherapy.* American Society for Microbiology, Washington, D.C.

28. Lacy, M. K., W. Lu, X. Xu, P. R. Tessier, D. P. Nicolau, R. Quintiliani, and C. H. Nightingale. 1999. Pharmacodynamic comparisons of levofloxacin, ciprofloxacin, and ampicillin against *Streptococcus pneumoniae* in an in vitro model of infection. *Antimicrob. Agents Chemother.* **43**:672–677.

29. Leggett, J. E., S. Ebert, B. Fantin, and W. A. Craig. 1991. Comparative dose-effect relations at several dosing intervals for beta-lactam, aminoglycoside and quinolone antibiotics against gram-negative bacilli in murine thigh-infection and pneumonitis models. *Scand. J. Infect. Dis. Suppl.* **74**:179–184.

30. Leggett, J. E., B. Fantin, S. Ebert, K. Totsuka, B. Vogelman, W. Calame, H. Mattie, and W. A. Craig. 1989. Comparative antibiotic dose-effect relations at several dosing intervals in murine pneumonitis and thigh-infection models. *J. Infect. Dis.* **159**:281–292.

31. Lister, P. D., and C. C. Sanders. 1999. Pharmacodynamics of levofloxacin and ciprofloxacin against *Streptococcus pneumoniae*. *J. Antimicrob. Chemother.* **43**:79–86.

32. Lutsar, I., I. R. Friedland, L. Wubbel, C. C. McColg, H. S. Jafrir, W. Ng, F. Ghaffar, and G. H. McCracken, Jr. 1998. Pharmacodynamics of gatifloxacin in cerebrospinal fluid in experimental resistant pneumococcal meningitis. *Antimicrob. Agents Chemother.* **42**:2650–2655.

33. MacGowan, A., and K. Bowker. 2002. Developments in PK/PD: optimizing efficacy and prevention of resistance. A critical review of PK/PD in in vitro models. *Int. J. Antimicrob. Agents* **19**:291–298.

34. MacGowan, A., and K. E. Bowker. 2001. The magnitude of the pharmacodynamic parameters which predict fluoroquinolone antibacterial effect and emergence of resistance are not uniform for all species, abstr. A-441. *In Abstracts of the 41th Interscience Conference on Antimicrobial Agents and Chemotherapy.* American Society for Microbiology, Washington, D.C.

35. Marchbanks, C. R., J. R. McKiel, D. H. Gilbert, N. J. Robillard, B. Painter, S. H. Zinner, and M. N. Dudley. 1993. Dose ranging and fractionation of intravenous ciprofloxacin against Pseudomonas aeruginosa and Staphylococcus aureus in an in vitro model of infection. *Antimicrob. Agents Chemother.* **37**:1756–1763.

36. Meinl, B., J. M. Hyatt, A. Forrest, S. Chodosh, and J. J. Schentag. 2000. Pharmacokinetic/pharmacodynamic predictors of time to clinical resolution in patients with acute bacterial exacerbations of chronic bronchitis treated with a fluoroquinolone. *Int. J. Antimicrob. Agents* **16**:273–280.

37. Odenholt, I. 2001. Pharmacodynamic effects of subinhibitory antibiotic concentrations. *Int. J. Antimicrob. Agents* **17**:1–8.

38. Odenholt, I., T. Cars, and E. Lowdin. 2000. Pharmacodynamic studies of trovafloxacin and grepafloxacin in vitro against gram-positive and gram-negative bacteria. *J. Antimicrob. Chemother.* **46**:35–43.

39. Pankuch, G., M. R. Jacobs, P. C. Appelbaum. 2002. Post-antibiotic effect of garenoxacin against gram-positive and -negative organisms, abstr. A-496. *In Abstracts of the 42th Interscience Conference on Antimicrobial Agents and Chemotherapy.* American Society for Microbiology, Washington, D.C.

40. Peloquin, C. A., T. J. Cumbo, D. E. Nix, M. F. Sands, J. J. Schentag. 1989. Evaluation of intravenous ciprofloxacin in patients with nosocomial lower respiratory tract infections. *Arch. Intern. Med.* **149**:2269–2273.

41. Preston, S. L., G. L. Drusano, A. L. Berman, C. L. Fowler, A. T. Chow, B. Dornseif, V. Reichl, J. Natarajan, and M. Corrado. 1998. Pharmacodynamics of levofloxacin: a new paradigm for early clinical trials. *JAMA* **279**:125–129.

42. Rodruguez-Cerrato, V., F. Ghaffar, and F. Saavedra, et al. 2001. BMS-284756 in experimental cephalosporin-resistant pneumococcal meningitis. *Antimicrob. Agents Chemother.* **45**:3098–3103.

43. Sindelar, G., X. Zhao, A. Liew, Y. Dong, T. Lu, J. Zhou, J. Domagala, and K. Drlica. 2000. Mutant prevention concentration as a measure of fluoroquinolone potency against mycobacteria. *Antimicrob. Agents Chemother.* **44**:3337–3343.

44. Tam, V. H., A. Louie, and M. R. Deziel, et al. 2001. Pharmacodynamics of BMS-284756 in counter-selecting resistance in a hollow-fiber system, abstr. A-442. *In Abstracts of the 41th Interscience Conference on Antimicrobial Agents and Chemotherapy.* American Society for Microbiology, Washington, D.C.

45. Tam, V. H., A. Louie, M. R. Deziel, et al. 2002. AUC/MIC ratio of a quinolone is predictive of emergence of resistance in *Pseudomonas aeruginosa*: in vitro–in vivo correlation, abstr. A-1213 *In Abstracts of the 42th Interscience Conference on Antimicrobial Agents and Chemotherapy.* American Society for Microbiology, Washington, D.C.

46. Thomas, J. K., A. Forrest, S. M. Bhavani, J. M. Hyatt, A. Cheng, C. H. Ballow, and J. J. Schentag. 1998. Pharmacodynamic evaluation of factors associated with the development of bacterial resistance in acutely ill patients during therapy. *Antimicrob. Agents Chemother.* **42**:521–527.

47. Trampuz, A., M. Wenk, Z. Rajacic, and W. Zimmerli. 2000. Pharmacokinetics and pharmacodynamics of levofloxacin against Streptococcus pneumoniae and Staphylococcus aureus in human skin blister fluid. *Antimicrob. Agents Chemother.* **44**:1352–1355.

48. Vogelman, B. S., S. Gudmundsson, J. Turnidge, J. E. Leggett, and W. A. Craig. 1988. The in vivo post antibiotic effect in a thigh infection in neutropenic mice. *J. Infect. Dis.* **157**:287–298.

49. Vogelman, B. S., S. Gudmundsson, J. Leggett, J. Turnidge, S. Ebert, and W. A. Craig. 1988. Correlation of antimicrobial pharmacokinetic parameters with therapeutic efficacy in an animal model. *J. Infect. Dis.* **158**:831–847.

50. Vostrov, S. N., O. V. Kononenko, I. Y. Lubenko, S. H. Zinner, and A. A. Firsov. 2000. Comparative pharmacodynamics of gatifloxacin and ciprofloxacin in an in vitro dynamic model: prediction of equiefficient doses and the breakpoints of the area under the curve/MIC ratio. *Antimicrob. Agents Chemother.* **44**:879–884.

51. Zinner, S. H., K. Simmons, and D. Gilbert. 2000. Comparative activities of ciprofloxacin and levofloxacin against Streptococcus pneumoniae in an in vitro dynamic model. *Antimicrob. Agents Chemother.* **44**:773–774.

III. CLINICAL APPLICATIONS

Quinolone Antimicrobial Agents, 3rd ed.
Edited by David C. Hooper and Ethan Rubinstein
© 2003 ASM Press, Washington, D.C.

Chapter 9

Treatment of Urinary Tract Infections

KALPANA GUPTA, KURT NABER, AND WALTER STAMM

EPIDEMIOLOGY AND CLINICAL DEFINITIONS OF URINARY TRACT INFECTION

Urinary tract infections (UTIs) are among the most common reasons for an outpatient office visit and for antimicrobial usage among adult patients. UTIs occur most frequently in young adult women, affecting up to 50% of women at some time during their lifetime. Approximately 30% of women who experience a UTI will have recurrent episodes of UTI, often within 3 months of the original episode. With advancing age, UTI incidence in males increases and approaches the rate seen in postmenopausal women, primarily due to prostate disease. It has been estimated that up to half of all men suffer from symptoms of prostatitis at some time in their lives. In the early 1900s, prostatitis resulted in 2 million office visits per year in the United States, rivaling the number of visits for benign prostatic hypertrophy at the time. It is the most common urological diagnosis in men younger than 50 years of age and the third most common urological diagnosis in men older than 50 years of age (14). It has been clearly demonstrated that patients diagnosed with chronic prostatitis experience a quality-of-life impact similar to patients suffering from myocardial infarction, angina, or Crohn's disease (97). Thus, UTI is a significant health care issue for both men and women. The fluoroquinolones play a major role in the management of this common bacterial infection.

UTIs comprise several clinical syndromes defined by the clinical setting, host characteristics, and anatomic portion of the urinary tract involved. The major syndromes include cystitis, prostatitis, pyelonephritis, recurrent UTI, catheter-associated UTI, and asymptomatic bacteriuria. Cystitis is clinically defined as acute onset of dysuria, urinary frequency and/or urgency, generally without associated fever. Suprapubic pain and hematuria may be present. This syndrome comprises the vast majority of UTIs seen in the outpatient setting and is most common in otherwise healthy women. Clinically, pyelonephritis presents with fever and flank pain with or without symptoms of cystitis. Nausea, vomiting, and abdominal pain may be present. Prostatitis presents differently depending on whether it is acute or chronic in nature. Acute prostatitis presents with acute onset of perineal and abdominal pain, fever, dysuria, urgency, obstructive symptoms, and pain on defecation. Chronic prostatitis should be suspected in any male with recurrent UTIs. Obstructive voiding symptoms may be present between UTIs. Catheter-associated UTI is a very common nosocomial infection and may present with symptoms of cystitis or more severe systemic symptoms of sepsis. Asymptomatic bacteriuria detected on routine screening urine cultures is usually not of clinical significance except in certain patient populations such as pregnant women, renal transplant and other immunocompromised patients, and prior to genitourinary instrumentation.

The classification of UTI into uncomplicated versus complicated infection is important both for understanding the pathogenesis of disease and for diagnostic and management strategies. Acute cystitis or pyelonephritis in an otherwise healthy adult woman with no known abnormalities of the urinary tract is classified as uncomplicated. UTIs occurring in men, elderly or pregnant women, children, and patients who are hospitalized or have comorbid conditions are typically considered to be complicated. Recent data suggest that young adult men can also have an episode of UTI that is not related to an underlying anatomic or physiologic abnormality of the urinary tract, (i.e., is uncomplicated). This syndrome may be seen in men who have sex with men or in men with human immunodeficiency virus infection with a CD4 count less than 200 (33). The majority of UTIs in men, however, occur in older

Kalpana Gupta and Walter Stamm • Department of Medicine, Division of Allergy & Infectious Diseases, University of Washington School of Medicine, 1959 NE Pacific Street, BB1221, Mailstop 356523, Seattle, WA 98195. **Kurt G. Naber** • Urologic Clinic, Hospital St. Elisabeth, D-94315 Straubing, Germany.

males with prostatic hypertrophy or indwelling urinary catheters. UTIs in postmenopausal women are quite common and often are not associated with definable abnormalities of the urinary tract system. In general, these can be considered uncomplicated. However, if there are comorbid conditions or the presence of a urinary catheter, the UTI should be classified as complicated. UTIs in pregnant women are considered complicated because of the physiologic changes during pregnancy which increase the risk of upper UTI, as well as the potential for adverse outcomes for the mother and fetus, which have been associated with UTI.

IN VITRO ACTIVITY

The in vitro activity of the fluoroquinolones against members of the *Enterobacteriaceae* makes them excellent candidates for treatment of urinary tract infections. The spectrum of etiologic organisms in uncomplicated UTI is highly predictable, with *Escherichia coli* accounting for 75 to 90% of isolates, *Staphylococcus saprophyticus* accounting for 5 to 15% of isolates, and *Klebsiella* spp., *Proteus* spp., enterococci, and other organisms accounting for 5 to 10% of isolates. In complicated UTIs, there is a wider spectrum of organisms as well as an increased likelihood of antimicrobial resistance. *E. coli* is still the predominant gram-negative organism, but *Klebsiella* spp., *Proteus* spp., *Serratia* spp., *Citrobacter* spp., *Acinetobacter* spp., *Morganella* spp., and *Pseudomonas aeruginosa* are also frequently isolated. Gram-positive bacteria such as enterococci and *Staphylococcus aureus* as well as yeast are also common pathogens in complicated UTI.

The main problem affecting the intrinsically excellent in vitro activity of fluoroquinolones against most urinary pathogens is the development of antimicrobial resistance to these agents. In uncomplicated cystitis, very little development of fluoroquinolone resistance has occurred in the United States, as evidenced by regional as well as national data (26, 27, 78). Outside of North America, however, resistance to the quinolones is quite high, even among community-acquired UTI pathogens (25). It is likely that these resistant strains causing uncomplicated UTI will become more widespread during the next few years.

The susceptibility of pathogens causing complicated UTIs varies depending on the individual institution or region being studied. In general, fluoroquinolone resistance is an important consideration in these infections (41). Thus, although the inherent in vitro activity of the fluoroquinolones against UTI

pathogens is generally very good, increased antimicrobial resistance is making use of these agents in the urinary tract more problematic.

PHARMACOLOGY OF QUINOLONE AGENTS IN THE URINARY TRACT

Since the fluoroquinolones are usually administered orally for this indication, the serum drug concentrations, half-life, and amount excreted as active drug by the kidney, which reflects bioavailability and renal handling, are the most important pharmacokinetic parameters for the treatment of UTIs. It can be seen that the renal excretion varies widely between substances (Table 1). Renal excretion is highest ($\geq$75% of a dose) with gatifloxacin (80%), levofloxacin (84%), lomefloxacin (75%), and ofloxacin (81%). An intermediate excretion rate (40 to 74%) is seen with ciprofloxacin (43%), enoxacin (53%), and fleroxacin (67%), and rather low excretion (<40%) is seen with gemifloxacin (28%), moxifloxacin (20%), norfloxacin (20%), pefloxacin (14%) and sparfloxacin (10%). Penetration into prostatic tissue and prostatic secretions also contributes to efficacy in prostatitis.

According to pharmacodynamic studies the fluoroquinolones exhibit concentration depending killing (18). The antibacterial activity of fluoroquinolones in urine is reduced as compared with nutrient broth. The activity in urine depends on the

Table 1. Selected pharmacokinetic parameters of oral fluoroquinolones[a]

Substance	Dose (mg)	Peak serum concn (mg/liter)	Serum half-life (h)	Urinary excretion of parent drug (%)
Group 1				
Norfloxacin	400	1.5[98]	3.2[98]	20[30]
Pefloxacin	400	3.2[4]	10.5[4]	14 + 18(N)[30]
Group 2				
Enoxacin	400	3.1[99]	4.9[99]	53[96]
Fleroxacin	400	4.4[94]	9.2[94]	67[60]
Ofloxacin	400	4.2[59]	5.4[59]	81[59]
Lomefloxacin	400	5.2[8]	8.1[8]	75[8]
Ciprofloxacin	500	2.6[10]	4.2[10]	43[10]
Group 3				
Levofloxacin	500	5.2[12]	7.4[12]	84[53]
Sparfloxacin	200	1.6[49]	17[49]	10[49]
Group 4				
Gatifloxacin	400	3.4[86]	8[86]	80[85]
Moxifloxacin	400	2.5[87]	13.1[87]	20[2]
Gemifloxacin*	320	1.3[52]	6.1[52]	28[52]

[a] Superscripts denote reference number; *, not registered yet; (N), norfloxacin. Table adapted from reference 55 with permission from Elsevier.

urine pH and contents of various solutes, mainly cations (54). In addition, in complicated UTI biofilm infection may play an important role in which the susceptibility of the pathogens is several folds reduced as compared with planktonic or pure culture cells (16). In an experimental study it was shown that 32- to 64-fold higher concentrations than that of the minimal bactericidal concentrations of levofloxacin or ciprofloxacin, respectively, were required to eradicate a strain of *P. aeruginosa* in a catheter-associated biofilm infection (23).

In order to combine the pharmacokinetic properties and the antibacterial activity, the ex vivo urinary bactericidal titers of various fluoroquinolones were determined in comparative studies for healthy volunteers. If the urinary bactericidal titers are used as pharmacodynamic parameters, oral dosages of fluoroquinolones exhibiting comparable urinary antibactericidal activity against the main uropathogens could be considered pharmacologically equivalent dosages, which are shown in Table 2.

ROLE OF QUINOLONE AGENTS IN TREATMENT OF UTI

Numerous clinical studies have evaluated the efficacy and safety of the fluoroquinolones in the treatment of UTI. The wide variety of drugs and dosing regimens used makes the results from these studies difficult to compare. Even studies evaluating the same two drugs are difficult to compare because they often include different study populations and/or definitions for bacteriuria, cure, and relapse. Despite these issues, some general themes clearly emerge when studies are stratified by the clinical UTI syndrome being evaluated.

Table 2. Equivalent dosages of oral fluoroquinolones for the treatment of urinary tract infections

Treatment	Fluoroquinolone	Dose (mg)
Low dosage	Norfloxacin	400 b.i.d.
	Enoxacin	200 b.i.d.
	Ofloxacin	100 b.i.d.
	Ciprofloxacin	125 (100) b.i.d.
Standard dosage	Enoxacin	400 b.i.d.
	Ofloxacin	200 b.i.d.
	Ciprofloxacin	250 b.i.d.
	Levofloxacin	250 once daily
	Gatifloxacin	200 once daily
High dosage	Ciprofloxacin	500[a] b.i.d.
	Levofloxacin	500[a] once daily
	Gatifloxacin	400 once daily

[a] Dosage can be increased if necessary.

Acute Uncomplicated Cystitis

The use of fluoroquinolones for treatment of acute uncomplicated cystitis remains controversial, not because of concern over the efficacy of these agents in UTI, but due to potential emergence of resistance among pathogens causing UTI (and more serious invasive infections) with the increased use of fluoroquinolones. However, the increasing rates of resistance to trimethoprim and trimethoprim-sulfamethoxazole (SXT) (the accepted first-line agents for treatment of acute uncomplicated cystitis) in many areas have resulted in the need for alternative agents for treatment of UTI, including acute uncomplicated cystitis. In a recent evidence-based guideline published by the Infectious Diseases Society of America, the main alternative agents to SMT included the fluoroquinolones, nitrofurantoin, or fosfomycin (93). The β-lactam agents were not considered to be viable alternatives for treatment of acute uncomplicated cystitis because of high levels of antimicrobial resistance, low efficacy, and in some cases increased rate of side effects with this class of drugs. The fluoroquinolones were the only class of drug found to have efficacy equal to SXT in a 3-day regimen. A selected group of randomized clinical trials comparing fluoroquinolones to SXT for treatment of acute cystitis is shown in Table 3.

As seen in Table 3, the bacterial eradication rates with the fluoroquinolones are roughly equal to those achieved with SXT, regardless of the dosage strength, frequency, or duration of therapy with the fluoroquinolone. The short-term cure rates with fluoroquinolones range from 85 to 100% and for SXT range from 81 to 100%. The long-term cure rates (defined differently for many studies) are also similar. An important caveat is that some of the studies included patients who were unlikely to have uncomplicated cystitis, i.e., males or hospitalized patients. However, even in these studies, the cure rates did not differ markedly between SXT and the specific fluoroquinolone tested. Studies that evaluated single-dose therapy were not included in this table since single-dose therapy for acute uncomplicated cystitis is no longer advocated due to low efficacy rates. However, many studies have reported reasonable efficacy rates with single-dose regimens of the fluoroquinolones, especially those with long half-lives. Unlike infections caused by *E. coli* or other aerobic gram-negative rods, single-dose treatment of *S. saprophyticus* infections with fluoroquinolones often does result in high failure rates. Since it is the causative uropathogen in 5 to 15% of young women with acute uncomplicated cystitis, single-dose regimens of fluoroquinolones are not recommended (93).

Table 3. Comparative studies of fluoroquinolones versus SXT for acute uncomplicated cystitis[a]

Reference	Regimens	Short-term bacterial eradication rates (%)	Long-term bacterial eradication rates (%)	Study population
3	Ofloxacin 200 mg q.d. × 3 d	84.8	NA	>90% women with AUC
	SXT DS b.i.d. × 7 d	81.5		
85	Ofloxacin 200 mg q.d. × 5 d	91.8	78.7	Outpatients with cystitis, 12% males
	Trimethoprim 200 mg b.i.d. × 5 d	80.7*	72.2	
	SXT DS b.i.d. × 5 d	80.9*	75.9	
7	Ofloxacin 100 mg b.i.d. × 3 d	92	4	Women with AUC
	SXT DS b.i.d. × 3 d	88	15	
32	Ofloxacin 200 mg b.i.d. × 3 d	96	88	Woman with AUC
	Ofloxacin 200 mg b.i.d. × 7 d	91	86	
	Ofloxacin 300 mg b.i.d. × 7 d	96	100	
	SXT DS b.i.d. × 7 d	93	88	
31	Ofloxacin 200 mg q.d. × 3 d	92	89	Women with AUC
	SXT DS b.i.d. × 7 d	95	98*	
24	Lomefloxacin 400 mg q.d. × 5 d	100	83	80–92% women
	SXT DS b.i.d. × 7 d	87	80	
29	Ciprofloxacin 250 mg b.i.d. × 10 d	100	7	Women with AUC
	SXT b.i.d. × 10 d	94	18	
46	Ciprofloxacin 100 mg b.i.d. × 3 d	94	89	Women with AUC
	Ofloxacin 200 mg b.i.d. × 3 d	97	87	
	SXT DS b.i.d. × 3 d	93	84	
37	Ciprofloxacin 100 mg b.i.d. × 3 d	88	91	Women with AUC
	SXT DS b.i.d. × 7 d	93	79	
	NTF 100 mg b.i.d. × 7 d	86	82*	
88	Norfloxacin 400 mg b.i.d. × 3 d	96	91	>90% females with AUC
	SXT b.i.d. × 10 d	100	95	
90	Norfloxacin 200 mg b.i.d. × 7 d	98	88	>90% women
	Norfloxacin 400 mg b.i.d. × 7 d	98	89	
	SXT DS b.i.d. × 7 d	99	88	

[a] DS, double strength; NA, not available. q.d., once a day; NTF, nitrofurantoin. Asterisk indicates $P < 0.05$ for comparison with the fluoroquinolone tested.

Studies comparing fluoroquinolone regimens to other antimicrobials used for treatment of acute uncomplicated cystitis are found less frequently in the literature. Studies comparing a β-lactam to the quinolones have had varying results, likely because the spectrum of the β-lactam used varies from study to study. In a pooled analysis of two large multicenter treatment trials, pivmecillinam 200 mg twice a day (b.i.d.) × 7 days demonstrated equal bacterial eradication rates to norfloxacin 400 mg b.i.d. × 3 days at early follow-up (64). Pivmecillinam 400 mg b.i.d. × 3 days resulted in significantly lower bacterial eradication rates. Other studies have compared cefixime and cefuroxime axetil to fluoroquinolone regimens and did not find a statistically significant difference in bacterial eradication rates, although small sample sizes limited the power of statistical comparisons (11, 58, 74). Only a few studies have compared single-dose fosfomycin with a multidose fluoroquinolone regimen (9, 19, 40). The majority of these studies demonstrated equal bacterial eradication rates between the two drugs, although a meta-analysis of two studies demonstrated that adverse

events were more frequent with fosfomycin (93). Few studies have directly compared nitrofurantoin to a fluoroquinolone. Two of these trials found equivalence in early bacterial eradication rates whereas a third demonstrated a slight advantage for the quinolone tested, ofloxacin (37, 44, 83).

Thus, in summary, ample data clearly support the efficacy and safety of fluoroquinolones for treatment of acute uncomplicated cystitis. The cure rates are similar to (and in some cases better than) those achieved with SXT. In locales with a high prevalence of SXT resistance, bacteriologic and clinical cure rates with SXT are only in the range of 40 to 50%, significantly lower than what would be expected with a fluoroquinolone (72). Comparison with other UTI antimicrobials is not as well studied, but none of the studies we reviewed demonstrated lower efficacy with use of a fluoroquinolone as compared with a β-lactam, nitrofurantoin, or fosfomycin. Thus, the use of a fluoroquinolone for acute uncomplicated cystitis depends on balancing issues such as safety, cost, cost-effectiveness, prevalence of SXT resistance in the local area, and concern over propagation of antibiotic resistance in the community. From a cost-effectiveness perspective, the efficacy and safety of these agents makes them as cost-effective as SXT, at least as demonstrated in one clinical trial (34). Whether short-course use of fluoroquinolones for the treatment of uncomplicated UTI actually contributes significantly to the development of antibiotic resistance in the community is difficult to assess, although fluoroquinolones used in longer courses have clearly been associated with fluoroquinolone-resistant uropathogens (21, 35).

The choice among fluoroquinolones for treatment of acute uncomplicated cystitis is becoming increasingly difficult as the number of available agents increases. However, the added benefit of gram-positive, atypical, and anaerobic coverage afforded by many of the newer quinolones is of little value in treatment of acute uncomplicated cystitis because, as noted above, the distribution of uropathogens in this syndrome is quite predictably weighted toward facultative gram-negative rods. Thus, use of a quinolone with mainly gram-negative activity and a proven safety profile seems to be the prudent choice for acute uncomplicated cystitis. The option of once-daily dosing of some of the newer fluoroquinolones is a potential advantage when compliance is an issue. Table 4 shows some of the many studies comparing different fluoroquinolones for treatment of acute uncomplicated cystitis. The problem of different doses of varying durations makes interstudy comparison difficult, but, in general, most of the studies found equivalence between the fluoroquinolones tested. Notably, ciprofloxacin resulted in higher bacterial eradication rates than cinoxacin or sparfloxacin (the latter is not approved for treatment

of UTI). Two newer fluoroquinolones, gatifloxacin and gemifloxacin, have been demonstrated to be equivalent to ciprofloxacin in terms of bacterial eradication of susceptible pathogens (55). The extensive experience and demonstrated safety and efficacy with ciprofloxacin and levofloxacin and the minimal benefit associated with use of newer fluoroquinolones for treatment of acute cystitis argues for the continued use of ciprofloxacin and levofloxacin for this indication.

Acute Pyelonephritis

The use of quinolones for treatment of acute pyelonephritis is appealing because of the high concentrations achieved by most agents in this class in renal tissue. There are few randomized controlled studies evaluating fluoroquinolones for the treatment of pyelonephritis. Most studies demonstrate that these agents are equivalent or superior to other antimicrobials such as β-lactams, gentamicin, and SXT (Table 5). Many of these studies, however, include both men and women and inpatients and outpatients. Thus, few clearly evaluate treatment for acute uncomplicated pyelonephritis. The study by Talan et al. was limited to pyelonephritis occurring in women who had no other urinary tract abnormalities and were amenable to outpatient oral therapy (89). In this multicenter study, a 7-day course of ciprofloxacin was superior to a 14-day course of SXT (Table 5) in terms of bacterial eradication at the short-term follow-up. Most of the failures in the SXT-treated group occurred in women with SXT-resistant strains. On the basis of data from this and other studies, the Infectious Disease Society of

Table 4. Comparative trials of fluoroquinolones for acute uncomplicated cystitis[a]

Reference	Regimen	Short-term bacterial eradication rate (%)	Long-term bacterial eradication rate (%)	Study population
22	Ciprofloxacin 250 mg b.i.d. × 10 d	83	80	>90% women with uncomplicated UTI
	Cinoxacin 500 mg b.i.d. × 10 d	71	73	
28	Sparfloxacin 400 mg q.d. × 1 d	92	81	Women with AUC
	Sparfloxacin × 3 d (400/200/200 mg)	93	89	
	Ciprofloxacin 250 mg b.i.d. × 7 d	97	93	
69	Gatifloxacin 200 mg q.d. × 3 d	95	NA	Women with AUC
	Ciprofloxacin 100 mg b.i.d. × 3 d	93		
65	Lomefloxacin 400 mg q.d. × 3 d	97	87	Women with AUC
	Norfloxacin 400 mg b.i.d. × 3 d	95	90	
63	Lomefloxacin 400 mg q.d. × 3 d	88	81	Women with AUC
	Lomefloxacin 400 mg q.d. × 7 d	93	82	
	Norfloxacin 400 mg b.i.d. × 7 d	93	85	
46	Ciprofloxacin 100 mg b.i.d. × 3 d	94	89	Women with AUC
	Ofloxacin 200 mg b.i.d. × 3 d	97	87	

[a] q.d., once a day; NA, not available.

Table 5. Fluoroquinolone treatment trials for pyelonephritis[a]

Reference	Regimens	Short-term bacterial eradication rates (%)	Long-term bacterial eradication rates (%)	Study population
77	Levofloxacin 250 q.d. × 10–14 d	95	87	Mixed gender and in/out patients
	Ciprofloxacin 500 b.i.d. × 10 d	94	93	
	Lomefloxacin 400 q.d. × 14 d	95	—	
50	Lomefloxacin 400 q.d. × 14 d	100	80	Mixed gender and in/out patients
	SXT DS b.i.d. × 14 d	89*	67*	
80	Norfloxacin 400 b.i.d. × 14 d	98	87	Mixed gender and in/out patients
	Cefadroxil 1 g b.i.d. × 14 d	65*	48*	
44	Ofloxacin 200 b.i.d. × 7 d	85	NA	Mixed gender
	SXT DS b.i.d. × 7 d	69		
89	Ciprofloxacin 500 b.i.d. × 7 d	99	85	Women with AUP
	SXT DS b.i.d. × 14 d	89*	74	

[a]—, combined rate for ciprofloxacin and lomefloxacin; NA, not available; q.d., once a day. Asterisk indicates $P \leq 0.05$ for comparison with fluoroquinolone.

America guidelines recommend the use of a fluoro-quinolone as first-line empiric therapy for acute uncomplicated pyelonephritis. Administration of the first dose parenterally followed by oral therapy is probably reasonable for women who are well enough to be treated in the outpatient setting. Women with nausea, vomiting, hypotension, severe pain, or uncertain diagnosis should be hospitalized for initial parenteral therapy for 2 to 3 days until improvement occurs and oral therapy can be used. SXT is a reasonable alternative if the infecting organism is known to be susceptible to this drug. Amoxicillin plus gentamicin or amoxicillin/clavulanic acid should be reserved for cases when a gram stain suggests infection with a gram-positive organism. Treatment of complicated cases of pyelonephritis is discussed in the section on complicated UTI.

UTI in the Elderly

Use of fluoroquinolones for treatment of UTI in elderly women deserves special mention because these UTIs are often complicated due to the presence of comorbid conditions or anatomical abnormalities and because the potential for adverse side effects or drug interactions may be higher in this population. Raz and Rozenfeld compared the use of a 3-day regimen of ofloxacin with a 7-day regimen of cephalexin for treatment of UTI occurring in postmenopausal women (75). The ofloxacin regimen resulted in significantly higher bacterial eradication rates both at the short- (77 versus 64%) and long-term (74 versus 61%) follow-up visits. In addition, the ofloxacin regimen was cheaper than the cephalexin regimen. Adverse events were not significantly different

between the two treatment groups. In another multi-center study comparing 7-day regimens of ciprofloxacin (250 mg twice daily) with ofloxacin (200 mg twice daily) for treatment of uncomplicated cystitis in a predominantly postmenopausal population, bacterial eradication at 5–9 days posttreatment was achieved in 90 and 87% of the women, respectively (73). There was no significant difference in the rate of adverse events, with gastrointestinal and nervous system abnormalities being the most common complaints in both treatment groups. Thus, studies demonstrate that the fluoroquinolones are relatively well tolerated and efficacious in elderly women. The slightly lower cure rates seen in this population as compared with the studies in premenopausal women may be related to differences in the microbial species and resistance profiles of the causative uropathogens. A national laboratory survey demonstrated that women older than 50 years of age were more likely to have enterococci and other non-*E. coli* gram-negative rods as the causative uropathogen. In addition, overall susceptibility of uropathogens to the fluoroquinolones was somewhat lower in the older women, mainly because of the higher prevalence and resistance of enterococci in this age group (26).

Complicated UTI

The broad range of clinical conditions and patient populations encompassed by the term complicated UTI makes it difficult to generalize about treatment. However, the fluoroquinolones are often cited as the drugs of choice for these infections because of their in vitro activity and efficacy against most organisms isolated in these settings. Numerous studies compare treatment regimens for complicated UTI, and despite marked variations in study populations, most demonstrate similarly high cure rates with the fluoroquinolones (17, 67, 68, 70). However, the treatment of complicated UTIs caused by *P. aeruginosa* deserves special comment.

P. aeruginosa is a commonly isolated organism in complicated UTI, and the fluoroquinolones have the unique advantage of being the only available oral therapy with activity against this organism. Unfortunately, *P. aeruginosa* resistance to the fluoroquinolones can occur readily, and thus use of a fluoroquinolone with excellent in vitro activity and in a high dose is critical for bacterial eradication (55, 62). Among the currently available fluoroquinolones, ciprofloxacin has the best in vitro activity against *P. aeruginosa*. Ciprofloxacin should be used at 500 or 750 mg twice daily, and levofloxacin should be given at a dose of at least 500 mg daily for treatment of *P. aeruginosa* UTI. The MICs of the newer fluoroquinolones for pseudomonal strains are, in general, higher than the MICs of ciprofloxacin, ofloxacin, and levofloxacin, making the newer fluoroquinolones less attractive for treatment of pseudomonal UTI (57).

The newer fluoroquinolones tend to have better activity against gram-positive organisms and thus may have a unique role in treatment of UTIs because of staphylococci and enterococci. Gemifloxacin, moxifloxacin, and trovafloxacin, however, do not achieve high urinary concentrations, and thus the use of these newer quinolones is not indicated for treatment of complicated UTI (57). Gatifloxacin is mainly renally excreted and may be reasonable for use in complicated UTI if the infecting organism is susceptible.

Prostatitis

In the past, prostatitis was most frequently classified on the basis of the results of the bacteriologic

Table 6. NIH/National Institute of Diabetes and Digestive and Kidney Diseases classification of prostatitis (1995)

Category	Classification
I	Acute bacterial prostatitis
II	Chronic bacterial prostatitis
III	Chronic pelvic pain syndrome (CPPS)
IIIA	CPPS: inflammatory
IIIB	CPPS: noninflammatory
IV	Asymptomatic inflammatory prostatitis

localization patterns obtained by the four-glass specimens technique (47). Because of lack of knowledge concerning epidemiology, pathophysiology, diagnosis, and treatment of prostatitis, the National Institutes of Health (NIH) of the United States started an international initiative. A new classification system (82) was suggested as a first step that provides uniform definitions of the various types of prostatitis to facilitate collaborative research. The NIH/National Institute of Diabetes and Digestive and Kidney Diseases proposed this new classification system in 1995, which was reaffirmed in 1998 (Table 6) (67a).

Despite reports that less than 10% of prostatitis cases are caused by bacterial infection (95), a much higher proportion of men diagnosed with prostatitis receive antimicrobials. Antibiotic therapy is recommended for acute bacterial prostatitis and chronic bacterial prostatitis; it is debatable in patients with inflammatory chronic pelvic pain syndrome (6). Because of their favorable pharmacokinetic properties the fluoroquinolones can be considered drugs of choice. Several clinical studies with quinolones have been published (61). The results are difficult to compare, however, because not all workers used the Meares and Stamey technique for diagnosis. The duration of treatment (which should last for a minimum of 2 to 4 weeks) and the follow-up period differed tremendously. Only a few studies had a follow-up period of at least 6 months (Table 7).

Table 7. Fluoroquinolones in the treatment of chronic bacterial prostatitis with a follow-up of at least 6 months[a]

Quinolone	Daily dosage (mg)	Duration of therapy (days)	Evaluable patients (n)	Bacteriological eradication (%)	Duration of follow-up (months)
Norfloxacin	800	28	14	64	6
Norfloxacin	4–800	174	42	60	8
Ofloxacin	400	14	21	67	12
Ciprofloxacin	1,000	14	15	60	12
Ciprofloxacin	1,000	28	16	63	21–36
Ciprofloxacin	1,000	60–150	7	86	12
Ciprofloxacin	1,000	28	34	76	6
Ciprofloxacin	1,000	28	78	72	6
Lomefloxacin	400	28	75	63	6

[a]Adapted from reference 61 by permission of Oxford University Press.

Norfloxacin, ofloxacin, and ciprofloxacin produced bacteriologic eradication rates of 60 to 86%. Because relapse is the main problem in chronic prostatitis, the follow-up period must be sufficiently long to state that the patient is cured. First clinical results with fluoroquinolones are promising, at least in patients with chronic bacterial prostatitis due to *E. coli* and other members of the *Enterobacteriaceae*. The therapeutic role of these drugs, however, needs to be defined by controlled studies and comparison with SXT. To achieve comparable results an internationally accepted protocol should be utilized. Such a protocol was propagated at the 3rd International Symposium on Clinical Evaluation of Drug Efficacy in UTI (56).

ROLE OF QUINOLONES IN PREVENTION OF UTI

Recurrent UTI in Women

As mentioned above, recurrent UTI is a common problem among pre- and postmenopausal women. In women who have frequent recurrences, strategies such as avoiding use of a diaphragm-spermicide for contraception and repleting estrogen should be used routinely. If these measures are not feasible or do not result in a reduction of UTI recurrences to less than three per year, antimicrobial prophylaxis is warranted. Several antimicrobial agents have been shown to be highly effective in reducing UTI recurrence rates to almost 0% when administered in low doses either postcoitally, thrice weekly, or daily (20). SXT, trimethoprim alone, and nitrofurantoin are among the most commonly used drugs for this purpose. The fluoroquinolones are also highly effective for this purpose, but in general are not the drugs of choice because of their expense and potential toxicity in pregnant women (71). Of the fluoroquinolones, the ones most commonly studied for prophylaxis include norfloxacin and ciprofloxacin. Norfloxacin was demonstrated to be significantly better than placebo in reducing the incidence of recurrent UTIs (0 versus 67%) over a 1-year period (66). Ciprofloxacin has been shown to be effective in a daily as well as postcoital regimen (48). More recent studies have evaluated once-weekly dosing of pefloxacin and fleroxacin (not available in the United States) and found these agents to be equally as effective in preventing recurrent UTI (43). A weekly regimen of 800 mg of pefloxacin has also been found to be equal in efficacy to a daily regimen of 125 mg of ciprofloxacin (43). None of these studies demonstrated the emergence of quinolone-resist-

ant *Enterobacteriaceae*, even after 12 months of prophylaxis. However, two breakthrough infections due to ciprofloxacin-resistant enterococcal and staphylococcal species were reported in the trial by Melekos et al. (48). As SXT resistance becomes more widespread among community-acquired *E. coli* UTI, use of fluoroquinolones for prophylaxis will likely increase.

Urological Surgery

Multiple studies have been published regarding the efficacy or cost-effectiveness of antimicrobial prophylaxis prior to procedures involving instrumentation of the urinary tract. In patients who have nonsterile urine prior to the procedure or who have a risk of endocarditis, use of perioperative antibiotics is standard practice (81). Among patients not meeting these criteria, use of perioperative antibiotics for prophylaxis of UTI remains controversial (83, 91). If prophylactic antibiotics are given, fluoroquinolones are often used because of their high bioavailability and long half-life. Studies have shown that prophylaxis with an oral fluoroquinolone (ciprofloxacin being the one most commonly studied) prior to transurethral urological procedures or transrectal biopsy of the prostate gland is efficacious in reducing the number of postprocedure UTIs as compared with no therapy or placebo (1, 38). A single oral dose of 500 mg of ciprofloxacin has been shown to be equivalent in efficacy to intravenous cefotaxime and cefazolin, as well as more cost-effective than the latter drug (13, 42, 84). In another trial, six doses of 500 mg of ciprofloxacin resulted in a post-prostate biopsy symptomatic UTI rate of 0.3% as compared with a rate of 1.7% among patients receiving only four doses of the same regimen (39). Rates of UTI in this study were lower than those reported in the single-dose studies above, but differences in the definition of UTI probably accounts for some of this decrease. The appropriate duration of prophylaxis remains to be defined, but is often dictated by the duration of postprocedure catheterization.

At least two studies have demonstrated that antibiotic prophylaxis prior to extracorporeal shock-wave lithotripsy for management of urinary tract stones does not reduce the number of postprocedure UTIs as long as the preprocedure urine is proven to be sterile. (5, 36). Obviously, in the setting of positive urine cultures prior to the procedure, antibiotic therapy is necessary (45).

Patients undergoing renal transplantation are at high risk of UTI and subsequent complications such as bacterial infection or rejection of the transplanted kidney. Thus, prophylaxis with SXT is often used for several months after transplantation. SXT has the added advantage of providing prophylaxis against other opportunistic infections such as *Pneumocystis carinii* and *Nocardia asteroides* and is less expensive to administer than a fluoroquinolone. In patients who cannot take SXT, use of a fluoroquinolone should be considered. Ciprofloxacin has been shown to be highly effective and well tolerated for UTI prophylaxis in this population (51).

Catheter-Associated UTI

Catheterization of the bladder is associated with high rates of bacteriuria, most of which are asymptomatic. The two strategies accepted for prevention of catheter-associated UTI include maintaining a closed drainage system and removing the catheter as soon as possible. Antimicrobial prophylaxis with a fluoroquinolone has also been demonstrated to be quite effective in decreasing and or delaying the onset of catheter-associated UTIs. However, emergence of resistant organisms almost predictably occurs with prolonged use of antimicrobials in catheterized patients, and thus routine usage of antimicrobial prophylaxis is not recommended. However, in selected patients who are at increased risk of morbidity due to UTI, such as renal transplant patients or those undergoing urologic surgery, use of prophylactic antibiotics during short-course catheterization may be of benefit (79, 92). When antibiotics are used for short-term catheterization, fluoroquinolones are very useful agents because of their activity and bioavailability. In addition, preliminary studies have demonstrated that ciprofloxacin may prevent bacterial adhesion and biofilm formation on urologic devices such as ureteral and prostatic stents (15, 76).

CONCLUSIONS

The pharmacokinetics, spectrum of activity, and bioavailability of the fluoroquinolones continue to make them highly attractive for treatment of infections involving the urinary tract. However, cost and development of antimicrobial resistance are two issues that need to be considered before choosing these agents over the other therapeutic agents that are available for UTI. Their use for treatment of uncomplicated cystitis or for prophylaxis of recurrent UTIs in women should be reserved for cases in which use of alternative agents is precluded by resistance patterns or patient factors. Fluoroquinolones have emerged as the drugs of choice for treatment of uncomplicated pyelonephritis and com-

plicated UTI, with the caveat that some of the newer quinolones that have lower renal excretion should be avoided for these infections. The fluoroquinolones are highly effective for management of both acute and chronic bacterial prostatitis and should be considered the drug of choice for these infections. Hopefully the need for antimicrobial therapy of UTI will diminish with better understanding of the pathogenesis of UTI and the development of non-antibiotic-based prevention strategies.

REFERENCES

1. **Aron, M., T. P. Rajeev, and N. P. Gupta.** 2000. Antibiotic prophylaxis for transrectal needle biopsy of the prostate: a randomized controlled study. *Br. J. Urol. Int.* **85:**682–685.
2. **Balfour J. A. B., and L. R. Wiseman.** 1999. Moxifloxacin. *Drugs* **57:**363–373.
3. **Basista, M. P.** 1991. Randomized study to evaluate efficacy and safety of ofloxacin vs. trimethoprim and sulfamethoxazole in treatment of uncomplicated urinary tract infection. *Urology* **37**(Suppl.):21–27.
4. **Barre J., G. Houin, and J. P. Tillement.** 1984. Dose-dependent pharmacokinetic study of pefloxacin, a new antibacterial agent, in humans. *J. Pharm. Sci.* **73:**1379–1382.
5. **Bierkens, A. F., A. J. Hendrikx, K. E. Ezz el Din, J. J. de la Rosette, A. Horrevort, W. Doesburg, and F. M. Debruyne.** 1997. The value of antibiotic prophylaxis during extracorporeal shock wave lithotripsy in the prevention of urinary tract infections in patients with urine proven sterile prior to treatment. *Eur. Urol.* **31:**30–35.
6. **Bjerklund Johansen T. E., R. N. Grüneberg, J. Guibert, A. Hofstetter, B. Lobel, K. G. Naber, J. Palou Redorta, and P. J. van Cangh.** 1998. The role of antibiotics in the treatment of chronic prostatitis: a consensus statement. *Eur. Urol.* **34:**457–466.
7. **Block, J. M., R. A. Walstad, A. Bjertnaes, P. E. Hafstad, M. Holte, I. Ottemo, P. L. Svarva, T. Rolstad, and L. E. Peterson.** 1987. Ofloxacin versus trimethoprim-sulphamethoxazole in acute cystitis. *Drugs* **34:**100–106.
8. **Blum, R.A., R. W. Schultz, and J. J. Schentag.** 1990. Pharmacokinetics of lomefloxacin in renally compromised patients. *Antimicrob. Agents Chemother.* **34:**2364–2368.
9. **Boerema, J. B. J., and F. T. C. Willems.** 1990. Fosfomycin trometamol in a single dose versus norfloxacin for seven days in the treatment of uncomplicated urinary infections in general practice. *Infection* **18:**S80–S87.
10. **Brittain, D. C., B. E. Scully, M. J. McElrath, R. Steinman, P. Labthavikul, and H. Neu.** 1985. The pharmacokinetics and serum and urine bactericidal activity of ciprofloxacin. *J. Clin. Pharmacol.* **25:**82–88.
11. **Brumfitt, W., J. M. T. Hamilton-Miller, and S. Walker.** 1993. Enoxacin relieves symptoms of recurrent urinary infections more rapidly than cefuroxime axetil. *Antimicrob. Agents Chemother.* **37:**1558–1559.
12. **Chien S. C., M. C. Rogge, L. G. Gisclon, C. Curtin, F. Wong, J. Natarajan, R. R. Williams, C. L. Fowler, W. K. Cheung, and A. T. Chow.** 1997. Pharmacokinetic profile of levofloxacin following once-daily 500-milligram oral or intravenous doses. *Antimicrob. Agents Chemother.* **41:**2256–2280.
13. **Christiano, A. P., C. M. P. Hollowell, H. Kim, J. Kim, R. Patel, G. T. Bales, and G. S. Gerber.** 2000. Double-blind

randomized comparison of single-dose ciprofloxacin versus intravenous cefazolin in patients undergoing outpatient endourologic surgery. *Urology* 55:182–185.

14. Collins M. M., R. S. Stafford, M. P. O'Lary, and M. J. Barry. 1998. How common is prostatitis? A national survey of physician visits. *J. Urol.* 159:1224–1228.

15. Cormio, L., P. La Forgia, A. Siitonen, M. Ruutu, P. Tormala, and M. Talja. 1997. Immersion in antibiotic solution prevents bacterial adhesion on biodegradable prostatic stents. *Br. J. Urol.* 79:409–413.

16. Costerton, J. W. 1999. Introduction to biofilm. *Int. J. Antimicrob. Agents* 11:217–222.

17. Cox, C. E. 1992. A comparison of the safety and efficacy of lomefloxacin and ciprofloxacin in the treatment of complicated or recurrent urinary tract infections. *Am. J. Med.* 92:82S–86S.

18. Craig, W. A. 1998. Pharmacokinetic/pharmacodynamic parameters: rationale for antibacterial dosing of mice and men. *Clin. Infect. Dis.* 26:1–12.

19. de Jong, Z., F. Pontonnier, and P. Plante. 1991. Single-dose fosfomycin trometamol (Monuril) versus multiple-dose norfloxacin: results of a multicenter study of females with uncomplicated urinary tract infections. *Urol. Int.* 46:344–348.

20. Engel, J. D., and A. J. Schaeffer. 1998. Evaluation of and antimicrobial therapy for recurrent urinary tract infections in women. *Urol. Clin. N. Am.* 25:685–701.

21. Ena, J., M. M. Lopez-Perezagua, C. Martinez-Peinado, M. A. Cia-Barrio, and I. Ruiz-Lopez. 1998. Emergence of ciprofloxacin resistance in Escherichia coli isolates after widespread use of fluoroquinolones. *Diagn. Microbiol. Infect. Dis.* 30:103–107.

22. Goldstein, E. J. C., R. M. Kahn, M. L. Alpert, B. P. Ginsberg, F. L. Greenway, and D. M. Citron. 1987. Ciprofloxacin versus cinoxacin in therapy of urinary tract infections. *Am. J. Med.* 82:284–287.

23. Goto, T., Y. Nakane, M. Nishida, and Y. Ohi. 1999. Bacterial biofilms and catheters in experimental urinary tract infection. *Int. J. Antimicrob. Agents* 11:227–232.

24. Guibert, J., and M. H. Capron. 1992. Uncomplicated urinary tract infections: lomefloxacin versus trimethoprim/sulphamethoxazole. *J. Int. Med. Res.* 20:467–474.

25. Gupta, K., T. M. Hooton, and W. E. Stamm. 2001. Increasing antimicrobial resistance and the management of uncomplicated community-acquired urinary tract infections. *Ann. Intern. Med.* 135:41–50.

26. Gupta, K., D. F. Sahm, D. Mayfield, and W. E. Stamm. 2001. Antimicrobial resistance among uropathogens that cause community- acquired urinary tract infections in women: a nationwide analysis. *Clin. Infect. Dis.* 33:89–94.

27. Gupta, K., D. Scholes, and W. E. Stamm. 1999. Increasing prevalence of antimicrobial resistance among uropathogens causing acute uncomplicated cystitis in women. *JAMA* 281:736–738.

28. Henry, D. C., R. C. Nenad, A. Iravani, A. D. Tice, D. L. Mansfield, D. J. Magner, M. B. Dorr, and G. H. Talbot. 1999. Comparison of sparfloxacin and ciprofloxacin in the treatment of community-acquired acute uncomplicated urinary tract infection in women. *Clin. Ther.* 21:966–981.

29. Henry, N. K., H. J. Schultz, N. C. Grubbs, S. M. Muller, D. M. Ilstrup, and W. R. Wilson. 1986. Comparison of ciprofloxacin and co-trimoxazole in the treatment of uncomplicated urinary tract infection in women. *J. Antimicrob. Chemother.* 18:103–106.

30. Hofbauer, H., K. G. Naber, M. Kinzig-Schippers, F. Sörgel, C. Rustige-Wiedemann, B. Wiedemann, A. Reiz, and M.

31. Hooton, T. M., C. Johnson, C. Winter, L. Kuwamura, M. E. Rogers, P. L. Roberts, and W. E. Stamm. 1991. Single-dose and three-day regimens of ofloxacin versus trimethoprim-sulfamethoxazole for acute cystitis in women. *Antimicrob. Agents Chemother.* 35:1479–1483.

32. Hooton, T. M., R. H. Latham, E. S. Wong, C. Johnson, P. Roberts, and W. E. Stamm. 1989. Ofloxacin versus trimethoprim-sulfamethoxazole for treatment of acute cystitis. *Antimicrob. Agents Chemother.* 33:1308–1312.

33. Hooton, T. M., and W. E. Stamm. 1997. Diagnosis and treatment of uncomplicated urinary tract infection. *Infect. Dis. Clin. N. Am.* 11:551–581.

34. Hooton T. M., C. Winter, F. Tiu, and W. E. Stamm. 1995. Randomized comparative trial and cost analysis of 3-day antimicrobial regimens for treatment of acute cystitis in women. *JAMA.* 273:41–45.

35. Horcajada, J. P., J. Vila, A. Moreno-Martinez, J. Ruiz, J. A. Martinez, M. Sanchez, E. Soriano, and J. Mensa. 2002. Molecular epidemiology and evolution of resistance to quinolones in *Escherichia coli* after prolonged administration of ciprofloxacin in patients with prostatitis. *J. Antimicrob. Chemother.* 49:55–59.

36. Ilker, Y., L. N. Turkeri, V. Korten, T. Tarcan, and A. Akdas. 1995. Antimicrobial prophylaxis in management of urinary tract stones by extracorporeal shock-wave lithotripsy: is it necessary? *Urology* 46:165–167.

37. Iravani, A., I. Klimberg, C. Briefer, C. Munera, S. F. Kowalsky, R. M. Echols, and the Urinary Tract Infection Group. 1999. A trial comparing low-dose, short-course ciprofloxacin and standard 7 day therapy with co-trimoxazole or nitrofurantoin in the treatment of uncomplicated urinary tract infection. *J. Antimicrob. Chemother.* 43:67–75.

38. Isen, K., B. Kupeli, Z. Sinik, S. Sozen, and I. Bozkirli. 1999. Antibiotic prophylaxis for transrectal biopsy of the prostate: a prospective randomized study of the prophylactic use of single dose oral fluoroquinolone versus trimethoprim-sulfamethoxazole. *Int. Urol. Nephrol.* 31:491–495.

39. Janoff, D. M., D. W. Skarecky, C. E. McLaren, and T. E. Ahlering. 2000. Prostate needle biopsy infection after four or six dose ciprofloxacin. *Can. J. Urol.* 7:1066–1069.

40. Jardin, A. 1990. A general practitioner muticenter study: fosfomycin trometamol single dose versus pipemidic acid multiple dose. *Infection* 18:S89–S93.

41. Jones, R. N., K. C. Kugler, M. A. Pfaller, P. L. Winokur, and the Sentry Surveillance Group, North America. 1999. Characteristics of pathogens causing urinary tract infections in hospitals in North America: results from the sentry antimicrobial surveillance program. *Diagn. Microbial. Infect. Dis.* 35:55–63.

42. Klimberg, I. W., G. H. Malek, C. E. Cox, A. L. Patterson, E. Whalen, S. F. Kowalsky, and R. M. Echols. 1999. Single-dose oral ciprofloxacin compared with cefotaxime and placebo for prophylaxis during transurethral surgery. *J. Antimicrob. Chemother.* 43:77–84.

43. Krcmery, S., J. Hromec, M. Tvrdikova, M. Hassan, and D. Gulla. 1999. Newer quinolones in the long term prophylaxis of recurrent urinary tract infections (UTI). *Drugs* 58:99–102.

44. Ludwig, G., and H. Pauthner. 1987. Clinical experience with ofloxacin in upper and lower urinary tract infections a comparison with co-trimoxazole and nitrofurantoin. *Drugs* 34:95–99.

45. Martin, T. V., and R. E. Sosa. 1998. Shock wave lithotripsy, p. 2735. *In* P. C. Walsh, A. B. Retik, E. D. Vaughan, and A.

J. Wein (ed.). *Campbell's Urology*, 7th ed. W. B. Saunders Company, Philadelphia, Pa.

46. McCarty, J. M., G. Richard, W. Huck, R. M. Tucker, R. L. Tosiello, M. Shan, A. Heyd, and R. M. Echols. 1999. A randomized trial of short-course ciprofloxacin, ofloxacin, or trimethoprim/sulfamethoxazole for the treatment of acute urinary tract infection in women. Ciprofloxacin Urinary Tract Infection Group. *Am. J. Med.* **106:**292–299.

47. Meares E. M., and T. A. Stamey. 1968. Bacteriologic localisation patterns in bacterial prostatitis and urethritis. *Invest. Urol.* **5:**492–518.

48. Melekos, M. D., H. W. Asbach, E. Gerharz, I. E. Zarakovitis, K. Weingaertner, and K. G. Naber. 1997. Post-intercourse versus daily ciprofloxacin prophylaxis for recurrent urinary tract infections in premenopausal women. *J. Urol.* **157:**935–939.

49. Montay G., R. Bruno, J. J. Thebault, J. C. Verginol, D. Chonsard, M. Ebmeier, and J. Galliot. 1990. Dose-dependent pharmacokinetic study of sparfloxacin in healthy young volunteers, abstr. 1248. *Program and Abstracts of the 30th Interscience Conference on Antimicrobial Agents and Chemotherapy*. American Society for Microbiology, Washington, D.C.

50. Mouton, Y., F. Ajana, C. Chidiac, M. H. Capron, P. Home, and A. Masquelier. 1992. Multicenter study of lomefloxacin and trimethoprim/sulfamethoxazole in the treatment of uncomplicated acute pyelonephritis. *Am. J. Med.* **92:**87S–90S.

51. Moyses, N. M., R. S. Costa, M. A. Reis, A. S. Ferraz, L. T. Saber, M. E. Batista, V. Muglia, T. M. Garcia, and J. F. Figueiredo. 1997. Use of ciprofloxacin as a prophylactic agent in urinary tract infectious in renal transplant recipients. *Clin. Transplant.* **11:**446–452.

52. Naber C. K., M. Hammer, M. Kinzig-Schippers, C. Sauber, F. Sörgel, A. Fairless, E. Bygate, K. Machka, and K. G. Naber. 2001. Urinary excretion and bactericidal activities of gemifloxacin and ofloxacin after a single oral dose in healthy volunteers. *Antimicrob. Agents Chemother.* **45:**3524–3530.

53. Naber, C. K., M. Hammer, M. Kinzig-Schippers, F. Sörgel, and K. G. Naber. 2000. Urinary excretion and bactericidal activity of levofloxacin versus ciprofloxacin in healthy volunteers after a single oral dose of 500mg, poster 10920. *In 9th International Congress on Infectious Dis.*

54. Naber, K. G. 1997. Antibacterial activity of antibacterial agents in urine: an overview of applied methods, p. 74–83. *In* T. Bergan (ed.), *Urinary Tract Infections*. Infectiology, Basel, Switzerland.

55. Naber, K. G. 2001. Which fluoroquinolones are suitable for the treatment of urinary tract infections? *Int. J. Antimicrob. Agents* **17:**331–341.

56. Naber, K. G., and H. Giamarellou. 1994. Proposed study design in prostatitis. *Infection* **22**(Suppl. 1):59–60.

57. Naber, K. G., K. Hollauer, D. Kirchbauer, and W. Witte. 2000. In vitro activity of gatifloxacin compared with gemifloxacin, moxifloxacin, trovafloxacin, ciprofloxacin and ofloxacin against uropathogens cultured from patients with complicated urinary tract infections. *Int. J. Antimicrob. Agents* **16:**239–243.

58. Naber, K. G., and E. M. W. Koch. 1993. Cefuroxime axetil versus ofloxacin for short-term therapy of acute uncomplicated lower urinary tract infections in women. *Infection.* **21:**34–45.

59. Naber, K. G., C. K. Naber, M. Hammer, M. Kinzig-Schippers, F. Sörgel, A. Fairless, and E. Bygate. 1999. Pharmacokinetics and penetration of gemifloxacin versus ofloxacin into prostate secretion and ejaculate after single oral dosing in volunteers, poster 92. *37th Annual Meeting of the Infectious Diseases Society of America*. Infectious Diseases Society of America, Philadelphia, Pa.

60. Naber, K. G., U. Theuretzbacher, M. Kinzing, O. Savov, and F. Sörgel. 1998. Urinary excretion and bactericidal activities of a single oral dose of 400 milligrams of fleroxacin versus a single oral dose of 800 milligrams of pefloxacin in healthy volunteers. *Antimicrob. Agents Chemother.* **42:**1659–1665.

61. Naber, K. G., and W. Weidner 2000. Chronic prostatitis: an infectious disease? *J. Antimicrob. Chemother.* **46:**157–161.

62. Nakano, M., M. Yasuda, S. Yokoi, Y. Takahashi, S. Ishihara, and T. Deguchi. 2001. In vivo selection of pseudomonas aeruginosa with decreased susceptiilities to fluoroquinolones during fluoroquinolone treatment of urinary tract infection. *Urology* **58:**125–128.

63. Neringer R., A. Forsgren, C. Hansson, B. Ode. 1992. Lomefloxacin versus norfloxacin in the treatment of uncomplicated urinary tract infections: three-day versus seven-day treatment. The South Swedish Lolex Study Group. *Scand. J. Infect. Dis.* **24:**773–780.

64. Nicolle, L. E. 2000. Pivmecillinam in the treatment of urinary tract infections. *J. Antimicrob Chemother.* **46**(Suppl. 1):35–39.

65. Nicolle, L. E., J. DuBois, A. Y. Martel, G. K. M. Harding, S. D. Shafran, and J. M. Conly. 1993. Treatment of acute uncomplicated urinary tract infections with 3 days of lomefloxacin compared with treatment with 3 days of norfloxacin. *Antimicrob. Agents Chemother.* **37:**574–579.

66. Nicolle, L. E., G. K. Harding, M. Thompson, J. Kennedy, B. Urias, and A. Ronald. 1989. Prospective, randomized, placebo-controlled trial of norfloxacin for the prophylaxis of recurrent urinary tract infection in women. *Antimicrob. Agents Chemother.* **33:**1032–1035.

67. Nicolle, L. E., T. J. Louie, J. Dubois, A. Martel, G. K. M. Harding, and C. P. Sinave. 1994. Treatment of complicated urinary tract infections with lomefloxacin compared with that with trimethoprim-sulfamethoxazole. *Antimicrob. Agents Chemother.* **38:**1368–1373.

67a. Nickel, J. C., L. M. Nyberg, and M. Hennenfent. 1999. Research guidelines for chronic prostatitis: consensus report from the first National Institutes of Health International Prostatitis Collaborative Network. *Urology* **54:**229–233.

68. Peng, M. Y. 1999. Randomized, double-blind, comparative study of levofloxacin and ofloxacin in the treatment of complicated urinary tract infections. *J. Microbiol. Immunol. Infect.* **32:**33–39.

69. Perry, C. M., J. A. Barman Balfour, and H. M. Lamb. 1999. Gatifloxacin. *Drugs* **58:**691–696.

70. Pisani, E., R. Bartoletti, A. Trinchieri, and M. Rizzo. 1996. Lomefloxacin versus ciprofloxacin in the treatment of complicated urinary tract infections: a multicenter study. *J. Chemother.* **8:**210–213.

71. Raz, R., and S. Boger. 1991. Long-term prophylaxis with norfloxacin versus nitrofurantoin women with recurrent urinary tract infection. *Antimicrob. Agents Chemother.* **35:**1241–1242.

72. Raz, R., B. Chazan, Y. Kennes, R. Colodner, E. Rottensterich, M. Dan, I. Lavi, W. Stamm, and the Israeli Urinary Tract Infection Group. 2002. Empiric use of TMP/SMX in the treatment of women with uncomplicated UTIs, in a geographical area with a high prevalence of TMP/SMX-resistant uropathogens. *Clin. Infect. Dis.* **34:**1165–1169.

73. Raz, R., K. G. Naber, C. Raizenberg, Y. Rohana, I. Unamba-Oparah, G. Korfman, and I. Yaniv. 2000. Ciprofloxacin 250 mg twice daily versus ofloxacin 200 mg twice daily in the treatment of complicated urinary tract infections in women. *Eur. J. Clin. Microbiol. Infect. Dis.* **19:**327–331.

74. Raz, R., E. Rottensterich, Y. Leshem, and H. Tabenkin.

1994. Double-blind study comparing 3-day regimens of cefixime and ofloxacin in treatment of uncomplicated urinary tract infections in women. *Antimicrob. Agents Chemother.* **38:**1176–1177.

75. **Raz, R., and S. Rozenfeld.** 1996. 3-day course of ofloxacin versus cefalexin in the treatment of urinary tract infections in postmenopausal women. *Antimicrob. Agents Chemother.* **40:**2200–2201.

76. **Reid, G., M. Habash, D. Vachon, J. Denstedt, J. Riddell, and M. Beheshti.** 2001. Oral fluoroquinolone therapy results in drug adsorption on ureteral stents and prevention of biofilm formation. *Int. J. Antimicrob. Agents* **17:**317–320.

77. **Richard, G. A., I. N. Klimber, C. L. Fowler, S. Callery-D'Amico, and S. S. Kim.** 1998. Levofloxacin versus ciprofloxacin versus lomefloxacin in acute pyelonephritis. *Urology* **52:**51–55.

78. **Sahm, D. F., C. Thornsberry, D. C. Mayfield, M. E. Jones, and J. A. Karlowsky.** 2001. Multidrug-resistant urinary tract isolates of *Escherichia coli:* prevalence and patient demographics in the United States in 2000. *Antimicrob. Agents Chemother.* **45:**1402–1406.

79. **Saint, S., and B. Lipsky.** 1999. Preventing catheter-related bacteriuria: Should we? Can we? How? *Arch. Intern. Med.* **159:**800–808.

80. **Sandberg, T., G. Englund, K. Lincoln, and L. G. Nilsson.** 1990. Randomised double-blind study of norfloxacin and cefadroxil in the treatment of acute pyelonephritis. *Eur. J. Clin. Mircrobiol. Infect. Dis.* **9:**317–323.

81. **Schaeffer, A. J.** 1998. Antimicrobial prophylaxis for transurethral procedures, p. 561. *In* P. C. Walsh, A. B. Retik, E. D. Vaughan, and A. J. Wein (ed.). *Campbell's Urology*, 7th ed. W. B. Saunders Company, Philadelphia, Pa.

82. **Schaeffer, A. J.** Prostatitis: US perspective. *Int. J. Antimicrob. Agents* **11:**205–211.

83. **Schneider, R. E.** 1982. Single-blind comparison of cinoxacin and nitrofurantoin in the treatment of urinary tract infection. *Clin. Ther.* **4:**390–394.

84. **Sieber, P. R., F. M. Rommel, V. E. Agusta, J. A. Breslin, H. W. Huffnagle, and L. E. Harpster.** 1997. Antibiotic prophylaxis in ultrasound guided transrectal prostate biopsy. *J. Urol.* **157:**2199–2200.

85. **Spencer, R. C., and T. P Cole.** 1992. Ofloxacin versus trimethoprim and co-trimoxazole in the treatment of uncomplicated urinary tract infection in general practice. *Br. J. Clin. Pract.* **46:**30–33.

86. **Stahlberg, H. J., K. G. Göhler, M. Guillaume, and A. Mignot.** 1997. Multiple-dose pharmacokinetics and excretion balance of gatifloxacin, a new fluoroquinolone antibiotic, following oral administration to healthy caucasian volunteers, abstr. A 71. *Program and Abstracts of the 37th Interscience Conference on Antimicrobial Agents and Chemotherapy.* American Society for Microbiology, Washington, D.C.

87. **Stass, H. H., A. Dalhoff, D. Kubitza, and G. Ahr.** 1998. Pharmacokinetic, safety, and tolerability of ascending single doses of moxifloxacin, a new 8-methoxyquinolone, administered to healthy subjects. *Antimicrob. Agents Chemother.* **42:**2060–2065.

88. **Stein, G. E., N. Mummaw, E. J. C. Goldstein, E. J. Boyko, L. B. Reller, T. O. Kurtz, K. Miller, and C. E. Cox.** 1987. A multicenter comparative trial of three-day norfloxacin vs. ten-day sulfamethoxazole and trimethoprim for the treatment of uncomplicated urinary tract infections. *Arch. Intern. Med.* **147:**1760–1762.

89. **Talan, D. A., W. E. Stamm, T. M. Hooton, G. J. Moran, T. Burke, A. Iravani, J. Reuning-Scherer, and D. A. Church.** 2000. Comparison of ciprofloxacin (7 days) and trimethoprim-sulfamethoxazole (14 days) for acute uncomplicated pyelonephritis in women: a randomized trial. *JAMA* **283:**1583–1590.

90. **The Urinary Tract Infection Study Group.** 1987. Coordinated multicenter study of norfloxacin versus trimethoprim-sulfamethoxazole treatment of symptomatic urinary tract infections. *J. Infect. Dis.* **155:**170–177.

91. **Tsugawa, M., K. Monden, Y. Nasu, H. Kumon, and H. Ohmori.** 1998. Prospective randomized comparative study of antibiotic prophylaxis in urethrocystoscopy and urethrocystography. *Int. J. Urol.* **5:**441–443.

92. **Warren, J. W.** 2001. Catheter-associated urinary tract infections. *Int. J. Antimicrob. Agents* **17:**299–303.

93. **Warren, J. W., E. Abrutyn, J. R. Hebel, J. R. Johnson, A. J. Schaeffer, and W. E. Stamm.** 1999. Guidelines for antimicrobial treatment of uncomplicated acute bacterial cystitis and acute pyelonephritis in women. Infectious Diseases Society of America (IDSA). *Clin. Infect. Dis.* **29:**745–758.

94. **Weidekamm, E, R. Portmann, K. Suter, C. Partos, D. Dell, and P. W. Lucker.** 1987. Single- and multiple- dose pharmacokinetics of fleroxacin, a trifluorinated quinolone in humans. *Antimicrob. Agents Chemother.* **31:**1909–1914.

95. **Weidner W., H. G. Schiefer, H. Krauss, C. H. Jantos, H. J. Fredrich, and M. Altmannsberger.** 1991. Chronic prostatitis: a thorough search for etiologically involved microorganisms in 1.461 patients. *Infection* **19**(Suppl. 3):119–125.

96. **Well, M., K. G. Naber, M. Kinzig-Schippers, and F. Sörgel.** 1998. Urinary bactericidal activity and pharmacokinetics of enoxacin versus norfloxacin and ciprofloxacin in healthy volunteers after a single oral dose. *Int. J. Antimicrob. Agents* **10:**31–38.

97. **Wenninger, K., J. R. Heiman, I. Rothman, J. P. Berghuis, and R. E. Berger.** 1996. Sickness impact of chronic nonbacterial prostatitis and its correlates. *J. Urol.* **155:**965–968.

98. **Wise, R., D. Lister, C. A. M. McNulty, D. Griggs, and J. M. Andrews.** 1986. The comparative pharmacokinetics of five quinolones. *J. Antimicrob. Chemother.* **18**(Suppl. D): 71–81.

99. **Wolf, R., R. Eberl, A. Dundy, N. Mertz, T. Chang, J. R. Goulet, and J. Latts.** 1984. The clinical pharmacokinetics and tolerance of enoxacin in healthy volunteers. *J. Antimicrob. Chemother.* **14:**63–69.

Quinolone Antimicrobial Agents, 3rd ed.
Edited by David C. Hooper and Ethan Rubinstein
© 2003 ASM Press, Washington, D.C.

Chapter 10

Use of Quinolones for Treatment of Sexually Transmitted Diseases

ROSANNA W. PEELING AND ALLAN R. RONALD

Bacterial sexually transmitted diseases (STDs) are a global public health problem. The annual incidence of bacterial STDs exceeds 100,000,000 (156). Unrecognized, asymptomatic, or latent infections may make this number closer to 200,000,000. Table 1 depicts the bacterial STDs that are discussed in this chapter and identifies acute presentations and sequelae.

Bacterial STDs, specifically those caused by *Chlamydia trachomatis* and *Neisseria gonorrhoeae*, are responsible for serious morbidity in women including pelvic inflammatory disease, ectopic pregnancy, tubal infertility, chronic pelvic pain, neonatal infection, and increased risks of acquiring or transmitting human immunodeficiency virus (HIV) (48). The incidence of these sequelae are increasing dramatically in some societies with particular consequence to reproductive health in women and the well being of their offspring (24).

Programs to control STDs are different from other infectious diseases for the following reasons.

- Individuals and societies stigmatize and often denigrate individuals with these infections. Also, these infections tend to occur more commonly among individuals who are socioeconomically disadvantaged, and consequently health programs for STDs are given a lower priority in many societies.
- STDs are largely transmitted by individuals who are asymptomatic and usually unaware of their infection.
- A core group of vulnerable individuals or "high-frequency transmitters" are responsible for maintaining these infections in society through their frequent changes of sexual partners and their social mixing patterns. Effective treatment removes them from the chain of transmission and may prevent many individuals from being infected (20).

- The sequelae of these infections usually occur after an interval of months to years and may not be linked to previous episodes of STDs by either health care providers or the patient.
- Many treatment programs depend on syndrome recognition with treatment based on probabilities of one or more pathogens being present. In as many as 30% of patients, more than one bacterial pathogen is present, requiring concurrent treatment.
- Frequently treatment is empiric because laboratory confirmation is not available or delayed.
- An individual with an STD requires education and counseling with regard to risky sexual behavior and contact tracing as well as effective treatment.
- Some bacterial STDs, specifically *N. gonorrhoeae* and *Haemophilus ducreyi*, have rapidly developed resistance to a wide variety of treatment regimens. Both plasmid-mediated and chromosomally mediated resistance occurs. Strategies to prevent the emergence of resistance to newer agents, particularly the quinolones, need to be considered in their initial clinical evaluation and subsequent use.
- Conventional STDs, specifically chancroid and perhaps genital herpes, syphilis, and gonococcal and chlamydial infections, are implicated as cofactors in the transmission of HIV (6, 48). As a result, efforts to control and, if possible, markedly reduce the incidence of these infections are mandated by the importance of strategies to slow the sexual spread of HIV infection (73).

IDEAL DRUGS FOR BACTERIAL STDs

No treatment regimen meets all expectations. However, critiera are being established that can be

Rosanna W. Peeling • The Sexually Transmitted Diseases Diagnostics Initiative, The World Health Organization, Geneva, Switzerland.
Allan R. Ronald • Division of Infectious Diseases, St. Boniface Hospital, 409 Tache Avenue, Winnipeg, Manitoba, Canada R2H 2A6.

Table 1. Clinical manifestations of bacterial STDs

STD pathogen	Illness	Manifestation(s) in:		
		Males	Females	Infants
Neisseria gonorrhoeae	Acute illness	Urethritis Conjunctivitis Proctitis Epididymitis	Cervicitis Endometritis Urethritis Conjunctivitis Proctitis Salpingitis Perihepatitis	Conjunctivitis
	Sequelae	Urethralitis Stricture	Ectopic pregnancy Tubal infertility Pelvic pain syndrome	Blindness
Chlamydia trachomatis[a]	Acute illness	Urethritis Conjunctivitis Proctitis Epididymitis Lymphogranuloma venereum[b]	Cervicitis Urethritis Conjunctivitis Proctitis Salpingitis Endometritis Perihepatitis Lymphogranuloma venereum[b]	Conjunctivitis Pneumonia
	Sequelae	Reiter's syndrome	Reiter's syndrome Pelvic pain syndrome Ectopic pregnancy Tubal infertility	
Treponema pallidum	Acute illness	Genital ulcers	Genital ulcers	Congenital syphilis
	Sequelae	Proctitis	Proctitis	Late manifestation of congenital syphilis
		Secondary & tertiary syphilis	Secondary & tertiary syphilis	
Haemophilus ducreyi		Genital ulcer with buboswith	Genital ulcer with buboswith	None
Mycoplasma hominis		None proven	Possible PID Postpartum pyrexia	None proven
Mycoplasma genitalium		Urethritis	Endometritis	
Ureaplasma urealyticum		Probable urethritis	None proven	Pneumonia
Bacterial vaginosis associated organisms		None	Bacterial vaginosis	None

[a] Complications of pregnancy are not included.
[b] Limited to unique serovars of *C. trachomatis*.

used to judge the potential therapeutic value of proposed regimens. Many of these arise from unique features of bacterial STDs. At present they can be summarized as follows:

- A single dose can be prescribed and administered so that cure is not dependent on patient compliance.
- Oral administration is possible with predictable results in all patients.
- Affordable costs that are not a deterrent to individual or government purchases.
- Wide distribution in the body, particularly on mucosal surfaces, to ensure predictable eradication of the pathogen not only at the genital site but also at other sites in which it may reside. This is especially important for patients with gonococcal infections who may have concurrent rectal or pharyngeal infection.

- The overlapping presentations of *N. gonorrhoeae* and *C. trachomatis* make syndrome diagnosis and treatment essential. Effectiveness against each of these pathogens is essential.
- Cure of incubating syphilis in patients presenting with urethritis or other genital syndromes. *Treponema pallidum* has an incubation period of several weeks before serologic evidence or clinical illness is apparent. Regimens for gonococcal infections such as amoxicillin that cure incubating *T. pallidum* infection have been considered to be advantageous.
- The probability of cure should be sufficiently high that follow-up cultures are not necessary. For gonococcal infection, this essentially means cure rates of at least 98%.
- The regimens need to be safe because they will usually be administered in outpatient settings and often prescribed by individuals other than

physicians. They should be safe for pregnant and lactating women as well as for adolescents and infants. The quinolones are specifically contraindicated in pregnancy, and while breast-feeding as well as during childhood.

- The regimen can be used for empiric treatment of contacts who are usually asymptomatic and uncertain of the necessity of treatment.
- Resistance does not appear either during treatment or as a result of an epidemiological shift in bacterial populations.

DURATION OF TREATMENT

During the 1970s, studies by Jaffe et al. (70) showed that the major determinant of cure for gonococcal infection was the MIC for *N. gonorrhoeae* and the length of time that the concentration of the therapeutic agent remained above the MIC. A level in serum of about four times the MIC for 10 h was required for penicillin to cure gonococcal urethritis. Similar studies for *H. ducreyi* showed that antibacterial levels need to exceed the MIC for 36 to 48 h to cure chancroid (43). Recent studies have demonstrated that concentration-dependent bactericidal activity allows some antiinfective agents to be much more effective if the levels substantially exceed the MIC for the infecting organism. The quinolones in particular are an example of this phenomenen. As a result, the quinolones that are well absorbed with levels in plasma/tissue 10 to 100 times the MIC for the organism kill more rapidly than do the β-lactams which lack "concentration-dependent" killing activity (87, 88, 90). This has made it possible for some of the quinolones to be excellent drugs for single-dose treatment of a variety of infections including *N. gonorrhoeae* and *H. ducreyi*. In a study of 14 patients, *N. gonorrhoeae* was eliminated from the urogenital tract and urine within 4 h, and from semen by 24 h after treatment with a single oral dose of 500 mg of ciprofloxacin (56).

The minimal period of therapy for chlamydial infections has not been adequately determined, but most regimens are prescribed for 7 to 10 days. At least two studies demonstrated that a 5-day course of treatment with quinolones resulted in an excess of treatment failures (79, 96).

GUIDELINES FOR THE TREATMENT OF STDS

Recommendations for the treatment of STDs have been published by public health agencies in the United States, Canada, and United Kingdom and, more recently, by the World Health Organization (7, 26, 61, 155). In the most recent guidelines, the clinical management of all STDs was updated and recommended treatment regimens were identified. A significant number of publications are now identifying the role of the quinolones for bacterial STDs.

In the United States, guidelines for the design and conduct of clinical trials of therapeutic agents for STDs and other infectious diseases have been established (57). These enable both pharmaceutical companies and investigators to design more appropriate microbiologic and clinical treatment trials with outcomes that meet the expectations of patients and their care providers.

CHLAMYDIA TRACHOMATIS INFECTION

Introduction

The biphasic life cycle of *C. trachomatis* presents unique challenges for antimicrobial therapy. The infectious extracellular form, the elementary body, is metabolically inert and is therefore not susceptible to antimicrobial agents whose activity requires DNA or protein synthesis. The intracellular reticulate body multiplies inside a membrane-bound inclusion in the host cell. An antimicrobial agent must therefore gain access to the multiplying chlamydia through the host cell and cross the inclusion membrane. The life cycle of chlamydiae is 48 to 72 h, considerably longer than that of *N. gonorrhoeae*, hence requiring that drug levels be maintained above the MIC for several days. This requirement is supported by the study of Kawada et al. in which 42% of 67 patients with chlamydial urethritis treated for 5 days with ofloxacin remained culture positive compared with only 3% of 95 patients treated for 10 days (79). Mikamo et al. found that 56% of 18 women treated with a 5-day regimen of levofloxacin at 300 mg thrice daily remained culture positive on follow-up compared with 12% of 33 women and 11% of 35 women treated with 7- and 14-day regimens at the same dosage respectively (96). However, a prolonged regimen often leads to inadequate compliance because of symptomatic resolution prior to microbiological cure.

About one-third of chlamydial infections lead to complications in women (25). Failure to eradicate *C. trachomatis* completely in symptomatic women or to detect and treat infection in asymptomatic women may permit latent or persistent infections, which have been associated with adverse long-term sequelae of pelvic inflammatory disease, ectopic pregnancy, and tubal infertility (34, 123). A population-based study in Seattle, Wash., has demonstrated the cost-effectiveness of screening and treating cervical chlamydial infections in the prevention of pelvic inflammatory disease (119). The goals of curing the infection, interrupting transmission, and preventing sequelae in the upper genital tract are all essential outcomes of treatment for genital chlamydial infections.

Microbiological Studies

Standardized procedures for *in vitro* antimicrobial susceptibility testing for chlamydia have not been widely accepted. Parameters that can give rise to variability in results have been reviewed (44, 134). Inoculum size, time of antimicrobial addition, and definition of end points (minimum inhibitory and bactericidal concentrations) must be standardized. Above all, studies to determine the relevance of these values to immediate and long-term therapeutic outcomes are required.

The range of MICs at which 90% of the isolates tested are inhibited (MIC_{90}s) of the quinolones and other relevant therapeutic agents against *C. trachomatis* are shown in Table 2. The more recent fluoroquinolones, such as ofloxacin, sparfloxacin, levofloxacin, grepafloxacin, and moxifloxacin, are clearly superior to norfloxacin, ciprofloxacin, fleroxacin, and pefloxacin. However, both fleroxacin and pefloxacin have a longer serum half-life (10 to 12 h) and may be able to sustain activity against *C. trachomatis* with appropriate dosing. The therapeutic ratio for each quinolone, estimated as a ratio of its estimated serum or tissue concentration to the mean in vitro activity, suggests that ofloxacin, sparfloxacin, levofloxacin, and moxifloxacin achieve adequate tissue to MIC ratios (Table 2).

Although true resistance has not been reported for *C. trachomatis* to date, resistance to the fluoroquinolones can be selected in vitro by exposing a reference strain to four passages in culture in the presence of ofloxacin and sparfloxacin at subinhibitory concentrations of 0.5 and 0.015 mg/liter respectively (35). The mutants exhibit high-level resistance mapped to the quinolone resistance-determining region (QRDR) of the *gyrA* gene with a Ser-83 to Ile substitution.

Heterotypic resistance for *C. trachomatis* was first reported by Jones et al. in isolates from patients who failed treatment with tetracycline (74). Heterotypic resistance is a phenomenon where the resistance phenotype is manifested by a small proportion of organisms in a population. A large inoculum is required to demonstrate its presence. Isolates

Table 2. In vitro activity of quinolones and other agents against *Chlamydia trachomatis*[a]

Quinolones	MIC_{90} range (μg/ml)	Estimated therapeutic ratio
Ciprofloxacin	0.25–2.0	1
Fleroxacin	0.5–2.0	1–2
Grepafloxacin	0.06–0.125	8–16
Lomefloxacin	0.5–4.0	<1
Levofloxacin	0.5–1.0	1–4
Moxifloxacin	0.03–0.125	8–16
Norfloxacin	4.0–16.0	<1
Ofloxacin	0.5–2.0	1–2
Pefloxacin	2.0–8.0	1
Rosoxacin	5.0–40.0	<1
Sparfloxacin	0.01–0.05	8–16
Other agents		
Azithromycin	0.03–0.125	>8
Erythromycin	0.063–0.25	4–8
Doxycycline	0.015–0.5	4–8

[a] Data from references 15, 38, 42, 45, 63, 81, 93, 109, 116, 117, 124, 135.

from Jones' study were resistant to tetracycline, doxycycline, erythromycin, sulfamethoxasole, and clindamycin but sensitive to rifampin and ofloxacin. In a follow-up study to determine the clinical significance of heterotypic resistance in *C. trachomatis*, the authors examined 270 isolates from the same clinic, collected between 1984 and 1989 (120). Heterotypic resistance was found in up to 69% of isolates each year, and patients with this pattern of resistance were more likely to fail therapy. Heterotypic resistance to the quinolones was recently reported in three patients whose isolates were resistant to doxycycline, azithromycin, and ofloxacin at concentrations >4.0 mg/liter (127). In vitro, it has been shown that a small proportion of *C. trachomatis* strains can survive high concentrations of doxycycline, azithromycin, and ofloxacin (134). Dreses-Werringloer et al. showed that a small proportion of *C. trachomatis* can survive in an altered state or persistent form in cell culture in the presence of 0.5 to 2 mg/liter of ofloxacin and ciprofloxacin (40). The persistent form showed reduced synthesis of structural proteins such as the major outer membrane protein, but normal levels of the 60-kDa heat shock protein, chsp-60. In this persistent form, the organism is nonculturable but remains viable, because it can resume normal growth after the quinolone is removed from cell culture. Human immune response to chsp-60 has been correlated with the development of reproductive sequelae such as pelvic inflammatory disease, ectopic pregnancy, and infertility (19, 21, 94). The clinical significance of heterotypic resistance and the relevance of MICs to the immediate and long-term therapeutic outcomes of *C. trachomatis* infection require further study.

A fascinating study in a mouse model of *C. trachomatis* salpingitis found that mice treated with sparfloxacin had normal fertility following recovery (141). This outcome was significantly better than that in mice treated with ofloxacin or minocycline.

Clinical Studies

New treatment regimens for *C. trachomatis* must at least show equivalence to established regimens. For the past two decades, a tetracycline, specifically doxycycline, has been the regimen most frequently chosen for treating *C. trachomatis*. Reasonably large clinical trials have shown that adequate cure rates comparable with those with doxycycline can be achieved with ofloxacin. The cure rates achieved with a 7-day course of twice daily dosing of ofloxacin have ranged between 90 and 100% (Table 3). Ofloxacin is now an alternate regimen for treatment of chlamydial infection in both the Canadian and U.S. treatment guidelines (26). Norfloxacin, enoxacin, lomefloxacin, and ciprofloxacin are inadequate choices and should not be prescribed for treating patients with proven or possible *C. trachomatis* infection.

Although once daily therapy with fleroxacin is reported to be effective for chlamydial infections, the adverse reaction rate has made it less useful (54) (Table 3). The more recent quinolones have not been as well studied, particularly in once daily dosing. Mikamo

et al. evaluated the efficacy of levofloxacin at an oral dosage of 300 mg thrice daily for various periods in 86 women with cervical chlamydial infection (96). The eradication rate was 44, 88, and 89% and the recurrence rate was 50, 0, and 0% for regimens of 5, 7, and 14 days, respectively. Phillips et al. conducted a multicenter double-blind randomized study of men with nongonococcal urethritis comparing the efficacy of oral sparfloxacin with doxycycline (107). The microbiologic cure rate was 97% (64/66 patients) for a regimen of 200 mg of sparfloxacin on day 1 followed by 100 mg for days 2 to 7, compared with 96% (73/76 patients) for doxycycline at 200 mg once daily for 7 days. A 7-day regimen of grepafloxacin, 400 mg once daily appears to be as effective as oral doxycycline, 100 mg twice daily for women with chlamydia cervicitis (95). The microbiologic cure rates were 96% (78/81 patients) for grepafloxacin and 99% (72/73 patients) for doxycycline. The once daily dosing for quinolones offers an advantage in terms of patient compliance.

The follow-up periods in clinical trials vary. Ideally cultures should be obtained at 1 week, 4 weeks, and 8 weeks after completion of treatment to ensure cure and to identify reinfections. Late-treatment failures have been documented when follow-up continues for longer than a week but unfortunately reinfections become difficult to distinguish from relapse. Also, the long-term reproductive health following treatment of acute or asymptomatic chlamydial infections has not been well established, and more long-term studies are needed.

Table 3. Treatment trials of oral quinolones for genital chlamydial infections

Drug/dosage (mg)	Location (reference)	Infection site[a]	Microbiologic cure rate (%)
Fleroxacin			
400 × 7 d	Austria (128)	U, C	21/22 (95)
	Norway (54)	U, C	6/10 (60)
600 × 7 d	United States (92)	U, C	100/104 (97) vs doxycycline[b] 122/129 (95)
600 × 7 d	Finland (72)	U, C	45/48 (94) vs doxycycline[b] 33/34 (97)
800 × 7 d	United States (110)	U	10/10 (100)
Ofloxacin[c]			
300 b.i.d. × 7 d	United States (16)	U	15/18 (83) vs doxycycline[b] 10/10 (100)
	United Kingdom (82)	U, C	38/38 (100) vs doxycycline[b] 28/28 (100)
300 b.i.d. × 7 d	United States (98)		23/24 (96) vs. doxycycline[b] 17/18 (100)
300 b.i.d. × 7 d	United States (46)	C	20/20 (100) vs doxycycline[b] 18/20 (90)
Levofloxacin			
300 t.i.d. × 5 d	Japan (96)	C	8/18 (44)
300 t.i.d. × 7 d			29/33 (88)
300 t.i.d. × 14 d			31/35 (89)
Sparfloxacin			
200 day 1,	Europe (107)	U	59/67 (88) vs doxycycline[b] 73/76 (96)
+ 100 day 2–3			
+ 100 day 2–7		U	64/66 (97)
Grepafloxacin			
400 × 7 d	United States (95)	C	78/81 (96) vs doxycycline[b] 72/73 (99)

[a] U, urethra; C, cervix.
[b] All doxycycline regimens are 100 mg b.i.d. × 7 days.
[c] b.i.d., twice a day; t.i.d., three times a day.

No studies are yet published in which the quinolones have been used to treat lymphogranuloma venereum.

Summary

Ofloxacin is a proven effective therapeutic agent in men and women for *C. trachomatis* when prescribed for at least 7 days. Limited studies suggest that fleroxacin, levofloxacin, and sparfloxacin may also be acceptable as alternate agents, but larger clinical studies are required to confirm their efficacy. Other new quinolones, specifically moxifloxacin and grepafloxacin, have not been actively studied with sufficiently large numbers of patients to determine whether they are adequate treatment for *C. trachomatis* infections.

GONOCOCCAL INFECTION

Introduction

The quinolones were found to be excellent drugs for the treatment of gonococcal infection. Cure rates approached 100% for most fluoroquinolones, with ciprofloxacin being the most widely used drug (42, 113). Many of these studies included large numbers of gonococcal strains that were penicillinase-producing (PPNG) or tetracycline-resistent (TRNG) (22, 139). The ease of single-dose oral administration, together with the safety and efficacy of the quinolones for the treatment of gonococcal infection, permitted treatment strategies to reduce rapidly the prevalence of gonococcal infection from populations at increased risk, specifically sex workers and their clients.

Despite this encouraging scenario, the development of quinolone resistance by the gonococci during the past decade has now altered our ability to use these agents with the expectation of uniformly satisfactory outcomes (71, 139).

Microbiological Studies

The in vitro activity of the fluoroquinolones against *N. gonorrhoeae* is depicted in Table 4. Ciprofloxacin is extremely active with a MIC_{90} of 0.001 to 0.06 when it was first introduced in the 1980s with serum level to MIC_{90} ratios of 50 to 100. By the mid-1990s, the MIC_{90} for ciprofloxacin has increased almost 100-fold to 0.125 to 0.5 mg/liter in parts of Asia. Although somewhat less so, fleroxacin and ofloxacin also are active in vitro. Sparfloxacin and the more recent quinolones are also effective in

Table 4. In vitro activity of quinolones versus *Neisseria gonorrhoeae*[a]

Drug	Estimated MIC_{90} range (µg/ml)	Therapeutic ratios
Before 1990[b]		
Ciprofloxacin	0.001–0.1	50–100
Fleroxacin	0.002–0.06	20–100
Lomefloxacin	0.008–0.063	10–100
Norfloxacin	0.0015–0.5	10–100
Ofloxacin	0.004–0.1	10–100
Pefloxacin	0.008–0.06	10–100
Sparfloxacin	0.001–8.0	
After 1990[c]		
Ciprofloxacin	0.004–8.0	1–>100
Gatifloxacin	0.002–0.5	4–>100
Gemifloxacin	0.008–0.125	4–>100
Grepafloxacin	0.004–0.5	4–>100
Levofloxacin	0.002–2.0	1–>100
Moxifloxacin	0.001–0.5	2–>100

[a] Data from references 12, 27, 52, 65, 75, 99, 121, 124, 132, 135, 138.
[b] MICs performed on fully susceptible strains mostly from industrialized countries.
[c] MICs performed on varying proportions of fully susceptible strains and strains resistant to ciprofloxacin or of decreased susceptibility to quinolones.

vitro and have serum to MIC_{90} ratios in excess of 100. Although unproven, it is possible that these high ratios of serum to maximum MIC for gonococci prevent the emergence of resistance due to gonococcal mutants that require multiple-step mutations to survive in the presence of the fluoroquinolones (58).

Clinical Studies

Single-dose ciprofloxacin in studies conducted in many parts of the world was shown to be as effective as any other treatment regimen for gonococcal infections (Table 5). Other quinolones, including fleroxacin, norfloxacin, ofloxacin, sparfloxacin, and levofloxacin, also achieved microbiologic cure rates approaching 100%. These drugs became agents of choice in most of the world for suspected or possible gonococcal infection including for syndromic treatment regimens (102). Unfortunately, with the rapid emergence of quinolone-resistant *N. gonorrhoeae* (QRNG) in Asia, ciprofloxacin must be abandoned.

Table 6 shows quinolone treatment trials in the QRNG era. A study in 105 female sex workers in the Philippines showed that ciprofloxacin efficacy was only 68% among isolates with reduced susceptibility to ciprofloxacin, including 49% with ciprofloxacin MIC of >4.0 mg/liter (5). The National Committee for Clinical Laboratory Standards has defined suceptibility as an MIC <0.125 mg/liter, decreased susceptibility as 0.125 to <2 mg/liter and resistance as greater than or equal to 2 mg/liter for the activity of quinolones against *N. gonorrhoeae*. Studies to deter-

Table 5. Treatment trials of oral quinolones for gonococcal infections up to 1996

Drug, dosage[a]	Location (reference)	Microbiologic cure rates (%)	Comments
Ciprofloxacin, 250 mg	Zambia (22)	83/83 (100)	31% PPNG, 25% CMRNG, all men
Ceftriaxone, 250 mg i.m.		81/82 (99)	37% PPNG, 23% CMRNG, all men
Ciprofloxacin, 500 mg	Kenya (102)	33/34 (97)	All women
Ceftriaxone, 250 mg i.m.		20/21 (95)	All women
Ciprofloxacin, 250 mg		79/79 (100)	All men, 67% PPNG
Kanamycin, 2 g i.m.		56/57 (84)	All men
Amoxicillin 3 g,		74/78 (95)	All men
AMC 500/250 mg + probenicid 1 g			
Penicillin 4.8 MU,		63/68 (93)	All men
AMC 500/250 + probenecid 1 g			
Ciprofloxacin			
100 mg	Belgium (8)	25/25 (100)	20 men, 5 women
250 mg		22/22 (100)	17 men, 5 women
Ciprofloxacin, 250 mg	United Kingdom (122)	59/59 (100)	All women
Ciprofloxacin, 250 mg	United States (64)	3/93 (100)	All women
Ceftriaxone, 250 mg i.m.		83/84 (99)	
Ciprofloxacin, 500 mg p.o.	United States (142)	171/171 (100)	Men, PPNG eradicated in 34/34 (100%)
		118/119 (99)	Women, PPNG eradicated in 32/32 (100%)
Cefuroxime, 1,000 mg		154/166 (93)	Men, PPNG eradicated in 35/36 (97%)
		114/118 (97)	Women, PPNG eardicated in 21/22 (96%)
Fleroxacin, 400 mg	Finland (86)	48/48 (100)	All men
Penicillin G, 2.4×10^6 units		48/48 (100)	All men
i.m. + probenecid, 1 g			
Fleroxacin, 400 mg	United States (126)	154/155 (99)	Men
Ceftriaxone, 250 mg i.m.		156/156 (100)	
		127/128 (99)	Women
		108/108 (100)	
Norfloxacin, 800 mg	Thailand (103)	94/94 (100)	PPNG: 142 men and 97 women treated and cured
	Singapore	145/145 (100)	Non-PPNG: 142 men and 97 women treated and cured
Spectinomycin, 2 g i.m.		82/82 (100)	PPNG: 144/145 men treated and cured
		159/161 (99)	Non-PPNG: 97/98 women treated and cured
Ofloxacin, 400 mg	Malaysia (112)	43/43 (100)	
Ofloxacin, 400 mg	United Kingdom (114)	50/50 (100)	39 men, 11 women
Ofloxacin, 400 mg	United States (125)	49/49 (100)	44% PPNG, 22% TRNG
			36 men, 13 women
Ofloxacin, 300 mg b.i.d. × 7 d	United States (16)	30/30 (100)	10% PPNG, all men
Doxycycline, 100 mg b.i.d. × 7 d		32/34 (94)	
Ofloxacin, 400 mg	United States (30)	47/47 (100)	34–36% PPNG, 27 men, 20 women
Ceftriaxone, 250 mg i.m.		42/42 (100)	25 men, 17 women
Pefloxacin, 800 mg	The Netherlands (143)	35/35 (100)	9% PPNG, all men
Cefotaxime, 1 g i.m.		32/32 (100)	

[a] i.m., intramuscular; p.o., orally; AMC, amoxicillin-clavulanic acid. Boldface type indicates a quinolone.

mine the relationship between in vitro susceptibility and clinical outcome of quinolone treatment show that the treatment failure rate is 1 to 4% in patients with MICs below 0.125 mg/liter, 8 to 12% for MICs of 0.125 to <2, 18 to 37% for MIC of >2 to 4, and 37 to 47% in patients whose isolates had MIC of 8 mg/liter or greater (5, 77, 111).

Studies with the more recent quinolones, such as gatifloxacin and grepafloxacin, showed microbiologic cure rates of 99 to 100% (Table 6; 65, 132). No treatment failures with gatifloxacin were reported for isolates with reduced susceptibility to ciprofloxacin (<0.5 mg/liter). The MICs of gatifloxacin for these isolates were 0.125 and 0.25 mg/liter, respectively. In this study, 9 of 20 women coinfected with C. trachomatis remained culture positive at follow-up (132). Empirical treatment of genital chlamydial infection must be combined with gonococcal treatment because a single oral dose of any quinolone is inadequate to cure chlamydial infection.

Studies in both men and women have shown gonococcal eradication not only from genital sites but also from the pharynx and the rectum (Table 7; 28, 64, 65, 125, 126, 142).

Table 6. Treatment trials of oral quinolones for gonococcal infections, 1997 to 2001

Drug, dosage (mg)[a]	Location (reference)	Microbiologic cure rates (%)	Comments
Ciprofloxacin, 500	Philippines (5)	48/72 (68)	49% of isolates had MIC ≥4.0 mg/liter
Cefixime, 400		25/26 (96)	
Gatifloxacin			
400	United States (132)[b]	116/117 (99)	Men
		100/101 (99)	Women
600		122/122 (100)	Men
		103/104 (99)	Women
Ofloxacin, 400		55/55 (100)	Men
		55/55 (100)	Women
Grepafloxacin, 400	United States (65)	147/149 (99)	All men, 47% PPNG, 21% TRNG
Cefixime, 400		145/150 (97)	
Sparfloxacin, 200	International (99)	96/97 (99)	Men
Ciprofloxacin, 250		92/94 (98)	

[a] Boldface type indicates a quinolone.
[b] >99% of the men and 98% of women in the study had isolates that were fully susceptible to quinolones.

The newer quinolones do not appear to have any advantage over ciprofloxacin. At present there is no reason to use them preferentially over ciprofloxacin in areas where ciprofloxacin resistance is not prevalent.

The Epidemiology of Resistance

The emergence of gonococci with decreased susceptibility to the quinolones initially noted in the Philippines in the late 1980s, and quickly spreading throughout much of Asia and now globally, has thwarted the continuing choice of the quinolones for the treatment of proven or suspected gonococcal infections (53, 71, 139). In the Phillipines, ciprofloxacin-resistant *N. gonorrhoeae* strains increased from 12% in 1994 to 73% in 1997 (139). High-level ciprofloxacin resistance (MIC, >4 mg/liter) in commercial sex workers increased from 9% in 1994 to 49% in 1997. In Hong Kong, the first

Table 7. Treatment trials of oral quinolones for gonococcal infections at other body sites

Drug, dose[a]	Study location (reference)	Microbiologic cure rate (%)	
		Pharynx	Rectum
Ciprofloxacin, 250 mg	United Kingdom (28)	3/3 (100)	4/4 (100)
Ciprofloxacin, 500 mg, p.o.	United States (142)	Men:8/8 (100)	1/1 (100)
		Women:13/13 (100) 25/25	(100)
Cefuroxime, 1,000 mg		Men:4/10 (40)	1/1 (100)
		Women:9/12 (75)	29/30 (97)
Ciprofloxacin, 250 mg	United States (64)	5/5 (100)	20/20 (100)
Ceftriaxone, 250 mg i.m.		6/6 (100)	21/21 (100)
Fleroxacin, 400 mg, p.o.	United States (126)	Men:5/5 (100)	2/2 (100)
		Women: 7/7 (100)	20/20 (100)
Ceftriaxone, 250 mg i.m.		Women: 9/9 (100)	24/24 (100)
Gatifloxacin			
400 mg	United States (132)	Men:3/3 (100)	
		Women: 5/5 (100)	20/20 (100)
600 mg		Men: 5/5 (100)	
		Women:14/14 (100)	16/16 (100)
Ofloxacin, 400 mg		Men:1/1 (100)	
		Women: 3/3 (100)	7/7 (100)
Grepafloxacin, 400 mg	United States (65)	8/8 (100)	1/1 (100)
Cefixime, 400 mg		10/12 (83)	3/3 (100)
Ofloxacin, 400 mg	United States(87)	6/7 (86)	12/12 (100)
Amoxicillin, 3 g + probenecid, 1 g		3/5 (60)	11/12 (92)
Ofloxacin, 400 mg	United States (30)	1/1(100)	2/2 (100)
Ceftriaxone, 250 mg i.m.		3/3(100)	5/6 (83)

[a] p.o., orally; i.m., intramuscularly. Boldface type indicates a quinolone.

reports of decreased ofloxacin susceptibility appeared in 1990, 2 years after the introduction of ofloxacin as a first-line drug for the treatment of gonococcal infection (77). From 1992 to 1994, *N. gonorrhoeae* strains with an ofloxacin MIC greater than 1 mg/liter increased from 0.5 to 10.4% in 1994 (77). In many industrialized countries, sporadic reports of decreased susceptibility of the gonococci to quinolones first appeared between 1991 and 1997. Characterization of these strains showed large numbers of phenotypes and genotypes suggesting sporadic importation of these strains from Asia (85, 139). Since 1998, the number of quinolone-resistant isolates of *N. gonorrhoeae* has increased dramatically in most industrialized countries, but these strains belong to fewer genotypes indicating either the importation of fewer strains or the endemic spread of quinolone-resistant strains (139).

In Asia, as many as one-quarter to one-half of gonococci are now resistant to quinolones (QRNG). Initially (1990 to 1994), with low-level and intermediate-level resistance, the quinolones continued to effectively treat 80 to 95% of patients despite the substantial 10-fold or greater increase in MIC. However, with the emergence of high-level quinolone resistance, treatment failure in 40 to 70% of patients now occurs routinely and has quickly reduced the value of the quinolones (5, 83).

In most industrialized countries, programs are underway to detect QRNG and to immediately ensure that they do not become widely disseminated as epidemic strains. This approach has worked reasonably well, and at present QRNG account for less than 2% of isolates (85, 139). However, if history with penicillin resistance can be expected to repeat itself, this will probably be a "losing battle" as quinolone-resistant isolates become the dominant strains in most resource-limited countries and spread continues to other countries. Fortunately, this has not yet occurred in most regions of Africa.

The emergence of fluoroquinolone resistance in Hong Kong from 1992 to 1994 has been associated with a rapid decline in PPNG from 26% in early 1993 to 4% in late 1994 and TRNG from 4.5 to 2.1% (78). Because quinolones can cure some plasmids, it is interesting to speculate that quinolone use might have eliminated these plasmids conferring penicillin resistance.

Mechanisms of Resistance

Recent studies have demonstrated the genetic basis of gonococcal resistance. Resistance is chromosomally mediated and, as yet, there is no evidence of plasmid-mediated quinolone resistance in *N. gon-*

orrhoeae. Among isolates from patients, quinolone resistance in the gonococcus may arise from one of several mutations in the genes encoding the DNA gyrase (*gyrA* or *gyrB*) or the topoisomerase IV *parC* gene. Quinolone resistance can also arise from the genes regulating drug diffusion through the outer-membrane porin proteins or active efflux of drug. Resistance is likely a stepwise process in which each mutation progressively decreases susceptibility by approximately eightfold (118). Mutations, in particular those involving genes that regulate drug diffusion, may confer cross-resistance to other quinolones or structurally unrelated antibiotics. Mutations involving the drug targets are more likely to give rise to dichotomous resistance patterns where the resistance is restricted to the drug involved in the selection. Low-level quinolone resistance has been correlated with single mutations in the QRDR of the *gyrA* or *gyrB* gene (130, 137). The increase in resistance is usually 2- to 10-fold, and it occurs at a very low frequency of between 10^{-8} and 10^{-9}. Further resistance is difficult to develop in vitro, and organisms with stable resistance to 0.1 µg/ml of ciprofloxacin have not selected in the laboratory.

Apart from selection of mutants, the gonococci can acquire the resistance genotype from a resistant gonococcal strain by transformation, a process in which DNA from a donor strain is taken up and recombined into the DNA of the recipient strain (129). Corkill et al. showed that in vitro ciprofloxacin resistance could be transferred to other gonococci which share the same porin protein type (29). The transformants showed a 20-fold increase in MICs from <0.003 to 0.064 µg/ml. However, this was 10-fold less than that of the parent strain. Resistance to tetracycline and chloramphenicol was not cotransferred with ciprofloxacin resistance, suggesting that these resistance genes are not linked (29). The uptake of ciprofloxacin was reduced in resistant strains, and this reduction was enhanced by further exposure to subinhibitory concentrations of ciprofloxacin. This finding suggests that the mechanism for controlling intracellular drug concentrations has at least several components that can be altered by mutation or induction. The protein 1-B is the porin which acts as the diffusion pathway through the outer membrane for the quinolones and mutations of this protein are a possible mechanism for slowing quinolone diffusion (29).

It is probable that mutants for which the ciprofloxacin MICs are below 0.1 µg/ml, selected during therapy, would presumably be killed following "a usual" therapeutic dose of ciprofloxacin. However, resistance could be postulated to occur in two scenarios. First, if patients are reinfected while quinolone levels are falling, these very low drug levels may select for strains with small increases in MICs. This occurrence would be most likely in individuals who have frequent reinfections or individuals who use the quinolones for prophylaxis against gonococcal infection. Second, the quinolones with lower serum to MIC ratios such as norfloxacin, rosoxacin, and enoxacin may more readily select low-level incremental resistance. This possibility is of particular concern because the experience to date suggests that use of these quinolones has been associated with the emergence of resistance. Additional studies should be done to determine whether quinolones with therapeutic ratios of less than 10 are appropriate choices to treat gonococcal infection.

Resistance emerging in clinical settings appears to be stable, and MIC as high as 32 µg/ml for ciprofloxacin have been reported from patient isolates (5). Patients infected with these organisms will fail treatment with ciprofloxacin. Table 8 shows examples of how high-level resistance phenotypes can be selected after treatment with various quinolones. It appears from these case reports that treatment of patients with *N. gonorrhoeae* which already have mutations in the *gyrA* or *parC* genes and decreased susceptibility to quinolones will allow the selection of additional mutations that confer high-level resistance (133). Multiple mutations in the QRDR, especially those containing a Ser-91 or Asp-95 substitution in the *gyrA* gene and a Ser-88 or Glu-91 in the *parC* gene, will result in isolates with MICs 40- to 200-fold higher than the pretreatment isolate (37, 138, 150). Although studies have shown reasonable efficacy using a single oral dose of 250 mg of ciprofloxacin, this lower dose may increase the risk of treatment failure in those patients with gonococci with decreased susceptibility to quinolones. Continued use of quinolones in areas with

decreased susceptibility may hasten the selection of high-level resistance phenotypes which may confer cross-resistance to structurally unrelated antibiotics such as the cephalosporins and tetracyclines (37). Monitoring of susceptibility patterns in different geographic areas and networks to disseminate information in a timely manner are essential to the control of gonococcal infections worldwide.

Lessons Learned from the Emergence of QRNG

What lessons are to be learned from the emergence of QRNG and its subsequent global spread? Will the widespread use of the quinolones result in the rapid appearance of resistance, or is the emergence of resistance an isolated rare phenomenon that will be sporadic and perhaps unimportant? Can the development of resistance be prevented by the use of quinolones with very high therapeutic ratios of serum drug levels to MIC_{90}? Are there any other ways of thwarting the emergence of resistance among the quinolones other than restricting their use? Could resistance have been prevented with better guidelines for treatment, e.g, if gonococcal infection had more restricted use of the quinolones (49)? Would the use of quinolones that had very low MICs specific for gonococci compared with ciprofloxacin permitted the emergence of resistance? Is much of the resistance due to the use of nalidixic acid, norfloxacin, and other quinolones that were less adequate and permitted resistance to emerge to all the quinolones? Concerns have also been raised about a possible contribution to resistance from use of counterfeit versions of fluoroquinolones with low potency in some developing countries.

Once resistance was detected, could resources have been used to limit its occurrence in resource-lim-

Table 8. Treatment regimens and the development of quinolone-resistant phenotypes[a]

Quinolone (reference), dose	Time of administration	Mutations		MIC (µg/ml)	
		gyrA	*parC*	tx drug	CPFX
Sparfloxacin (136), 100 mg t.i.d. × 5 days	Pre-tx	Ser91 to Phe Asp95 to Asn	Ser88 to Pro	0.25	0.5
	Post-tx	Ser91 to Phe Asp95 to Asn	Ser88 to Pro **Glu91 to Gly**	4.0[b]	4.0
Rufloxacin (150), 400 mg, single dose	Pre-tx	Asp95 to Asn		0.25	0.003
	Post-tx	Asp95 to Asn **Ser91 to Phe**		8.0	>0.12
Ofloxacin (37), 200 mg t.i.d. × 5 days	Pre-tx	Ser91 to Phe	Ser87 to Ile	1.0	0.25
	Post-tx	Ser91 to Phe	Ser87 to Ile	8.0[c]	1.00

[a] tx, treatment; CPFX, ciprofloxacin; bold type under mutations indicates new amino acid substitution in posttreatment isolate.
[b] Reduced susceptibility to structurally unrelated antibiotics and a fourfold decrease in sparfloxacin accumulation level were noted in the posttreatment isolate.
[c] Decreased susceptibility to cephalosporins was noted.

ited countries and prevent its continuing clonal distribution? What will be the incidence of introduction and spread within industrialized countries? Will conventional strategies for STD control, including surveillance for QRNG, prevent large endemic foci from occurring and becoming dominant in industrialized countries? At what level of prevalence does empiric therapy with quinolones become too great a risk for treatment of the individual patient? Are QRNG equivalent to quinolone-susceptible strains with regard to their epidemiologic and/or clinical virulence?

The loss of these agents is a tragedy and has importance with regard to our continuing efforts to maintain gonococcal prevalence at a low rate. It is a blow to our control strategies for gonococcal infection and for the routine inclusion of the quinolones in regimens to treat syndromically patients with urethritis, cervicitis, epididimitis, and pelvic inflammatory disease. The widespread use of quinolones aided STD control programs during the early 1990s in Thailand, Kenya, and other societies where their use was followed by a substantial reduction in both prevalence and incidence of gonococcal infections.

At least six reasons can be identified for the emergence of QRNG, and their individual contributions to the sum are not well understood. However, they should each be considered in all regions of the world in which quinolone resistance has not yet become a significant problem. Among the reasons we would include:

1. The use of quinolones such as nalidixic acid, rosoxacin, norfloxacin, enoxacin, lomefloxacin, and others with less in vitro effectiveness compared with ciprofloxacin for *N. gonorrhoeae*. There can be a 10- to 100-fold difference in quinolone MICs between ciprofloxacin and many of the other agents. Should we be introducing initiatives to insist that only ciprofloxacin or equally active quinolones be used for the treatment of gonococcal infections and for patients with clinical syndromes in which gonococcal treatment is indicated?

2. Has the use of very low doses of ciprofloxacin facilitated the emergence of resistance? In early studies, patients were treated with 100 mg with high cure rates (8). In retrospect, this choice of dosage appears unfortunate (58).

3. Is the widespread use of quinolones for treatment of many nongonococcal infections and their availability without prescription in some countries contributing the emergence of resistance?

4. Is the use of ciprofloxacin for empiric periodic treatment of commercial sex workers creating a setting in which resistance emerges as the level of ciprofloxacin falls and patients are exposed to gono-

cocci with low-level resistance? This occurrence very well may be the mechanism by which incremental resistance has occurred within most societies.

5. Is the lack of effective programs for STD control contributing in an important way to the spread of clonal resistance when it occurs? How can this problem best be resolved within all societies with varying resources of STD control programs?

6. Would it be effective for the quinolones to be restricted whenever low level and/or intermediate resistance appears within a society to forestall the occurrence of high-level quinolone resistance? Should each country or region have periodic surveys of resistance with the goal to attempt to control quinolone use in order to prevent the emergence of high-level resistance?

Strategies to make global decisions about antimicrobial use have not proven to be successful in the past. Although we should be very concerned about the emergence and spread of quinolone-resistant *N. gonorrhoeae*, it is unlikely that we can make a significant impact and do anything other than generally slow the emergence and spread of quinolone-resistant clones. More research in this area should be an urgent priority.

In industrialized countries, strategies to slow the increasing prevalence of high-level quinolone-resistant *N. gonorrhoeae* through case finding and intensive control measures will likely be successful, at least in the short term. These strategies should be pursued with enthusiasm and resources. In the meantime, ongoing surveillance for resistance must occur using sensitive and relatively simple techniques. Low-level resistance to the quinolones can be detected by screening with a 30-μg nalidixic acid disk during routine disk diffusion susceptibility testing (144). Gonococci with any level of resistance to any of the quinolones will show no zone around the 30-μg nalidixic acid disk.

The opportunities for interventions are more difficult in resource-limited societies. Cultures are only occasionally obtained and susceptibilities are rarely performed. In many of these countries, quinolones are being prescribed for a wide variety of infections with the probability that strains will be selected with increasing resistance and that these gonococcal clones will spread widely within patient populations. Klausner et al. showed that self-medication is correlated with the finding of resistant strains in commercial sex workers in the Phillipines (83).

Finally, will any of the new quinolones, including those still being investigated within the laboratory, enable us to reverse this trend? At present, there is limited evidence that complete susceptibility with MIC levels comparable with those routinely present in 1990 will be achieved with new quinolones in the future. However, efforts should continue to identify new quinolones effective against QRNG. Although the mechanism of action of quinolones is not entirely understood, it is likely that a two-step process is involved: the conversion of the topoisomerase-quinolone-DNA complex to an irreversible form and the generation of a double-strand break by denaturation of the topoisomerase to block bacterial replication (66, 118). Quinolones with similar activities against both targets may be less likely to select resistance.

Summary

The fluoroquinolones, especially ciprofloxacin, were effective single-dose therapeutic agents for *N. gonorrhoeae*. The emergence of resistance in the 1990s and its rapid spread throughout most of Asia with introduction of high-level resistance into every society is an immense tragedy. Strategies to prevent the emergence of resistance and to slow the spread of these isolates by utilizing global and regional networks already established for the monitoring of penicillin resistance should be a priority.

NONSPECIFIC URETHRITIS AND CERVICITIS AND THE GENITAL MYCOPLASMAS

Introduction

Nonspecific urethritis (NSU) in males and mucopurulent cervicitis (MPC) in females are elusive diseases to diagnose and treat. The initial diagnosis of NSU is, in most instances, made on the basis of a clinical presentation of dysuria and urethral discharge and a Gram stain in which no gram-negative diplococci are apparent, with at least 10 to 15 polymorphonuclear leukocytes (PMNs) per high-power field. In 30 to 50% of patients, cultures for *C. trachomatis* will be positive (67, 131, 148). In a minority of patients, usually less than 10%, herpes simplex virus, *Trichomonas vaginalis*, or urinary tract pathogens such as *Escherichia coli* are the etiologic agents. Although *Mycoplasma hominis* can be isolated from about 20% of patients with urethritis, no significant differences in isolation rates are noted between patients and controls. Antimicrobial agents with little or no activity against *M. hominis* are as effective in the treatment of NSU as antiinfective drugs that are active against *M. hominis*. The etiologic role of *Ureaplasma urealyticum* in NSU remains controversial. The most convincing studies are based on quantitative culture of *U. urealyticum*.

Although qualitative studies suggest that if sexual activity is controlled, patients with NSU and controls will each have a 50% isolation rate for *U. urealyticum*, placebo-controlled studies show improved outcomes if antiinfective agents that eradicate *U. urealyticum* are prescribed.

Studies have shown that the syndromes of NSU and MPC are sexually transmitted despite our failure to culture either *N. gonorrhoeae* or *C. trachomatis*. In several studies, between 13 and 25% of patients with NSU have had *Mycoplasma genitalium* isolated (36, 50, 68, 89). In a recent study from West Africa, *M. genitalium* was found in 10% of 659 men with urethral discharge, 18% of 209 men with urethral discharge negative for *N. gonorrhoeae* and *C. trachomatis*, and in 9% of 339 controls who had no symptoms (105). In this study the authors concluded that *M. genitalium* is an etiologic agent of urethritis.

Very few and very small clinical trials have evaluated the usefulness of the quinolones for *M. genitalium*. At present, we can make no recommendation about their usefulness. Philips et al. compared the efficacy and safety of sparfloxacin versus doxycycline in the treatment of NSU in men in a multicenter, double-blind randomized study (107). A 7-day regimen of sparfloxacin (200 mg on day 1 followed by 100 mg on days 2 to 7) eradicated *C. trachomatis* in 64 of 66 patients (97%) and *U. urealyticum* in 31 of 40 patients (78%) compared with 96% (73/76 patients) and 81% (38/47 patients), respectively, for a 7-day regimen of doxycycline at 200 mg once daily.

Microbiological Studies

The fluoroquinolones have limited in vitro efficacy against *M. hominis*, *U. urealyticum*, or *M. genitalium* (Table 9). The MICs are difficult to interpret but they are in the range in which many pathogens are not effectively treated with fluoroquinolones.

Table 9. In vitro activity of quinolones against *Mycoplasma hominis* and *Ureaplasma urealyticum*[a]

Quinolone	MIC$_{90}$ range (μg/ml)	
	M. hominis	*U. urealyticum*
Ciprofloxacin	0.5–4.0	0.5–32.0
Fleroxacin	4.0	4
Grepafloxacin	0.015–0.05	0.12–1.0
Levofloxacin	1.0	1.0
Lomefloxacin	4.0–8.0	8.0
Moxifloxacin	0.03–0.125	
Norfloxacin	8.0–32.0	
Ofloxacin	0.25–2.0	0.5–8.0
Rosoxacin	0.5–≥62.0	
Sparfloxacin	0.125–1.0	0.125–2.0

[a] Data from references 10, 39, 59, 63, 80, 93, 117, 140, 146, 152, and 153.

Clinical Studies

Clinical trials for NSU are summarized in Table 10. The satisfactory clinical response is the resolution of symptoms and signs with fewer than 5 PMN/high-power field in the urethral smear on a return visit (67). Unfortunately most trials have focused on the isolation of *M. hominis* or *U. urealyticum* (148, 151). At present, the evidence argues that neither of these pathogens is the etiologic cause of urethritis and presumably treatment should not be directed toward them. On the other hand, only very limited trials have been performed with *M. genitalium*. As a result, no recommendation with regard to use of the quinolones can be made.

Summary

The uncertain etiologies of sexually transmitted nonspecific urethritis and cervicitis other than *C. trachomatis* make definitive clinical studies difficult. However, the recent evidence that *M. genitalium* is an etiologic agent and responsible for urethritis and mucopurulent cervicitis, is an opportunity to perform well designed studies to determine the effectiveness of the quinolones for these patients. These syndromes can be persistent and lead patients to seek many treatments. At present, no recommendation can be made with regard to the use of the quinolones for the treatment of these syndromes.

CHANCROID AND *HAEMOPHILUS DUCREYI*

Introduction

Chancroid is endemic in many developing countries. Impressive evidence links genital ulcerative disease, particularly chancroid, to increased heterosexual transmission of HIV-1 and -2 (73). As a result, strategies to control chancroid with effective regimens are increasingly important.

Penicillin and ampicillin, the tetracyclines, the sulfonamides, and trimethoprim are now all ineffective in many parts of the world because of the emergence of resistance (14). Erythromycin, selected cephalosporins, amoxicillin with clavulanic acid, and the fluoroquinolones are now the agents of choice for treating chancroid (9).

Treatment regimens for chancroid have recently been further complicated by studies that report an increased failure rate in HIV-positive patients (145). A regimen such as ceftriaxone, prescribed as a single injection of 250 mg, cured essentially all patients. In a recent study of chancroid, the microbiologic cure rate was only 60% in circumcised HIV-positive patients, and fewer than one-half of uncircumcised HIV-positive patients were cured (145).

As a result, both antimicrobial resistance and increasing HIV seroprevalence in many populations in which chancroid is endemic make alternate treatment regimens a priority.

Microbiological Studies

The MICs of most of the fluoroquinolones for *H. ducreyi* have been reported (Table 11). The MIC$_{90}$ for *H. ducreyi* in most instances is similar to those of other very susceptible gram-negative organisms such as *N. gonorrhoeae* or *H. influenzae*. The strains are homogenous with essentially all strains susceptible to a narrow range of fluoroquinolone concentrations. To date, no resistance to any of the quinolones has been reported. *H. ducreyi* usually develops resistance to antibacterial agents through the acquisition of

Table 10. Treatment of nongonococcal urethritis and cervicitis

Drug, dosage[a]	Location (reference)	Cure rates (%)			
		C. trachomatis	*U. urealyticum*	*M. hominis*	Clinical
Ofloxacin, 200 mg b.i.d. × 7 days	Denmark (69)	36/43(84)			40/43(93)
Erythromycin, 500 mg b.i.d. × 7 days		24/31(77%)			43/51(84)
Ofloxacin, 200 mg b.i.d. × 7 days	Sweden and Denmark (100)	46/46(100)	6/6(100)	1/3(33)	(84)
Erythromycin, 500 mg b.i.d. × 7 days		34/36(94)	9/10(90)	0/5(0)	(77)
Ofloxacin, 300 mg b.i.d. × 7 days	United States (98)	23/24(96)	3/4(75)		12/14 (86)
Doxycycline, 100 mg b.i.d. × 7 days		18/18(100)	9/11(82)		12/12(100)
Ofloxacin, 400 mg × 7 d	United Kingdom (82)	38/38(100)			36/43 (84)
Doxycycline, 100 mg b.i.d. × 7 days		28/28(100)			31/40 (78)
Sparfloxacin, 200 mg day 1	Europe (107)				
+ 100 mg day 2–3		59/67 (88)	43/50 (86)		159/195 (82)
+ 100 mg day 2–7		64/66 (97)	31/40 (78)		173/201 86)
Doxycycline, 200 mg once daily × 7 days		73/76 (96)	38/47 (81)		176/212 (83)

[a] b.i.d., twice a day. Boldface type indicates a quinolone.

Table 11. Activity of quinolones and other agents against
Haemophilus ducreyi[a]

Quinolone	MIC range (µg/ml)
Nalidixic acid	8.0–32.0
Ciprofloxacin	0.007–0.016
Fleroxacin	0.008–0.25
Lomefloxacin	0.03
Norfloxacin	0.12–0.25
Ofloxacin	0.03–0.06
Pefloxacin	0.06–0.12
Rosoxacin	0.004–0.12

[a] Data from references 1, 14, 63, 84, and 124.

plasmids containing genes mediating resistance. Chromosomal quinolone resistance mutations in *H. ducreyi* have not been studied. However, ongoing monitoring of *H. ducreyi* resistance to antimicrobial agents must continue, in particular, in patients treated with the fluoroquinolones to determine whether incremental resistance by mutations of DNA gyrase will occur.

Clinical Studies

The quinolones have been investigated in clinical studies with chancroid (Table 12). In all studies, the quinolones have cured almost all patients with chancroid. However, only therapeutic agents with a prolonged half-life can be expected to cure chancroid with single-dose therapy.

Ciprofloxacin is effective as single-dose therapy if 0.5 or 1 g is used as the initial dose (9, 11, 13, 41,

90, 101). Fleroxacin is also effective as a single-dose regimen of either 200 or 400 mg (88, 97, 108).

No studies have been published on the efficacy of the fluoroquinolones in the sexual contacts of patients with chancroid. At present, treatment with a regimen similar to that used for the index case should be prescribed for all sexual contacts of patients with chancroid.

Summary

The quinolones are the agents of first choice for patients with chancroid. The ability to prescribe single-dose oral regimens, the lack of evidence for emergence of resistance, and the growing significance of programs to control chancroid all support the choice of these agents. The evidence that short courses of therapy may occasionally be less effective in patients who are coinfected with HIV requires ongoing investigation to determine which regimens are optimal for these patients.

GRANULOMA INGUINALE (DONOVANOSIS)

Granuloma inguinale is a cause of genital ulceration in some parts of the world, including Southeast Asia, India, Australia, and South Africa. Trimethroprim sulfamethoxazole has been the drug of choice.

In a recent study, granuloma inguinale in three patients was treated with a 14-day regimen of ciprofloxacin 500 mg twice daily with excellent results (2). Further studies are needed.

Table 12. Treatment of *Haemophilus ducreyi* infection: clinical trials

Drug, dosage[a]	Location (reference)	Microbiologic cure rate (%)[b]
Ciprofloxacin, 500 mg	Thailand (13)	43/43 (100)
Ciprofloxacin		
500 mg	Kenya (101)	39/41 (95)
500 b.i.d. × 3 days		40/40 (100)
Ciprofloxacin, 500 mg b.i.d. × 3 days	India (41)	15/15 (100)
Erythromycin, 500 mg q.i.d. × 7 days		15/15 (100)
Co-trimoxazole		8/15 (53)
Ciprofloxacin		
250 mg × 5 days	Malawi (11)	90/104 (87)
500 mg, single-dose		75/85 (88)
Erythromycin, 500 mg t.i.d. × 7 d		99/111 (89)
Fleroxacin		
200 mg	Kenya (88)	23/25 (92)
400 mg		19/23 (83)
400 mg	Kenya (108)	39/40 (98)
Rosoxacin		
300 mg	Kenya (55)	17/28 (61)
150 mg b.i.d. × 3 days		38/40 (95)

[a] b.i.d., twice a day; q.i.d., four times a day; t.i.d., three times a day. Boldface type indicates a quinolone.
[b] Microbiologic cure was achieved in 8/11 (73%) HIV-1 seropositive patients vs 35/37 (95%) of HIV-1 seronegative patients ($P = 0.07$).

PELVIC INFLAMMATORY DISEASE (PID)

Introduction

This syndrome is usually diagnosed and treated empirically, because microbiologic results are not available or inadequate. It is estimated that about one million women are treated for PID each year in the United States (24). Substantial epidemiologic and microbiologic evidence argues for the importance of *N. gonorrhoeae* and *C. trachomatis* in 50 to 60% of women with this diagnosis. As a result, the empiric therapeutic regimen must provide excellent antibacterial activity against both these pathogens as well as broad-spectrum coverage in selected patients for the *Enterobacteriaceae* and on occasion, anaerobes (60, 62, 104, 106). In many areas of the world, more than 20% of isolates are PPNG, and all women with PID should be treated with regimens effective against PPNG. Also, at least 20% of patients investigated by laparoscopic examinations have been erroneously diagnosed as having PID. Although laparoscopic diagnosis is now usually required for patients entered into clinical trials, it is not a routine practice (106).

An important therapeutic goal apart from the treatment of clinical symptoms is to preserve fertility by preventing further long-term complications of tubal obstruction and ectopic pregnancy. Most studies have not conducted adequate follow-up in patients and long-term sequelae and fertility outcome or prognosis are not determined. The approach of a second-look laparoscopy should be evaluated (17). Brumsted et al. (18) examined the reproductive outcome, in a retrospective study, of women treated for PID. Of the 27 women who attempted to conceive, 9 (33%) had an intrauterine pregnancy while 15 (56%) remained involuntarily childless. Three (11%) had tubal damage that resulted in an ectopic pregnancy during an average duration of 4.9 years after PID (18).

The current standard regimens for PID include ceftriaxone plus doxycycline with or without metronidazole, cefoxitin, or cefotetan plus doxycycline, or clindamycin plus gentamicin. All of these regimens provide reasonably adequate coverage for both *N. gonorrhoeae* and *C. trachomatis*. Since 1999, ofloxacin with or without metronidazole has also been suggested to be an adequate treatment regimen and achieves excellent levels in tissue (26, 51).

Clinical Studies

Ciprofloxacin has been prospectively studied in numerous randomized clinical trials and appears to provide adequate cure rates for patients with both *N. gonorrhoeae* and *C. trachomatis* (4, 33). However, the variable clinical efficacy of ciprofloxacin for *C. trachomatis* precludes this agent from being used as a single quinolone for patients with PID. Also the emergence and spread of resistance to the quinolones among *N. gonorrhoeae* make it mandatory that the quinolones be used only if it is known that at least 95% of *N. gonorrhoeae* in the population are susceptible to the quinolones.

Ofloxacin has been an adequate therapeutic regimen and the randomized clinical trials with this agent are summarized in Table 13. Essentially all patients with pretreatment cultures positive for *N. gonorrhoeae* had negative posttreatment cultures, and more than 90% of patients with cultures positive for *C. trachomatis* were cured (46). The new "respiratory" quinolones such as moxifloxacin have potential efficacy against both *N. gonorrhoeae* and *C. trachomatis* and could be used for PID. However, no large studies have been published to date.

M. genitalium is now emerging as a probable important cause of endometritis. Although requiring confirmation, it is probable that *M. genitalium* accounts for 5 to 20% of patients with PID in many settings. Its treatment remains uncertain and clinical trials are required.

Combinations of the quinolones with agents active against anaerobes have been investigated and they appear to be effective, but at present the evidence that an anaerobic drug must be added to the quinolones for the treatment of PID remains uncertain. However, the predictable absorption after oral administration of a quinolone such as ofloxacin, together with its limited side effects, makes this drug, either alone or in combination with metronidazole or clindamycin, a very attractive regimen for the outpatient treatment of mild to moderately severe PID. Well designed clinical trials with long-term follow-up to assess reproductive function remain a priority.

Summary

The quinolones, specifically those with increased activity against *C. trachomatis*, are useful agents for the treatment of PID. Unfortunately the emergence and widespread clonal-resistant *N. gonorrhoeae* are now limiting the usefulness of this regimen, and only if the prevalence of high-level quinolone resistance in a community is less than 5% can these regimens be prescribed with confidence of an immediate excellent response and satisfactory long-term outcomes.

Table 13. Pelvic inflammatory disease trials: comparative studies

Drug, dosage[a]	Location (reference)	Clinical		Microbiologic cure rates[b] (%)	
		Diagnosis	Cure rate (%)	Gonococcal	Chlamydial
Ciprofloxacin					
300 mg i.v.	United States (4)	Clinical criteria	10/10 (100)	7/7 (100)	11/12 (92)
750 mg p.o. b.i.d.					
Clindamycin, 900 mg i.v.,			13/15 (87)	4/6 (67)	6/7 (86)
450 mg p.o. q.i.d. + gentamicin, 1.5 mg/kg					
Ciprofloxacin, 300 mg i.v., 750 mg p.o.	United States (33)	Clinical criteria	31/33 (94)	22/22 (100)	6/7 (86)
Clindamycin, 600 mg i.v. + gentamicin,					
300 mg p.o. × 2–5 days (14 days for					
both regimens)			34/35 (97)	22/22 (100)	6/6 (100)
Ciprofloxacin					
200 mg i.v.	Finland (62)	Laparoscopy	15/16 (94)	3/3* (100)	6/6 (100)
750 mg p.o. × 14 d					
Doxycycline, 100 mg i.v.,			14/20 (70)	2/3* (67)	3/3 (100)
150 mg + metronidazole 500 mg i.v.,					
400 mg × 14 days t.i.d.					
Ciprofloxacin, 750 mg p.o. b.i.d. × 10 d	Germany (47)	Laparoscopy	18/22 (82)	1/1 (100)	8/9 (89)
Ciprofloxacin + metronidazole	Germany (47)	Clinical criteria	(92)		
Cefoxitin 2g i.m. + doxycycline			(87)		
100 mg p.o. b.i.d. × 10 days					
Ofloxacin, 200 mg b.i.d. × 3 wks.	France (76)	Clinical criteria	58/60 (97)		60/60 (100)
+ amoxicillin-clavulanic acid (1 g b.i.d.)		(84 endometritis, 34 salpingitis)			
Doxycycline 100 mg b.i.d.			56/58 (97)		56/58 (97)
+ amoxicillin-clavulanic acid (1 g b.i.d.)					
Ofloxacin, 400 mg b.i.d. × 10 days	United States (91)	Clinical criteria	122/128 (95)	47/47 (100)	18/18 (100)
Cefoxitin (2 g i.m.) + doxycycline			112/121 (93)	23/23 (100)	15/17 (88)
100 mg b.i.d. × 10 days					
Ofloxacin, 400 mg i.v. q12h + 400 mg	United States (104)	Laparoscopy	61/70 (87)	4/4 (100)	13/13 (100)
p.o. q12h × 10–14 days					

[a] Boldface type indicates a quinolone.
[b] Asterisks indicate coinfection with *C. trachomatis*.

EPIDIDYMITIS

Epididymitis occurs in about 1% of men with urethritis and is equivalent to ascending genital infection in women. The majority of infections, before the age of 50 years, are due to *C. trachomatis* or *N. gonorrhoeae*. In older men, urinary tract pathogens become the predominent etiologic agent. Anaerobic pathogens are uncommon.

The fluoroquinolones are potentially excellent therapeutic choices for epididymitis because of their favorable pharmacokinetics and broad-spectrum activity. Few clinical studies have been reported to date. Costa et al. studied the use of 800 mg of pefloxacin for 21 or 42 days in the treatment of 20 patients with acute epididymitis (32). A rapid clinical response was evident in all men. There was no relapse in 18 patients followed up for a year, although small epididymal nodules persisted in 25% of men. There was no significant difference related to the duration of therapy. Weidner et al. successfully treated nongonococcal epididymitis with ofloxacin (154).

SYPHILIS

The quinolones are not effective in animal models of *T. pallidum*. Veller-Fornasa et al. (149) reported the failure of a 3-day course of ofloxacin (100 mg/kg) to suppress *T. pallidum* in experimentally infected rabbits. This lack of efficacy was confirmed by Une et al. (147). At present, there is no evidence to suggest that the quinolones will have any role in the treatment of *T. pallidum* infection. Presumably patients coinfected with *T. pallidum* and another pathogen and treated with a quinolone will continue to have unmodified *T. pallidum* infection. This limitation should be considered in all patients at risk of syphilis.

BACTERIAL VAGINOSIS

The rationale for the treament of bacterial vaginosis (BV) is increasing as the microbiology of BV is better understood. BV appears to result from a shift of endogenous vaginal flora from hydrogen peroxide producing lactobacilli to anaerobes and, presumably, to *Gardnerella vaginalis*. Therapy with quinolone agents, such as ciprofloxacin, norfloxacin, and ofloxacin, has not been promising because of their poor in vitro activity against anaerobes (115). A review of MICs against *G. vaginalis* showed that MICs of rosoxacin, ciprofloxacin, ofloxacin, and enoxacin are in the range of 1.0 to 32 mg/liter. A clinical trial involving 27 women culture-positive for *G. vaginalis* showed that clinical cure was achieved in 70, 70, and 40% of women treated with 7-day courses of ciprofloxacin (500 mg b.i.d.), ofloxacin (300 mg b.i.d.), and norfloxacin (400 mg b.i.d.) (3). A clinical trial of ciprofloxacin 500 mg twice daily showed that although clinical cure was achieved in 17 of 22 women after 7 days, clue cells persisted in 11 patients, suggesting persistence of infection (23). Covino compared ofloxacin (300 mg twice daily for 7 days) with oral metronidazole (500 mg twice daily for 7 days) in a randomized double-blind trial in 27 women (31). Microbiologic failure was observed in 57% treated with ofloxacin and 8% treated with metronidazole ($P = 0.01$).

CONCLUSIONS

The quinolones are assuming a significant role in the management of patients with STDs. Their efficacy for gonococcal infection and chancroid is well established. Ofloxacin, levofloxacin, and perhaps sparfloxacin provide equivalence to doxycycline for the treatment of *C. trachomatis* infections. Presumably, syndromes such as PID, epididymitis, nonspecific urethritis, cervicitis, and possibly granuloma inguinale will be well managed by quinolones, either alone or in combination with drugs effective against anaerobes. However, at present there are still too few large clinical trials to identify the quinolones as the drugs of choice for any of these syndromes. The quinolones are not effective for syphilis or for bacterial vaginosis. No studies have yet been reported in which the quinolones have been used for either lymphogranuloma venereum or granuloma inguinale.

The quinolones are restricted by proscription against their use in adolescents and in women who are pregnant or at significant risk of pregnancy.

The role of the quinolones in strategic efforts to control STDs, particularly *N. gonorrhoeae* and perhaps to a lesser extent *C. trachomatis*, requires further study.

REFERENCES

1. Abeck, D., A. P. Johnson, Y. Dangor, and R. C. Ballard. 1988. Antibiotic susceptibilities and plasmid profiles of *Haemophilus ducreyi* isolates from southern Africa. *J. Antimicrob. Chemother.* **22**:437–444.

2. Ahmed, B. A., and A. Tang. 1996. Successful treatment of donovanosis with ciprofloxacin. *Genitourin. Med.* **72**:73–74.

3. Alegente, G., B. Marchi, F. Mugnaini, L. Toscano, and F. De Lalla. 1989. Treatment of *Gardnerella vaginalis* syndrome with new quinolones: preliminary results. *Rev. Infect. Dis.* **11**(Suppl. 5):S1308.

4. Apuzzio, J. J., R. Stankiewicz, V. Ganesh, S. Jain, Z. Kaminski, and D. Louria. 1989. Comparison of parenteral ciprofloxacin with clindamycin-gentamicin in the treatment of pelvic infection. *Am. J. Med.* **87**(Suppl 5A):148S–151S.

5. Aplasca de los Reyes, R. M., V. P. Mesola, J. D. Klausner, R. Manalastas, T. Wi, C. U. Tuszon, G. Dallabetta, W. L. H. Whittington, and K. K. Holmes. 2001. A randomised trial of ciprofloxacin versus cefixime for the treatment of gonorrhea after rapid emergence of gonococcal ciprofloxacin resistance in the Philippines. *Clin. Infect. Dis.* **32**:1313–1318.

6. Aral, S. O., and K. K. Holmes. 1991. Sexually transmitted diseases in the AIDS era. *Sci. Am.* **264**:62–69.

7. Association of Genitourinary Medicine and the Medical Society for the Study of Venereal Diseases. 1999. National Guidelines for the management of sexually transmitted diseases. *Sex. Transm. Infect.* **75**(Suppl. 1).

8. Avonts, D., L. Fransen, J. Vielfont, A. Stevens, K. Hendrick, and P. Piot. 1988. Treating uncomplicated gonococcal infection with 250 mg or 100 mg ciprofloxacin in a single oral dose. *Genitourin. Med.* **64**:134.

9. Ballard, R. C., M. O. Duncan, H. G. Fehler, Y. Dangor, F. L. Exposto, A. S. Latif. 1989. Treating chancroid: summary of studies in southern Africa. *Genitourin. Med.* **65**:54–57.

10. Bebear, C. M., H. Renaudin, A. Bryskier, and C. Bebear. 2000. Comparative activities of telithromycin (HMR 3647), levofloxacin and other antimicrobial agents against human mycoplasmas. *Antimicrob. Agents Chemother.* **44**:1980–1982.

11. Behets, F. M., G. Liomba, G. Lule, G. Dallabetta, I. F. Hoffman, Hamilton, S. Moeng, and M. S. Cohen. 1995. Sexually transmitted diseases and human immunodeficiency control in Malawi: a field study of genital ulcers. *J. Infect. Dis.* **171**:451–455.

12. Biedenbach, D. J., R. N. Jones, M. L. Beach, M. S. Barrett, D. M. Johnson, M. A. Pfaller, and G. V. Doern. 1999. In vitro antimicrobial activity of gatifloxacin against *N. gonorrhoeae* and *H influenzae*. *Drugs* **58**(Suppl. 2):178–179.

13. Bodhidatta, L., D. N. Taylor, A. Chitwarakorn, K. Kuvanont, and P. Echeverria. 1988. Evaluation of 500- and 1,000-mg doses of ciprofloxacin for the treatment of chancroid. *Antmicrob. Agents Chemother.* **32**:723–725.

14. Bogaerts, J., L. Kestens, W. Martinez Tello, J. Akingeneye, V. Mukantabana, J. Verhaegen, E. Van Dyck, and P. Piot. 1995. Failure of treatment for chancroid in Rwanda is not related to Human Immunodeficiency Virus infection: in vitro resistance to *Haemophilus ducreyi* to trimethoprim-sulfamethoxazole. *Clin. Infect. Dis.* **20**:924–930.

15. Borsum, T., L. Dannevig, G. Storvold, and K. Melby. 1990. *Chlamydia trachomatis*: in vitro susceptibility of genital and ocular isolates to some quinolones, amoxicillin and azithromycin. *Chemotherapy* **36**:407–415.

16. Boslego, J. W., C. B. Hicks, R. Greenup, R. J. Thomas, H. A. Wiener, J. Ciak, and E. C. Tramont. 1988. A prospective randomized trial of ofloxacin vs. doxycycline in the treatment of uncomplicated male urethritis. *Sex. Transm. Dis.* **15**:186–191.

17. Brihmer, C., I. Kallings, C. E. Nord, and J. Brundin. 1989. Second look laparoscopy: evaluation of two different antibiotic regimens after treatment of acute salpingitis. *Eur. J. Obstet. Gynecol. Reprod. Biol.* **30**:263–274.

18. **Brumsted, J. R., P. M. Clifford, S. T. Nakajima, and M. Gibson.** 1988. Reproductive outcome after medical management of complicated pelvic inflammatory disease. *Fertil. Steril.* **50:**667–669.

19. **Brunham, R. C., I. W. Maclean, B. Binns, and R. Peeling.** 1985. *Chlamydia trachomatis:* its role in tubal infertility. *J. Infect. Dis.* **152:**1275–1282.

20. **Brunham, R. C., and F. A. Plummer.** 1990. A general model of sexually transmitted disease epidemiology and its implications for control. *Med. Clin. N. Am.* **74:**1339–1352.

21. **Brunham, R. C., R. W. Peeling, I. W. Maclean, M. L. Kosseim, and M. Paraskevas.** 1992. *Chlamydia trachomatis*-associated ectopic pregnancy: serologic and histologic correlates. *J. Infect. Dis.* **165:**1076–1081.

22. **Bryan, J. P., S. K. Hira, W. Brady, N. Luo, C. Mwale, G. Mpoko, R. Krieg, E. Siwiwaliondo, C. Reichart, C. Waters, and P. L. Perine.** 1990. Oral ciprofloxacin versus ceftriaxone for the treatment of urethritis from resistant *Neisseria gonorrhoeae* in Zambia. *Antimicrob. Agents Chemother.* **34:**819–822.

23. **Carmona O., S. Hernandez-Gonzalez, and R. Kobelt.** 1987. Ciprofloxacin in the treatment of non-specific vaginitis. *Am. J. Med.* **82**(Suppl. 4A):321–323.

24. **Cates, W., R. T. Rolfs, and S. Aral.** 1990. Sexual transmitted diseases, pelvic inflammatory disease, and infertility: an epidemiologic update. *Epidemiol. Rev.* **12:**199–220.

25. **Cates, W., and J. N. Wasserheit.** 1991. Genital chlamydial infections: epidemiology and reproductive sequelae. *Am. J. Obstet. Gynecol.* **164:**1771–1781.

26. **Centers for Disease Control and Prevention.** 2002. Guidelines for treatment of sexually transmitted diseases. *Morb. Mortal. Wkly. Rep.* **51**(RR-6):1–78. Web access: http://www.cdc.gov/nchstp/dstd/1998_STD_Guidelines.

27. **Clendennen, T. E. III, C. S. Hames, E. S. Kees, F. C. Price, W. J. Rueppel, A. B. Andrada, G. E. Espinosa, G. Kabrerra, and F. S. Wignall.** 1992. In vitro antibiotic susceptibilities of *Neisseria gonorrhoeae* isolates in the Philippines. *Antimicrob. Agents Chemother.* **36:**277–282.

28. **Coker, D. M., I. Ahmed-Jushuf, O. P. Arya, J. S. Chessbrough, and B. C. Pratt.** 1989. Evaluation of single dose ciprofloxacin in the treatment of rectal and pharyngeal gonorrhoea. *J. Antimicrob. Chemother.* **24:**271–272.

29. **Corkill, J. E., A. Percival, and M. Lind.** 1991. Reduced uptake of ciprofloxacin in a resistant strain of *Neisseria gonorrhoeae* and transformation of resistance to other strains. *J. Antimicrob. Chemother.* **28:**601–604.

30. **Covino, J. M., M. Cummings, B. Smith, S. Benes, K. Draft, and W. M. McCormack.** 1990. Comparison of ofloxacin and ceftriaxone in the treatment of uncomplicated gonorrhea caused by penicillinase-producing and non-penicillinase-producing strains. *Antimicrob. Agents Chemother.* **34:**148–149.

31. **Covino, J. M., J. R. Black, M. Cummings, S. Smith, B. Zwickl, and W. M. McCormack.** 1993. Comparative evaluation of ofloxacin and metronidazole in the treatment of bacterial vaginosis. *Sex. Transm. Dis.* **20:**262–264.

32. **Costa, P., J. F. Louis, N. Mottet, H. Navratil, M. Favier, E. Jarroux, and A. Boccanfuso.** 1991. Acute epididymitis and pefloxacin in mono-antibiotic therapy. *Eur. J. Clin. Microbiol. Infect. Dis.* **Special issue:** 626–627.

33. **Crombleholme, W. R., J. Schachter, M. Ohm-Smith, J. Luft, R. Whidden, and R. L. Sweet.** 1989. Efficacy of single-agent therapy for the treatment of acute pelvic inflammatory disease with ciprofloxacin. *Am. J. Med.* **87**(Suppl. 5A):142S–147S.

34. **Dean, D., R. J. Suchland, and W. E. Stamm.** 2000. Evidence for long-term cervical persistence of *Chlamydia trachomatis* by *omp1* genotyping. *J. Infect. Dis.* **182:**909–916.

35. **Dessus-Babus, S., C. M. B'b'ar, A. Charron, C. B'b'ar, and B. de Barbeyrac.** 1998. Sequencing of gyrase and topoisomerase IV quinolone-resistance-determining regions of *Chlamydia trachomatis* and characterization of quinolone-resistant mutants obtained *in vitro*. *Antimicrob. Agents Chemother.* **42:**2474–2481.

36. **Deguchi, T., H. Komeda, and M. Yasuda.** 1995. *Mycoplasma genitalium* in nongoncocal urethritis. *Int. J. STD AIDS* **6:**144–145.

37. **Deguchi, T., I. Saito, M. Tanaka, K. Sato, K. Deguchi, M. Yasuda, M. Nakano, Y. Nishino, E. Kanematsu, S. Ozeki, and Y. Kawada.** 1997. Fluoroquinolone treatment failure in gonorrhea. *Sex. Transm. Dis.* **24:**247–250.

38. **Donati, M., F. Rumpianesi, F. Marchetti, V. Smabri, and R. Cevenini.** 1998. Comparative in vitro activity of levofloxacin against Chlamydia spp. *J. Antimicrob. Chemother.* **48:**670–671.

39. **Dosa, E., E. Nagy, W. Falk, I. Szoke, and U. Ballies.** 1999. Evaluation of the E test for susceptibility testing of *Mycoplasma hominis* and *Ureaplasma urealyticum*. *J. Antimicrob. Chemother.* **43:**575–578.

40. **Dreses-Werringloer, U., I. Padubrin, B. Jürgens-Saathoff, A. P. Hudson, H. Zeidler, and L. Köhler.** 2000. Persistence of *Chlamydia trachomatis* is induced by ciprofloxacin and ofloxacin *in vitro*. *Antimicrob. Agents Chemother.* **44:**3288–3297.

41. **D'Souza, P., R. Pandhi, N. Khanna, A. Rattan, and R. S. Misra.** 1998. A comparative study of therapeutic response of patients with clinical chancroid to ciprofloxacin, erythromycin, and cotrimoxasole. *Sex. Transm. Dis.* **25:**293–295.

42. **Dubois, J., and V. Fontaine.** 1988. In vitro activity of fleroxacin against urinary tract and genital tract pathogens. *J. Antimicrob. Chemother.* **22**(Suppl. D):31–34.

43. **Dylewski, J., H. Nsanze, L. D'Costa, L. Slaney, and A. R. Ronald.** 1985. Trimethoprimsulfamoxazole in the treatment of chancroid comparison of two single dose treatment regimens with a five day regimen. *J. Antimicrob. Chemother.* **16:**103–110.

44. **Ehret, J. M., and F. N. Judson.** 1988. Susceptibility testing of *Chlamydia trachomatis:* from eggs to monoclonal antibodies. *Antimicrob. Agents Chemother.* **32:**1295–1299.

45. **Endtz, H., J. M. Ossewaarde, P. J. G. M. van de Korput, and H. T. Weiland.** 1989. In vitro activity of eight quinolones against *Chlamydia trachomatis*. *Rev. Infect. Dis.* **11**(Suppl. 5):S1278.

46. **Faro, S., M. G. Martens, M. Maccato, H. A. Hammill, S. Roberts, and G. Riddle.** 1991. Effectiveness of ofloxacin in the treatment of *Chlamydia trachomatis* and *Neisseria gonorrhoeae* cervical infection. *Am. J. Obstet. Gynecol.* **164:**1380–1383.

47. **Fishbach, F., R. Deckardt, H. Graeff, and W. Busch.** 1991. Comparison of ciprofloxacin/metronidazole versus cefoxitin/doxycycline in the treatment of pelvic inflammatory disease. *Eur. J. Clin. Microbiol. Infect. Dis.* **Special issue:**402–403.

48. **Fleming, D. T., and J. N. Wasserheit.** 1999. From epidemiological synergy to public health policy and practice: the contribution of other sexually transmitted diseases to sexual transmission of HIV infection. *Sex. Transm. Infect.* **75:**3–17.

49. **Friesen, T. R., and R. J. Mangi.** 1990. Inappropriate use of oral ciprofloxacin. *JAMA* **264:**1438–1440.

50. **Gambini, D., I. Decleva, L. Lupica, M. Ghislanzoni, M. Cusini, and E. Alessi.** 2000. *Mycoplasma genitalium* in males with nongonococcal urethritis:prevalence and clinical efficacy of eradication. *Sex. Transm. Dis.* **27:**226–229.

51. Gerding, G. N., and J. A. Hitt. 1989. Tissue penetration of the new quinolones in humans. *Rev. Infect. Dis.* **11**(Suppl. 5):S1046–S1057.

52. Gransden, W. R., C. A. Warren, I. Phillips, M. Hodges, and D. Barlow. 1990. Decreased susceptibility of *Neisseria gonorrhoeae* to ciprofloxacin. *Lancet.* **335**:51.

53. Gransden, W. R., C. Warren, and I. Phillips. 1991. 4-Quinolone-resistant *Neisseria gonorrhoeae* in the United Kingdom. *J. Med. Microbiol.* **34**:23–27.

54. Gundersen, T., and F. Zahm. 1989. Fleroxacin in the treatment of urogenital infections caused by *Chlamydia trachomatis*: a pilot study. *Rev. Infect. Dis.* **11**:S1278.

55. Haase, D. A., J. O. Ndinya-Achola, R. A. Nash, L. J. D'Costa, D. Hazlett, S. Lubwama, H. Nsanze, and A. R. Ronald. 1986. Clinical evaluation of rosoxacin for the treatment of chancroid. *Antimicrob. Agents Chemother.* **30**:39–41.

56. Haizlip, J., S. F. Isbey, H. A. Hamilton, A. E. Jerse, P. A. Leone, R. H. Davis, and M. S. Cohen. 1995. Time required for elimination of Neisseria gonorrhoeae from the urogenital tract in men with symptomatic urethritis: comparison of oral and intramuscular single-dose therapy. *Sex. Transm. Dis.* **22**:145–148.

57. Handsfield, H. H., J. A. McCutchan, L. Corey, and A. R. Ronald. 1992. Special issues in clinical trials of new anti-infective drugs for the treatment of sexually transmitted diseases. *Clin. Infect. Dis.* **15**(Suppl. 1):596–598.

58. Handsfield, H. H. 1996. Antibiotic-resistant Neisseria gonorrhoeae: the calm before another storm? *Ann. Intern. Med.* **125**:507–509.

59. Hannan, P. C., and G. Woodnutt. 2000. In vitro activity of gemifloxacin (SB 265805; LB 20304a) against human mycoplasmas. *J. Antimicrob. Chemother.* **45**:367–369.

60. Hasselquist, M. B., and S. Hillier. 1991. Susceptibility of upper tract isolates from women with pelvic inflammatory disease to ampicillin, cefpodoxime, metronidazole and doxycycline. *Sex. Transm. Dis.* **18**:146–149.

61. Health Canada. 1998. *Canadian Guidelines for the Management of Sexually Transmitted Diseases.* http://www.hc-sc.gc.ca/hpb/lcdc/publicat/std98

62. Heinonen, P. K., K. Teisala, R. Aine, and A. Miettinen. 1989. Intravenous and oral ciprofloxacin in the treatment of proven pelvic inflammatory disease. A comparison with doxycycline and metronidazole. *Am. J. Med.* **87**(Suppl. 5A):152S–156S.

63. Hoban, D., P. DeGagne, and E. Witwicki. 1989. In vitro activity of lomefloxacin against *Chlamydiatrachomatis, Neisseria gonorrhoeae, Haemophilusducreyi, Mycoplasmahominis,* and *Ureaplasmaurealyticum. Diagn. Microbiol. Infect. Dis.* **12**(Suppl. 3):83S–86S.

64. Hook, E. W., III, R. B. Jones, D. H. Martin, G. A. Bolan, T. F. Mroczkowski, T. M. Neumann, J. J. Haag, and R. Echols. 1993. Comparison of ciprofloxacin and ceftriaxone as single-dose therapy for uncomplicated gonorrhea in women. *Antimicrob. Agents Chemother.* **37**:1670–1673.

65. Hook, E. W., III, W. McCormack, D. Martin, R. Jones, K. Bean, and A. Maroli. 1997. Comparison of single-dose oral grepafloxacin with cefixime for treatment of uncomplicated gonorrhea in men. *Antimicrob. Agents Chemother.* **41**:1843–1845.

66. Hooper, D. C. Mechanisms of action of antimicrobials: focus on the quinolones. *Clin. Infect. Dis.* **32**(Suppl. 1):S9–S15.

67. Hooton, T. M., M. E. Rogers, T. G. Medina, L. E. Kuwamura, C. Ewers, P. L. Roberts, and W. E. Stamm. 1990. Ciprofloxacin compared with doxycycline for non-

gonococcal urethritis. Ineffectiveness against *Chlamydia trachomatis* due to relapsing infection. *JAMA* **264**:1418–1421.

68. Horner, P. J., C. R. Gilroy, B. J. Thomas, R. O. M. Naidoo, and D. Taylor-Robinson. 1993. Association of *Mycoplasma gentialium* with acute nongonococcal urethritis. *Lancet* **342**:582–585.

69. Ibsen, H. H. W., B. R. Moller, L. Halkier-Sorensen, and E. From. 1989. Treatment of nongonococcal urethritis: comparison of ofloxacin and erythromycin. *Sex. Transm. Dis.* **16**:32–35.

70. Jaffe, H. W., A. L. Schroeter, G. H. Reynolds, A. A. Zaidi, J. E. Martin, Jr., and J. D. Thayer. 1979. Pharmacokinetic determinants of penicillin cure of gonococcal urethritis. *Antimicrob. Agents Chemother.* **15**:587–591.

71. Jephcott, A. E., and A. Turner A. 1990. Ciprofloxacin resistance in gonococci. *Lancet* **335**:165.

72. Jeskanen, L., and A. Lassus 1991. Fleroxacin (Ro 23–6240) versus doxycycline in the treatment of chlamydial urethritis and/or cervicitis. *Eur. J. Clin. Microbiol. Infect. Dis.* **Special Issue**:457–458.

73. Jha, P., J. D. Nagelkerke, E. N. Ngugi, J. V. Prasada Rao, B. Willbond, S. Moses, and F. A. Plummer. 2001. Public health. Reducing HIV transmission in developing countries. *Science* **292**:224–225.

74. Jones, R. B., B. Van Der Pol, D. H. Martin, and M. K. Shepard. 1990. Partial characterization of *Chlamydia trachomatis* isolates resistant to multiple antibiotics. *J. Infect. Dis.* **162**:1309–1315.

75. Jones, R. N., L. M. Deshpande, M. E. Erwin, M. S. Barrett, and M. L. Beach. 2000. Anti-gonococcal activity of gemifloxacin against fluoroquinolone-resistant strains and a comparison of agar dilution and Etest methods. *J. Antimicrob. Chemother.* **45**(Suppl. 1):67–70.

76. Judlin, P., C. Scheffler, M. Dailloux, and P. Landes. 1991. Shorter duration of treatment in chlamydial pelvic infections with ofloxacin-amoxicillin-clavulanate, compared with doxycycline-amoxicillin-clavulanate. *Eur. J. Clin. Microbiol. Infect. Dis.* **Special Issue**: p. 314–315.

77. Kam, K. M., K. K. Lo, L. Y. Chong, W. F. Au, P. Y. Wong, and M. M. Cheung. 1999. Correlation between *in vitro* quinolone susceptibility of *Neisseria gonorrhoeae* and outcome of treatment of gonococcal urethritis with single-dose ofloxacin. *Clin. Infect. Dis.* **28**:1165–1166.

78. Kam, K. M., K. K. Lo, N. K. Ho, and M. M. Cheung. 1995. Rapid decline in penicillinase-producing *Neisseria gonorrhoeae* in Hong Kong associated with emerging 4-fluoroquinolone resistance. *Genitourin. Med.* **71**:141–144.

79. Kawada, Y. 1989. Multicentre study of ofloxacin for non-gonococcal urethritis in Asia. *Rev. Infect. Dis.* **11**(Suppl. 5):S1318–S1319.

80. Kenny, G. E., T. M. Hooton, M. C. Roberts, F. D. Cartwright, and J. Hoyt. 1989. Susceptibilities of genital mycoplasmas to the newer quinolones as determined by the agar dilution method. *Antimicrob. Agents Chemother.* **33**:103–107.

81. Kimura, M., T. Kishimoto, Y. Niki, and R. Soejima. 1993. In vitro and in vivo antichlamydial activities of newly developed quinolone antimicrobial agents. *Antimicrob. Agents Chemother.* **37**:801–803

82. Kitchen, V. S., C. Donegan, H. Ward, B. Thomas, J. R. Harris, and D. Taylor-Robinson. 1990. Comparison of ofloxacin with doxycycline in the treatment of non-gonococcal urethritis and cervical chlamydial infection. *J. Antimicrob. Chemother.* **26**(Suppl. D):99–105.

83. Klausner, J. D., M. Aplasca, V. P. Mesola, G. Bolan, W. L. Whittington, and K. K. Holmes. 1999. Correlates of gono-

coccal infection and of antimicrobial-resistant Neisseria gonorrhoeae among female sex workers, Republic of Philippines, 1996–1997. *J. Infect. Dis.* **179**:729–733.

84. **Knapp, J. S., A. F. Back, A. F. Babat, D. Taylor, and R. J. Rice.** 1993. Antimicrobial Susceptibility of isolates of *Haemophilus ducreyi* from Thailand and the United States to currently recommended and newer agents for the treatment of chancroid. *Antimicrob. Agents Chemother.* **37**:1552–1555.

85. **Knapp, J. S., K. K. Fox, D. L. Trees, and W. L. Whittington.** 1997. Fluoroquinolone resistance in *Neisseria gonorrhoeae*. *Emerg. Infect. Dis.* **3**:33–39.

86. **Lassus, A., O. V. Renkonen, J. Ellmen.** 1988. Fleroxacin versus standard therapy in gonococcal urethritis. *J. Antimicrob. Chemother.* **22**(Suppl. D):223–225.

87. **Lutz, F. B., Jr.** 1989. Single-dose efficacy of ofloxacin in uncomplicated gonorrhea. *Am. J. Med.* **87**:69S–74S.

88. **MacDonald, K. S., D. W. Cameron, L. D'Costa, J. O. Ndinya-Achola, F. A. Plummer, and A. R. Ronald.** 1989. Evaluation of fleroxacin (RO 23-6240) as single-oral-dose therapy of culture-proven chancroid in Nairobi, Kenya. *Antimicrob. Agents Chemother.* **33**:612–614.

89. **Maeda, S., M. Tamaki, K. Kojima, T. Yoshida, H. Ishiko, M. Yasuda, and T. Deguchi.** 2001. Association of Mycoplasma genitalium persistence in the urethra with recurrence of non-gonococcal urethritis. *Sex. Transm. Dis.* **28**:472–476.

90. **Malonza, I. M., M. W. Tyndall, J. O. Ndinya-Achola, I. Maclean, S. Omar, K. S. MacDonald, J. Perriens, K. Orle, F. A. Plummer, A. R. Ronald, and S. Moses.** 1999. A randomised double-blind placebo-controlled trial of single-dose ciprofloxacin versus erthromycin for the treatment of chancroid in Nairobi, Kenya. *J. Infect. Dis.* **180**:1886–1893.

91. **Martens, M. G., S. Gordon, D. R. Yarborough, S. Faro, D. Binder, and A. Berkeley.** 1993. Multicenter randomised trial of ofloxacin versus cefoxitin and doxycycline in outpatient treatment of pelvic inflammatory disease. *South. Med. J.* **86**:604–610.

92. **Martin, D. H., T. F. Mroczkowski, T. Richelo, P. St. Clair, and S. Pizzuti.** 1991. Randomized double-blind study of fleroxacin and doxycycline for the treatment of *Chlamydia trachomatis* genital tract infections. *Eur. J. Clin. Microbiol. Infect. Dis.* Special Issue:458–459.

93. **Martin, D. H., C. L. Cammarata, and D. Grubb.** 1991. In vitro activity of sparfloxacin (CI-978, AT-4140), ofloxacin, doxycycline, and tetracycline versus genital tract mycoplasmas and *Chlamydia trachomatis*. *Eur. J. Clin. Microbiol. Infect. Dis.* Special issue:563–564.

94. **Mabey, D., and R. W. Peeling.** 1999. Heat shock protein expression and immunity in chlamydial infections. *Infect. Dis. Obstet. Gynecol* **7**:72–79.

95. **McCormack, W. M., D. H. Martin, E. W. Hook, and R. B. Jones.** 1998. Daily oral grepafloxacin vs. twice daily oral doxycycline in the treatment of Chlamydia trachomatis endocervical infection. *Infect. Dis. Obstet. Gynecol.* **6**:109–115.

96. **Mikamo, H., Y. Sato, Y. Hayasaki, Y. X. Hua, and T. Tamaya.** 2000. Adequate levofloxacin treatment schedules for uterine cervicitis caused by Chlamydia trachomatis. *Chemotherapy* **46**:150–152.

97. **Miller, S. D., F. da L. Exposto, Y. Dangor, S. Kaka, H. G. Fehler, and H. J. Koornhof.** 1989. A dose finding study of fleroxacin in the treatment of chancroid. *Rev. Infect. Dis.* **11**(Suppl. 5):S1310–S1311.

98. **Mogabgab, W. J., B. Holmes, M. Murray, R. Beville, F. B. Lutz, and K. J. Tack.** 1990. Randomized comparison of ofloxacin and doxycycline for chlamydia and ureaplama urethritis and cervicitis. *Chemotherapy* **36**:70–76.

99. **Moi, H., P. Morel, B. Gianotti, D. Barlow, I. Phillips, and C. Jean.** 1996. Comparative efficacy and safety of single oral doses of sparfloxacin versus ciprofloxacin in the treatment of acute gonococcal urethritis in men. *J. Antimicrob. Chemother.* **37**(Suppl. A):115–122.

100. **Moller, B. R., B. Herrmann, H. H. Ibsen, L. Halkier-Sorensen, E. From, and P.-A. Mardh.** 1990. Occurrence of *Ureaplasma urealyticum* and *Mycoplasma hominis* in non-gonococcal urethritis before and after treatment in a double-blind trial of ofloxacin versus erythromycin. *Scand. J. Infect. Dis.* **68**(Suppl.):31–34.

101. **Naamara, W., F. A. Plummer, R. Greenblatt, L. J. D'Costa, J. O. Ndinya-Achola, and A. R. Ronald.** 1987. Treatment of chancroid with ciprofloxacin: a prospective, randomized clinical trial. *Am. J. Med.* **82**:S317–S320.

102. **Ndinya-Achola, O., F. A. Odhiambo, P. Wambugu, L. Slaney, M. Bosire, J. Kimata, M. Malisa, F. Plummer, and A. R. Ronald.** 1991. Ciprofloxacin treatment of gonoccocal infections in Nairobi, Kenya, abstr. P-20-258. *Proceedings of the 9th Meeting of the International Society of Sexually Transmitted Diseases Research.*

103. **Panikabutra, K., C. T. Lee, B. Ho, and P. Bamberg.** 1988. Single dose oral norfloxacin or intramuscular spectinomycin to treat gonorrhoea (PPNG and non-PPNG infections): analysis of efficacy and patient preference. *Genitourin. Med.* **64**:235–240.

104. **Peipert J. F., R. L. Sweet, C. K. Walker, J. Krahn, and K. Rielly-Gauvin.** 1999. Evaluation of ofloxacin in the treatment of laparoscopically documented acute pelvic inflammatory disease (salpingitis). *J. Infect. Dis. Obstet. Gynecol.* **7**:138–144.

105. **Pepin, J., F. Sobela, S. Deslandis, M. Alary, K. Wegner, N. Khonde, F. Kintin, A. Kamuragiye, M. Sylla, P.-J. Zerbo, E. Baganizi, A. Kone, F. Kane, B. Masse, P. Viens, and E. Frost.** 2001. Etiology of uethral discharge in west Africa: the role of *Mycoplasma genitalium* and *Trichomonas vaginalis*. *Bull. W.H.O.* **79**:118–126.

106. **Peterson, H. B., C. K. Walker, J. G. Kahn, A. E. Washington, D. A. Eschenbach, and S. Faro.** 1991. Pelvic inflammatory disease: key treatment issues and options. *JAMA* **266**:2605–2612.

107. **Phillips, I., C. Dimian, D. Barlow, H. Moi, E. Stolz, W. Weidner, and E. Perea.** 1996. A comparative study of two different regimens of sparfloxacin versus doxycycline in the treatment of non-gonococcal urethritis in men. *J. Antimicrob. Chermother.* **37**:123–134.

108. **Plourde, P. J., L. J. D'Costa, E. Agoki, J. Ombette, J. O. Ndinya-Achola, L. A. Slaney, A. R. Ronald, and F. A. Plummer.** 1991. A randomized double-blind study of the efficacy of fleroxacin vs. trimethoprim-sulfamethoxazole in female prostitutes with culture-proven chancroid. *J. Infect. Dis.* **165**:949–952.

109. **Poutiers, F., S. Bessu-Babus, F. Leblanc, C. Bebear, and B. de Barbeyrac.** 1999. In vitro activity of grepafloxacin against Chlamydia trachomatis. *Drugs* **58**(Suppl. 2):404–405.

110. **Pust, R. A., H. R. Ackenheil-Koppe, W. Weidner, and H. Meier-Ewert.** 1988. Clinical efficacy and tolerance of fleroxacin in patients with urethritis caused by *Chlamydia trachomatis*. *J. Antimicrob. Chemother.* **22**(Suppl. D):227–230.

111. **Rahman, M., A. Alam, K. Nessa, S. Nahar, D. K. Dutta, L. Yasmin, S. Monira, Z. Sultan, S. A. Khan, and M. J. Albert.** 2001. Treatment failure with the use of ciprofloxacin for gonorrhea correlates with the prevalence of fluoroquinolone-resistant *Neisseria gonorrhoeae* strains in Bangladesh. *Clin. Infect. Dis.* **32**:884–889.

112. Rajakumar, M. K., Y. F. Ngeow, B. S. Khor, and K. F. Lim. 1988. Ofloxacin, a new quinolone for the treatment of gonorrhea. *Sex. Transm. Dis.* **15:**25–26.

113. Ramirez, C. A., J. L. Bran, C. R. Mejia, and J. F. Garcia. 1985. Open, prospective study of the clinical efficacy of oral ciprofloxacin. *Antimicrob. Agents Chemother.* **28:**128–132.

114. Richmond, S. J., M. N. Bhattacharyya, H. Maiti, F. H. Chowdhurry, R. M. Stirland, and J. A. Tooth. 1998. The efficacy of ofloxacin against infection caused by *Neisseria gonorrhoeae* and *Chlamydia trachomatis*. *J. Antimicrob. Chemother.* **22**(Suppl. C):149–153.

115. Ridgway, G. L. 1995. Quinolones in sexually transmitted diseases: global experience. *Drugs* **49**(Suppl. 2):115–122.

116. Ridgway, G. L. 1997. Treatment of chlamydial genital infection. *J. Antimicrob. Chemother.* **40:**311–314.

117. Ridgway, G. L., H. Salman, M. J. Robbins, C. Dencer, and D. Felmingham. 1997. The in-vitro activity of grepafloxacin against Chlamydia spp., Mycoplasma spp., *Urealplasma urealyticum* and Legionella spp. *J. Antimicrob. Chemother* **40**(Suppl. A):31–34.

118. Sanders, C. C. 2001. Mechanisms responsible for cross-resistance and dichotomous resistance among the quinolones. *Clin. Infect. Dis.* **32**(Suppl. 1):S1–S8.

119. Scholes, D., A. Stergachis, F. E. Heidrich, H. Andrilla, K. K. Holmes, and W. E. Stamm. 1996. Prevention of pelvic inflammatory disease by screening for cervical chlamydial infection. *N. Engl. J. Med.* **334:**1362–1366.

120. Schmid, G., B. Van Der Pol, R. B. Jones, and R. Johnson. 2001. Further investigating the clinical importance of heterotypic antimicrobial resistance in *Chlamydia trachomatis*. *Int. J. STD & AIDS* **12:**41.

121. Schwarez, S. K., J. M. Zenilman, D. Schnell, J. S. Knapp, E. Hook, S. Thompson, F. N. Judson, and K. K. Holmes. 1990. The gonococcal isolate surveillance project. National Surveillance of Antimicrobial Resistance in *Neisseria gonorrhoeae. JAMA* **264:**1413–1417.

122. Shanmugaratnam, K., M. S. Sprott, R. S. Pattman, A. M. Kearns, and P. G. Watson. 1989. Single dose ciprofloxacin to treat women with gonorrhoea. *Genitourin. Med.* **65:**129.

123. Shepard, M. K., and R. B. Jones. 1989. Recovery of *Chlamydia trachomatis* from endometrial and fallopian tube biopsies in women with infertility of tubal origin. *Fertil. Steril.* **52:**232–238.

124. Slaney, L., H. Chubb, A. Ronald, and R. Brunham. 1990. In vitro activity of azithromycin, erythromycin, ciprofloxacin and norfloxacin against *Neisseria gonorrhoeae, Haemophilus ducreyi*, and *Chlamydia trachomatis. J. Antimicrob. Chemother.* **25**(Suppl. A):1–5.

125. Smith, B. L., M. C. Cummings, J. M. Covino, S. Benes, K. Draft, and W. M. McCormack. 1991. Evaluation of ofloxacin in the treatment of uncomplicated gonorrhea. *Sex. Transm. Dis.* **18:**18–20.

126. Smith, B. L., W. J. Mogabgab, Z. A. Dalu, R. B. Jones, J. M. Douglas, H. H. Handsfield, E. W. Hook, B. L. Vinear, J. W. Shands, and W. M. McCormack. 1993. Multicenter trial of fleroxacin versus ceftriaxone in the treatment of uncomplicated gonorrhea. *Am. J. Med.* **94:**81S–84S.

127. Somani, J., V. B. Bhullar, K. A. Workowski, C. E. Farshy, and C. M. Black. 2000. Multiple drug-resistant *Chlamydia trachomatis* associated with clinical treatment failure. *J. Infect. Dis.* **181:**1421–1427.

128. Soltz-Szots, J., S. Schneider, and H. Mailer. 1989. Efficacy of and tolerance to fleroxacin in the treatment of chlamydia urethritis and cervicitis. *Rev. Infect. Dis.* **11:**S1280–S1281.

129. Stein, D. C. 1991. Transformation of *Neisseria gonorrhoeae*: physical requirements of transforming DNA. *Can. J. Microbiol.* **37:**345–349.

130. Stein, D. C., R. J. Danaher, and T. M. Cook. 1991. Characterization of a *gyr*B mutation responsible for low-level nalidixic acid resistance in *Neisseria gonorrhoeae. Antimicrob. Agents Chemother.* **35:**622–626.

131. Stein, G. E., and L. D. Saravolatz. 1989. Randomized clinical study of ofloxacin and doxycycline in the treatment of nongonococcal urethritis and cervicitis. *Rev. Infect. Dis.* **11:**S1277.

132. Stoner, B. P., J. M. Douglas, D. H. Martin, E. W. Hook, P. Leone, W. M. McCormack, T. F. Mroczkowki, R. Jones, J. Yang, and T. Baumgartner. 2000. Single dose gatifloxacin compared with ofloxacin for the treatment of uncomplicated gonorrhea. *Sex. Transm. Dis.* **28:**136–142.

133. Su, X., and I. Lind. 2001. Molecular basis of high-level ciprofloxacin resistance in *Neisseria gonorrhoeae* strains isolated in Denmark from 1995 to 1998. *Antimicrob. Agents Chemother.* **45:**117–123.

134. Suchland, R. J., W. M. Geisler, J. C. Lara, and W. E. Stamm. 2001. Evaluation of methodologies and cell lines for antibiotic susceptibility testing of Chlamydia spp., poster C-286. *Procdings of the Annual Meeting of the American Society for Microbiology.* American Society for Microbiology, Washington, D.C.

135. Talbot, H., and B. Romanowski. 1989. In vitro activities of lomefloxacin, tetracycline, penicillin, spectinomycin, and ceftriaxone against *Neisseria gonorrhoeae* and *Chlamydia trachomatis. Antimicrob. Agents Chemother.* **33:**2049–2051.

136. Tanaka, M., H. Nakayama, M. Haraoka, T. Nagafuji, T. Saika, and I. Kobayashi. 1998. Analysis of quinolone resistance mechanisms in a sparfloxacin-resistant clinical isolate of *Neissseria gonorrhoeae. Sex. Transm. Dis.* **25:**489–493.

137. Tanaka, M., T. Matsumoto, M. Sakumoto, K. Takahashi, T. Saika, I. Kabayashi, J. Kumazawa, and the Pazufloxacin STD group. 1998. Reduced clinical efficacy of pazufloxacin against gonorrhea due to high prevalence of quinolone-resistant isolates with the *gyr*A mutation. *Antimicrob. Agents Chemother.* **42:**579–582.

138. Tanaka, M., H. Nakayama, M. Haraoka, T. Saika, I. Kobayashi, and S. Naito. 2000. Antimicrobial resistance of *Neisseria gonorrhoeae* and high prevalence of ciprofloxacin-resistant isolates in Japan, 1993 to 1998. *J. Clin. Microbiol.* **38:**521–525.

139. Tapsall, J. 2001. *Antimicrobial Resistance in Neisseria gonorrhoeae*, WHO/CDS/CSR/2001.3. World Health Organization, Geneva, Switzerland.

140. Taylor-Robinson, D., and C. Bebear. 1997. Antibiotic susceptibilities of mycoplasmas and treatment of mycoplasma infections. *J. Antimicrob. Chemother.* **40:**622–630.

141. Thomas, D., J. Orfila, and E. Bissac. 1995. Evaluation of the activity of different quinolones in the experimental chlamydia salpingitis mouse model. *Drugs* **49**(Suppl. 2):261–263.

142. Thorpe, E. M., J. R. Schwebke, E. W. Hook III, A. Rompalo, W. M. McCormack, K. Mussari, G. C. Giguere, and J. J. Collins. 1996. Comparison of single-dose cefuroxime axetil with ciprofloxacin in treatment of uncomplicated gonorrhea caused by penicillinase-producing and non-penicillinase producing *Neisseria gonorrhoeae* strains. *Antimicrob. Agents Chemother.* **40:**2775–2780.

143. Tio, T. T., I. R. Sindhunata, J. H. T. Wagenvoort, A. F. Angulo, L. Habbema, and M. F. Michel, E. Stolz. 1990. Pefloxacin compared with cefotaxime for treating men with uncomplicated gonococcal urethritis. *J. Antimicrob. Chemother.* **22**(Suppl. B):141–146.

144. Turner, A., A. E. Jephcott, and K. R. Gough. 1991. Laboratory detection of ciprofloxacin resistant *Neisseria gonorrhoeae. J. Clin. Pathol.* **44:**169–170.

145. Tyndall M., M. Malisa, F. A. Plummer, J. Ombetti, J. O. Ndinya-Achola, and A. R. Ronald. 1993. Fleroxacin in the treatment of chancroid: an open study in men seropositive or seronegative for the human immunodeficiency virus type 1. *Am. J. Med.* *94*(Suppl. 3A):85S–88S.

146. Ulmann, U., S. Schubert, and R. Krause. 1999. Comparative in-vitro activity of levofloxacin, other fluoroquinolones, doxycycline and erythromycin against *Ureaplasma urealyticum* and *Mycoplasma hominis.* *J. Antimicrob. Chemother.* *43*(Suppl. C):33–36.

147. Une, T., R. Nakajima, T. Otani, K. Katami, Y. Osada, and M. Otani. 1987. Lack of effectiveness of ofloxacin against experimental syphilis in rabbits. *Forsch. Klin. Lab.* *37*:1048–1041.

148. van der Willigen, A. H., A. A. Polak-Vogelzang, L. Habbema, and J. H. Wagenvoort. 1988. Clinical efficacy of ciprofloxacin versus doxycycline in the treatment of nongonococcal urethritis in males. *Eur. J. Clin. Microbiol. Infect. Dis.* *7*:658–661.

149. Veller-Fornasa, C., M. Tarantello, R. Cepriani, L. Gurerra, and A. Peserico. 1987. Effect of ofloxacin on *Treponema pallidum* in incubating experimental syphilis. *Genitourin. Med.* *63*:214.

150. Vila, J., L. Olmos, J. Ballesteros, J. A. Vasquez, M. J. Gimenez, F. Marco, and L. Aguilar. 1997. Development of in vivo resistance after quinolone treatment of gonococcal urethritis. *J. Antimicrob. Chemother.* *39*:841.

151. Vilata, J. J., J. Garcia-De-Lomas, J. Sanchez, A. Lloret, M. Evole, and J. M. Nogueira. 1989. A double-blind randomized study comparing two ofloxacin regimens vs. minocycline in the treatment of nongonococcal urethritis. *Rev. Infect. Dis.* *11*(Suppl. 5):S1285–S1286.

152. Waites, K. B., L. B. Duffy, T. Schmidt, D. Crabb, M. S. Pate, and G. H. Cassel. 1999. In vitro susceptibilities of *Mycoplasma pneumoniae, Mycoplasma hominis, Ureaplasma urealyticum* to sparfloxacin and PD 127391. *Antimicrob. Agents Chemother.* *43*:2571–2573.

153. Waites, K. B., K. C. Canupp, and G. E. Kenny. 1999. Susceptibilities of Mycoplasma *hominis* to moxifloxacin by E-test and agar dilution. *Drugs* *58*(Suppl. 2):406–407.

154. Weidner, W., H. G. Schiefer, and C. Garbe. 1987. Acute nongonococcal epididymitis. Aetiological and therapeutic aspects. *Drugs* *34*(Suppl. 1):111–117.

155. **World Health Organization.** 2001. *Guidelines for the Management of Sexually Transmitted Infections.* WHO/HIV_AIDS/2001.01. World Health Organization, Geneva, Switzerland.

156. **World Health Organization.** *Global Prevalence and Incidence of Selected Curable Sexually Transmitted Infections: Overview and Estimates.* WHO/HIV.AIDS/2001.02. World Health Organization, Geneva, Switzerland.

Quinolone Antimicrobial Agents, 3rd ed.
Edited by David C. Hooper and Ethan Rubinstein
© 2003 ASM Press, Washington, D.C.

Chapter 11

Treatment and Prophylaxis of Gastroenteritis

MICHAEL L. BENNISH

Quinolone antimicrobial agents have been mainstays of the treatment of bacterial gastrointestinal infections since their introduction into clinical use in the 1980s. The older quinolone agent nalidixic acid was sparingly used in the treatment of enteric infections (102), with its primary use being for treatment of multiply resistant *Shigella* infections in poor countries (199). Because of its modest efficacy for this indication, however (99), and the rapid development of resistance (23, 46, 106, 188, 222), nalidixic acid was never widely used outside of developing countries.

In contrast, a confluence of factors led to the fluoroquinolones being quickly adopted into clinical use for treatment of enteric bacterial infections (128). The fluoroquinolones have much greater in vitro activity against *Enterobacteriaceae* than nalidixic acid (46, 85), while achieving similar concentrations in serum; there were a large number of well-conducted clinical trials showing efficacy of the fluoroquinolones for enteric infections, thus providing an empiric basis for therapy; the quinolones have a high therapeutic to toxicity ratio; and finally, the emergence of widespread resistance among bacterial enteric pathogens to ampicillin and trimethoprim-sulfamethoxazole, the agents that had been the treatment of choice for many enteric infections necessitated the use of other drugs (23, 106, 155, 209, 247).

Experience with fluoroquinolones in treating enteric infections is primarily with the older fluoroquinolone agents ciprofloxacin, ofloxacin, and norfloxacin. The newer quinolone agents, though having the potential advantage of longer serum half-lives, usually are modestly less active in vitro against bacterial enteric pathogens (70, 71) and have primarily been evaluated and promoted for respiratory tract infections (109).

This chapter reviews the characteristics of the quinolones that make them useful for the treatment of enteric infections, and the role of these agents in treating enteric infections.

IN VITRO ACTIVITY AGAINST BACTERIAL ENTERIC PATHOGENS

When first introduced, the fluoroquinolones were highly active against all bacterial enteric pathogens (26, 36, 85, 87, 210) and 50 to >100 times more active than the older quinolone agent nalidixic acid (Table 1) (93, 135). Ciprofloxacin was the most active of the agents, with its activity in general being two to four times greater than that of other fluoroquinolones (26, 43, 70, 83, 85, 87, 93, 135, 165, 236). Because of the initial exquisite susceptibility of all bacterial enteropathogens to the fluoroquinolone agents, with drug concentrations at the site of infection often being 100-fold or more in excess of the MIC of the organism, the differences in activity between the fluoroquinolones probably had little clinical significance. With the increase in the prevalence of enteric pathogens with diminished susceptibility to the fluoroquinolones, the differences in activity between drugs in this class may now have greater clinical importance (29). Given that few if any clinical studies directly compared two fluoroquinolones, the relative advantages (if any) of the different fluoroquinolones have to be inferred from in vitro studies and differences in pharmacologic properties.

Strains with diminished susceptibility or frank resistance to fluoroquinolones have now been reported for most enteric pathogens (Table 2) (180). Among *Enterobacteriaceae* frank resistance to nalidixic acid (MIC > 32 µg/ml) usually results from a single mutation in the *gyrA* gene coding DNA gyrase, the latter being the target of quinolones. Although such mutations are usually associated with a 10-fold or greater increase in MICs to the fluoroquinolones, MICs generally remain below the 2 to 4 µg/ml concentrations that are considered the breakpoints for resistance to the fluoroquinolones (110, 193, 227). Clinical response to these isolates with

Michael L. Bennish • Africa Centre for Health and Population Studies, Mtubatuba, South Africa.

Table 1. Representative in vitro activity of quinolone agents against common bacterial enteric pathogens from largely susceptible strains of pathogens[a]

Agent and organism	MIC 90% (μg/ml)	MIC lowest-highest values (μg/ml)
Nalidixic acid		
Campylobacter jejuni	8	2–16
Enterotoxigenic *Escherichia coli*	2	0.125–2
Nontyphoid *Salmonella* spp.	8	4->128
Salmonella enterica serovar Typhi	4	2–8
Shigella spp.	4	1–4
Vibrio cholerae	0.5	0.125–1
Yersinia enterocolitica	2	0.5->128
Ciprofloxacin		
C. jejuni	0.25	0.016–0.25
Enterotoxigenic *E. coli*	≤0.015	≤0.015
Nontyphoid *Salmonella* spp.	0.016	0.008–0.016
S. enterica serovar Typhi	0.03	0.008–0.03
Shigella spp.	0.015	0.008–0.03
V. cholerae O1	0.004	0.002–0.015
Y. enterocolitica	0.03	≤0.015–0.25
Ofloxacin		
C. jejuni	0.78	<0.097–1.56
Enterotoxigenic *E. coli*	<0.097	<0.097–0.195
Nontyphoid *Salmonella* spp.	0.25	0.03–2
S. enterica serovar Typhi	0.06	0.03–0.12
Shigella spp.	0.06	0.03–0.12
V. cholerae	0.015	0.008–0.015
Y. enterocolitica	0.12	0.03–0.5

[a]For *C. jejuni*, data are from reference 84 for nalidixic acid and ciprofloxacin and from reference 86 for ofloxacin; for enterotoxigenic *E. coli* data are from reference 209 for nalidixic acid, from reference 35 for ciprofloxacin, and from reference 86 for ofloxacin; for nontyphoid *Salmonella* spp., *S. enterica* serovar Typhi, *Shigella* spp., and *V. cholerae* from reference 70; for *Y. enterocolitica*, from reference 71.

diminished susceptibility has been varied. For *Salmonella enterica* serovar Typhi, (227), and possibly for *Shigella dysenteriae* type 1 (24), successful therapy of strains with diminished susceptibility requires a longer duration or therapy, higher dosages, or both. High-level resistance (MIC > 4 μg/ml) to fluoroquinolones among *Enterobacteriaceae* usually results from two or more mutations in the *gyrA* gene (47), and clinical response to such frankly resistant isolates is likely to be poor. The use of older nonfluorinated quinolones can select for single mutants, presumably increasing the risk of double mutants occurring (231). Thus, the continued use of nalidixic acid in developing countries, as recommended by the World Health Organization for the treatment of dysentery (12), is concerning both because nalidixic acid is less effective than the fluoroquinolones, and because it may increase the risk of high-level fluoroquinolone resistance developing.

The problem of fluoroquinolone resistance has been most pronounced for *Campylobacter jejuni* (113, 147, 177, 228), which had the highest initial MICs of fluoroquinolones (85, 106, 165, 236).

Resistance among other enteric pathogens has developed more slowly (74, 106, 113, 225, 166). *Campylobacter* infection is a zoonosis, and the rapid development of resistance among *Campylobacter* may result in part from the extensive veterinary use of quinolones, especially in poultry production (62, 63, 196, 213, 235). Resistance has also developed while receiving therapy in as many as 10 to 20% of patients with *Campylobacter* treated with a fluoroquinolone (61, 208, 253, 255). Quinolone use in veterinary practice has also been associated with the development and spread of resistance in nontyphoidal *Salmonella* (11, 140, 148, 149).

Development of resistance has profound implication for clinical practice. The fluoroquinolones are no longer useful for the treatment of *C. jejuni* infections, and in a retrospective study in Denmark infection with a quinolone-resistant strain of *S. enterica* serovar Typhimurium was associated with an approximate fivefold increase in the risk of death when compared with a pan-susceptible strain (104).

As is almost always the case with bacterial resistance, there is marked geographic variability in the prevalence of resistance (75). Decisions about the utility of the quinolones in individual infections must be based on local surveillance. Screening with nalidixic acid has been found to be useful in detecting strains that have intermediate susceptibility to the fluoroquinolones, but are not frankly resistant based on the National Committee for Clinical Laboratory Standards breakpoint of ≥4 μg/ml for resistant isolates (97)

PHARMACOLOGIC PROPERTIES OF IMPORTANCE IN TREATING ENTERIC INFECTIONS

In addition to their good in vitro activity, the fluoroquinolones are well absorbed after oral administration, even in patients with diarrhea (20, 22, 27, 120, 123, 129). The option for oral administration is important for a disease that, at least in industrialized countries, is rarely life threatening, and in which patients are alert enough to take oral medication. In the tropics, where diarrheal disease remains a major killer, (21, 25, 195), facilities for giving parenteral therapy are often not available, and thus oral administration is a necessity.

Serum drug concentrations after oral administration in patients with diarrhea are 1 to 5 μg/ml, depending on the quinolone used and the dosage given (22, 27, 29, 121, 123, 129). Concentrations in stool are manyfold higher than those in serum (22, 121, 123, 129), a consequence of both incomplete absorption and trans-intestinal elimination of drug

Table 2. Recent reports of susceptibility of enteric pathogens to the fluoroquinolones

Author (reference)	Country	Dates of isolation	Organism (*n*)	Rates of resistance[a]
Chu (46)	Hong Kong	1994–1995	*Shigella flexneri* (94)	60% to NA, 2% to CIP
			Shigella sonnei (38)	3% to NA, 0% of CIP
Vila (240)	Tanzania	1998	Enteroaggregative *E. coli* (65)	2% to NA, 0% to CIP
			Enterotoxigenic *E. coli* (44)	2% to NA, 0% to CIP
			Enteropathogenic *E. coli* (21)	0% to both NA and CIP
Chitnis (45)	India	1998–1999	*S. enterica* serovar Typhi (50)	60% to CIP
Threllfall (226)	England	1999	*S. enterica* serovar Typhi (179)	23% to NA and diminished susceptibility to CIP (0.38–0.75 µg/ml)
Thwaites (228)	England	1997	*C. jejuni* (5,401)	15% to NA, 10% to CIP
Smith (213)	United States, Minnesota	1998	*C. jejuni* (~800)	Approximately 10% to both NA and CIP
Hakanen (97)	Finland	1995–1997	Domestically acquired *S. enterica* serovar Typhimurium (154)	1% to both NA and CIP
			Foreign-acquired *S. enterica* serovar Typhimurium (34)	24% to NA, 15% to CIP
			Domestically acquired *S. enterica* serovar Enteritidis (75)	No resistance to NA or CIP
			Foreign-acquired *S. enterica* serovar Enteritidis (163)	4% to NA, 1% to CIP
Sáenz (196)	Spain	1997–1998	*C. jejuni* (537)	75% to NA
Prats (180)	Spain	1995–1998	*Salmonella* sp. (832)	11% to NA; <1% to CIP
			S. sonnei (30)	3% to NA, all susceptible to CIP
			S. flexneri (19)	5% to NA, all susceptible to CIP
Shapiro (209)	Kenya	1997–1998	*S. dysenteriae* type 1 (22)	2% to NA, 0% of CIP
			S. flexneri (51)	2% to NA, 0% to CIP
			Non-typhi *Salmonella* (29)	7% to NA, 0% to CIP
			45 *V. cholerae* O1	100% of 4 tested for NA, 0% to CIP
Isenbarger (112)	Thailand and Vietnam	1996–1999	Enterotoxigenic *E. coli* isolates from Thailand (203)	3% to NA, 2% to CIP
			Enterotoxigenic *E. coli* from Vietnam (112)	<1% for NA and CIP
			Salmonella sp. from Thailand (696)	21% to NA, <1% to CIP
			Salmonella sp. from Vientam (30)	0% to NA or CIP
			Shigella spp. from Thailand (175)	<1% to nalidixic acid, 0% to ciprofloxacin
			Shigella spp. from Vietnam (305)	<1% to NA, 0% to CIP
			C. jejuni from Thailand	72% to NA (489 isolates) 75% to CIP (426 isolates)
			C. jejuni from Vietnam (71)	1% to NA and CIP

[a] NA, nalidixic acid; CIP, ciprofloxacin.

(92, 157, 182–184, 191, 192). Trans-intestinal elimination may account for up to 25% of all excreted drug for some quinolones. Enterotoxins of *Vibrio cholerae* and *Escherichia coli* may further increase trans-intestinal elimination (156, 158).

Serum drug concentrations are usually >100-fold the MIC for most susceptible strains of enteric pathogens, and 10-fold or more the MIC for most strains that are resistant to nalidixic acid and have diminished susceptibility to fluoroquinolones (Table 3) (22, 24, 29, 121, 123, 129). Given that the quinolones are thought to have concentration-dependent bactericidal activity (259), these high concentrations relative to the MIC for enteric pathogens are likely an important determinant of their clinical efficacy. Concentrations in stool can be many thousandfold in excess of the MIC for the infecting enteric pathogen (Table 3) (22, 24, 86, 121, 123, 129, 130, 172). The quinolones leave the anaerobic gut flora relatively unchanged, thus also hopefully leaving colonization resistance intact (172, 173).

The relative importance of concentrations of drug in serum or stool depends on the enteric pathogen. For noninvasive pathogens, such as *V. cholerae*, intraluminal concentrations of drug are the critical determinant of success. For pathogens that invade the gut epithelium or can become systemically invasive, such as *Shigella* or *Salmonella*, serum, tissue, and intracellular drug concentrations are the more important determinant of success.

Table 3. Concentrations of ciprofloxacin in serum and stool of patients infected with *Shigella* or *V. cholerae*

Group (reference)	Dose of ciprofloxacin	Concn (μg/ml) in serum	Multiple of MIC for infecting strain of pathogen	Concn (μg/ml) in stool	Multiple of MIC for infecting strain of pathogen
60 adults with *S. dysenteriae* or *S. flexneri* infection (22)	500 mg every 12 h for 5 days	Peak: 1.50 Trough: 0.65	615 258	Day 3: 359 Day 5: 410	>1,000 >1,000
33 children with *S. dysenteriae* or *S. flexneri* infection (71% of *Shigella* resistant to nalidixic acid) (195)	10 mg/kg of body weight every 12 h for 5 days	Peak: 1.42 Trough: 0.16	11 1.8	Day 2: 156 Day 4: 154 Day 6: 18	>200 >200 >100
20 adults with *V. cholerae* infection (115)	1g single dose	Peak: 2.2	882	Peak: 21	>5,000

The relatively long half-life of the fluoroquinolones allows for once or twice daily dosing schedules (109). This property is a major advantage, especially in developing countries, where compliance can be especially problematic. The long half-life, combined with the very good activity against susceptible strains, has allowed successful use of quinolones for single-dose therapy of cholera and traveler's diarrhea (121, 197) and for shortened courses of therapy for shigellosis (one to three doses for infections with species other than *Shigella dysenteriae* type 1) (24) and for typhoid fever (163). The bioavailability of quinolones is not markedly affected by food intake, a crucial issue in the tropics where malnourished patients with diarrhea need to eat frequently.

In adults and in children, the quinolones are well tolerated, especially when given for the short courses used for treating enteric infections (22, 24, 27, 29, 121, 123, 129, 136). Nausea, anorexia, and diarrhea, which are the most commonly reported side effects of the quinolones, are hard to distinguish from the underlying disease in patients with diarrhea. In comparative studies of patients with diarrhea, nausea and other gastrointestinal complaints have not been more common in the quinolone-treated group. Other reported side effects of quinolones, including central nervous system alterations, have been rare in patients treated for diarrhea.

The safety of quinolones in children has remained a concern because, in juveniles of selected animal species, quinolones damage the articular cartilage of weight-bearing joints (37). Arthropathy in animals occurs at per kilogram per body weight doses similar in magnitude to those used in humans. Arthropathy has not been demonstrated in studies of children treated with quinolones for diarrhea or other acute infections (30, 31, 37, 40, 126, 129, 179, 199, 200, 229, 243, 244). Most of these studies have had relatively short follow-up (weeks to months), had a limited numbers of patients, and relied on clinical evaluation to assess arthropathy, rather than on

more sensitive indicators such as magnetic resonance imaging. Thus a small risk of the quinolones causing arthropathy, especially if the clinical manifestations of the arthropathy were to occur only years after the administration of the drug, cannot be ruled out. With increasing use of quinolones in children, larger retrospective studies have also not demonstrated an increased risk of tendon or joint disorders in children who have taken quinolones when compared with other antimicrobials (260). There are a limited number of case reports of quinolones causing arthralgia when used for longer periods. The majority of these have been in children with cystic fibrosis, which is known to be associated with arthralgia, or with the prolonged use of pefloxacin, which is the most potent of the quinolones in initiating arthropathy in animals (37). The arthralgia almost always has reversed on stopping the use of the quinolone agent (37).

Because of the uncertainty about whether quinolones cause arthropathy in children most clinicians in industrialized countries have not used it for non-life-threatening indications, such as diarrhea. In poor countries, where diarrhea is often a life-threatening illness, and because of the high prevalence of resistance to other agents, there has been much greater use of the quinolones. Depending on the pattern of resistance, in much of the developing world quinolones are first-line therapy for *Shigella* and *S. enterica* serovar typhi infections in children (12).

TREATMENT OF SPECIFIC CLINICAL CONDITIONS AND INFECTIONS

Fluoroquinolones—primarily ciprofloxacin and ofloxacin—are currently in routine use for the treatment of infections with *Shigella*, *S. enterica* serovar Typhi, severe or invasive infections with nontyphoid *Salmonella*, and for traveler's diarrhea. Because of widespread resistance, they are no longer useful for the treatment of *Campylobacter* infections.

This section reviews the indications for quinolone use in specific enteric infections or clinical conditions.

Empiric Therapy of Acute Diarrhea

Although most treatment studies have focused on patients with identifiable clinical syndromes associated with an enteric pathogen, most patients with diarrhea in industrialized countries present with nonspecific diarrhea. The utility of the fluoroquinolone agents for empiric therapy of diarrhea has been examined in at least five prospective, placebo-controlled studies in industrialized countries (54, 86, 164, 176, 253) (Table 4), and in at least three studies conducted completely or primarily in developing countries (38, 50, 138). Patients enrolled in these studies have been heterogeneous. In the five studies in industrialized countries the duration of diarrhea has ranged from 2 to 7 days (86, 164). The proportion of persons who had recently traveled outside the country where the study was conducted ranged from 1% (86) to 79% (253), and bacterial pathogens were identified in 33% (86) to 100% (176).

Four of the five studies have shown modest but significant reductions in diarrhea duration in the fluoroquinolone-treated group compared with placebo (Table 4). This reduction was one day in two studies (86, 253), 1.4 days in another study (176), and 2.4 days in the study that showed the greatest effect (54). The percent reduction in diarrhea duration after initiation of treatment ranged from 29 to 52%. Microbiologic outcome has been disappointing. *Campylobacter* resistance developed while receiving norfloxacin therapy in 6 of 69 patients in one study (253), and in 2 of 10 patients taking ciprofloxacin in another study (86). The four studies that provided information all showed an effect on pathogen excretion during or at the end of fluoroquinolone administration, undoubtedly representing suppression of growth because of remaining high stool concentrations of drugs. This salutary effect, at least for *Salmonella*, was largely lost when samples were taken in the weeks after therapy. *Salmonella* excretion was prolonged with norfloxacin treatment in one study (253), unchanged in one study of ciprofloxacin (54), and one study of ofloxacin (164), and reduced in one study of ciprofloxacin (175). There were too few (two) patients with *Salmonella* infection treated with ciprofloxacin in the fifth study to judge the effect of therapy (86).

The differences between studies make it difficult to reach a consensus about the role of empiric fluoroquinolone therapy for community-acquired diarrhea in industrialized countries. On the basis of the successful use of fluoroquinolones in treating traveler's diarrhea, when therapy is usually initiated early in the course of illness, there is reason to think that patients with acute diarrhea in industrialized countries who received early treatment would benefit the most. The study in which patients had the shortest duration of illness, however, was the only one that did not show a reduction in diarrhea duration (164). Another study that stratified by illness duration, however, found those treated within 48 h of onset derived the greatest benefit (253).

The studies that showed the greatest effect were those that may have had the sickest patients (54, 176). Based on that observation, some have recommended empiric use of fluoroquinolones for severe disease, often defined as more than four stools per day with associated symptoms (88). Such recommendations have drawn strong objections as not being cost-effective or as encouraging inappropriate use that will increase the prevalence of resistance in both pathogens and commensal flora (39, 112, 131, 221). A consensus statement from the British Society for the Study of Infection recommended against empiric therapy of acute gastroenteritis, estimating that the cost of ciprofloxacin for routine empiric therapy would be £24,000,000 annually in the United Kingdom (69). This group did suggest that empiric therapy with a fluoroquinolone might be warranted in the elderly or in those with dysentery. The Infectious Disease Society of America guidelines recommend, ". . .for patients with febrile diarrheal illnesses, especially those believed to have moderate to severe invasive disease, empirical treatment should be considered. . ." (94). Physicians, however, are likely to treat more often than is recommended by current guidelines. In one study, half of all patients admitted to the hospital with diarrhea received empirical ciprofloxacin, and the use of drug did not correlate with pathogen recovery (128).

Since the studies quoted above were conducted, two important changes have occurred. One is the marked increase in the prevalence of *Campylobacter* resistant to fluoroquinolones, which is now a worldwide phenomenon (64, 77, 78, 80, 106, 113, 151, 180, 194, 196, 211, 213, 228). This increase in resistance makes it unlikely that quinolones would still show the modest benefit they originally did in the four studies (all of which showed benefit) that included a large number of patients with *Campylobacter* infection (54, 86, 175, 253).

The second important change is research suggesting increased risk for the development of hemolytic-uremic syndrome (HUS) when patients with Shiga toxin producing *E. coli* (STEC) receive antimicrobials, especially quinolone agents. In exper-

Table 4. Studies of quinolones for empiric therapy of acute diarrhea in industrialized countries[a]

Author (reference), year	Where conducted	Study design	Quinolone dosage regimen	Comparator drug	Patient population and pathogens isolated	Clinical outcome	Bacteriologic outcome
Pichler (176), 1987	Austria	Randomized, double-blind	Ciprofloxacin, 500 mg q12h × 5 days	Placebo	76 adults > 19 yr with acute diarrhea <14 d admitted to hospital. Mean duration 4.3 days. All had bacterial infection; 37 Salmonella, 30 C. jejuni, 9 Shigella.	Diarrhea duration 1.5 days in ciprofloxacin group vs. 2.9 days in placebo group ($P < 0.001$).	3 wk after end of therapy 3/38 in ciprofloxacin group culture positive vs 12/36 in placebo group ($P < 0.001$)
Goodman (85), 1990	United States	Randomized, double-blind	Ciprofloxacin, 500 mg q12h × 5 days q12h × 5 days	Placebo or trimethoprim-sulfamethoxazole (800/160 mg)	173 adults with acute diarrhea ≤7 days, treated on presentation. Mean duration ≈4 days. 33% with bacterial infection: 32 C. jejuni, 16 Shigella, 13 Salmonella, 15 rotavirus	Diarrhea duration 2.4 days in ciprofloxacin group vs. 3.4 days in placebo group ($P < 0.005$); no significant difference between trimethoprim-sulfamethoxazole group and placebo group.	Bacteriologic eradication reported in 14 of 17 taking ciprofloxacin; 12 of 25 taking trimethoprim-sulfamethoxazole; and 4 of 19 taking placebo ($P < 0.001$ for ciprofloxacin compared with other two groups).
Wiström (253), 1992	Sweden	Randomized, double-blind	Norfloxacin, 400 mg q12h × 5 days	Placebo	511 persons > 11 yr with acute diarrhea < 6 days. Average duration, 2.8 days. 79% had traveled outside of Sweden in previous 6 wk. 51% with bacterial infection: 146 Campylobacter, 82 nontyphoid Salmonella, 18 Shigella	Median diarrhea duration 3 days in norfloxacin group and 4 days in the placebo group ($P = 0.02$). For patients with Campylobacter, the duration was 3 and 5 days, respectively ($P = 0.05$); for Salmonella 5 and 7 days ($P > 0.2$); for Shigella 2 and 3.5 days ($P > 0.2$).	7 to 12 days after completing therapy, Salmonella excretion rate in the norfloxacin group (32 of 39) was higher than in the placebo group (17 of 33, $P = 0.006$) and Campylobacter excretion was lower (17 of 56 vs. 32 of 64, $P = 0.03$). Shigella excretion rate was not significantly different (0 of 10 vs. 2 of 7, $P = 0.2$)

198

Study	Country	Design	Treatment	Comparison	Patient population	Clinical outcome	Microbiologic outcome
Noguerado (164), 1995	Spain	Randomized, double-blind	Ofloxacin, 400 mg as a single dose	Placebo	114 persons >15 yr with diarrhea ≤48 h. Mean duration 25 h. 62% with bacterial infection; 65 nontyphoid *Salmonella*; 5 *C. jejuni*; 1 each *Shigella* or *Aeromonas hydrophila*.	Diarrhea duration 2.6 days in ofloxacin group vs. 3.4 days in placebo group ($P = 0.1$) No significant difference in duration when only those with pathogen identified compared. Fever was shorter in ofloxacin group than in placebo group (0.6 vs. 1.1 day; $P = 0.02$).	At 48 h, 32% of ofloxacin group originally with enteric pathogen still culture positive vs. 59% in placebo group ($P = 0.002$). At 15 days, 23% vs. 29% ($P = 0.6$).
Dryden (54), 1996	United Kingdom	Randomized, double-blind	Ciprofloxacin, 500 mg b.i.d. × 5 days	Placebo	162 adults >18 yr with diarrhea (>4 stools/day for ≥3 days; upper duration limit not noted. Mean duration, 4.4 days. Bacterial pathogens in 85%; 74 *Campylobacter*; 51 *Salmonella*; 12 *Shigella*	Diarrhea duration 2.2 days in ciprofloxacin group vs. 4.6 days in placebo group ($P < 0.001$).	Pathogen present at end of treatment in 10/69 patients in ciprofloxacin groups vs. 44/67 in placebo group ($P < 0.0001$); at 6 wk respective values 8/67 vs. 8/65 ($P = 0.9$)

---

[a] Abbreviations: q12h, every 12 h; b.i.d., twice a day.

imental animal studies quinolones have been shown to increase the amount of Shiga toxin produced during STEC infection (1, 262). Both retrospective and a single prospective study found that antimicrobial treatment of patients infected with Shiga toxin producing *E. coli* increases the risk of developing HUS (170, 212, 257), though patients in those studies were predominantly treated with β-lactam or sulfa agents. Infection with STEC is increasingly common, especially in North America (13), and the clinical syndrome is not always so distinctive that patients with this infection could be excluded from empiric treatment on the basis of clinical features (28).

Studies of empiric fluoroquinolone therapy for acute diarrheal illness have not been conducted in children in industrialized countries. This presumably reflects, in part, the assumption that gastroenteritis in children is more likely to be caused by a viral infection (68) and the continued concerns about quinolone toxicity in children.

Two studies of empiric therapy of acute diarrhea using norfloxacin or fleroxacin were conducted primarily in developing countries and had a plurality of patients infected with *V. cholerae* or *Vibrio parahaemolyticus* (38, 138). Both showed clinical and microbiologic efficacy. A third study, conducted in Mexico, enrolled both residents and expatriates and found no significant effect of enoxacin when compared with placebo (50).

Traveler's Diarrhea

Treatment

All of the fluoroquinolone agents studied—ciprofloxacin (66, 197, 220, 252), norfloxacin (143, 224, 254), ofloxacin (55, 65), and fleroxacin (215)—have proven effective in shortening the duration and intensity of diarrhea when given to travelers with diarrhea. Treatment studies have demonstrated that illness duration after therapy can be shortened 25 to 75%, with most studies noting a duration of illness of 24 to 36 h after therapy is initiated (55, 66, 143, 174, 197, 215, 220) compared with 72 h or longer in the placebo groups.

The more consistent and more dramatic effect of fluoroquinolones on traveler's diarrhea when compared with empiric therapy of acute diarrhea in industrialized countries may be attributable to many factors. A large proportion (25% or more in most studies [55, 66, 143, 215], as high as 57% in one study [35, 220]) of travelers' diarrhea is caused by infection with enterotoxigenic *E. coli* (115), which is known to respond to antimicrobial therapy. Therapy is self-administered in most studies and thus is begun quite early in illness. Compliance among a motivated group of usually highly educated travelers is likely to be high.

Most studies have not had enough patients with *Campylobacter* or *Salmonella* to analyze separately the efficacy of empiric fluoroquinolone therapy in subsets of patients with these infections. In one study that did, 10 patients infected with *Salmonella* and treated with norfloxacin (400 mg twice daily for 3 days) had a mean duration of diarrhea of 1.1 days versus 4.1 days in the 13 patients in the placebo group ($P < 0.01$), and 11 patients infected with *C. jejuni* had a mean duration of diarrhea of 1.8 days compared with 5.0 days in the 10 patients in the placebo group ($P < 0.01$) (143). A separate study showed efficacy of ofloxacin treatment in a subset of patients infected with *Shigella* (55) and another in patients with enteroaggregative *E. coli* (82).

The fluoroquinolones do not appear to be better than trimethoprim-sulfamethoxazole (66, 224) or nonabsorbable agents (56) for treatment of traveler's diarrhea when infections are due to susceptible strains (2). This is not surprising, given that the predominant cause of traveler's diarrhea, enterotoxigenic *E. coli*, is not an invasive pathogen, and any agent that attains high intraluminal concentrations and to which *E. coli* is susceptible is likely to be effective.

In most parts of the developing world that have been studied, however, trimethoprim–sulfamethoxazole-resistant enteric pathogens are common (>25% of all isolates from recent studies of traveler's diarrhea) (84, 224, 239–242, 252, 254). The fluoroquinolones, in a single dose, have thus become the drugs of choice for treating traveler's diarrhea. Proven options for single-dose therapy include ciprofloxacin, 500 mg to 1 g (174, 197), 400 mg ofloxacin (65), or 400 mg of fleroxacin (215). Single-dose therapy is also likely to be effective even for *Shigella* infections, for which a single 1-g dose has been shown to be effective in infections with non-*S. dysenteriae* type 1 serotypes (24).

Studies of the antimotility agent loperamide given in addition to fluoroquinolones have given divergent results, with two studies showing no or modest benefit (174, 220), and another study showing considerable benefit when given with single-dose ofloxacin (65).

There have been no studies of fluoroquinolone treatment of children with traveler's diarrhea, and little is known about the epidemiology of traveler's diarrhea in children. As with empiric fluoroquinolone therapy of acute diarrhea in children in industrialized countries, this lack of study reflects lingering concerns about possible joint toxicity of the quinolones, and perhaps the belief that children who travel are more likely to be infected with viral agents rather than the bacterial pathogens to which their elders fall prey.

Prophylaxis of traveler's diarrhea

The efficacy of antimicrobial prophylaxis of traveler's diarrhea was well established by studies conducted starting in the 1970s with doxycycline, and then with trimethoprim-sulfamethoxazole (187). There have been at least six studies of fluoroquinolone prophylaxis of traveler's diarrhea (103, 116, 169, 181, 206, 256). All studies examined either norfloxacin or ciprofloxacin given once daily. The duration of prophylaxis in these studies ranged from 1 to 4 weeks. All six studies showed efficacy in reducing the incidence of diarrhea. The protection afforded by prophylaxis in these studies ranged from 76 to 100%, similar to what is found using nonquinolone agents (103). No major side effects of therapy were reported. In the two studies that reported on it, there was no increase in quinolone-resistant fecal flora (116, 256).

Despite the evident efficacy of prophylactic fluoroquinolones in preventing traveler's diarrhea, enthusiasm for its routine use has been limited. Reasons for this include the efficacy of early initiation of treatment in reducing the severity of diarrhea if it does occur, concerns about the development of resistance, concerns that travelers who take succor in the prophylactic drug will not use elementary precautions in avoiding high-risk food, the cost of the drug, and concerns about how to manage the patient if diarrhea does occur. Still, if someone is going to a particularly high-risk area for a short time, prophylaxis with a fluoroquinolone is likely to markedly diminish the risk of traveler's diarrhea.

Campylobacter jejuni

Even under the best of circumstances—early initiation of treatment, infection with susceptible strains—there is limited evidence that any antimicrobial has benefit in the treatment of *Campylobacter* enteritis.

Initial clinical studies conducted with erythromycin, both in children and adults, showed no or minimal clinical benefit of the treatment of *Campylobacter* enteritis (10, 141, 189). Benefit in these three studies might have been obscured by initiation of antimicrobial therapy late in the course of illness (5.6 days in one study) (10) or because of a high rate of coinfection with additional pathogens in another study (189). The one controlled study that showed benefit provided empiric erythromycin treatment to 170 children in Peru with inflammatory

diarrhea (201). In the subset of 28 children infected with *C. jejuni*, the subsequent duration of diarrhea was 2.4 days in the erythromycin-treated group and 4.2 days in the placebo group.

Because of their greater in vitro potency compared with erythromycin, the fluoroquinolones were expected to become standard treatment for campylobacteriosis (85). This expectation has not been realized for at least two reasons: lack of evidence from controlled trials that the fluoroquinolones are effective in treating *Campylobacter* infections, and rapid development of resistance to the fluoroquinolone agents (8).

Despite *Campylobacter* being the most common or the second most common (after *Salmonella*) enteric pathogen identified in the United States in recent years (13, 145), designing good controlled studies of *Campylobacter* enteritis is difficult. The lack of a distinctive clinical presentation does not allow a cohort of solely *Campylobacter*-infected individuals to be assembled. Reported series of patients in clinical trials treated with quinolones are all subsets of larger studies, either of travelers or persons with acute diarrhea in industrialized countries.

In the studies of empiric therapy in industrialized countries with sufficient patients with *Campylobacter* infection to allow analysis, one showed a decrease in duration of diarrhea after initiation of ciprofloxacin treatment (500 mg twice a day [b.i.d.] $\times$ 5 days) from 2.2 days in 11 patients in the placebo group to 1.1 days in the 19 patients in the ciprofloxacin group ($P < 0.01$) (176). In a study of norfloxacin (400 mg b.i.d. for 5 days), 69 patients receiving norfloxacin had diarrhea lasting 3 days after initiation of treatment compared with 5 days in 77 patients who received placebo ($P = 0.05$) (253). A third study showed no effect of therapy in 40 patients (85% of whom were infected with *Campylobacter*) who recieved lomefloxacin (400 mg once daily for 5 days) compared with 44 patients (89% infected with *Campylobacter*) who received placebo (61). All of the 36 *Campylobacter* isolates from patients in the lomefloxacin treatment group that were tested on admission were susceptible to this agent; following therapy, 7 (19%) had become resistant (61). One study of 42 travelers to Thailand who had *Campylobacter* infection and were treated with either ciprofloxacin or azithromycin found no difference between the two drugs in clinical outcome despite half the isolates being resistant in vitro to ciprofloxacin(127). This suggests that neither agent was effective.

The marked increase in resistance to the fluoroquinolones among *Campylobacter* (62–64, 75, 77, 78, 80, 106, 113, 127, 144, 151, 154, 180, 196, 211,

213, 228), including the high rate of development of resistance while on therapy (86, 258), has made their possible utility for empiric treatment of this infection a moot point. The prevalence of resistance is too high to allow their use for empiric therapy, for which a macrolide should be used if *Campylobacter* is suspected and the prescriber is convinced of the efficacy of therapy for this indication. Treatment of severe, documented infections should be guided by the antimicrobial susceptibility of the isolate.

Escherichia coli

Of the five diarrheagenic types of *E. coli*—enterotoxigenic, enteroinvasive, enterohemorrhagic, enteroaggregative, and enteropathogenic—evidence for the utility of the fluoroquinolones for treatment is available only for enterotoxigenic *E. coli*, with more limited evidence for its utility in enteroaggregative *E. coli*. As with *Campylobacter,* there is rarely a unique clinical picture for the diarrheagenic *E. coli* infections. Enterotoxigenic *E. coli* infection, the most common type worldwide, presents as nonspecific watery diarrhea that is difficult to distinguish from common viral causes of watery diarrhea. The nonspecific nature of the clinical illness, along with the lack of a rapid diagnostic test, makes it difficult to assemble a cohort for treatment studies. Thus evidence for the utility of the quinolones in treating *E. coli* infection has come from subsets of *E. coli*-infected patients enrolled in studies of empiric therapy, in this case, studies of traveler's diarrhea as discussed above.

Of the studies of empiric therapy of traveler's diarrhea that separately reported on the efficacy of treatment in patients with enterotoxigenic *E. coli*, one found a diarrhea duration after initiation of therapy of 33 h in 23 patients treated with 500 mg of ciprofloxacin b.i.d. for 5 days versus 84 h in 24 patients who received placebo ($P < 0.001$) (66). Another found a duration of diarrhea after initiation of treatment of 26 h in 22 patients given 300 mg of ofloxacin twice daily compared with 66 h in 26 patients who received placebo ($P < 0.05$), though in this same study the reduction achieved in the 18 patients who took 5 days of twice-daily ofloxacin (36 h) did not differ significantly from the placebo group (55). In a third study eight patients who received 400 mg of norfloxacin twice daily and were infected with enterotoxigenic *E. coli* had a diarrhea duration after treatment initiation of 1.0 day versus 3.1 days in 18 patients who received placebo (143).

One study of traveler's diarrhea examined a subset of patients infected with enteroaggregative *E. coli* and found a reduction in diarrhea duration after

initiation of therapy from 55 h in 16 patients who received placebo to 35.3 h in patients who received ciprofloxacin (500 mg twice daily for 3 days) ($P = 0.05$). There was no significant difference in stool frequency between the two groups (5.6 versus 7.5 stools).

In a study of chronic diarrhea associated with enteroaggregative *E. coli* infection in 24 HIV-infected adults in the United States, stool frequency decreased from 5.0 stools per day to 2.4 stools per day while receiving treatment with 500 mg of ciprofloxacin twice daily for 7 days ($P = 0.02$) (251). Seventy-nine percent of patients reported resolution or improvement of their diarrhea. Enteroaggregative *E. coli* could not be isolated from any patient 2 weeks after the initiation of therapy (in this study with a cross-over design, that meant that some were just completing ciprofloxacin therapy, and some had completed therapy 7 days previously) (251).

There is no evidence of the utility of the fluoroquinolones in enteroinvasive *E. coli* diarrhea (which is uncommon), enteropathogenic diarrhea (which is probably common but not often identified), or enterohemorrhagic *E. coli*. The latter presents with a somewhat distinctive pattern (though there is overlap with *Campylobacter*, *Shigella*, and *Salmonella* infection). There has been reluctance to conduct clinical trials of antimicrobials for this infection because, as discussed above, evidence exists that antimicrobial treatment might increase the risk of development of HUS (257). There is also evidence from in vitro and animal studies that treatment with ciprofloxacin, or other antimicrobials that damage DNA or inhibit its replication, increase Shiga toxin production by inducing bacteriophages that encode for the toxin (124, 125, 142, 262). It is Shiga toxin that is thought crucial for development of HUS during STEC infections.

Vibrio cholerae

Severe cholera is an immediately recognizable disease. No other illness causes such voluminous diarrhea and such rapid and profound diarrhea if untreated. Fluid replacement is the cornerstone of therapy; antimicrobial therapy, by reducing the duration and volume of diarrhea by half, is an important adjunct. This was first demonstrated in the early 1960s in a series of studies conducted with tetracycline at the Cholera Research Laboratory in Bangladesh (133, 134).

There have been only a limited number of randomized trials (some with quite small numbers of patients) examining the utility of fluoroquinolone agents in cholera (33, 38, 53, 57, 91, 120, 121, 150,

233). But because the efficacy of antimicrobial therapy in cholera had been well established before the fluoroquinolones became available, and because the results of the studies conducted to date (with norfloxacin, ciprofloxacin, or ofloxacin) have been so clear, fluoroquinolones now have an established role in the treatment of cholera.

In one study in Calcutta, India, 13 *V. cholerae*-infected patients treated with 400 mg of norfloxacin twice daily for 5 days had a significantly ($P < 0.05$) shorter duration of diarrhea after initiation of therapy than 12 patients receiving placebo (19.2 h versus 29.3 h) and less stool output (1,979 ml versus 3,507 ml) (32). A much larger double-blind study from Peru compared 100 patients who received 250 mg of ciprofloxacin once daily with 102 patients who received 500 mg of tetracycline four times daily, both for 3 days (91). Duration of diarrhea after initiation of therapy (51 h versus 48 h) and stool volume (219 versus 193 ml/kg body weight) were similar (91).

In a study of 15 patients given 500 mg of ciprofloxacin twice daily for 3 days in comparison with four other regimens, patients given ciprofloxacin had a watery stool output after initiation of therapy (155 ml/kg body weight) similar to 15 patients each given 3 days of treatment with erythromycin (221 ml/kg), nalidixic acid (246 ml/kg), or pivamdinocillin (212 ml/kg), and significantly less than 12 patients treated with tetracycline (293 ml/kg) (120). The latter were all infected with tetracycline-resistant *V. cholerae* O1 (120).

Two studies have examined single-dose ciprofloxacin therapy in cholera. One open-label randomized study of 74 adults with *V. cholerae* O1 infection in Turkey found a single 1-g dose of ciprofloxacin equivalent to two 500-mg doses of ciprofloxacin given on the same day and 100 mg of doxycycline given twice daily for 3 days in reduction of diarrhea volume, and superior to the doxycycline group in reducing diarrhea duration (233). A randomized, double-blind study conducted in Bangladesh compared a single 1-g dose of ciprofloxacin to a single 300-mg dose of doxycycline in 130 adults infected with *V. cholerae* O1 and 130 adults infected with *V. cholerae* O139 (121). Therapy was clinically successful (defined as cessation of diarrhea by 48 h after initiation of therapy) in 94% of the *V. cholerae* O1-infected patients who received ciprofloxacin versus 73% of the patients who received doxycycline ($P = 0.003$); in the *V. cholerae* O139-infected patients the rate of cure was 92% in each group. Bacteriologic success, defined as the absence of *V. cholerae* from cultures of stools after study day 2, was achieved in 95% of the *V.*

cholerae O1 patients treated with ciprofloxacin versus 69% of patients receiving doxycycline ($P < 0.001$); the respective proportions for the *V. cholerae* O139-infected patients were 98% and 79%, respectively ($P = 0.002$). In the *V. cholerae* O1 patient group the lower rate of clinical and bacteriologic success was attributable to the 27 patients in the doxycycline group infected with tetracycline-resistant strains of *V. cholerae*; therapy failed clinically in 14 of these patients.

A single study examining the efficacy of ciprofloxacin in preventing cholera in household contacts of persons with cholera found that a single 250-mg dose given within 24 h of the index case presenting was not successful in either preventing infection with *V. cholerae* O1 or the development of diarrhea (60).

To date, *V. cholerae* O1 or O139 strains resistant to the fluoroquinolones have not been reported. This lack of resistance, combined with the simplicity and efficacy of the single-dose ciprofloxacin regimen, make this a treatment of choice for cholera, along with other drugs, doxycycline and azithromycin, known to be effective in single-dose therapy of cholera (122).

Shigella

Nalidixic acid was the first quinolone agent evaluated for the treatment of shigellosis (99, 101, 199). The initial study found nalidixic acid largely ineffective for treating shigellosis (99); two subsequent studies both demonstrated efficacy (101, 199). Because of its much lower in vitro activity when compared with the fluoroquinolones, and the rapid development of resistance, especially among *S. dysenteriae* type 1 isolates (23), the role for nalidixic acid is treatment of shigellosis is limited (198).

Numerous studies have examined the utility of the fluoroquinolones (most commonly ciprofloxacin and norfloxacin) for treating shigellosis (19, 22, 24, 31, 34, 51, 79, 90, 123, 129, 139, 153, 190, 200, 243). Because the efficacy of antimicrobial therapy is well established in bacillary dysentery and because untreated disease can have substantial morbidity and mortality (21, 100), all of these studies compared a fluoroquinolone with an alternative therapy (nalidixic acid, trimethoprim-sulfamethoxazole, pivamdinocillin, ceftriaxone, or azithromycin), rather than placebo. In all studies the fluoroquinolone agents were as effective (19, 51, 90, 123, 129), or more effective bacteriologically (139, 190, 200, 243), or more effective bacteriologically and clinically (22, 34), than the comparator drug. Studies of empiric fluoroquinolone therapy of diarrhea that included a placebo control and sufficient number of patients infected with *Shigella* to allow analysis reconfirmed the efficacy of antimicrobial treatment of this illness (38, 138).

Most studies have examined fluoroquinolone therapy of 3 to 5 days duration (24, 34, 51, 123, 129, 139, 190, 200). Shorter courses of therapy, a single 800-mg dose of norfloxacin in adults (19, 90), a single 1-g dose of ciprofloxacin, or two 1-g doses of ciprofloxacin given 24 h apart (24), or two doses of 7.5 mg of ofloxacin given on 1 day to children (243), have all been effective in treating *Shigella* infections caused by nondysenteriae type 1 strains of *Shigella*. In the single study of short-course therapy in which large numbers of patients with *S. dysenteriae* type 1 (the most virulent serotype of *Shigella*) were enrolled, short-course therapy was inferior to 5-day therapy (six treatment failures of 25 patients in the one- or two-dose treatment groups, no treatment failures in the 10-dose treatment groups) (24). The inferior clinical response in short-course therapy in *S. dysenteriae* type 1 patients when compared with short-course therapy for patients infected with other serotypes of *Shigella* enrolled in the study may have been because of the greater severity of disease in *S. dysenteriae* type 1-infected patients, or because the median ciprofloxacin MICs for the *S. dysenteriae* type 1 isolates were more than 10 times those for isolates of other serotypes (0.06 μg/ml versus ≤0.004 μg/ml).

There have been at least five studies of fluoroquinolones (ciprofloxacin, norfloxacin, ofloxacin) in childhood shigellosis (31, 129, 200, 243, 263). None have noted arthropathy attributable to drug therapy. In one study in adults loperamide in addition to ciprofloxacin improved outcome without increasing toxicity (153).

Nontyphoid *Salmonella*

Fluoroquinolones have at least four potential uses in the treatment of nontyphoid *Salmonella*. These are reducing the duration of diarrheal illness, treating severe or invasive disease, decreasing the duration of excretion of *Salmonella*, and eradicating the organism in long-term carriers of *Salmonella*.

There is limited evidence from controlled clinical trials on which to base a firm recommendation for the use of fluoroquinolones for these four different indications. Placebo-controlled studies of the effect of treatment on the course of diarrheal illness have given contradictory results. Three studies have shown no effect of fluoroquinolone therapy on the clinical course of illness (38, 164, 204); two have

shown modest reductions (from 5 to 3 days, and from 3.4 to 1.9 days) in the duration of diarrhea (175, 253).

Also, the evidence on the utility of fluoroquinolones for reducing the duration of fecal excretion of *Salmonella* is contradictory. Most studies that have included cultures obtained after therapy had been stopped for 72 h or more have found either no effect of fluoroquinolone therapy on *Salmonella* excretion (41, 160, 164, 178, 204), or a prolongation of excretion (253). Prolonging therapy to 10 or 14 days does not seem to increase the rate of eradication (160, 246). Studies finding decreased duration of excretion are limited (176). Given the marginal clinical efficacy of fluoroquinolones for uncomplicated salmonellosis and the lack of bacteriologic efficacy, there seems to be no role for routine use of the fluoroquinolones for this indication.

Treatment of severe and invasive disease, or infections in immunocompromised hosts, has not been subject to clinical trials. Practice is based on many years of clinical experience in treating *Salmonella* with a variety of different antimicrobials for these indications, as well as case reports on the efficacy of fluoroquinolones for these indications (15, 67, 105, 111, 161). The very good in vitro activity of fluoroquinolones against most non-typhi *Salmonella* makes them useful for treating *Salmonella* in the immunocompromised host or for invasive disease.

The difficulty of assembling large numbers of established, chronic *Salmonella* carriers has made controlled clinical trials of fluoroquinolones for this indication difficult. Most case reports suggest that prolonged treatment with fluoroquinolones can reduce chronic carriage (52, 137, 186, 202); however, there may be a publication bias for cases in which treatment was successful in eradicating carriage. Fluoroquinolones have also been used, with reported success, to control outbreaks of *Salmonella* (4).

There is increasing resistance among non-typhi *Salmonella* to the quinolones (Table 4). In industrialized countries the risk of acquiring a resistant infection is particularly high for those who have recently traveled to a developing country (96, 98).

Typhoid fever

Numerous randomized, controlled studies, and reports of series of patients, have documented the efficacy of first nalidixic acid (102), and then the fluoroquinolones in achieving clinical and bacteriologic cure in patients with enteric fever caused either by *S. enterica* serovar Typhi or *S. enterica* serovar Paratyphi (3, 5–7, 9, 14, 40, 42, 44, 48, 49, 59, 81,

95, 119, 146, 162, 163, 185, 205, 207, 214, 223, 229, 230, 232, 234, 237, 244, 249, 250, 261). In a number of these studies the fluoroquinolone agent achieved better clinical results (40, 95, 230, 249), or better clinical and microbiologic results (214), when compared with trimethoprim-sulfamethoxazole (95) or with a cephalosporin (40, 214, 230, 249).

Before the fluoroquinolones became available, standard treatment regimens for the treatment of typhoid fever were 10 to 14 days. The very good in vitro potency of the quinolones, and their good intracellular activity (171) (S. enterica serovar Typhi is an intracellular pathogen), tempted several investigators to evaluate shorter courses of therapy—ranging from 2 to 7 days—for treating enteric fever (Table 5). In these trials short courses of therapy have been as effective as longer courses of therapy. Stopping therapy after 2 days, when the majority of patients are still febrile, is, if not counterintuitive, discomforting for most clinicians, and most would still treat for a minimum of 5 to 7 days.

As with Shigella, Campylobacter, and nontyphoid strains of Salmonella, the fluoroquinolone MICs for isolates of S. enterica serovar Typhi or S. enterica serovar Paratyphi that are resistant to nalidixic acid will be increased 10-fold or more, with resultant MICs being in the range of 0.125 to 2.0 µg/ml (44, 227, 248). The prevalence of such strains has been reported with alarmingly increasing frequency (33 to 90% of all isolates) from the Indian subcontinent (45, 114, 118), Southeast Asia (168), central Asia (152), and in travelers returning to Europe (225–227).

Infection with nalidixic acid-resistant strains impairs the clinical response to treatment with a fluoroquinolone. In a retrospective comparison from Vietnam of 150 patients treated with short (2 or 3 day) courses of ofloxacin, 18 patients infected with nalidixic acid-resistant strains had a higher rate of clinical failure (50 versus 3%, $P < 0.0001$) than 132 patients infected with susceptible strains, and a longer duration of fever (156 h versus 84 h, $P = 0.001$) (248). These high rates of clinical failure did not correlate with microbiologic response, because microbiologic failure occurred in only one patient infected with a nalidixic acid-resistant strain (248). Other series have also reported diminished clinical efficacy of fluoroquinolones in treating nalidixic acid-resistant strains of S. enterica serovar Typhi or Paratyphi (44, 58, 163). Resistance remains circumscribed geographically, with little quinolone resistance (or in some areas even resistance to older agents) being reported from Latin America or Africa (216).

Two studies with long-term follow-up have examined the utility of fluoroquinolones for eradicating chronic carriage of S. enterica serovar Typhi. In a comparative, blinded study, 11 of 12 persons receiving 400 mg of norfloxacin twice daily for 28 days had eradication of the organism, compared with 1 of 12 persons treated with placebo ($P < 0.01$) (89). In an uncontrolled study S. enterica serovar Typhi eradication was achieved in 10 of 12 persons treated with 750 mg of ciprofloxacin twice daily for 28 days (73).

Other enteric infections or conditions

Yersinia enterocolitica strains remain almost universally susceptible to the fluoroquinolones (72, 217, 219). The efficacy of antimicrobial therapy in Yersinia infection is uncertain, either for the enteritis or for invasive or immunologic sequelae (107, 108). Because most Y. enterocolitica remain susceptible to older, less expensive agents (219), there is little need to use a fluoroquinolone if treatment is initiated.

Aeromonas is increasingly considered a cause of diarrhea. Isolates remain uniformly susceptible to the fluoroquinolones (70, 76, 117, 167, 203), and case reports suggest clinical benefit from using fluoroquinolones (132, 159). As with Yersinia, because most strains remain susceptible to a variety of other less expensive agents, if therapy is initiated there is little need to use a quinolone. Plesiomonas shigelloides is another putative cause of gastroenteritis, strains of which are almost all susceptible to quinolones (17, 218). There is little evidence that antimicrobial therapy is indicated for this infection, however (94, 245). Ciprofloxacin has also been evaluated for treatment of chronic diarrhea in HIV-infected patients with the protozoan agents Isospora belli and Cyclospora cayetanensis, in which it was less effective than trimethoprim-sulfamethoxazole (238).

In controlled trials, nalidixic acid was found ineffective in 46 children with chronic diarrhea in India (18), but norfloxacin was effective in reducing stool frequency in 9 of 10 adult patients with small bowel overgrowth syndrome and chronic diarrhea (16).

SUMMARY

The fluoroquinolones, after more than 15 years in clinical use, remain among the drugs of choice for treating traveler's diarrhea, invasive or severe salmonellosis, enteric fever due to S. enterica serovar Typhi or S. enterica serovar Paratyphi, cholera, and shigellosis (Table 6). The development of resistance has, however, limited their usefulness for treating Campylobacter infections, and threatens their usefulness for treating enteric fever.

Table 5. Efficacy in comparative trials of short courses of fluoroquinolones in treating enteric fever[a]

Author (reference) year	Where conducted	Study design	Quinolone dosage regimen	Comparator drug	Patients enrolled	Clinical outcome	Bacteriologic outcome
Sarma (205), 1991	India	Open, randomized	Norfloxacin, 400 mg q12h × 7 days	Chloramphenicol, 15 mg/kg q6h until defervescence, then 13 mg/kg t.i.d. until day 14	40 adults	Mean time to defervescence 88 h in norfloxacin group, 124 h in chloramphenicol group. No relapses	Not reported
Smith (214), 1994	Vietnam	Open, randomized	Ofloxacin, 200 mg b.i.d. × 5 days	Ceftriaxone 3 g i.v. daily × 3 d	47 adults	Mean time to defervescence 81 h in ofloxacin group, 196 h in ceftriaxone group ($P < 0.0001$). Cure rate 100% in ofloxacin group, 72% in ceftriaxone group ($P = 0.01$).	100% in ofloxacin group, 92% in ceftriaxone group ($P = $ NS)
Tran (230), 1994	Vietnam	Open, randomized	Fleroxacin, 400 mg single daily dose × 7 days	Ceftriaxone 2 g i.v. daily × 5 days	31 adults	Mean time to defervescence 81 h in fleroxacin group, 160 h in ceftriaxone group, $P = 0.02$). Clinical cure 100% in fleroxacin group, 87% in ceftriaxone group ($P = $ NS)	100% in fleroxacin group, 93% in ceftriaxone group ($P = $ NS)
Nelwan (162), 1995	Indonesia	Open, randomized	Ciprofloxacin, 500 mg b.i.d. × 3 days	Ciprofloxacin, 500 mg b.i.d. ×6 days	59 adults	Clinical failure 14% in 3-day group, 0% in 6-day group ($P = 0.14$). One relapse in 3-day group.	89% cure rate in 3-day group, 94% in 6-day group ($P = $ NS)
Vinh (243), 1996	Vietnam	Open, randomized	Ofloxacin, 7.5 mg/kg b.i.d. × 2 days	Ofloxacin, 7.5 mg/kg t.i.d. × 3 days	100 children 1–15 yr	Mean time to defervescence 107 h in the 2-day group; 100 h in the 3-day group ($P = $ NS). Clinical cure rate 89% in 2-day group vs. 96% in the 3-day group ($P = $ NS). No relapses.	100% microbiologic cure in 2-day group; 98% in 3-day group ($P = $ NS)

Reference, year	Location	Design	Treatment 1	Treatment 2	No. of patients	Defervescence/clinical results	Cure rate
Ünal (232), 1996	Turkey	Open, randomized	Pefloxacin, 400 mg b.i.d. × 5 days	Pefloxacin, 400 mg b.i.d. × 7 days	46 adults	Mean time to defervescence, 3.1 days in 5-day group, 3.4 days in 7-day group (P = NS). One relapse in 5-day group.	96% in 5-day group, 100% in 7-day group (P = NS)
Agalar (3), 1997	Turkey	Open, randomized	Ciprofloxacin, 500 mg b.i.d. × 7 days	Ciprofloxacin, 750 mg b.i.d. × 10 days	50 adults	84% rate of cure in 7-day group vs. 96% in 10-day group (P = NS).	100% cure rate in both groups
Nguyen (163), 1997	Vietnam	Open, randomized	Ofloxacin, 7.5 mg/kg b.i.d. × 2 days	Ofloxacin, 5 mg/kg b.i.d. × 3 days	107 adults	Mean time to defervescence 97 h in both groups	100% in 2-day group, 98% in 3-day group
Girgis (80), 1999	Egypt	Open, randomized	Ciprofloxacin, 500 mg b.i.d. × 7 days	Azithromycin, 1 g on day 1, then 500 mg/d × 4 days	64 adults	Mean time to defervescence 3.3 days in ciprofloxacin group, 3.8 days in azithromycin group. No relapses	Cure rate in 100% in ciprofloxacin group, 97% in azithromycin group
Cao (39), 1999	Vietnam	Open, randomized	Ofloxacin, 5 mg/kg b.i.d. × 5 days	Cefixime, 10 mg/kg × 7 days	82 children <15 yr	Mean time to defervescence, 105 h in ofloxacin group; 204 h in cefixime group (P < 0.0001); clinical cure 97% in ofloxacin group, 75% in cefixime group (P = 0.002)	Microbiologic cure 100% in ofloxacin group, 95% in cefixime group (P = NS)
Chinh (43) 2000	Vietnam	Open, randomized	Ofloxacin, 200 mg b.i.d. × 5 days	Azithromycin, 1 g daily × 5 days	88 adults	Mean time to defervescence 134 h in ofloxacin group, 130 hours in azithromycin group (P = NS). Two relapses in ofloxacin group, none in azithromycin group	Cure rate 96% in ofloxacin group, 98% in azithromycin group (P = NS)

[a] Abbreviations: q12h, every 12h; b.i.d., twice a day; q6h, every 6h; t.i.d., three times a day; i.v., intravenously.

Table 6. Cost in Bangladesh and the United States of current regimens useful for the treatment of adults with bacterial diarrhea

Drug	Dose regimen and amount of drug	Cost in Bangladesh[a]	Percent of daily gross per capita national income in Bangladesh[b]	Cost in the United States[c]	Percent of daily gross per capita national income in the United States[b]
Ampicillin	500 mg q6h × 5 days	$2.61	258	$9.99	12
Azithromycin	500 mg day 1, then 250 mg daily × 4 days	$1.91	189	$42.99	50
Ciprofloxacin	500 mg q12h × 5 days	$2.43	241	$41.98	49
Doxycycline	300 mg single dose (for cholera)	$0.10	10	$2.10	2
Ofloxacin	400 mg ofloxacin q12h × 5 days	$2.61	258	$47.85	56
Trimethoprim-sulfamethoxazole	160/800 mg q12h × 5 days	$0.35	35	$10.99	13

[a] Prices are based on state-regulated prices for Bangladesh, which does not observe international patent rights on medications. Costs are calculated on the basis of the least number of tablets or smallest bottle of suspension required for treatment.
[b] Gross national income is from the World Bank (*http://www.worldbank.org/data/countrydata/countrydata.html*). Annual gross national income per capita in Bangladesh is $370, or $1.01 per day, and in the United States is $31,400 per year, or $86.03 per day.
[c] United States costs are from costs to patients posted on the website of a drugstore chain (*www.walgreens.com*).

Table 7. Treatment options for ciprofloxacin and ofloxacin in enteric infections where their efficacy is well established[a]

Infection	Adult dosage	Pediatric dosage
Traveler's diarrhea	Ciprofloxacin, 500 mg–1 g as single dose	Not evaluated
	Ofloxacin, 400–800 mg as single dose	
S. enterica serovar Typhi or Paratyphi	Ciprofloxacin, 500 mg twice daily for 5–7 days	Ciprofloxacin, 10 mg/kg twice daily for 5–7 days
	Ofloxacin, 400 mg twice daily for 5–7 days	Ofloxacin, 7.5 mg/kg twice daily for 5–7 days[b]
Shigella	Ciprofloxacin, 500 mg twice daily for 3 days	Ciprofloxacin, 10 mg/kg twice daily for 5–7 days
	Ofloxacin, 400 mg twice daily for 3 days	Ofloxacin, 7.5 mg/kg twice daily for 5–7 days
V. cholerae O1 or O129	Ciprofloxacin, 1 g as a single dose	Not evaluated
	Ofloxacin, 800 mg as a single dose	

[a] Ciprofloxacin and ofloxacin are selected as representative members of the fluoroquinolones with which there is the greatest experience treating these infections. Other fluoroquinolones with activities similar to those of these agents are likely to be efficacious.
[b] Longer courses of therapy or alternative agents may be required for treatment of strains with diminished susceptibility to fluoroquinolones (MICs, 0.125 to 1.0 µg/ml).

Although concerns about toxicity initially limited their use for treating childhood diarrhea, the age group with the highest incidence of infection, increasing experience has found little evidence of short- or long-term toxicity when these drugs are used for treatment of diarrhea.

The vast burden of diarrheal disease is borne by persons living in poor countries in Africa, Asia, and Latin America. Because most of the quinolones remain on patent, the costs of drug remain high, thereby limiting access to these agents where they are most needed. When quinolones are produced or procured off patent, their cost is much reduced, though often still prohibitively expensive for the poor (Table 7).

Since the introduction of the fluoroquinolones there have been no other classes of agents introduced that have their advantages for treating enteric infections. Continuing to benefit from the quinolones will require judicious use to halt (or if possible reverse) the development of resistance and to ensure that they are affordable to those persons in developing countries who need them most.

REFERENCES

1. Acheson, D. W., and C. L. Sears. 2001. Dangers of empiric oral ciprofloxacin in the treatment of acute inflammatory diarrhea in children. *Pediatr. Infect. Dis. J.* **20:**817–818.
2. Adachi, J. A., L. Ostrosky-Zeichner, H. L. DuPont, and C. D. Ericsson. 2000. Empirical antimicrobial therapy for traveler's diarrhea. *Clin. Infect. Dis.* **31:**1079–1083.
3. Agalar, C., S. Usubutun, E. Tutuncu, and R. Turkyilmaz. 1997. Comparison of two regimens for ciprofloxacin treatment of enteric infections. *Eur. J. Clin. Microbiol. Infect. Dis.* **16:**803–806.
4. Ahmad, F., G. Bray, R. W. Prescott, S. Aquilla, and N. F. Lightfoot. 1991. Use of ciprofloxacin to control a Salmonella outbreak in a long-stay psychiatric hospital. *J. Hosp. Infect.* **17:**171–178.
5. Ahmed, A., N. Salahuddin, T. Ahsan, S. Afsar, N. Nasir, S. Farooqui, A. N. Chaoudri, M. A. Akhtar, I. Agha, and N. Nagi. 1992. Enoxacin in the treatment of typhoid fever. *Clin. Ther.* **14:**825–828.
6. Ait-Khaled, A., L. Zidane, A. Amrane, and R. Aklil. 1990. The efficacy and safety of pefloxacin in the treatment of typhoid fever in Algeria. *J. Antimicrob. Chemother.* **26:**181–186.
7. Alam, M. N., S. A. Haq, K. K. Das, P. K. Baral, M. N. Mazid, R. U. Siddique, K. M. Rahman, Z. Hasan, M. A. Khan, and P. Dutta. 1995. Efficacy of ciprofloxacin in

enteric fever: comparison of treatment duration in sensitive and multidrug-resistant Salmonella. *Am. J. Trop. Med. Hyg.* **53:**306–311.

8. Allos, B. M. 2001. Campylobacter jejuni infections: update on emerging issues and trends. *Clin. Infect. Dis.* **32:**1201–1206.

9. Alsoub, H., A. K. Uwaydah, I. Matar, M. Zebeib, and K. M. Elhag. 1997. A clinical comparison of typhoid fever caused by susceptible and multidrug-resistant strains of Salmonella typhi. *Br. J. Clin. Pract.* **51:**8–10.

10. Anders, B. J., B. A. Lauer, J. W. Paisley, and L. B. Reller. 1982. Double-blind placebo controlled trial of erythromycin for treatment of Campylobacter enteritis. *Lancet.* **1:**131–132.

11. Angulo, F. J., K. R. Johnson, R. V. Tauxe, and M. L. Cohen. 2000. Origins and consequences of antimicrobial-resistant nontyphoidal Salmonella: implications for the use of fluoroquinolones in food animals. *Microb. Drug Resist.* **6:**77–83.

12. Anonymous. 1995. Guidelines for the control of epidemics due to *Shigella dysenteriae* type 1 WHO/CDR/95.4. World Health Organization, Geneva, Switzerland.

13. Anonymous. 2002. Preliminary FoodNet data on the incidence of foodborne illnesses—selected sites, United States, 2001. *Morb. Mortal. Wkly. Rep.* **51:**325–329.

14. Arnold, K., C. S. Hong, R. Nelwan, I. Zavala-Trujillo, A. Kadio, M. A. Barros, and S. de Garis. 1993. Randomized comparative study of fleroxacin and chloramphenicol in typhoid fever. *Am. J. Med.* **94:**195S-200S.

15. Asperilla, M. O., R. A. Smego, Jr., and L. K. Scott. 1990. Quinolone antibiotics in the treatment of Salmonella infections. *Rev. Infect. Dis.* **12:**873–889.

16. Attar, A., B. Flourie, J. C. Rambaud, C. Franchisseur, P. Ruszniewski, and Y. Bouhnik. 1999. Antibiotic efficacy in small intestinal bacterial overgrowth-related chronic diarrhea: a crossover, randomized trial. *Gastroenterology.* **117:**794–797.

17. Auckenthaler, R., M. Michea-Hamzehpour, and J. C. Pechere. 1986. In-vitro activity of newer quinolones against aerobic bacteria. *J. Antimicrob. Chemother.* **17:**29–39.

18. Bahl, R., N. Bhandari, M. K. Bhan, M. Saxena, and A. Bagati. 1996. Efficacy of antimicrobial treatment in non-dysenteric persistent diarrhoea in a community setting. *Acta Paediatr.* **85:**1290–1294.

19. Bassily, S., K. C. Hyams, N. A. el-Masry, Z. Farid, E. Cross, A. L. Bourgeois, E. Ayad, and R. G. Hibbs. 1994. Short-course norfloxacin and trimethoprim-sulfamethoxazole treatment of shigellosis and salmonellosis in Egypt. *Am. J. Trop. Med. Hyg.* **51:**219–223.

20. Beckebaum, S., J. Bircher, and H. Gallenkamp. 1996. Bioavailability of ciprofloxacin in patients with acute infectious diarrhoe. *Eur. J. Clin. Pharmacol.* **50:**511–512.

21. Bennish, M. L., J. R. Harris, B. J. Wojtyniak, and M. Struelens 1990. Death in shigellosis: incidence and risk factors in hospitalized patients. *J. Infect. Dis.* **161:**500–506.

22. Bennish, M. L., M. A. Salam, R. Haider, and M. Barza. 1990. Therapy for shigellosis. II. Randomized, double-blind comparison of ciprofloxacin and ampicillin. *J. Infect. Dis.* **162:**711–716.

23. Bennish, M. L., M. A. Salam, M. A. Hossain, J. Myaux, E. H. Khan, J. Chakraborty, F. Henry, and C. Ronsmans. 1992. Antimicrobial resistance of Shigella isolates in Bangladesh, 1983–1990: increasing frequency of strains multiply resistant to ampicillin, trimethoprim-sulfamethoxazole, and nalidixic acid. *Clin. Infect. Dis.* **14:**1055–1060.

24. Bennish, M. L., M. A. Salam, W. A. Khan, and A. M. Khan. 1992. Treatment of shigellosis: III. Comparison of one- or

two-dose ciprofloxacin with standard 5-day therapy. A randomized, blinded trial. *Ann. Intern. Med.* **117:**727–734.

25. Bennish, M. L., and B. J. Wojtyniak 1991. Mortality due to shigellosis: community and hospital data. *Rev. Infect. Dis.* **13:**S245–S251.

26. Bergan, T., S. Lolekha, M. K. Cheong, C. L. Poh, S. Doencham, and D. Charoenpipop. 1988. Effect of recent antibacterial agents against bacteria causing diarrhoea. *Scand. J. Infect. Dis. Suppl.* **56:**7–10.

27. Bergan, T., S. Lolekha, M. K. Cheong, C. L. Poh, and S. Patancharoen. 1988. Consequences of diarrhoeal disease on the pharmacokinetics of norfloxacin. *Scand J. Infect. Dis. Suppl.* **56:**11–3.

28. Besser, R. E., P. M. Griffin, and L. Slutsker. 1999. Escherichia coli O157:H7 gastroenteritis and the hemolytic uremic syndrome: an emerging infectious disease. *Annu. Rev. Med.* **50:**355–367.

29. Bethell, D. B., N. P. Day, N. M. Dung, C. McMullin, H. T. Loan, D. T. Tam, L. T. Minh, N. T. Linh, N. Q. Dung, H. Vinh, A. P. MacGowan, L. O. White, and N. J. White. 1996. Pharmacokinetics of oral and intravenous ofloxacin in children with multidrug-resistant typhoid fever. *Antimicrob Agents Chemother.* **40:**2167–2172.

30. Bethell, D. B., T. T. Hien, L. T. Phi, N. P. Day, H. Vinh, N. M. Duong, N. V. Len, L. V. Chuong, and N. J. White. 1996. Effects on growth of single short courses of fluoroquinolones. *Arch. Dis. Child.* **74:**44–46.

31. Bhattacharya, K., M. K. Bhattacharya, D. Dutta, S. Dutta, M. Deb, A. Deb, K. P. Das, H. Koley, and G. B. Nair. 1997. Double-blind, randomized clinical trial for safety and efficacy of norfloxacin for shigellosis in children. *Acta. Paediatr.* **86:**319–320.

32. Bhattacharya, M. K., G. B. Nair, D. Sen, M. Paul, A. Debnath, A. Nag, D. Dutta, P. Dutta, S. C. Pal, and S. K. Bhattacharya. 1992. Efficacy of norfloxacin for shigellosis: a double-blind randomised clinical trial. *J. Diarrhoeal. Dis. Res.* **10:**146–150.

33. Bhattacharya, S. K., M. K. Bhattacharya, P. Dutta, D. Dutta, S. P. De, S. N. Sikdar, A. Maitra, A. Dutta, and S. C. Pal. 1990. Double-blind, randomized, controlled clinical trial of norfloxacin for cholera. *Antimicrob. Agents. Chemother.* **34:**939–940.

34. Bhattacharya, S. K., M. K. Bhattacharya, P. Dutta, D. Sen, R. Rasaily, A. Moitra, and S. C. Pal. 1991. Randomized clinical trial of norfloxacin for shigellosis. *Am. J. Trop. Med. Hyg.* **45:**683–687.

35. Bouckenooghe, A. R., Z. D. Jiang, F. J. De La Cabada, C. D. Ericsson, and H. L. DuPont. 2002. Enterotoxigenic Escherichia coli as cause of diarrhea among Mexican Adults and US Travelers in Mexico. *J. Travel Med.* **9:**137–140.

36. Bryan, J. P., C. Waters, J. Sheffield, R. E. Krieg, P. L. Perine, and K. Wagner 1990. In vitro activities of tosufloxacin, temafloxacin, and A-56620 against pathogens of diarrhea. *Antimicrob. Agents Chemother.* **34:**368–370.

37. Burkhardt, J. E., J. N. Walterspiel, and U. B. Schaad. 1997. Quinolone arthropathy in animals versus children. *Clin. Infect. Dis.* **25:**1196–1204.

38. Butler, T., S. Lolekha, C. Rasidi, A. Kadio, P. L. del Rosal, H. Iskandar, E. Rubinstein, and G. Pastore. 1993. Treatment of acute bacterial diarrhea: a multicenter international trial comparing placebo with fleroxacin given as a single dose or once daily for 3 days. *Am. J. Med.* **94:**187S-194S.

39. Cadamy, A. R. 1997. Treating diarrhoea. Patients must be educated about which symptoms require treatment. *Br. Med. I. J.* **315:**1378.

40. Cao, X. T., R. Kneen, T. A. Nguyen, D. L. Truong, N. J. White, and C. M. Parry. 1999. A comparative study of

ofloxacin and cefixime for treatment of typhoid fever in children. The Dong Nai Pediatric Center Typhoid Study Group. *Pediatr. Infect. Dis. J.* **18**:245–248.

41. Carlstedt, G., P. Dahl, P. M. Niklasson, K. Gullberg, G. Banck, and G. Kahlmeter. 1990. Norfloxacin treatment of salmonellosis does not shorten the carrier stage. *Scand. J. Infect. Dis.* **22**:553–556.

42. Chew, S. K., E. H. Monteiro, Y. S. Lim, and D. M. Allen. 1992. A 7-day course of ciprofloxacin for enteric fever. *J. Infect.* **25**:267–271.

43. Chin, N. X., and H. C. Neu. 1984. Ciprofloxacin, a quinolone carboxylic acid compound active against aerobic and anaerobic bacteria. *Antimicrob. Agents Chemother.* **25**:319–326.

44. Chinh, N. T., C. M. Parry, N. T. Ly, H. D. Ha, M. X. Thong, T. S. Diep, J. Wain, N. J. White, and J. J. Farrar. 2000. A randomized controlled comparison of azithromycin and ofloxacin for treatment of multidrug-resistant or nalidixic acid-resistant enteric fever. *Antimicrob. Agents Chemother.* **44**:1855–1859.

45. Chitnis, V., D. Chitnis, S. Verma, and N. Hemvani. 1999. Multidrug-resistant Salmonella typhi in India. *Lancet* **354**:514–515.

46. Chu, Y. W., E. T. Houang, D. J. Lyon, J. M. Ling, T. K. Ng, and A. F. Cheng. 1998. Antimicrobial resistance in Shigella flexneri and Shigella sonnei in Hong Kong, 1986 to 1995. *Antimicrob. Agents Chemother.* **42**:440–443.

47. Conrad, S., M. Oethinger, K. Kaifel, G. Klotz, R. Marre, and W. V. Kern. 1996. gyrA mutations in high-level fluoroquinolone-resistant clinical isolates of *Escherichia coli.* *J. Antimicrob. Chemother.* **38**:443–455.

48. Cristiano, P., L. Imparato, C. Carpinelli, F. Lauria, M. R. Iovene, M. F. Corrado, P. Maio, and C. Imperatore. 1995. Pefloxacin versus chloramphenicol in the therapy of typhoid fever. *Infection* **23**:103–106.

49. Cristiano, P., G. Morelli, V. Briante, M. R. Iovene, F. Simioli, and P. Altucci. 1989. Clinical experience with pefloxacin in the therapy of typhoid fever. *Infection* **17**:86–87.

50. de la Cabada, F. J., H. L. DuPont, K. Gyr, and J. J. Mathewson. 1992. Antimicrobial therapy of bacterial diarrhea in adult residents of Mexico—lack of an effect. *Digestion* **53**:134–141.

51. De Mol, P., T. Mets, R. Lagasse, J. Vandepitte, A. Mutwewingabo, and J. P. Butzler. 1987. Treatment of bacillary dysentery: a comparison between enoxacin and nalidixic acid. *J. Antimicrob. Chemother.* **19**:695–698.

52. Diridl, G., H. Pichler, and D. Wolf. 1986. Treatment of chronic salmonella carriers with ciprofloxacin. *Eur. J. Clin. Microbiol.* **5**:260–261.

53. Doganci, L., H. Gun, M. Baysallar, A. Albay, E. Cinar, and T. Haznedaroglu 1995. Short-term quinolones for successful eradication of multiply resistant Vibrio cholerae in adult patients. *Scand. J. Infect. Dis.* **27**:425–426.

54. Dryden, M. S., R. J. Gabb, and S. K. Wright. 1996. Empirical treatment of severe acute community-acquired gastroenteritis with ciprofloxacin. *Clin. Infect. Dis.* **22**:1019–1025.

55. DuPont, H. L., C. D. Ericsson, J. J. Mathewson, and M. W. DuPont. 1992. Five versus three days of ofloxacin therapy for traveler's diarrhea: a placebo-controlled study. *Antimicrob. Agents Chemother.* **36**:87–91.

56. DuPont, H. L., Z. D. Jiang, C. D. Ericsson, J. A. Adachi, J. J. Mathewson, M. W. DuPont, E. Palazzini, L. M. Riopel, D. Ashley, and F. Martinez-Sandoval. 2001. Rifaximin versus ciprofloxacin for the treatment of traveler's diarrhea: a

randomized, double-blind clinical trial. *Clin. Infect. Dis.* **33**:1807–1815.

57. Dutta, D., S. K. Bhattacharya, M. K. Bhattacharya, A. Deb, M. Deb, B. Manna, A. Moitra, A. K. Mukhopadhyay, and G. B. Nair. 1996. Efficacy of norfloxacin and doxycycline for treatment of vibrio cholerae 0139 infection. *J. Antimicrob. Chemother.* **37**:575–581.

58. Dutta, P., U. Mitra, S. Dutta, A. De, M. K. Chatterjee, and S. K. Bhattacharya. 2001. Ceftriaxone therapy in ciprofloxacin treatment failure typhoid fever in children. *Indian J. Med. Res.* **113**:210–213.

59. Dutta, P., R. Rasaily, M. R. Saha, U. Mitra, S. K. Bhattacharya, M. K. Bhattacharya, and M. Lahiri. 1993. Ciprofloxacin for treatment of severe typhoid fever in children. *Antimicrob. Agents Chemother.* **37**:1197–1199.

60. Echevarria, J., C. Seas, C. Carrillo, R. Mostorino, R. Ruiz, and E. Gotuzzo. 1995. Efficacy and tolerability of ciprofloxacin prophylaxis in adult household contacts of patients with cholera. *Clin. Infect. Dis.* **20**:1480–1484.

61. Ellis-Pegler, R. B., L. K. Hyman, R. J. Ingram, and M. McCarthy. 1995. A placebo controlled evaluation of lomefloxacin in the treatment of bacterial diarrhoea in the community. *J. Antimicrob. Chemother.* **36**:259–263.

62. Endtz, H. P., R. P. Mouton, T. van der Reyden, G. J. Ruijs, M. Biever, and B. van Klingeren. 1990. Fluoroquinolone resistance in Campylobacter spp isolated from human stools and poultry products. *Lancet* **335**:787.

63. Endtz, H. P., G. J. Ruijs, B. van Klingeren, W. H. Jansen, T. van der Reyden, and R. P. Mouton. 1991. Quinolone resistance in campylobacter isolated from man and poultry following the introduction of fluoroquinolones in veterinary medicine. *J. Antimicrob. Chemother.* **27**:199–208.

64. Engberg, J., F. M. Aarestrup, D. E. Taylor, P. Gerner-Smidt, and I. Nachamkin. 2001. Quinolone and macrolide resistance in Campylobacter jejuni and C. coli: resistance mechanisms and trends in human isolates. *Emerg. Infect. Dis.* **7**:24–34.

65. Ericsson, C. D., H. L. DuPont, and J. J. Mathewson. 1997. Single dose ofloxacin plus loperamide compared with single dose or three days of ofloxacin in the treatment of traveler's diarrhea. *J. Travel Med.* **4**:3–7.

66. Ericsson, C. D., P. C. Johnson, H. L. Dupont, D. R. Morgan, J. A. Bitsura, and F. J. de la Cabada. 1987. Ciprofloxacin or trimethoprim-sulfamethoxazole as initial therapy for travelers' diarrhea. A placebo-controlled, randomized trial. *Ann. Intern. Med.* **106**:216–220.

67. Esposito, S., G. B. Gaeta, D. Galante, and D. Barba. 1985. Successful treatment with ciprofloxacin of Salmonella typhimurium infection in an immunocompromised host. *Infection* **13**:288.

68. Essers, B., A. P. Burnens, F. M. Lanfranchini, S. G. Somaruga, R. O. von Vigier, U. B. Schaad, C. Aebi, and M. G. Bianchetti. 2000. Acute community-acquired diarrhea requiring hospital admission in Swiss children. *Clin. Infect. Dis.* **31**:192–196.

69. Farthing, M., R. Feldman, R. Finch, R. Fox, C. Leen, B. Mandal, P. Moss, D. Nathwani, F. Nye, A. Percival, R. Read, L. Ritchie, W. T. Todd, and M. Wood. 1996. The management of infective gastroenteritis in adults. A consensus statement by an expert panel convened by the British Society for the Study of Infection. *J. Infect.* **33**:143–152.

70. Felmingham, D., and M. J. Robbins. 1992. In vitro activity of lomefloxacin and other antimicrobials against bacterial enteritis pathogens. *Diagn. Microbiol. Infect. Dis.* **15**:339–343.

71. Felmingham, D., M. J. Robbins, K. Ingley, I. Mathias, H.

Bhogal, A. Leakey, G. L. Ridgway, and R. N. Gruneberg. 1997. In-vitro activity of trovafloxacin, a new fluoroquinolone, against recent clinical isolates. *J. Antimicrob. Chemother.* **39**:43–49.

72. Fernandez-Roblas, R., F. Cabria, J. Esteban, J. C. Lopez, I. Gadea, and F. Soriano. 2000. In vitro activity of gemifloxacin (SB-265805) compared with 14 other antimicrobials against intestinal pathogens. *J. Antimicrob. Chemother.* **46**:1023–1027.

73. Ferreccio, C., J. G. Morris, Jr., C. Valdivieso, I. Prenzel, V. Sotomayor, G. L. Drusano, and M. M. Levine 1988. Efficacy of ciprofloxacin in the treatment of chronic typhoid carriers. *J. Infect. Dis.* **157**:1235–1239.

74. Frost, J. A., A. Kelleher, and B. Rowe. 1996. Increasing ciprofloxacin resistance in salmonellas in England and Wales 1991–1994. *J. Antimicrob. Chemother.* **37**:85–91.

75. Garcia-Rodriguez, J. A., M. J. Fresnadillo, M. I. Garcia, E. Garcia-Sanchez, J. E. Garcia-Sanchez, and I. Trujillano. 1995. Multicenter Spanish study of ciprofloxacin susceptibility in gram-negative bacteria. The Spanish Study Group on Quinolone Resistance. *Eur. J. Clin. Microbiol. Infect. Dis.* **14**:456–459.

76. Garcia-Rodriguez, J. A., J. E. Garcia Sanchez, M. I. Garcia Garcia, M. J. Fresnadillo, I. Trujillano, and E. Garcia Sanchez 1994. In-vitro activity of four new fluoroquinolones. *J. Antimicrob. Chemother.* **34**:53–64.

77. Gaudreau, C., and H. Gilbert. 1998. Antimicrobial resistance of clinical strains of Campylobacter jejuni subsp. jejuni isolated from 1985 to 1997 in Quebec, Canada. *Antimicrob. Agents Chemother.* **42**:2106–2108.

78. Gaunt, P. N., and L. J. Piddock. 1996. Ciprofloxacin resistant Campylobacter spp. in humans: an epidemiological and laboratory study. *J. Antimicrob. Chemother.* **37**:747–757.

79. Gendrel, D., J. L. Moreno, M. Nduwimana, C. Baribwira, and J. Raymond. 1997. One-dose treatment with pefloxacin for infection due to multidrug-resistant Shigella dysenteriae type 1 in Burundi. *Clin. Infect. Dis.* **24**:83.

80. Gibreel, A., E. Sjogren, B. Kaijser, B. Wretlind, and O. Skold. 1998. Rapid emergence of high-level resistance to quinolones in Campylobacter jejuni associated with mutational changes in gyrA and parC. *Antimicrob. Agents Chemother.* **42**:3276–3278.

81. Girgis, N. I., T. Butler, R. W. Frenck, Y. Sultan, F. M. Brown, D. Tribble, and R. Khakhria. 1999. Azithromycin versus ciprofloxacin for treatment of uncomplicated typhoid fever in a randomized trial in Egypt that included patients with multidrug resistance. *Antimicrob. Agents Chemother.* **43**:1441–1444.

82. Glandt, M., J. A. Adachi, J. J. Mathewson, Z. D. Jiang, D. DiCesare, D. Ashley, C. D. Ericsson, and H. L. DuPont. 1999. Enteroaggregative Escherichia coli as a cause of traveler's diarrhea: clinical response to ciprofloxacin. *Clin. Infect. Dis.* **29**:335–338.

83. Goldstein, F. W., J. C. Chumpitaz, J. M. Guevara, B. Papadopoulou, J. F. Acar, and J. F. Vieu. 1986. Plasmidmediated resistance to multiple antibiotics in Salmonella typhi. *J. Infect. Dis.* **153**:261–266.

84. Gomi, H., Z. D. Jiang, J. A. Adachi, D. Ashley, B. Lowe, M. P. Verenkar, R. Steffen, and H. L. DuPont. 2001. In vitro antimicrobial susceptibility testing of bacterial enteropathogens causing traveler's diarrhea in four geographic regions. *Antimicrob. Agents Chemother.* **45**: 212–216.

85. Goodman, L. J., R. M. Fliegelman, G. M. Trenholme, and R. L. Kaplan. 1984. Comparative in vitro activity of ciprofloxacin against Campylobacter spp. and other bacterial enteric pathogens. *Antimicrob. Agents Chemother.* **25**:504–506.

86. Goodman, L. J., G. M. Trenholme, R. L. Kaplan, J. Segreti, D. Hines, R. Petrak, J. A. Nelson, K. W. Mayer, W. Landau, G. W. Parkhurst, et al. 1990. Empiric antimicrobial therapy of domestically acquired acute diarrhea in urban adults. *Arch. Intern. Med.* **150**:541–546.

87. Goossens, H., P. De Mol, H. Coignau, J. Levy, O. Grados, G. Ghysels, H. Innocent, and J. P. Butzler. 1985. Comparative in vitro activities of aztreonam, ciprofloxacin, norfloxacin, ofloxacin, HR 810 (a new cephalosporin), RU28965 (a new macrolide), and other agents against enteropathogens. *Antimicrob. Agents Chemother.* **27**:388–392.

88. Gorbach, S. L. 1997. Treating diarrhoea. *Br. Med. J.* **314**:1776–1777.

89. Gotuzzo, E., J. G. Guerra, L. Benavente, J. C. Palomino, C. Carrillo, J. Lopera, F. Delgado, D. R. Nalin, and J. Sabbaj. 1988. Use of norfloxacin to treat chronic typhoid carriers. *J. Infect. Dis.* **157**:1221–1225.

90. Gotuzzo, E., R. A. Oberhelman, C. Maguina, S. J. Berry, A. Yi, M. Guzman, R. Ruiz, R. Leon-Barua, and R. B. Sack. 1989. Comparison of single-dose treatment with norfloxacin and standard 5-day treatment with trimethoprim-sulfamethoxazole for acute shigellosis in adults. *Antimicrob. Agents Chemother.* **33**:1101–1104.

91. Gotuzzo, E., C. Seas, J. Echevarria, C. Carrillo, R. Mostorino, and R. Ruiz. 1995. Ciprofloxacin for the treatment of cholera: a randomized, double-blind, controlled clinical trial of a single daily dose in Peruvian adults. *Clin. Infect. Dis.* **20**:1485–1490.

92. Griffiths, N. M., B. H. Hirst, and N. L. Simmons. 1994. Active intestinal secretion of the fluoroquinolone antibacterials ciprofloxacin, norfloxacin and pefloxacin; a common secretory pathway? *J. Pharmacol. Exp. Ther.* **269**:496–502.

93. Gruneberg, R. N., D. Felmingham, M. D. O'Hare, M. J. Robbins, K. Perry, R. A. Wall, and G. L. Ridgway. 1988. The comparative in-vitro activity of ofloxacin. *J. Antimicrob. Chemother.* **22**:9–19.

94. Guerrant, R. L., T. Van Gilder, T. S. Steiner, N. M. Thielman, L. Slutsker, R. V. Tauxe, T. Hennessy, P. M. Griffin, H. DuPont, R. B. Sack, P. Tarr, M. Neill, I. Nachamkin, L. B. Reller, M. T. Osterholm, M. L. Bennish, and L. K. Pickering. 2001. Practice guidelines for the management of infectious diarrhea. *Clin. Infect. Dis.* **32**:331–351.

95. Hajji, M., N. el Mdaghri, M. Benbachir, K. M. el Filali, and H. Himmich. 1988. Prospective randomized comparative trial of pefloxacin versus cotrimoxazole in the treatment of typhoid fever in adults. *Eur. J. Clin. Microbiol. Infect. Dis.* **7**:361–363.

96. Hakanen, A., P. Kotilainen, P. Huovinen, H. Helenius, and A. Siitonen. 2001. Reduced fluoroquinolone susceptibility in Salmonella enterica serotypes in travelers returning from Southeast Asia. *Emerg. Infect. Dis.* **7**:996–1003.

97. Hakanen, A., P. Kotilainen, J. Jalava, A. Siitonen, and P. Huovinen. 1999. Detection of decreased fluoroquinolone susceptibility in Salmonellas and validation of nalidixic acid screening test. *J. Clin. Microbiol.* **37**:3572–3577.

98. Hakanen, A., A. Siitonen, P. Kotilainen, and P. Huovinen. 1999. Increasing fluoroquinolone resistance in salmonella serotypes in Finland during 1995–1997. *J. Antimicrob. Chemother.* **43**:145–148.

99. Haltalin, K. C., J. D. Nelson, and H. T. Kusmiesz. 1973. Comparative efficacy of nalidixic acid and ampicillin for severe shigellosis. *Arch. Dis. Child.* **48**:305–312.

100. Haltalin, K. C., J. D. Nelson, R. Ring III, M. Sladoje, and L. V. Hinton. 1967. Double-blind treatment study of shigellosis comparing ampicillin, sulfadiazine, and placebo. J. Pediatr. 70:970–981.

101. Hansson, H. B., G. Barkenius, S. Cronberg, and I. Juhlin. 1981. Controlled comparison of nalidixic acid or lactulose with placebo in shigellosis. Scand. J. Infect. Dis. 13:191–193.

102. Hassan, A., M. F. Wahab, Z. Farid, and A. S. el-Rooby. 1970. Treatment of typhoid and paratyphoid fever with nalidixic acid. J. Trop. Med. Hyg. 73:145–147.

103. Heck, J. E., J. L. Staneck, M. B. Cohen, L. S. Weckbach, R. A. Giannella, J. Hawkins, and R. Tosiello. 1994. Prevention of Travelers' Diarrhea: ciprofloxacin versus trimethoprim/sulfamethoxazole in adult volunteers working in Latin America and the Caribbean. J. Travel Med. 1:136–142.

104. Helms, M., P. Vastrup, P. Gerner-Smidt, and K. Molbak. 2002. Excess mortality associated with antimicrobial drug-resistant Salmonella typhimurium. Emerg. Infect. Dis. 8:490–495.

105. Heseltine, P. N., D. M. Causey, M. D. Appleman, M. L. Corrado, and J. M. Leedom. 1988. Norfloxacin in the eradication of enteric infections in AIDS patients. Eur. J. Cancer Clin. Oncol. 24:S25–S8.

106. Hoge, C. W., J. M. Gambel, A. Srijan, C. Pitarangsi, and P. Echeverria. 1998. Trends in antibiotic resistance among diarrheal pathogens isolated in Thailand over 15 years. Clin. Infect. Dis. 26:341–345.

107. Hoogkamp-Korstanje, J. A.. 1987. Antibiotics in Yersinia enterocolitica infections. J. Antimicrob. Chemother. 20:123–131.

108. Hoogkamp-Korstanje, J. A., H. Moesker, and G. A. Bruyn. 2000. Ciprofloxacin v placebo for treatment of Yersinia enterocolitica triggered reactive arthritis. Ann. Rheum. Dis. 59:914–917.

109. Hooper, D. C. 2000. New uses for new and old quinolones and the challenge of resistance. Clin. Infect. Dis. 30:243–254.

110. Horiuchi, S., Y. Inagaki, N. Yamamoto, N. Okamura, Y. Imagawa, and R. Nakaya. 1993. Reduced susceptibilities of Shigella sonnei strains isolated from patients with dysentery to fluoroquinolones. Antimicrob. Agents Chemother. 37:2486–2489.

111. Hung, C. C., S. M. Hsieh, C. F. Hsiao, M. Y. Chen, and W. H. Sheng. 2001. Risk of recurrent non-typhoid Salmonella bacteraemia after early discontinuation of ciprofloxacin as secondary prophylaxis in AIDS patients in the era of highly active antiretroviral therapy. AIDS 15:645–647.

112. Inglesfield, J. W. 1997. Treating diarrhoea. Advocating widespread use of antimicrobial agents has economic implications. Br. Med. J. 315:1379.

113. Isenbarger, D. W., C. W. Hoge, A. Srijan, C. Pitarangsi, N. Vithayasai, L. Bodhidatta, K. W. Hickey, and P. D. Cam. 2002. Comparative antibiotic resistance of diarrheal pathogens from Vietnam and Thailand, 1996–1999. Emerg. Infect. Dis. 8:175–180.

114. Jesudason, M. V., B. Malathy, and T. J. John. 1996. Trend of increasing levels of minimum inhibitory concentration of ciprofloxacin to Salmonella typhi Indian. J. Med. Res. 103:247–249.

115. Jiang, Z. D., B. Lowe, M. P. Verenkar, D. Ashley, R. Steffen, N. Tornieporth, F. von Sonnenburg, P. Waiyaki, and H. L. DuPont. 2002. Prevalence of enteric pathogens among international travelers with diarrhea acquired in Kenya (Mombasa), India (Goa), or Jamaica (Montego Bay). J. Infect. Dis. 185:497–502.

116. Johnson, P. C., C. D. Ericsson, D. R. Morgan, H. L. Dupont, and F. J. Cabada. 1986. Lack of emergence of resistant fecal flora during successful prophylaxis of traveler's diarrhea with norfloxacin. Antimicrob. Agents Chemother. 30:671–674.

117. Kampfer, P., C. Christmann, J. Swings, and G. Huys. 1999. In vitro susceptibilities of Aeromonas genomic species to 69 antimicrobial agents. Syst. Appl. Microbiol. 22:662–669.

118. Kapil, A., S. Sood, N. R. Dash, B. K. Das, and P. Seth. 1999. Ciprofloxacin in typhoid fever. Lancet 354:164.

119. Khan, M. A., Z. Hayat, and A. Sadick. 1994. Ofloxacin in the treatment of typhoid fever resistant to chloramphenicol and amoxicillin. Clin. Ther. 16:815–818.

120. Khan, W. A., M. Begum, M. A. Salam, P. K. Bardhan, M. R. Islam, and D. Mahalanabis. 1995. Comparative trial of five antimicrobial compounds in the treatment of cholera in adults. Trans. R. Soc. Trop. Med. Hyg. 89:103–106.

121. Khan, W. A., M. L. Bennish, C. Seas, E. H. Khan, A. Ronan, U. Dhar, W. Busch, and M. A. Salam. 1996. Randomised controlled comparison of single-dose ciprofloxacin and doxycycline for cholera caused by Vibrio cholerae 01 or 0139. Lancet 348:296–300.

122. Khan, W. A., D. Saha, A. Rahman, M. A. Salam, J. Bogaerts, and M. L. Bennish. Randomised, double-blinded comparison of single-dose azithromycin and 12 dose, 3-day erythromycin therapy for childhood cholera Lancet, in press.

123. Khan, W. A., C. Seas, U. Dhar, M. A. Salam, and M. L. Bennish. 1997. Treatment of shigellosis. V. Comparison of azithromycin and ciprofloxacin. A double-blind, randomized, controlled trial. Ann. Intern. Med. 126:697–703.

124. Kimmitt, P. T., C. R. Harwood, and M. R. Barer. 1999. Induction of type 2 Shiga toxin synthesis in Escherichia coli O157 by 4-quinolones. Lancet 353:1588–1589.

125. Kimmitt, P. T., C. R. Harwood, and M. R. Barer. 2000. Toxin gene expression by shiga toxin-producing Escherichia coli: the role of antibiotics and the bacterial SOS response. Emerg. Infect. Dis. 6:458–465.

126. Kubin, R. 1993. Safety and efficacy of ciprofloxacin in paediatric patients—review. Infection 21:413–421.

127. Kuschner, R. A., A. F. Trofa, R. J. Thomas, C. W. Hoge, C. Pitarangsi, S. Amato, R. P. Olafson, P. Echeverria, J. C. Sadoff, and D. N. Taylor. 1995. Use of azithromycin for the treatment of Campylobacter enteritis in travelers to Thailand, an area where ciprofloxacin resistance is prevalent.Clin. Infect. Dis. 21:536–541.

128. Laing, R. B., C. Lee, and C. L. Leen. 1996. An audit of the clinical features and use of antimicrobials in adult diarrhoea. J. Infect. 32:17–21.

129. Leibovitz, E., J. Janco, L. Piglansky, J. Press, P. Yagupsky, H. Reinhart, I. Yaniv, and R. Dagan. 2000. Oral ciprofloxacin vs. intramuscular ceftriaxone as empiric treatment of acute invasive diarrhea in children. Pediatr. Infect. Dis. J. 19:1060–1067.

130. Leigh, D. A., B. Walsh, K. Harris, P. Hancock, and G. Travers. 1988. Pharmacokinetics of ofloxacin and the effect on the faecal flora of healthy volunteers. J. Antimicrob. Chemother. 22:115–125.

131. Leung, D., and P. Venkatesan. 1997. Treating diarrhoea. More evidence is needed that widespread use of quinolones will benefit patients. Br. Med. J. 315:1379.

132. Liao, W. C., and M. S. Cappell. 1989. Treatment with ciprofloxacin of Aeromonas hydrophila associated colitis in a male with antibodies to the human immunodeficiency virus. J. Clin. Gastroenterol. 11:552–554.

133. Lindenbaum, J., W. B. Greenough, and M. R. Islam. 1967. Antibiotic therapy of cholera. Bull. W. H. O. 36:871–883.

134. Lindenbaum, J., W. B. Greenough, and M. R. Islam. 1967. Antibiotic therapy of cholera in children. *Bull. W. H. O.* 37:529–538.

135. Ling, J., K. M. Kam, A. W. Lam, and G. L. French. 1988. Susceptibilities of Hong Kong isolates of multiply resistant Shigella spp. to 25 antimicrobial agents, including ampicillin plus sulbactam and new 4-quinolones. *Antimicrob. Agents. Chemother.* 32:20–23.

136. Lipsky, B. A., and C. A. Baker. 1999. Fluoroquinolone toxicity profiles: a review focusing on newer agents. *Clin. Infect. Dis.* 28:352–364.

137. Loffler, A., and H. Grafvon Westphalen. 1986. Successful treatment of chronic Salmonella excretor with ofloxacin. *Lancet* 1:1206.

138. Lolekha, S., S. Patanacharoen, B. Thanangkul, and S. Vibulbandhitkit. 1988. Norfloxacin versus co-trimoxazole in the treatment of acute bacterial diarrhoea: a placebo controlled study. *Scand. J. Infect. Dis. Suppl.* 56:35–45.

139. Lolekha, S., S. Vibulbandhitkit, and P. Poonyarit. 1991. Response to antimicrobial therapy for shigellosis in Thailand. *Rev. Infect. Dis.* 13:S342–S346.

140. Malorny, B., A. Schroeter, and R. Helmuth. 1999. Incidence of quinolone resistance over the period 1986 to 1998 in veterinary Salmonella isolates from Germany. *Antimicrob. Agents Chemother.* 43:2278–2282.

141. Mandal, B. K., M. E. Ellis, E. M. Dunbar, and K. Whale. 1984. Double-blind placebo-controlled trial of erythromycin in the treatment of clinical campylobacter infection. *J. Antimicrob. Chemother.* 13:619–623.

142. Matsushiro, A., K. Sato, H. Miyamoto, T. Yamamura, and T. Honda. 1999. Induction of prophages of enterohemorrhagic Escherichia coli O157:H7 with norfloxacin. *J. Bacteriol.* 181:2257–2260.

143. Mattila, L., H. Peltola, A. Siitonen, H. Kyronseppa, I. Simula, and M. Kataja. 1993. Short-term treatment of traveler's diarrhea with norfloxacin: a double-blind, placebo-controlled study during two seasons. *Clin. Infect. Dis.* 17:779–782.

144. McDermott, P. F., S. M. Bodeis, L. L. English, D. G. White, R. D. Walker, S. Zhao, S. Simjee, and D. D. Wagner. 2002. Ciprofloxacin resistance in Campylobacter jejuni evolves rapidly in chickens treated with fluoroquinolones. *J. Infect. Dis.* 185:837–840.

145. Mead, P. S., L. Slutsker, V. Dietz, L. F. McCaig, J. S. Bresee, C. Shapiro, P. M. Griffin, and R. V. Tauxe. 1999. Food-related illness and death in the United States. *Emerg. Infect. Dis.* 5:607–625.

146. Meskin, S., M. S. Jacob, R. Macaden, J. S. Keystone, P. E. Kozarsky, A. N. Ramachadran, and B. Metchock. 1992. Short-course treatment of typhoid fever with ciprofloxacin in south India. *Trans. R. Soc. Trop. Med. Hyg.* 86:446–447.

147. Mirelis, B., E. Miro, F. Navarro, C. A. Ogalla, J. Bonal, and G. Prats. 1993. Increased resistance to quinolone in Catalonia, Spain. *Diagn. Microbiol. Infect. Dis.* 16:137–139.

148. Molbak, K., D. L. Baggesen, F. M. Aarestrup, J. M. Ebbesen, J. Engberg, K. Frydendahl, P. Gerner-Smidt, A. M. Petersen, and H. C. Wegener. 1999. An outbreak of multidrug-resistant, quinolone-resistant Salmonella enterica serotype typhimurium DT104. *N. Engl. J. Med.* 341:1420–1425.

149. Molbak, K., P. Gerner-Smidt, and H. C. Wegener. 2002. Increasing quinolone resistance in Salmonella enterica serotype Enteritidis. *Emerg. Infect. Dis.* 8:514–515.

150. Moolasart, P., B. Eampokalap, and S. Supaswadikul. 1998. Comparison of the efficacy of tetracycline and norfloxacin in the treatment of acute severe watery diarrhea. *Southeast. Asian. J. Trop. Med. Public Health.* 29:108–111.

151. Moore, J. E., M. Crowe, N. Heaney, and E. Crothers. 2001. Antibiotic resistance in Campylobacter spp. isolated from human faeces (1980–2000) and foods (1997–2000) in Northern Ireland: an update. *J. Antimicrob. Chemother.* 48:455–457.

152. Murdoch, D. A., N. Banatvaia, A. Bone, B. I. Shoismatulloev, L. R. Ward, E. J. Threlfall, and N. A. Banatvala. 1998. Epidemic ciprofloxacin-resistant Salmonella typhi in Tajikistan. *Lancet* 351:339.

153. Murphy, G. S., L. Bodhidatta, P. Echeverria, S. Tansuphaswadikul, C. W. Hoge, S. Imlarp, and K. Tamura. 1993. Ciprofloxacin and loperamide in the treatment of bacillary dysentery. *Ann. Intern. Med.* 118:582–586.

154. Murphy, G. S., Jr., P. Echeverria, L. R. Jackson, M. K. Arness, C. LeBron, and C. Pitarangsi. 1996. Ciprofloxacin-and azithromycin-resistant Campylobacter causing traveler's diarrhea in U.S. troops deployed to Thailand in 1994. *Clin. Infect. Dis.* 22:868–869.

155. Murray, B. E., T. Alvarado, K. H. Kim, M. Vorachit, P. Jayanetra, M. M. Levine, I. Prenzel, M. Fling, L. Elwell, G. H. McCracken, et al. 1985. Increasing resistance to trimethoprim-sulfamethoxazole among isolates of Escherichia coli in developing countries. *J. Infect. Dis.* 152:1107–1113.

156. Musafija, A., A. Barzilai, J. Ramon, and E. Rubinstein. 1998. Effect of cholera toxin on intestinal elimination of ciprofloxacin in rabbits. *Antimicrob. Agents Chemother.* 42:473–474.

157. Musafija, A., J. Ramon, Y. Shtelman, G. Yoseph, B. Rubinovitz, S. Segev, and E. Rubinstein. 2000. Trans-epithelial intestinal elimination of moxifloxacin in rabbits. *J. Antimicrob. Chemother.* 45:803–805.

158. Musafija, A., Y. Shtelman, J. Ramon, M. Volk, S. Segev, and E. Rubinstein. 2001. The effect of Escherichia coli heat-stable toxin on the trans-epithelial intestinal elimination of ciprofloxacin in the rabbit. *J. Antimicrob. Chemother.* 47:697–699.

159. Nathwani, D., R. B. Laing, G. Harvey, and C. C. Smith. 1991. Treatment of symptomatic enteric aeromonas hydrophila infection with ciprofloxacin. *Scand. J. Infect. Dis.* 23:653–654.

160. Neill, M. A., S. M. Opal, J. Heelan, R. Giusti, J. E. Cassidy, R. White, and K. H. Mayer. 1991. Failure of ciprofloxacin to eradicate convalescent fecal excretion after acute salmonellosis: experience during an outbreak in health care workers. *Ann. Intern. Med.* 114:195–199.

161. Nelson, M. R., D. C. Shanson, D. A. Hawkins, and B. G. Gazzard. 1992. Salmonella, Campylobacter and Shigella in HIV-seropositive patients. *AIDS* 6:1495–1498.

162. Nelwan, R. H., Hendarwanto, I. Zulkarnain, J. Gunawan, I. Supandiman, H. Yusuf, P. Soedjana, and A. Syahroni. 1995. A comparative study of short course ciprofloxacin treatment in typhoid and paratyphoid fever. *Drugs* 49:463–465.

163. Nguyen, T. C., T. Solomon, X. T. Mai, T. L. Nguyen, T. T. Nguyen, J. Wain, S. D. To, M. D. Smith, N. P. Day, T. P. Le, C. Parry, and N. J. White. 1997. Short courses of ofloxacin for the treatment of enteric fever. *Trans. R. Soc. Trop. Med. Hyg.* 91:347–349.

164. Noguerado, A., I. Garcia-Polo, T. Isasia, M. L. Jimenez, P. Bermudez, J. Pita, and R. Gabriel. 1995. Early single dose therapy with ofloxacin for empirical treatment of acute gastroenteritis: a randomised, placebo-controlled double-blind clinical trial. *J. Antimicrob. Chemother.* 36:665–672.

165. O'Hare, M. D., D. Felmingham, G. L. Ridgway, and R. N. Gruneberg. 1985. The comparative in vitro activity of twelve

4-quinolone antimicrobials against enteric pathogens. *Drugs Exp. Clin. Res.* **11**:253–257.

166. Olsen, S. J., E. E. DeBess, T. E. McGivern, N. Marano, T. Eby, S. Mauvais, V. K. Balan, G. Zirnstein, P. R. Cieslak, and F. J. Angulo. 2001. A nosocomial outbreak of fluoroquinolone-resistant salmonella infection. *N. Engl. J. Med.* **344**:1572–1579.

167. Olsson-Liljequist, B., and R. Mollby. 1990. In vitro activity of norfloxacin and other antibacterial agents against gastrointestinal pathogens isolated in Sweden. *APMIS* **98**:150–155.

168. Parry, C., J. Wain, N. T. Chinh, H. Vinh, and J. J. Farrar. 1998. Quinolone-resistant Salmonella typhi in Vietnam. *Lancet* **351**:1289.

169. Parry, H., A. J. Howard, O. P. Galpin, and S. P. Hassan. 1994. The prophylaxis of travellers' diarrhoea; a double blind placebo controlled trial of ciprofloxacin during a Himalayan expedition. *J. Infect.* **28**:337–338.

170. Pavia, A. T., C. R. Nichols, D. P. Green, R. V. Tauxe, S. Mottice, K. D. Greene, J. G. Wells, R. L. Siegler, E. D. Brewer, D. Hannon, et al. 1990. Hemolytic-uremic syndrome during an outbreak of Escherichia coli O157:H7 infections in institutions for mentally retarded persons: clinical and epidemiologic observations. *J. Pediatr.* **116**:544–551.

171. Pechere, J. C. 1993. Quinolones in intracellular infections. *Drugs* **45**:29–36.

172. Pecquet, S., A. Andremont, and C. Tancrede. 1987. Effect of oral ofloxacin on fecal bacteria in human volunteers. *Antimicrob. Agents Chemother.* **31**:124–125.

173. Pecquet, S., S. Ravoire, and A. Andremont. 1990. Faecal excretion of ciprofloxacin after a single oral dose and its effect on faecal bacteria in healthy volunteers. *J. Antimicrob. Chemother.* **26**:125–129.

174. Petruccelli, B. P., G. S. Murphy, J. L. Sanchez, S. Walz, R. DeFraites, J. Gelnett, R. L. Haberberger, P. Echeverria, and D. N. Taylor. 1992. Treatment of traveler's diarrhea with ciprofloxacin and loperamide. *J. Infect. Dis.* **165**:557–560.

175. Pichler, H., G. Diridl, and D. Wolf. 1986. Ciprofloxacin in the treatment of acute bacterial diarrhea: a double blind study. *Eur. J. Clin. Microbiol.* **5**:241–243.

176. Pichler, H. E., G. Diridl, K. Stickler, and D. Wolf. 1987. Clinical efficacy of ciprofloxacin compared with placebo in bacterial diarrhea. *Am. J. Med.* **82**:329–332.

177. Piddock, L. J. 1995. Quinolone resistance and Campylobacter spp. *J. Antimicrob. Chemother.* **36**:891–898.

178. Pitkajarvi, T., E. Kujanne, I. Sillantaka, and J. Lumio. 1996. Norfloxacin and Salmonella excretion in acute gastroenteritis—a 6-month follow-up study. *Scand. J. Infect. Dis.* **28**:177–180.

179. Pradhan, K. M., N. K. Arora, A. Jena, A. K. Susheela, and M. K. Bhan. 1995. Safety of ciprofloxacin therapy in children: magnetic resonance images, body fluid levels of fluoride and linear growth. *Acta. Paediatr.* **84**:555–560.

180. Prats, G., B. Mirelis, T. Llovet, C. Munoz, E. Miro, and F. Navarro. 2000. Antibiotic resistance trends in enteropathogenic bacteria isolated in 1985–1987 and 1995–1998 in Barcelona. *Antimicrob. Agents Chemother.* **44**:1140–1145.

181. Rademaker, C. M., I. M. Hoepelman, M. J. Wolfhagen, H. Beumer, M. Rozenberg-Arska, and J. Verhoef. 1989. Results of a double-blind placebo-controlled study using ciprofloxacin for prevention of travelers' diarrhea. *Eur. J. Clin. Microbiol. Infect. Dis.* **8**:690–694.

182. Ramon, J., M. Ben-Haim, M. Shabtai, and E. Rubinstein. 2001. Transepithelial intestinal excretion of ciprofloxacin in humans. *Clin. Infect. Dis.* **32**:822–823.

183. Ramon, J., S. Dautrey, R. Farinoti, C. Carbon, and E. Rubinstein. 1996. Excretion of ciprofloxacin into the large bowel of the rabbit. *Antimicrob. Agents Chemother.* **40**:11–13.

184. Ramon, J., S. Dautrey, R. Farinoti, C. Carbon, and E. Rubinstein. 1994. Intestinal elimination of ciprofloxacin in rabbits. *Antimicrob. Agents Chemother.* **38**:757–760.

185. Rathish, K. C., M. R. Chandrashekar, and C. N. Nagesha. 1995. An outbreak of multidrug resistant typhoid fever in Bangalore. *Indian J. Pediatr.* **62**:445–448.

186. Reid, T., and C. Smith. 1987. Ciprofloxacin treatment of chronic Salmonella excretors. *Chemioterapia* **6**:485–486.

187. Rendi-Wagner, P., and H. Kollaritsch. 2002. Drug prophylaxis for travelers' diarrhea. *Clin. Infect. Dis.* **34**:628–633.

188. Ries, A. A., J. G. Wells, D. Olivola, M. Ntakibirora, S. Nyandwi, M. Ntibakivayo, C. B. Ivey, K. D. Greene, F. C. Tenover, S. P. Wahlquist, et al. 1994. Epidemic Shigella dysenteriae type 1 in Burundi: panresistance and implications for prevention. *J. Infect. Dis.* **169**:1035–1041.

189. Robins-Browne, R. M., M. K. Mackenjee, M. N. Bodasing, and H. M. Coovadia. 1983. Treatment of Campylobacter-associated enteritis with erythromycin. *Am. J. Dis. Child.* **137**:282–285.

190. Rogerie, F., D. Ott, J. Vandepitte, L. Verbist, P. Lemmens, and I. Habiyaremye. 1986. Comparison of norfloxacin and nalidixic acid for treatment of dysentery caused by Shigella dysenteriae type 1 in adults. *Antimicrob. Agents Chemother.* **29**:883–886.

191. Rubinstein, E., S. Dautrey, R. Farinoti, L. St Julien, J. Ramon, and C. Carbon. 1995. Intestinal elimination of sparfloxacin, fleroxacin, and ciprofloxacin in rats. *Antimicrob. Agents Chemother.* **39**:99–102.

192. Rubinstein, E., L. St Julien, J. Ramon, S. Dautrey, R. Farinotti, J. F. Huneau, and C. Carbon. 1994. The intestinal elimination of ciprofloxacin in the rat. *J. Infect. Dis.* **169**:218–221.

193. Ruiz, J., J. Gomez, M. M. Navia, A. Ribera, J. M. Sierra, F. Marco, J. Mensa, and J. Vila. 2002. High prevalence of nalidixic acid resistant, ciprofloxacin susceptible phenotype among clinical isolates of Escherichia coli and other Enterobacteriaceae. *Diagn. Microbiol. Infect. Dis.* **42**:257–261.

194. Ruiz, J., P. Goni, F. Marco, F. Gallardo, B. Mirelis, T. Jimenez De Anta, and J. Vila. 1998. Increased resistance to quinolones in Campylobacter jejuni: a genetic analysis of gyrA gene mutations in quinolone-resistant clinical isolates. *Microbiol. Immunol.* **42**:223–226.

195. Ryan, E. T., U. Dhar, W. A. Khan, M. A. Salam, A. S. Faruque, G. J. Fuchs, S. B. Calderwood, and M. L. Bennish. 2000. Mortality, morbidity, and microbiology of endemic cholera among hospitalized patients in Dhaka, Bangladesh. *Am. J. Trop. Med. Hyg.* **63**:12–20.

196. Saenz, Y., M. Zarazaga, M. Lantero, M. J. Gastanares, F. Baquero, and C. Torres. 2000. Antibiotic resistance in Campylobacter strains isolated from animals, foods, and humans in Spain in 1997–1998. *Antimicrob. Agents Chemother.* **44**:267–271.

197. Salam, I., P. Katelaris, S. Leigh-Smith, and M. J. Farthing. 1994. Randomised trial of single-dose ciprofloxacin for travellers' diarrhoea. *Lancet* **344**:1537–1539.

198. Salam, M. A., and M. L. Bennish. 1991. Antimicrobial therapy for shigellosis. *Rev. Infect. Dis.* **13**:S332–S341.

199. Salam, M. A., and M. L. Bennish. 1988. Therapy for shigellosis. I. Randomized, double-blind trial of nalidixic acid in childhood shigellosis. *J. Pediatr.* **113**:901–907.

200. Salam, M. A., U. Dhar, W. A. Khan, and M. L. Bennish. 1998. Randomised comparison of ciprofloxacin suspension

and pivmecillinam for childhood shigellosis. *Lancet* 352:522–527.

201. Salazar-Lindo, E., R. B. Sack, E. Chea-Woo, B. A. Kay, Z. A. Piscoya, R. Leon-Barua, and A. Yi. 1986. Early treatment with erythromycin of Campylobacter jejuni-associated dysentery in children. *J. Pediatr.* 109:355–360.

202. Sammalkorpi, K., J. Lahdevirta, T. Makela, and T. Rostila. 1987. Treatment of chronic Salmonella carriers with ciprofloxacin. *Lancet* 2:164–165.

203. San Joaquin, V. H., R. K. Scribner, D. A. Pickett, and D. F. Welch. 1986. Antimicrobial susceptibility of Aeromonas species isolated from patients with diarrhea. *Antimicrob. Agents Chemother.* 30:794–795.

204. Sanchez, C., E. Garcia-Restoy, J. Garau, F. Bella, N. Freixas, M. Simo, J. Lite, P. Sanchez, E. Espejo, E. Cobo, et al. 1993. Ciprofloxacin and trimethoprim-sulfamethoxazole versus placebo in acute uncomplicated Salmonella enteritis: a double-blind trial. *J. Infect. Dis.* 168:1304–1307.

205. Sarma, P. S., and P. Durairaj. 1991. Randomized treatment of patients with typhoid and paratyphoid fevers using norfloxacin or chloramphenicol. *Trans. R. Soc. Trop. Med. Hyg.* 85:670–671.

206. Scott, D. A., R. L. Haberberger, S. A. Thornton, and K. C. Hyams. 1990. Norfloxacin for the prophylaxis of travelers' diarrhea in U.S. military personnel. *Am. J. Trop. Med. Hyg.* 42:160–164.

207. Secmeer, G., G. Kanra, G. Figen, O. Akan, M. Ceyhan, and Z. Ecevit. 1997. Ofloxacin versus co-trimoxazole in the treatment of typhoid fever in children. *Acta Paediatr. Jpn.* 39:218–221.

208. Segreti, J., T. D. Gootz, L. J. Goodman, G. W. Parkhurst, J. P. Quinn, B. A. Martin, and G. M. Trenholme. 1992. High-level quinolone resistance in clinical isolates of Campylobacter jejuni. *J. Infect. Dis.* 165:667–670.

209. Shapiro, R. L., L. Kumar, P. Phillips-Howard, J. G. Wells, P. Adcock, J. Brooks, M. L. Ackers, J. B. Ochieng, E. Mintz, S. Wahlquist, P. Waiyaki, and L. Slutsker. 2001. Antimicrobial-resistant bacterial diarrhea in rural western Kenya. *J. Infect. Dis.* 183:1701–1704.

210. Shungu, D. L., E. Weinberg, and H. H. Gadebusch. 1983. In vitro antibacterial activity of norfloxacin (MK-0366, AM-715) and other agents against gastrointestinal tract pathogens. *Antimicrob. Agents Chemother.* 23:86–90.

211. Sjogren, E., G. B. Lindblom, and B. Kaijser. 1997. Norfloxacin resistance in Campylobacter jejuni and Campylobacter coli isolates from Swedish patients. *J. Antimicrob. Chemother.* 40:257–261.

212. Slutsker, L., A. A. Ries, K. Maloney, J. G. Wells, K. D. Greene, and P. M. Griffin. 1998. A nationwide case-control study of Escherichia coli O157:H7 infection in the United States. *J. Infect. Dis.* 177:962–966.

213. Smith, K. E., J. M. Besser, C. W. Hedberg, F. T. Leano, J. B. Bender, J. H. Wicklund, B. P. Johnson, K. A. Moore, and M. T. Osterholm. 1999. Quinolone-resistant Campylobacter jejuni infections in Minnesota, 1992–1998. Investigation Team. *N. Engl. J. Med.* 340:1525–1532.

214. Smith, M. D., N. M. Duong, N. T. Hoa, J. Wain, H. D. Ha, T. S. Diep, N. P. Day, T. T. Hien, and N. J. White. 1994. Comparison of ofloxacin and ceftriaxone for short-course treatment of enteric fever. *Antimicrob. Agents Chemother.* 38:1716–1720.

215. Steffen, R., R. Jori, H. L. DuPont, J. J. Mathewson, and D. Sturchler. 1993. Efficacy and toxicity of fleroxacin in the treatment of travelers' diarrhea. *Am. J. Med.* 94:182S–186S.

216. Stephens, I., and M. M. Levine. 2002. Management of typhoid fever in children. *Pediatr. Infect. Dis. J.* 21:157–158.

217. Stock, I., B. Henrichfreise, and B. Wiedemann. 2002. Natural antibiotic susceptibility and biochemical profiles of Yersinia enterocolitica-like strains: Y. bercovieri, Y. mollaretii, Y. aldovae and 'Y. ruckeri.' *J. Med. Microbiol.* 51:56–69.

218. Stock, I., and B. Wiedemann. 2001. Natural antimicrobial susceptibilities of Plesiomonas shigelloides strains. *J. Antimicrob. Chemother.* 48:803–811.

219. Stolk-Engelaar, V. M., J. F. Meis, J. A. Mulder, F. L. Loeffen, and J. A. Hoogkamp-Korstanje. 1995. In-vitro antimicrobial susceptibility of Yersinia enterocolitica isolates from stools of patients in The Netherlands from 1982–1991. *J. Antimicrob. Chemother.* 36:839–843.

220. Taylor, D. N., J. L. Sanchez, W. Candler, S. Thornton, C. McQueen, and P. Echeverria. 1991. Treatment of travelers' diarrhea: ciprofloxacin plus loperamide compared with ciprofloxacin alone. A placebo-controlled, randomized trial. *Ann. Intern. Med.* 114:731–734.

221. Taylor, S. J. 1997. Treating diarrhoea. Proposals are irresponsible and impractical. *Br. Med. J.* 315:1377–1378.

222. Thomas, M. E., and N. Datta. 1969. Emergence of Shigella sonnei resistant to kanamycin and to nalidixic acid, without exposure to these drugs. *J. Med. Microbiol.* 2:457–461.

223. Thomsen, L. L., and A. Paerregaard. 1998. Treatment with ciprofloxacin in children with typhoid fever. *Scand. J. Infect. Dis.* 30:355–357.

224. Thornton, S. A., S. F. Wignall, M. E. Kilpatrick, A. L. Bourgeois, C. Gardiner, R. A. Batchelor, D. H. Burr, J. J. Oprandy, P. Garst, and K. C. Hyams. 1992. Norfloxacin compared to trimethoprim/sulfamethoxazole for the treatment of travelers' diarrhea among U.S. military personnel deployed to South America and West Africa. *Mil. Med.* 157:55–58.

225. Threlfall, E. J., A. Graham, T. Cheasty, L. R. Ward, and B. Rowe. 1997. Resistance to ciprofloxacin in pathogenic Enterobacteriaceae in England and Wales in 1996. *J. Clin. Pathol.* 50:1027–1028.

226. Threlfall, E. J., and L. R. Ward. 2001. Decreased susceptibility to ciprofloxacin in Salmonella enterica serotype typhi, United Kingdom. *Emerg. Infect. Dis.* 7:448–450.

227. Threlfall, E. J., L. R. Ward, J. A. Skinner, H. R. Smith, and S. Lacey. 1999. Ciprofloxacin-resistant Salmonella typhi and treatment failure. *Lancet* 353:1590–1591.

228. Thwaites, R. T., and J. A. Frost. 1999. Drug resistance in Campylobacter jejuni, C coli, and C lari isolated from humans in north west England and Wales, 1997. *J. Clin. Pathol.* 52:812–814.

229. Tran, T. H., D. B. Bethell, T. T. Nguyen, J. Wain, S. D. To, T. P. Le, M. C. Bui, M. D. Nguyen, T. T. Pham, A. L. Walsh, et al. 1995. Short course of ofloxacin for treatment of multidrug-resistant typhoid. *Clin. Infect. Dis.* 20:917–923.

230. Tran, T. H., M. D. Nguyen, D. H. Huynh, T. T. Nguyen, S. D. To, T. P. Le, and K. Arnold. 1994. A randomized comparative study of fleroxacin and ceftriaxone in enteric fever. *Trans. R. Soc. Trop. Med. Hyg.* 88:464–465.

231. Truong, Q. C., S. Ouabdesselam, D. C. Hooper, N. J. Moreau, and C. J. Soussy. 1995. Sequential mutations of gyrA in Escherichia coli associated with quinolone therapy. *J. Antimicrob. Chemother.* 36:1055–1059.

232. Unal, S., M. Hayran, S. Tuncer, D. Gur, O. Uzun, M. Akova, and H. E. Akalin. 1996. Treatment of enteric fever with pefloxacin for 7 days versus 5 days: a randomized clinical trial. *Antimicrob. Agents Chemother.* 40:2898–2900.

233. Usubutun, S., C. Agalar, C. Diri, and R. Turkyilmaz. 1997. Single dose ciprofloxacin in cholera. *Eur. J. Emerg. Med.* 4:145–149.

234. Uwaydah, A. K., H. al Soub, and I. Matar. 1992. Randomized prospective study comparing two dosage regimens of ciprofloxacin for the treatment of typhoid fever. *J. Antimicrob. Chemother.* **30**:707–711.

235. Van Looveren, M., G. Daube, L. De Zutter, J. M. Dumont, C. Lammens, M. Wijdooghe, P. Vandamme, M. Jouret, M. Cornelis, and H. Goossens. 2001. Antimicrobial susceptibilities of Campylobacter strains isolated from food animals in Belgium. *J. Antimicrob. Chemother.* **48**:235–240.

236. Vanhoof, R., J. M. Hubrechts, E. Roebben, H. J. Nyssen, E. Nulens, J. Leger, and N. De Schepper. 1986. The comparative activity of pefloxacin, enoxacin, ciprofloxacin and 13 other antimicrobial agents against enteropathogenic microorganisms. *Infection.* **14**:294–298.

237. Velmonte, M. A., and C. S. Montalban. 1988. Norfloxacin in the treatment of infections caused by Salmonella typhi. *Scand. J. Infect. Dis. Suppl.* **56**:46–48.

238. Verdier, R. I., D. W. Fitzgerald, W. D. Johnson, Jr., and J. W. Pape. 2000. Trimethoprim-sulfamethoxazole compared with ciprofloxacin for treatment and prophylaxis of Isospora belli and Cyclospora cayetanensis infection in HIV-infected patients. A randomized, controlled trial. *Ann. Intern. Med.* **132**:885–888.

239. Vila, J., J. Gascon, S. Abdalla, J. Gomez, F. Marco, A. Moreno, M. Corachan, and T. Jimenez de Anta. 1994. Antimicrobial resistance of Shigella isolates causing traveler's diarrhea. *Antimicrob. Agents Chemother.* **38**:2668–2670.

240. Vila, J., M. Vargas, C. Casals, H. Urassa, H. Mshinda, D. Schellemberg, and J. Gascon. 1999. Antimicrobial resistance of diarrheagenic Escherichia coli isolated from children under the age of 5 years from Ifakara, Tanzania. *Antimicrob. Agents Chemother.* **43**:3022–3024.

241. Vila, J., M. Vargas, J. Ruiz, M. Corachan, M. T. Jimenez De Anta, and J. Gascon. 2000. Quinolone resistance in enterotoxigenic Escherichia coli causing diarrhea in travelers to India in comparison with other geographical areas. *Antimicrob. Agents Chemother.* **44**:1731–1733.

242. Vila, J., M. Vargas, J. Ruiz, M. Espasa, M. Pujol, M. Corachan, M. T. Jimenez de Anta, and J. Gascon. 2001. Susceptibility patterns of enteroaggregative Escherichia coli associated with traveller's diarrhoea: emergence of quinolone resistance. *J. Med. Microbiol.* **50**:996–1000.

243. Vinh, H., J. Wain, M. T. Chinh, C. T. Tam, P. T. Trang, D. Nga, P. Echeverria, T. S. Diep, N. J. White, and C. M. Parry. 2000. Treatment of bacillary dysentery in Vietnamese children: two doses of ofloxacin versus 5-days nalidixic acid. *Trans. R. Soc. Trop. Med. Hyg.* **94**:323–326.

244. Vinh, H., J. Wain, T. N. Vo, N. N. Cao, T. C. Mai, D. Bethell, T. T. Nguyen, S. D. Tu, M. D. Nguyen, and N. J. White. 1996. Two or three days of ofloxacin treatment for uncomplicated multidrug-resistant typhoid fever in children. *Antimicrob. Agents Chemother.* **40**:958–961.

245. Visitsunthorn, N., and P. Komolpis. 1995. Antimicrobial therapy in Plesiomonas shigelloides-associated diarrhea in Thai children. *Southeast Asian J. Trop. Med. Public Health* **26**:86–90.

246. Voltersvik, P., A. Halstensen, N. Langeland, A. Digranes, L. E. Peterson, T. Rolstad, and C. O. Solberg. 2000. Eradication of non-typhoid salmonellae in acute enteritis after therapy with ofloxacin for 5 or 10 days. *J. Antimicrob. Chemother.* **46**:457–459.

247. Voogd, C. E., C. S. Schot, W. J. van Leeuwen, and B. van Klingeren. 1992. Monitoring of antibiotic resistance in shigellae isolated in The Netherlands 1984–1989. *Eur. J. Clin. Microbiol. Infect. Dis.* **11**:164–167.

248. Wain, J., N. T. Hoa, N. T. Chinh, H. Vinh, M. J. Everett, T. S. Diep, N. P. Day, T. Solomon, N. J. White, L. J. Piddock, and C. M. Parry. 1997. Quinolone-resistant Salmonella typhi in Viet Nam: molecular basis of resistance and clinical response to treatment. *Clin. Infect. Dis.* **25**:1404–1410.

249. Wallace, M. R., A. A. Yousif, G. A. Mahroos, T. Mapes, E. J. Threlfall, B. Rowe, and K. C. Hyams. 1993. Ciprofloxacin versus ceftriaxone in the treatment of multiresistant typhoid fever. *Eur. J. Clin. Microbiol. Infect. Dis.* **12**:907–910.

250. Wang, F., X. J. Gu, M. F. Zhang, and T. Y. Tai. 1989. Treatment of typhoid fever with ofloxacin. *J. Antimicrob. Chemother.* **23**:785–788.

251. Wanke, C. A., J. Gerrior, V. Blais, H. Mayer, and D. Acheson. 1998. Successful treatment of diarrheal disease associated with enteroaggregative Escherichia coli in adults infected with human immunodeficiency virus. *J. Infect. Dis.* **178**:1369–1372.

252. Wistrom, J., L. O. Gentry, A. C. Palmgren, M. Price, C. E. Nord, A. Ljungh, and S. R. Norrby. 1992. Ecological effects of short-term ciprofloxacin treatment of travellers' diarrhoea. *J. Antimicrob. Chemother.* **30**:693–706.

253. Wistrom, J., M. Jertborn, E. Ekwall, K. Norlin, B. Soderquist, A. Stromberg, R. Lundholm, H. Hogevik, L. Lagergren, G. Englund, et al. 1992. Empiric treatment of acute diarrheal disease with norfloxacin. A randomized, placebo-controlled study. Swedish Study Group. *Ann. Intern. Med.* **117**:202–208.

254. Wistrom, J., M. Jertborn, S. A. Hedstrom, K. Alestig, G. Englund, B. Jellheden, and S. R. Norrby. 1989. Short-term self-treatment of travellers' diarrhoea with norfloxacin: a placebo-controlled study. *J. Antimicrob. Chemother.* **23**:905–913.

255. Wistrom, J., and S. R. Norrby. 1995. Fluoroquinolones and bacterial enteritis, when and for whom? *J. Antimicrob. Chemother.* **36**:23–39.

256. Wistrom, J., S. R. Norrby, L. G. Burman, R. Lundholm, B. Jellheden, and G. Englund. 1987. Norfloxacin versus placebo for prophylaxis against travellers' diarrhoea. *J. Antimicrob. Chemother.* **20**:563–574.

257. Wong, C. S., S. Jelacic, R. L. Habeeb, S. L. Watkins, and P. I. Tarr. 2000. The risk of the hemolytic-uremic syndrome after antibiotic treatment of Escherichia coli O157:H7 infections. *N. Engl. J. Med.* **342**:1930–1936.

258. Wretlind, B., A. Stromberg, L. Ostlund, E. Sjogren, and B. Kaijser. 1992. Rapid emergence of quinolone resistance in Campylobacter jejuni in patients treated with norfloxacin. *Scand. J. Infect. Dis.* **24**:685–686.

259. Wright, D. H., G. H. Brown, M. L. Peterson, and J. C. Rotschafer. 2000. Application of fluoroquinolone pharmacodynamics. *J. Antimicrob. Chemother.* **46**:669–683.

260. Yee, C. L., C. Duffy, P. G. Gerbino, S. Stryker, and G. J. Noel. 2002. Tendon or joint disorders in children after treatment with fluoroquinolones or azithromycin. *Pediatr. Infect. Dis. J.* **21**:525–529.

261. Yousaf, M., and A. Sadick. 1990. Ofloxacin in the treatment of typhoid fever unresponsive to chloramphenicol. *Clin. Ther.* **12**:44–47.

262. Zhang, X., A. D. McDaniel, L. E. Wolf, G. T. Keusch, M. K. Waldor, and D. W. Acheson. 2000. Quinolone antibiotics induce Shiga toxin-encoding bacteriophages, toxin production, and death in mice. *J. Infect. Dis.* **181**:664–670.

263. Zimbasa, S. G. Three day, six dose ciprofloxacin therapy of S. dysenteriae type 1 infections in children. *Pediatr. Infect. Dis. J.*, in press.

Quinolone Antimicrobial Agents, 3rd ed.
Edited by David C. Hooper and Ethan Rubinstein
© 2003 ASM Press, Washington, D.C.

Chapter 12

Treatment of Intra-Abdominal Infections

JOSEPH S. SOLOMKIN

Antibiotic therapy has assumed an increasingly important role in the management of intra-abdominal infections because of the replacement of surgical extirpation of inflamed and infected tissue by minimally invasive or percutaneous drainage procedures. This less morbid approach has become possible only because of the potency of currently available antimicrobials. Such procedures leave abscess walls, inflamed peritoneum, and intramural bowel inflammation in place, structures that contain high densities of microorganisms.

Many classes of antimicrobial agents and combination regimens have been subjected to prospective trial, generally as a means to obtain regulatory approval of the agent for use in these infections. Quinolones have only recently been so studied, but considerable information about the utility of these agents is available because the studies that have been performed have generally followed guidelines of the Infectious Diseases Society of America and the U.S. Food and Drug Administration (29).

This review describes the key findings of clinical trials performed to date and then describes settings in which these agents may be the preferred antimicrobials. The primary questions remaining about these agents center on their activity against anaerobic organisms. A parallel concern is the risk of resistance of community organisms through quinolone usage for other conditions. Acquisition of resistance by colonic anaerobes for patients receiving quinolone therapy seems to be common.

THE MICROBIOLOGY OF COMMUNITY-ACQUIRED INTRA-ABDOMINAL INFECTION

The organisms encountered in intra-abdominal infections are listed in Table 1. Table 1 details three studies in which very detailed bacteriology was per-

formed. In two, separate anaerobic specimen processing was used. These data provide a complete picture of the antimicrobial spectrum sought in an agent or combination of agents to be utilized for intra-abdominal infections.

There is little debate that "appropriate therapy" is active against the facultative and aerobic gram-negatives encountered in these infections. It is worthwhile making the case for aggressive anti-anaerobic therapy, particularly against *Bacteroides fragilis* and other *Bacteroides* species. Nguyen and colleagues conducted a prospective multicenter observational study of 128 patients with *Bacteroides* bacteremia (23). Outcome was correlated with results of in vitro susceptibility testing of *Bacteroides* isolates recovered from blood and/or nonblood sites, determined with use of three end points: mortality at 30 days, clinical response (cure versus failure), and microbiological response (eradication versus persistence). The mortality rate among patients who received inactive therapy (45%) was higher than among patients who received active therapy (16%; $P = 0.04$). Clinical failure (82%) and microbiological persistence (42%) were higher for patients who received inactive therapy than for patients who received active therapy (22 and 12%, respectively; $P = 0.0002$ and 0.06, respectively). The authors concluded that in vitro activity of agents directed at *Bacteroides* species reliably predicts outcome.

CLINICAL TRIALS TO ESTABLISH EFFICACY OF QUINOLONE THERAPY IN INTRA-ABDOMINAL INFECTION

Four quinolones have been examined in clinical trials for intra-abdominal infections: ciprofloxacin, trovafloxacin, clinafloxacin, and pefloxacin (9, 13, 20, 30, 31). These agents have considerable activity against the gram-negative facultative and aerobic

Joseph S. Solomkin • Division of Trauma and Critical Care, Department of Surgery, 231 Albert B. Sabin Way, Cincinnati, OH 45267-0558.

Table 1. Organisms identified in three recently completed clinical trials in intra-abdominal infections[a]

Parameter	Cip/Imi	Clina/Imi	Erta/PipTazo
No. of patients	330	312	396
% Facultative/aerobic gram-negatives	81	84	83
% any anaerobes	50	67	
% any gram-positive cocci	61	67	50
% of organisms identified			
Escherichia coli	59	68	70
Klebsiella species	19	16	13
Pseudomonas aeruginosa	12	15	13
Proteus species	7	6	4
Enterobacter species	5	5	5
Citrobacter species	5	4	
Other gram-negative organisms	12	8	12
Bacteroides fragilis	31	32	36
Bacteroides thetaiotaomicron		19	20
Bacteroides uniformis		14	11
Bacteroides vulgatus		9	7
Bacteroides distasonis		8	11
Bacteroides ovatus			11
Other *Bacteroides*	11	13	17
Clostridium species	12	20	33
Prevotella species		14	10
Peptostreptococci	9	18	16
Fusobacterium	2	11	7
Eubacterium spp.		15	18
Other anaerobes	12	24	19
Streptococci	16	58	22
Streptococcus viridans	17		8
β-Hemolytic streptococci	5		
Staphylococcus aureus	5	5	2
Other staphylococci	4		6
Coagulase-negative staphylococci	6		
Enterococcus, not speciated	17	2	12
Enterococcus faecalis	4	13	11
Enterococcus faecium	2	4	3
Enterococcus avium		6	
Group D streptococcus	5		

[a] Data from references 30, 31, and 31a. Cip/Imi, ciprofloxacin-imipenem; Clina/Imi, clinafloxacin-imipenem; Erta/Pip Tazo, ertapenem-piperacillin-tazobactam.

organisms commonly encountered in intra-abdominal infections (4, 32, 33). An additional benefit of quinolone therapy is the availability of oral congeners for conversion from initial intravenous to completion oral therapy. This has been studied in two trials with ciprofloxacin-metronidazole regimens and one with trovafloxacin.

PEFLOXACIN-METRONIDAZOLE VERSUS GENTAMICIN-METRONIDAZOLE

Two hundred seventy-one patients with intra-abdominal infection were enrolled in an open, randomized comparative trial (1): 136 patients were enrolled in the pefloxacin/metronidazole group and 135 were enrolled in the gentamicin/metronidazole group. Patients received intravenously (i.v.) either pefloxacin (400 mg twice daily after an 800-mg loading dose) or gentamicin (1.4 mg/kg of body weight every 8–24 h depending on the renal function). Metronidazole was given to both groups as a 500-mg intravenous infusion three times a day. Eighty-seven patients were excluded from the efficacy analysis, principally because of unproven infection, previous antimicrobial therapy, or treatment duration less than 3 days. Ninety-four of 104 patients receiving pefloxacin-metronidazole (90.4%) were cured or improved, and there were two failures and eight relapses. In the gentamicin-metronidazole group, 64 of 80 patients (80.0%) were cured or improved, while there were three failures, nine relapses, and two deaths. The use of gentamicin as the sole agent with activity against aerobic gram-negative bacteria, however, may be problematic in intra-abdominal infections because anaerobic conditions may reduce its activity.

CIPROFLOXACIN-METRONIDAZOLE VERSUS IMIPENEM-CILASTATIN

The first North American trial of a quinolone for complicated intra-abdominal infections was performed in the mid-1990s (30). There was considerable evidence justifying a trial of ciprofloxacin in intra-abdominal infections. The agent had been available for several years and had been used parenterally in Europe for some years.

This agent has a large volume of distribution and penetrates well into most tissue compartments, including the peritoneal cavity (12, 27). Furthermore, this and other quinolones are concentrated within leukocytes, a phenomenon that may contribute to their delivery to intra-abdominal sites of infection. Recent in vitro and animal studies have explored the activity of a quinolone-based regimen for intra-abdominal infections (8, 34), and i.v. ciprofloxacin therapy has been found clinically effective for other serious gram-negative infections (15). Finally, the agent had considerable activity against the facultative and aerobic gram-negative organisms commonly seen in intra-abdominal infections. Ciprofloxacin has little activity against *B. fragilis* and needs to be combined with an antianaerobic agent for empirical treatment of intra-abdominal infections.

This study was designed to examine the efficacy of i.v. therapy and to explore conversion of therapeutic regimens to oral administration. To perform a randomized, double-blind study including patients treated with i.v. agents and patients treated with sequential i.v./oral (p.o.) agents, three randomization groups were created. All three groups initially received i.v. therapy: two received ciprofloxacin plus metronidazole (CIP/MTZ i.v. and CIP/MTZ i.v./p.o.) and the other group received imipenem-cilastatin (IMI i.v.). Ciprofloxacin i.v. was administered at a dosage of 400 mg every 12 h along with metronidazole 500 mg every 6 h. Imipenem-cilastatin was administered at a dosage of 500 mg every 6 h. Patients receiving imipenem-cilastatin also received a placebo infusion every 12 h.

The criteria for providing patients with p.o. treatment were restoration of oral intake and an initially favorable clinical response. Patients randomized to the groups referred to as CIP/MTZ i.v. or IMI i.v. received i.v. ciprofloxacin plus metronidazole or i.v. imipenem-cilastatin, respectively. If selected for p.o. therapy, these patients received p.o. placebo and continued active i.v. therapy. Patients randomized to the group referred to as CIP/MTZ i.v./p.o. initially received i.v. ciprofloxacin plus metronidazole, followed by p.o. ciprofloxacin plus p.o. metronidazole and i.v. placebo if selected for p.o. treatment. Oral ciprofloxacin was given at a dosage of 500 mg every 12 h and p.o. metronidazole was administered 500 mg every 6 h.

The organisms encountered are listed in Table 1. One or more gram-negative isolates were found in 269 patients, and anaerobes were found in 161 patients. Mixed gram-negative and anaerobic infections were found in 127 patients, and 27 patients had only aerobic gram-positive isolates.

In vitro resistance to either regimen was uncommon and was primarily encountered with gram-positive organisms. For imipenem-cilastatin, three *Proteus mirabilis* isolates were found to be resistant, as were one *P. aeruginosa*, one *Enterobacter aerogenes*, and one *Morganella morganii*. Forty-nine of 315 patients (15%) without resistant isolates failed, compared with 6 of 15 patients (40%) with organisms resistant to the therapy given ($P = 0.02$).

OUTCOMES

The overall clinical success rates for each arm in the intent-to-treat analysis were 82% (182/222) for CIP/MTZ i.v., 84% (183/219) for CIP/MTZ i.v./p.o., and 82% (189/230) for IMI i.v. The clinical success rates for valid patients were 80% (89/111), 81% (92/113), and 84% (98/117) for CIP/MTZ i.v., CIP/MTZ i.v./p.o., and IMI i.v., respectively. The success rates for CIP/MTZ i.v. and IMI i.v. valid patients were statistically equivalent.

OUTCOME RESULTS: ORAL THERAPY GROUP

One hundred fifty-five of the 330 valid patients (47%) received p.o. treatment as part of the study protocol. Patients initially randomly assigned to the CIP/MTZ i.v./p.o. group received active p.o. therapy ($n = 46$). One hundred seventy-five patients of the 340 valid patients were not given oral treatment, and of these, 39 patients were treatment failures. The major reasons patients were not given oral therapy were absent bowel function ($n = 126$), physician discretion ($n = 9$), and no improvement ($n = 8$).

Only 2 of 46 patients who received active p.o. treatment were considered clinical failures. One failed because of a wound infection identified after discharge, and the other failed because of treatment with nonprotocol therapy at discharge without documented infection. Six of 55 IMI i.v.-treated patients given p.o. placebo and continued active i.v. therapy were considered clinical failures. All developed abscesses and underwent either operative (3) or percutaneous (3) drainage. This difference was not statistically significant ($P = 0.2854$). Six of 54 CIP/MTZ i.v. patients who received p.o. placebo and continued CIP/MTZ i.v. failed. Two developed wound infections, three developed abscesses drained percutaneously, and one received poststudy antibiotic treatment without documented infection. No patients assigned to either active or placebo oral therapy died.

For all valid patients given oral agents, active or placebo, the average duration of all therapy was 8.5 ± 3.6 days, including 4.0 ± 3.0 days of p.o. treatment. The total duration of treatment for groups who received i.v./p.o. therapy and i.v. therapy alone was the same for both groups.

As one would expect, there were several differences in study entry characteristics that were helpful in predicting patients who would be given p.o. therapy. Patients chosen to receive p.o. treatment were on average less acutely ill than those who were not given p.o. treatment. Patients receiving p.o. therapy had a mean APACHE II score on study entry of 8.1 ± 4.9 versus a mean of 10.9 ± 8.1 for patients not receiving p.o. treatment ($P < 0.0001$). Age was also considerably different between the two groups. Patients not receiving p.o. agents had a mean age of 55.46 ± 10.9, vs. 49.7 ± 8.1 for those given p.o. therapy ($P = 0.0076$). Finally, the diagnostic mix was considerably different. Forty percent of patients given p.o. therapy had appendicitis, compared with 17% of those not given p.o. therapy.

MICROBIOLOGIC CORRELATES OF TREATMENT FAILURE

We analyzed microbiology results for the 30 patients undergoing intervention for recurrent abscesses or peritonitis; 25 had microbiology results reported. The organisms which were found in failures are described in Table 2. Ten of these patients harbored enterococcal isolates, but in only four were persisting organisms. Thirteen treatment failures of the 113 patients receiving imipenem had gram-negative isolates, and nine were persisting from the initial study entry procedure. Four patients of the 217 CIP/MTZ i.v. or i.v./p.o. patients had persisting gram negatives. The data suggest that persistence of gram-negative organisms was more common in the imipenem-treated patients who subsequently failed. This post hoc analysis was reexamined in a trial comparing clinafloxacin with imipenem (see below).

CIPROFLOXACIN-METRONIDAZOLE VERSUS PIPERACILLIN-TAZOBACTAM

The results of the ciprofloxacin-metronidazole versus imipenem study described above were largely confirmed in a follow-on study comparing ciprofloxacin-metronidazole to piperacillin-tazobactam (9). This study report, however, did not follow standard definitions, and critical data items were not reported. These problems interfere with interpretation of the study.

The study was a multicenter, randomized, double-blind trial involving 459 patients. Initial i.v. therapy

Table 2. The microbiology of treatment failure from two trials with quinolones for intra-abdominal infections[a]

Parameter	Clinafloxacin ($n = 27$ of 150)	Imipenem ($n = 32$ of 162)	Ciprofloxacin ($n = 33$ of 217)	Imipenem ($n = 22$ of 113)
No. valid failures undergoing reintervention	16	22	16	14
No. valid failures with positive cultures at intervention for failure	14	18	12	13
No. of organisms identified:				
Escherichia coli	1	7	2	6
Pseudomonas aeruginosa	2	3	0	2
Other gram-negatives[b]	3	7	3	3
Enterococcus faecalis	2	5	0	0
Enterococcus faecium		3	0	0
Enterococcus spp.	1	6	7	3
Streptococcus spp.	3	2	5	8
Staphylococcus aureus	0	0	0	2
Coagulase-negative staphylococci	0	3	0	4
Bacteroides fragilis	4	8	1	1
Bacteroides spp	4	6		
Other anaerobes	3	5	1	1

[a] Data from references 30 and 31.
[b] *Klebsiella* spp., *Citrobacter freundii*, *Morganella morganii*, *Proteus* spp., *Serratia marcescens*, *Enterobacter cloacae*, *Citrobacter freundii*, *Stenotrophomonas maltophilia*.

consisted of ciprofloxacin (400 mg every 12 h) plus metronidazole 500 mg every 6 h or piperacillin-tazobactam 3.375 g every 6 h. Clinically improved i.v.-treated patients could be switched to oral therapy after 48 h. Patients initially treated with CIP + MET were given oral ciprofloxacin (500 mg every 12 h) and metronidazole. Patients initially treated with PIP/TAZO were given placebo tablets and continued on i.v. PIP/TAZO. If antibiotics were still required at the time of hospital discharge, patients could be given antibiotics in an unmasked fashion. Fully 30% of patients received such unmasked treatment. Most of these patients, regardless of their randomized therapy, received ciprofloxacin (59/85, 70%) and metronidazole (55/85, 65%). In addition, prescribed drugs included amoxicillin-clavulanic acid (11/85, 13%) and unspecified other treatment in 15/85, 18%. This was a confounding variable. It is not clear, for example, how many of these patients were considered treatment failures simply because their attending physicians prescribed nonprotocol discharge medication. Provision of antibacterials in the posttherapy follow-up period is described as a basis for failure for this study.

This point is of considerable importance in that a significant difference in outcome was noted. Overall clinical response was the primary efficacy measurement. A total of 282 patients (151 CIP + MET, 131 PIP/TAZO) were valid for efficacy. Overall clinical resolution rates were statistically superior for CIP + MET (74%) compared with PIP/TAZO (63%). Of the evaluable patients, 64% CIP+MET and 57% PIP/TAZO patients were considered candidates for oral therapy. In patients who received oral therapy, corresponding success rates were 69/81 (85%) for CIP+MET versus 28/39 (70%), ($P = 0.028$). For patients with appendicitis, success rates were 89% (24/27) for CIP+MET versus 68% (19/28) for PIP/TAZO patients.

Patients had a mean APACHE II score of 9.6. The most common diagnoses were appendicitis (33%), other intra-abdominal infection (29%), and abscess without specification of the organ source (25%). Postsurgical wound infection rates were significantly lower in CIP + MET (11%) versus PIP/TAZO patients (19%). Mean length of stay was 14 days for CIP + MET and 17 days for PIP/TAZO patients.

The claim of superiority here is difficult to assess because data describing bases for failure are not provided. Further, the nonstandard disease reporting definitions make this study difficult to compare with others. Finally, the failure rates observed in general and with PIP/TAZO in particular are markedly different from the other studies done with quinolones and the even larger number done with PIP/TAZO.

STUDIES WITH CLINAFLOXACIN AND TROVAFLOXACIN

Newer fluoroquinolones with increased in vitro activity against anaerobes are under study and include levofloxacin, clinafloxacin, sparfloxacin, trovafloxacin, grepafloxacin, and sitafloxacin. Of these, clinafloxacin and trovafloxacin have completed clinical trials, and trials with moxifloxacin and sitafloxacin are in various stages of progress. The in vitro activity of various quinolones is provided in Table 3.

CLINAFLOXACIN STUDY

We have performed a similarly designed study (without oral arms) comparing clinafloxacin with imipenem-cilastatin (31). For the modified intention to treat groups, 219 of 259 clinafloxacin-treated patients (84%) were considered successes, as were 219 of 270

Table 3. Reported susceptibilities of anaerobic bacteria to quinolones[a]

Species	MIC (μg/ml)							
	Ciprofloxacin	Ofloxacin	Sparfloxacin	Clinafloxacin	Gatifloxacin	Grepafloxacin	Trovafloxacin	Moxifloxacin
Bacteroides fragilis	16	16	2	2	1	8	0.5	0.5
Clostridium perfringens	1–4	4	1	1	1	1	0.5	0.5
Eubacterium lentum	1	1					0.25	0.25
Peptostreptococcus spp.	0.5–4	1		1		2	0.5	0.25
Prevotella bivia	8–16	8			8	16	1	2
Prevotella disiens	1	2				2	1	0.5
Fusobacterium spp.	4	4		0.5		2	0.5	0.5

[a] Data are taken from reference 36.

imipenem-cilastatin-treated patients (81%). Of the 150 valid patients treated with clinafloxacin (82%) 123 were considered treatment successes, as were 130 of the 162 (80%) treated with imipenem.

Thirty-nine valid patients failed and underwent either operative or percutaneous drainage. Fourteen clinafloxacin-treated patients had positive cultures at reintervention: 11 abscess cultures, 1 peritonitis fluid culture, and 2 wound cultures. Eighteen imipenem/cilastatin-treated patients had positive cultures: 14 from abscesses, 1 from peritonitis fluid, and 3 from wound cultures.

There were substantially more gram-negative bacteria recovered from treatment failures initially treated with imipenem-treated patients (Table 2). The most common was *Escherichia coli*, followed by *Pseudomonas aeruginosa*, and three *Proteus* species and *M. morganii*. The ratios of patients with gram-negative bacteria to patients with any positive culture indicated that this difference was marginally significant, with $P = 0.0626$. There was no such significance for gram-positive organisms, $P = 0.2635$.

The basis for the persistence of gram-negative organisms in imipenem treatment failures is unclear. We are concerned that the dose of imipenem used in the current trial, 500 mg every 6 h, may be relatively low given the need to achieve effective antibiotic levels in peritoneal fluid. This finding is similar to that reported in those studies of imipenem/cilastatin which used doses of 500 mg and provided information on the microbiology of treatment failure (3, 5, 6). In two studies performed by the Swedish Multicenter Study Group using either imipenem or meropenem at 500 mg every 8 h, even higher failure rates were encountered (7, 24). Penetration of imipenem and ciprofloxacin into the peritoneal cavity has been studied in patients undergoing elective laporotomy (10, 11, 35). These data show achievement of antibiotic concentrations related to the dose administered and approximating 60% of simultaneously studied levels in plasma. No data are available regarding penetration of either imipenem or ciprofloxacin into the inflamed peritoneum.

The basis for this limited efficacy is unclear. Many of the persisting isolates were highly susceptible to imipenem. We suspect this effect might be due to the relatively low levels of imipenem in plasma when dosed at 500 mg. Levels of imipenem or other anti-infectives have not been measured in the residual inflamed tissue after appropriate intervention, and this tissue is most likely the initiating site of recurrent abscess. Studies performed with 1-g doses of carbapenems did not find a similar high level of persisting gram negatives (6, 13, 17). These data support the use of the microbiology of treatment failure as a surrogate endpoint.

TROVAFLOXACIN

The efficacy of alatrofloxacin followed by oral trovafloxacin was compared with the standard regimen of i.v. imipenem-cilastatin followed by oral amoxicillin-clavulanic acid in a prospective, multicenter, double-blind trial (14). Patients were randomly selected to receive either 300 mg of alatrofloxacin daily followed by 200 mg of oral trovafloxacin daily or 1 g of imipenem-cilastatin intravenously three times daily followed by 500 mg of oral amoxicillin-clavulanic acid three times daily for up to 14 days after surgical intervention of a documented intra-abdominal infection. Efficacy was assessed at the end of therapy and at follow-up (day 30). At the end of the study, cure or improvement occurred in 83% (129/156) and 84% (127/152) of clinically evaluable patients in the trovafloxacin and comparative groups, respectively. Pathogen eradication rates, adverse-event profiles, and significant laboratory abnormalities were comparable between groups. APACHE II scores (6.4 and 7.0 in the two groups) were sufficiently low that good outcomes would be predicted in both treatment arms.

It is highly likely that other quinolones could be used with equal efficacy to ciprofloxacin. Levofloxacin, gatifloxicin, and moxifloxacin have sufficiently broad gram-negative activity to be useful, likely in combination with metronidazole. It is also useful to note that metronidazole has a half-life sufficiently long to allow once daily dosing (18, 19, 21, 26, 28).

ARE QUINOLONES SUFFICIENT THERAPY FOR ANAEROBES?

Anaerobic bacteria play an important role in the pathogenicity of mixed aerobic-anaerobic infections, such as intra-abdominal, obstetric-gynecologic, and diabetic foot infections. Exchange of antimicrobial resistance genetic elements has been shown among anaerobes for the agents cefoxitin, imipenem, clindamycin, tetracycline, chloramphenicol, and metronidazole (2).

The area of greatest concern with quinolones is the rapid development of resistance by anaerobes, in particular, *B. fragilis*. The most common mechanism for this appears to be mutation on the DNA gyrase A target. In one study of resistant *Bacteroides*, 44 clinafloxacin-resistant and -susceptible fecal and clinical isolates of the *B. fragilis* group (eight *B. fragilis*, three *Bacteroides ovatus*, five *Bacteroides thetaiotaomicron*, six *Bacteroides uniformis*, and 22 *Bacteroides vulgatus*) and six ATCC strains of the *B. fragilis* group were analyzed (25). Susceptibility to ciprofloxacin, levofloxacin, moxifloxacin, and clinafloxacin was determined. Sequencing of the *gyrA* quinolone resistance-determining region located between amino acid residues equivalent to Ala-67 through Gln-106 in *E. coli* revealed substitutions at positions 82 ($n = 15$) and 86 ($n = 8$). Strains with Ser82Leu substitutions ($n = 13$) were highly resistant to all quinolones tested. Mutations in other positions of gyrA were also frequently found in quinolone-resistant and -susceptible isolates.

This finding appears to have clinical substance. In one study, 12 healthy volunteers received clinafloxacin orally, 200 mg twice daily for 7 days (26). Fecal specimens were collected at defined intervals before, during, and after the administration. Oral administration of clinafloxacin resulted in high drug levels in feces (mean value, 176.2 mg/kg on day 7) and pronounced microbiologic disturbances. The aerobic microflora were eradicated in 11 of the 12 subjects, and the anaerobic microflora were strongly suppressed during administration. There was a significant emergence of clinafloxacin-resistant *Bacteroides* spp. strains (MIC, ≥ 4 mg/ml) during administration. The MICs remained elevated 2 weeks after discontinuation of the antibiotic.

Rates of resistance to these antibiotics in clinical populations are increasing. In an ongoing surveillance study, 16.4% of 1,220 clinical *B. fragilis* group strains from 19 European countries were considered resistant to moxifloxacin, with MICs of 4 μg/ml (M. Hedberg, Karolinska Institute, Sweden; cited in reference 25).

USE OF QUINOLONES IN POSTOPERATIVE INFECTIONS

One issue with these agents is whether they are suitable for postoperative intra-abdominal infections, infections that typically have a more resistant nosocomial flora, including *P. aeruginosa*, *Enterobacter* spp., and β-lactamase-producing *Klebsiella*. Montravers and colleagues retrospectively studied 100 patients with postoperative peritonitis (22). The organisms encountered are detailed in Table 4. The adequacy of empirical treatment was determined by means of culture and susceptibility data obtained at the time of reoperation, and the effect of such treatment on outcome was evaluated.

One hundred antibiotic-resistant pathogens were isolated from 70 patients, of whom 45% died; by comparison, mortality among those from whom susceptible organisms were isolated was 16% ($P <$ 0.05). Inadequate empirical treatment was administered to 54 patients and was associated with poorer

Table 4. Gram-negative organisms identified in 100 patients with postoperative peritonitis[a]

Organism	n (of 100 patients)
E. coli	53
Proteus/Morganella	25
Pseudomonas aeruginosa	21
Klebsiella	14
Enterobacter cloacae	10
Acinetobacter/Citrobacter/Serratia	10

[a] Data from reference 22.

outcome ($P \leq 0.05$). The outcome of postoperative peritonitis is affected by the choice and adequacy of the initial empirical antibiotic therapy. Late changes in antibiotic therapy based on culture results did not affect outcome when the initial regimen was inadequate. The profile of quinolones would seem appropriate for coverage of gram-negative aerobes found in these infections and in some cases might reduce the need for multidrug regimens.

CONCLUSIONS

The safety and efficacy of quinolone-based regimens in intra-abdominal infections has been clearly documented in clinical trials and is supported by the pharmacodynamics of these agents. The agents currently available likely do not have sufficient activity against anaerobes, and in particular *Bacteroides* spp., to be used alone. Rather, combination therapy with metronidazole appears appropriate.

REFERENCES

1. 1990. A randomized multicentre trial of pefloxacin plus metronidazole and gentamicin plus metronidazole in the treatment of severe intra-abdominal infections. Report from a Swedish Study Group. *J. Antimicrob. Chemother.* **26**(Suppl. B):173–180.

2. **Aldridge, K. E., D. Ashcraft, K. Cambre, C.L. Pierson, S. G. Jenkins, and J. E. Rosenblatt.** 2001. Multicenter survey of the changing in vitro antimicrobial susceptibilities of clinical isolates of *Bacteroides fragilis* group, *Prevotella*, *Fusobacterium*, *Porphyromonas*, and *Peptostreptococcus* species. *Antimicrob. Agents Chemother.* **45**:1238–1243.

3. **Barie, P. S., N. V. Christou, E. P. Dellinger, W. R. Rout, H. H. Stone, and J. P. Waymack.** 1990. Pathogenicity of the enterococcus in surgical infections. *Ann. Surg.* **212**:155–159.

4. **Bauernfeind, A.** 1993. Comparative in-vitro activities of the new quinolone, Bay y 3118, and ciprofloxacin, sparfloxacin, tosufloxacin, CI-960 and CI-990. *J. Antimicrob. Chemother.* **31**:505–522.

5. **Brismar, B., J. E. Akerlund, S. Sjostedt , C. Johansson, A. Tornqvist, B. Backstrand, H. Bang, L. Andaker, R. O. Gustafsson, N. Darle, M. Angeras, A. Falk, G. Tunevall, B. Kasholm-Tengve, T. Skau, P. O. Nystrom, T. Gasslander, A. Hagelback, B. Olsson-Liljequist, A. E. Eklund, and C. E.**

Nord. 1996. Biapenem versus imipenem/cilastatin in the treatment of complicated intra-abdominal infections: report from a Swedish Study Group. *Scand. J. Infect. Dis.* **28**:507–512.

6. Brismar, B., A. S. Malmborg, G. Tunevall, V. Lindgren, L. Bergman, L. O. Mentzing, P. O. Nystrom, S. Ansehn, B. Backstrand, T. Skau, L. Andaker, P. O. Gustafsson, B. Kasholm-Tengve, L. Sjoberg, B. Olsson-Liljequist, A. E. Eklund, and C. E. Nord. 1995. Meropenem versus imipenem/cilastatin in the treatment of intra-abdominal infections. *J. Antimicrob. Chemother.* **35**:139–148.

7. Brismar, B., A. S. Malmborg, G. Tunevall, B. Wretlind, L. Bergman, L. O. Mentzing, P. O. Nystrom, E. Kihlstrom, B. Backstrand, and T. Skau. 1992. Piperacillin-tazobactam versus imipenem-cilastatin for treatment of intra-abdominal infections. *Antimicrob. Agents Chemother.* **36**:2766–2773.

8. Brook, I. 1993. In vivo efficacies of quinolones and clindamycin for treatment of infections with Bacteroides fragilis and/or Escherichia coli in mice: correlation with in vitro susceptibilities. *Antimicrob. Agents Chemother.* **37**:997–1000.

9. Cohn, S. M., P. A. Lipsett, T. G. Buchman, W. G. Cheadle, J. W. Milsom, S. O'Marro, A. E. Yellin, S. Jungerwirth, E. V. Rochefort, D. C. Haverstock, and S. F. Kowalsky. 2000. Comparison of intravenous/oral ciprofloxacin plus metronidazole versus piperacillin/tazobactam in the treatment of complicated intraabdominal infections. *Ann. Surg.* **232**:254–262.

10. Dan, M., F. Serour, and F. Poch 1992. Penetration of ciprofloxacin into human peritoneal tissue following a single oral dose of 750 milligrams. *J. Chemother.* **4**:27–29.

11. Dan, M., T. Zuabi, C. Quassem, and H. H. Rotmensch. 1992. Distribution of ciprofloxacin in ascitic fluid following administration of a single oral dose of 750 milligrams. *Antimicrob. Agents Chemother.* **36**:677–678.

12. Davis, R. L., J. R. Koup, J. Williams-Warren, A. Weber, and A. L. Smith. 1985. Pharmacokinetics of three oral formulations of ciprofloxacin. *Antimicrob. Agents Chemother.* **28**:74–77.

13. Donahue, P. E., D. L. Smith, A. E. Yellin, S. J. Mintz, F. Bur, and D. R. Luke. 1998. Trovafloxacin in the treatment of intra-abdominal infections: results of a double-blind, multicenter comparison with imipenem/cilastatin. Trovafloxacin Surgical Group. *Am. J. Surg.* **176**(Suppl. 6A):53S-61S.

14. Donahue, P. E., D. L. Smith, A. E. Yellin, S. J. Mintz, F. Bur, and D. R. Luke. 1998. Trovafloxacin in the treatment of intra-abdominal infections: results of a double-blind, multicenter comparison with imipenem/cilastatin. Trovafloxacin Surgical Group. *Am. J. Surg.* **176**(Suppl. 6A):53S-61S.

15. Fink, M. P., Snydman, D. R. Niederman, M. S. Leeper, K. V. Jr., Johnson, R. H. Heard, S. O. R. G. Wunderink, J. W. Caldwell, J. J. Schentag, and G. A. Siami. For the severe Pneumonia Study Group. 1994. Treatment of severe pneumonia in hospitalized patients: results of a multicenter, randomized, double-blind trial comparing intravenous ciprofloxacin with imipenem-cilastatin. The Severe Pneumonia Study Group. *Antimicrob. Agents Chemother.* **38**:547–557.

16. Reference deleted.

17. Geroulanos, S. J. 1995. Meropenem versus imipenem/cilastatin in intra-abdominal infections requiring surgery. Meropenem Study Group. *J. Antimicrob. Chemother.* **36**(Suppl. A):191–205.

18. Lamp, K. C., C. D. Freeman, N. E. Klutman, and M. K. Lacy. 1999. Pharmacokinetics and pharmacodynamics of the nitroimidazole antimicrobials. *Clin. Pharmacokinet.* **36**:353–373.

19. Lau, A. H., K. Emmons, and R. Seligsohn. Pharmacokinetics of intravenous metronidazole at different dosages in healthy subjects. *Int. J. Clin. Pharmacol. Ther. Toxicol.* **29**:386–390.

20. Luke, D. R., and J. Peterson. 1999. Treatment of complicated intra-abdominal infections: comparison of the tolerability and safety of intravenous/oral trovafloxacin versus intravenous imipenem/cilastatin switching to oral amoxycillin/clavulanic acid. *Int. J. Clin. Pract.* **53**:166–173.

21. Martin, C., B. Sastre, M. N. Mallet, B. Bruguerolle, J. P. Brun, P. De Micco, and F. Gouin. 1991. Pharmacokinetics and tissue penetration of a single 1,000-milligram, intravenous dose of metronidazole for antibiotic prophylaxis of colorectal surgery. *Antimicrob. Agents Chemother.* **35**:2602–2605.

22. Montravers, P., R. Gauzit, C. Muller, J. P. Marmuse, A. Fichelle, and J. M. Desmonts. 1996. Emergence of antibiotic-resistant bacteria in cases of peritonitis after intraabdominal surgery affects the efficacy of empirical antimicrobial therapy. *Clin. Infect. Dis.* **23**:486–494.

23. Nguyen, M. H., V. L. Yu, A. J. Morris, L. McDermott, M. W. Wagener, L. Harrell and D. R. Snydman. 2000. Antimicrobial resistance and clinical outcome of Bacteroides bacteremia: findings of a multicenter prospective observational trial. *Clin. Infect. Dis.* **30**:870–876.

24. Nord, C. E., P. O. Nystrom, and B. Brismar. 1994. A comparative trial for intraabdominal infections of meropenem. *Intersci. Conf. Antimicrob. Agents Chemother.* American Society for Microbiology, Washington, D. C.

25. Oh, H., N. El Amin, T. Davies, P. C. Appelbaum, and C. Edlund. 2001. gyrA mutations associated with quinolone resistance in Bacteroides fragilis group strains. *Antimicrob. Agents Chemother.* **45**:1977–1981.

26. Oh, H., C. E. Nord, L. Barkholt, M. Hedberg, and C. Edlund. 2000. Ecological disturbances in intestinal microflora caused by clinafloxacin, an extended-spectrum quinolone. *Infection.* **28**:272–277.

27. Paradis, D., F. Vallee, S. Allard, C. Bisson, N. Daviau, C. Drapeau, F. Auger, and M. LeBel. 1992. Comparative study of pharmacokinetics and serum bactericidal activities of cefpirome, ceftazidime, ceftriaxone, imipenem, and ciprofloxacin. *Antimicrob. Agents Chemother.* **36**:2085–2092.

28. Plaisance, K. I., R. Quintiliani, and C. H. Nightingale. 1998. The pharmacokinetics of metronidazole and its metabolites in critically ill patients. *J. Antimicrob. Chemother.* **21**:195–200.

29. Solomkin, J. S., D. L. Hemsell, R. Sweet, F. Tally, and J. Bartlett. 1992. Evaluation of new anti-infective drugs for the treatment of intraabdominal infections. Infectious Diseases Society of America and the Food and Drug Administration. *Clin. Infect. Dis.* **15**(Suppl. 1):S33–S42.

30. Solomkin, J. S., H. H. Reinhart, E. P. Dellinger, J. M. Bohnen, O. D. Rotstein, S. B. Vogel, H. H. Simms, C. S. Hill, H. S. Bjornson, D. C. Haverstock, H. O. Coulter, and R. M. Echols. 1996. Results of a randomized trial comparing sequential intravenous/oral treatment with ciprofloxacin plus metronidazole to imipenem/cilastatin for intra-abdominal infections. The Intra-Abdominal Infection Study Group. *Ann. Surg.* **223**:303–315.

31. Solomkin, J. S., S. E. Wilson, N. V. Christou, O. D. Rotstein, E. P. Dellinger, R. S. Bennion, R. Pak, and K. Tack. 2001. Results of a clinical trial of clinafloxacin versus imipenem/cilastatin for intraabdominal infections. *Ann. Surg.* **233**:79–87.

31a. Solomkin, J. S., A. E. Yellin, O. D. Rotstein. 2003. Results of a double-blind, randomized comparative phase III trial of ertapenem vs piperacillin/tazobactam in the treatment of complicated intraabdominal infections. *Ann. Surg.* **237**:235–245.

32. **Stratton, C.** 1992. Fluoroquinolone antibiotics: properties of the class and individual agents. *Clin. Ther.* **14:**347–375.

33. **Thadepalli, H., M. B. Bansal, B. Rao, R. See, S. K. Chuah, R. Marshall and V. K. Dhawan.** 1988. Ciprofloxacin: in vitro, experimental, and clinical evaluation. *Rev. Infect. Dis.* **10:**505–515.

34. **Whiting, J. L., N. Cheng, A. W. Chow.** 1987. Interactions of ciprofloxacin with clindamycin, metronidazole, cefoxitin, cefotaxime, and mezlocillin against Gram-positive and Gram-negative anaerobic bacteria. *Antimicrob. Agents Chemother.* **31:**1379–1382.

35. **Wise, R., I. A. Donovan, M. R. Lockley, J. Drumm, and J. M. Andrews.** 1986. The pharmacokinetics and tissue penetration of imipenem. *J. Antimicrob. Chemother.* **18**(Suppl. E):93–101.

36. **Zhanel, G. G., K. Ennis, L. Vercaigne, A. Walkty, A. S. Gin, J. Embil, H. Smith, and D. J. Hoban.** 2002. A critical review of the fluoroquinolones: focus on respiratory infections. *Drugs* **62:**13–59.

Quinolone Antimicrobial Agents, 3rd ed.
Edited by David C. Hooper and Ethan Rubinstein
© 2003 ASM Press, Washington, D.C.

Chapter 13

Treatment of Community-Acquired Respiratory Tract Infections

PETER BALL AND LIONEL MANDELL

The use of quinolones in respiratory tract infection (RTI) has developed from unpromising origins. The new agents of the 1990s and the millennium are now being referred to as "respiratory" quinolones because of in vitro, pharmacodynamic, and clinical justification, supported by a large clinical trial database in both community-acquired pneumonia (CAP) and acute exacerbations of chronic bronchitis (AECB). This contrasts with the position in the 1980s, when their use was considered by many to be malpractice. This largely related to a perceived lack of potency against the pneumococcus, which varied considerably between members of the class. Thus, ciprofloxacin and ofloxacin had MICs at which 90% of the isolates tested are inhibited (MIC90s), which, between published series, ranged from 0.5 to 4 mg/liter—the latter clearly marginal—and pefloxacin, enoxacin, and lomefloxacin MICs ranged from 2 to 16 mg/liter—the latter clearly resistant. Nevertheless, despite criticism of use in CAP on the basis of potency, ciprofloxacin and ofloxacin actually gave good results in early clinical trials in CAP (24, 15). The landmark study of ciprofloxacin in severely ill, hospitalized patients, predominantly those in the intensive care unit who were also ventilated, gave significantly superior clinical results to imipenem and did much to rehabilitate this agent (61).

Nevertheless, use in community-acquired infections was punctuated by reports of failure in pneumococcal disease (95), although, on review, many such failures were due to inadequate dosage and absorptive interactions (15), and yet others occurred after oral therapy in severely ill patients who clearly warranted alternative treatment. Currently, significant resistance to second-generation agents, such as ciprofloxacin and levofloxacin, is beginning to appear (31, 83, 84) and clinical failures are being recorded due to such strains (82, 156). Arguments over second-generation drugs are fast becoming superfluous because of the availability of moxifloxacin, gatifloxacin, and agents submitted for licensing, e.g., gemifloxacin, which have improved potency and pharmacodynamic properties and which give excellent clinical results in both CAP and AECB. However, there is a lack of data on fluoroquinolone-treated infections caused by penicillin/macrolide-resistant *Streptococcus pneumoniae* and, at the end of 2001, levofloxacin remained the only quinolone licensed in the United States for use in drug-resistant pneumococcal disease. Although the incidence of pneumococcal disease may, in the future, be influenced by the availability of the 23-valent capsular polysaccharide vaccine, which has had a substantial effect on incidence, morbidity, and mortality in subjects aged 65 years or older (36), there is an increasing need for replacement of standard β-lactam and macrolide therapy. At the millennium, the "respiratory" quinolones appeared well placed to fill that requirement.

Certain agents from the 1990s, which had improved potency against the pneumococcus and which included temafloxacin, sparfloxacin, trovafloxacin, grepafloxacin, and clinafloxacin, have been withdrawn or suspended from use on toxicological grounds, but data on these compounds is included to illustrate the potential of the "respiratory" quinolones.

CAP

CAP is a potentially lethal infection with significant impact on both individuals and society as a whole. It is currently the sixth leading cause of death in the United States, the estimated 3 to 4 million cases occurring annually resulting in more than 600,000 hospitalizations and 64 million days of restricted activity (113).

Peter Ball • School of Biomedical Sciences, University of St. Andrews, Fife, Scotland, United Kingdom. **Lionel Mandell** • Division of Infectious Diseases, McMaster University, Hamilton, Ontario L8V 1C3, Canada.

A number of differing pathogens cause CAP, which is not a homogeneous clinical entity. The etiology must be considered in the context of a variety of factors, including the sites of acquisition of infection (community versus nursing home) and care (outpatient, inpatient, or nursing home), the immune status of the patient, and the presence of comorbid illness. Polymicrobial infection may be present in any given patient, the overall incidence of mixed infection ranging from 2.7 to 10% (54, 108, 112).

The predominant pathogen of CAP is *S. pneumoniae*. A meta-analysis of 7,000 cases of etiologically proven cases of pneumonia revealed that *S. pneumoniae* accounts for two thirds of all cases and a similar proportion of fatalities (60). Atypical pathogens, such as *Mycoplasma pneumoniae*, *Chlamydia pneumoniae,* and *Legionella* species are also important. A recent study of more than 2,700 hospitalized patients with CAP ranked these pathogens second, third, and fourth of all etiologic agents meeting the criteria for a "definite" diagnosis (109). In selected cases, aerobic gram-negative rods may also play a role (54, 123).

A number of management issues are unique to this disease. Despite investigation, a specific pathogen cannot be found in up to one-half of cases, even in tertiary-care-level university hospitals. At the time of initiation of treatment, limitations in diagnostic methods impose major uncertainties as to the nature of the potential pathogen(s). In general, diagnostic evaluation may be both clinical (patient history, physical examination, chest radiograph, sputum gram stain, and blood and sputum cultures) (24) and invasive and/or quantitative (bronchoscopic techniques, pleural fluid aspiration and, in selected cases, lung biopsy) (15). Clinical methodology is insensitive and lacks specificity, while invasive or quantitative methods require special expertise and laboratory support and are costly. In routine clinical practice in the United Kingdom, pathogen(s) are identified in only 25% of cases of CAP and such data result in modification of antibiotic treatment in just 10% of cases (162).

Before initiation of therapy, the need for hospital admission must be assessed. This has significant economic implications; the cost of inpatient care exceeds that of outpatient treatment by a factor of 15 to 20, and hospital management accounts for most of the estimated 4 billion dollars spent annually on CAP in the United States. In many cases it is immediately apparent whether a patient can be treated at home or requires admission to the hospital or to the intensive care unit (ICU). In others it may not be obvious just how ill the patient is (or may become) and whether he or she should be admitted to the hospital. Validated prognostic scores and outcome measures can assist physicians with the site-of-care decision, may minimize unnecessary hospital admissions, and may identify those who will benefit from hospital care in the ward or ICU. They have a significant impact on antibiotic choices. Although not originally developed for triage, the most widely used prognostic tool is that of Fine and his colleagues, published in 1997 (59). This two-step rule identifies patients at low risk for mortality and has been adopted by the Infectious Diseases Society of America (IDSA) and the Joint Guidelines prepared by the Canadian Infectious Disease Society and the Canadian Thoracic Society (CIDS-CTS) (28, 104).

Treatment of CAP

Appropriate choices of antibiotic(s) for CAP have generated considerable discussion, and a number of learned bodies have developed guidelines to assist physicians (4, 28, 52, 80, 102, 104). However, the existence of four separate and distinct sets of guidelines in North America alone highlights the degree of controversy associated with the topic (4, 28, 80, 104). Detailed discussion of guidelines is beyond the scope of this chapter, but comments regarding the inclusion of fluoroquinolones are appropriate.

The original guidelines, published in North America in 1993 by the Canadian Infectious Disease Society (CIDS) and the American Thoracic Society (ATS), suggested macrolides as first-choice therapy for outpatients (105, 116). This was unrelated to potential pneumococcal penicillin resistance (at that time uncommon) but reflected concerns about the increasingly apparent role of atypical pathogens. Recently, the fluoroquinolones have assumed a more important role, partly relating to multidrug (β-lactam, macrolide, and other) resistance among pneumococci and to the potential importance of gram-negative rods in selected patients and the recent licensing of the more active "respiratory" fluoroquinolones. Fluoroquinolones refer primarily to three currently available agents: levofloxacin, gatifloxacin and moxifloxacin. Before reviewing each of these agents it is worth considering their pharmacokinetics (PK) and pharmacodynamics (PD).

PK-PD Parameters in Relation to Therapy

PK and PD parameters, which correlate with efficacy, differ among the major antibiotic classes. Time above MIC correlates best with the efficacy of β-lactams, with most macrolides, and with clindamycin. However, for aminoglycosides and fluoroquinolones, drugs that exhibit concentration-dependent killing, the ratios of area under the curve (AUC)/MIC and maximum concentration of drug in serum (C_{max})/MIC correlate best with efficacy (see chapter 8). The AUC/MIC is an integrated PD measurement that defines regimens as a ratio of drug exposure to MIC and allows comparisons of various agents.

The most relevant PD-related outcome measures are bacterial eradication and clinical response. For fluoroquinolones, most PD parameters including AUC/MIC ratios (81,86,140) and C_{max}/MIC ratios (131,132) correlate with these outcomes. Resistance emergence may also be predicted by PK/PD analyses. For example, in nosocomial lower respiratory tract infections, an AUC/MIC of <100 was associated with a significant increase in emergence of resistance, the probability of a pathogen remaining susceptible for a 2-week period being <20% if the AUC/MIC was <100 as opposed to 85% if the AUC/MIC exceeded 100 (150). Any rise in MIC or inadequacies of dosage or absorption lowers the AUC/MIC ratio and predisposes to resistance emergence, a powerful argument for use of the most effective agents available at appropriate dosage.

The breakpoint AUC/MIC ratio of 125, generally considered predictive of success or failure, was derived from a study of gram-negative pathogens in which tobramycin, cefmenoxime, and ciprofloxacin AUC/MICs were studied over a range of MICs (139). As AUC/MIC increases to levels greater than 250, resistance emergence is less common, and pathogens are eliminated more rapidly. Sixty percent of patient cultures become culture-negative on day 1 of treatment (65). The application of this general principle from infections caused by gram-negative to those caused by gram-positive pathogens is under discussion. In an in vitro model of the bactericidal characteristics and PD profiles of levofloxacin, ciprofloxacin, and ampicillin, against four isolates of *S. pneumoniae*, the range of effective AUIC values was 30 to 55, values considerably less than 125 (93). A recent comprehensive review of in vitro and ex vivo models of pneumococcal infection found most to

indicate positive outcomes at AUC/MIC values of 20 to 50, thus explaining the paradox of certain fluoroquinolones, such as levofloxacin, which failed to attain AUC/MIC ratios in keeping with previously recommended levels (125 or greater) yet proved highly effective in human infection (164). Arguably, tissue or tissue fluid penetration may be a more reliable, although little investigated, predictor of outcomes. Ratios of fluoroquinolone concentrations in either epithelial lining fluid or alveolar macrophages to the MICs of CAP pathogens are substantial (Table 1).

The "Respiratory" Fluoroquinolones

Data on the published clinical trials in CAP of oral and parenteral quinolones, both current and past, are summarized in Tables 2 and 3. Responses in pneumococcal infections are detailed in Table 4. For the currently available agents and those in development, the data are discussed further below.

Levofloxacin

Levofloxacin, the L-enantiomer of ofloxacin, has improved potency against pneumococci (MIC_{90}, 1 to 2mg/liter) and is available in both intravenous (i.v.) and oral (p.o.) formulations. For pneumonia, levofloxacin C_{max}/MIC ratios of 12 or greater predict clinical efficacy (131, 132). These are almost invariably achieved in routine practice, although rising pneumococcal MICs in some countries may compromise this position (31, 82, 84, 156). Clinical studies with levofloxacin (i.v./p.o. switch) have yielded excellent results, in some cases superior to standard agents such as ceftriaxone ± erythromycin, including >98% response in atypical disease (57). Similarly equivalent responses were found in comparison with amoxicillin-clavulanate (30). Pneumococcal eradication rates were 100% in both studies. Levofloxacin produced outcomes equivalent to ceftriaxone in more severely ill patients with CAP (118) and satisfactory responses in bacteremic patients (71).

Table 1. Peak quinolone concentrations in serum and in pulmonary tissues, fluids, and cells

Fluoroquinolone	Dose (mg)	C_{max}(mg/liter) in serum	Concn (mg/liter) in:			Reference
			Bronchial mucosa	Epithelial lining fluid	Alveolar macrophage	
Moxifloxacin	400	3.3	5.5	24.4	61.8	145
Gatifloxacin	400	3.2	5.32	6.16	77.3	146
Trovafloxacin	200	1.4	1.52	3	19.1	147
Grepafloxacin	400	1.82	5.32	27.1	278	148
Sparfloxacin	400/200	1.2	4.4	15	53.7	149
Levofloxacin	500	4.9	6.5	9	41.9	150

Table 2. Results of oral quinolone therapy for CAP

Agents compared	Dosage (mg)/frequency (h)/duration (d)	Clinical success at end of study (%)	Bacteriological efficacy/eradication (%)	Reference
Sparfloxacin	400/200/24/10	112/136 (89)	77/86 (89.5)	151
Amoxicillin	1,000/8/10–14	118/150 (84.5)	69/80 (86)	
		Evaluables at EOS[a]	Efficacy at EOS	
Grepafloxacin	600/24/7–10	87/114 (76)	32/36 (89)	79
Amoxicillin	500/8/7–10	85/111 (74)	32/45 (71)	
		Evaluables at EOS	Eradication at EOS	
Trovafloxacin	200/24/7–10	125/138 (91)	79/86 (92)	49
Amoxicillin	1,000/8/7–10	119/147 (81)	72/87 (83)	
		$P = 0.01$	Eradication at EOS	
Moxifloxacin	400/24/10	143/160 (89.5)	63/70 (90)	48
Amoxicillin	1,000/8/10	159/178 (89.5)	65/78 (83)	
		Evaluables at EOS	Eradication at EOT[b]	
Trovafloxacin	200/24/7–10	120/135 (89)	50/53 (94.5)	152
Clarithromycin	500/12/7–10	124/144 (86)	53/59 (90)	
		Evaluables at EOS	Eradication at EOS	
Moxifloxacin	400/24/10	184/194 (95)	106/110 (94)	47
Clarithromycin	500/12/10	178/188 (95)	100/104 (93)	
		Evaluables at EOS	Eradication at EOT	
Gatifloxacin	400/24/7–14	181/191 (95)	98	57
Clarithromycin	500/12/7–14	177/190 (93)	93	
		Evaluables at EOS	Efficacy at EOS	
Gemifloxacin	320/24/7–14	228/238 (95.8)	94/100 (94)	61
Trovafloxacin	200/24/7–14	218/233 (93.6)	85/90 (94.4)	
		Evaluables at EOT	Eradication at EOT	

[a] EOS, end of study.
[b] EOT, end of treatment.

Nevertheless, more extensive use of levofloxacin (and other earlier agents such as ciprofloxacin), may generate single-step resistance mutations and could prime resistance to more potent (double target, parC and gyrA) quinolones, which then require only a single further mutation to develop high-level resistance (87). Reports of pneumococcal fluoroquinolone resistance from Canada, the United States, and the Far East (31, 46, 83, 84) are now being followed by (so far) isolated reports of clinical failures of levofloxacin therapy in meningitis (163) and pneumonia (40). Strains that develop both parC and gyrA mutations also have raised MICs for 8-methoxyquinolones (moxifloxacin and gatifloxacin) and for gemifloxacin, and spread may occur rapidly to other patients (156). Risk factors for levofloxacin-resistant infections include prior exposure to fluoroquinolones, chronic obstructive pulmonary disease, and institutional acquisition (82, 84).

Moxifloxacin

A once-daily 8-methoxyquinolone, currently only available p.o., but with an i.v. formulation soon to be released, has excellent potency against respiratory pathogens, including a pneumococcal MIC_{90} of 0.12 to 0.25 mg/liter. Peak serum concentrations are at least 15 to 25 times the pneumococcal MIC, and the AUC values average 200–400 mg/liter. h (161), thus easily exceeding the PD parameters predictive of favorable outcomes.

Moxifloxacin has been highly effective in CAP. Compared with clarithromycin, bacterial eradication rates were 94 and 93% (100% for S. pneumoniae) and response rates in atypical infections were 96 and 99%, respectively (63). Comparison with amoxicillin 1 g every 8 h demonstrated an apparent improvement in eradication rate of 90 versus 83% (127), consistent with trovafloxacin, which resulted in better clinical results: 91 versus 81% for amoxicillin ($P = 0.01$) and higher bacteriological eradication rates: 92 versus 83% (151).

A meta-analysis of moxifloxacin trials identified four deaths among 701 patients (0.57%) compared with 12 among 705 comparator-treated patients (1.70%; $P = 0.045$). Thirty-nine (5.6%) moxifloxacin-treated patients required hospital admission compared with 43 (6.1%) patients receiving comparators (114).

The i.v. derivative has been investigated in both North American and European studies (Table 3) (68,

Table 3. Results of parenteral quinolone therapy for CAP

Agents compared	Dosage (mg or g)/ frequency (h)/and duration in days (d)	Clinical success at end of study (%)	Bacteriological efficacy/ eradication (%)	Reference
Levofloxacin i.v. to p.o vs. Ceftriaxone i.v. and/or Cefuroxime p.o. ± erythromycin (either arm)	500 mg/24/7–14 1–2 g/12/24 500 mg/12 h/both 7–14	217/226 (96) 207/230 (90) at 5–7d post-Rx:[a] CI[b] significant	125/128 (98) 122/144 (85) at 5–7 d post-Rx: CI significant	38
Levofloxacin i.v. to p.o. vs. Ceftriaxone (severe infections)	500 mg/12 h/median, 9 d 4 g/24 h/median 8 d	112/127 (87) 120/139 (86) at 2–5d post-Rx	71/82 (87) 92/108 (85) At 2–5 d post-Rx	40
Trovafloxacin i.v. to p.o. vs.	200 mg/24 h/7–10 d	136/159 (86) (10/10 DRSP)	65/77 (84.5)	153
Ceftriaxone i.v. and/or Cefpodoxime p.o. ± erythromycin (either arm)	1g/24 h/followed by 200 mg/12 h/7–10 d Evaluables at EOS	138/169 (82)[c] Eradication of selected pathogens	72/85 (85)	
Gatifloxacin i.v. to p.o. vs.	400 mg/24 h/7–14 d	96/99 (97)	69/71 (97) (18/19 *S. pneumoniae*)	54
Ceftriaxone i.v. ± erythromycin i.v. to p.o. clarithromycin	1–2g/24 h/7–14 d	96/106 (91) Evaluables at EOT[d]	73/79 (92) (20/21 *S. pneumoniae*)	
Gatifloxacin i.v. to p.o./p.o. vs. Levofloxacin i.v. to p.o./p.o.	400 mg/24 h/7–14 d 500 mg/24 h/7–14 d	156/163 (96) 166/176 (94) Evaluables at EOT	122/125 (98) (12/12 *S. pneumoniae*) 106/114 (93) (14/18 *S. pneumoniae*)	56
Moxifloxacin i.v. to p.o. vs. Amoxicillin-clavulanate ± Clarithromycin	400 mg/24 h/7–14 d	241/258 (93) 239/280 (85) Evaluables at EOT	(94) (39/39 *S. pneumoniae*) (82) (26/32 *S. pneumoniae*)	51
Moxifloxacin i.v. to p.o. vs. Trovafloxacin/levofloxacin i.v. to p.o.	400 mg/24 h/7–14 d	157/182 (86) 161/180 (89)	66/80 (83) (40/45 *S. pneumoniae*) 70/78 (90) (40/44 *S. pneumoniae*) (91)	53

[a] Rx, treatment.
[b] CI, confidence interval.
[c] EOS, end of study.
[d] EOT, end of treatment.

69). In North America, comparison with trovafloxacin (replaced by levofloxacin once trovafloxacin was recognized to cause rare, but serious adverse events), revealed that, despite disproportionately more severely ill patients being included in the moxifloxacin arm, these agents were equivalent (69). In Europe, moxifloxacin therapy was superior to treatment with amoxicillin-clavulanate (68).

Gatifloxacin

Gatifloxacin, also a once daily 8-methoxyquinolone, has similar potency (pneumococcal MIC$_{90}$, 0.25 to 0.5 mg/liter) and is available in both i.v. and p.o. formulations. In hospitalized patients, using an i.v./p.o. switch regimen, gatifloxacin (400 mg once daily) gave cure rates of 97% (in comparison with 91% for ceftriaxone), pneumococcal eradication rates of 95% for both groups, and 100% suc-

cess in atypical infections (62). A further comparison with ceftriaxone demonstrated i.v./p.o. gatifloxacin therapy to reduce duration in ICU and hospital length of stay (66) and an i.v./p.o. switch comparison with levofloxacin resulted in cure rates of 96 versus 94% and bacterial eradication rates of 98% (*S. pneumoniae* 100%) versus 93% (148). Oral gatifloxacin alone proved equal to clarithromycin, demonstrating success rates of 95 versus 93% in evaluable patients and 92 versus 89% in those with severe disease (135).

The most recently published study about hospitalized CAP patients (49) compared i.v./p.o. gatifloxacin versus i.v. ceftriaxone with or without i.v. erythromycin switching to oral clarithromycin and served as a cost-effectiveness analysis. Clinical response rates of 98 and 92% (bacterial eradication rates, 97 versus 92%) for gatifloxacin and control, respectively, were reported. The geometric mean cost

Table 4. Clinical efficacy and bacteriological eradication rates in selected trials of pneumococcal CAP

Fluoroquinolone	Efficacy (%)	Eradication (%)	Reference
Levofloxacin vs.	30/30 (100)	30/30 (100)	38
Ceftriaxone/cefuroxime	31/33 (94)	31/32 (97)	
	5–7 days posttherapy		
Sparfloxacin vs.	125/146 (85.5)	Not stated	154
Amoxicillin + ofloxacin	106/124 (85.5)		
	33–47 days after commencing therapy		
Sparfloxacin vs.	71/80 (89)	Not stated	151
Amoxicillin	59/65 (91)		
	39–41 days after commencing therapy		
Sparfloxacin vs.	25/26 (96)	Not stated	78
Roxithromycin	14/15 (93)		
Grepafloxacin vs.	15/18 (83)	20/20 (100)	79
Amoxicillin	6/12 (50)	13/13 (100)	
Trovafloxacin vs.	20/21 (95)	20/20 (100)	49
Amoxicillin	21/24 (87)	17/21 (81)[a]	
	35 days after commencing therapy		
Trovafloxacin vs.	11/12 (92)	11/12 (92)	152
Clarithromycin	13/15 (87)	13/15 (87)	
	28–35 days after commencing therapy		
Moxifloxacin vs.	49/58 (84.5)	43/48 (90)	48
Amoxicillin	53/65 (81.5)	39/46 (85)	
	31–38 days after commencing therapy		
Moxifloxacin vs.	112/120 (93.5)	Not stated	73
Amoxicillin and clarithromycin	68/77 (88)		
	3–5 days after commencing therapy		
Gatifloxacin vs.	Not stated	12/12 (100)	56
Levofloxacin		14/18 (78)	
Gatifloxacin vs.	Not stated	18/19 (95)	54
Ceftriaxone		20/21 (95)	
Gemifloxacin vs.	Not stated	18/18 (100)	61
Trovafloxacin		14/15 (93)	

[a] No significant difference.

per patient was $5,109 for gatifloxacin and $6,164 for ceftriaxone ($P = 0.011$) (49).

Gemifloxacin

Gemifloxacin, a fluoronaphthyridone currently under development, has greatly enhanced pneumococcal potency (MIC_{90}, 0.03 mg/liter). To date, most clinical trial results are presented only in abstract form, but indicate in both outpatient and inpatient settings that gemifloxacin p.o. (320 mg once daily) is equal to control regimens, including amoxicillin/clavulanate 1 g/125 mg. p.o. three times a day and ceftriaxone i.v. switch to cefuroxime p.o. ± macrolide, respectively (97, 100). In the outpatient study, gemifloxacin was given for only 7 days while the comparator was given for 10 days; in the inpatient study oral gemifloxacin was used throughout, indicating possible logistical and economic advantages over parenteral therapy.

The currently published study (56), which had a sample size of 573 patients and comprised 73% outpatients and 27% inpatients, randomized patients to receive either gemifloxacin (320 mg once daily) or trovafloxacin (200 mg once daily). Both drugs were given p.o. throughout. Overall clinical analysis reported equivalent success rates of 95.8% for gemifloxacin and 93.6% for trovafloxacin. However, the intention-to-treat analysis showed gemifloxacin to be significantly superior (87.6% success) to trovafloxacin (81.1%) (95% confidence interval [CI] 0.5 to 12.4), possibly the only published instance in which one fluoroquinolone has proven superior to another.

Pharmacoeconomic Analyses of Fluoroquinolone Therapy

During the early 1990s, ciprofloxacin and ofloxacin rapidly became agents of choice for sequential i.v. to p.o. switch therapy (76, 124, 133). For example, i.v. to p.o. ofloxacin therapy was highly effective in nosocomial and CAP (125) and sequential therapy using oral ciprofloxacin substitution after initial i.v. therapy reduced drug hospitalization costs by up to 45 and 20%, respectively

(124). Compared with ceftazidime in nosocomial and severe pneumonia, ciprofloxacin i.v./p.o. therapy reduced costs by $500 per treatment (65) and compared with imipenem, significantly reduced post-treatment days in hospital, further antibiotic costs, and repeat hospitalizations (73).

Recent studies, initially utilizing levofloxacin as part of a critical pathway in comparison with standard care of CAP (107) and as formulary choice in hospital (106) demonstrated cost advantages relating to fewer admissions, length of stay, and overall cost. For gatifloxacin, use indicated a reduction in geometric mean cost per patient versus ceftriaxone and the cost-effectiveness ratios (mean cost per expected success) were $5236/1 and $7047/1 for gatifloxacin and ceftriaxone respectively (49).

The use of such monotherapy versus combination treatment has obvious logistic and pharmacoeconomic advantages. Reduction in length of stay has a significant impact on overall cost of treatment, but prevention of admissions has the greatest effect by avoiding hospital costs entirely.

The Role of Fluoroquinolones in CAP

Ultimately, the role for the fluoroquinolones in CAP must be defined. In doing so, the following issues should be kept in mind:

1. The etiological agent(s) are rarely recognized at the start of treatment.
2. Polymicrobial infection is more common than previously appreciated.
3. Inappropriate initial treatment of severe CAP is associated with a significantly higher risk of death (98).
4. Pneumococcal infections are associated with increasing risk of resistance to penicillin, to macrolides, or to both (plus other potential agents).

The problem of resistance to both penicillins and macrolides is one that is inexorably increasing. The phenotypic expression of resistance corresponds to genetic alterations resulting from either horizontal acquisition of genetic information or from mutations in the bacterial genome. The emergence of resistance to penicillin among S. pneumoniae isolates represents a gradual reduction in in vitro susceptibility and is due solely to the presence of low-affinity penicillin-binding proteins. Macrolide resistance, on the other hand, can occur either by target site modification (high-level resistance) or by an efflux pump (low-level resistance).

A disturbing phenomenon is the known association of pneumococcal resistance to penicillin with reduced susceptibility to other drugs such as macrolides, lincosamides, and streptogramins. In the United States, 58.9 and 74.5% of pneumococcal blood and respiratory isolates, respectively, are also macrolide resistant (D. Sahm, personal communication). For S. pneumoniae strains with MICs of 2 and 4 mg/liter, there are reports of increases in mortality and complications (29, 48, 55, 153) and there are recent reports of clinical macrolide failures involving both low- and high-level resistant isolates from both United States and Europe, respectively (16, 67, 70, 90, 128). Taken alone, such reports may not be sufficient to convince physicians that fluoroquinolones should be substituted. However, a review of the randomized controlled trials by the CIDS-CTS, IDSA, and ATS CAP Guideline committees revealed that 4 of the 14 studies comparing a fluoroquinolone with a comparator regimen showed a statistically significant improvement in clinical and/or bacteriologic outcome for the fluoroquinolone agent (57, 120, 122, 151). Two fluoroquinolones, trovafloxacin and moxifloxacin, also demonstrated a reduction in mortality (114, 152). With trovafloxacin the difference was not statistically significant, but with moxifloxacin, it was. Trovafloxacin has to all intents and purposes been withdrawn from use because of severe adverse reactions, but moxifloxacin is now increasingly used more widely.

The fluoroquinolones do not play a prominent role in the CAP guidelines from the British Thoracic Society (102). They are not indicated for first line treatment but are listed as possible alternatives for CAP patients treated in the hospital who are "not severe" or "severe." In both cases a fluoroquinolone with some enhanced pneumococcal activity is recommended. For the not-severe group levofloxacin 500 mg o.d. p.o. is suggested, while for the severe group levofloxacin 500 mg twice a day i.v. or p.o. plus benzylpenicillin 1.2 g once a day i.v. is recommended.

A review of North American CAP Guidelines from 1993 to the present reveals recommendations for macrolides or doxycycline for outpatients and a second- to third-generation cephalosporin and a macrolide for hospitalized ward patients (4, 27, 28, 80, 104, 105, 116). With the exception of the CDC statement all recent North American guidelines have recommended the fluoroquinolones for selected outpatients, hospitalized ward patients, and the 2% of patients admitted to the ICU (4, 28, 104). For outpatients the IDSA suggests that a fluoroquinolone may be the preferred choice for older patients or those with comorbidity. The ATS suggests that a fluoroquinolone alone or a β-lactam plus macrolide or doxycycline may be used for outpatients with cardiopulmonary disease and/or other modifying factors, while the CIDS-CTS Guidelines recommend fluoroquinolones as potentially ideal for patients with chronic obstructive pulmonary disease who have recently received other antimicrobials or steroids. Such patients are at greater risk of infection with penicillin and/or macrolide-resistant pneumococci.

For hospitalized patients in general wards, the IDSA, CIDS-CTS, and ATS recommend a cephalosporin or β-lactam–β-lactamase inhibitor plus a macrolide or a fluoroquinolone as monotherapy. The Canadian document alone recommends a fluoroquinolone as first choice. The ATS in contrast to the others suggests that a macrolide alone may be used (i.v. azithromycin) for patients with no cardiopulmonary disease and no modifying factors. Interestingly, the Centers for Disease Control and Prevention document alone excludes fluoroquinolones from a first-line role in outpatients and hospitalized ward patients. It is also the only North American guideline that is not evidence based.

For patients admitted to the ICU, all four groups recommend a β-lactam plus a fluoroquinolone or macrolide. None was willing to recommend a fluoroquinolone as monotherapy: there are no well-designed studies that have addressed this problem. Additionally, the CIDS-CTS Guideline recommended a fluoroquinolone alone (or amoxicillin-clavulanate plus a macrolide) as first choice in patients who are treated in the nursing home.

In summary, fluoroquinolones may be used:

1. as first-line agents for treatment of
    a. outpatients at risk of penicillin- and/or macrolide-resistant pneumococcal disease and
    b. patients in nursing homes,
2. for monotherapy for CAP patients hospitalized on a medical ward, and
3. for treatment of severe CAP in the ICU in combination with a β-lactam.

Analysis of bacteriologic results according to specific pathogens has shown that the quinolones, in particular, agents such as levofloxacin, moxifloxacin, gatifloxacin, and gemifloxacin, are at least comparable with control drugs for the treatment of infections caused by *S. pneumoniae*, *H. influenzae*, and other common pathogens. They may also be the drugs of choice for legionellosis (44). One abstract reported an overall clinical success rate of 89% for 28 patients with *Legionella* spp. pneumonia, 15 of whom were treated with gemifloxacin (320 mg p.o. o.d.) and 13 with trovafloxacin (200 mg p.o. o.d) (138).

PHARYNGITIS

Of the various community-acquired RTIs, pharyngitis is one of the most common and carries a significant burden of illness. Referred to by laymen as a "sore throat" it affects an area bounded by the pharynx, hypopharynx, tonsils, and uvula, and it may be caused by a wide variety of bacterial, viral, and miscellaneous pathogens. Of the infections described in this chapter, pharyngitis is the only one affecting the upper respiratory tract and it is responsible for 200 physician visits per 1,000 population annually (11).

To a large extent, the determination of the etiologic agent will depend on the diagnostic methods used, the time of year (winter versus summer), and the age group and its characteristics, e.g., children in day care versus free living adults. Most infections are viral; many do not require treatment, and, for most, there is no specific treatment available. Among bacterial causes, the single most important pathogen is the group A β-hemolytic streptococcus (GABHS) (*Streptococcus pyogenes*). GABHS accounts for 15 to 30% of cases in children and 5 to 10% of cases in adults (91, 130). It may be associated with local invasive complications (peritonsillar abscess) and postinfectious sequelae, including acute rheumatic fever and acute glomerulonephritis.

Other treatable bacterial pathogens include *Neisseria gonorrhoeae* and *Corynebacterium diphtheriae*. The atypical pathogens *Mycoplasma pneumoniae* and *Chlamydia pneumoniae* are associated with pharyngitis, but their importance remains to be determined. Gonococcal pharyngitis should be suspected (but not exclusively) in younger sexually active individuals. Infections are often asymptomatic but may present with sore throat and cervical lymphadenitis or, rarely, more distant complications, such as endocarditis. Coinfection (possibly at other sites) with *T. pallidum*, *C. trachomatis*, and human immunodeficiency virus should be excluded.

The main purpose of diagnostic testing is to distinguish cases caused by GABHS from those of viral etiology. Identification of cases caused by GABHS allows therapeutic intervention, which reduces transmission to close contacts and prevents suppurative complications such as peritonsillar abscess as well as acute rheumatic fever (38, 39, 45, 144). Gonococcal pharyngitis is the only situation in which current fluoroquinolones would be used in pharyngitis.

Fluoroquinolone Use in Pharyngitis

Fluoroquinolones have high in vitro potency against *N. gonorrhoeae*, including strains that produce β-lactamase and are resistant to other drugs. Many have proved successful as single-dose therapy for treatment of uncomplicated anogenital infection. However, there are no randomized, controlled trials of fluoroquinolones in pharyngeal gonococcal infection. One study randomized patients with anal or pharyngeal gonorrhea to receive either 200 or 400 mg of enoxacin twice daily for 2 days. All anal and 12 of 13 pharyngeal infections were eradicated (91). Another reported the results of ciprofloxacin use (250 mg p.o. twice a day) in 25 patients with acute bacterial pharyngotonsillitis who failed to respond to previous courses of antibiotics (51). A favorable clinical response was seen in 92% of patients (15 resolutions, seven improvements). The pathogens included a variety of gram-positive and gram-negative organisms, including *Staphylococcus aureus*, streptococci, and *Proteus vulgaris*, *Escherichia coli*, *Serratia marcescens*, and *Pseudomonas aeruginosa*.

Fluoroquinolones have no significant role to play in pharyngitis. Their use should be limited to cases of gonorrhea in which infection with a β-lactamase producing pathogen is suspected and in selected cases unresponsive to prior antibiotic therapy because of resistance or low concentrations of drug in pharyngeal tissue.

ACUTE BRONCHITIS

Acute bronchitis is primarily a viral or noninfective, pollution-related entity which occurs in patients with normal airways and, as such, does not routinely justify antibiotic therapy (58, 72). Undoubtedly, some cases may prove to be caused by infection with *C. pneumoniae*, but these too are usually self-limiting. Therefore, prescribing is more likely to initiate and perpetuate resistance than benefit the patient (16). Patient demands are often blamed for the continued over-prescribing of antibiotics in this area (157), and a large-scale survey of prescribing habits in acute LRTI found family practitioners to consider antibiotics indicated in only 1% of those in whom patients pressure was the main influence on the prescribing decision (103). Explanations, verbal or printed, given at the time of withholding therapy may significantly reduce this pressure (58, 79, 103).

Nevertheless, antibiotics continue to be prescribed in considerable quantities—a phenomenon for which, in an age of evidence-based medicine, there is little evidence, most of it contradictory, that antibiotics have any effect. An evaluation of all published trials of antibiotic therapy of AB (121) found no benefits from doxycycline therapy and, in poorly validated studies, only slight benefits for erythromycin or TMP-SMZ. Two subsequent meta-analyses failed to find agreement as to the overall value of antibiotic therapy (53, 143), but these and other studies have suggested value in specific patient groups—possibly those with underlying physical signs and the possibility of coexistent bacterial parenchymal lung disease, e.g., latent pneumonia (12).

The very definition of such patients is the pivotal decision point to prescribe or withhold antibiotics (12, 58). Typical patients might apparently include those with lower respiratory tract signs, those aged 55 years or older and who have frequent (persistent) cough and malaise (12). However, such groups are poorly defined and may well include patients with early pneumonia (12), who would certainly justify treatment but, by providing positive results, might skew opinion toward unnecessary use of antibiotics in those who do not.

Thus, in the absence of recognized epidemics of influenza (with secondary staphylococcal bronchitis) or acute bronchitis caused by *Mycoplasma* or *C. pneumoniae*, antibiotics will continue to be used empirically and, in the most part, inappropriately. Persistent symptoms may justify antibiotic prescription in apparently acute bronchial infections, and recent population surveys suggest that up to half of such patients may have asthma or early chronic bronchitis (149). The latter could justify therapy and, thus, there may be groups of patients in whom antibiotic therapy of "acute bronchitis" is appropriate. However, there is little evidence on which to base a rational prescribing decision and no trials of fluoroquinolones in this "indication."

ACUTE EXACERBATIONS OF CHRONIC BRONCHITIS

Despite initially gloomy prognostications in respect to second-generation agents, such as ciprofloxacin, largely relating to perceptions of suboptimal antipneumococcal potency, the quinolones have become agents of choice for AECB in patients with more advanced disease (17), in which gram-negative pathogens (*Haemophilus influenzae*, *Enterobacteriaceae*, and *P. aeruginosa*) predominate (50). They have been incorporated into many guidelines worldwide (14, 22, 88). The new agents, which have markedly enhanced potency and clinical efficacy against pneumococci, obviate previous arguments for their avoidance.

Chronic bronchitis can be defined as persistent cough with purulent sputum production for at least 2 to 3 months in 2 to 3 consecutive years, usually in the winter months and subject to periodic exacerbations (22). The latter are associated with bacterial infection in probably 50 to 70% of cases, and there is general agreement that quinolones:

1. are indicated in:
   a. substantive exacerbations of AECB (2, 8, 17, 26, 75, 117, 137),
   b. AECB in patients with risk factors for poor outcome (18, 21, 141),
2. reducing relapse rates and prolonging the infection free interval (IFI) or time to the next exacerbation (18, 22, 35, 141),
3. improving quality of life (1, 10, 78).

However, there is surprisingly little evidence that, in the short term, quinolones, which have excellent pharmacodynamic attributes, secondary to excellent concentration in bronchial mucosa (Table 1), give better outcomes than standard agents, such as the β-lactams and macroazalides. This is largely a function of trial design (23,111), which is beginning to change, current studies linking better bacterial eradication with lower relapse rates, longer infection-free interval, reduced costs, and increased quality of life (20, 78, 89).

As might be expected from the potency of quinolones against *H. influenzae*, the major pathogen of AECB (17), studies of the original second-generation agents proved encouraging both in terms of short-term outcome and in prolongation of the IFI. Personal analyses of overall clinical trial data gave clinical and bacteriological response rates of 96 and 87%, respectively, for ciprofloxacin (15) and 95 and 84% for ofloxacin (24). Ciprofloxacin became a drug of choice for more severe exacerbations in various guidelines for the management of AECB (14, 88).

However, the relative inactivity of these agents against the pneumococcus, the cause of a significant minority of AECB, resulted in response rates of 72% for ciprofloxacin and similarly suboptimal rates for ofloxacin. Temafloxacin, the first agent available with significantly improved activity against the pneumococcus, dramatically improved overall cure and eradication rates to 97 and 98%, respectively (25). A very large study of sparfloxacin gave identical clinical results to amoxicillin-clavulanate: 87 versus 89%, but suggested bacterial eradication to be superior: 88 versus 78%, although the pneumococcal eradication rates were 82 and 86%, respectively (3). Finally, although less intrinsically potent, levofloxacin, which penetrates very effectively into respiratory tissues and fluids, has given excellent results in AECB, including patients with severe disease (Table 5).

The Third Generation Quinolones

The development of 8-methoxyquinolones and fluoronaphthyridones, while retaining characteristic quinolone potency against *H. influenzae* and *Moraxella catarrhalis*, led to a dramatic increase in activity against *S. pneumoniae*. These agents also attain high concentrations in bronchial tissues (Table 1). Reawakened interest in the class as broad-spectrum respiratory antibiotics has resulted in an extensive clinical trial program, the results of which are summarized in Table 5.

Achieving pharmacodynamic thresholds for LRTIs may improve clinical outcomes, enhance bacterial eradication and prevent, or at least delay, emergence of bacterial resistance (140). These conclusions mostly derive from patients with pneumonia, but PD studies may also assist in optimizing choices and dosages of antibiotics for AECB. Thus, for grepafloxacin, dosage resulting in AUC/MIC_{24h} values >175 gave a probability of cure of 98% compared with 71% ($P = 0.01$) for $AUIC_{24h}$ values <75 (64). Comparative AUC/MIC studies with other quinolones have not been reported. However, overall clinical efficacy has clearly been established (Table 5), and it is difficult to see what advantages could be discerned when, in routine patients, all present studies suggest excellent clinical response. The true differences may only become apparent either by investigating severe exacerbations by nontraditional outcomes (23, 111) or, as trends to resistance become established, in AECBs caused by pathogens with raised quinolone MICs.

Treatment Duration and Response to Therapy

There has been a recent trend, perhaps market driven, to shorten the duration of antibiotic therapy of AECB. As shown in Table 5, most of the latter trials have investigated 5- to 7-day fluoroquinolone courses, and most have shown equivalence with comparator courses of 7- to 10-day duration. However, there has been little comparison of differing durations of treatment for specific individual agents. Where there has, the outcome may not support ever briefer periods of treatment. For example, *H. influenzae* eradication rates for 5-day grepafloxacin therapy were 68% compared with 79% for 10-day treatment (94). However, for moxifloxacin, 5- and 10-day courses were equivalent, giving 94 to 95% cure and eradication (32). There may be some differences between the quinolone class and other agents, such as macrolides, in rate of response to treatment. Patients in the United States receiving moxifloxacin felt better, experienced symptom relief, and returned to normal activities more quickly than a group receiving azithromycin (92). In Germany, a similar study involving comparison with roxithromycin, clarithromycin, and azithromycin showed advan-

Table 5. Results of oral quinolone therapy for acute exacerbations of chronic bronchitis

Fluoroquinolone and comparator	Dosage (mg)/frequency (h)/duration in days (d)	Clinical success (%)/ method of analysis	Bacterial eradication (%)/ rate for *H. influenzae* (%)	Reference
Levofloxacin vs.	500/24/7–10	108/137 (79)	82/107 (77), 83	132
Cefuroxime axetil	250/12/7–10	88/134 (66) Evaluables at EOS[a]	68/114 (60), 56	
Levofloxacin vs.	500/24/7		28/41 (68.5)	155
Cefuroxime axetil	250/12/7		20/42 (47.5) Combined clinical and bacterial success rate 1 wk after Rx	
Levofloxacin vs.	500/24/5–7	141/154 (92)	97/103 (94)	156
Cefaclor	250/12/7–10	142/155 (92) Not stated	77/89 (87)	
Sparfloxacin vs.	200/100/24 h	151/173 (87)	75/85 (88), 100	125
Amoxicillin-clavulanate	625/8/both for 7–14	158/178 (89) Evaluables at EOS	62/79 (78.5), 73	
Grepafloxacin vs.	400/24/5 or 400/24/10	113/156 (72) 127/157 (81)	64/99 (64), 68 66/98 (66), 79	127
Clarithromycin	250/12/10	117/160 (73) Evaluable at EOS	70/124 (56.5), 54	
Trovafloxacin vs.	200/24/5	87/113 (77)	71/76 (93.5), 90	157
Amoxicillin	500/8/5	86/109 (79) Evaluable at EOS	62/74 (84), 70	
Trovafloxacin vs.	200/24/5	103/113 (91)	49/49 (100), 97	158
Amoxicillin-Clavulanate	500/125/8/5	97/110 (88) Evaluable at EOS	52/60 (87), 78	

[a] EOS, end of study.
[b] Rx, treatment.

tages to moxifloxacin in terms of fever, chest pain, dyspnoea and painful cough, particularly in the early phase of treatment (101). This might support shorter courses of therapy in milder exacerbations.

Severe Exacerbations

The response in patients with risk factors for poor outcome is not frequently studied, but this is a prime area of interest for fluoroquinolones. High-dose (750 mg twice a day) ciprofloxacin failed to demonstrate significant differences with clarithromycin in complicated/severe exacerbations (9) and comparison of levofloxacin with cefuroxime axetil also showed no significant differences overall. Subset, risk factor-directed analysis resulted in higher (but not statistically superior) success rates for levofloxacin in patients with a peak flow rate of less than 300 liters/min, those in hospital, and those receiving either steroids or theophylline (142). Moxifloxacin was clinically equivalent to clarithromycin (89 versus 88%) in evaluable patients (159) but superior in bacterial eradication (77 versus 62%) and in infections due to *H. influenzae* (eradication 52.3%, presumed eradication 38.6 versus 9.3% and 44.2% respectively). A subanalysis of patients with risk factors found excess failure rates of

6% with moxifloxacin and 22% with clarithromycin in patients with coexistent cardiopulmonary disease, but the difference was not significant (159).

Prolongation of the Infection Free Interval

Studies of prolongation of the IFI have consistently shown fluoroquinolones to be superior to other agents (17, 35), but interclass comparisons are largely between studies and have included historical controls. More recently, Chodosh and colleagues (33, 34) compared ciprofloxacin with both cefuroxime axetil and clarithromycin, all administered for 14 days. Initial clinical response was identical (93 versus 90% and 90 versus 82%, respectively, in evaluable patients). Bacterial eradication with ciprofloxacin was better than with either cefuroxime axetil (96 versus 82%, $P < 0.01$) or clarithromycin (91 versus 77%, $P = 0.01$). However, in contrast to earlier findings with oral cephalosporins such as cefaclor (35), there was no difference in the IFI after cefuroxime (178 days) and ciprofloxacin (146 days; $P = 0.37$) or, despite the tantalizing disparity in figures, between clarithromycin (51 days) and ciprofloxacin (142 days; $P = 0.15$). A single study of temafloxacin versus ciprofloxacin showed IFIs of 235 and 209 days, respectively (35), but no studies have been reported on sparfloxacin, levofloxacin, or trovafloxacin.

Most recently the GLOBE study (20,158) of gemifloxacin and clarithromycin showed a trend to superior bacterial eradication by gemifloxacin (86.7 versus 73.1%) at end of treatment and a significant difference by week 4 to 5 (82 versus 62%: $P < 0.05$) with a related, significant difference in relapse rates over the ensuing period of 26 weeks (29% for gemifloxacin and 41.5% for clarithromycin: $P = 0.016$) (158). Hospitalization rates were 2.3% and 6.25% respectively ($P = 0.059$).

However, it may be more relevant in future studies to measure exacerbation-symptom-free intervals when comparing classes and agents. It is clear that quality of life assessments indicate return of clinical features and normal functions to base may take weeks to months after the index exacerbation. If this is influenced by choice of agent, then measurement of the interval between return to base line and the next AECB could be a more relevant comparator (23). Equally, longer-term follow-up (latest trials compare only 6-month periods) is required to assess the true effects of relapse reduction on overall costs, not only hospitalization rates. Further, the apparently relentless progress of disease might be dramatically altered by reduction in exacerbation frequency (7, 23, 146).

Costs of Therapy

Analytical models certainly indicate that fluoroquinolones are cost-effective in patients with more severe disease (154) and the CHEST study clearly demonstrated in patients with multiple risk factors that ciprofloxacin was beneficial in comparison with usual care both in terms of cost and quality of life assessments (74). A retrospective review (47) showed "third-line" agents, (ciprofloxacin, azithromycin, and amoxicillin-clavulanate) to be superior to "first-line" therapy (amoxicillin, cotrimoxazole, tetracyclines) in various respects:

- Failure rate: 7 versus 19% ($P < 0.05$)
- Hospitalization rate: 5.3 versus 18% ($P < 0.02$)
- Infection-free interval: 17 versus 34 weeks ($P < 0.005$)

Acquisition costs for the "improved" agents were significantly greater, but the overall cost of therapy for each AECB episode was US$942 for first-line therapy and US$542 for "improved" agents (47). The cost of clinical failure, linked to failure of bacterial eradication (17, 126), especially in respect of hospitalization (110), may be the most important aspect of treatment choice (155). Quinolones may be superior to other classes both in this respect and IFI

duration; this may well be a class attribute, for reasons as yet undefined. However, comparative data among the quinolones are largely lacking, and such studies as are presented are heavily criticized. For example, the Canadian comparison of admission rates for AECB over 1 year between Quebec (quinolones allowed and 24% reduction in admissions achieved) and Saskatchewan (quinolones proscribed and no difference observed) has never achieved publication in a peer-reviewed Journal. Similarly, a pharmacoeconomic study comparing moxifloxacin favorably with levofloxacin in terms of post-AECB workplace costs (99) might be difficult for formulary and guideline committees to interpret appropriately.

CONCLUSIONS

A decade ago, the reader of the first edition of this reference work might have concluded that the fluoroquinolones offered major advances in the management of many infections below the diaphragm but few above it. Molecular manipulation has now resulted in safe agents with markedly improved potency, notably, but not only, against the pneumococcus, which are appropriate for use in community-acquired lower respiratory infections (16). Perhaps, the next 10 years will see the third-generation agents secure a significant role in standard therapy of CAP and AECBs, as have their forebears, in gram-negative infections. It is to be hoped that nascent pneumococcal fluoroquinolone resistance can be stemmed prior to this event. The methods by which this might be achieved continue to be debated (16).

REFERENCES

1. Adams, S. G., J. Melo, M. Luther, and A. Anzueto. 2000. Antibiotics are associated with lower relapse rates in outpatients with acute exacerbations of COPD. *Chest* 117:1345–1352.
2. Allegra, L., C. Grassi, E. Grossi, E. Pozzi, F. Blasi, D. Frigerio, and A. Nastri. 1991. Ruolo degli antibiotici nel trattamento delle riacutizza della bronchite cronica. *Ital. J. Chest. Dis.* 45:38–48.
3. Allegra, L., N. Konietzko, P. Leophonte, J. Hosie, R. Pauwels, J. N. Guyen, and P. Petitpretz. 1996. Comparative safety and efficacy of sparfloxacin in the treatment of acute exacerbations of chronic obstructive pulmonary disease: a double-blind, randomised, parallel, multicentre study. *J. Antimicrob. Chemother.* 37(Suppl. A):93–104.
4. American Thoracic Society. 2001. Guidelines for the management of adults with community-acquired pneumonia: diagnosis, assessment of severity, antimicrobial therapy and prevention. *Am. J. Respir. Crit. Care Med.* 163:1730–1754.
5. Andrews, J. M., D. Honeybourne, G. Jevons, N. P. Brenwald, B. Cunningham, and R. Wise. 1997.

Concentrations of trovafloxacin in bronchial mucosa, epithelial lining fluid, alveolar macrophages and serum after administration of single or multiple oral doses in patients undergoing fibre-optic bronchoscopy. *J. Antimicrob. Chemother.* **39:**797–802.

6. **Andrews, J. M., D. Honeybourne, G. Jevons, N. P. Brenwald, B. Cunningham, and R. Wise.** 1997. Concentrations of levofloxacin (HR 355) in the respiratory tract following a single oral doses in patients undergoing fibre-optic bronchoscopy. *J. Antimicrob. Chemother.* **40:**573–577.

7. **Anie, K., K. Lowton, and P. W. Jones.** 1997. Changes in health status following an acute exacerbation of chronic bronchitis. *Eur. Respir. J.* **10**(Suppl. 25):148S.

8. **Anthonisen, N. R., J. Manfreda, C. P. W. Warren, E. S. Hershfield, G. K. M. Harding, and N. A. Nelson.** 1987. Antibiotic therapy in exacerbations of chronic obstructive pulmonary disease. *Ann. Intern. Med.* **106:**196–204.

9. **Anzueto, A., M. S. Niederman, and G. S. Tillotson.** 1998. Etiology, susceptibility and treatment of acute bacterial exacerbations of complicated chronic bronchitis in the primary care setting: ciprofloxacin 750 mg bid versus clarithromycin 500 mg bid. *Clin. Ther.* **27:**722–729.

10. **Anzueto, A., J. A. Rizzo, and R. F. Grossman.** 1999. The infection free interval: its use in evaluating antimicrobial treatment of acute exacerbations of chronic bronchitis. *Clin. Infect. Dis.* **28:**1344–1345.

11. **Armstrong, G. L., and R. W. Pinner.** 1999. Outpatient visits for infectious diseases in the United States, 1980 through 1996. *Arch. Intern. Med.* **159:**2531–2536.

12. **Arroll, B., and B. Kenealy.** 2001. Antibiotics for acute bronchitis. *Brit. Med. J.* **322:**939–940.

13. **Aubier, M., H. Lode, and G. Gialdroni-Grassi, J. Huchon, J. Hosie, N. Legakis, C. Reganey, S. Segev, R. Vester, W. J. Wijnands, and N. Tolstuchow.** 1996. Sparfloxacin for the treatment of community acquired pneumonia: a pooled data analysis of two studies. *J. Antimicrob. Chemother.* **37**(Suppl. A):73–82.

14. **Balgos, A. A., and the Consensus Group.** 1998. Guidelines for the role of antibiotics in acute exacerbations of chronic bronchitis in the Asia Pacific region: report and recommendations of a consensus group. *Med. Prog.* **25:**29–38.

15. **Ball, A. P., and G. S. Tillotson.** 1995. Lower respiratory tract infection therapy: the role of ciprofloxacin. *J. Int. Med. Res.* **23:**315–327.

16. **Ball, P., F. Baquero, O. Cars, and the Consensus Group on Resistance and Prescribing in Respiratory Tract Infection.** Antibiotic therapy of community respiratory tract infections: strategies for optimal outcomes and minimized resistance emergence. *J. Antimicrob. Chemother.,* in press.

17. **Ball, P., S. Chodosh, R. Grossman, G. Tillotson, and R. Wilson.** 2000. Causes, epidemiology and treatment of bronchial infections. *Infect. Med.* **17:**186–198.

18. **Ball, P., J. M. Harris, D. Lowson, G. Tillotson, and R. Wilson.** 1995. Acute infective exacerbations of chronic bronchitis. *Q. J. Med.* **88:**61–68.

19. **Ball, P., R. Wilson, L. Mandell, and the 069 Study Group.** 2001. Efficacy of gemifloxacin in acute exacerbations of chronic bronchitis: a randomised, double-blind comparison with trovafloxacin. *J. Chemother.* **13:**288–298.

20. **Ball, P., R. Wilson, L. Mandell, and the Globe Study group.** 2000. Gemifloxacin long term outcomes in bronchitis exacerbations (Globe) study—an assessment of health outcome benefits in AECB patients following 5 days gemifloxacin therapy, abstr. 812. *Program and Abstracts of the 40*th *Interscience Conference on Antimicrobial Agents and Chemotherapy.* American Society for Microbiology, Washington, D.C.

21. **Ball, P.** 2000. Acute exacerbations of chronic bronchitis. *Curr. Opin. Infect. Dis.* **13:**171–176.

22. **Ball, P.** 2000. Acute exacerbations of chronic bronchitis: in search of a definition, p. 24–35. *In* L. Allegra, F. Blasi (ed.), *Mechanisms and Management of COPD Exacerbations.* Springer-Verlag, Milan, Italy.

23. **Ball, P.** 2000. Future antibiotic trials. *Semin. Respir. Infect.* **15:**82–89.

24. **Ball, P.** 1990. Overview of experience with ofloxacin in respiratory tract infection. *Scan. J. Infect. Dis. Suppl.* **68:**56–63.

25. **Ball, P.** 1991. The role of temafloxacin in the community: an overview. *J. Antimicrob. Chemother.* **28**(Suppl. C):121–130.

26. **Banerjee, D., and D. Honeybourne.** 1999. The role of fluoroquinolones in chronic obstructive pulmonary disease. *Curr. Opin. Infect. Dis.* **12:**543–547.

27. **Bartlett, J. G., R. F. Breiman, L. A. Mandell, and T. M. File, Jr.** 1998. Community-acquired pneumonia in adults: guidelines for management. *Clin. Infect. Dis.* **26:**811–838.

28. **Bartlett, J. G., S. F. Dowell, L. A. Mandell, and T. M. File, Jr., D. M. Musher, and M. J. Fire.** 2000. Practice guidelines for the management of community-acquired pneumonia in adults. *Clin. Infect. Dis.* **31:**347–382.

29. **Buckingham, S. C., S. P. Brown, and V. H. Joaquin.** 1998. Break-through bacteremia and menigitis during treatment parenterally with cephalosporins for pneumococcal pneumonia. *J. Pediatr.* **132:**174–176.

30. **Carbon, C., H. Ariza, W. J. Rabie, C. R. Salvarezza, D. Elkharrat, M. Rangaraj, and P. Decosta.** 1999. Comparative study of levofloxacin and amoxycillin-clavulanic acid in adults with mild-to-moderate community-acquired pneumonia. *Clin. Microbiol. Infect.* **5:**724–732.

31. **Chen, D. K., A. McGreer, J. C. de Azavedo, D. E. Low, and the Canadian Bacterial Surveillance Network.** 1999. Decreased susceptibility of *Streptococcus pneumoniae* to fluoroquinolones in Canada. *N. Engl. J. Med.* **341:**233–239.

32. **Chodosh, S., C. A. DeAbate, D. Haverstock, and the Bronchitis Study Group.** 2000. Short course moxifloxacin therapy for treatment of acute bacterial exacerbations of chronic bronchitis. *Respir. Med.* **94:**18–27.

33. **Chodosh, S., A. Schreurs, G. Siami, and the Bronchitis Study Group.** 1998. Efficacy of oral ciprofloxacin vs. clarithromycin for treatment of acute bacterial exacerbations of chronic bronchitis. *Clin. Infect. Dis.* **27:**730–738.

34. **Chodosh, S., A. Schreurs, G. Siami, and the Bronchitis Study Group.** 1998. Randomised, double bind study of ciprofloxacin and cefuroxime axetil for treatment of acute bacterial exacerbations of chronic bronchitis. *Clin. Infect. Dis.* **27:**733–739.

35. **Chodosh, S.** 1991. Treatment of acute exacerbations of chronic bronchitis: state of the art. *Am. J. Med.* **91**(Suppl 6A):87S–92S.

36. **Christenson, B., P. Lundbergh, J. Hedlund, and A. Ortquist.** 2001. Effects of a large scale intervention with influenza and 23-valent pneumococcal vaccination in adults aged 65 years or older: a prospective study. *Lancet* **357:**1008–1011.

37. **Cook, P. J., J. M. Andrews, R. Wise, D. Honeybourne, H. Moudgil.** 1995. Concentrations of OPC-17116 (grepafloxacin), a new fluoroquinolone antibacterial in serum and lung compartments. *J. Antimicrob. Chemother.* **35:**317–326.

38. **Cooper RJ, Hoffman JR, Bartlett JG, R. E. Besser, R. Gonzales, J. M. Hickner, and M. A. Sande.** 2001. Principles of appropriate antibiotic use for acute pharyngitis in adults: background. *Ann. Intern. Med.* **134:**509–517.

39. Dajani, A., K. Taubert, P. Ferrieri, G. Peter, and S. Shulman. 1995. Treatment of acute streptococcal pharyngitis and prevention of rheumatic fever: a statement for health professionals. *Pediatrics* **96**:758–764.

40. Davidson, R., R. Cavalcanti, J. L. Brunton, D. J. Bast, J. C. S. de Azavedo, P. Kibsey, C. Fleming, and D. E. Low. 2001. Levofloxacin treatment failures of pneumococcal pneumonia in association with resistance. *N. Engl. J. Med.*, in press.

41. Davies, B. I., and F. P. V. Maesen. 1999. Clinical effectiveness of levofloxacin in patients with acute purulent exacerbations of chronic bronchitis: the relationship with in vitro activity. *J. Antimicrob. Chemother.* **43**(Suppl. C):83–90.

42. DeAbate, C. A., C. P. Mathew, J. H. Warner, A. Heyd, D. Church. 2000. The safety and efficacy of short course (5-day) mocifloxacin vs. azithromycin in the treatment of patients with acute exacerbations of chronic bronchitis. *Respir. Med.* **94**:1029–1037.

43. DeAbate, C. A., R. A. McIvor, P. McElvaine, K. Skuba, and P. F. Pierce. Gatifloxacin vs. cefuroxime axetil in patients with acute exacerbations of chronic bronchitis. 1999. *J. Respir. Dis.* **20**(Suppl. 11):S23–S29.

44. Dedicoat, M., and P. Venkatesan. 1999. The treatment of Legionnaire's disease. *J. Antimicrob. Chemother.* **43**:747–752.

45. Denny, F. W. Effect of treatment on streptococcal pharyngitis: is the issue really settled? 1985. *Pediatr. Infect. Dis.* **4**:352–354.

46. Despande, L. M., and R. N. Jones. 2000. Antimicrobial activity of advanced-spectrum fluoroquinolones tested against more than 2000 contemporary bacterial isolates of species causing community-acquired respiratory tract infections in the United States (1999). *Diagn. Microbiol. Infect. Dis.* **37**:139–142.

47. Destache, C. J., N. Dewan, W. J. O'Donohue, J. C. Campbell, and Angelillo. 1999. Clinical and economic considerations in the treatment of acute exacerbations of chronic bronchitis. *J. Antimicrob. Chemother.* **43**(Suppl. A):107–113.

48. Dowell, S. F., T. Smith, K. Leversedge, and J. Snitzer. 1999. Pneumonia treatment failure associated with highly resistant pneumococci. *Clin. Infect. Dis.* **29**:462–463.

49. Dresser, L. D., M. S. Niederman, and J. A. Paladino. 2001. Cost-effectiveness of gatifloxacin vs ceftriaxone with a macrolide for the treatment of community-acquired pneumonia. *Chest.* **119**:1439–1448.

50. Eller, J., A. Ede, T. Schaberg, M. S. Niederman, H. Mauch, and H. Lode. 1998. Infective exacerbations of chronic bronchitis: relation between bacteriologic etiology and lung function. *Chest.* **113**:1542–1548.

51. Esposito, S., G. D'errico, C. Montanaro. 1990. Oral ciprofloxacin for treatment of acute bacterial pharyngotonsillitis. *J. Chemother.* **2**:108–112.

52. European Respiratory Society. 1998. Guidelines for management of adult community-acquired lower respiratory tract infections. ERS Task Force Report. *Eur. Respir. J.* **11**:986–991.

53. Fahey, T., N. Stocks, and T. Thomas. 1998. Quantitative systematic review of randomised controlled trials comparing antibiotic with placebo for acute cough in adults. *Brit. Med. J.* **316**:906–910.

54. Fang, G. D., M. Fine, J. Orloff, D. Arisumi, V. L. Yu, W. Kapoor, J. T. Grayston, S. P. Wang, R. Kohler, R. R. Muder, et al. 1990. New and emerging etiologies for community-acquired pneumonia with implications for therapy: a prospective multicenter study of 359 cases. *Medicine* **69**:307–316.

55. Feikin, D., A. Schuchat, M. Kolczak, N. L. Barrett, L. H. Harrison, L. Lefkowitz, A. McGeer, M. M. Farley, D. J. Vugian, C. Lexau, K. R. Stefonek, J. E. Patterson, and J. H. Jorgensen. 2000. Mortality from invasive pneumococcal pneumonia in the era of antibiotic resistance, 1995–1997. *Am. J. Public Health* **90**:223–229.

56. File, T. M., B. Schlemmer, J. Garau, M. Cupo, C. Young, and the 049 Clinical Study Group. 2001. Efficacy and safety of gemifloxacin in the treatment of community-acquired pneumonia: a randomized, double-blind comparison with trovafloxacin. *J. Antimicrob. Chemother.* **48**:67–74.

57. File, T. M., J. Segreti, L. Dunbar, R. Player, R. Kohler, R. R. Williams, C. Kojak, and A. Rubin. 1997. A multicenter, randomised study comparing the efficacy and safety of intravenous and/or oral levofloxacin versus ceftriaxone and/or cefuroxime axetil in treatment of adults with community-acquired pneumonia. *Antimicrob. Agents Chemother.* **41**:1967–1972.

58. File, T.M. 1999. Acute bronchitis: indication for antibiotic avoidance. *Curr. Opin. Infect. Dis.* **12**:111–113.

59. Fine, M. J., T. E. Auble, D. M. Yealy, B. H. Hanusa, L. A. Weissfeld, D. E. Singer, C. M. Coley, T. J. Morrie, and W. N. Kapoor. 1997. A prediction rule to identify low-risk patients with community-acquired pneumonia. *N. Engl. J. Med.* **336**:243–250.

60. Fine, M. J., M. A. Smith, C. A. Carson, S. S. Muthan, S. S. Sankey, L. A. Weissfeld, and W. N. Kapoor. 1996. Prognosis and outcomes of patients with community-acquired pneumonia. *JAMA* **275**:134–141.

61. Fink, M. P., D. R. Snydman, M. S. Niederman, K. V. Leeper, Jr., R. H. Johnson, S. O. Heard, R. G. Wunderink, J. W. Caldwell, J. J. Schentag, G. A. Siami, et al. 1994. Treatment of severe pneumonia in hospitalised patients: results of a multicenter, randomised, double blind trial comparing intravenous ciprofloxacin with imipenem-cilastatin. *Antimcrob. Agents Chemother.* **38**:547–557.

62. Fogarty, C., M. E. Dowell, W. T. Ellison, et al. 1999.Treating community-acquired pneumonia in hospitalized patients: gatifloxacin vs ceftriaxone/clarithromycin. *J. Respir. Dis.* **20**(Suppl):S60–S69.

63. Fogarty, C., C. Grossman, J. Williams, and the Community-acquired Pneumonia Study Group. 1999. Efficacy and safety of moxifloxacin vs clarithromycin for community-acquired pneumonia. *Infect. Med.* **16**:748–763.

64. Forrest, A., S. Chodosh, M. A. Amantea, D. A. Coillins, J. J. Schentag. 1997. Pharmacokinetics and pharmacodynamics of oral grepafloxacin in patients with acute bacterial exacerbations of chronic bronchitis. *J. Antimicrob. Chemother.* **40**(Suppl. A):45–57.

65. Forrest, A., D. E. Nix, C. H. Ballow, T. F. Goss, M. C. Birmingham, J. J. Schentag. 1993. Pharmacodynamics of intravenous ciprofloxacin in seriously ill patients. *Antimicrob. Agents Chemother.* **37**:1073–1081.

66. Gallagher. 1999. Abstr. 2246. *Intersci. Conf. Antimicrob. Agents Chemother.* American Society for Microbiology, Washington, D. C.

67. Garau, J., J. R. Lonks, L. Gomez, M. Xercavins, and A. A. Medeiros. 2000. Failure of macrolide therapy in patients with bacteremia due to macrolide resistant streptococcus pneumoniae, abstr. N709. *In 5th International Conference on Macrolides, Azalides and Streptogramins.*

68. Garau, J. 2001. Data presented at the 5th International Moxifloxacin Symposium.

69. Garau, J. 2001. Data presented at the 5th International Moxifloxacin Symposium.

70. Garau, J. 2001. Clinical failures: the tip of the iceberg? *Respir. Med.*, **95**(Suppl. A):S3–S11.

71. Geddes, A. M., M. Thaler, S. Schonwald, M. Harkonen, F. Jacobs, and I. Nowotny. 1999. Levofloxacin in the empirical treatment of patients with suspected bacteraemia/sepsis: comparison with imipenem/cilastatin in an open randomised trial. *J. Antimicrob. Chemother.* **44:**799–810.

72. Gonzalez, R., J. F. Steiner, and M. A. Sande. 1997. Antibiotic prescribing for adults with colds, upper respiratory tract infection and bronchitis by ambulatory care physicians. *JAMA* **278:**901–904.

73. Graham, E., E. Whalen, M. E. Smith, et al. 1994. Comparison of costs between ciprofloxacin and imipenem for the treatment of severe pneumonia in hospitalised patients. *Pharmacotherapy* **14:**370–371.

74. Grossman, R., J. Mukherjee, D. Vaughan, and the Canadian Ciprofloxacin Health Economic Study Group. 1998. A 1 year community-based health economic study of ciprofloxacin vs. usual antibiotic treatment in acute exacerbations of chronic bronchitis. *Chest* **113:**131–141.

75. Grossman, R. 1997. The role of fluoroquinolones in respiratory tract infections. *J. Antimicrob. Chemother.* **40**(Suppl. A):59–62.

76. Guay, D. R. 1993. Sequential antimicrobial therapy: a realistic approach to cost containment? *Pharmacoeconomics* **3:**341–344.

77. Habib, M. P., L. O. Gentry, G. Rodriguez-Gomez, et al. 1998. Multicenter randomised study comparing efficacy and safety of oral levofloxacin and cefaclor in treatment of acute bacterial exacerbations of chronic bronchitis. *Infect. Dis. Clin. Pract.* **7:**101–109.

78. Halpern, M. T., C. S. Palmer, M. Zodet, J. M. Kirsch, and the Globe Study Group. 2001. Cost effectiveness of gemifloxacin versus clarithromycin in the treatment of AECB: the Globe study. *J. Antimicrob. Chemother.* **47**(Suppl. S1):43.

79. Hamm, R. M., R. J. Hicks and D. A. Bemben. 1996. Antibiotics and respiratory infections: are patients more satisfied when expectations are met? *J. Fam. Pract.* **43:**56–62.

80. Heffelfinger, J. D., S. F. Dowell, J. H. Jorgensen, K. P. Klugman, L. R. Mabry, D. M. Musher, J. F. Plouffe A. Rakowsky, A. Schuchat, and C. G. Whitney. 2000. Management of community-acquired pneumonia in the era of pneumococcal resistance: A report from the Drug-Resistant *Streptococcus pneumoniae* Therapeutic Working Group. *Arch. Intern. Med.* **160:**1399–1408.

81. Highet, V. S., A. Forrest, C. H. Ballow, J. J. Scentag. 1999. Antibiotic dosing issues in lower respiratory tract infection: population-derived area under inhibitory curve is predictive of efficacy. *J. Antimicrob. Chemother.* **43**(Suppl. A):55–63.

82. Ho, P. L., R. W. H. Yung, D. N. C. Tsang, T. L. Que, M. Ho, W. H. Seto, T. K. Ng, W. C. Yam, and W. W. Ng. 2001. Increasing resistance of Streptococcus pneumonia to fluoroquinolones: results of a Hong Kong multi-centre study in 2000. *J. Antimicrob. Chemother.* **48:**659–665.

83. Ho, P. L., T. L. Que, D. N. Tsang, T. K. Ng, K. H. Chow, and W. H. Seto. 1999. Emergence of fluoroquinolone resistance among multiply resistant strains of *Streptococcus pneumoniae* in Hong Kong. *Antimicrobial. Agents and Chemother.* **43:**1310–1313.

84. Ho, P. L., W. S. Tse, K. W. T. Tsang, T. K., Kwok, T. K. Ng, V. C. Cheng, and R. M. Chan. 2000. Risk factors for acquisition of levofloxacin-resistant *Streptococcus pneumoniae:* a case control study. *Clin. Infect. Dis.* **32:**701–707.

85. Honeybourne, D., D. Banerjee, J. Andrews, and R. Wise. 2001. Concentrations of gatifloxacin in plasma and pulmonary compartments following a single 400 mg oral dose in patients undergoing fibre-optic bronchoscopy. *J. Antimicrob. Chemother.* **48:**63–66.

86. Hyatt, J. M., A. B. Luzier, A. Forrest, C. W. Ballow, and J. J. Schentag. 1997. Modeling the response of pneumonia to antimicrobial therapy. *Antimicrob. Agents Chemother.* **41:**1269–1274.

87. Janoir, C., V. Zeller, M. D. Kitzis, N. J. Moreua, and L. Gutmann. 1996. High level fluoroquinolone resistance in *Streptococcus pneumoniea* requires mutations in par C and gyr A. *Antimicrob. Agents Chemother.* **40:**2760–2764.

88. Jardim ,J. R. for Consenso Latinamerico. 1997. Consenso Latinamerico sobre infecciones en bronquitis cronica. *Rev. Panam. Infectol.* **1:**1–19.

89. Jones, P., S. Spencer, and the Globe Study Group. 2001. Greater improvement in health status of smokers and ex-smokers treated for AECB with gemifloxacin versus clarithromycin: the Globe Study. *J. Antimicrob. Chemother.* **47**(Suppl. S1):43.

90. Kelley, M. A., D. J. Weber, P. Gilligan, M. S. Cohen. 2000. Break-through pneumococcal bacteremia in patients being treated with azithromycin and clarithromycin. *Clin. Infect. Dis.* **31:**1008–1011.

91. Komaroff, A. L., T. M. Pass, M. D. Aronson, C. T. Ervin, S. Cinetin, R. N. Winickoff, and W. T. Branch, Jr. 1986. The prediction of streptococcal pharyngitis in adults. *J. Gen. Intern. Med.* **1:**1–7.

92. Kreis, S. R., N. Herrera, N. Golzar, and the Therapeutic Circles Bronchitis Study Group. 2000. A comparison of moxifloxacin and azithromycin in the treatment of acute exacerbations of chronic bronchitis. *J. Clin. Outcomes Manage.* **7:**33–37.

93. Lacy, M. K., W. Lu, X. Xu, P. R. Tessier, D. P. Nicolau, R. Quintiliani, and C. H. Nightingale. 1999. Pharmacodynamic comparisons of levofloxacin, ciprofloxacin, and ampicillin against *Streptococcus pneumoniae* in an in vitro model of infection. *Antimicrob. Agents Chemother.* **43:**672–777.

94. Langan, C. E., P. Zuck, F. Vogel, A. McIvor, W. Peirzchala, M. Smakal, H. Staley and C. Marr. 1999. Randomised, double blind study of short course (5 day) grepafloxacin versus 10d clarithromycin in patients with acute bacterial exacerbations of chronic bronchitis. *J. Antimicrob. Chemother.* **44:**515–523.

95. Lee, B. L., A. M. Padula, R. C. Kimbrough, S. R. Jones, R. E. Chaisson, J. Mills, M. A. Sande. 1997. Infectious complications with respiratory pathogens despite ciprofloxacin. *N. Engl. J. Med.* **325:**520–521.

96. Leophonte, P., R. J. T. Baldwin, and N. Pluck. 1998. Trovafloxacin versus amoxicillin-clavulanic acid in the treatment of acute exacerbations of chronic bronchitis. *Eur. J. Clin. Microbiol. Infect. Dis.* **17:**434–440.

97. Leophonte, P., B. Schlemmer, F. Goldstein, J. Garau, E. Rouffiac, and The Gemifloxacin 011 Study Group. Efficacy and safety of once daily gemifloxacin (GEMI) for the treatment of community-acquired pneumonia (CAP) of suspected pneumococcal origin. French Meeting.

98. Leroy, O., C. Santre, and C. Beuscart. 1995. A 5-year study of severe community-acquired pneumonia with emphasis on prognosis in patients admitted to an ICU. *Intensive Care. Med.* **21:**24–31.

99. Li-McLeod, J., and E. M. Perfetto. 2001. Workplace costs associated with acute exacerbation of chronic bronchitis: a comparison of moxifloxacin and levofloxacin. *Managed Care Interface* **February:** 505.

100. Lode, H., T. File, L. Mandell, P. Ball, R. Pypstra, and The 185 Gemifloxacin Study Group. 2001. Comparative efficacy of oral gemifloxacin (GEM) and intravenous ceftriaxone (CTX) followed by oral cefuroxime (CFU) (± macrolide) in the treatment of community-acquired pneumonia (CAP). American College of Chest Physicians.

101. Lorenz, J., I. M. Thate-Waschke, O. Mast, R. Kubin, R. Rychlik, T. Pfeil, D. Daniel, and G. S. Tillotson. 2001. Treatment outcomes in acute exacerbations of chronic bronchitis: comparison of macrolides and moxifloxacin from the patients perspective. *J. Int. Med. Res.* **29:**74–86.

102. Macfarlane, J., T. Boswell, G. Douglas, et al. 2001. The British Thoracic Society Guidelines for the Management of Community-acquired Pneumonia in Adults. *Thorax* **56.**

103. Macfarlane, J., W. Holmes, R. Macfarlane, and N. Britten. 1997. Influence of patients expectations on antibiotic management of acute lower respiratory tract illness in general practice: questionnaire study. *Br. Med. J.* **315:**1211–1214.

104. Mandell, L. A., T. H. Marrie, R. F. Grossman, A. W. Chow, and R. H. Hyland, and the Canadian Community-Acquired Pneumonia Working Group. 2000. Canadian guidelines for the initial management of community-acquired pneumonia: an evidence-based update by the Canadian Infectious Disease Society and the Canadian Thoracic Society. *Clin. Infect. Dis.* **31:**383–421.

105. Mandell, L. A., M. S. Niederman. 1993. The Canadian Community-acquired Pneumonia Consensus Conference Group, Antimicrobial treatment of community-acquired pneumonia in adults: a conference report. *Can. J. Infect. Dis.* **4:**25–28.

106. Marras, T. K., L. Lee-Pack, L. Jamieson, and C. K. Chan. 2001. Effect of new guidelines and a respiratory quinolone on clinical outcomes in hospitalised patients with community-acquired pneumonia. *J. Antimicrob. Chemother.* **47**(Suppl. S1):44–45.

107. Marrie, T. J., C. Y. Lau, S. Wheeler, C. J. Wong, M. K. Vandervoort, B. G. Feagan, and the Capital Study Investigators. 2000. A controlled trial of a critical pathway for treatment of community acquired pneumonia. *JAMA* **283:**749–755.

108. Marrie, T. J. 1994. Community-acquired pneumonia. *Clin. Infect. Dis.* **18:**501–515.

109. Marston, B. J., J. F. Plouffe, T. M. File, Jr., B. A. Hackman, S. J. Salstrom, H. B. Lipman, M. S. Kolczak, and R. F. Breiman. 1997. Incidence of community-acquired pneumonia requiring hospitalization. *Arch. Intern. Med.* **277:**1214–1218.

110. McGuire, A. 1998. Burden and cost of LRTI: a methodologic overview. *Infect. Med.* **15**(Suppl. E):26–33.

111. Miravitles, M. 2000. Designing future clinical trials for exacerbations of chronic bronchitis, pp 88–89. *In* L. Allegra, and F. Blasi (ed.), Mechanisms and Management of COPD Exacerbations. Springer-Verlag, Milan, Italy.

112. Moine, P., J.-B. Vercken, S. Chevret, C. Chastang, and P. Gajdos. 1994. Severe community-acquired pneumonia: Etiology, epidemiology and prognostic factors. *Chest* **105:**1487–1495.

113. National Centre for Health Statistics. 1998. National Hospital Discharge Survey: Annual Summary 1996. *Vital Health Stat.* **13:**1–225.

114. Niederman, M., D. Church, J. Kaufmann, and M. Springsklee. 2000. Does appropriate antibiotic treatment influence outcome in community acquired pneumonia? *Respir. Med.* **94**(Suppl. A):A14.

115. Niederman, M., S. Traub, W. T. Ellison, and D. J. Williams. Comparison of IV alatrofloxacin/oral trovafloxacin with IV ceftriaxone/oral cefpodoxime in hoispitalised patients with community acquired pneumonia. *Am. J. Resp. Crit. Care Med.*, in press.

116. Niederman, M. S., J. B. Bass, Jr., G. D. Campbell, A. M. Fein, R. F. Grossman, L. A. Mandell, T. J. Marrie, G. A. Sarosi, A. Torres, and V. L. Yu. 1993. American Thoracic Society Guidelines for the initial management of adults with community-acquired pneumonia: diagnosis, assessment of severity, and initial antimicrobial therapy. American Thoracic Society. Medical Section of the American Lung Association. *Am. Rev. Respir. Dis.* **148:**1418–1426.

117. Niederman, M. S. 2000. Infection and antibiotic treatment in acute exacerbations of chronic bronchitis, p. 73–87. *In* L. Allegra and F. Blasi, (ed.) *Mechanisms and Management of COPD Exacerbations.* Springer-Verlag, Milan, Italy.

118. Norrby, S. R., W. Petermann, P. A. Willcox, N. Vetter, and E. Salewski. 1998. A comparative study of levofloxacin and ceftriaxone in the treatment of hospitalised patients with pneumonia. *Scand. J. Infect. Dis.* **30:**397–404.

119. O'Doherty, B., and R. Daniel. 1998. Treatment of acute exacerbations of chronic bronchitis: comparison of trovafloxacin and amoxicillin in a multicentre, double blind, double dummy study. *Eur. J. Clin. Microbiol. Infect. Dis.* **17:**441–446.

120. O'Doherty, B., D. A. Dutchman, R. Pettit, et al. 1997. Randomized, double-blind, comparative study of grepafloxacin and amoxycillin in the treatment of patients with community-acquired pneumonia. *J. Antimicrob. Chemother.* **40**(Suppl. A):73–81.

121. Orr, P. H., K. Scherer, A. MacDonald, and M. E. K. Moffat. 1993. Randomised placebo-controlled trials of antibiotics for acute bronchitis: a critical review of the literature. *J. Fam. Pract.* **36:**507–512.

122. Ortqvist, A., M. Valtonen, and O. Cars, et al. 1996. Oral empiric treatment of community-acquired pneumonia: a multicentre, double-blind, randomized study comparing sparfloxacin with roxithromycin. *Chest* **110:**1499–1506.

123. Pachon, J., M. D. Prados, F. Capote, J. A. Cuello, J. Garnacho, and A. Verano. 1990. A. Severe community-acquired pneumonia: Etiology, prognosis and treatment. *Am. Rev. Respir. Dis.* **142:**369–373.

124. Paladino, J. A., H. E. Sperry, J. M. Backes, J. A. Gelber, D. J. Serrianne, T. J Cumbo, and J. J. Schentag. 1991. Clinical and economic evaluation of oral ciprofloxacin after an abbreviated course of intravenous antibiotics. *Am. J. Med.* **91:**462–470.

125. Paladino, J. A. 1995. Pharmacoeconomic comparison of sequential IV/oral ciprofloxacin versus ceftazidime in the treatment of nosocomial pneumonia. *Can. J. Hosp. Pharm.* **48:**276–283.

126. Pechere, J. C. 1998. Modeling and predicting clinical outcomes of antibiotic therapy. *Infect. Med.* **15**(Suppl. E):46–54.

127. Petipretz, P., P. Arvis, M. Mavel, J. Moita, J. Ureueta, and CAP₅ Moxifloxacin Study Group. 2001. Oral moxifloxacin vs high-dosage amoxicillin in the treatment of mild to moderate community-acquired, suspected pneumococcal pneumonia in adults. *Chest* **119:**185–195.

128. Pihlajamaki, M., P. Kotilainen, T. Kaurila, T. Klaukka, E. Palva, and P. Huovinen. 2001. Macrolide resistant Streptococcus pneumoniae and use of antimicrobial agents. *Clin. Infect. Dis.* **33:**483–488.

129. Portier, H., T. May, A. Proust, and the French Study Group. 1996. Comparative efficacy of sparfloxacin in comparison with amoxycillin plus ofloxacin in the treatment of community acquired pneumonia. *J. Antimicrob. Chemother.* **37**(Suppl. A):83–91.

130. Poses, R. M., R. D. Cebul, M. Collins, and S. S. Fager. 1985. The accuracy of experienced physician's probability estimates for patients with sore throats: implications for decision making. *JAMA* **254:**925–929.

131. Preston, S. L., G. L. Drusano, A. L. Berman, et al. 1998. Levofloxacin population pharmacokinetics and creation of a

demographic model for prediction of individual drug clearance in patients with serious community-acquired infection. *Antimicrob. Agents Chemother.* **42**:1098–1104.

132. Preston, S. L., G. L. Drusano, A. L. Berman, C. L. Fowler, A. J. Chow, B. Dornseif, V. Reichl, J. Natarajan, F. A. Wong, and M. Corrado. 1998. Pharmacodynamics of levofloxacin: a new paradigm for early clinical trials. *JAMA* **279**:125–129.

133. Quintilliani, R., and C. Nightingale. 1994. Transitional antibiotic therapy. *Infect. Dis. Clin. Pract.* **3**(Suppl. 3):S161–S167.

134. Ramirez, A., J. Molina, A. Dolmann, et al. 1999. Gatifloxacin treatment in patients with acute exacerbations of chronic bronchitis: clinical trial results. *J. Respir. Dis.* **20**(Suppl. 11):S30–S9.

135. Ramirez, J. A., T.-H. Nguyen, G. Tellier, et al. 1999. Treating community-acquired pneumonia with once daily gatifloxacin vs twice daily clarithromycin. *J. Respir. Dis.* **20**(Suppl.):S40–48.

136. Romanowski, B., J. S. Hardy, M. S. Rafter, J. Draker. Enoxacin in the therapy of anal and pharyngeal gonococcal infections. *Sex. Transm. Dis.* Vol. 16, No. **4**:190–191.

137. Saint, S., S. Bent, E. Vittinghof, D. Grady. 1995. Antibiotics in chronic obstructive pulmonary disease exacerbations: a meta-analysis. *JAMA* **273**:957–960.

138. Santos, J., B. Siquier, J. Duran, J. Custardoy, A. Gil-Aguado, C. Garcia-Rey, L. Aguilar and The 049 CAP Collaborative Study Group. 2001. Usefulness of new quinolones in the treatment of *Legionella* pneumonia: a report of 28 cases. *Progr. Abstr. 41st Intersci. Conf. Antimicrob. Agents Chemother.* American Society for Microbiology, Washington, D.C.

139. Schentag, J. J., D. E. Nix and M. H. Adelman. 1991. Mathematical examination of dual individualization principles (I): relationships between AUC above MIC and area under the inhibitory curve for cefmenoxime, ciprofloxacin, and tobramycin. *DICP Ann. Pharmacother.* **25**:1050–1057.

140. Schentag, J. J. 2000. Clinical pharmacology of the fluoroquinolones: studies in human dynamic/kinetic models. *Clin. Infect. Dis.* **31**(Suppl. 2):S40–S44.

141. Sethi, S. 1999. Infectious exacerbations of chronic bronchitis: diagnosis and management. *J. Antimicrob. Chemother.* **43**(Suppl. A):97–105.

142. Shah, P. M., F. P. V. Maesen, A. Dolmann, N. Vetter, E. Fiss, and R. Wesch. 1999. Levofloxacin versus cefuroxime axetil in the treatment of acute exacerbation of chronic bronchitis: results of a randomised, double-blind study. *J. Antimicrob. Chemother.* **43**:529–539.

143. Smucny, J., T. Fahey, L. Becker, R. Glazier, and W. McIsaac. Antibiotics for acute bronchitis (Cochrane Review). *In Cochrane Collaboration.* Cochrane Database System Revision 2000. 4:CD000245.

144. Snellman, L. W., H. J. Stang, J. M. Stang, D. R. Johnson, and E. L. Kaplan. 1993. Duration of positive throat cultures for group A streptococci after initiation of antibiotic therapy. *Pediatrics* **91**:1166–1170.

145. Soman, A., D. Honeybourne, J. Andrews, G. Jevons, and R. Wise. 1999. Concentrations of moxifloxacin in serum and pulmonary compartments following a single 400 mg dose in patients undergoing fibre-optic bronchoscopy. *J. Antimicrob. Chemother.* **44**:835–838.

146. Spencer, S., K. Anie, and P. W. Jones. 1999. Annual rate of health status decline in COPD patients is significantly related to frequency of acute exacerbations. *Eur. Respir. J.* **14**(Suppl. 30):19S.

147. Sullivan, J., J. Gezon, J. Herrod, et al. A randomized double blind trial of trovafloxaxcin versus clarithromycin in community acquired pneumonia.

148. Sullivan, J. G., A. D. McElroy, R. W. Honsinger, et al. 1999. Treating community-acquired pneumonia with once-daily gatifloxacin vs once-daily levofloxacin. *J. Respir. Dis.* **20**.

149. Thiadens, H. A., G. H. de Bock, F. W. Dekker, J. A. Huysman, J. C. van Houwelingen, M. P. Springer, and D. S. Postma. 1998. Identifying asthma and chronic obstructive pulmonary disease in patients with persistent cough presenting to general practitioners: descriptive study. *Br. Med. J.* **316**:1286–1290.

150. Thomas, J. K., A. Forrest, S. M. Bhavnani, J. M. Hyatt, A. Cheng, C. H. Ballow, and J. J. Schentag. 1998. Pharmacodynamic evaluation of factors associated with the development of bacterial resistance in acutely ill patients during therapy. *Antimicrob. Agents Chemother.* **42**:521–527.

151. Tremolieres, F., F. de Kock, N. Pluck, and R. Daniel. 1998. Trovafloxacin versus high dose amoxicillin (1g three times daily) in the treatment of community-acquired bacterial pneumonia. *Eur. J. Clin. Microbiol. Infect. Dis.* **17**:447–453.

152. 1997. Trovafloxacin Abstract Reduced Mortality. *Intersci. Conf. Antimicrob. Agents Chemother.* American Society for Microbiology, Washington, D.C.

153. Turret, G. L., S. Blum, B. A. Fazal, J. E. Justman, E. E. Telzak. 1999. Penicillin resistance and other predictors of mortality in pneumococcal bacteremia in a population with high HIV seroprevalence. *Clin. Infect. Dis.* **29**:321–327.

154. Van Barlingen, H. J. J., M. J. C. Nuijten, T. Volmer et al. 1998. Model to evaluate the cost-effectiveness of different antibiotics in the management of acute bacterial exacerbations of chronic bronchitis in Germany. *J. Med. Econ.* **1**:210–218.

155. Vogel, F. 1998. Cost benefits from improving clinical outcome. *Infect. Med.* **15**(Suppl. E):61–67.

156. Weiss, K., C. Restieri, R. Gauthier, M. Laverdière, A. McGeer, R. J. Davidson, L. Kilburn, D. J. Bast, J. de Azavedo, and D. E. Low. 2001. A nosocomial outbreak of fluoroquinolone-resistant *Streptococcus pneumoniae.* *Clin. Infect. Dis.* **33**, 517–522.

157. Weiss, M. C., R. Fitzpatrick, D. K. Scott, and M. J. Goldacre. 1996. Pressures on the general practitioner and decisions to prescribe. *Fam. Pract.* **13**:432–438.

158. Wilson, R., P. Ball, and L. Mandell, and the Globe Study Group. 2000. Efficacy of once daily gemifloxacin (GEMI) for 5 days compared with twice daily clarithromycin (CLARI) for 7 days in the treatment of AECB, abstr. 815. *Prog. Abstr. 40th Intersci. Conf. Antimicrob. Agents Chemother.* American Society for Microbiology, Washington, D.C.

159. Wilson, R., R. Kubin, I. Ballin, K. M. Deppermann, H. P. Bassaris, P. Leophonte, A. J. Schreurs, A. Torres, and B. Sommerauer. 1999. Five day moxifloxacin therapy compared with 7 day clarithromycin therapy for the treatment of acute exacerbations of chronic bronchitis. *J. Antimicrob. Chemother.* **44**:501–513.

160. Wise, R., and D. Honeybourne. 1996. A review of the penetration of sparfloxacin into the lower respiratory tract and sinuses. *J. Antimicrob. Chemother.* **37**(Suppl. A):57–63.

161. Wise, R. 1999. A review of the clinical pharmacology of moxifloxacin, a new 8-methoxyquinolone, and its potential relation to therapeutic efficacy. *Clin. Drug. Invest.* **17**:365–387.

162. Woodhead, M. A., J. Arrowsmith, R. Chamberlain-Webber, et al. 1991. The value of routine microbial investigation in community-acquired pneumonia. *Respir. Med.* **85**:313–317.

163. Wortmann, G. W., and S. P. Bennett. 1999. Fatal meningitis due to levofloxacin-resistant *Streptococcus pneumoniae.* *Clin. Infect. Dis.* **29**:1599–1600.

164. Wright, D. H., G. H. Brown, M. L. Peterson, and J. C. Rotschafer. 2000. Application of fluoroquinolone pharmacodynamics. *J. Antimicrob. Chemother.* **46**:669–684.

Quinolone Antimicrobial Agents, 3rd ed.
Edited by David C. Hooper and Ethan Rubinstein
© 2003 ASM Press, Washington, D.C.

Chapter 14

Treatment of Infections of the Ears, Nose, and Throat and Nasal Carriage

JENNIFER RUBIN GRANDIS AND VICTOR L. YU

The availability of quinolones represents an important therapeutic option for certain otolaryngologic infectious conditions. The advantages of quinolones include the oral or topical routes of administration, the low toxicity profile, and the excellent penetration into nasal secretions, saliva, and bone (4). Despite the widespread use of quinolones to treat infections of the ears, nose, and throat, well-controlled studies are uncommon.

MALIGNANT (NECROTIZING) EXTERNAL OTITIS

Malignant (necrotizing) external otitis is an invasive infection of the external auditory canal and skull base, whose typical host is the elderly patient with diabetes mellitus. *Pseudomonas aeruginosa* is nearly always the causative organism (>98% of cases) (60), although widespread use of quinolones may make its isolation difficult. Since both aging and diabetes mellitus are associated with abnormalities of small blood vessels, we and others have hypothesized that microangiopathy in the ear canal may predispose elderly diabetics to malignant external otitis (7, 60). However, no direct relationship has been delineated between the degree of glucose intolerance and disease susceptibility (60). Several studies have reported an increased pH in diabetic cerumen, which may contribute to the development of malignant external otitis (3).

Fewer than 20 pediatric cases have been reported in the literature, making this a rare disease in children. In contrast to the clinical picture in adults, children are more apt to be immunocompromised on the basis of malignancy and malnutrition. Although no deaths have been reported, children tend to be more toxic with their illness, as illustrated by reports of fever, leukocytosis, and *P. aeruginosa* bacteremia (62). Increasing reports of malignant external otitis

in patients with AIDS implicate a compromised immune system as a predisposing factor in this disease (31, 43, 46, 54, 56, 57, 65, 78). These patients tend to be younger and are not diabetic compared with the classic patient with malignant external otitis. Six of the seven patients have been adults and none had diabetes. *Aspergillus fumigatus* was isolated in three cases.

Antipseudomonal antimicrobials are the mainstay of therapy for malignant external otitis. Before the development of systemic agents, the mortality from this disease approximated 50% with frequent recurrences (7). Introduction of parenteral antipseudomonal pencillins reduced the mortality to 20% (71). Prolonged combination parenteral therapy for this disease was associated with long-term hospitalization and renal and vestibular toxicity, in addition to the morbidity of the disease itself. Quinolone agents, especially ciprofloxacin, have essentially revolutionized the treatment of malignant external otitis, and oral quinolones have generally replaced combination therapy with aminoglycosides and antipseudomonal beta-lactam antibiotics in the treatment of this disease. Their activity against *P. aeruginosa*, the oral route of administration, and high penetration into soft tissues and bone have eliminated the need for prolonged hospitalization (22, 25, 36, 69, 79). In addition, the dose of ciprofloxacin does not require adjustment in the elderly patient with renal failure (27, 80). With the introduction of quinolones, the cure rate has increased to 90%, with few adverse effects reported. Ciprofloxacin (750 mg twice a day) remains the antibiotic of choice, although no comparative trials have been reported (26, 29, 35, 37, 45, 59, 63). Despite the rapid relief of symptoms (pain and otorrhea), prolonged treatment for 6 to 8 weeks is generally recommended, as indicated for an osteomyelitis. Although used prior to the development of antipseudomonal antibiotics, surgery plays no role in

Jennifer Rubin Grandis • Department of Otolaryngology, University of Pittsburgh, Pittsburgh, PA 15213.   Victor L. Yu •
Infectious Disease Section, VA Medical Center, University of Pittsburgh, Pittsburgh, PA 15240.

the treatment of this disease. Debridement and/or biopsy to rule out cancer are the only indicated surgical procedures. Hyperbaric oxygen has been used on occasion with mixed results and may be considered as an adjuvant treatment for refractory cases (10, 39, 40, 41, 68).

Laboratory parameters are generally unaffected in malignant external otitis, with the exception of an elevated erythrocyte sedimentation rate (ESR). We have found the ESR to be a useful way of monitoring disease activity and response to therapy (60). In one study, the ESR fell from a mean pretreatment value of 81 mm/h (range, 41 to 138 mm/h) to a mean value of 18 mm/h (range, 3 to 45 mm/h) (59). The utility of nuclear imaging studies is evolving. Bone scanning with technetium Tc 99m, where the radionuclide tracer accumulates at sites of osteoblastic activity, is very sensitive in making the diagnosis. However, the bone scan never normalizes, rendering the study unamenable to follow-up, and there are reports of positive bone scans in simple external otitis (38). Quantitative bone scanning may be able to distinguish simple from malignant external otitis and demonstrate disease resolution (72). Gallium (^{67}Ga) citrate scanning seems to be more specific than bone scanning because of incorporation of the radioisotope into granulocytes and bacteria. Although several studies have reported that gallium scanning can be used to monitor disease activity, others have noted that normal scans can be found in patients with recurrent disease (18, 20, 48, 49). Several studies suggest that the combination of ^{67}Ga and computerized tomography (CT) as single-photon emission CT scanning is useful in the diagnosis and follow-up examination of these patients (1, 24, 72).

Anatomic imaging modalities allow for both anatomic localization of disease as well as the assessment of disease resolution. CT scanning is ideal for the assessment of bone erosion. In a prospective study, we determined that the presence of bone erosion and/or soft-tissue in the subtemporal region was helpful in making the diagnosis of malignant external otitis (58). Although the bone did not remineralize, resolution of the soft-tissue component did correlate with disease activity. To compare CT with magnetic resonance imaging, we performed a long-term prospective study in seven patients with malignant external otitis, and found that magnetic resonance imaging was slightly better at demonstrating medial skull base disease because of its ability to delineate changes in the fat content of the marrow (23).

With the advent and widespread use of quinolones for all ear infections, patients with malignant external otitis are being diagnosed and treated earlier in the course of the disease, thus changing the

clinical spectrum of this infection. These individuals with "limited-MEO" may present with a lower or even normal ESR and no evidence of bone destruction on anatomic imaging studies. It is important to maintain a high index of suspicion when the typical host presents with otalgia that is out of proportion to findings on physical examination. Furthermore, a history of ear irrigation (usually for cerumen impaction) should be sought because of the association between malignant external otitis and water exposure (15, 61).

AURICULAR PERICHONDRITIS

Perichondritis of the auricle caused by *P. aeruginosa* can occur in burn patients as well as patients with malignant external otitis. Because of the excellent soft-tissue penetration of quinolones such as ciprofloxacin, they are ideal agents for treating this disease. Oral ciprofloxacin has been used successfully for individuals with auricular perichondritis (47). Potential limitations of oral quinolones for the treatment of soft-tissue infections of the auricle is suggested by reports of phototoxic lesions induced by quinolones in the auricular skin of mouse models (66).

TREATMENT OF CHRONIC EAR DISEASE

Chronic inflammatory conditions of the ear must be carefully separated into infectious versus noninfectious etiologies as well as consideration of the site of the disease process under scrutiny. Specifically, the status of the external ear canal, middle ear and tympanic membrane, presence of cholesteatoma, and prior mastoid surgery are all important parameters in delineating the condition under investigation. Early reports on the use of quinolones for ear disease other than malignant external otitis often grouped patients with different disease processes together, thus confounding interpretation of the results (21, 51, 73). Increasingly, studies have defined the populations under investigation more precisely and have compared the efficacy of fluoroquinolones with another drug, or untreated controls. The high concentrations of orally administered ciprofloxacin into the middle ear mucosa and cortical bone of the mastoid process supports its use in the treatment of chronic otitis media (42).

In an early study, oral ciprofloxacin (500 mg twice a day for 2 weeks) was given to 19 patients with many ear conditions, including chronic otitis media, an infected mastoid cavity, cholesteatoma, or chronic external otitis (51). Limitations of this study included the failure to control for the use of topical antibiotics, absence of posttreatment cultures, and a relatively short follow-up period. The overall cure rate was 58%; however, patients with cholesteatoma had a lower response rate. Using a similarly heterogeneous patient population with chronic ear disease, Van deHeyning treated 59 patients with a higher dose of ciprofloxacin (750 mg twice a day) with similar rates of clinical and bacteriologic cures (77). Patients with cholesteatoma benefited from surgical intervention in addition to antimicrobial therapy. Although the authors recommended the use of perioperative ciprofloxacin as prophylaxis in otologic surgery, the need for any antibiotic in this setting has never been clearly determined.

Topical quinolones are now widely available and used commonly for ear diseases, often prior to obtaining cultures. The efficacy of topical ciprofloxacin was explored in one study where 232 patients with chronic suppurative otitis media were randomized in a nonblinded, multicenter study to receive topical ciprofloxacin (0.2% solution in single-dose containers) or the commonly used combination of polymyxin B, neomycin, and hydrocortisone in suspension (44). Although this study found that the two treatments were equally effective, an earlier trial demonstrated significantly less active disease in patients who had received the ofloxacin eardrops (75). Ciprofloxacin was found to be equivalent to topical tobramycin for the treatment of chronic suppurative otitis media without cholesteatoma (16). However, an earlier study suggested that topical ciprofloxacin was superior to gentamicin for chronic ear disease (76). Since aminoglycosides have demonstrated evidence of ototoxicity, it would be prudent to utilize a topical quinolone for the treatment of otorrhea in the setting of a perforated tympanic membrane. Although not a comparative trial, another study demonstrated efficacy of topical ciprofloxacin in 80 patients with chronic suppurative otitis media (32). Few careful dosing studies have been performed. It appears that 125 μg of ciprofloxacin per ml was as effective as 250 μg/ml in eradicating otorrhea as long as it was administered for at least 14 days (2). With 1-month follow-up, the treatments showed equivalent bacteriologic and clinical cure rates.

The role of the oral quinolones for the treatment of chronic otitis media remains undetermined. Studies have demonstrated the safety and efficacy of systemic ciprofloxacin (13, 19, 30). In a randomized trial, oral ciprofloxacin was shown to be superior to amoxicillin/clavulanic acid for the treatment of chronic suppurative otitis media (34). However, the benefit of oral ciprofloxacin in addition to the topical preparation has not been demonstrated. One study examined 60 patients with chronic otitis media randomized to receive oral ciprofloxacin alone (250 mg twice a day for 5 to 10 days), topical ciprofloxacin alone (3 drops containing 250 μg of ciprofloxacin per ml in saline solution twice a day), or oral plus topical ciprofloxacin twice a day (12). Although the follow-up period was only 14 days, topical ciprofloxacin alone appeared to be more efficacious than the oral drug alone or in combination with topical therapy. Such results confirm the clinical impression that topical antimicrobials for external otitis are often sufficient, and oral antibiotics are not required. In addition, chronic otorrhea is primarily a disease of children (often after insertion of tympanostomy tubes), for whom the use of systemic ciprofloxacin is currently not approved because of the possible deleterious effects on developing joints and cartilage. Topical quinolones are unlikely to be absorbed and lead to systemic toxicities, making them ideal therapeutic agents for the treatment of otorrhea in the pediatric population. In fact, topical ciprofloxacin has been demonstrated to be effective and safe for children with otorrhea after tympanostomy tube placement (14). A survey of in vitro and in vivo antimicrobial activity of topical ofloxacin compared with other ototopical agents concluded that ofloxacin otic solution was effective in eradicating the bacterial pathogen from the infection site. However, it was equivalent to older, less costly agents for simple external otitis in children (33).

Cumulative evidence supports the utility of quinolones for treatment of chronic ear infections with multiresistant bacterial. While there is little justification for the use of quinolones as first-line agents in the treatment of simple external otitis or acute or serous otitis media, their efficacy and lack of ototoxicity support the administration of quinolones for cases of chronic otitis, especially when the tympanic membrane is not intact. The benefit of oral quinolones in addition to topical preparations in chronic otitis media with otorrhea has not been defined. Further randomized studies are required that outline rigorous criteria for entry, specify the disease process being studied, and evaluate objective end points. Without supporting data, it would be prudent to initiate treatment with a topical quinolone if *P. aeruginosa* or other gram-negative bacilli are isolated from ear drainage. An oral agent may be indicated in the setting of persistent drainage despite ototopical therapy, severe symptoms, or the development of complications.

TREATMENT OF ACUTE PHARYNGOTONSILLITIS

Quinolones have no role in the treatment of pharyngitis. Several studies have examined the efficacy of fluoroquinolones for acute pharyngotonsillitis. Amoxicillin (250 mg three times a day) was compared with ofloxacin (200 mg three times a day) and found to be equally effective (64). Other studies have not used comparative control groups and have generally found that the quinolones were well tolerated and effective (12, 28, 64). Despite the general success reported in these studies, there is little rationale for using fluoroquinolones as first-line agents in acute or chronic tonsillitis, given the availability of other, less costly agents.

NASAL CARRIAGE OF BACTERIA

Neisseria meningitidis

Ciprofloxacin has excellent in vitro activity against Neisseria meningitidis, and its concentration in nasal secretions exceeds the MIC_{90} of strains of this organism by 70-fold (52). Concentrations in nasal secretions were as high as 0.4 μg/ml (mean, about 0.14 μg/ml) or approximately 10% of that in serum, while the MIC_{90}s for N. meningitidis strains was about 0.004 μg/ml. In large surveys of antibiotic resistance in invasive isolates of N. meningitidis, quinolone susceptibility remained excellent, although extremely rare instances of decreased susceptibility have been reported (74). In one survey of 1,434 strains of N. meningitidis isolated from patients with invasive meningococcal disease in Australia during a six-year period, only one isolate had decreased quinolone susceptibility (67). In an outbreak of meningococcal disease in Canada, isolates of moderately penicillin-resistant N. meningitidis (defined as MIC ≥ 0.04 ug/ml) were 100% susceptible to ciprofloxacin (5).

Short courses of ciprofloxacin (2 to 5 days) at doses of 250 to 500 mg twice a day have been effective in eradicating meningococcal carriage in chronic nasal carriers (53, 55). A single oral dose of 750 mg of ciprofloxacin was evaluated in a placebo-controlled, double-blind trial of healthy volunteers (11). One dose proved to be effective in eradicating the organism in 96% of volunteers at 7 and 21 days after therapy. Of note, one of the volunteers who was treated successfully carried a minocycline-resistant strain. In rural Africa, 1,878 children (ages 2 to 18 years) and adults of contacts of patients with meningococcal-meningitis were evaluated in a prospective randomized study of meningococcal carriage. Ciprofloxacin (91.1%) was comparable with rifampin (94.7%) in eradicating carriage.

Ciprofloxacin has now been added as an acceptable alternative to rifampin for chemoprophylaxis in selected populations in the 1997 Guidelines for Prevention of Meningococcal Disease (6).

Staphylococcus aureus

Ciprofloxacin in nasal secretions was insufficient to inhibit either methicillin-sensitive or methicillin-resistant S. aureus strains (9). In a study of staphylococcal nasal carriage in hemodialysis patients given 750 mg of ciprofloxacin a day for 6 days, 54% were free of staphylococci 1 day after therapy; however, the number of Staphylococcus carriers declined to only 27% 4 weeks later (8). Prolonged use of ciprofloxacin has proven to be relatively ineffective in eradicating carriage by methicillin-resistant S. aureus, and emergence of resistance in vitro following such therapy has been commonplace (50, 70).

SUMMARY

Infections of the ear, nose, and throat are among the most common outpatient maladies in the world. Oral quinolones are the drugs of choice for the treatment of disease caused by P. aeruginosa, including malignant external otitis and auricular perichondritis. Topical quinolones are the ideal agent for chronic suppurative otitis media and otorrhea through a tympanic membrane perforation. However, systemic quinolones for nonnecrotizing otitis media are not indicated. Similarly, there appears to be little rationale for the use of quinolones as initial therapy for otitis media, sinusitis, or pharyngotonsillitis. In fact, pneumococcal bacteremia following ciprofloxacin therapy for acute otitis media has been reported (17).

REFERENCES

1. **Amorosa, L., G. C. Modugno, and A. Pirodda.** 1996. Malignant external otitis: review and personal experience. *Acta Otolaryngol. Suppl.* 521:3–16.
2. **Asian, A.** 1998. A new dosage regimen for topical application of ciprofloxacin in the management of chronic suppurative otitis media. *Otolaryngol. Head Neck Surg.* 118:883–885.
3. **Barrow, H. N., and M. J. Levenson.** 1992. Necrotizing 'malignant' external otitis caused by Staphylococcus epidermidis. *Arch. Otolaryngol. Head Neck Surg.* 118:94–96.
4. **Barza, M.** 1988. Pharmacokinetics and efficacy of the new quinolones in infections of the eye, ear, nose, and throat. *Rev. Infect. Dis.* 10(Suppl 1):S241–S247.
5. **Blondeau, J. M., and Y. Yaschuk.** 1995. In vitro activities of ciprofloxacin, cefotaxime, ceftriaxone, chloramphenicol, and rifampin against fully susceptible and moderately penicillin-resistant Neisseria meningitidis. *Antimicrob. Agents Chemother.* 39:2577–2579.
6. **Centers for Disease Control and Prevention.** 1997. Control and prevention of meningococcal disease: recommendations of the Advisory Committee on Immunization Practices (ACIP). *Morb. Mortal. Wkly. Rep.* 46(RR-5):1–10.

7. Chandler, J. R. 1968. Malignant external otitis. *Laryngoscope* 78:1257–1294.

8. Chow, J. W., and V. L. Yu. 1992. Failure of oral ciprofloxacin in suppressing *Staphylococcus aureus* carriage in hemodialysis patients. *J. Antimicrob. Chemother.* 29:88–89.

9. Darouiche, R., B. Perkins, B. D. Musher, R. Hamill, and S. Tsai. 1990. Levels of rifampin and ciprofloxacin in nasal secretions; correlation with MIC 90 and eradication of nasopharyngeal carriage of bacteria. *J. Infect. Dis.* 162:1124–1127.

10. Davis, J. C., G. A. Gates, C. Lerner, M. G. Davis, Jr., J. T. Mader, and A. Dinesman. 1992. Adjuvant hyperbaric oxygen in malignant external otitis. *Arch. Otolaryngol. Head Neck Surg.* 118:89–93.

11. Dworzack, D. L., C. C. Sanders, E. A. Horowitz, J. Allais, M. Sookpranee, W. E. Sanders, and F. M. Ferraro. 1988. Evaluation of single-dose ciprofloxacin in the eradication of *Neisseria meningitidis* from nasopharyngeal carriers. *Antimicrob. Agents Chemother.* 32:1740–1741.

12. Esposito, S., G. D'Errico, and C. Montanaro. 1990. Topical and oral treatment of chronic otitis media with ciprofloxacin. A preliminary study. *Arch. Otolaryngol. Head Neck Surg.* 116:557–559.

13. Fombeur, J. P., S. Barrault, G. Koubbi, J. N. Laurier, D. Ebbo, F. Lecomte, N. Sorrel, and S. Dobler. 1994. Study of the efficacy and safety of ciprofloxacin in the treatment of chronic otitis. *Chemotherapy* 40(Suppl. 1):29–34.

14. Force, R. W., M. C. Hart, S. A. Plummer, D. A. Powell, and M. C. Nahata. 1995. Topical ciprofloxacin for otorrhea after tympanostomy tube placement. *Arch. Otolaryngol. Head Neck Surg.* 121:880–884.

15. Ford, G. R., and R. G. Courteney-Harris. 1990. Another hazard of ear syringing: malignant external otitis. *J. Laryngol. Otol.* 104:709–710.

16. Fradis, M., A. Brodsky, J. Ben-David, I. Srugo, J. Larboni, and L. Podoshin. 1997. Chronic otitis media treated topically with ciprofloxacin or tobramycin. *Arch. Otolaryngol. Head Neck Surg.* 123:1057–1060.

17. Frieden, T. R., and R. J. Mangi. 1990. Inappropriate use of oral ciprofloxacin. *JAMA* 264:1438–1440.

18. Garty, I., G. Rosen, and Y. Holdstein. 1985. The radionuclide diagnosis, evaluation and follow-up of malignant external otitis (MEO). The value of immediate blood pool scanning. *J. Laryngol. Otol.* 99:109–115.

19. Gehanno, P. 1997. Multicenter study of the efficacy and safety of oral ciprofloxacin in the treatment of chronic suppurative otitis media in adults. The French Study Group. *Otolaryngol. Head Neck Surg.* 117:83–90.

20. Gherini, S. G., D. E. Brackmann, and W. G. Bradley. 1986. Magnetic resonance imaging and computerized tomography in malignant external otitis. *Laryngoscope* 96:542–548.

21. Giamarellou, H., N. Galanakis, E. Daphnis, H. Stephanou, and P. Sfikakis. 1988. Treating acute and choronic otitis with ciprofloxacin: a step forward a better prognosis? *Rev. Infect. Dis.* 10(Suppl. 1):S248.

22. Gilbert, D. N., A. D. Tice, P. K. Marsh, P. C. Craven, and L. C. Preheim. 1987. Oral ciprofloxacin therapy for chronic contiguous osteomyelitis caused by aerobic gram-negative bacilli. *Am. J. Med.* 82(Suppl. 4A):254–258.

23. Grandis, J. R., H. D. Curtin, and V. L. Yu. 1995. Necrotizing (malignant) external otitis: prospective comparison of CT and MR imaging in diagnosis and follow-up. *Radiology* 196:499–504.

24. Hardoff, R., S. Gips, N. Uri, A. Front, and A. Tamir. 1994. Semiquantitative skull planar and SPECT bone scintigraphy in diabetic patients: differentiation of necrotizing (malignant) external otitis from severe external otitis. *J. Nucl. Med.* 35:411–415.

25. Hessen, M. T., M. J. Ingerman, D. H. Kaufman, P. Weiner, J. Santoro, O. M. Korzeniowski, J. Boscia, M. Topiel, L. M. Bush, D. Kaye, and M. Levison. 1987. Clinical efficacy of ciprofloxacin therapy for gram-negative bacillary osteomyelitis. *Am. J. Med.* 82(Suppl. 4A):262–265.

26. Hickey, S. A., G. R. Ford, A. F. O'Connor, S. J. Eykyn, and P. H. Sonksen. 1989. Treating malignant otitis with oral ciprofloxacin. *Br. Med. J.* 299:550–551.

27. Hirata, C. A., D. R. Guay, W. M. Awni, D. J. Stein, and P. K. Peterson. 1989. Steady-state pharmacokinetics of intravenous and oral ciprofloxacin in elderly patients. *Antimicrob. Agents Chemother.* 33:1927–1931.

28. Iwasawa, T. 1984. Fundamental and clinical studies of DL-8280 in the otorhinolaryngologic field. *Chemotherapy (Tokyo)* 32(Suppl. 1):1001–1012.

29. Joachims, H. Z., J. Danino, and R. Raz. 1988. Malignant external otitis: treatment with fluoroquinolones. *Am. J. Otolaryngol.* 9:102–105.

30. Kasemsuwan, L., and P. Clongsuesuek. 1997. A double blind, prospective trial of topical ciprofloxacin versus normal saline solution in the treatment of otorrhoea. *Clin. Otolaryngol. Allied Sci.* 22:44–46.

31. Kielhofner, M., R. L. Atmar, R. J. Hamill, and D. M. Musher. 1992. Life-threatening Pseudomonas aeruginosa infections in patients with human immunodeficiency virus infection. *Clin. Infect. Dis.* 14:403–411.

32. Kiris, M., M. Berktas, E. Egeli, and A. Kutluhan. 1998. The efficacy of topical ciprofloxacin in the treatment of chronic suppurative otitis media. *Entechnology* 77:904–905.

33. Klein, J. O. 2001. In vitro and in vivo antimicrobial activity of topical ofloxacin and other ototopical agents. *Pediatr. Infect. Dis. J.* 20:102–103.

34. Legent, F., P. Bordure, C. Beauvillain, and P. Berche. 1994. Controlled prospective study of oral ciprofloxacin versus amoxycillin/clavulanic acid in chronic suppurative otitis media in adults. *Chemotherapy* 40(Suppl. 1):16–23.

35. Leggett, J. M., and K. Prendergast. 1988. Malignant external otitis: the use of oral ciprofloxacin. *J. Laryngol. Otol.* 102:53–54.

36. Lesse, A. J., C. Freer, R. A. Salata, J. B. Francis, and W. M. Scheld. 1987. Oral ciprofloxacin therapy for gram-negative bacillary osteomyelitis. *Am. J. Med.* 82(Suppl. 4A):247–253.

37. Levenson, M. J., S. C. Parisier, J. Dolitsky, and G. Bindra. 1991. Ciprofloxacin: drug of choice in the treatment of malignant external otitis (MEO). *Laryngoscope* 101:821–824.

38. Levin, W. J., J. H. Shary III, L. T. Nichols, and F. E. Lucente. 1986. Bone scanning in severe external otitis. *Laryngoscope* 96:1193–1195.

39. Lucente, F. E., S. C. Parisier, and P. M. Som. 1983. Complications of the treatment of malignant external otitis. *Laryngoscope* 93:279–281.

40. Lucente, F. E., S. C. Parisier, P. M. Som, and L. M. Arnold. 1982. Malignant external otitis: a dangerous misnomer? *Otolaryngol. Head Neck Surg.* 90:266–269.

41. Mader, J. T., and J. T. Love. 1982. Malignant external otitis. Cure with adjunctive hyperbaric oxygen therapy. *Arch. Otolaryngol.* 108:38–40.

42. Massias, L., P. Buffe, B. Cohen, Y. Cudennec, P. Gehanno, O. Sterkers, and R. Farinotti. 1994. Study of the distribution of oral ciprofloxacin into the mucosa of the middle ear and the cortical bone of the mastoid process. *Chemotherapy* 40(Suppl. 1):3–7.

43. McElroy, E. A., Jr., and G. L. Marks. 1991. Fatal necrotizing otitis externa in a patient with AIDS. *Rev. Infect. Dis.* 13:1246–1247.

44. Miro, N. 2000. Controlled multicenter study on chronic suppurative otitis media treated with topical applications of

ciprofloxacin 0.2% solution in single-dose containers or combination of polymyxin B, neomycin, and hydrocortisone suspension. *Otolaryngol. Head Neck Surg.* **123**:617–623.

45. Morrison, G. A., and C. M. Bailey. 1988. Relapsing malignant otitis externa successfully treated with ciprofloxacin. *J. Laryngol. Otol.* **102**:872–876.

46. Munoz, A., and E. Martinez-Chamorro. 1998. Necrotizing external otitis caused by Aspergillus fumigatus: computed tomography and high resolution magnetic resonance imaging in an AIDS patient. *J. Laryngol. Otol.* **112**:98–102.

47. Noel, S. B., P. Scallan, M. C. Meadors, T. J. Meek, Jr., and G. A. Pankey. 1989. Treatment of Pseudomonas aeruginosa auricular perichondritis with oral ciprofloxacin. *J. Dermatol. Surg. Oncol.* **15**:633–637.

48. Ostfeld, E., M. Segal, and B. Czernobilsky. 1981. Malignant external otitis: early histopathologic changes and pathogenic mechanism. *Laryngoscope* **91**:965–970.

49. Parisier, S. C., F. E. Lucente, P. M. Som, S. Z. Hirschman, L. M. Arnold, and J. D. Roffman. 1982. Nuclear scanning in necrotizing progressive "malignant" external otitis. *Laryngoscope* **92**:1016–1019.

50. Peterson, L., J. Quick, B. Jensen, S. Homann, and S. Johnson. 1990. Emergence of ciprofloxacin resistance in nosocomial methicillin-resistant staphylococcus aureus isolation; resistance during ciprofloxacin plus rifampin therapy for methicillin-resistant *S. aureus* colonization. *Arch. Intern. Med.* **150**:2151–2155.

51. Piccirillo, J. F., and S. M. Parnes. 1989. Ciprofloxacin for the treatment of chronic ear disease. *Laryngoscope* **99**:510–513.

52. Piercy, E. A., R. Bawdon, and M. P. A. Mac-Kowiak. 1989. Penetration of ciprofloxacin into saliva and nasal secretion and effect of the drug on the oropharyngeal flora of all subjects. *Antimicrob. Agents Chemother.* **33**:1645–1646.

53. Pugsley, M. P., D. L. Dworzack, J. Roccaforte, C. C. Sanders, J. Bakken, and W. E. Sanders. 1988. An open study of the efficacy of a single dose of ciprofloxacin in eliminating the chronic nasopharyngeal carriage of Neisseria meningitidis. *J. Infect. Dis.* **157**:852–853.

54. Reiss, P., R. Hadderingh, L. J. Schot, and S. A. Danner. 1991. Invasive external otitis caused by Aspergillus fumigatus in two patients with AIDS. *AIDS* **5**:605–606.

55. Renkonen, O. V., A. Sivonen, and R. Visakorpi. 1987. Effect of ciprofloxacin on carrier rate of Neisseria meningitidis in army recruits in Finland. *Antimicrob. Agents Chemother.* **31**:962–963.

56. Ress, B. D., M. Luntz, F. F. Telischi, T. J. Balkany, and M. L. Whiteman. 1997. Necrotizing external otitis in patients with AIDS. *Laryngoscope* **107**:456–460.

57. Rivas Lacarte, M. P., and F. Pumarola Segura. 1990. [Malignant otitis externa and HIV antibodies. A case report]. *An. Otorrinolaringol. Ibero Am.* **17**:505–512.

58. Rubin, J., H. D. Curtin, V. L. Yu, and D. B. Kamerer. 1990. Malignant external otitis: utility of CT in diagnosis and follow-up. *Radiology* **174**:391–4.

59. Rubin, J., G. Stoehr, V. L. Yu, R. R. Muder, A. Matador, and D. B. Kamerer. 1989. Efficacy of oral ciprofloxacin plus rifampin for treatment of malignant external otitis. *Arch. Otolaryngol. Head Neck Surg.* **115**:1063–1069.

60. Rubin, J., and V. L. Yu. 1988. Malignant external otitis: insights into pathogenesis, clinical manifestations, diagnosis, and therapy. *Am. J. Med.* **85**:391–398.

61. Rubin, J., V. L. Yu, D. B. Kamerer, and M. Wagener. 1990. Aural irrigation with water: a potential pathogenic mechanism for inducing malignant external otitis? *Ann. Otol. Rhinol. Laryngol.* **99**:117–119.

62. Rubin, J., V. L. Yu, and S. E. Stool. 1988. Malignant external otitis in children. *J. Pediatr.* **113**:965–970.

63. Sade, J., R. Lang, S. Goshen, and R. Kitzes-Cohen. 1989. Ciprofloxacin treatment of malignant external otitis. *Am. J. Med.* **87**(Suppl. 5A):138S–141S.

64. Sasaki, T., T. Unno, T. Tomiyamo, O. Yamai, and T. Iwasawa. 1984. Evaluation of clinical effectiveness and safety of dl-8280 in acute lacunar tonsillitis. *Otol. Fukuoka* **30**:484–513.

65. Scott, G. B., B. E. Buck, J. G. Leterman, F. L. Bloom, and W. P. Parks. 1984. Acquired immunodeficiency syndrome in infants. *N. Engl. J. Med.* **310**:76–81.

66. Shimoda, K., M. Yoshida, N. Wagai, S. Takayama, and M. Kato. 1993. Phototoxic lesions induced by quinolone antibacterial agents in auricular skin and retina of albino mice. [see comments]. *Toxicol. Pathol.* **21**:554–561.

67. Shultz, T. R., J. W. Tapsall, P. A. White, and P. J. Newton. 2000. An invasive isolate of Neisseria meningitidis showing decreased susceptibility to quinolones. *Antimicrob. Agents Chemother.* **44**:1116.

68. Shupak, A., E. Greenberg, R. Hardoff, C. Gordon, Y. Melamed, and W. S. Meyer. 1989. Hyperbaric oxygenation for necrotizing (malignant) otitis externa. *Arch. Otolaryngol. Head Neck Surg.* **115**:1470–1475.

69. Slama, T. G., J. Misinski, and S. Sklar. 1987. Oral ciprofloxacin therapy for osteomyelitis caused by aerobic gran-negative bacilli. *Am. J. Med.* **82**:S259–S261.

70. Smith, S. M., R. H. K. Eng, and F. Tomang-Tecson. 1990. Epidemiology of ciprofloxacin resistance among patients with methicillin-resistant *Staphyloccus aureus*. *J. Antimicrob. Chemother.* **26**:567–572.

71. Soliman, A. E. 1978. A rare case of malignant otitis externa in a non-diabetic patient. *J. Laryngol. Otol.* **92**:811–812.

72. Stokkel, M. P., R. P. Takes, B. L. van Eck-Smit, and R. J. Baatenburg de Jong. 1997. The value of quantitative gallium-67 single-photon emission tomography in the clinical management of malignant external otitis. *Eur. J. Nucl. Med.* **24**:1429–1432.

73. Sundberg, L., and T. Eden. 1990. Penetration of enoxacin into middle ear effusion. *Acta Otolaryngol.* **109**:438–443.

74. Tapsall, J. W., T. Shultz, E. Limnios, R. Munro, J. Mercer, R. Porritt, J. Griffith, G. Hogg, G. Lum, A. Lawrence, D. Hansman, P. Collignon, P. Southwell, K. Ott, M. Gardam, C. J. Richardson, J. Bates, D. Murphy, and H. Smith. 2001. Surveillance of antibiotic resistance in invasive isolates of Neisseria meningitidis in Australia 1994–1999. *Pathology* **33**:359–361.

75. Tong, M., J. Woo, and C. v. Hasselt. 1996. A double-blind comparative study of ofloxacin otic drops versus neomycin-polymyxin B-hydrocortisone otic drops in the medical treatment of chronic suppurative otitis media. *J. Laryngol. Otol.* **110**:309–314.

76. Tutkun, A., A. Ozagar, A. Koc, C. Batman, C. Uneri, and M. A. Sehitoglu. 1995. Treatment of chronic ear disease. Topical ciprofloxacin vs topical gentamicin. *Arch. Otolaryngol. Head Neck Surg.* **121**:1414–1416.

77. Van de Heyning, P. H., S. R. Pattyn, and H. D. Valcke. 1986. Ciprofloxacin in oral treatment of ear infections. *Pharm. Weekbl. Sci.* **8**:63–66.

78. Weinroth, S. E., D. Schessel, and C. U. Tuazon. 1994. Malignant otitis externa in AIDS patients: case report and review of the literature. *Ear Nose Throat J.* **73**:772–778.

79. Wise, R., and I. A. Donovan. 1987. Tissue penetration and metabolism of ciprofloxacin. *Am. J. Med.* **82**(Suppl. 4A):103–107.

80. Wiseman, L. R., and J. A. Balfour. 1994. Ciprofloxacin. A review of its pharmacological profile and therapeutic use in the elderly. *Drugs Aging* **4**:145–173.

Quinolone Antimicrobial Agents, 3rd ed.
Edited by David C. Hooper and Ethan Rubinstein
© 2003 ASM Press, Washington, D.C.

Chapter 15

Treatment of Osteomyelitis and Septic Arthritis

LOUIS BERNARD, FRANCIS WALDVOGEL, AND DANIEL LEW

Patients with osteomyelitis require a surgical approach associated with long-term antibiotic prophylaxis. Apart from rifampin and quinolones, antibiotics penetrate badly into bone, and their levels are usually quite low a few hours after administration when compared with levels in serum. To achieve an acceptable cure rate, parenteral antibiotic treatment has to be administered during several weeks. Fluoroquinolones present several advantages due to their good oral biodisponibility; their penetration of bone at concentrations high enough to inhibit most strains of *Enterobacteriaceae*, *Pseudomonas* spp., and an important percentage of *Staphylococcus aureus*; and their relatively few toxic effects (1, 35, 36).

During the past decade, more extensive experience has been acquired in the use of quinolones for the treatment of osteomyelitis and septic arthritis (13, 18, 20, 29, 51, 55, 64). Additional extensive experience has been gained in experimental models using newer agents, or combination therapy. This review summarizes the current knowledge of the use of quinolones in the treatment of osteomyelitis and septic arthritis.

GENERAL CONSIDERATIONS OF OSTEOMYELITIS

The identification of the causative organisms of osteomyelitis is essential for diagnosis and treatment. It is important to obtain deep specimens, in particular by bone biopsy, for microbiological and pathological analysis. Infection is diagnosed if a pathogen is recovered from the surgical specimen, in conjunction with (i) purulence noted at the time of surgery and/or (ii) histological evidence of infection.

It is important to distinguish between acute and chronic osteomyelitis, and osteomyelitis associated with peripheral vascular disease, such as diabetes. Acute infection is defined by the occurrence of symptoms of ≤4 weeks duration with an absence of bone destruction, and is often associated with bacteremia. It is predominantly diagnosed in prepubertal children as a complication of bacteremia, usually located in the metaphyseal area of long bones (tibia and femur), or in the vertebrae in adults. Chronic infection diagnosis is established by the persistence of symptoms for >4 weeks. It is most often diagnosed in adults secondary to trauma and is usually associated with an open fracture, contiguous infections such as decubitus ulcers, or after surgery, in particular, the insertion of prostheses. Diabetic patients typically have osteomyelitis of the feet associated with peripheral vascular disease (37, 62).

It is important to distinguish between acute and chronic osteomyelitis, and osteomyelitis associated with a foreign-body implant because the surgical and medical treatments differ. The classification proposed by one of the authors of this review several years ago was to separate hematogenous osteomyelitis from osteomyelitis secondary to a contiguous focus of infection, with or without vascular insufficiency (62). An alternative classification which is perhaps more useful to surgeons was proposed by Cierny and colleagues and takes into consideration the anatomic nature of infection: stage 1, intramedullary osteomyelitis (infected intramedullary rod); stage 2, superficial osteomyelitis; stage 3, localized osteomyelitis (full-thickness, cortical sequestration, or sequelae); and stage 4, diffuse osteomyelitis (fracture with nonunion, prosthesis infected); as well as the quality of the host and treatment and prognosis factors (7). Patients with foreign-body implants are particularly at risk because of a high susceptibility to infection and the necessity to remove the prosthesis to achieve cure.

MICROBIOLOGICAL ASPECTS OF OSTEOMYELITIS

The specific organism isolated in bacterial osteomyelitis is often associated with the age of the

Louis Bernard, Francis Waldvogel, and Daniel Lew • Infectious Diseases Division and Medical Clinic II, Department of Medicine, Geneva University Hospitals, 24 Rue Micheli-du-Crest, 1211 Geneva, Switzerland.

patient, a common clinical presentation (i.e., trauma or recent surgery), and the presence or absence of vascular insufficiency. *S. aureus* is found in most patients with acute hematogenous osteomyelitis. *Staphylococcus epidermidis, S. aureus, Pseudomonas aeruginosa, Enterobacteriaceae (Serratia marcescens* and *Escherichia coli)* are commonly isolated in patients with chronic osteomyelitis (5). Methicillin-resistant *S. aureus* (MRSA) is often involved in acute nosocomial infection of arthroplasty. In chronic infection of arthroplasty, *S. epidermidis* and streptococci infections are usually isolated but, increasingly, *Propionibacterium* spp. (3) infections are reported. In the case of vascular insufficiency, particularly that associated with diabetes, the microbiology of osteomyelitis is complex and involves several microorganisms (*S. aureus*, anaerobes, streptococci, and gram-negative rods) (37) (Table 1).

During osteomyelitis treatment, antibiotic concentrations should be effective to achieve levels in joint fluid or bone exceeding the MICs for isolated microorganisms during significant periods. Concentrations of newer quinolones achieved in human bone appear satisfactory, exceeding the MIC_{90} against *Enterobacteriaceae* and a significant proportion of staphylococci and *P. aeruginosa*. However, older quinolones do not achieve this goal (due to their inefficacy) against streptococci and anaerobes.

EXPERIMENTAL OSTEOMYELITIS AND ARTHRITIS

In view of the lack of well-performed, large-scale clinical trials on the use of quinolones for osteomyelitis in humans, data obtained from animal studies remain extremely valuable and permit a comparison with different therapy groups.

In past reviews, several experimental studies have indicated that gram-negative infections such as *E. coli* arthritis or *P. aeruginosa* osteomyelitis

showed impressive 95% cure rates. These latter results were tempered by the demonstration that a significant percentage of the *Pseudomonas* isolated during therapy had important increases in their MIC. These excellent results obtained in experimental animal infections correlated well with the results obtained in humans (22) and emphasize the importance of preliminary experiments in animals to determine optimal therapy in humans. More recent animal studies have attempted to study the role of quinolones in staphylococcal infections as well as infections in the presence of prosthetic material. Several studies have shown excellent results with quinolones in experimental osteomyelitis and/or osteoarthritis (36).

The Rabbit Model

The rabbit model of *P. aeruginosa* chronic osteomyelitis has the relative advantage of assessing the rate of negative microbiological cultures after 3 to 4 weeks of therapy. In a rather classical paper, Norden and Shinners showed an excellent activity of ciprofloxacin compared with a poor activity of tobramycin (50). Similar results were obtained by Bayer et al. in a rabbit model of acute *E. coli* arthritis where ciprofloxacin was compared with gentamicin (1). In a recent study, Shirtliff et al. (58) showed an inferior efficacy of levofloxacin to nafcillin in the treatment of methicillin-susceptible *S. aureus* osteomyelitis in rabbits. The inferior efficacy of levofloxacin may be due to its pharmacokinetic profile given that it was almost undetectable in bone after 12 h.

The Rat Model

The rat model of chronic osteomyelitis is a more difficult therapeutic model because no cure is achievable and results are expressed by changes in the number of microorganisms per gram of bone. Two interesting studies were performed in the rat model of chronic osteomyelitis due to MRSA (length of thera-

Table 1. Spectrum of microorganisms responsible for osteomyelitis in adults

Microorganism	Acute osteomyelitis[a]	Chronic osteomyelitis[b]	Osteomyelitis and diabetes[c]	Infected orthopedic implant[d]
Staphylococcus aureus	+++	++	++	++
Staphylococcus epidermidis	−	+	+	+++
Gram-negative rods	++	++	+	−
Streptococci	(+)	+	+	+
Anaerobes	(+)	+	++	+
Candida species	(+)	−	−	−

[a] Frequently single culture.
[b] Frequently mixed culture.
[c] Frequently mixed culture with anaerobes.
[d] Frequently single culture.

py, 21 to 30 days). In a study by Henry et al., van-comycin performed poorly, ciprofloxacin had an intermediate activity, and the best results were obtained by the addition of rifampin to both regimens (27). Similarly, in a study by Dworkin et al., vancomycin and the quinolones ciprofloxacin and pefloxacin were ineffective when given alone, but their combination with rifampin gave highly satisfactory results (15). In a recent study by Monzon et al., cefuroxime demonstrated the best activity in reducing the number of bacteria in biofilms adhering to implants relative to vancomycin, tobramycin, and ciprofloxacin (45).

Models with the Presence of a Foreign Implant

Additional studies of therapy in the presence of foreign implants, representing a much more difficult experimental situation, have been performed by various groups. Bouchenaki et al. have studied the prophylactic activity of various quinolones in a guinea pig model of *S. aureus* foreign-body infections (2). Ciprofloxacin and ofloxacin in single doses demonstrated poor efficacy but this could be improved by the administration of a second dose. Lucet et al. have studied the role of fleroxacin, vancomycin, and rifampin alone or in combination for the short therapy (1 week) of a chronic staphylococcal foreign-body infection. The combination of fleroxacin-rifampin proved to be the optimal therapy both to decrease bacterial cell counts as well as to prevent development of resistance to rifampin (40). Chuard et al. (6) extended these studies by prolonging the antimicrobial therapy for 3 weeks. Although fleroxacin-rifampin continued to prove efficient and sterilized the fluid surrounding the prosthesis, surface-attached bacteria could still be detected. In contrast, the triple combination of vancomycin-fleroxacin-rifampin proved highly efficient and sterilized the surface of the implants in most cases (6). Cremieux et al. have demonstrated the efficacy of sparfloxacin, in addition to its autoradiographic distribution pattern, in the rabbit model of *S. aureus* joint prosthesis infection. The radiographic levels of sparfloxacin detected were higher around the prosthesis than those of pefloxacin and those in the control group (9). These results underscore the importance of an antimicrobial with prolonged half-life in the prevention and/or therapy of infection associated with foreign bodies. The above-mentioned studies indicate that quinolone-rifampin combination regimens may offer a nonparenteral option for the treatment of chronic osteomyelitis caused by *S. aureus*, even in the presence of foreign implants. Combination therapy with quinolones, rifampin, and other antimicrobials may prove to be a successful approach in the future.

Penetration of Quinolones into Bone by Using Experimental Drug-Carrier Systems

Several recent studies show interesting results concerning the potential utilization of quinolones in local drug-carrier systems that allow high local antibiotic concentrations to be achieved. These studies show good bone concentrations of quinolones using cement beads in rabbits with biodegradable delivery systems containing ofloxacin, pefloxacin, or ciprofloxacin. Also used as carriers were polylactides-coglycolides or biodegradable polymers containing quinolones in the rabbit model. The experimental drug carriers had been tested in the prophylaxis and therapy of experimental bone infection. Nicolau et al. showed the usefulness of this prophylaxis in acute *S. aureus* osteomyelitis in the rabbit with absorbable ofloxacin-impregnated beads (46). These rabbits had lower infection rates as compared with the control group. Nie et al. showed good therapeutic efficacy by the use of a bioabsorbable polymer for the delivery of ofloxacin during experimental osteomyelitis treatment in rabbits (47). Both ofloxacin polymer in the presence or absence of systemic ofloxacin improved the rates of sterilization of *Pseudomonas* infection.

Kanellakopoulou et al. have demonstrated the efficacy of biodegradable systems for the local release of pefloxacin in the treatment of *S. aureus* osteomyelitis in the rabbit model. A 99.9% decrease in the viable count of bacteria was achieved by day 12 with complete bacterial eradication on day 33 (32).

Fractures Exposed to Quinolones

An experimental investigation performed at the Mayo Clinic by Huddleston et al. (31) suggests that fractures exposed to ciprofloxacin may compromise the clinical course of fracture healing. Fracture calluses in the animals treated with ciprofloxacin showed abnormalities in the cartilage morphology and a significant decrease in the number of chondrocytes compared with the controls (31). The clinical significance of this finding remains to be shown.

Concentration of Quinolones in Human Bone

Different clinical studies have assessed the concentration reached by quinolones (ciprofloxacin, pefloxacin, and ofloxacin) in human bone (43, 44, 65). Most were performed in patients undergoing total hip arthroplasty and, in some cases, in those treated for bone infection.

Although these measurements have several methodological problems (methods of extraction, blood contamination, different kinetics of bone to serum), they are useful because they provide an estimate of levels achievable in bone and allow comparison with the MIC of infecting microorganisms. However, it should be noted that most of the studies were performed with "normal" bone, and few data are available in the presence of infection. The values achieved were proportional to the dose of quinolone given. The ratio of peak bone to peak serum drug concentrations ranged between 0.25 and 0.66 for various quinolones. With peak concentrations between 1 and 2 μg/μg for the most frequently used quinolones (ciprofloxacin and ofloxacin, while higher levels were obtained with pefloxacin), the levels in bone were significantly higher than the MIC_{90} for *Enterobacteriaceae* and within the range of susceptibility of many staphylococci but not all *Pseudomonas* spp. When compared with previous data on concentrations of β-lactams or cephalosporins in bone, quinolone concentrations were in the therapeutic range (8, 12, 16).

Clinical Studies

Several elements play a role in the difficulty in evaluating the efficacy of treatment during osteomyelitis. First, adequate surgical debridement is a major factor for the success of therapy, and its adequacy is often difficult to assess. Second, the removal of infected foreign material also is a major determinant of outcome. Adequate concentrations of the antibiotic must be maintained in bone for prolonged periods, i.e., at least 4 to 6 weeks for acute infections and often much longer for chronic infection. Even this approach does not guarantee success because of potential differential distribution of the antibiotic in different parts of the bone (cortex, medulla, and periosteum). In addition, the specific physiochemical conditions of a focus of osteomyelitis and arthritis with a low pH will increase the MIC of quinolones. Finally, the presence of dead bone and foreign material will lead to failure if a combined surgical (debridement and removal of foreign material) and medical approach is not applied. Clinical success is defined as the resolution of all signs and symptoms of active disease at the end of therapy and after a significantly long posttreatment observation period (40, 46).

Treatment of Chronic Osteomyelitis with Quinolones

Several recent reviews of the use of various agents in the therapy of osteomyelitis have reported that among the quinolones presently available, ciprofloxacin, ofloxacin, and pefloxacin have been used most often in large series of patients with bacterial osteomyelitis.

Nonprospective and Open Studies

Most of the studies performed so far with quinolones are open, nonprospective (or sequential), and noncomparative. In these studies, the most frequently identified bacterial organism was *S. aureus*. Ciprofloxacin has been the most widely used quinolone for bacterial osteomyelitis. The usual dosage was 750 mg twice daily for periods usually ranging from 6 weeks to several months. Tolerance was good; 28% of patients were reported to have adverse effects, but most were minor (nausea, alteration in liver enzymes, or rash). Rates of clinical success after follow-up ranging from 2 to 21 months indicate 56% cure, 11% improvement, and 32% failure (10, 24, 27–30, 45, 54, 56, 59, 60, 61, 66).

Pefloxacin was given in few studies. The usual dosage was 400 mg every 8 h with a duration of treatment of between 2 and 6 months. Eighty-two percent of patients had minor adverse effects that allowed continuation of treatment; in the two studies where adverse effects were reported, the rates of clinical success for follow-up ranged from 2 to 84 months with 80% cure, 3% improvement, and 17% failure (34).

Ofloxacin was given to 341 patients in three open studies (21, 33, 57). The usual dosage was 200 mg every 8 to 12 h. Average duration of treatment was three to six weeks. Tolerance was excellent, with only 2% reporting secondary effects. The rate of clinical success after a follow-up of 6 months was 89%. The microbial group with the highest failure rate was *Pseudomonas* spp.

More recently, Greenberg et al. (25) have analyzed the efficacy and safety of three oral fluoroquinolones (levofloxacin, lomefloxacin, and ciprofloxacin) for the treatment of 27 patients with chronic osteomyelitis. The average duration therapy was 60.6 days and the average follow-up without antibiotic was 11.8 months. Therapy was effective for levofloxacin in 9 of 15 patients (60%), lomefloxacin, 5 of 7 patients (71%), and ciprofloxacin, 2 of 5 patients (40%). Another recent study by Ortega et al. (52) analyzed the tolerability and safety of levofloxacin for long-term treatment of ten patients with prosthetic joint infections and five with chronic osteomyelitis. The mean duration of therapy was 3.6 months, and levofloxacin was well tolerated, but efficacy of treatment was not provided.

Comparative Studies

Although well performed, most of the comparative studies reported are too small to allow any statistical conclusions to be made. Cumulative data analysis of four studies in which oral ciprofloxacin, usually given as 750 mg every 12 h (total number of patients treated, 94), was compared with various parenteral antibiotic combinations (total number of patients treated, 91) shows that patients treated with ciprofloxacin had 81% success, 2% improvement, and 17% failure. In the group with various parenteral therapies, the success and failure rates were 85 and 15%, respectively. Adverse effects with parenteral antibiotics were frequently severe (16%) and included phlebitis and leukopenia.

Differences between the two treatment groups, however, did not reach statistical significance. To demonstrate the equivalence ($P < 0.05$) between the two treatment arms in a well-designed clinical trial would require the involvement of at least 392 patients in each group, assuming a cure rate of 80% ($\pm 10\%$) with a study power of 0.8 (11, 17, 19, 20, 25, 34, 39).

In a recent small study, Gomis et al. (23) reported a prospective, randomized comparison of oral ofloxacin and intravenous imipenem-cilastatin for the treatment of 32 patients with chronic osteomyelitis. Oral ofloxacin therapy was as effective as parenteral therapy with intravenous imipenem-cilastatin.

Quinolones and Diabetic Osteomyelitis

Although quite popular for the treatment of chronic osteomyelitis, data on the use of quinolones for this type of infection are sparse. In the presence of severe vascular disease, failure is common regardless of the antibiotic regimen used. An open study by Peterson et al. in 29 patients treated with ciprofloxacin showed a successful outcome of 65% after 1 year (54). These good results were tempered by the study of Nix et al. (48), which showed a successful outcome in only 7 of 24 patients (29%), after a one-year follow-up. Lipsky et al. reported a 71% success rate with ofloxacin in 21 patients with diabetic osteomyelitis (38).

Open Fracture Wounds

Patzakis et al. (53) analyzed a prospective, randomized study comparing ciprofloxacin with cefamandole and gentamicin in open fracture wounds. They showed a high failure rate for ciprofloxacin in the type III open fracture group, with the wounds being five times more likely to become infected than in the combination therapy group.

Treatment of infected orthopedic implants

On the basis of considerable experience from animal experiments as previously described, Drancourt et

al. analyzed a prospective cohort of 47 evaluable patients with *Staphylococcus*-infected orthopedic implants treated with oral rifampin (900 mg/day) plus ofloxacin (600 mg/day). Hip prostheses were treated for 6 months, and the prosthesis was removed after 5 months of therapy if it was unstable. Knee prostheses or bone plates were treated for 9 and 6 months, respectively, with all the prostheses removed after 6 and 3 months. The overall success rate was 74%. Eight failures were related to resistant bacteria. In 13 of 21 patients cured, the prosthesis was not removed, whereas in 23 of 26 patients cured, the prosthesis was removed (14). In two studies, Zimmerli et al. (67) treated early staphyloccocal orthopedic device-related infection with oral ciprofloxacin in the presence or absence of rifampin in a double-blind, randomized trial. Thirty-three patients with stable orthopedic device infection (hip and knee prostheses, or internal fixation) underwent surgery without removal of the prosthesis. After an initial 2 weeks of flucloxacillin or vancomycin therapy (with rifampin or placebo), patients were treated from 3 to 6 months (6 months for knee) with ciprofloxacin (500 mg twice daily orally) and rifampin (900 mg per day orally), or placebo (instead of rifampin). In the presence of rifampin, a 100% success rate was demonstrated for the 12 *S. aureus*-infected patients. In the group treated with ciprofloxacin and placebo, four failures in the *S. aureus*-infected patients were observed and one failure in the four cases of *S. epidermidis* disease was observed (63). In the latter case, the strain was identified as identical to the initial infecting microorganism by typing and showed the development of ciprofloxacin resistance. Brouqui et al. (4) attempted to treat *P. aeruginosa*-infected prostheses with ciprofloxacin in combination with ceftazidime, which was administered for 6 weeks followed by oral ciprofloxacin for an extended period. Interestingly, combination therapy cured 9 of 9 patients with infected osteosynthetic material and 4 of 5 patients with a hip or knee prosthesis (4).

These data continue to indicate that a minority of prosthetic infections can be cured by quinolone-containing regimens without prosthesis removal. However, these studies also suggest that antibiotic therapy for *S. aureus* infections may assist the surgeon, possibly allowing one-step exchange arthroplasty after treatment with ciprofloxacin plus rifampin by substantially reducing the number of residual organisms at the time of replacement of the prosthesis.

SUMMARY

An analysis of publications on the topic of quinolones and osteomyelitis during the last 10 or more years allows several conclusions, which are summarized below.

1. Animal models have shown the following characteristics:
   • excellent penetration of quinolones into bone;
   • excellent results in osteomyelitis due to gram-negative rods;
   • in combination with rifampin, good results in osteomyelitis due to staphylococci, even in the presence of a foreign body;
   • in the presence of a foreign body, excellent results with triple therapy (addition of vancomycin to a quinolone and to rifampin), even against surface-adherent MRSA.

2. Concentrations of quinolones in human bone appear satisfactory with levels achieved that are higher than the MIC_{90} for *Enterobacteriaceae*, in the range of MIC_{90} for methicillin-sensitive staphylococci and above the MIC for a significant proportion of strains of *P. aeruginosa*.

3. Unfortunately, most of the clinical studies performed with quinolones in osteomyelitis are open, often without clear definition, thus indicating a bias in selection and follow-up of these patients (42, 49).

4. In a specific situation, such as diabetic osteomyelitis, use of antimicrobials with a wider spectrum (in combinations that include antianaerobe coverage) appears to be a wise recommendation at present.

5. A few good comparative studies have been performed, but the number of patients recruited was low and, therefore, no statistical conclusion could be drawn from individual trials. Combining the results of all the studies of ciprofloxacin compared with parenteral therapy (>90 patients in each arm) suggests success rates of more than 80% for both arms.

6. Microbiological analysis of osteomyelitis cases treated with oral ciprofloxacin shows success rates of 92% for *Enterobacteriaceae* (and even higher if one excludes cases of *Serratia* infection), 72% for *P. aeruginosa*, and 75% for *S. aureus*. Analysis of the data revealed osteomyelitis due to *P. aeruginosa* or *S. aureus* to be associated with a fourfold increase in failure rate (odds ratio, 3.85; 95% confidence interval, 1.97 to 7.50, $P < 0.001$) compared with osteomyelitis due to other pathogens (36).

7. In the case of osteomyelitis due to *Enterobacteriaceae*, the success rates are so good that no further trials appear necessary.

8. For osteomyelitis due to *S. aureus* or *P. aeruginosa*, and in particular in the presence of a foreign body, well-performed comparative studies with more classical parenteral therapy appear necessary. These studies should be performed in a sufficiently high number of patients to allow statistical conclusions.

9. The combination of quinolones with rifampin for the treatment of staphylococcal osteomyelitis appears promising. Further studies in this area should be encouraged to confirm these results and to evaluate newer quinolones with more potent antistaphylococcal activity.

Overall, oral quinolones offer several advantages when compared with parenteral antibiotics, in particular, shorter hospital stay, lower cost, and no adverse effects due to the use of an intravenous line. It can be concluded that oral quinolones have contributed to significant progress in the treatment of osteomyelitis and septic arthritis, which still remain complicated and difficult to treat.

REFERENCES

1. Bayer, A. S., D. Norman, and D. Anderson. 1985. Efficacy of ciprofloxacin in experimental arthritis caused by *Escherichia coli*—in vitro-in vivo correlations. *J. Infect. Dis.* **152**:811–816.

2. Bouchenaki, N., P. E. Vaudaux, E. Huggler, F. A. Waldvogel, and D. P. Lew. 1990. Successful single-dose prophylaxis of *Staphylococcus aureus* foreign body infections in guinea pigs by fleroxacin. *Antimicrob. Agents Chemother.* **34**:21–24.

3. Bouza, E., and P. Munoz. 1999. Micro-organisms responsible for osteoarticular infections. *Baillieres Best Pract. Res. Clin. Rheumatol.* **13**:21–35.

4. Brouqui, P., M. C. Rousseau, A. Stein, M. Drancourt, and D. Raoult. 1995. Treatment of *Pseudomonas aeruginosa*-infected orthopedic prostheses with ceftazidime-ciprofloxacin antibiotic combination. *Antimicrob. Agents Chemother.* **39**:2423–2425.

5. Carek, P. J., L. M. Dickerson, and J. L. Sack. 2001. Diagnosis and management of osteomyelitis. *Am. Fam. Physician* **63**:2413–2412.

6. Chuard, C., M. Herrmann, P. Vaudaux, F. A., Waldvogel, and D. P. Lew. 1991. Successful therapy of experimental chronic foreign-body infection due to methicillin-resistant Staphylococcus aureus by antimicrobial combinations. *Antimicrob. Agents Chemother.* **35**:2611–2616.

7. Cierny, G., J. T. Mader, and H. Pennick. 1985. A clinical staging system of adult osteomyelitis system. *Contemp. Orthop.* **10**:17–37.

8. Coignard, S., C. Renard, and A. Lortat-Jacob. 1986. Diffusion de la pefloxacine dans le tissu osseux humain. *Méd. Mal. Infect.* **7**:471–474.

9. Cremieux, A. C., A. S. Mghir, R. Bleton, M. Manteau, N. Belmatoug, L. Massias, L. Garry, N. Sales, B. Maziere, and C. Carbon. 1996. Efficacy of sparfloxacin and autoradiographic diffusion pattern of [^{14}C]sparfloxacin in experimental *Staphylococcus aureus* joint prosthesis infection. *Antimicrob. Agents Chemother.* **40**:2111–2116.

10. Dan, M., Y. Siegman Igra, S. Pitlik, and R. Raz. 1990. Oral ciprofloxacin treatment of *Pseudomonas aeruginosa* osteomyelitis. *Antimicrob. Agents Chemother.* **34**:849–852.

11. Defino, H. L. A., J. E. Moretti, and A. E. Rodrigues-Fuentes. 1992. Comparative study of the efficacy of pefloxacin versus cephalotin/cephalexin + gentamicin in the treatment of post-traumatic or post-surgical osteomyelitis. *Rev. Bras. Med.* **49**:785–790.

12. Dellamonica, P., E. Bernard, H. Etesse, and R. Garraffo. 1986. The diffusion of pefloxacin into bone and the treatment of osteomyelitis. *J. Antimicrob. Chemother.* **17**(Suppl. B):93–102.

13. Desplaces, N., and J. F. Acar. 1988. New quinolones in the treatment of joint and bone infections. *Rev. Infect. Dis.* **10**(Suppl. 1):S179–S183.

14. Drancourt, M., A. Stein, J. N. Argenson, A. Zannier, G. Curvale, and D. Raoult. 1993. Oral rifampin plus ofloxacin for treatment of *Staphylococcus*-infected orthopedic implants. *Antimicrob. Agents Chemother.* **37**:1214–1218.

15. Dworkin, R., G. Modin, S. Kunz, R. Rich, O. Zak, and M. Sande. 1990. Comparative efficacies of ciprofloxacin, pefloxacin, and vancomycin in combination with rifampin in a rat model of methicillin-resistant *Staphylococcus aureus* chronic osteomyelitis. *Antimicrob. Agents Chemother.* **34**:1014–1016.

16. Fong, I.W., W. H. Ledbetter, A. C. Vandenbroucke, M. Simbul, and V. Rahm. 1986. Ciprofloxacin concentrations in bone and muscle after oral dosing. *Antimicrob. Agents Chemother.* **29**:405–408.

17. Galanakis, N., H. Giamarellou, T. Moussas, E. Dounis. 1997. Chronic osteomyelitis caused by multi-resistant gram-negative bacteria: evaluation of treatment with newer quinolones after prolonged follow-up. *J. Antimicrob. Chemother.* **39**:241–246.

18. Garcia Rosario, L. N., and C. H. Ramirez Ronda. 1990. The use of ciprofloxacin in patients with osteomyelitis associated with vascular insufficiency. *Bol. Assoc. Med. P. R.* **82**:125–128.

19. Gentry, L. O., and G. G. Rodriguez. 1990. Oral ciprofloxacin compared with parenteral antibiotics in the treatment of osteomyelitis. *Antimicrob. Agents Chemother.* **34**:40–43.

20. Gentry, L. O. 1991. Oral antimicrobial therapy for osteomyelitis. *Ann. Intern. Med.* **114**:986–987.

21. Gentry, L. O., and G. G. Rodriguez. 1991. Ofloxacin versus parenteral therapy for chronic osteomyelitis. *Antimicrob. Agents Chemother.* **35**:538–541.

22. Gilbert, D. N., A. D. Tice, P. K. Marsh, P. C. Craven, and L. C. Preheim. 1987. Oral ciprofloxacin therapy for chronic contiguous osteomyelitis caused by aerobic gram-negative bacilli. *Am. J. Med.* **82**:254–258.

23. Gomis, M., J. Barberan, B. Sanchez, S. Khorrami, J. Borja, and J. Garcia-Barbal. 1999. Oral ofloxacin versus parenteral imipenem-cilastatin in the treatment of osteomyelitis. *Rev. Esp. Quimioter* **12**:244–9.

24. Greenberg, R. N., D. J. Kennedy, P. M. Reilly, K. L. Luppen, W. J. Weinandt, M. R. Bollinger, F. Aguirre, F. Kodesch, A. M. Saeed. 1987. Treatment of bone, joint, and soft-tissue infections with oral ciprofloxacin. *Antimicrob. Agents Chemother.* **31**:151–155.

25. Greenberg, R. N., M. T. Newman, S. Shariaty, and R. W. Pectol. 2000. Ciprofloxacin, lomefloxacin, or levofloxacin as treatment for chronic osteomyelitis. *Antimicrob. Agents Chemother.* **44**:164–166.

26. Greenberg, R. N., A. D. Tice, P. K. Marsh, P. C. Craven, P. M. Reilly, M. Bollinger, and W. J. Weinandt. 1987. Randomized trial of ciprofloxacin compared with other antimicrobial therapy in the treatment of osteomyelitis. *Am. J. Med.* **82**:266–269.

27. Henry, N. K., M. S. Rouse, A. L. Whitesell, M. E. McConnell, and W. R. Wilson. 1987. Treatment of methicillin-resistant *Staphylococcus aureus* experimental osteomyelitis with ciprofloxacin or vancomycin alone or in combination with rifampin. *Am. J. Med.* **82**:73–75.

28. Hessen, M. T., M. J. Ingerman, D. H. Kaufman, M. T. Hessen, M. J. Ingerman, D. H. Kaufman, P. Weiner, J.

Santoro, O. M. Korzeniowski, J. Boscia, M. Topiel, L. M. Bush, and D. Kaye.. 1987. Clinical efficacy of ciprofloxacin therapy for gram-negative bacillary osteomyelitis. *Am. J. Med.* **82**:262–265.

29. Hessen, M. T., and M. E. Levison. 1989. Ciprofloxacin for the treatment of osteomyelitis: a review. *J. Foot Surg.* **28**:100–105.

30. Hoogkamp-Korstanje, J. A., H. A. van Bottenburg, J. van Bruggen, J. S. Davidson, S. J. Detmar, W. de Graaf, J. Rijnks, J. F. Ypma, D. F. de Zwart. 1989. Treatment of chronic osteomyelitis with ciprofloxacin. *J. Antimicrob. Chemother.* **23**:427–432.

31. Huddleston, P. M., J. M. Steckelberg, A. D. Hanssen, M. S. Rouse, M. E. Bolander, and R. Patel. 2000. Ciprofloxacin inhibition of experimental fracture healing. *J. Bone Joint Surg.* **82**:161–173.

32. Kanellakopoulou, K., N. Galanakis, E. J. Giamarellos-Bourboulis, C. Rifiotis, K. Papakostas, A. Andreopoulos, E. Dounis, P. Karagianakos, H. Giamarellou. 2000. Treatment of experimental osteomyelitis caused by methicillin-resistant *Staphylococcus aureus* with a biodegradable system of lactic acid polymer releasing pefloxacin. *J. Antimicrob. Chemother.* **46**:311–314.

33. Ketterl, R., T. Beckurts, B. Stubinger, and B. Claudi. 1988. Use of ofloxacin in open fractures and in the treatment of posttraumatic osteomyelitis. *J. Antimicrob. Chemother.* **22**(Suppl C):S159–S166.

34. Ketterl, R., W. Wittwer, and T. Beckurts. 1995. Ofloxacin zur antibiotikatherapie bei der chronischen posttraumatischen Osteitis. *Med. Welt.* **46**:505–511.

35. Lew, D. P., and F. A. Waldvogel. 1993. Use of quinolones for treatment of osteomyelitis and septic arthritis, p. 371–379. *In* D. C. Hooper and J. S. Wolfson (ed.), *Quinolone Antimicrobial Agents*, 2nd ed. American Society for Microbiology, Washington, D.C.

36. Lew, D. P., and F. A. Waldvogel. 1999. Quinolones and osteomyelitis: state-of-the-art. *Drugs.* **4958**(Suppl. 2):S85100–S91110.

37. Lew, D. P., and F. A. Waldvogel. 1997. Osteomyelitis. *N. Engl. J. Med.* **336**:999–1007.

38. Lipsky, B. A., P. D. Baker, G. C. Landon, and R. Fernau. 1997. Antibiotic therapy for diabetic foot infections: comparison of two parenteral-to-oral regimens. *Clin. Infect. Dis.* **24**:643–648.

39. Lipsky, B. A. 1997. Osteomyelitis of the foot in diabetic patients. *Clin. Infect. Dis.* **25**:1318–1326.

40. Lucet, J. C., M. Herrmann, P. Rohner, R. Auckenthaler, F. A. Waldvogel, and D. P. Lew. 1990. Treatment of experimental foreign body infection caused by methicillin-resistant Staphylococcus aureus. *Antimicrob. Agents Chemother.* **34**:2312–2317.

41. Mader, J. T., J. S. Cantrell, and J. Calhoun. 1990. Oral ciprofloxacin compared with standard parenteral antibiotic therapy for chronic osteomyelitis in adults. *J. Bone Joint Surg.* **72**:104–110.

42. Mader, J. T., C. Norden, J. D. Nelson, and G. B. Calandra. 1992. Evaluation of new anti-infective drugs for the treatment of osteomyelitis in adults. Infectious Diseases Society of America and the Food and Drug Administration. *Clin. Infect. Dis.* **15**(Suppl. 1):S155–S16.

43. Meissner, A., and K. Borner. 1993. Konzentration von Ciprofloxacin im Knochengewebe Concentration of Ciproloxacin in Bone Tissue. *Akt. Traumatol.* **23**:80–84.

44. Meissner, A., K. Borner, and P. Koeppe. 1990. Concentrations of ofloxacin in human bone and in cartilage. *J. Antimicrob. Chemother.* **26**(Suppl. D):69–74.

45. Monzon, M., F. Garcia-Alvarez, A. Lacleriga, E. Gracia, J. Leiva, C. Oteiza, and B. Amorena. 2001. A simple infection

model using pre-colonized implants to reproduce rat chronic *Staphylococcus aureus* osteomyelitis and study antibiotic treatment. *J. Orthop. Res.* **19**:820–826.

46. **Nicolau, D. P., L. Nie, P. R. Tessier, H. P. Kourea, and C. H. Nightingale.** 1998. Prophylaxis of acute osteomyelitis with asorbable ofloxacin-impregnated beads. *Antimicrob. Agents Chemother.* **42**:840–842.

47. **Nie, L., D. P. Nicolau, P. R. Tessier, H. P. Kourea, B. D. Browner, and C. H. Nightingale.** 1998. Use of a bioabsorbable polymer for the delivery of ofloxacin during experimental osteomyelitis treatment. *J. Orthop. Res.* **16**:76–79.

48. **Nix, D. E., T. J. Cumbo, P. Kuritzky, J. M. DeVito, J. J. Schentag.** 1987. Oral ciprofloxacin in the treatment of serious soft tissue and bone infections. Efficacy, safety, and pharmacokinetics. *Am. J. Med.* **82**:146–153.

49. **Norden, C., J. D. Nelson, J. T. Mader, and G. B. Calandra.** 1992. Evaluation of new anti-infective drugs for the treatment of infectious arthritis in adults. Infectious Diseases Society of America and the Food and Drug Administration. *Clin. Infect. Dis.* **15**(Suppl. 1):S167–S171.

50. **Norden, C. W., and E. Shinners.** 1995. Ciprofloxacin as therapy for experimental osteomyelitis caused by *Pseudomonas aeruginosa. J. Infect. Dis.* **151**:291–294.

51. **Norrby, S. R.** 1989. Ciprofloxacin in the treatment of acute and chronic osteomyelitis: a review. *Scand. J Infect. Dis. Suppl.* **60**(Suppl.):S74–S78.

52. **Ortega, M., A. Soriano, S. Garcia, M. Almela, J. L. Alvarez, X. Tomas, J. Mensa, and E. Soriano.** 2000. Tolerability and safety of levofloxacin long-term treatment. *Rev. Esp. Quimioter* **13**:263–266.

53. **Patzakis, M. J., R. S. Bains, J. Lee, L. Shepherd, G. Singer, R. Ressler, F. Harvey, and P. Holtom.** 2000. Prospective, randomized, double-blind study comparing single-agent antibiotic therapy, ciprofloxacin, to combination antibiotic therapy in open fracture wounds. *J. Orthop. Trauma.* **14**:529–533.

54. **Peterson, L. R., L. M. Lissack, K. Canter, C. E. Fasching, C. Clabots, D. N. Gerding.** 1989. Therapy of lower extremity infections with ciprofloxacin in patients with diabetes mellitus, peripheral vascular disease, or both. *Am. J. Med.* **86**:801–808.

55. **Rissing, J. P.** 1997. Antimicrobial therapy for chronic osteomyelitis in adults: role of the quinolones. *Clin. Infect. Dis.* **25**:1327–1333.

56. **Schlichting, C., C. Branger, J. M. Fournier, W. Witte, A. Boutonnier, C. Wolz, P. Goullet, and G. Doring.** 1993. Typing of *Staphylococcus aureus* by pulsed-field gel electrophoresis, zymotyping, capsular typing, and phage typing: resolution of clonal relationships. *J. Clin. Microbiol.* **31**:227–232.

57. **Seibold, R., and A. Betz.** 1991. Treatment of posttraumatic osteitis with intravenous ofloxacin. *Clin. Ther.* **13**:457–459.

58. **Shirtliff, M. E., J. H. Calhoun, and J. T. Mader.** 2001. Comparative evaluation of oral levofloxacin and parenteral nafcillin in the treatment of experimental methicillin-susceptible *Staphylococcus aureus* osteomyelitis in rabbits. *J. Antimicrob. Chemother.* **48**:253–258.

59. **Swedish Study Group.** 1988. Therapy of acute and chronic gram-negative osteomyelitis with ciprofloxacin. *J. Antimicrob. Chemother.* **22**:221–228.

60. **Trujillo, I. Z., G. Valladares, and A. Nava.** 1993. Ciprofloxacin in the treatment of chronic osteomyelitis in adults. *Drugs* **45**(Suppl. 3):S454–S455.

61. **Waldvogel, F. A.** 1989. Use of quinolones for the treatment of osteomyelitis and septic arthritis. *Rev. Infect. Dis.* **11**:S1259–S1263

62. **Waldvogel, F. A., G. Medoff, and M. N. Swartz.** 1970. Osteomyelitis: a review of clinical features, therapeutic considerations and unusual aspects. *N. Engl. J. Med.* **29**:260–6.

63. **Widmer, A. F., A. Gaechter, P. E. Ochsner, and W. Zimmerli.** 1992. Antimicrobial treatment of orthopedic implant-related infections with rifampin combinations. *Clin. Infect. Dis.* **14**:1251–1253.

64. **Wispelwey, B., and W. M. Scheld.** 1990. Ciprofloxacin in the treatment of *Staphylococcus aureus* osteomyelitis. A review. *Diagn. Microbiol. Infect. Dis.* **13**:169–171.

65. **Wittmann, D. H., and E. Kotthaus.** 1986. Further methodological improvement in antibiotic bone concentration measurements: penetration of ofloxacin into bone and cartilage. *Infection* **14**(Suppl. 4):S270–S273

66. **Yamaguti, A., C. Trevisanello, I. M. Lobo, M. C. Carvano, M. L. Bortoletto, M. L. Silva, R. Brasil Filho, G. C. Levi, and J. S. Mendonca.** 1993. Oral ciprofloxacin for treatment of chronic osteomyelitis. *Int. J. Clin. Pharmacol. Res.* **13**:75–79.

67. **Zimmerli, W., A. F. Widmer, M. Blatter, R. Frei, P. E. Ochsner.** 1998. Foreign-body infection (FBI) study group. Role of rifampin for treatment of orthopedic implant-related staphylococcal infections—a randomized controlled trial. *JAMA* **279**:1537–1541.

Quinolone Antimicrobial Agents, 3rd ed.
Edited by David C. Hooper and Ethan Rubinstein
© 2003 ASM Press, Washington, D.C.

Chapter 16

Treatment of Experimental and Human Bacterial Endocarditis with Quinolone Antimicrobial Agents

THUAN P. LE, MICHAEL R. YEAMAN, AND ARNOLD S. BAYER

The efficacy evaluations of newly developed antimicrobial agents in relevant animal and ex vivo models of infection (e.g., tissue culture) have been an important transitional link between the in vitro activity and human utility of such drugs. A review of the in vitro activity spectra of both new and existing quinolones suggests that these agents might be useful for the therapy of selected patients with bacterial endocarditis (BE), an important human infection. In particular, the newer generations of fluoroquinolone agents possess in vitro activity spectra encompassing organisms associated with particularly recalcitrant forms of BE, including *Staphylococcus aureus* (both methicillin-susceptible [MSSA] and methicillin-resistant [MRSA] strains), *Pseudomonas aeruginosa* (1, 31), and *Coxiella burnetii* (70, 98). The latter forms of BE have been associated with relatively poor clinical outcomes when treated with standard antimicrobial regimens (55, 73).

Experimental animal models of BE provide rigorous tests of the efficacy of any antimicrobial regimen. In experimental BE, infection is induced in rabbits or rats by placing a polyethylene catheter across a heart valve (e.g., aortic or tricuspid) to induce marantic (sterile) endocarditis, which is then followed by seeding of the sterile vegetation with a large bacterial challenge usually administered intravenously (37). The catheter is generally secured in place for the duration of the study. This procedure reliably induces BE in catheterized animals, with infected vegetations containing >10^7 to 10^9 bacteria/g of tissue. Effective antimicrobial agents must sterilize vegetations containing high bacterial densities in the presence of an indwelling foreign body. In addition to a mechanical barrier to antibiotic penetrations provided by the vegetation, many of the organisms in the interstices of the experimental vegetation appear to be in a metabolically inactive phase of growth (stationary [29]), making the efficacy of

cell wall-active antibiotics problematic in the treatment of BE.

Newer quinolone antibiotics appear particularly promising for the treatment of BE because they possess in vitro features that circumvent the above-mentioned therapeutic problems. First, the newer quinolones do not exhibit a pronounced inoculum effect in vitro (an effect seen with many aminoglycosides and β-lactams [87]), and they often remain bactericidal at challenge inocula of ~10^6 to 10^8 CFU/ml, depending on the organism (5, 11, 78). Second, although strain specific, the newer quinolones in some circumstances exert bactericidal activity against stationary-phase bacteria in vitro (100). Third, the newer quinolones remain relatively active at acidic pH, a microenvironment found with metastatic abscesses complicating BE (e.g., renal abscesses) (4, 5). Fourth, quinolones distribute well throughout experimental cardiac vegetations (26). Fifth, quinolones often exhibit concentration-dependent killing kinetics in vivo, such that increases in administered doses result in roughly proportional increases in bacterial killing (42); and finally, quinolones appear to act synergistically with host-defense cells such as leukocytes.

This chapter concentrates predominantly on a detailed analysis of the results of quinolone treatment protocols in discriminative animal models of BE that may be relevant to the treatment of human BE. In addition, the available literature on the efficacy of quinolones in human BE is summarized.

RELEVANT TISSUE PENETRATION OF NEWER-GENERATION QUINOLONES IN BE

An interesting study by Endtz et al. (32) compared the in vitro activities of a panel of fluoroquinolones with bacterial isolates from patients with

Thuan P. Le • Division of Pediatric Infectious Diseases, Harbor-UCLA Medical Center, 1124 West Carson St., E-6, Torrance, CA 90509. **Michael R. Yeaman and Arnold S. Bayer** • Division of Adult Infectious Diseases, Harbor-UCLA Medical Center, 1000 West Carson St., Bldg. RB2, Torrance, CA 90509.

endocarditis, as compared with isolates from patients with other bloodstream infections. Isolates included MSSA and MRSA, viridans group streptococci, and enterococci. In this analysis, most of the quinolones tested demonstrated generally good activity against many of the isolates studied. The relative rank in MICs at which 90% of the isolates tested are inhibited (MIC_{90}) of fluoroquinolones tested (in order of greatest activity) was trovafloxacin > sparfloxacin > ciprofloxacin = ofloxacin > pefloxacin. For example, trovafloxacin was 4- to 64-fold more active than ciprofloxacin against a comparative panel of isolates. These results underscore that the therapeutic efficacy of a fluoroquinolone results from a combination of its activity against the specific pathogen, as well as its ability to penetrate into relatively complex biomatrices such as platelet-fibrin clots that make up the infected cardiac vegetation.

As noted above, infected cardiac vegetations represent a nidus of infection in which reduced antibiotic penetration (due to mechanical barriers) and high densities of bacteria combine to present special problems in the therapy of BE. However, data from experimental BE models and from human pharmacokinetic studies suggest that quinolones may be potentially useful in the prophylaxis and/or treatment of human BE. For example, Contrepois et al. (25) showed that pefloxacin, given intravenously at 15 mg/kg of body weight, achieved peak levels of ~20 and 40 μg/g in the aortic valves of healthy rabbits and those with *Escherichia coli* BE, respectively. Moreover, when this dose was repeated every 12 h, intravegetation *E. coli* titers in animals with BE were significantly reduced compared with untreated controls. In contrast, our laboratory previously demonstrated that pefloxacin penetrated poorly into the vegetations of animals with aortic BE due to MRSA. After single intravenous doses of 20 or 40 mg/kg, mean peak concentrations within aortic vegetations were ~1.5 and 3 μg/g, respectively (6). These intravegetation concentrations were significantly lower than those typically achieved after a single intravenous dose of vancomycin (15 mg/kg). These differences in the abilities of pefloxacin and vancomycin to penetrate MRSA-infected aortic vegetations were also mirrored in vivo (i.e., vancomycin caused a more rapid decline in intravegetation MRSA densities than did pefloxacin at both dose regimens). Disparities in the levels of drug achieved within vegetations in the latter study, as compared with that of Contrepois et al. may relate either to differences in the route of administration (intravenous infusion [25] versus intravenous bolus [6]), or to methods of preparing vegetations for tissue drug assays (i.e., in the latter study, vegetations were care-

fully dried after removal to evaporate extravascular fluid contamination).

As a corollary to the investigations above, Brion et al. (19) studied the penetration of pefloxacin into abnormal cardiac valves of humans undergoing open heart surgery for prosthetic valve insertion. They showed that a single 800-mg intravenous dose of pefloxacin achieved mean peak levels of ~2 to 9 μg/g in such valves 4 to 24 h after infusion. Additionally, the mean ratios of valve-to-plasma pefloxacin concentrations were often >1.0, suggesting complete penetration from the vascular to the tissue compartment. Moreover, the levels of pefloxacin in vegetations were well above the pefloxacin minimal bactericidal concentrations (MBCs) for 90% of the valvular pathogens tested, including viridans group streptococci, enterococci, MRSA, MSSA, and *P. aeruginosa*. Carbon et al. (21) have also demonstrated that quinolones are rapidly bactericidal in experimental BE, and also induce prolonged in vivo postantibiotic effects, allowing for long intervals between dosing without the loss of efficacy. Cremieux et al. studied the diffusion of ^{14}C-labeled temafloxacin within cardiac vegetations using quantitative autoradiography (26). These investigators used a left-sided rabbit model of nutritionally variant streptococcal BE, receiving either radiolabeled temafloxacin (8 μg/ml concentration in serum) or radiolabeled penicillin (20 μg/ml concentration in serum). Temafloxacin distributed homogeneously throughout the vegetations, and also demonstrated a superior in vitro time-kill curve compared with penicillin; moreover, both agents reduced mean bacterial counts in vegetations to equivalent levels. Collectively, these pharmacokinetic and pharmacodynamic data from human patients and from the experimental BE model suggest that, in selected circumstances, newer-generation quinolones with long half-lives penetrate sufficiently into BE lesions to be useful in the prophylaxis or treatment of human BE.

EFFICACY OF NEWER-GENERATION QUINOLONES IN EXPERIMENTAL BE

A tabular summary of published data on various quinolone agents in experimental BE models is presented in Table 1.

Staphylococcus aureus

Pohlod et al. (66) demonstrated that fleroxacin, ciprofloxacin, and difloxacin were active in vitro against human BE isolates of MRSA and MSSA, with MICs for 90% of strains of ≤1.0 μg for these agents.

Table 1. Summary of in vivo activity of fluoroquinolones in animal endocarditis models[a]

Organism (references)	Agents	Comparator	Efficacy outcomes
MSSA (22, 34, 86)	Pefloxacin (P)	Cephalothin (Ct)	P = Ct
	Ciprofloxacin (C)	Nafcillin (N)	C = N
	Levofloxacin (L)	Flucoxacillin (F)	L = F
MRSA (9, 22, 34, 39, 49, 51, 86)	Pefloxacin (P)	Vancomycin (V)	P = V
	Ciprofloxacin (C)	Vancomycin (V)	C = V
	Enoxacin (E)	Vancomycin (V)	E = V
	Trovafloxacin (T)	Vancomycin (V)	T = V
	Trovafloxacin (T)	Vancomycin (V)	T = V
	Trovafloxacin (T)	Vancomycin (V)	T = V
		Ampicillin-sulbactam (U)	T = U
	Levofloxacin (L)	Vancomycin (V)	L = V
MRSE (51, 75)	Ciprofloxacin (C)	Vancomycin (V)	C > V
	Trovafloxacin (T)	Vancomycin (V)	T = V
VRE (59, 68, 91, 99)	Ciprofloxacin (C)	Rifampin (R)/gentamicin (G)	R = R+C = R+C+G
	Ciprofloxacin (C)	Novobiocin (N)	C+N > N
	Ciprofloxacin (C)	Ampicillin (A)	C+ P < P+G
	Clinafloxacin (Cl)	± Penicillin (P)	Cl+P> Cl alone or P alone
VGS (24, 33, 65)	Sparfloxacin (S)	Ceftriaxone (Cx)	S < Cx
	Trovafloxacin (T)	Penicillin (P)	T < P
	Levofloxacin (L)	Penicillin (P)	L < P
P. aeruginosa (5, 8, 47, 92)	Ciprofloxacin (C)	Ceftazidime (Cd)	C > Cd
	Ciprofloxacin (C)	Azlocillin (A)	C = A
	Pefloxacin (P)	Ceftazidime (Cd)	P > Cd
	Pefloxacin (P)	± Fosfomycin (F)	P + F > P
	Ciprofloxacin (C)	± Fosfomycin (F)	C + F > C
Enterobacteriaceae (16)	Enoxacin (E)	± Cefoperazone (Cp)	E > Cp
	Difloxacin (D)	± Fosfomycin (F)	D > Cp

[a]VGS, viridans group streptococci; VRE, vancomycin-resistant enterococci.

Furthermore, these investigators did not detect selection or emergence of resistance in vitro among isolates after exposure to fleroxacin, amifloxacin, or ofloxacin, whereas resistance in these isolates did follow exposure to other quinolone drugs.

Sullam et al. (86) compared pefloxacin with cephalothin in experimental MSSA BE, and with vancoymcin in MRSA BE. Cephalothin and pefloxacin were equally effective in reducing MSSA-induced mortality and intravegetation densities as compared with untreated controls. Likewise, both pefloxacin and vancomycin significantly reduced mortality and vegetation densities due to MRSA, as compared with untreated controls. In a similar study, Carpenter et al. (22) confirmed that ciprofloxacin was as effective as nafcillin in experimental MSSA aortic BE, and as effective as vancomycin in experimental MRSA aortic BE, in reducing intravegetation staphylococcal densities. Kaatz et al. (49) also demonstrated equivalent efficacies of intravenously administered ciprofloxacin and vancomycin in reducing intravegetation MRSA densities as compared with untreated controls. They also confirmed significant reductions in BE-related intrarenal and intrasplenic MRSA abscesses when either ciprofloxacin or vancomycin was used. Moreover,

Kaatz et al. (49, 50) showed that multiple-dose pharmacokinetics of ciprofloxacin in infected animals were markedly different from those that were predicted from single-dose pharmacokinetics in uninfected rabbits. Of particular importance were the higher-than-predicted peak serum ciprofloxacin levels in rabbit BE after multiple-drug doses. This difference was postulated to be related to a decreased clearance of ciprofloxacin due to BE-induced renal dysfunction. Lastly, no ciprofloxacin resistance was noted among MRSA organisms that survived in cardiac vegetations (49).

The development of ciprofloxacin resistance in vivo during treatment of experimental BE has been well documented (50, 53). In these studies, ciprofloxacin-resistant clones of *S. aureus* were observed in 12.5% of all animals treated (50). The mechanisms of ciprofloxacin resistance in *S. aureus* strains recovered from experimental BE have been investigated (50, 53). Two such isolates have exhibited decreased ciprofloxacin-mediated inhibition of DNA synthesis, suggesting mutations in DNA gyrase (23). The results were similar to previously reported patterns of resistance among animals with quinolone-resistant pseudomonal BE. A third strain possessed an upregulated, energy-dependent quinolone efflux mechanism, which was independent of alterations in the *gyrA* gene product (the A subunit of DNA gyrase) and was transferable to a ciprofloxacin-sensitive *E. coli* host by means of a 2.7-kb chromosomal fragment. Resistance to fleroxacin among MSSA isolates has also been reported in experimental BE (52).

Maserati and colleagues compared the efficacies of sparfloxacin and vancomycin in experimental BE in rabbits caused by MRSA (62). Animals received 25 mg/kg dosing of either agent, although the MIC of sparfloxacin against the challenge strain was approximately 10-fold less than that of vancomycin. Yet no difference was observed between the efficacies of these agents after 4 days of therapy. Moreover, the combination of sparfloxacin and vancomycin yielded no improvement as compared with either agent alone in reducing tissue MRSA density. Similarly, Gilbert et al. studied the comparative efficacies of an orally administered quinolone (enoxacin) versus intravenously administered vancomycin in MRSA aortic valve BE in rabbits (39). These investigators observed that both agents significantly lowered intravegetation MRSA densities during the 5-day treatment period as compared with untreated controls, although the in vivo bactericidal effect of enoxacin occurred earlier than that of vancomycin (at 3 versus 5 days of treatment). Our laboratory has also examined the efficacies of intravenously administered pefloxacin (40 or 80 mg/kg/day) and vancomycin (30 mg/kg/day) in experimental MRSA aortic BE (6). Our results with pefloxacin differ from those of Gilbert et al. (39). As in this latter study, a high-dose regimen of pefloxacin and vancomycin significantly lowered intravegetation MRSA densities after 6 days of treatment as compared with densities in untreated controls. We observed, however, that the onset of bactericidal activity in vivo was more rapid with vancomycin than with pefloxacin. Significant reductions in intravegetation MRSA densities were seen by the third day of treatment only among vancomycin recipients. We examined various pharmacokinetic and pharmacodynamic parameters that might account for the superior effect of vancomycin compared with pefloxacin in this model. The in vitro and ex vivo (i.e., intravegetation) postantibiotic effects against the infecting MRSA strain were virtually identical for pefloxacin and vancomycin. Moreover, the trough bactericidal titers in serum were significantly more profound with pefloxacin. Of interest, despite the superior pharmacokinetic properties of pefloxacin in serum, the penetration of vancomycin in vegetations exceeded that of pefloxacin by 7- to 11-fold. This finding supports the concept of Gengo et al. (38) that suggests that levels of antimicrobial

agents achievable in vegetations may correlate better with therapeutic outcome in experimental BE than levels in serum.

Boscia et al. (17) reported the comparative efficacies of oral difloxacin and enoxacin versus parenteral cefazolin in experimental MSSA aortic valve BE in rabbits. Difloxacin therapy yielded significantly greater reductions of intravegetation bacterial densities than did enoxacin treatment, presumably reflecting the longer serum elimination half-life and higher achievable levels of difloxacin in serum. These workers have also reported that enoxacin and vancomycin had equivalent therapeutic efficacies in treating experimental MRSA BE (39).

More recently, Entenza et al. demonstrated the efficacy of levofloxacin against MSSA and MRSA in experimental BE without the selection of levofloxacin resistance, as described previously with ciprofloxacin (34). In MRSA BE caused by ciprofloxacin-susceptible MRSA, a 3-day levofloxacin regimen sterilized valvular vegetations from 19 of 20 animals, as compared with 8 of 13 for the vancomycin-treated group and 0 of 11 for the control group.

Recently, we evaluated trovafloxacin's activity against MRSA BE in comparison with vancomycin and ampicillin-sulbactam (9). Trovafloxacin was the most rapidly bactericidal agent in vivo. Kim et al. (57) demonstrated that trovafloxacin had efficacy similar to vancomycin in rabbits with left-sided MRSA BE. Of note, the intramuscular administration of vancomycin at a 50-mg/kg dose yielded relatively low peak concentrations compared with those achieved with intravenous (i.v.) administration. In addition, only ciprofloxacin-susceptible MRSA strains were tested. Kaatz et al. confirmed the efficacy of trovafloxacin in MRSA BE, showing equivalent clearance of bacteremia and reduction in vegetation and other target tissue bacterial counts as compared with vancomycin (51). In these studies, no resistance to trovafloxacin developed in vivo in any target tissue.

Staphylococcus epidermidis

Rouse et al. (75) studied the efficacy of ciprofloxacin in methicillin-resistant *S. epidermidis* (MRSE) experimental BE. These investigators evaluated ciprofloxacin (alone or with rifampin) in comparison with teicoplanin or vancomycin (alone or in combination with gentamicin, rifampin, or both). Their data showed that ciprofloxacin alone was more effective at reducing intravegetation MRSE densities than vancomycin alone or in combination with gentamicin. Regimens of ciprofloxacin-rifampin, vancomycin-gentamicin (with or without rifampin) were equally efficacious in reducing intravegetation MRSE densities and were the most active regimens studied.

The treatment of experimental MRSE BE with quinolones was also studied in our laboratory using trovafloxacin. Trovafloxacin, vancomycin, and ampicillin-sulbactam all significantly reduced vegetation MRSE counts to an equivalent degree, as compared with untreated controls (9). In contrast to what we had observed with MRSA, the efficacy of trovafloxacin was not clearly superior to that of vancomycin. This may have been related to the fact that the vancomycin MIC for the MRSE was eightfold less than that of the MRSA strain.

P. aeruginosa

BE due to *P. aeruginosa* remains an important infection among parenteral drug abusers in the United States (73, 82). Experiences in treating this infection in humans and experimental animals have emphasized the difficulties in achieving cures with aminoglycoside-β-lactam regimens alone, especially with left-sided valve involvement (12, 73). Such regimens have been limited by primary drug failures, bacteriologic relapses, and the development of antibiotic resistance in vivo (12, 48, 73).

Our laboratory and others have reported on the efficacies of newer quinolones in experimental *P. aeruginosa* BE. For example, Ingerman et al. examined the relative efficacies of ciprofloxacin versus ceftazidime or cefipime, with and without gentamicin, in the rat model of aortic *P. aeruginosa* BE (47). In vitro, ciprofloxacin exhibited a significantly faster onset of bactericidal action against the infecting pseudomonal strain than did either β-lactam regimen (with or without the addition of gentamicin). These investigators confirmed that ciprofloxacin, but not the β-lactams, exerted a persistent suppression of pseudomonal growth in vitro ("postantibiotic effect") for at least 2.5 h after a brief exposure (2 h) to the drug. In vivo, ciprofloxacin therapy produced significantly greater reductions in pseudomonal bacterial densities within vegetations and more sterile vegetations than any of the β-lactam regimens. This therapeutic difference occurred despite the β-lactam agents being present within infected vegetations at concentrations above the MBCs for periods similar to those observed in the ciprofloxacin-treated animals. This study confirmed the importance of pharmacodynamic parameters such as postantibiotic effect and time-above-MBC at the tissue infection site as dual determinants of the outcome of β-lactam therapy in experimental BE (38).

Our laboratory has also examined the efficacy of ciprofloxacin in rabbit models of experimental tri-

cuspid and aortic valve BE caused by *P. aeruginosa* (5, 8, 10). Comparator drug regimens included combinations of an aminoglycoside (amikacin or netilmicin) with an antipseudomonal penicillin (azlocillin), which were synergistically active against the infecting bacterial strain in vitro. In tricuspid valve BE, ciprofloxacin and the combination of amikacin and azlocillin were equally effective in reducing pseudomonal densities in vegetations as compared with untreated controls. Also, these regimens were equivalent in preventing posttherapy bacteriologic relapse, a substantial problem in the therapy of human pseudomonal BE (8). Moreover, no development of resistance to ciprofloxacin, amikacin, or azlocillin was observed in vivo. The addition of amikacin did not enhance the outcome of ciprofloxacin monotherapy, despite the frequently additive bactericidal effects of such combinations in vitro (43). In aortic valve BE, ciprofloxacin was significantly more effective than a combination of netilmicin-azlocillin in sterilizing vegetations, reducing pseudomonal densities within vegetations, and preventing posttherapy bacteriologic relapses. In contrast, the ciprofloxacin and netilmicin-azlocillin regimens were equally effective in sterilizing renal abscesses. Resistance to azlocillin, but not to ciprofloxacin or netilmicin, was occasionally seen among *P. aeruginosa* strains isolated from cardiac vegetations during the second week of treatment. Development of resistance to β-lactams (e.g., ceftazidime) in the second week of therapy has been noted previously using this model and has been associated with the selection of stably derepressed mutants with constitutive, chromosomally regulated overproduction of type Id β-lactamases (12). Therefore, the ability of the aminoglycoside-β-lactam combination to sterilize renal abscesses, but not vegetations, suggests differential penetration of these agents into these respective tissues. Strunk et al. (85) have also confirmed in experimental BE models that ciprofloxacin was as effective as the synergistically active combination of tobramycin-azlocillin in reducing intrarenal and intravegetation pseudomonal densities as well as in rendering these tissues sterile. Moreover, none of the surviving bacteria from renal tissue or vegetations were resistant to the relevant study drug. Microbiologic relapses were less likely to occur after ciprofloxacin therapy than after tobramycin-azlocillin, although this trend did not reach statistical significance. The equivalent efficacies of the quinolone and the aminoglycoside-β-lactam regimens in the latter study (85) are in contrast to the inferior outcome with similar regimens in our study of aortic BE cited above, possibly relating to differences in the experimental models utilized. For example, in the study by Strunk et al. (85), the catheter was removed approximately 1 h after its placement across the aortic valve and the injection of the pseudomonal inoculum through the catheter; in contrast, in our study, the catheter remained within the left ventricle for the duration of the study while the pseudomonal inoculum was given intravenously. It seems likely that the persistent presence of the foreign body adversely affected the ability of the aminoglycoside-β-lactam regimen to eradicate *P. aeruginosa* from vegetations.

Our laboratory also reported on the efficacy of pefloxacin in experimental aortic valve *P. aeruginosa* BE (7). Pefloxacin was compared with a high-dose combination of amikacin-ceftazidime that exhibited bactericidal synergy against the infecting pseudomonal strain in vitro. Pefloxacin and the combination regimen each significantly reduced bacterial densities within vegetations as compared with untreated controls. As seen in our previous models of aortic pseudomonal BE treated with β-lactams, bacteria isolated from vegetations after 2 weeks of therapy exhibited ceftazidime resistance related to the constitutive overproduction of β-lactamase (5, 12). Morever, as opposed to experiences with ciprofloxacin therapy in this model, intravegetation isolates from pefloxacin recipients showed significant increases (four- to eightfold) in pefloxacin MICs as early as the fourth day of therapy. Among these pefloxacin-resistant variants, increases in ciprofloxacin MICs, as well as pleiotropic resistance to ticarcillin and chloramphenicol, but not to amikacin, ceftazidime, or tetracycline, were also exhibited. Because the MIC increases for our strain were similar to to those caused in *E. coli* by *cfxB*, *nfxB*, or *norB* gene mutations associated with decreased porin protein OmpF (45, 46), it appeared that altered drug permeability might be the underlying mechanism of resistance in our strain. In collaboration with Chamberland et al. (23), we subsequently showed that the major mechanisms of quinolone resistance in these pefloxacin-resistant variants were the result of at least two distinct alterations of the drug target ("target insensitivity" and altered DNA gyrase). Although a drug permeability defect was also noted, increased pefloxacin MICs correlated most closely with the 50% inhibitory concentrations for inhibition of DNA synthesis.

Experiments with combination therapy to prevent the emergence of resistance were subsequently performed by Xiong et al. using ciprofloxacin and pefloxacin, with and without fosfomycin, in experimental aortic valve BE caused by multidrug-susceptible or multidrug-resistant *P. aeruginosa* (92). Initiating treatment at 12 h versus 48 h postinfection facilitated a comparison of the impact of early versus later treatment, it was observed that early treatment

with ciprofloxacin and fosfomycin was better than ciprofloxacin alone; moreover, pefloxacin and fosfomycin were better than pefloxacin alone, irrespective of the MIC susceptibility profiles of the infecting strain of *Pseudomonas*. In the late treatment arm, there were no significant improvements of combination therapy as compared with monotherapy with either ciprofloxacin or pefloxacin.

Similar to the studies described above, Papadakis et al. (64) have examined the efficacies of a panel of fluoroquinolones against *P. aeruginosa* in an experimental model of BE. In these studies, the efficacies of ofloxacin, pefloxacin, ciprofloxacin, enoxacin, or fleroxacin administered intramuscularly were compared with that of amikacin. Enoxacin and ciprofloxacin were equivalent, and superior, to all other agents tested in reducing tissue bacterial burden, or sterilizing vegetations. In contrast, fleroxacin exhibited relatively weak activity as compared with other quinolones. Some fluoroquinolones may interfere with the antipseudomonal activities of other agents. For example, Bugnon et al. (20) demonstrated that pefloxacin reduced the bactericidal effect of fosfomycin against *P. aeruginosa* in a rabbit model of BE, negatively affecting the ability of the combination of agents to reduce bacterial vegetation densities.

During the past two decades, several β-lactamase-resistant, extended-spectrum cephalosporins have been in wide clinical use (e.g., cefotaxime, ceftriaxone, and ceftazidime). Recently, increasing numbers of reports have documented the emergence of resistance to these agents by selection of mutants with derepressed β-lactamase overproduction (48, 67, 77, 79); in addition, several of these multiply β-lactam-resistant strains have exhibited cross-resistance to aminoglycosides (67). This resistance phenomenon has been seen most commonly among bacterial genera within the expanded spectrum of these newer β-lactams, especially *Enterobacter*, *Serratia*, and *Pseudomonas* species (77); by comparison, the quinolones generally retain good in vitro efficacy against these β-lactam-resistant mutants. We utilized the experimental aortic valve BE model to evaluate the efficacy of ciprofloxacin against such strains in vivo (11). The infecting strain was a multiply β-lactam-resistant *P. aeruginosa* variant derepressed for constitutive β-lactamase (type Id) overproduction (13). Ciprofloxacin significantly lowered pseudomonal densities within vegetations and rendered significantly more animals blood culture-negative and with sterile vegetations than did ceftazidime.

Enterobacter aerogenes

Enterobacter species rarely cause human BE but are relatively common causes of serious nosocomial infections among patients in intensive care units (18). Boscia et al. (16, 17) performed two studies to evaluate the use of oral quinolone agents in *Enterobacter aerogenes* aortic BE as a critical test of drug efficacy in this difficult model of hematogenously disseminated infection. These investigators first compared oral enoxacin with intramuscular cefoperazone in *Enterobacter* endocarditis (17). In vitro, both enoxacin and cefoperazone exerted a rapid and substantial bactericidal effect against the infecting *Enterobacter* strain. However, high-dose oral enoxacin (100 mg/kg administered every 6 h) was significantly better at reducing intravegetation bacterial densities than was lower-dose enoxacin (25 mg/kg given every 6 h) or cefoperazone (60 mg/kg given every 6 h intramuscularly). These findings suggested that the longer half-life of enoxacin (~3 h) versus that of cefoperazone (~1 h) probably contributed to the therapeutic differences observed. In a similar study, Boscia et al. (16) compared the efficacies of two oral quinolones, enoxacin and difloxacin, with that of parenterally administered cefoperazone in a experimental aortic BE model caused by *E. aerogenes*. As in their previous study, all three agents were active in vitro against the infecting *Enterobacter* strain, although difloxacin exhibited the most rapid and complete killing of this strain in time-kill experiments. Difloxacin (100 mg/kg given orally every 12 h) was significantly better at reducing intravegetation *Enterobacter* densities than was enoxacin (given at the same dose regimen) or cefoperazone. The authors again ascribed the superior efficacy of difloxacin to its longer half-life (~3.5 h) compared with those of enoxacin (~2.3 h) and cefoperazone (~0.6 h). They also concluded that the relatively inferior outcome of enoxacin therapy, compared with that of their prior study, was related to differences in the enoxacin-dosing intervals utilized in the two studies (every 6 h versus every 12 h).

E. coli

Only limited investigations into the efficacy of quinolone agents in experimental BE caused by *E. coli* have been conducted. However, Contrepois et al. (25) reported on the efficacy of 3 days of pefloxacin therapy given at 30 mg/kg/day intramuscularly for experimental *E. coli* aortic valve BE. This regimen significantly lowered intravegetation *E. coli* densities compared with untreated controls; unfortunately, these investigators did not include a comparative therapy group for pefloxacin.

Viridans Group Streptococci (VGS)

The VGS are the most frequent cause of native-valve BE. The recent emphasis on single daily dose,

short-duration, and outpatient-based therapy regimens for VGS BE (e.g., ceftriaxone-based [35, 36, 81]) has suggested that quinolones might be potential agents for such infections, particularly among patients allergic to β-lactams. Entenza et al. compared the efficacy of sparfloxacin versus ceftriaxone in rat models of aortic valve BE caused by *Streptococcus sanguis* and *Streptococcus mitis* (33). The MICs of ceftriaxone were generally lower than those of sparfloxacin for the penicillin-susceptible strains, ranging from 0.032 to 0.064 µg/ml versus 0.25 to 0.50 µg/ml, respectively. Animals were given continuous infusion of all antibiotics over a 3 to 5-day period. After 3 days of treatment, sparfloxacin was less effective than ceftriaxone in sterilizing vegetations and reducing bacterial vegetation densities in BE caused by penicillin-susceptible VGS strains. When treatment was extended to 5 days, both regimens were equally effective. Thus, sparfloxacin exerted a slower in vivo bactericidal effect than ceftriaxone in this model of BE.

Chambers et al. studied the efficacy of levofloxacin in experimental aortic valve BE in rabbits caused by penicillin-susceptible and -resistant VGS (24). The levofloxacin MICs for these strains were 0.5 and 2 µg/ml, respectively. However, despite these serum-achievable MICs, levofloxacin was ineffective against either VGS strain after 3 days of treatment in this model. Recently, trovafloxacin was studied in a similar model of VGS BE (65). As above, the in vitro activity of trovafloxacin against the infecting VGS strains was not predictive of its activity in vivo in experimental BE (i.e., trovafloxacin exerted no substantive impact intravegetation clearance of VGS despite an in vitro trovafloxacin MIC and MBC of 0.25 and 1 µg/ml, respectively). In contrast, we have recently demonstrated good in vivo efficacy of a new-generation quinolone against VGS. Our laboratory (58) evaluated the efficacy of BMS-284756, a novel desfluoro (F-6)-quinolone, against *S. sanguis* in a right-sided rabbit BE model. After a 4-day treatment course, BMS-284756 (20 mg/kg/day i.v.) was comparable to ampicillin (50 mg/kg three times a day given intramuscularly) in terms of VGS clearance from tricuspid valve vegetations and embolic pulmonary abscesses.

Studies of the chemoprophylactic efficacy of quinolones in BE have been reported recently by Katsarolis et al. against experimental VGS BE using trovafloxacin bioavailability (56). Trovafloxacin (15 mg/kg) was given in either a single-dose or two-dose intravenous prophylactic regimen and was compared to ampicillin (40 mg/kg). In this study, trovafloxacin exhibited a rapid rate of elimination from rabbit serum and poor distribution within the vegetation at the time of bacterial challenge. Despite pharmacokinetic variations among rabbits as compared with humans, the two-dose trovafloxacin regimen was able to protect all animals from VGS BE.

Enterococci

The increased prevalence of multidrug resistance among clinical enterococcal isolates has stimulated evaluation of fluoroquinolones to treat infections caused by such strains. However, monotherapy with fluoroquinolones has generally demonstrated both poor in vitro and in vivo activity against enterococci (59, 68, 90, 91, 99). Whitman et al. studied ciprofloxacin in combination with gentamicin and/or rifampin in an experimental model of vancomycin- and ampicillin-resistant *Enterococcus faecium* BE (91). Left-sided aortic valve BE was induced with an *E. faecium* strain for which the MICs were as follows: ciprofloxacin, 3.1 μg/ml; rifampin, 0.1 μg/ml; gentamicin, 12.5 μg/ml; vancomycin, 500 μg/ml; ampicillin, 250 μg/ml; and streptomycin, >2,000 μg/ml. After 5 days of therapy, the mean bacterial counts in vegetations showed that the rifampin-alone group, ciprofloxacin-rifampin group, and the ciprofloxacin-rifampin-gentamicin group were statistically equivalent, and significantly lower than those of the untreated group, the ciprofloxacin-alone group, and the gentamicin-alone group.

In similar studies, Quale et al. and Landman et al. evaluated the therapy of *E. faecium* BE utilizing ciprofloxacin-novobiocin (68), ciprofloxacin-ampicillin (59), or clinafloxacin-penicillin (99) regimens. In vitro, ciprofloxacin-novobiocin showed synergy in time-killed assays, as compared with ciprofloxacin monotherapy. However, the ciprofloxacin-novobiocin combination exerted only a modest in vivo effect as compared with monotherapy regimens. Kidney bacterial counts were dramatically lower in the combination group compared with untreated controls or either ciprofloxacin or novobiocin alone, suggesting possible efficacy in enterococcal genital-urinary infections. Quinolone-β-lactam combination therapies have also been disappointing in experimental enterococcal BE (59). Newer quinolones, such as clinafloxacin, have demonstrated some in vivo efficacy in experimental enterococcal BE; however, efficacy was predominantly seen at high serum clinafloxacin levels, which may not be tolerated or practical in humans (99).

Coxiella burnetii (Agent of Q Fever)

Chronic Q fever BE is an important and often devastating form of valvular infection, which is prevalent and endemic in many countries (e.g., Scotland, Australia, New Zealand, and the entire Mediterranean area). The response of this infection to medical therapy alone has been generally poor, and cardiac valve replacement has frequently been necessary for radical cure. Progress toward understanding the fundamental pathogenetic mechanisms of *C. burnetii*-induced BE has been difficult, largely because of the obligate intracellular nature of this pathogen. There is no experimental animal model of Q fever BE; however, an in vitro tissue-culture model of persistent infection of various cell types by *C. burnetii* has been developed (3, 74). This model system has been used extensively to generate information concerning the efficacies of a variety of the new quinolones against several *C. burnetii* isolates implicated in distinct clinical syndromes, including BE (71, 94, 96, 97).

Of importance, a correlation has been detected between specific Q fever clinical disease syndromes (i.e., acute versus chronic Q fever) and isolate antibiotic susceptibility profiles, with isolates from patients with acute Q fever being consistently more susceptible to quinolones and other antibiotics than isolates implicated in chronic Q fever (96). Moreover, the process of persistent infection itself appears to result in decreased *C. burnetii* susceptibility to quinolone and other antibiotics, since organisms infecting cells for ≤30 days exhibit significantly lower quinolone MICs than the same isolates infecting cells, for ≥400 days. For this reason, rapid *C. burnetii* antibiotic susceptibility assays such as the shell vial technique, in which organisms typically infect host cells for ≤10 days prior to susceptibility testing (72), provide information pertaining only to acute infection, and therefore are difficult to interpret in the context of chronic disease.

The above-mentioned model system of intracellular *C. burnetii* infection has demonstrated that several quinolone antibiotics (i.e., ciprofloxacin, ofloxacin, pefloxacin, norfloxacin, and difloxacin) are significantly more effective than tetracyclines (tetracycline, doxycycline) in controlling persistent *C. burnetii* infection in vitro (71, 95, 96, 97). Sparfloxacin has also been demonstrated to exert an inhibitory effect on *C. burnetii* within acutely infected host cells in vitro (69). In addition, studies evaluating the efficacies of combinations of quinolones with other antibiotics have revealed evidence of in vitro synergy against *C. burnetii* strains (96), prompting the use of quinolones in combination with rifampin in the treatment of Q fever BE.

Some recent studies have suggested that certain quinolone antibiotics are bactericidal versus *C. burnetii*. Such bactericidal action is evidenced by quinolone-induced reductions in intracellular bacterial counts within host cells that occurs more rapidly than would be expected by host cell elimination of statically inhibited organisms or by dilution of static parasite burden via host cell division (96). Other studies have attempted to differentiate potential bacteriostatic and bactericidal actions of quinolones against *C. burnetii* through the use of cycloheximide treatment to prevent infected host cell division, followed by exposure to quinolone antibiotics (72). Quinolones do not lead to the complete elimination of *C. burnetii* from infected, cycloheximide-inhibited host cells in such studies. However, the effects of cycloheximide-induced host cell inhibition as they relate to the intracellular metabolic activity of the obligate parasite *C. burnetii* are not well understood. More substantive information is required to address the specific actions of quinolone antibiotics against *C. burnetii*.

Potential mechanisms that may account for differential antibiotic susceptibilities among *C. burnetii* isolates have also been examined. Although Samuel et al. have correlated plasmid type with clinical Q fever syndromes caused by distinct isolates of *C. burnetii* (76), differences in plasmid repertoire have not accounted for the observed differences in quinolone susceptibilities of these isolates. Rather, differential susceptibilities to quinolone antibiotics in *C. burnetii* isolates from acute versus chronic Q fever appear to be the result of differences in drug accumulation (93).

USE OF QUINOLONES IN HUMAN BE

Although quinolone antibiotics have not been utilized as primary therapy in human BE, the use of such agents has been studied in selective patient groups with human BE. A tabular summary of published data on various quinolone agents in human BE is presented in Table 2.

Staphylococcus aureus

The largest clinical experience with quinolones in the treatment of human BE has involved therapy of *S. aureus* BE. Dworkin et al. described 10 intravenous-drug addicts with right-sided (tricuspid valve) *S. aureus* BE who were treated with a predominantly oral regimen of ciprofloxacin (750 mg twice daily) plus rifampin (600 mg/day) for 3 to 4 weeks, following a short-course of initial intravenous administration (30); all 10 patients were cured of their infections. This study was an open, nonrandomized evaluation, and the excellent results prompted a larger, prospective, randomized trial comparing oral ciprofloxacin plus rifampin versus nafcillin plus gentamicin in addict-related, right-sided *S. aureus* BE (44). Out of 573 febrile drug addicts initially screened, 90 had evidence of right-sided BE, with 44 evaluable by the end of the trial. The high attrition rate was mainly due to patient withdrawal from study or antibiotic protocol violations. The oral ciprofloxacin-rifampin group exhibited a cure rate of 95% (18/19) versus 88% (22/25) for the standard IV arm.

Despite these encouraging results, concern remains about the utility of the quinolones, especially as single agents, in the therapy of invasive staphylococcal infections (88). The recent report of the failure of ciprofloxacin in controlling right-sided BE illustrates the propensity of *S. aureus* to develop resistance to this class of drugs in vivo, when the drug is used as

Table 2. Summary of activity of fluoroquinolones in human bacterial endocarditis

Organism (Reference)	Agents	Trial type	Patients (n)	Cure rates
MSSA (30)	Ciprofloxacin-rifampin	Right-sided *S. aureus* endocarditis, open/non-randomized	10	100%
	Ciprofloxacin-rifampin versus i.v. standard of care	Right-sided *S. aureus* endocarditis, prospective/randomized	43 (evaluable)	95% Cipro-rifampin combination, 88% nafcillin-gentamicin combination
Pseudomonas aeruginosa (27, 89)	Ciprofloxacin	Case report	3	33%
Coxiella burnetii (70, 98)	Ciprofloxacin	Case report	1	100%
	Ofloxacin-doxycycline	Prospective/randomized	14	50% with 4 wks treatment; 100% with 4 yrs treatment
Actinobacillus (2)	Ciprofloxacin	Case report	1	100%
Brucella (54)	Pefloxacin	Case report	1	0%

a single-drug regimen in a "high inoculum" clinical infection such as BE (40). For example, within 11 days of oral ciprofloxacin therapy in one patient (used in this patient because of suspected β-lactam allergy), the causative *S. aureus* isolate exhibited an eightfold increase in ciprofloxacin MIC (2 to 16μg/ml), and a fourfold increase (4 to 16 μg/ml) in ciprofloxacin MBC. High-level ciprofloxacin resistance has now been observed among MRSA strains in many medical centers (80). Although less well documented, quinolone resistance among MSSA isolates may also be increasing. As noted before, development of ciprofloxacin resistance in experimental BE has been observed (49, 50, 53). Findings such as these have given rise to the suggestion that rifampin may largely contribute to both the clinical efficacy of the ciprofloxacin-rifampin synergy observed, as well as the prevention of development of ciprofloxacin resistance (15, 27). Similarly, fluoroquinolones may enhance the efficacy of conventional antistaphylococcal regimens in the treatment of staphylococcal endocarditis. For example, Berrington and coworkers demonstrated that the addition of moxifloxacin converted a failing conventional treatment regimen to one that proved curative (14).

P. aeruginosa and Other Gram-Negative Bacilli

A literature review over the past 20 years has revealed three cases of *P. aeruginosa* BE treated with quinolone regimens. Daikos et al. (27) reported their experiences with oral quinolone therapy in two such patients. One patient was an intravenous-drug addict with refractory mitral valve BE, despite two mitral valve replacements and three courses of combination, parenteral antipseudomonal regimens. Oral ciprofloxacin therapy, with daily doses between 1 and 2 g, was continued for 3.5 months (total dose, 150 g). Blood cultures were sterilized during therapy, and fever abated. However, the patient expired with fulminant pseudomonal BE approximately 1 month after a reduction in the dosage of ciprofloxacin, necessitated by drug-induced hepatitis. At autopsy, mitral vegetations contained enormous densities of *P. aeruginosa* ($\sim 10^8$ CFU/g of tissue).

A second patient, who had a permanent cardiac pacemaker, developed mural BE due to *P. aeruginosa*. He failed treatment with parenteral antipseudomonal agents and was treated with 1.5 g of oral ciprofloxacin per day for nearly 2 years, with sterilization of blood cultures and partial abatement of fever. The patient, however, failed a test-of-cure after 1 year of therapy during a planned discontinuation of the drug. A rapid recrudescence of pseudomonal bacteremia and fever occurred, and

progressive biventricular heart failure and anemia developed. At postmortem examination, right ventricular mural BE, as well as tricuspid and aortic valvular BE, was seen, with vegetation bacterial densities of $\sim 10^5$ CFU/g noted. Selective increases in the ciprofloxacin MIC by four- to eightfold were demonstrated for pseudomonal isolates after quinolone therapy in both patients, without increases in the MICs of other classes of antibiotics.

Uzun et al. treated a 40-year-old patient with *P. aeruginosa* prosthetic valve BE involving both mitral and aortic valve prostheses (89). Given only medical management as an option, ciprofloxacin plus ceftazidime were given for 6 weeks, after which oral ciprofloxacin (1 g/day) was given for 36 months. The patient improved clinically from his New York Heart Association functional class III to class II, and remained blood culture negative without any drug-related side effects.

Other cases of nonpseudomonal gram-negative bacterial prosthetic valve BE have been reported. Ciprofloxacin was utilized in a 76-year-old patient with prosthetic mitral valve BE due to *Actinobacillus actinomycetemcomitans* (2). This patient completed an 8-week course of oral ciprofloxacin (1.5 g/day) with clinical resolution of infection. Pefloxacin in combination with rifampin has also been used to treat a patient with *Brucella melitensis*-induced BE on a Starr-Edwards aortic valve prosthesis (54). This antimicrobial combination failed to prevent periannular abscess formation and prosthesis deterioration, necessitating subsequent valve replacement as a result of persistent infection and hemodynamic impairment. Fluoroquinolone-resistant *B. melitensis* was subsequently recovered from the infected prosthesis. Following placement of the new valve, continued dual antibiotic therapy with pefloxacin-rifampin led to apyrexia and overall clinical improvement. Similarly, fluoroquinolones have proved effective against BE due to other gram-negative pathogens, including *Salmonella* (Goerre et al. [41]) and *Haemophilus* (Dawson and White [28]).

Q Fever

As noted above, Q fever BE has been associated with a high mortality rate due to cardiac failure, despite cardiac valve resection and prosthetic valve replacement in conjunction with prolonged antibiotic therapy. However, on the basis of the in vitro findings outlined previously (84, 85, 95, 96), quinolone antibiotics alone and in combination with rifampin or doxycycline are now being utilized in the medical management of chronic Q fever BE. Yebra et al. (98) used oral ciprofloxacin (500 mg twice daily) in the treatment of chronic Q fever BE in an elderly patient with prior aortic valve replacement. Within 12 weeks of such therapy, this patient became afebrile, and his phase I complement-fixing-anti-*C. burnetii* antibody titer dropped from 1:1,024 to 1:128. One year later, the patient was asymptomatic, while continuing on ciprofloxacin therapy.

Quinolone antibiotics have also been shown to enhance substantially the efficacy of doxycycline in controlling chronic Q fever BE (60). In a study comparing doxycycline alone versus doxycycline–co-trimoxazole, doxycycline-ofloxacin (200 and 400 mg/day, respectively), or doxycycline-pefloxacin (200 and 400 mg/day, respectively), doxycycline-pefloxacin led to the most significant reduction in mortality versus its comparators. However, quinolone therapy did not statistically diminish the need for eventual cardiac valve replacement because of hemodynamic insufficiency. Moreover, the combined doxycycline-quinolone regimens did not lead to an eradication of *C. burnetii* organisms from cardiac valve tissue at the time of surgery, despite up to 12 months of treatment. Therefore, it is generally felt that the duration for all oral regimens for chronic *C. burnetii* BE should be at least 24 to 36 months, and overall management of the disease may include eventual cardiac valve replacement for progressive valvular incompetence. Such prolonged antibiotic therapy appears warranted prior to valve replacement surgery in this infection for several important reasons. First, autopsy data (63, 83) have suggested that valvular infection seen in chronic Q fever BE generally may involve all four valves histopathologically, despite the dominance of one valve (typically the aortic) in the clinical presentation. Secondly, a recent, large series of operated patients with Q fever BE emphasized the necessity of longer-term medical therapy in patients with this infection (59a). In this study, the investigators confirmed the predominantly subendothelial targeting of valves by *C. burnetii* (versus traditional vegetation in non-Q-fever BE). In addition, in those patients receiving <1 year of medical therapy, active *C. burnetii* infection was confirmed by PCR, tissue culture, and immunohistochemistry. In contrast, those patients receiving >1 year of therapy had a substantially lower detection rate of active *C. burnetii* valvulitis. Moreover, patients with chronic Q fever BE may have concomitant Q fever hepatitis that may serve as a nidus for subsequent hematogenous seeding of a valve prosthesis.

Raoult et al., comparing two regimens containing doxycycline plus either ofloxacin or hydroxychloroquine, performed the largest recent therapeutic trial of patients with Q fever BE (70). A total of 14 patients were treated with doxycycline and ofloxacin, which resulted in one death, seven relapses, one ongoing treatment, and five cures. In the comparator arm of 21 patients (doxycycline plus hydroxychloroquine), there was one death, two ongoing treatment courses, and seventeen cures. The two regimens had identical mortality rates, frequency of valve surgery, and drug-regimen tolerance. The mean duration of treatment was 55 versus 31 months in the doxycycline-ofloxacin versus comparator groups, respectively. The authors concluded that using hydroxychloroquine was more efficacious than adding ofloxacin to the standard doxycycline regimen; this was felt to be related to the efficacy of hydroxychloroquine in alkalinizing the *C. burnetii*-infected phagolysosome, making the organism more susceptible to killing by doxycycline (61).

Despite the efficacy of fluoroquinolones in treating Q fever endocarditis as described above, there is growing concern regarding quinolone resistance even among strains normally associated with acute disease. For example, Spyridaki et al. (84) recently showed that pefloxacin resistance in vitro results from a transition mutation (G to A) leading to alteration of the *gyrA* gene sequence. Two pefloxacin-resistant strains possessed this mutation, while 10 pefloxacin-sensitive strains did not. Such mutations have been implicated, but not yet proven, in cases of chronic Q fever endocarditis that are refractory to long-term quinolone therapy, alone or in combination.

SUMMARY

Quinolones have generally performed well in experimental animal models of BE, including both early generation agents (ciprofloxacin), as well as newer-generation fluoroquinolones (e.g., levofloxacin). Studies have demonstrated that ciprofloxacin is equal to or more effective than synergistically active combinations of aminoglycosides and β-lactams in the treatment of experimental *P. aeruginosa* BE. However, reports documenting the development of increases in the MICs to older quinolone agents (e.g., ciprofloxacin) during the therapy of human and experimental pseudomonal BE are disturbing.

The newer quinolones (e.g., levofloxacin and trovafloxacin) also appear to be highly active in vivo against both MSSA and MRSA strains in experimental BE models. Their efficacy appears to be roughly equivalent to that of standard antimicrobial regimens, such as vancoymcin for MRSA BE, or semisynthetic penicillins or cephalosporins for MSSA BE. However, the hepatotoxicity of trovafloxacin makes its current clinical utility problematic. Moreover, the human toxicities of sparfloxacin and temafloxacin curtailed their clinical development. To date, there is only limited experience with the quinolones in human *S. aureus* BE, although they appear promising in selected cases of right-sided BE, particularly when combined with rifampin. Despite these encouraging preliminary results, the development of quinolone resistance in vivo is a growing concern in the therapy of experimental MSSA or MRSA BE, although few of the clinical studies have systematically examined this phenomenon. Moreover, preliminary data suggest the utility of the newer quinolone antibiotics in the prophylaxis of VGS BE (56); such data need to be confirmed further. With respect to the therapy of VGS and enterococcal BE, although quinolones have exhibited promising in vitro data in combination therapy, in vivo activity in experimental BE is relatively poor. In vitro studies have prompted the evaluation of newer quinolone antibiotics alone and in combination with doxycycline for the treatment of chronic Q fever BE. However, doxycycline-hydroxy-chloroquine combinations may have advantages to doxycycline-quinolone regimens in treatment of infection due to quinolone-resistant strains.

REFERENCES

1. Auckenthaler, R., M. Michea-Hamzehpour, and J. C. Pechere. 1986. In-vitro activity of newer quinolones against aerobic bacteria. *J. Antimicrob. Chemother.* **17**(Suppl. B):29–39.

2. Babinchak, T. J. 1995. Oral ciprofloxacin therapy for prosthetic valve endocarditis due to Actinobacillus actinomycetemcomitans. *Clin. Infect. Dis.* **21**:1517–1518.

3. Baca, O. G., and D. Paretsky. 1983. Q fever and *Coxiella burnetii*: a model for host-parasite interactions. *Microbiol. Rev.* **47**:127–149.

4. Bauernfeind, A., and C. Petermuller. 1983. In vitro activity of ciprofloxacin, norfloxacin and nalidixic acid. *Eur. J. Clin. Microbiol.* **2**:111–115.

5. Bayer, A. S., I. K. Blomquist, and K. S. Kim. 1986. Ciprofloxacin in experimental aortic valve endocarditis due to *Pseudomonas aeruginosa*. *J. Antimicrob. Chemother.* **17**:641–649.

6. Bayer, A. S., D. P. Greenberg, and J. Yih. 1988. Correlates of therapeutic efficacy in experimental methicillin-resistant *Staphylococcus aureus* endocarditis. *Chemotherapy* **34**:46–55.

7. Bayer, A. S., L. Hirano, and J. Yih. 1988. Development of beta-lactam resistance and increased quinolone MICs during therapy of experimental *Pseudomonas aeruginosa* endocarditis. *Antimicrob. Agents Chemother.* **32**:231–235.

8. Bayer, A. S. and K. S. Kim. 1986. In vivo efficacy of azlocillin and amikacin versus ciprofloxacin with and without amikacin in experimental right-sided endocarditis due to *Pseudomonas aeruginosa*. *Chemotherapy* **32**:364–373.

9. Bayer, A. S., C. Li, and M. Ing. 1998. Efficacy of trovafloxacin, a new quinolone antibiotic, in experimental staphylococcal endocarditis due to oxacillin-resistant strains. *Antimicrob. Agents Chemother.* **42**:1837–1841.

10. Bayer, A. S., P. Lindsay, J. Yih, L. Hirano, D. Lee, and I. K. Blomquist. 1986. Efficacy of ciprofloxacin in experimental aortic valve endocarditis caused by a multiply beta-lactam-resistant variant of *Pseudomonas aeruginosa* stably derepressed for beta-lactamase production. *Antimicrob. Agents Chemother.* **30**:528–531.

11. Bayer, A. S., D. Norman, and D. Anderson. 1985. Efficacy of ciprofloxacin in experimental arthritis caused by *Escherichia coli*—in vitro-in vivo correlations. *J. Infect. Dis.* **152**:811–816.

12. Bayer, A. S., D. Norman, and K. S. Kim. 1985. Efficacy of amikacin and ceftazidime in experimental aortic valve endocarditis due to *Pseudomonas aeruginosa*. *Antimicrob. Agents Chemother.* **28**:781–785.

13. Bayer, A. S., J. Peters, T. R. Parr, Jr., L. Chan, and R. E. Hancock. 1987. Role of beta-lactamase in in vivo development of ceftazidime resistance in experimental *Pseudomonas aeruginosa* endocarditis. *Antimicrob. Agents Chemother.* **31**:253–258.

14. Berrington, A. W., R. J. Koerner, J. D. Perry, H. H. Bain, and F. K. Gould. 2001. Treatment of *Staphylococcus aureus* endocarditis using moxifloxacin. *Int. J. Med. Microbiol.* **291**:237–239.

15. Bignardi, G. E. 1989. Ciprofloxacin resistance and staphylococcal endocarditis. *Lancet* **ii**:1526.

16. Boscia, J. A., W. D. Kobasa, and D. Kaye. 1987. Comparison of difloxacin, enoxacin, and cefoperazone for treatment of experimental *Enterobacter aerogenes* endocarditis. *Antimicrob. Agents Chemother.* **31**:458–460.

17. Boscia, J. A., W. D. Kobasa, and D. Kaye. 1985. Enoxacin compared with cefoperazone for the treatment of experimental *Enterobacter aerogenes* endocarditis. *Antimicrob. Agents Chemother.* **27**:708–711.

18. Bouza, E., M. Garcia de la Torre, A. Erice, E. Loza, J. M. Diaz-Borrego, and L. Buzon. 1985. *Enterobacter* bacteremia. An analysis of 50 episodes. *Arch. Intern. Med.* **145**:1024–1027.

19. Brion, N., A. Lessana, F. Mosset, J. J. Lefevre, and G. Montay. 1986. Penetration of pefloxacin in human heart valves. *J. Antimicrob. Chemother.* **17**(Suppl. B):89–92.

20. Bugnon, D., G. Potel, Y.Q. Xiong, J. Caillon, D. Navas, C. Gras, M.F. Kergueris, P. Le Conte, F. Jehl, D. Baron, and H. Drugeon. 1997. Bactericidal effect of pefloxacin and fosfomycin against *Pseudomonas aeruginosa* in a rabbit endocarditis model with pharmacokinetics of pefloxacin in humans simulated in vivo. *Eur. J. Clin. Microbiol. Infect. Dis.* **16**:575–580.

21. Carbon, C. 1990. Impact of the antibiotic dosage schedule on efficacy in experimental endocarditis. *Scand. J. Infect. Dis. Suppl.* **74**:163–172.

22. Carpenter, T. C., C. J. Hackbarth, H. F. Chambers, and M. A. Sande. 1986. Efficacy of ciprofloxacin for experimental endocarditis caused by methicillin-susceptible or -resistant strains of *Staphylococcus aureus*. *Antimicrob. Agents Chemother.* **30**:382–384.

23. Chamberland, S., A. S. Bayer, T. Schollaardt, S. A. Wong, and L. E. Bryan. 1989. Characterization of mechanisms of quinolone resistance in *Pseudomonas aeruginosa* strains isolated in vitro and in vivo during experimental endocarditis. *Antimicrob. Agents Chemother.* **33**:624–634.

24. Chambers, H. F., Q. Xiang, Liu, L. L. Chow, and C. Hackbarth. 1999. Efficacy of levofloxacin for experimental aortic-valve endocarditis in rabbits infected with *viridans group streptococcus* or *Staphylococcus aureus*. *Antimicrob. Agents Chemother.* **43**:2742–2746.

25. Contrepois, A., C. Daldoss, B. Pangon, J. J. Garaud, M. Kecir, C. Sarrazin, J. M. Vallois, and C. Carbon. 1984.

Pefloxacin in rabbits: protein binding, extravascular diffusion, urinary excretion and bactericidal effect in experimental endocarditis. *J. Antimicrob. Chemother.* 14:51–57.

26. Cremieux, A. C., A. Saleh-Mghir, J. M. Vallois, B. Maziere, M. Muffat-Joly, C. Devine, A. Bouvet, J. J. Pocidalo, and C. Carbon. 1992. Efficacy of temafloxacin in experimental *Streptococcus adjacens* endocarditis and autoradiographic diffusion pattern of ¹⁴C temafloxacin in cardiac vegetations. *Antimicrob. Agents Chemother.* 36:2216–2221.

27. Daikos, G. L., S. B. Kathpalia, V. T. Lolans, G. G. Jackson, and E. Fosslien. 1988. Long-term oral ciprofloxacin: experience in the treatment of incurable infective endocarditis. *Am. J. Med.* 84:786–790.

28. Dawson, S. J., and L. A. White. 1992. Treatment of *Haemophilus aphrophilus* endocarditis with ciprofloxacin. *J. Infect.* 24:317–320.

29. Durack, D. T. and P. B. Beeson. 1972. Experimental bacterial endocarditis. II. Survival of a bacteria in endocardial vegetations. *Br. J. Exp. Pathol.* 53:50–53.

30. Dworkin, R. J., B. L. Lee, M. A. Sande, and H. F. Chambers. 1989. Treatment of right-sided *Staphylococcus aureus* endocarditis in intravenous drug users with ciprofloxacin and rifampicin. *Lancet* 2:1071–1073.

31. Eliopoulos, G. M., A. Gardella, and R. C. Moellering, Jr. 1984. In vitro activity of ciprofloxacin, a new carboxyquinoline antimicrobial agent. *Antimicrob. Agents Chemother.* 25:331–335.

32. Endtz, H. P., J. W. Mouton, J. G. den Hollander, N. van den Braak, and H. A. Verbrugh. 1997. Comparative in vitro activities of trovafloxacin (CP-99,219) against 445 Gram-positive isolates from patients with endocarditis and those with other bloodstream infections. *Antimicrob. Agents Chemother.* 41:1146–1149.

33. Entenza, J. M., M. Blatter, M. P. Glauser, and P. Moreillon. 1994. Parenteral sparfloxacin compared with ceftriaxone in treatment of experimental endocarditis due to penicillin-susceptible and -resistant streptococci. *Antimicrob. Agents Chemother.* 38:2683–2688.

34. Entenza, J. M., J. Vouillamoz, M. P. Glauser, and P. Moreillon. 1997. Levofloxacin versus ciprofloxacin, flucloxacillin, or vancomycin for treatment of experimental endocarditis due to methicillin-susceptible or -resistant *Staphylococcus aureus*. *Antimicrob. Agents Chemother.* 41:1662–1667.

35. Francioli, P., W. Ruch, and D. Stamboulian. 1995. Treatment of streptococcal endocarditis with a single daily dose of ceftriaxone and netilmicin for 14 days: a prospective multicenter study. *Clin. Infect. Dis.* 21:1406–1410.

36. Francioli, P. B. 1993. Ceftriaxone and outpatient treatment of infective endocarditis. *Infect. Dis. Clin. N. Am.* 7:97–115.

37. Freedman, L. R. and J. Valone Jr. 1979. Experimental infective endocarditis. *Prog. Cardiovasc. Dis.* 22:169–180.

38. Gengo, F. M., T. W. Mannion, C. H. Nightingale, and J. J. Schentag. 1984. Integration of pharmacokinetics and pharmacodynamics of methicillin in curative treatment of experimental endocarditis. *J. Antimicrob. Chemother.* 14:619–631.

39. Gilbert, M., J. A. Boscia, W. D. Kobasa, and D. Kaye. 1986. Enoxacin compared with vancomycin for the treatment of experimental methicillin-resistant *Staphylococcus aureus* endocarditis. *Antimicrob. Agents Chemother.* 29:461–463.

40. Gomez-Jimenez, J., E. Ribera, B. Almirante, O. Del Valle, A. Pahissa, and J. M. Martinez-Vazquez. 1989. Ciprofloxacin resistance and staphylococcal endocarditis. *Lancet* ii:1525–1526.

41. Goerre, S., R. Malinverni, and B. C. Aeschbacher. 1998. Successful conservative treatment of non-typhoid *Salmonella*

endocarditis involving a bioprosthetic valve. *Clin. Cardiol.* 21:368–370.

42. Hackbarth, C. J., H. F. Chambers, F. Stella, A. M. Shibl, and M. A. Sande. 1986. Ciprofloxacin in experimental *Pseudomonas aeruginosa* meningitis in rabbits. *J. Antimicrob. Chemother.* 18(Suppl. D):65–69.

43. Haller, I. 1985. Comprehensive evaluation of ciprofloxacin-aminoglycoside combinations against *Enterobacteriaceae* and *Pseudomonas aeruginosa* strains. *Antimicrob. Agents Chemother.* 28:663–666.

44. Heldman, A. W., T. V. Hartert, S. C. Ray, E. G. Daoud, T. E. Kowalski, V. J. Pompili, S. D. Sisson, W. C. Tidmore, K. A. vom Eigen, S. N. Goodman, P. S. Lietman, B. G. Petty, and C. Flexner. 1996. Oral antibiotic treatment of right-sided staphylococcal endocarditis in injection drug users: prospective randomized comparison with parenteral therapy. *Am. J. Med.* 101:68–76.

45. Hooper, D. C., J. S. Wolfson, E. Y. Ng, and M. N. Swartz. 1987. Mechanisms of action of and resistance to ciprofloxacin. *Am. J. Med.* 82:12–20.

46. Hooper, D. C., J. S. Wolfson, K. S. Souza, C. Tung, G. L. McHugh, and M. N. Swartz. 1986. Genetic and biochemical characterization of norfloxacin resistance in *Escherichia coli*. *Antimicrob. Agents Chemother.* 29:639–644.

47. Ingerman, M. J., P. G. Pitsakis, A. F. Rosenberg, and M. E. Levison. 1986. The importance of pharmacodynamics in determining the dosing interval in therapy for experimental pseudomonas endocarditis in the rat. *J. Infect. Dis.* 153:707–714.

48. Jimenez-Lucho, V. E., L. D. Saravolatz, A. A. Medeiros, and D. Pohlod. 1986. Failure of therapy in pseudomonas endocarditis: selection of resistant mutants. *J. Infect. Dis.* 154:64–68.

49. Kaatz, G. W., S. L. Barriere, D. R. Schaberg, and R. Fekety. 1987. Ciprofloxacin versus vancomycin in the therapy of experimental methicillin-resistant *Staphylococcus aureus* endocarditis. *Antimicrob. Agents Chemother.* 31:527–530.

50. Kaatz, G. W., S. L. Barriere, D. R. Schaberg, and R. Fekety. 1987. The emergence of resistance to ciprofloxacin during treatment of experimental *Staphylococcus aureus* endocarditis. *J. Antimicrob. Chemother.* 20:753–758.

51. Kaatz, G. W., S. M. Seo, J. R. Aeschlimann, H. H. Houlihan, R. C. Mercier, and M. J. Rybak. 1998. Efficacy of trovafloxacin against experimental *Staphylococcus aureus* endocarditis. *Antimicrob. Agents Chemother.* 42::254–256.

52. Kaatz, G. W., S. M. Seo, S. L. Barriere, L. M. Albrecht, and M. J. Rybak. 1991. Development of resistance to fleroxacin during therapy of experimental methicillin-susceptible *Staphylococcus aureus* endocarditis. *Antimicrob. Agents Chemother.* 35:1547–1550.

53. Kaatz, G. W., S. M. Seo, and C. A. Ruble. 1991. Mechanisms of fluoroquinolone resistance in *Staphylococcus aureus*. *J. Infect. Dis.* 163:1080–1086.

54. Kamoun, S., A. Hammami, S. Ben Hamed, M. M. Sahnoun, F. Elleuch, and M. Daoud. 1991. *Brucella* endocarditis on Starr aortic valve prosthesis. *Arch. Mal. Coeur Vaiss* 84:269–271.

55. Karchmer, A. W. 1985. Staphylococcal endocarditis. Laboratory and clinical basis for antibiotic therapy. *Am. J. Med.* 78:116–127.

56. Katsarolis, I., A. Pefanis, D. Iliopoulos, P. Siaperas, P. Karayiannakos, and H. Giamarellou. 2000. Successful trovafloxacin prophylaxis against experimental streptococcal aortic valve endocarditis. *Antimicrob. Agents Chemother.* 44:2564–2566.

57. Kim, Y. S., Q. Liu, L. L. Chow, H. F. Chambers, and M. G. Tauber. 1998. Comparative efficacy of trovafloxacin in

experimental endocarditis caused by ciprofloxacin-sensitive, methicillin-resistant *Staphylococcus aureus*. *Antimicrob. Agents Chemother.* **42**:3325–3327.

58. Kupferwasser, L. I., and A. S. Bayer. 2001. Efficacy of a new des-F(6) quinolone, BMS-284756, in the rabbit model of experimental right-sided endocarditis and lung abscess due to a microaerophilic *Streptococcus*, abstr. B-788 *Program and Abstracts of the 41st Interscience Conference on Antimicrobial Agents and Chemotherapy*. American Society for Microbiology, Washington, D.C.

59. Landman, D., J. M. Quale, N. Mobarakai, and M. M. Zaman. 1995. Ampicillin plus ciprofloxacin therapy of experimental endocarditis caused by multidrug-resistant *Enterococcus faecium*. *J. Antimicrob. Chemother.* **36**:253–258.

59a. Lepidi, H., P. Houpikian, Z. Liang, and D. Raoult. 2003. Cardiac valves in patients with Q fever with endocarditis: microbiological, molecular, and histologic studies. *J. Infect. Dis.* **187**:1097–1106.

60. Levy, P. Y., M. Drancourt, J. Etienne, J. C. Auvergnat, J. Beytout, J. M. Sainty, F. Goldstein, and D. Raoult. 1991. Comparison of different antibiotic regimens for therapy of 32 cases of Q fever endocarditis. *Antimicrob. Agents Chemother.* **35**:533–537.

61. Maurin, M., A. M. Benoliel, P. Bongrand, and D. Raoult. 1992. Phagolysosomal alkalinization and the bactericidal effect of antibiotics: the *Coxiella burnetii* paradigm. *J. Infect. Dis.* **166**:1097–1102.

62. Maserati, R., A. E. Cagni, and C. Segu. 1996. Sparfloxacin therapy for experimental endocarditis caused by methicillin-resistant *Staphylococcus aureus*. *Chemotherapy* **42**:133–139.

63. Palmer, S. R., and S. E. Young. 1982. Q-fever endocarditis in England and Wales, 1975–81. *Lancet* **2**:1448–1449.

64. Papadakis, J. A., G. Samonis, S. Maraki, J. Boutsikakis, V. Petrocheilou, and G. Saroglou. 2000. Efficacy of amikacin, ofloxacin, pefloxacin, ciprofloxacin, enoxacin, and fleroxacin in experimental left-sided *Pseudomonas aeruginosa* endocarditis. *Chemotherapy* **46**:116–121.

65. Piper, K. E., M. S. Rouse, K. L. Ronningen, J. M. Steckelberg, W. R. Wilson, and R. Patel. 2000. Trovafloxacin treatment of viridans group *Streptococcus* experimental endocarditis. *Antimicrob. Agents Chemother.* **44**:2554–2556.

66. Pohlod, D. J., L. D. Saravolatz, and M. M. Somerville. 1988. In-vitro susceptibility of staphylococci to fleroxacin in comparison with six other quinolones. *J. Antimicrob. Chemother.* **22**(Suppl. D):35–41.

67. Preheim, L. C., R. G. Penn, C. C. Sanders, R. V. Goering, and D. K. Giger. 1982. Emergence of resistance to beta-lactam and aminoglycoside antibiotics during moxalactam therapy of *Pseudomonas aeruginosa* infections. *Antimicrob. Agents Chemother.* **22**:1037–1041.

68. Quale, J. M., D. Landman, and N. Mobarakai. 1994. Treatment of experimental endocarditis due to multidrug resistant *Enterococcus faecium* with ciprofloxacin and novobiocin. *J. Antimicrob. Chemother.* **34**:797–802.

69. Raoult, D., P. Bres, M. Drancourt, and G. Vestris. 1991. In vitro susceptibilities of *Coxiella burnetii*, *Rickettsia rickettsii*, and *Rickettsia conorii* to the fluoroquinolone sparfloxacin. *Antimicrob. Agents Chemother.* **35**:88–91.

70. Raoult, D., P. Houpikian, H. Tissot Dupont, J. M. Riss, J. Arditi-Djiane, and P. Brouqui. 1999. Treatment of Q fever endocarditis: comparison of 2 regimens containing doxycycline and ofloxacin or hydroxychloroquine. *Arch. Intern. Med.* **159**:167–173.

71. Raoult, D., M. R. Yeaman, and and O. G. Baca. 1989. Susceptibiltiy of *Rickettsia* and *Coxiella burnetii* to quinolones. *Antimicrob. Agents Chemother.* **35**:2070–7077.

72. Raoult, D., H. Torres, and M. Drancourt. 1991. Shell-vial assay: evaluation of a new technique for determining antibiotic susceptibility, tested in 13 isolates of *Coxiella burnetii*. *Antimicrob. Agents Chemother.* **35**:2070–2077.

73. Reyes, M. P., and A. M. Lerner. 1983. Current problems in the treatment of infective endocarditis due to *Pseudomonas aeruginosa*. *Rev. Infect. Dis.* **5**:314–321.

74. Roman, M. J., P. D. Coriz, and O. G. Baca. 1986. A proposed model to explain persistent infection of host cells with *Coxiella burnetii*. *J. Gen. Microbiol.* **132**(Pt. 5):1415–1422.

75. Rouse, M. S., R. M. Wilcox, N. K. Henry, J. M. Steckelberg, and W. R. Wilson. 1990. Ciprofloxacin therapy of experimental endocarditis caused by methicillin-resistant *Staphylococcus epidermidis*. *Antimicrob. Agents Chemother.* **34**:273–276.

76. Samuel, J. E., M. E. Frazier, and L. P. Mallavia. 1985. Correlation of plasmid type and disease caused by *Coxiella burnetii*. *Infect. Immun.* **49**:775–779.

77. Sanders, C. C., and W. E. Sanders, Jr. 1983. Emergence of resistance during therapy with the newer beta-lactam antibiotics: role of inducible beta-lactamases and implications for the future. *Rev. Infect. Dis.* **5**:639–648.

78. Sanders, C. C., W. E. Sanders, Jr., and R. V. Goering. 1987. Overview of preclinical studies with ciprofloxacin. *Am. J. Med.* **82**:2–11.

79. Sanders, C. C., W. E. Sanders, Jr., R. V. Goering, and V. Werner. 1984. Selection of multiple antibiotic resistance by quinolones, beta-lactams, and aminoglycosides with special reference to cross-resistance between unrelated drug classes. *Antimicrob. Agents Chemother.* **26**:797–801.

80. Schaefler, S. 1989. Methicillin-resistant strains of *Staphylococcus aureus* resistant to quinolones. *J. Clin. Microbiol.* **27**:335–336.

81. Sexton, D. J., M. J. Tenenbaum, W. R. Wilson, J. M. Steckelberg, A. D. Tice, D. Gilbert, W. Dismukes, R. H. Drew, and D. T. Durack. 1998. Ceftriaxone once daily for four weeks compared with ceftriaxone plus gentamicin once daily for two weeks for treatment of endocarditis due to penicillin-susceptible streptococci. Endocarditis Treatment Consortium Group. *Clin. Infect. Dis.* **27**:1470–1474.

82. Shekar, R., T. W. Rice, C. H. Zierdt, and C. A. Kallick. 1985. Outbreak of endocarditis caused by *Pseudomonas aeruginosa* serotype O11 among pentazocine and tripelennamine abusers in Chicago. *J. Infect. Dis.* **151**:203–208.

83. Spelman, D. W. 1982. Q fever: a study of 111 consecutive cases. *Med. J. Aust.* **1**:547, 548, 551, 553.

84. Spyridaki, I., A. Psaroulaki, A. Aransay, E. Scoulica, and Y. Tselentis. 2000. Diagnosis of quinolone-resistant *Coxiella burnetii* by PCR-RFLP. *J. Clin. Lab. Anal.* **14**:59–63.

85. Strunk, R. W., J. C. Gratz, R. Maserati, and W. M. Scheld. 1985. Comparison of ciprofloxacin with azlocillin plus tobramycin in the therapy of experimental *Pseudomonas aeruginosa* endocarditis. *Antimicrob. Agents Chemother.* **28**:428–432.

86. Sullam, P. M., M. G. Tauber, C. J. Hackbarth, H. F. Chambers, K. G. Scott, and M. A. Sande. 1985. Pefloxacin therapy for experimental endocarditis caused by methicillin-susceptible or methicillin-resistant strains of *Staphylococcus aureus*. *Antimicrob. Agents Chemother.* **27**:685–687.

87. Thrupp, L. D. Susceptibiltiy testing of antibiotics in liquid media. p. 73–113. *In* V. Lorian (ed.), *Antibiotics in Laboratory Medicine*. The Williams & Wilkins Co., Baltimore, Md.

88. Trucksis, M., D. C. Hooper, and J. S. Wolfson. 1991. Emerging resistance to fluoroquinolones in staphylococci: an alert. *Ann. Intern. Med.* **114**:424–426.

89. Uzun, O., H. E. Akalin, S. Unal, M. Demircin, A. C. Yorgancioglu, and B. Ugurlu. 1992. Long-term oral ciprofloxacin in the treatment of prosthetic valve endocarditis due to *Pseudomonas aeruginosa*. *Scand. J. Infect. Dis.* 24:797–800.

90. Vazquez, J., M. B. Perri, L. A. Thal, S. A. Donabedian, and M. J. Zervos. 1993. Sparfloxacin and clinafloxacin alone or in combination with gentamicin for therapy of experimental ampicillin-resistant enterococcal endocarditis in rabbits. *J. Antimicrob. Chemother.* 32:715–721.

91. Whitman, M. S., P. G. Pitsakis, A. Zausner, L. L. Livornese, A. J. Osborne, C. C. Johnson, and M. E. Levison. 1993. Antibiotic treatment of experimental endocarditis due to vancomycin- and ampicillin-resistant *Enterococcus faecium*. *Antimicrob. Agents Chemother.* 37:2069–2073.

92. Xiong, Y. Q., G. Potel, J. Caillon, G. Stephant, F. Jehl, D. Bugnon, P. Le Conte, D. Baron, and H. Drugeon. 1995. Comparative efficacies of ciprofloxacin and pefloxacin alone or in combination with fosfomycin in experimental endocarditis induced by multidrug-susceptible and -resistant *Pseudomonas aeruginosa*. *Antimicrob. Agents Chemother.* 39:496–499.

93. Yeaman, M. R., and O. G. Baca. 1991. Mechanisms that may account for differential antibiotic susceptibilities among *Coxiella burnetii* isolates. *Antimicrob. Agents Chemother.* 35:948–954.

94. Yeaman, M. R., and O. G. Baca. 1990. Unexpected antibiotic susceptibility of a chronic isolate of *Coxiella burnetii*. *Ann. N. Y. Acad. Sci.* 590:297–305.

95. Yeaman, M. R., L. A. Mitscher, and O. G. Baca. 1987. In vitro susceptibility of *Coxiella burnetii* to antibiotics, including several quinolones. *Antimicrob. Agents Chemother.* 31:1079–1084.

96. Yeaman, M. R., M. J. Roman, and O. G. Baca. 1989. Antibiotic susceptibilities of two Coxiella burnetii isolates implicated in distinct clinical syndromes. *Antimicrob. Agents Chemother.* 33:1052–1057.

97. Yeaman, M. R., and O. G. Baca. 1990. Antibiotic susceptibility of *Coxiella burnetii*, p. 213–223. *In* T. J. Marrie (ed.), *Q fever*, vol. 1. *The Disease*. CRC Press, Inc., Boca Raton, Fla.

98. Yebra, M., J. Ortigosa, F. Albarran, and M. G. Crespo. 1990. Ciprofloxacin in a case of Q fever endocarditis. *N. Engl. J. Med.* 323:614.

99. Zaman, M. M., D. Landman, S. Burney, and J. M. Quale. 1996. Treatment of experimental endocarditis due to multidrug-resistant *Enterococcus faecium* with clinafloxacin and penicillin. *J. Antimicrob. Chemother.* 37:127–132.

100. Zeiler, H. J. 1985. Evaluation of the in vitro bactericidal action of ciprofloxacin on cells of *Escherichia coli* in the logarithmic and stationary phases of growth. *Antimicrob. Agents Chemother.* 28:524–527.

Quinolone Antimicrobial Agents, 3rd ed.
Edited by David C. Hooper and Ethan Rubinstein
© 2003 ASM Press, Washington, D.C.

Chapter 17

Treatment of Bacterial Meningitis and Other Central Nervous System Infections

ALLAN R. TUNKEL AND W. MICHAEL SCHELD

The fluoroquinolones have two important properties that suggest they may be appropriate agents for the treatment of central nervous system (CNS) infections: excellent in vitro activity against meningeal pathogens and good penetration into extravascular spaces, including cerebrospinal fluid (CSF). However, despite these favorable properties, the fluoroquinolones have been used infrequently to treat CNS infections. The fluoroquinolones have been studied most extensively in bacterial meningitis. The following sections review the epidemiology and etiology of bacterial meningitis, the in vitro activities of the fluoroquinolones against various meningeal pathogens, the therapeutic principles (i.e., CSF penetration and pharmacodynamics) for use of these agents in meningitis, and clinical results in both experimental animal models and humans to place in perspective the potential usefulness of the fluoroquinolones in the treatment and prevention of bacterial meningitis. The efficacy of the fluoroquinolones in the treatment of other CNS infections is also reviewed, where data are available on the utility of these agents.

EPIDEMIOLOGY AND ETIOLOGY OF BACTERIAL MENINGITIS

Bacterial meningitis is an illness that continues to have a high morbidity and mortality despite the availability of effective bactericidal antimicrobial agents. In a surveillance study of 13,974 cases of bacterial meningitis reported to the Centers for Disease Control and Prevention (CDC) from 27 states in the United States from 1978 through 1981 (77), the overall attack rate for bacterial meningitis was approximately 3.0 cases per 100,000 population; the majority of cases were caused by *Haemophilus influenzae* (48%), followed by *Neisseria meningitidis* (20%) and *Streptococcus*

pneumoniae (13%), with case fatality rates of 6.0, 10.3, and 26.3%, respectively. In a subsequent study involving five states (Missouri, New Jersey, Oklahoma, Tennessee, and Washington) and Los Angeles county (population of almost 34 million) (98), the overall incidence of bacterial meningitis was two to three times that of the previous report, with 77% of cases caused by *H. influenzae, N. meningitidis,* and *S. pneumoniae*. After the introduction of *H. influenzae* type b conjugate vaccines in the United States, another surveillance study was conducted during 1995 in laboratories serving all the acute care hospitals in 22 counties of four states (Georgia, Tennessee, Maryland, and California) and reported dramatic declines in the incidence of invasive *H. influenzae* type b disease (81); most cases (47%) of meningitis were caused by *S. pneumoniae,* followed by *N. meningitidis* (25%). These data indicate the importance of focusing on therapeutic and preventive interventions against these pathogens.

Bacterial meningitis also remains a significant problem in other parts of the world. In a review of all cases of purulent, nontuberculous meningitis in an isolation-fever hospital in Salvador, Brazil, for the decade 1973 to 1982, the three most common meningeal pathogens (*H. influenzae, N. meningitidis,* and *S. pneumoniae*) accounted for 72% of all cases and 70% of all deaths (8). The case fatality rate for meningitis caused by *H. influenzae* was 38% and that caused by *S. pneumoniae* was 59%, much higher than those encountered in the United States. The mortality for meningitis caused by members of the *Enterobacteriaceae* family was 86% in that survey, with more than half of the cases in children less than 24 months of age caused by *Salmonella* species, a rare cause of bacterial meningitis in the United States.

In addition to these unacceptable case fatality rates, recent antimicrobial susceptibility patterns of meningeal pathogens have documented resistance of

Allan R. Tunkel • Division of Infectious Diseases, Department of Medicine, Drexel University College of Medicine, 3300 Henry Avenue, Philadelphia, PA 19129. W. Michael Scheld • University of Virginia School of Medicine, P.O. Box 801342, Charlottesville, VA 22908-1342.

these microorganisms to many conventional antimicrobial agents. The therapy of meningitis caused by *S. pneumoniae* has been modified on the basis of trends in pneumococcal susceptibility patterns. In the past, pneumococci were uniformly susceptible to penicillin with MICs of ≤0.06 μg/ml. Numerous reports from the United States and throughout the world have now identified strains of pneumococci that are of intermediate resistance to penicillin (MIC range of 0.1 to 1.0 μg/ml), as well as strains that are highly resistant (MIC of ≥2.0 μg/ml) (9, 29, 35, 67, 88); in some areas of the United States, 25 to 30% of invasive pneumococcal isolates were found to have either intermediate- or high-level resistance to penicillin, with higher rates in other areas of the world. Strains of meningococci have also been identified that possess in vitro resistance to penicillin, reaching almost 50% of isolates in one hospital in Spain (70), although rates have been lower (3%) in the United States (34). β-Lactamase-producing strains of *H. influenzae* accounted for approximately 24% of CSF isolates in the United States in 1981 and for approximately 32% of CSF isolates in 1986 (77, 98). The etiologic agents of gram-negative bacillary meningitis (e.g., *Escherichia coli*, *Klebsiella pneumoniae*, and *Pseudomonas aeruginosa*) also have demonstrated increased resistance to standard antimicrobial agents, including expanded-spectrum cephalosporins (37, 44), particularly in the hospital setting. These data indicate the continued need to investigate the potential effectiveness of alternative antimicrobial agents for the therapy of bacterial meningitis.

IN VITRO ACTIVITY OF FLUOROQUINOLONES AGAINST MENINGEAL PATHOGENS

The in vitro activity of selected fluoroquinolones against meningeal pathogens is shown in Table 1 (30,

58, 60). The fluoroquinolones are extremely active in vitro against the gram-negative bacteria (e.g., *H. influenzae*, *N. meningitidis*, and *E. coli*) that cause acute bacterial meningitis. Ciprofloxacin is the most active fluoroquinolone against these organisms currently available in the United States and, in addition, it has the best in vitro activity of the fluoroquinolones against *P. aeruginosa*. The fluoroquinolones are also highly active in vitro against gram-negative pathogens rarely encountered in patients with bacterial meningitis (e.g., *Salmonella* species and other *Enterobacteriaceae*); these pathogens are associated with high mortality rates and are frequently resistant to other antimicrobial agents. Although the minimal bactericidal concentration (MBC) is more important than the MIC in determining the optimal response to antimicrobial therapy in patients with bacterial meningitis (see below), the concentrations in CSF achieved with these agents are, in general, about 4- to >50-fold higher than the MICs for 90% of the strains of gram-negative pathogens.

Although gram-negative pathogens are, in general, highly susceptible to the fluoroquinolones, gram-positive organisms are considerably less susceptible to older agents (e.g., ciprofloxacin and ofloxacin). However, newer agents (e.g., levofloxacin, gatifloxacin, moxifloxacin, trovafloxacin) have shown excellent in vitro activity against *S. pneumoniae* (59) and have been evaluated in experimental animal models of pneumococcal meningitis (see below). Of concern, however, are the recent reports of decreased susceptibility of the fluoroquinolones to *S. pneumoniae* (10). One group found that 5.5% of pneumococcal isolates in Hong Kong were resistant to levofloxacin (28), and one fatal case of meningitis caused by a levofloxacin-resistant *S. pneumoniae* has been reported (104). These data indicate the need to monitor in vitro pneumococcal susceptibility to these agents.

Table 1. In vitro activities of selected fluoroquinolones against major meningeal pathogens[a]

Organism	Representative MIC90 (range) (μg/ml)						
	Ciprofloxacin	Ofloxacin	Pefloxacin	Levofloxacin	Trovafloxacin	Grepafloxacin	Moxifloxacin
H. influenzae	≤0.008–≤0.06	≤0.06–0.5	0.06	0.025–0.06	0.015–0.03	0.008–0.0125	0.03–0.06
N. meningitidis	0.008–0.12	≤0.06–0.4	0.03		0.008	0.008	0.015
S. pneumoniae	2 (0.78–6.2)	2 (1–8)	12 (8–16)	1–3.13	0.125–0.25	0.12–0.4	0.12–0.25
E. coli	≤0.06 (≤0.01–0.25)	0.12 (0.02–1)	0.12–0.25	0.05–0.12	0.03–4	0.03–0.12	0.008
S. agalactiae	2 (0.5–4)	2 (2–4)	32	1–2	0.25–0.5	0.5	0.25–0.5
L. monocytogenes	2 (0.5–2)	2–4	6–8	1	0.25–0.5		0.5
P. aeruginosa	0.5 (0.25–8)	2 (2–>50)	2	2–50	1–8	0.5–>4	1–32
Salmonella species	≤0.06	0.12–0.25	0.12	0.12	0.03–12	0.06–0.12	0.062–0.13
S. aureus	0.5 (0.25–2)	0.5 (0.1–2)	0.5 (0.1–2)	0.5–0.8 (0.25–32)	0.03–4	0.12–>4	0.03–0.12

[a] Data from references 30, 58, and 60.

While several of the fluoroquinolones possess in vitro activity against staphylococci, including some methicillin-resistant strains, the concentrations of these agents that are achieved in CSF with systemic administration are barely equal to and usually do not exceed the MICs for these isolates. Furthermore, clinical experience with these agents in the therapy of staphylococcal meningitis is virtually nonexistent. For other gram-positive organisms that are important meningeal pathogens (e.g., *Streptococcus agalactiae*, *Listeria monocytogenes*), in vitro susceptibility of the currently available fluoroquinolones is marginal. Although some of the fluoroquinolones (e.g., ciprofloxacin, ofloxacin, levofloxacin, pefloxacin, sparfloxacin, clinafloxacin) have good in vitro activity against *L. monocytogenes* (50), a recent case report described a patient who developed *Listeria* meningitis while receiving ciprofloxacin therapy (26), indicating that further in vitro and in vivo studies are needed to evaluate these agents in the management of listeriosis.

BASIC THERAPEUTIC PRINCIPLES IN INFECTIONS OF THE CENTRAL NERVOUS SYSTEM

The definition of bacteriologic cure or response in patients with bacterial meningitis is based on bacteriologic eradication from CSF, and several factors determine whether bactericidal activity is achieved (2, 11, 48, 79, 93). The first factor relates to the penetration of the antimicrobial agent into CSF, which depends, to a great extent, on the status of the blood–brain barrier. Antimicrobial entry into CSF is also enhanced if the agent has a low molecular weight, low degree of ionization, high-lipid solubility, and low degree of protein binding. Furthermore, active transport systems in the cerebral capillaries and choroid plexi may remove some antimicrobial agents from the CSF to blood.

A second factor is the bactericidal activity of the antimicrobial agent within purulent CSF. This property is affected by the pH of CSF, because the bacteridical activity of some drugs (e.g., the aminoglycosides) may be diminished in an acidic environment; elevated protein concentrations in CSF which may decrease the activity of agents that are highly protein bound; metabolism of drugs in the CSF to inactive metabolites; influence of other drugs in CSF on bactericidal activity; and modification of bactericidal activity by the inoculum effect, in which the MIC of an antimicrobial agent against the infecting organism increases dramatically as the inoculum of the organism is increased. Rapid bacterial killing is also required for optimal therapy. Multiple studies in experimental animal models have shown that rapid

bacterial killing is observed in vivo only when CSF concentrations of β-lactams or aminoglycosides exceed the MBC by about 10- to 30-fold.

A final factor that may contribute to response to antimicrobial therapy in bacterial meningitis is pharmacodynamics, which relates to the time course of antimicrobial therapy at the site of infection (2, 48). An understanding of the pharmacodynamic properties of a single antimicrobial agent (which may be different in CSF because of poor penetration of CSF and low concentrations of antibody and complement in CSF) may be useful to determine a dosing regimen for optimal effectiveness. In general, two major patterns of antimicrobial activity have been described: time-dependent and concentration-dependent. In time-dependent killing, the bacterical activity of an antimicrobial agent depends on the time that its concentration exceeds the MIC. As stated above, the concentrations of β-lactams in CSF need to exceed the MBC by 10- to 30-fold to obtain the maximum bactericidal effect in experimental animal models of meningitis. However, peak antimicrobial concentrations in CSF and the time that the antimicrobial concentrations exceed the MBC ($T > MBC$) are interrelated, and it is likely in these studies that $T > MBC$ increased in parallel with peak concentrations in CSF. This pattern was recently studied in an experimental animal model of cephalosporin-resistant pneumococcal meningitis, in which ceftriaxone was administered at four different dosing regimens (45); the duration of time that the concentrations of ceftriaxone in CSF exceeded the MBC was the only parameter that independently correlated with the bacterial kill rate, and the maximal bacterial kill rate was achieved only when ceftriaxone concentrations in CSF exceeded the MBC for 95 to 100% of the dosing interval. In concentration-dependent killing, bacterial killing occurs over a wide range of antimicrobial concentrations and a prolonged recovery period (i.e., a postantibiotic effect) after drug concentrations fall below the MIC. This pattern is seen with the aminoglycosides. In an experimental animal model of *E. coli* meningitis, single-dose gentamicin therapy was as effective as divided dose regimens despite different times that gentamicin concentrations in CSF exceeded the MBC (1). The following sections review the importance of these factors in the use of the fluoroquinolones in bacterial meningitis.

Cerebrospinal Fluid Penetration of Fluoroquinolones

Animal models

As stated above, the penetration of an antimicrobial agent into CSF is an important factor in determining whether bactericidal activity is achieved in patients with bacterial meningitis. The fluoroquinolones have been evaluated in several experimental animal models to determine their entry into normal or purulent CSF (71, 76). Table 2 compares the penetration of several of the fluoroquinolones in CSF with those of conventional antimicrobial agents in the experimental rabbit model of bacterial meningitis.

Early experimental studies that examined the penetration of fluoroquinolones into CSF revealed that concentrations of pefloxacin in CSF were 76% of those in sera of dogs with experimental *Staphylococcus aureus* meningitis (4); penetration in healthy dogs was 44.6%. In another experimental canine model (92), a 1-h intravenous injection of either 12.5 or 25 mg of enoxacin per kg of body weight in uninfected animals produced average concentrations in CSF of 2.6 and 6.5 µg/ml, respective-

Table 2. Percent penetration of selected antimicrobial agents and fluoroquinolones into CSF of rabbits and humans with meningitis[a]

Antimicrobial agent	Percent penetration (range)	
	Rabbits	Humans
Penicillins		
Penicillin G	2.6–4.9	7.8
Ampicillin	12.1–18.4	4–65
Nafcillin	1.8–2.9	5–27
Piperacillin	15.7	22.7–32.0
Cephalosporins		
Cefotaxime	2.1–8.4	4–55
Ceftriaxone	2.7–12.0	1.5–16.0
Ceftazidime	7.6–11.1	14–45
Cefepime	16–22	10–11.8
Monobactams		
Aztreonam	22.9	5–17
Carbapenems		
Imipenem	3–13	10.6–41.0
Meropenem	6.4	10.7–21.0
Aminoglycosides		
Gentamicin	18.9–28.7	<1.0–2.5
Tobramycin	24.4–26.6	<1.0–0.9
Amikacin	19.0–35.5	20–34
Other Antimicrobial Agents		
Vancomycin	8.4–11.7	<1–53
Chloramphenicol	23.8–34.3	30–66
Rifampin	17.2–19.1	4–25
Fluoroquinolones		
Ciprofloxacin	15.0–27.5	6–37
Ofloxacin	20	28–87
Pefloxacin	46.0–51.3	52–58
Trovafloxacin	19–27	
Gatifloxacin	46–56	
Moxifloxacin	34–81	
Gemifloxacin	28–33	
Rufloxacin		72–84

[a] Data from references 2, 11, 48, 79, and 93. Values are calculated as (concentration in CSF/concentration in serum) × 100. These calculations are derived from peak concentrations, mean concentrations, or area-under-the-concentration curve.

ly, within 90 to 240 min; these corresponded to percent penetration values into CSF, as calculated by the area-under-the-curve method, of 33% (12.5 mg/kg of body weight dose) and 47% (25 mg/kg dose). In animals infected intracisternally with *S. aureus*, an intravenous dose of enoxacin (12.5 mg/kg) given 18 to 20 h later led to a peak concentration in CSF of 6.9 µg/ml (CSF penetration of 67.3%). In both uninfected and infected animals, the concentrations in CSF greatly exceeded the MICs of enoxacin (and other marketed fluoroquinolones) against meningococci and *H. influenzae*.

Pefloxacin has also been evaluated in an experimental rabbit model of *E. coli* meningitis (85). In uninfected rabbits, the percent penetration of pefloxacin into CSF after a 3-h infusion of 5, 15, or 30 mg/kg/h ranged from 26.4 to 39.2%. In animals with *E. coli* meningitis, the mean percent penetration of pefloxacin given at various dosages (1 to 30 mg/kg/h) for 7 h after an initial bolus was assessed 16 h after induction of meningitis. The mean percent penetration of pefloxacin into CSF was 51.3% in all rabbits with meningitis compared with percent penetration of 11.1% for cefotaxime (100 mg/kg/h) and 22.3% for chloramphenicol (60 mg/kg/h). In another animal study, the mean CSF pefloxacin concentrations (8.8 µg/ml) were 44.7% of serum pefloxacin concentrations (19.7 µg/ml) in three healthy dogs after 6 weeks of therapy (54).

Other fluoroquinolones have been examined with respect to CSF penetration in animal models of bacterial meningitis. In an experimental animal model of *P. aeruginosa* meningitis (27), the mean percent penetration of ciprofloxacin was 18.4% compared with 4.1% in uninfected rabbits. Similar findings have been observed in experimental animal models of gram-negative bacillary meningitis utilizing ciprofloxacin and ofloxacin (76, 87). Following a single intramuscular injection of ciprofloxacin (50 mg/kg) or ofloxacin (30 mg/kg), mean peak concentrations of ciprofloxacin and ofloxacin in CSF were 2.55 µg/ml (penetration in CSF of 27.5%) and 7.56 µg/ml (penetration in CSF of 20.0%), respectively. Fleroxacin has been evaluated in the rabbit model of *E. coli* meningitis (16), in which the mean percent penetrations of the drug into CSF of animals without meningitis were 46.5 and 71.8% after doses of 0.5 and 5 mg/kg/h, respectively; in animals with meningitis, the respective percent penetration values were 81.9 and 107%.

Taken collectively, these data suggest that as a class, newer fluoroquinolones penetrate into CSF in the presence of bacterial meningitis similarly to other agents (e.g., β-lactams; Table 1) that have proven useful for the therapy of this disease. Despite favorable penetration ratios, however, the absolute peak concentrations in CSF attained are marginal for the therapy of some forms of meningitis (see below) because of the low concentrations of quinolones in serum compared with those of β-lactam agents.

Humans

The percent penetration of the fluoroquinolones into human CSF has also been examined (Table 2). Pefloxacin was administered intravenously (7.5 or 15 mg/kg) or orally to 15 patients with meningitis or ventriculitis, 14 of whom were treated with a variety of other antimicrobial agents, from days 3 to 20 of illness (101). Two hours after the end of the third intravenous infusion or 4 h after the third oral ingestion, concentrations of pefloxacin in CSF were measured by high-performance liquid chromatography. The results revealed a variability in peak concentrations (6.8 to 16.0 μg/ml after a 7.5 mg/kg dose and 14.0 to 18.6 μg/ml after a 15 mg/kg dose). The percent penetration was good (Table 2), however, and appeared to persist beyond the point at which the meningitis was cured; concentrations of pefloxacin in CSF exceeded the MICs for most strains (except streptococci), especially when the higher dose was used. In another study (17), pefloxacin was administered as a single 400-mg intravenous dose for 1 h to nine patients with or without meningitis; CSF was sampled frequently through an external ventricular drain. Concentrations in CSF peaked at ~3 μg/ml 4 h later. The concentrations of pefloxacin in CSF and serum were maintained at 0.57 to 0.64 between 6 and 48 h after infusion, a finding that agrees with results of other studies. The apparent duration of transfer of pefloxacin from plasma into ventricular CSF was 1.26 h, with a CSF elimination half-life of 13.4 h (similar to the elimination half-life of pefloxacin from plasma).

The penetration of ciprofloxacin into noninflamed CSF was examined 48 h after oral ingestion of a single 500-mg tablet (40). Concentrations of ciprofloxacin in CSF ranged from 0.06 to 0.14 μg/ml, with a percent penetration into CSF (calculated as the area under the concentration curve of ciprofloxacin in CSF relative to the area under the concentration curve of ciprofloxacin in serum) of about 10%. Higher concentrations of ciprofloxacin in CSF (0.25 and 0.4 μg/ml) were observed in two patients with bacterial meningitis when concentrations were measured 2 to 3 h after oral ingestion. Similar results were obtained in a 65-year-old female without meningitis who had frequent sampling of CSF through an Ommaya intraventricular reservoir after a single 500-mg dose of ciprofloxacin (95), with

peak concentrations in serum and CSF of 3.5 and 0.15 μg/ml, respectively. In another study, three successive 200-mg doses of intravenous ciprofloxacin at 12-h intervals were administered to 23 patients with bacterial meningitis in addition to standard regimens (100). CSF sampling between days 2 and 4 of therapy and again between days 10 and 20, at 1 to 8 h after injection, revealed mean concentrations in CSF of 0.35 to 0.56 μg/ml and 0.15 to 0.27 μg/ml, respectively. Penetration, utilizing peak concentrations, ranged from 6.5 to 16.2% during the acute stage and from 4.0 to 9.9% during the late stage of the disease, suggesting that diffusion of the drug into CSF persists (but to a lesser extent) beyond the point at which meningitis is "cured." In addition, eight adult males hospitalized for reasons other than meningitis received three oral doses of ciprofloxacin at 750 mg every 12 h (49). They underwent lumbar punctures during myelography for lumbar disk disease. The mean ciprofloxacin concentration in CSF was 0.20 μg/ml, with a CSF/serum ratio of 0.082. The penetration of ciprofloxacin (200 mg intravenously for two doses given 12 h apart) into CSF was also studied in 25 patients with noninflamed meninges and in nine patients with inflamed meninges due to a variety of disorders (24). In the patients with noninflamed meninges, the ciprofloxacin concentrations in CSF varied from 0.038 to 0.178 μg/ml, with a CSF/plasma ratio of 0.038 to 0.40. In the nine patients with meningitis, the CSF/plasma ratio was markedly increased, ranging from 0.17 to 0.91, with the highest values observed at 7 and 9 h after dosing. However, in this study, the CSF was collected only once from each patient and at variable times, making it impossible to estimate a peak concentration in CSF and compare it with a peak concentration in plasma.

Several studies have investigated the penetration of ofloxacin into human CSF (94). In one report, ofloxacin was administered orally at a dosage of 200 mg twice daily for 2 to 8 days given to 17 patients with various neurologic disorders (90). At 1.5 and 12 h after dosing, samples of CSF and serum were obtained. Concentrations of 0.32 to 3.6 and 0.5 to 7.75 μg/ml were demonstrated in CSF and serum, respectively, at 1.5 h, and concentrations of 0.49 to 1.35 and 0.5 to 1.83 μg/ml were demonstrated in CSF and serum, respectively, at 12 h. The authors claimed the percent penetration to be 47% at 1.5 h and 87% at 12 h, although the original data are difficult to interpret. In a second study, nine patients with proved or presumed bacterial meningitis were treated with amoxicillin plus ofloxacin (200 mg orally twice daily for the first 5 days), and samples of CSF were obtained 2 to 12 h after dosing on days 2 and 5 (89). Concentrations of ofloxacin in CSF were generally 50 to 60% of those in serum. Ofloxacin was also evaluated in 12 patients with or without meningitis to whom a single 300-mg dose of ofloxacin was given orally (18); blood and CSF samples were analyzed 3 and 6 h later. The mean concentrations in plasma were 3.5 and 1.9 µg/ml after ingestion, respectively, while the mean concentrations in CSF were 1.4 µg/ml at 3 h and 0.7 µg/ml at 6 h after drug administration. In patients with purulent meningitis, mean concentrations in plasma and CSF were 2.5 and 0.7 µg/ml, respectively. In a study of cancer patients without meningitis (6), the penetration of ofloxacin in CSF (200-mg single dose) given orally or intravenously was assessed. Peak concentrations of ofloxacin in CSF (0.4 to 1.0 µg/ml) were observed 2 to 4 h after intravenous infusion or oral administration; peak concentrations in serum of 2.0 to 3.5 µg/ml were observed just after infusion, and concentrations of 1.7 to 4.0 µg/ml were documented 1 to 2 h after oral administration. Bactericidal titers against *N. meningitidis*, *H. influenzae*, and *E. coli* in CSF were high, whereas bactericidal titers against *S. aureus*, *L. monocytogenes*, and *S. pneumoniae* were low or nonexistent. In another study of 22 patients with purulent meningitis or ventriculitis treated with conventional antimicrobial therapy (62), three successive doses of ofloxacin (200 mg each) were infused at 12-h intervals during the acute stage of disease. The mean percent penetration into ventricular fluid, expressed as a ratio of areas under the curve for CSF and plasma over 0 to 12 h, was 73%.

Other fluoroquinolones have been examined for their penetration into human CSF. The mean concentration of temafloxacin in CSF in 30 patients without meningitis following two 600-mg doses given 12 h apart was 1.35 µg/ml, with a CSF/serum ratio of 0.38 (91). The mean CSF/serum ratios of sparfloxacin after a single 200-mg oral dose or 200 mg once daily for 3 days were 0.246 and 0.346, respectively (36). After intravenous infusion of alatrofloxacin, the alanyl-alanyl prodrug of trovafloxacin, into 12 healthy subjects, CSF/serum ratios ranged from 0.14 to 0.33 in the postdistribution phase from 5 to 24 h after infusion (13). Rufloxacin was also studied in 44 patients scheduled for lumbar puncture to determine the level of penetration of this orally administered agent into three groups of patients (55): those with normal CSF, those with aseptic meningitis, and those with bacterial meningitis. The mean rufloxacin concentrations in CSF and serum ranged from 0.57 to 0.84 depending on the study group; a higher, but not statistically significant, degree of penetration was observed in patients with

bacterial meningitis than in those patients with normal CSF or aseptic meningitis.

The fluoroquinolones may also reach potentially therapeutic concentrations in brain tissue. In the only reported study with humans, 30 patients received various regimens of pefloxacin prior to removal of a brain tumor (41). The concentrations of pefloxacin in brain tissue ranged from 3.28 to 4.50 µg/g versus concentrations in plasma of 5.05 to 10.22 µg/ml at the time of removal of brain tissue. In addition, pefloxacin concentrations were higher in tumor tissue than in the surrounding unaffected brain tissue (ratios of tumor/brain concentrations ranged from 1.57 to 3.16), although methods for correction of blood contamination in the samples were not mentioned in this report.

Pharmacodynamics

The fluoroquinolones exhibit pharmacokinetic and pharmacodynamic properties similar to the aminoglycosides. In experimental animal models of meningitis caused by *S. pneumoniae*, *E. coli*, and *P. aeruginosa*, increasing concentrations of fluoroquinolones in CSF have resulted in higher rates of bactericidal killing (27, 39, 47, 57). The postantibiotic effects of the fluoroquinolones with gram-negative bacilli are of moderate duration. However, features of both time and concentration dependence have been demonstrated with the fluoroquinolones in experimental animal models of meningitis. In two studies using the experimental animal models of pneumococcal meningitis (39, 47), the CSF concentrations of trovafloxacin and gatifloxacin needed to exceed the MBC for the entire dosing interval to achieve maximal bactericidal activity; divided dosing regimens of gatifloxacin appeared superior to single-dose regimens (47). By administration of gatifloxacin in divided doses, the peak concentrations in CSF and serum were lower and the time that the antimicrobial concentrations remained above the MBC (without changing the area-under-the-concentration-time curve) was extended. These findings are likely the result of the short (less than 2 h) postantibiotic effects of the fluoroquinolones against pneumococci in CSF.

EFFICACY OF FLUOROQUINOLONES IN ANIMAL MODELS

Many of the studies cited above that used fluoroquinolones in experimental models of bacterial meningitis also compared the bactericidal activities of these agents with those of several conventional antimicrobial agents. In an experimental rabbit model of *E. coli* meningitis (85), the rate of bacterial killing in animals treated with pefloxacin was only a mean of -0.37 $\log_{10}$ CFU/ml of CSF per hour at dosages of 1 to 15 mg/kg/h, and only 4 of 20 animals had sterile CSF at the end of drug infusion. In contrast, greater bacterial killing (-0.77 $\log_{10}$ CFU/ml of CSF per hour) was observed in animals receiving higher doses of pefloxacin (30 mg/kg/h), which was similar to that obtained with cefotaxime at doses simulating concentrations in serum commonly achieved in humans ($P > 0.1$). Bacterial killing in CSF with pefloxacin therapy at this higher dosage was superior to that obtained with chloramphenicol, with four of four CSF samples sterilized at the end of therapy (versus zero of two CSF samples sterilized with chloramphenicol). No pefloxacin-resistant colonies developed during therapy. However, this result (i.e., rate of eradication of *E. coli* from CSF equivalent to that with cefotaxime) required mean concentrations of pefloxacin in serum of 45.8 μg/ml, concentrations higher than those achievable in humans receiving standard regimens.

Ciprofloxacin has been evaluated in an experimental model of *P. aeruginosa* meningitis (27). The geometric mean MICs and MBCs against the test strain were 1 and 1 μg/ml for ciprofloxacin, 3.5 and 57 μg/ml for ceftazidime, and 0.8 and 2.6 μg/ml for tobramycin. The rate of bacterial killing in CSF was dose-dependent in ciprofloxacin-treated animals ($r = 0.74$; $P < 0.01$); the rate of killing at a ciprofloxacin dosage of 5 mg/kg/h was similar to that obtained with the combination of ceftazidime and tobramycin. However, these results required mean serum ciprofloxacin concentrations of 6.7 μg/ml, which corresponded to concentrations achievable in humans but were higher than those attainable when a dose of 750 mg was administered orally twice daily.

Ciprofloxacin and ofloxacin have also been evaluated in the experimental rabbit model of meningitis (75, 87). The results of therapy were assessed 6 h after the intracisternal inoculation of $10^{8.5}$ CFU of a β-lactamase-producing strain of *H. influenzae*. Although all untreated animals died, bacterial concentrations decreased 2.3 logs in 8 h in untreated animals, whereas bacterial concentrations in CSF decreased 6.9 and 7.2 logs in the ciprofloxacin- and ofloxacin-treated animals, respectively, during the 8-h infusion. These responses were significantly more rapid ($P < 0.01$) than those achieved with ampicillin or chloramphenicol against this β-lactamase-producing strain of *H. influenzae* and were similar to the results obtained with ceftriaxone in an experimental model of *E. coli* meningitis. In experimental *P. aeruginosa* meningitis, administration of ciprofloxacin,

ofloxacin, or ceftazidime 18 h after intracisternal inoculation of $10^{6.2}$ CFU led to a significant ($P < 0.01$) decrease in concentrations of bacteria in CSF compared with those in untreated animals, although the regimens did not differ from one another, producing a decline of only ~2 $\log_{10}$ CFU in bacterial concentrations over 8 h, a rate of killing much slower than that achieved against *H. influenzae* with the same duration of therapy at identical dosages. This slower rate of killing was presumably due to the lesser susceptibility of *P. aeruginosa* and the lower concentrations of ciprofloxacin achieved in serum (2.55 μg/ml) compared with those in other experimental model studies (27).

Trovafloxacin has excellent penetration into CSF and has been shown to have bactericidal activity in an experimental rabbit model of penicillin-resistant pneumococcal meningitis (39), an effect not altered by the coadministration of dexamethaxone. The combination of trovafloxacin and vancomycin was found to significantly ($P < 0.05$) increase the killing rate (mean decrease of -0.60 $\log_{10}$ CFU/ml per hour) in an experimental rabbit model of penicillin-resistant pneumococcal meningitis, a killing rate greater than when each agent was used alone (mean decrease of -0.39 $\log_{10}$ CFU/ml per hour for vancomycin and -0.33 $\log_{10}$ CFU/ml per hour for trovafloxacin) (68). Similar killing rates (mean decrease of -0.67 $\log_{10}$ CFU/ml per hour) were obtained with the combination of trovafloxacin and ceftriaxone against a penicillin-resistant pneumococcal strain (MIC = 4 μg/ml) (12), with greater killing rates than when either agent used alone or for the combination of vancomycin plus ceftriaxone (mean decrease of -0.53 $\log_{10}$ CFU/ml per hour), the combination most often used in clinical practice. These data suggest that the fluoroquinolones may have a role in combination with cell wall active antimicrobial agents when therapy of bacterial meningitis requires highly bactericidal activity (i.e., meningitis caused by penicillin-resistant pneumococci). Trovafloxacin has also been evaluated in an experimental rat model of *L. monocytogenes* meningoencephalitis (51) and was found to be more active that trimethoprim-sulfamethoxazole, but less active than the combination of amoxicillin plus gentamicin. This suggests that the new fluoroquinolones may be an effective alternative to trimethoprim-sulfamethoxazole in the therapy of *Listeria* meningitis in patients with β-lactam allergy, although further studies are needed before these agents can be recommended in patients with listeriosis.

Several of the other new fluoroquinolones have been evaluated in experimental animal models of meningitis. Moxifloxacin was shown to be as effective as ceftriaxone in the rabbit model of meningitis caused by a penicillin-sensitive pneumococcal strain (78); penetration into CSF was only slightly reduced by the coadministration of dexamethasone (from 3.8 to 3.3 μg/ml). Moxifloxacin has also shown efficacy in the therapy of penicillin-resistant pneumococcal meningitis (61) and was as effective as vancomycin and ceftriaxone in reduction of bacterial counts in CSF. Similar animal model results have been shown with gatifloxacin in experimental *E. coli* meningitis (46) and gemifloxacin in experimental pneumococcal meningitis (86). Finally, in a pneumococcal meningitis mouse model, clinafloxacin was compared with ceftriaxone against a penicillin-susceptible and a multidrug-resistant pneumococcal strain (84); ceftriaxone was the most active agent against the penicillin-susceptible isolate but showed a 30-fold decrease in potency against the resistant strain, whereas clinafloxacin was equally effective against both strains and was the most active against the penicillin-resistant pneumococcal isolate.

In the treatment of other CNS infections, few experimental studies have evaluated the efficacy of fluoroquinolones. Trovafloxacin has been evaluated in an experimental rat model of *S. aureus* brain abscess/cerebritis (56). Eighteen hours after intracranial injection of the organism, animals were treated subcutaneously with either ceftriaxone or trovafloxacin for 4 days. The results demonstrated no significant differences in bacterial clearance from the brain in animals treated with either ceftriaxone or trovafloxacin. These data indicate the potential usefulness of fluoroquinolones in treatment of brain abscess in humans (see below).

EFFICACY OF FLUOROQUINOLONES IN HUMANS

Meningitis

The fluoroquinolone antimicrobial agents have been used infrequently to treat bacterial meningitis in humans, and most of the available clinical data are represented by case reports rather than controlled clinical trials comparing the fluoroquinolones with standard therapy. An overview of the clinical efficacy of ciprofloxacin through 1986 in 3,981 patients (3) and an analysis of the new drug application and published clinical experience with ciprofloxacin in 2,018 patients (72) did not include any cases of bacterial meningitis. In another analysis of the results of ciprofloxacin therapy in 8,861 patients treated during clinical trials, among which 3,822 courses satisfied the standards of the Food and Drug Administration (74),

only three cases of meningitis (caused by *P. aeruginosa*, *S. aureus*, or *S. pneumoniae*) were identified; no clinical failures were noted, although no other details were reported.

Several isolated case reports subsequently suggested the potential benefits of the fluoroquinolones in the therapy of bacterial meningitis. For example, a 56-year-old male developed *P. aeruginosa* meningitis after a decompression laminectomy (52). Initial therapy with cefotaxime plus gentamicin was ineffective, but the patient made a complete recovery following combination therapy with ciprofloxacin (200 mg every 12 h) and tobramycin (120 mg every 8 h) administered intravenously for 14 days. A 78-year-old woman developed *Morganella morganii* meningitis following an L$_5$-S$_1$ laminectomy; the organism was eradicated by 7 days of intravenous pefloxacin therapy (800 mg every 12 h) (33). A premature infant born at 26 weeks of gestation developed a multidrug-resistant *P. aeruginosa* ventriculitis despite parenteral and ventricular therapy with netilmicin and colistin (32). The administration of ciprofloxacin (4 to 6 mg/kg/day for 28 days, with the last 14 days at the higher dose) and netilmicin (3.5 mg/kg/day administered systemically and 1 mg administered intraventricularly daily for 8 days) eradicated the infection, with no evidence of recurrence at a 3-month follow-up. In addition, oral ciprofloxacin was successfully utilized to prevent relapse in a patient with chronic pseudomonal meningitis (58). Ciprofloxacin has also been used to successfully treat a neonate with *Salmonella enterica* serovar Typhimurium meningitis after the patient experienced relapse caused by a chloramphenicol-resistant isolate that emerged during chloramphenicol therapy (65).

Data for several larger series in which patients with gram-negative meningitis were treated with fluoroquinolones have been published (Table 3). In one report (53), 11 adult patients with bacterial meningitis were treated with pefloxacin (400 mg two or three times daily or 800 mg twice daily). Pathogens isolated from CSF in these patients were *S. aureus* (two patients), *S. epidermidis* (one patient), *Bacillus cereus* (one patient), *E. coli* (three patients), *P. aeruginosa* (two patients), and *Acinetobacter calcoaceticus* (two patients). In patients completing therapy, the mean duration of treatment was 19 days (range, 8 to 45 days). Of seven patients treated with pefloxacin alone, six were cured, including one in whom pefloxacin followed previous successful therapy with thienamycin plus amikacin for pseudomonal meningitis. In another case, superinfection caused by a pefloxacin-resistant *Klebsiella* strain isolated from blood cultures occurred. In one patient, CSF cultures continued to grow *E. coli* despite 9 days of

Table 3. Results of clinical trials of fluoroquinolones in patients with bacterial meningitis[a]

Fluoroquinolone	No. of patients	Organism (no.)	No. of Patients			Reference
			Cured or improved	Relapsed	Failed	
Pefloxacin	11[b]	S. aureus (2), S. epidermidis (1), B. cereus (1), E. coli (3), P. aeruginosa (2), A. calcoaceticus (2)	8	1	1	53
Pefloxacin	16[c]	P. aeruginosa (5), A. calcoaceticus (4), K. pneumoniae (3), E. cloacae (2), C. diversus (1), Salmonella group C (1)	13	1	1	83
Ciprofloxacin	20	E. coli (6), P. mirabilis (3), K. pneumoniae (5), P. aeruginosa (2), E. cloacae (1), A. calcoaceticus (3)	18	0	2	80
Trovafloxacin	93[d]	N. meningitidis (93)	84	0	5	31
Ceftriaxone	97[d]	N. meningitidis (97)	87	0	6	
Ciprofloxacin	12	E. coli (2), S. enteritidis (1), A. calcoaceticus (1), S. aureus (4), E. faecalis (2), H. influenzae plus S. epidermidis (1), Acinetobacter species plus S. epidermidis (1)	10	1	1	42
Trovafloxacin	108	Not indicated	82[e]		22	69
Ceftriaxone + vancomycin	95		72[e]		16	

[a] Data from references 31, 42, 53, 69, 80, and 83; see text for complete details of these clinical trials, including drug dosages and concomitant use of other antimicrobial agents.
[b] One patient with a superinfection.
[c] One patient not accessible.
[d] Number of patients studied initially included 200, 100 receiving trovafloxacin and 100 receiving ceftriaxone.
[e] Clinical success 5 to 7 weeks after the end of treatment; data on relapse not indicated.

pefloxacin treatment; cure was then achieved with a combination of cefoxitin and dibekacin. Four patients received a combination of pefloxacin with either vancomycin (two patients), ceftazidime (one patient), or 5-flucytosine (one patient with suspected cryptococcosis). Three patients were apparently cured, and another relapsed at the end of treatment. Overall, 8 of 11 patients were cured, superinfection occurred in one, reinfection occurred in one, and one failed treatment.

In another trial (82), 10 patients with acute meningitis caused by gram-negative bacteria were treated with intravenous pefloxacin (mean daily dose of 19.61 mg/kg) for a mean period of 10 days. All patients had been previously treated ineffectively with a total of 23 courses of other agents (12 with β-lactams, 7 with aminoglycosides, and 4 with chloramphenicol). Organisms isolated included P. aeruginosa (three patients), A. calcoaceticus (three patients), K. pneumoniae (three patients, including one with a concomitant S. aureus isolate), and Citrobacter diversus (one patient). Of the 10 patients, seven were cured, one improved, one failed to respond, and one could not be assessed because of sudden death following an acute myocardial infarction. Of the seven patients who were cured, three

died as a result of their underlying diseases. Bacteriologic eradication of gram-negative bacteria was documented in nine of the CSF cultures, but a Klebsiella isolate was not eradicated in one patient, and S. aureus persisted in another patient. In another report, the same authors compiled data on 16 patients with acute meningitis (10 of whom were reported in the previous study) caused by gram-negative bacteria and treated with intravenous pefloxacin (800 mg twice daily in adult patients) for a mean period of 11 days (83). The causative organisms were P. aeruginosa (five patients), A. calcoaceticus (four patients), K. pneumoniae (three patients), Enterobacter cloacae (two patients), C. diversus (one patient), and Salmonella group C (one patient). Thirteen patients were cured or clinically improved, 12 were bacteriologically cured, one patient failed, one patient had reinfection, and one patient was not accessible.

In another study from Yugoslavia, ciprofloxacin (200 mg intravenously every 12 h for 10 days) was administered to 20 patients with gram-negative bacillary meningitis, which was most frequently associated with head trauma and neurosurgical procedures (80). In two patients, cefotaxime and penicillin G were also administered. Organisms isolated from

CSF included *E. coli*, *P. mirabilis*, *K. pneumoniae*, *P. aeruginosa*, *E. cloacae*, and *A. calcoaceticus*. Eighteen of twenty patients were apparently cured; in two patients, treatment was modified because a positive CSF culture was obtained after 48 h of therapy.

Trovafloxacin was compared with ceftriaxone in the treatment of epidemic meningococcal meningitis in children in Africa (31). Two hundred children were randomly assigned to receive trovafloxacin (3 mg/kg given orally or intravenously) or ceftriaxone (100 mg/kg intravenously or intramuscularly) for 5 days; 78% of the trovafloxacin patients received their full course of therapy as either an oral suspension or tablets. CSF cultures, latex agglutination, or polymerase chain reaction was positive for *N. meningitidis* in 86 and 81% of patients receiving trovafloxacin and ceftriaxone, respectively. The cure rate was 90.3% (84 of 93) for trovafloxacin and 89% (87 of 97) for ceftriaxone, with no relapses at the 4- to 6-week follow-up. Despite these promising results, concerns about liver toxicity related to trovafloxacin preclude its continued use in patients with bacterial meningitis. Furthermore, this study has only been published in abstract form.

In another series of nosocomial meningitis in 12 neonates, ciprofloxacin (in doses ranging from 10 to 60 mg/kg/day) was evaluated (42). Six of the infants presented with gram-negative meningitis (including two cases with mixed gram-positive and gram-negative infection), and six cases were attributable to gram-positive cocci. Ten patients were cured; of the two failures, one patient relapsed and one died. In two patients, reversible hydrocephalus appeared that responded to intraventricular punctures, and in seven children, there were no neurologic sequelae after a follow-up at 2 to 4 years. These reports demonstrate the potential efficacy of pefloxacin and ciprofloxacin in gram-negative meningitis, although more clinical data are needed to establish their precise roles in this life-threatening infection.

In a recent multicenter, randomized trial, trovafloxacin (administered as its intravenous prodrug alatrofloxacin) was compared with ceftriaxone ± vancomycin in children with bacterial meningitis (69). Of 203 fully evaluable patients, 108 were treated with trovafloxacin and 95 with ceftriaxone. At 5 to 7 weeks after the end of treatment, clinical success was equivalent in both groups (79% in those receiving trovafloxacin and 81% in those receiving ceftriaxone); similar results were seen in clinical success at the end of treatment and at 6 to 12 months after the end of treatment. At 24 to 36 h, bacterial eradication was 94% in patients receiving trovafloxacin and 96% in patients receiving ceftriaxone. Furthermore,

use of trovafloxacin was not associated with serious sequelae or joint abnormalities. These data support further evaluation of fluoroquinolones in the therapy of bacterial meningitis.

Numerous additional case reports have described the efficacy of the fluoroquinolones in the treatment of meningitis caused by *K. pneumoniae* (38, 43, 73), *E. cloacae* (14, 23), *E. coli* (25), *P. aeruginosa* (102), *Flavobacterium meningosepticum* (25), and *Xanthomonas* (*Stenotrophomonas*) *maltophilia* (22). In particular, the fluoroquinolones have shown excellent efficacy in meningitis caused by *Salmonella* species (5, 21, 97). The combination of ciprofloxacin plus a third-generation cephalosporin (either cefotaxime or ceftriaxone) has been suggested as an alternative regimen for the treatment of *Salmonella* meningitis (63). Although successful monotherapy with ciprofloxacin has been utilized in patients with *Salmonella* meningitis, because of the possibility of fluoroquinolone resistance in *Salmonella* and the lack of antagonism between these two agents, combined therapy has been advocated. Modification of therapy may then be indicated on the basis of in vitro susceptibility testing and clinical response.

Brain Abscess

The fluoroquinolones have been evaluated in patients with brain abscess. One patient was a male neonate with multiple brain abscesses caused by *S. enterica* serovar Enteritidis, in which the patient was initially treated with cefotaxime and chloramphenicol (99). However, on day 42 of treatment, computerized tomographic scanning showed abscess enlargement and development of communicating hydrocephalus. Therapy was changed to ciprofloxacin (10 mg/kg/day) for a total of 33 days and, on day 56, surgical drainage of the abscesses and ventricles was performed. Concentrations of ciprofloxacin in serum and abscess fluids were similar (0.1 to 2.8 μg/ml in serum, 0.1 to 1.6 μg/ml in the frontal abscess, and 0.1 to 2.7 μg/ml in the occipital abscess). Follow-up of the patient at 2 years of age showed normal physical and slightly delayed psychomotor development. In another infant with multiple cerebral abscesses caused by serovar Enteritidis, successful management included a prolonged course of antimicrobial therapy (cefotaxime plus ciprofloxacin at a dosage of 15 mg/kg/day), neurosurgical drainage, and long-term immunoglobulin supplements (103). Ciprofloxacin (750 mg orally twice daily for 4 months) was also utilized, following 3 weeks of intravenous therapy with cefotaxime, in an immunocompetent 43-year-old adult with an

S. enterica serovar Enteritidis brain abscess (7); 6 months after completion of therapy, the patient was considered cured. These case reports indicate that ciprofloxacin may have value in selected patients with brain abscess.

Chemoprophylaxis of Meningococcal Carriers

Although not directly pertinent to the treatment of bacterial meningitis, the risk of meningococcal disease among close (e.g., household) contacts of an index case during nonepidemic periods is ~3 in 1,000; this is ~500 to 1,000-fold higher than the background endemic rate (75). Close contacts of the index patient should receive chemoprophylaxis to eradicate nasopharyngeal carriage of meningococci. The current antimicrobial agent of choice in this situation is 600 mg of rifampin twice daily for 2 days in adults. However, there are problems with rifampin administration: (i) only 70 to 80% eradication rates of the organism from the nasopharynx are achieved, and this effect is transient; (ii) some adverse reactions occur; (iii) 2 days (four doses) of administration are necessary; and (iv) meningococcal resistance to rifampin has occasionally developed.

Recent reports suggest that ciprofloxacin is highly effective in eliminating *N. meningitidis* from the nasopharynx of patients carrying the organism (Table 4). Ciprofloxacin was shown to be efficacious among army recruits in Finland; a dose of 250 mg administered twice daily for 2 days eradicated meningococcal carriage from 96% of subjects versus only 13% of those given placebo (66). A single dose of ciprofloxacin (500 or 750 mg for adults) has also been shown in several reports to be effective in eliminating *N. meningitidis* from nasopharyngeal carriers (19, 20, 64), leading some to recommend ciprofloxacin for chemoprophylaxis for meningococcal disease in adults (96). Ciprofloxacin concentrations in nasal secretions have been shown to exceed the MIC for 90% of meningococcal and *H. influenzae* strains (15), suggesting that ciprofloxacin may also be effective in the elimination of nasopharyngeal

carriage of *H. influenzae*. However, no published trials support this suggestion.

SUMMARY AND CONCLUSIONS

The fluoroquinolone antimicrobial agents possess several properties that make them potential therapeutic agents for use in patients with bacterial meningitis. Their penetration into CSF is excellent, with remarkable agreement between values obtained in experimental animal models of meningitis and during therapy in humans. Compared with conventional antimicrobial agents utilized for the treatment of bacterial meningitis, the fluoroquinolones enter normal or purulent CSF more rapidly, with percent penetration values into purulent CSF of ~50% for enoxacin and pefloxacin and ~15 to 30% for ciprofloxacin and ofloxacin. However, despite this efficient penetration, concentrations in CSF are low, primarily because concentrations in serum are low after administration of conventional dosages. The concentrations achievable in CSF are directly correlated with the in vivo potency of each agent (i.e., higher rate of bacterial elimination from CSF as drug concentrations in CSF increase), and bactericidal activity in CSF correlates with in vitro potency, justifying the selective use of these agents in the therapy of bacterial meningitis caused by susceptible gram-negative bacteria, but not for meningitis caused by gram-positive organisms, pending further data. The currently available fluoroquinolones should never be used as first-line empiric therapy in patients with meningitis. The limited published literature on the use of fluoroquinolones in humans suggests that the primary area of usefulness of these agents in patients with bacterial meningitis is for therapy of multidrug-resistant gram-negative organisms (e.g., *P. aeruginosa*) or when the response to conventional β-lactam therapy is slow (e.g., meningitis caused by *Salmonella* species). In addition, the fluoroquinolones are relatively contraindicated in infants and children, the age groups accounting for many

Table 4. Evaluation of ciprofloxacin in eradication of *N. meningitidis* from nasopharyngeal carriers[a]

Treatment (no. of subjects)	Dose	Carrier reduction	Reference
Ciprofloxacin (56)	250 mg twice daily for 2 days	96% at day 8	66
Placebo (53)		13%	
Ciprofloxacin	750-mg single dose	96% at day 21	19
Placebo		9%	
Ciprofloxacin (12)	750-mg single dose	92% at day 14	64
Ciprofloxacin (336)	500-mg single dose	97% at day 14	20
Ciprofloxacin (104)	500-mg single dose	93% at weeks 6–9	

[a] Data from references 19, 20, 64, and 66.

cases of bacterial meningitis, although ciprofloxacin may be considered as appropriate in the treatment of serious pediatric infections when potential benefit outweighs the risk. Therefore, the fluoroquinolones have a limited role in the therapy of bacterial meningitis and will not supplant conventional antimicrobial regimens against the major meningeal pathogens. Ciprofloxacin appears promising for use in eradication of the meningococcal carrier state and may replace rifampin for this indication in adults and perhaps even in children. Although no clinical studies are currently available, the fluoroquinolones may also be effective in eliminating nasopharyngeal carriage of *H. influenzae*.

REFERENCES

1. Ahmed, A., M. M. Paris, M. Trujilo, S. M. Hickey, L. Wubbel, S. L. Shelton, and G. H. McCracken, Jr. 1997. Once-daily gentamicin therapy for experimental *Escherichia coli* meningitis. *Antimicrob. Agents Chemother.* **41**:49–53.

2. Andes, D. R., and W. A. Craig. 1999. Pharmacokinetics and pharmacodynamics of antibiotics in meningitis. *Infect. Dis. Clin. N. Am.* **13**:595–618.

3. Arcieri, G .E., E. Griffith, G. Gruenwaldt, A. Heyd, B. O'Brien, N. Becker, and R. August. 1987. Ciprofloxacin: an update on clinical experience. *Am. J. Med.* **46**(Suppl. 4A):381–386.

4. Armengaud, M., V. T. Tran, and B. DiConstanzo. 1983. Study of pefloxacin diffusion into serum and CSF in the dog, both with healthy meninges and during experimental meningitis, p. 23–28. *In Proceedings of the 13th International Congress on Chemotherapy.*

5. Bhutta, Z. A., B. J. Farooqui, and A. W. Sturm. 1992. Eradication of a multiple drug resistant *Salmonella paratyphi* A causing meningitis with ciprofloxacin. *J. Infect.* **25**:215–219.

6. Bitar, N., R. Claes, and P. Van der Auwera. 1989. Concentrations of ofloxacin in serum and cerebrospinal fluid of patients without meningitis receiving the drug intravenously and orally. *Antimicrob. Agents Chemother.* **33**:1686–1690.

7. Bonvin, P., T. Ejlertsen, and H. Dons-Jensen. 1998. Brain abscess caused by *Salmonella enteritidis* in an immunocompetent adult patient: successful treatment with cefotaxime and ciprofloxacin. *Scand. J. Infect. Dis.* **30**:632–634.

8. Bryan, J. P., H. R. de Silva, A. Tavares, H. Rocha, and W. M. Scheld. 1990. Etiology and mortality of bacterial meningitis in Northeastern Brazil. *Rev. Infect. Dis.* **12**:128–135.

9. Campbell, G. D., and R. Silberman. 1998. Drug-resistant *Streptococcus pneumoniae*. *Clin. Infect. Dis.* **26**:1188–1195.

10. Chen, D. K., A. McGeer, J. C. de Azavedo, and D. E. Low. 1999. Decreased susceptibility of *Streptococcus pneumoniae* to fluoroquinolones in Canada. *N. Engl. J. Med.* **341**:233–239.

11. Chowdhury, M. H., and A. R. Tunkel. 2000. Antibacterial agents in infections of the central nervous system. *Infect. Dis. Clin. N. Am.* **14**:391–408.

12. Cottagnoud, P., F. Acosta, M. Cottagnoud, K. Neftel, and M. G. Tauber. 2000. Synergy between trovafloxacin and ceftriaxone against penicillin-resistant pneumococci in the rabbit meningitis model and in vitro. *Antimicrob. Agents Chemother.* **44**:2179–2181.

13. Cutler, N. R., J. Vincent, S. S. Jhee, R. Teng, T. Wardle, G. Lucas, L. C. Dogolo, and J. J. Sramek. 1997. Penetration of trovafloxacin into cerebrospinal fluid in humans following intravenous infusion of alatrofloxacin. *Antimicrob. Agents Chemother.* **41**:1298–1300.

14. D'Antuono, V. S., and I. Brown. 1998. Successful treatment of *Enterobacter* meningitis with ciprofloxacin. *Clin. Infect. Dis.* **26**:206–207.

15. Darouiche, R., B. Perkins, D. Musher, R. Hamill, and S. Tsai. 1990. Levels of rifampin and ciprofloxacin in nasal secretions: correlation with MIC_{90} and eradication of nasopharyngeal carriage of bacteria. *J. Infect. Dis.* **162**:1124–1127.

16. Decazes, J. M., J. Mohler, A. Bure, J. M. Vallois, A. Meulemans, and J. Modai. 1989. Pharmacokinetics of fleroxacin and its metabolites in serum, cerebrospinal fluid, and brain of rabbits with and without experimental *Escherichia coli* meningitis. *Rev. Infect. Dis.* **11**:S1208–S1209.

17. Dow, J., J. Chazal, A. M. Frydman, P. Janny, R. Woehrle, F. Djebbar, and J. Gaillot. 1986. Transfer kinetics of pefloxacin into cerebrospinal fluid after one hour infusion of 400 mg in man. *J. Antimicrob. Chemother.* **17**(Suppl. B):81–87.

18. Drancourt, M., H. Gallais, D. Raoult, E. Estrangin, M. W. Mallet, and P. DeMicco. 1988. Ofloxacin penetration into cerebrospinal fluid. *J. Antimicrob Chemother.* **22**:263–265.

19. Dworzack, D. L., C. C. Sanders, E. A. Horowitz, J. M. Allais, M. Sookpranee, W. E. Sanders, Jr., and F. M. Ferraro. 1988. Evaluation of single-dose ciprofloxacin in the eradication of *Neisseria meningitidis* from nasopharyngeal carriers. *Antimicrob. Agents Chemother.* **32**:1740–1741.

20. Gaunt, P. N., and B. E. Lambert. 1988. Single dose ciprofloxacin for the eradication of pharyngeal carriage of *Neisseria meningitidis*. *J. Antimicrob. Chemother.* **21**:489–496.

21. Gille-Johnson, P., J. Kovamees, V. Lindgren, E. Aufwerber, and J. Struve. 2000. *Salmonella virchow* meningitis in an adult. *Scand. J. Infect. Dis.* **32**:431–433.

22. Girijaratnakumari, T., A. Raja, R. Ramani, B. Antony, and P. G. Shivananda. 1993. Meningitis due to *Xanthomonas maltophilia*. *J. Postgrad. Med.* **39**:153–155.

23. Goepp, J. G., C. K. K. Lee, T. Anderson, J. D. Dick, J. M. Stokoe, and J. Eiden. 1992. Use of ciprofloxacin in an infant with ventriculitis. *J. Pediatr.* **121**:303–305.

24. Gogos, C. A., T. G. Maraziotis, N. Papadakis, D. Beermann, D. K. Siamplis, and H. P. Bassaris. 1991. Penetration of ciprofloxacin into human cerebrospinal fluid in patients with inflamed and non-inflamed meninges. *Eur. J. Clin. Microbiol. Infect. Dis.* **10**:511–514.

25. Green, S. D. R., F. Ilunga, J. S. Cheesbrough, G. S. Tillotson, M. Hichens, and D. Felmingham. 1993. The treatment of neonatal meningitis due to gram-negative bacilli with ciprofloxacin: evidence of satisfactory penetration into the cerebrospinal fluid. *J. Infect.* **26**:253–256.

26. Grumback, N. M., E. Mylonakis, and E. J. Wing. 1999. Development of listerial meningitis during ciprofloxacin treatment. *Clin. Infect. Dis.* **29**:1340–1341.

27. Hackbarth, C. J., H. F. Chambers, F. Stella, A. M. Shibl, and M. A. Sande. 1986. Ciprofloxacin in experimental *Pseudomonas aeruginosa* meningitis in rabbits. *J. Antimicrob. Chemother.* **18**(Suppl. D):65–69.

28. Ho, P. L., T. L. Que, D. N. Tsang, T. K. Ng, K. H. Chow, and W. H. Seto. 1999. Emergence of fluoroquinolone resistance among multiply resistant strains of *Streptococcus pneumoniae* in Hong Kong. *Antimicrob. Agents Chemother.* **43**:1310–1313.

29. Hofmann, J., M. S. Cetron, M. M. Farley, W. S. Baughman, R. R. Facklam, J. A. Elliott, K. A. Deaver, and R. F. Breiman. 1995. The prevalence of drug-resistant *Streptococcus pneumoniae* in Atlanta. *N. Engl. J. Med.* **333:**481–486.

30. Hooper, D. C. 2000. Quinolones, p. 404–423. *In* G. L. Mandell, J. E. Bennett, and R. Dolin (ed.), *Principles and Practice of Infectious Diseases,* 5th ed. Churchill Livingstone, Philadelphia, Pa.

31. Hopkins, S., D. Williams, M. Dunne, L. Marinovich, M. Edeline, E. Utt, and A. I. Dutse. 1996. A randomized, controlled trial of oral or IV trovafloxacin vs. ceftriaxone in the treatment of epidemic meningococcal meningitis, abstr. LB21. *In Proceedings and Abstracts of the 36th Interscience Conference on Antimicrobial Agents and Chemotherapy.* American Society for Microbiology, Washington, D.C.

32. Isaacs, D. C., M. P. E. Slack, A. R. Wilkinson, and A. W. Westwood. 1986. Successful treatment of *Pseudomonas* ventriculitis with ciprofloxacin. *J. Antimicrob. Chemother.* **17:**535–538.

33. Isaacs, R. D., and R. B. Ellis-Pegler. 1987. Successful treatment of *Morganella morganii* meningitis with pefloxacin mesylate. *J. Antimicrob. Chemother.* **20:**769–770.

34. Jackson, L. A., F. C. Tenover, C. Baker, B. D. Plikaytis, M. W. Reeves, S. A. Stocker, R. E. Weaver, J. D. Wenger, and the Meningococcal Disease Study Group. 1994. Prevalence of *Neisseria meningitidis* relatively resistant to penicillin in the United States, 1991. *J. Infect. Dis.* **169:**438–441.

35. Jernigan, D. B., M. S. Cetron, R. F. Breiman. 1996. Minimizing the impact of drug-resistant *Streptococcus pneumoniae* (DRSP). A strategy from the DRSP working group. *JAMA* **275:**206–209.

36. Kawahara, K., M. Kawahara, T. Goto, and Y. Ohi. 1991. Penetration of sparfloxacin (AT-140) into human cerebrospinal fluid: a comparative study with five other fluoroquinolones. *Eur. J. Clin. Microbiol. Infect. Dis.* Special Issue:580–582.

37. Kaye, K., S., H. S. Fraimow, and E. Abrutyn. 2000. Pathogens resistant to antimicrobial agents: epidemiology, molecular mechanisms, and clinical management. *Infect. Dis. Clin. N. Am.* **14:**293–319.

38. Khaneja, M., J. Naprawa, A. Kumar, and S. Piecuch. 1999. Successful treatment of late-onset infection due to resistant *Klebsiella pneumoniae* in an extremely low birth weight infant using ciprofloxacin. *J. Perinatol.* **19:**311–314.

39. Kim, Y. S., Q. Liu, L. L. Chow, and M. G. Tauber. 1997. Trovafloxacin in treatment of rabbits with experimental meningitis caused by high-level penicillin-resistant *Streptococcus pneumoniae. Antimicrob. Agents Chemother.* **41:**1186–1189.

40. Kitzes-Cohen, R., A. Miler, A. Gilboa, and D. Harel. 1988. Penetration of ciprofloxacin into cerebrospinal fluid. *Rev. Infect. Dis.* **10:**S256–S257.

41. Korinek, A. M., G. Montay, A. Bianchi, M. Guggiari, R. Brob, and P. Viars. 1988. Penetration of pefloxacin into human brain tissue. *Rev. Infect. Dis.* **10:**S257.

42. Kremery, V., Jr., J. Filka, J. Uher, H. Kurak, T. Sagat, J. Tuharsky, I. Novak, T. Urbanova, K. Kralinsky, F. Mateicka, T. Kremeryova, L. Jurga, M. Sulcova, J. Stencl, and I. Krupova. 1999. Ciprofloxacin in treatment of nosocomial meningitis in neonates and in infants: report of 12 cases and review. *Diagn. Microbiol. Infect. Dis.* **35:**75–80.

43. Linder, N., R. Dagan, J. Kuint, N. Keler, G. Keren, and B. Reichman. 1994. Ventriculitis caused by *Klebsiella pneumoniae* successfully treated with pefloxacin in a neonate. *Infection* **22:**210–212.

44. Lu, C. H., W. N. Chang, and Y. C. Chuang. 1999. Resistance to third-generation cephalosporins in adult gram-negative bacillary meningitis. *Infection* **27:**208–211.

45. Lustar, I., A. Ahmed, I. R. Friedland, M. Trujillo, L. Wubbel, K. Olsen, and G. H. McCracken, Jr. 1997. Pharmacodynamics and bactericidal activity of ceftriaxone therapy in experimental cephalosporin-resistant pneumococcal meningitis. *Antimicrob. Agents Chemother.* **41:**2414–2417.

46. Lutsar, I., I. R. Friedland, H. S. Jafri, L. Wubbel, W. Ng, F. Ghaffar, and G. H. McCracken, Jr. 1999. Efficacy of gatifloxacin in experimental *Escherichia coli* meningitis. *Antimicrob. Agents Chemother.* **43:**1805–1807.

47. Lutsar, I., I. R. Friedland, L. Wubbel, C. C. McCoig, H. S. Jafri, W. Ng, F. Ghaffar, and G. H. McCracken, Jr. 1998. Pharmacodynamics of gatifloxacin in cerebrospinal fluid in experimental cephalosporin-resistant pneumococcal meningitis. *Antimicrob. Agents Chemother.* **42:**2650–2655.

48. Lutsar, I., G. H. McCracken, Jr., and I. R. Friedland. 1998. Antibiotic pharmacodynamics in cerebrospinal fluid. *Clin. Infect. Dis.* **27:**1117–1129.

49. McClain, J. B., J. Rhoads, and G. Krol. 1988. Cerebrospinal fluid concentrations of ciprofloxacin in subjects with uninflamed meninges. *J. Antimicrob. Chemother.* **21:**808–809.

50. Michelet, C., J. L. Avril, C. Arvieux, C. Jacquelinet, N. Vu, and F. Cartier. 1997. Comparative activities of new fluoroquinolones, alone or in combination with amoxicillin, trimethoprim-sulfamethoxazole, or rifampin, against intracellular *Listeria monocytogenes. Antimicrob. Agents Chemother.* **41:**60–65.

51. Michelet, C., S. L. Leib, D. Bentue-Ferrer, and M. G. Tauber. 1999. Comparative efficacies of antibiotics in a rat model of meningoencephalitis due to *Listeria monocytogenes. Antimicrob. Agents Chemother.* **43:**1651–1656.

52. Millar, M. R., M. A. Bransby-Zachary, D. S. Tompkins, P. M. Hawkey, and R. M. Gibson. 1986. Ciprofloxacin for *Pseudomonas aeruginosa* meningitis. *Lancet* **i:**325. (Letter.)

53. Modai, J. 1991. Potential role of fluoroquinolones in the treatment of bacterial meningitis. *Eur. J. Clin. Microbiol. Infect. Dis.* **10:**291–295.

54. Montay, G., Y. Goueffon, and F. Roquet. 1984. Absorption, distribution, metabolic fate, and elimination of pefloxacin mesylate in mice, rats, dogs, monkeys, and humans. *Antimicrob. Agents Chemother.* **25:**463–472.

55. Moretti, M. V., S. Pauluzzi, and M. Cesana. 2000. Penetration of rufloxacin into the cerebrospinal fluid in patients with inflamed and uninflamed meninges. *Antimicrob. Agents Chemother.* **44:**73–77.

56. Nathan, B. R., and W. M. Scheld. The efficacy of trovafloxacin versus ceftriaxone in the treatment of experimental brain abscess/cerebritis in the rat. *Life Sci.,* in press.

57. Nau, R., T. Schmidt, K. Kaye, J. L. Froula, and M. G. Tauber. 1995. Quinolone antibiotics in therapy of experimental pneumococcal meningitis in rabbits. *Antimicrob. Agents Chemother.* **41:**49–53.

58. Norrby, S. R. 1988. 4-Quinolones in the treatment of infections of the central nervous system. *Rev. Infect. Dis.* **10:**S253–S255.

59. Odland, B. A., R. N. Jones, J. Verhoef, A. Fluit, M. L. Beach, and the SENTRY Antimicrobial Surveillance Group. 1999. Antimicrobial activity of gatifloxacin (AM-1155, CG5501), and four other fluoroquinolones tested against 2,284 recent clinical strains of *Streptococcus pneumoniae* from Europe, Latin America, Canada, and the United States. *Diagn. Microbiol. Infect. Dis.* **34:**315–320.

60. O'Donnell, J. A., and S. P. Gelone. 2000. Fluoroquinolones. *Infect. Dis. Clin. N. Am.* **14:**489–513.

61. Ostergaard, C., T. K. Sorensen, J. D. Knudsen, and N. F. Moller. 1998. Evaluation of moxifloxacin, a new 8-methoxyquinolone, for treatment of meningitis caused by a

penicillin-resistant *Pneumococcus* in rabbits. *Antimicrob. Agents Chemother.* 42:1706–1712.

62. Pioget, J. C., M. Wolff, E. Singlas, M. J. Laisne, B. Clair, B. Regnier, and F. Vachon. 1989. Diffusion of ofloxacin into cerebrospinal fluid of patients with purulent meningitis or ventriculitis. *Antimicrob. Agents Chemother.* 33:933–936.

63. Price, E. H., J. de Louvois, and M. R. Workman. 2000. Antibiotics for *Salmonella* meningitis in children. *J. Antimicrob. Chemother.* 46:653–655.

64. Pugsley, M. P., D. L. Dworzack, J. S. Rocaforte, C. C. Sanders, J. S. Bakken, and W. E. Sanders, Jr. 1988. An open study of the efficacy of a single dose of ciprofloxacin in eliminating the chronic nasopharyngeal carriage of *Neisseria meningitidis. J. Infect. Dis.* 157:852–853. (Letter.)

65. Ragunathan, P. L., D. V. Potkins, J. G. Watson, A. M. Kearns, and A. Carroll. 1990. Neonatal meningitis due to *Salmonella typhimurium* treated with ciprofloxacin. *J. Antimicrob. Chemother.* 26:727–728.

66. Renkonen, O. V., A. Sivonen, and R. Visakorpi. 1987. Effect of ciprofloxacin on carrier rate of *Neisseria meningitidis* in army recruits in Finland. *Antimicrob. Agents Chemother.* 31:962–963.

67. Rocha, P., C. Baleeiro, and A. R. Tunkel. 2000. Impact of antimicrobial resistance on the treatment of invasive pneumococcal infections. *Curr. Infect. Dis. Rep.* 2:399–408.

68. Rodoni, D., F. Hanni, C. M. Gerber, M. Cottagnoud, K. Neftel, M. G. Tauber, and P. Cottagnoud. 1999. Trovafloxacin in combination with vancomycin against penicillin-resistant pneumococci in the rabbit meningitis model. *Antimicrob. Agents Chemother.* 43:963–965.

69. Saez-Llorens, X., C. McCoig, J. M. Feris, S. L. Vargas, K. P. Klugman, G. D. Hussey, R. W. Frenck, L. H. Falleiros-Carvalho, A. G. Arguedas, J. Bradley, A. C. Arrieta, E. R. Wald, S. Pancorbo, G. H. McCracken, Jr., and the Trovan Meningitis Study Group. 2002. Quinolone treatment for pediatric bacterial meningitis: a comparative study of trovafloxacin and ceftriaxone with or without vancomycin. *Pediatr. Infect. Dis. J.* 21:14–22.

70. Saez-Nieto, J. A., R. Lujan, S. Berron, J. Campos, M. Vinas, C. Fuste, J. A. Vazquez, Q. Y. Zhang, L. D. Bowler, J. V. Martinez-Suarez, and B. G. Spratt. 1992. Epidemiology and molecular basis of penicillin-resistant *Neisseria meningitidis* in Spain: a 5-year history (1985–1989). *Clin. Infect. Dis.* 14:394–402.

71. Sande, M. A., R. A. Brooks-Fournier, and J. L. Geberding. 1987. Efficacy of ciprofloxacin in animal models of infection: endocarditis, meningitis, and pneumonia. *Am. J. Med.* 82 (Suppl. 4A):63–66.

72. Sanders, W. E., Jr. 1988. Efficacy, safety, and potential economic benefits of oral ciprofloxacin in the treatment of infections. *Rev. Infect. Dis.* 10:528–543.

73. Sarkar, S., M. Singh, and A. Narang. 1993. Successful treatment of hospital acquired *Klebsiella pneumoniae* meningitis in a neonate with ciprofloxacin. *Indian Pediatr.* 30:913–914.

74. Schact, P., G. Arcieri, J. Branolte, H. Bruck, V. Chysky, E. Griffith, G. Gurenwald, R. Hullmann, C. A. Konopka, B. O'Brien, V. Rahm, T. Ryoki, A. Westwood, and H. Weuta. 1986. Worldwide clinical data on efficacy and safety of ciprofloxacin. *Infection* 16:S29–S43.

75. Scheld, W. M. 1989. Quinolone therapy for infections of the central nervous system. *Rev. Infect. Dis.* 4:74–83.

76. Scheld, W. M. 1991. Evaluation of quinolones in experimental animal models of infection. *Eur. J. Clin. Microbiol. Infect. Dis.* 10:275–290.

77. Schlech, W. F. III, J. I. Ward, J. D. Band, A. Hightower, D. W. Fraser, and C. V. Broome. 1985. Bacterial meningitis in the United States. The national bacterial meningitis surveillance study. *JAMA* 253:1749–1754.

78. Schmidt, H., A. Dalhoff, K. Stuertz, F. Trostdorf, V. Chen, O. Schneider, C. Kohlsdorfer, W. Bruck, and R. Nau. 1998. Moxifloxacin in the therapy of experimental pneumococcal meningitis. *Antimicrob. Agents Chemother.* 42:1397–1401.

79. Schmidt, T., and M. G. Tauber. 1993. Pharmacodynamics of antibiotics in the therapy of meningitis: infection model observations. *J. Antimicrob. Chemother.* 31:61–70.

80. Schonwald, S., I. Beus, M. Lisic, V. Car, and B. Gmajnicki. 1989. Brief report: ciprofloxacin in the treatment of gram-negative bacillary meningitis. *Am. J. Med.* 87(Suppl. 5A):248S–249S.

81. Schuchat, A., K. Robinson, J. D. Wenger, L. H. Harrison, M. Farley, A. L. Reingold, L. Lefkowitz, B. A. Perkins, for the Active Surveillance Team. 1997. Bacterial meningitis in the United States in 1995. *N. Engl. J. Med.* 337:970–976.

82. Segev, S., A. Barzilai, N. Rosen, G. Joseph, and E. Rubinstein. 1989. Pefloxacin treatment of meningitis caused by gram-negative bacteria. *Arch. Intern. Med.* 149:1314–1316.

83. Segev, S., N. Rosen, G. Joseph, H. Alpern Elran, and E. Rubinstein. 1990. Pefloxacin efficacy in gram-negative bacillary meningitis. *J. Antimicrob. Chemother.* 26(Suppl. B):187–192.

84. Shapiro, M. A., K. D. Donovan, and J. W. Gage. 2000. Comparative therapeutic efficacy of clinafloxacin in a pneumococcal meningitis mouse model. *J. Antimicrob. Chemother.* 45:489–492.

85. Shibl, A. M., C. J. Hackbarth, and M. A. Sande. 1986. Evaluation of pefloxacin in experimental *Escherichia coli* meningitis. *Antimicrob. Agents Chemother.* 29:409–411.

86. Smirnov, A., A. Wellmer, J. Gerber, K. Maier, S. Henne, and R. Nau. 2000. Gemifloxacin is effective in experimental pneumococcal meningitis. *Antimicrob. Agents Chemother.* 44:767–770.

87. Sobieski, M. W., and W. M. Scheld. 1985. Comparative activity of ciprofloxacin and ofloxacin in experimental *H. influenzae* meningitis, abstr. 216. *In Proceedings and Abstracts of the 25th Interscience Conference on Antimicrobial Agents and Chemotherapy.* American Society for Microbiology, Washington, D.C.

88. Song, J., N. Y. Lee, S. Ichiyama, R. Yoshida, Y. Hirakata, W. Fu, A. Chongthaleong, N. Aswapokee, C. H. Chiu, M. K. Lalitha, K. Thomas, J. Perera, T. T. Yee, F. Jamal, U. C. Warsa, B. X. Vinh, M. R. Jacobs, P. C. Appelbaum, C. H. Pai, and the ANSORP Study Group. 1999. *Streptococcus pneumoniae* in Asian countries: Asian Network for Surveillance of Resistant Pathogens (ANSORP). *Clin. Infect. Dis.* 28:1206–1211.

89. Stahl, J. P., J. Croize, M. A. Lefebvre, J. P. Bru, A. Guyot, D. Leduc, J. B. Fourtillan, and M. Micoud. 1986. Diffusion of ofloxacin into the cerebrospinal fluid in patients with bacterial meningitis. *Infection* 14:S254–S255.

90. Stubner, G., W. Weinrich, and U. Brands. 1986. Study of the cerebrospinal fluid penetration of ofloxacin. *Infection* 14:S250–S253.

91. Taeger, K., E. Wiethoff, G. Mahr, R. Seelmann, T. Lohr, and F. Sorgel. 1990. Penetration of temafloxacin into cerebrospinal fluid, abstr. 363. *In Proceedings 3rd International Symposium New Quinolones.*

92. Tho, T. V., A. Armengaud, and B. Davet. 1984. Diffusion of enoxacin into the cerebrospinal fluid in dogs with healthy meninges and with experimental meningitis. *J. Antimicrob. Chemother.* 14(Suppl. C):57–62.

93. Tunkel, A. R., and W. M. Scheld. 1989. Applications of therapy in animal models to bacterial infection in human disease. *Infect. Dis. Clin. N. Am.* 3:441–459.

94. Tunkel, A. R., and W. M. Scheld. 1991. Ofloxacin. *Infect. Control Hosp. Epidemiol.* **12:**549–557.

95. Valainis, G., D. Thomas, and G. Pankey. 1986. Penetration of ciprofloxacin into cerebrospinal fluid. *Eur. J. Clin. Microbiol.* **5:**206–207.

96. Visakorpi, R. 1989. Ciprofloxacin in meningococcal carriers. *Scand. J. Infect. Dis. Suppl.* **60:**108–111.

97. Visudhiphan, P., S. Chiemchanya, and A. Visutibhan. 1998. *Salmonella* meningitis in Thai infants: clinical case reports. *Trans. R. Soc. Trop. Med. Hyg.* **92:**181–184.

98. Wenger, J. D., A. W. Hightower, R. R. Facklam, S. Gaventa, C. V. Broome, and the Bacterial Meningitis Study Group. 1990. Bacterial meningitis in the United States, 1986: report of a multistate surveillance study. *J. Infect. Dis.* **162:**1316–1323.

99. Wessalowski, R., L. Thomas, J. Kivit, and T. Voit. 1993. Multiple brain abscesses caused by *Salmonella enteritidis* in a neonate: successful treatment with ciprofloxacin. *Pediatr. Infect. Dis. J.* **12:**683–688.

100. Wolff, M., L. Boutron, E. Singlas, B. Clair, J. M. Decazes, and B. Regnier. 1987. Penetration of ciprofloxacin into cerebrospinal fluid of patients with bacterial meningitis. *Antimicrob. Agents Chemother.* **31:**899–902.

101. Wolff, M., B. Regnier, C. Daldoss, M. Nkam, and F. Yachon. 1984. Penetration of pefloxacin into cerebrospinal fluid of patients with meningitis. *Antimicrob. Agents Chemother.* **26:**289–291.

102. Wong-Beringer, A., P. Beringer, and M. A. Lovett. 1997. Successful treatment of multidrug-resistant *Pseudomonas aeruginosa* meningitis with high-dose ciprofloxacin. *Clin. Infect. Dis.* **25:**936–937.

103. Workman, M. R., E. H. Price, and P. Bullock. 1999. *Salmonella* meningitis and multiple cerebral abscesses in an infant. *Int. J. Antimicrob. Agents* **13:**131–132.

104. Workmann, G. W., and S. P. Bennett. 1999. Fatal meningitis due to levofloxacin-resistant *Streptococcus pneumoniae*. *Clin. Infect. Dis.* **29:**1599–1600.

Chapter 18

Treatment of Eye Infections

MICHAEL H. MILLER AND MARTIN MAYERS

The quinolone antimicrobials are commonly prescribed as eye drops for the therapy of anterior eye infections such as conjunctivitis and keratitis. Ophthalmic drops containing 3 mg of norfloxacin, ciprofloxacin, ofloxacin, and levofloxacin per ml (0.3% solutions) are available. Ciprofloxacin 0.3% also comes as an ointment. Quinolones have good activity against most common ocular pathogens found in anterior infections, are well tolerated, and achieve therapeutic concentrations in tears, cornea, and the aqueous humor when given topically. Comparative outcome studies in animals with keratitis receiving quinolone eye drops generally show comparable or superior efficacy when compared with fortified antibiotic eye drops. Studies in humans with conjunctivitis or keratitis show equivalent outcomes; the exception is chlamydial conjunctivitis, in which quinolones appear to be superior to tetracycline. Systemically administered quinolones reach therapeutic concentrations in anterior ocular tissues, and combined topical and oral quinolone administration yield higher corneal and aqueous concentrations than topical therapy alone (23, 40, 111). No human studies have compared the use of intraocular or systemically administered quinolones for the treatment of posterior ocular infections (e.g., bacterial endophthalmitis), although intravitreal pefloxacin has been used in an uncontrolled study of bacterial endophthalmitis (82). In rabbits with endophthalmitis, systemically administered trovafloxacin shows efficacy against *Staphylococcus epidermidis* (85, 103). Animal studies show that the penetration of quinolones into the inflamed and uninflamed vitreous humor following systemic drug administration generally exceeds that of other antimicrobials. Depending on the quinolone studied, vitreal concentrations following systemic administration exceed the MICs for most organisms that cause endophthalmitis. Intraocular (IO) injection of antimicrobials is the administration route of choice for treat-

ing endophthalmitis in man. While the role of adjuvant therapy with systemically administered antimicrobials is uncertain, combination IO antibiotics and systemic therapy with quinolones has been used in the therapy of endophthalmitis (89, 106, 117).

Bacterial infections of the eye and contiguous tissues include conjunctivitis, keratitis, blepharitis, preseptal cellulitis, orbital cellulitis, cavernous sinus thrombosis, uveitis, and endophthalmitis. We limit our discussion to the use and pharmacology of quinolones for the treatment of bacterial infections of the conjunctiva (conjunctivitis), cornea (keratitis), and aqueous and vitreous humors (endophthalmitis).

OCULAR INFECTIONS, MICROBIOLOGY, AND RECOMMENDED THERAPY

Conjunctivitis is the most common bacterial infection of the eye and is also often caused by viruses. Although it causes local symptoms including irritation and tearing, it is rarely sight threatening and often resolves without antimicrobial therapy. Microbial etiologies in adults and children include both gram-positive and gram-negative bacteria. Streptococcus and staphylococcus isolates include viridans streptococci, *Streptococcus pneumoniae*, enterococci, group A streptococci, *S. epidermidis*, other coagulase-negative staphylococci, and *Staphylococcus aureus*. Gram-negative bacteria include *Haemophilus influenzae* and *Moraxella* sp., *Enterobacteriaceae, Pseudomonas aeruginosa,* and *Neisseria* spp. (both *N. gonorrhoeae* and *N. meningitidis*). Neonatal conjunctivitis is often caused by *N. gonorrhoeae* or *Chlamydia trachomatis* as well as the other pathogens listed above. In general, therapy of conjunctivitis consists of eye drops.

Bacterial keratitis is a relatively common infection that involves the cornea. Unlike conjunctivitis,

Michael H. Miller • Center for Immunology and Microbial Disease, Departments of Ophthalmology and Medicine, Albany Medical College, Albany, NY 12208. **Martin Mayers** • Department of Ophthalmology, Bronx Lebanon Medical Center, Albert Einstein College of Medicine, Bronx, NY 10457.

keratitis can cause vision loss and ulceration leading to perforation with potential loss of the eye. Microbial etiologies include *P. aeruginosa, S. aureus,* coagulase-negative *Staphylococcus, Streptococcus* sp., and *Enterobacteriaceae.* When possible, therapy should be tailored to the microbial etiology, and all patients with keratitis should be under the care of an ophthalmologist. In general, therapy consists of the frequent instillation of quinolone or antibiotic eye drops such as aminoglycosides or cephalosporins prepared as fortified solutions. Commercially available ophthalmic ointments, such as ciprofloxacin or bacitracin with or without polymyxin B and neomycin, are also available for treatment of bacterial keratitis. External drug-delivery devices (e.g., collagen shields and contact lenses) have been used to prolong drug exposure to the anterior eye structures but are not superior to the frequent instillation of antibiotic eye drops (6, 73, 130).

Although periocular injections function as a repository for antibiotic delivery to the conjunctiva and cornea, their utility is reserved for situations in which frequent topical instillation of antimicrobial drops cannot be performed. However, little experience has occurred with quinolones administered by this route. Combination therapy with systemic plus topical quinolones results in penetration into the cornea and aqueous humor that is often greater than penetration with topical agents alone (23, 40, 111).

Bacterial endophthalmitis is a sight-threatening inner eye infection that involves structures in the back of the eye (e.g., vitreous cavity, retina, and choroid) and anterior compartments (i.e., the anterior and posterior chambers). The posterior chamber is the space between the iris diaphragm and the anterior vitreous face (i.e., the lens and the spaces immediately contiguous). Most cases of bacterial endophthalmitis are exogenous and occur after intraocular surgery or perforating trauma. Endogenous endophthalmitis can occur secondary to bacteremia but is much less common than endophthalmitis from exogenous sources.

Postoperative endophthalmitis most commonly follows cataract surgery and occurs in approximately 1 of 1,000 patients. It can be subdivided into early and late infection. Patients with presumed postoperative endophthalmitis often have negative cultures. Organisms commonly causing early-onset postoperative endophthalmitis include coagulase-negative *S. aureus* and, less commonly, *Streptococcus* species, and assorted gram-negative bacteria. Delayed-onset postoperative endophthalmitis is often due to *Propionibacterium acnes,* coagulase-negative *Staphylococcus,* or fungi. Late endophthalmitis is caused by less invasive pathogens that are introduced

at the time of surgery. Postoperative entry of pathogens through a wound can also occur and is a particular problem following glaucoma filtration procedures. Postoperative endophthalmitis associated with glaucoma filtration surgery is a rapidly progressive sight-threatening infection commonly due to *Streptococcus* species including *S. pneumoniae,* group A streptococci and viridans streptococci, other gram-positive bacteria, and *Haemophilus* species. A particularly devastating form of endophthalmitis following trauma to the eye is caused by *Bacillus subtilis.*

The therapy of postoperative infectious endophthalmitis has been characterized in a large, multicenter, randomized study sponsored by the National Eye Institute, the Endophthalmitis Vitrectomy Study. Optimal therapy included the IO administration of antibiotics. Patients who presented with marked visual impairment also benefited from a vitrectomy (49). The antibiotics used intraocularly in the National Eye Institute, the Endophthalmitis Vitrectomy Study were vancomycin and amikacin. Vancomycin and amikacin were also used topically. While intravenous vancomycin and ceftazidime did not improve the outcome in patients randomly selected to receive systemic therapy, these antimicrobials exhibited poor penetration into noninflamed eyes. As a result, the potential role of adjuvant therapy with systemically administered antimicrobials that show better penetration into the vitreous humor such as the quinolones has not been addressed in human trials.

OCULAR PHARMACOLOGY

To understand the pharmacokinetics of quinolones in the eye it is important to consider anatomical and physiological features that have a bearing on ocular drug distribution. Conjunctivitis is a superficial infection that does not necessitate deeptissue penetration of antibiotic. Treatment of keratitis requires antibiotic penetration into the corneal stroma, and endophthalmitis requires penetration into the aqueous and vitreous humors.

The turnover of lacrimal fluid is approximately 20% per min and, following topical drug administration, reflex tearing also occurs. The volume of tear fluid is approximately 7 to 10 µl. Following topical administration of approximately 50 to 100 µl, most drug is immediately lost as overflow with a washout half-life of <5 min (99).

Corneal drug penetration of eye drops is necessary to treat bacterial keratitis. The corneal epithelium is approximately five cell layers thick with tight intercellular junctions. As a result, diffusion through the epithelial barrier is increased by lipophilicity. The corneal stroma is a loose, fluid-filled structure that does not impede the distribution of water-soluble medications (9). Entry into the corneal stroma following topical application is increased by inflammation and defects in the corneal epithelium.

Because of the rapid turnover of lacrimal fluid and reflex tearing, eye drops are formulated to contain very high drug concentrations and frequent dosing is necessary. Quinolone eye drop solutions contain 3,000 µg/ml, which is approximately 500- to 1,000-fold higher than concentrations that occur in the serum following oral or intravenous drug administration. Although for most eye drops no levels can be measured in the posterior chamber or vitreous humor, some penetration does occur with the quinolones.

Specialized barriers regulate drug distribution from the blood into protected compartments such as the eye and central nervous system. Systemically administered drugs often have poor access to the eye because of the blood-aqueous and blood-retinal barriers. The blood-ocular barrier (BOB) consists of tight endothelial junctions, which regulate transfer of medications according to molecular size, protein-binding affinity, lipophilicity, and degree of ionization (58, 87, 94, 107, 121, 138). Active transport systems also contribute to this barrier and regulate the effective penetration of a variety of antimicrobials, including quinolones (11, 15, 87).

Drug translocation is dependent on the functional anatomy and physiology of the eye as well as pharmacokinetics in the serum. The BOB is composed of three barriers: the corneal epithelial barrier (tear-corneal stroma barrier), retinal capillaries, and the retinal pigmented epithelium. The iris and ciliary body have fenestrated capillaries, whereas the pigment epithelium and endothelial cells of the retinal capillaries have tight intercellular junctions.

There are two major routes of antimicrobial elimination from the vitreous cavity, with ocular drug transfer occurring by both passive diffusion and active transport. Elimination by the anterior route is generally slow and requires diffusion through the vitreous body, entry into the aqueous humor, and drug elimination by bulk aqueous flow plus passive diffusion and efflux. Elimination by the posterior route is more rapid and involves diffusion through the vitreous body and passive diffusion and/or active efflux through the choroid and retina. However, many antimicrobials cannot pass through the retinal blood vessel endothelial cells or the retinal pigmented epithelium cells. Quinolones are eliminated via the posterior route. Following systemic administration, the concentrations of quinolones achieved in the pos-

terior eye depend on the competing rate constants describing uptake and efflux.

Inflammation due to infection or other causes alters the BOB by disrupting the tight junctions. Inflammation decreases the efflux rates for antimicrobials that are actively exported via the posterior route, such as the quinolones (86, 87) and penicillins (11). In contrast, for antibiotics that are not usually eliminated via the posterior route, inflammation increases the elimination via both the posterior and anterior routes (91). Inflammation also increases the penetration of systemically administered quinolones as well as other antimicrobials. The relative increase in the ocular penetration caused by inflammation is far greater for hydrophilic quinolones that penetrate poorly into the eye, such as ciprofloxacin, than for less hydrophilic quinolones that show better ocular penetration even without inflammation (86). For example, in rabbits with infection with *S. epidermidis* the penetration into the vitreous humor increased from 7 to 23% for ciprofloxacin and from 40 to 69% for trovafloxacin (86). Inflammation increased the mean ocular quinolone concentrations both by increasing entry and decreasing active efflux (71, 86).

The effects of the mode of quinolone administration (a single dose, multiple doses, or continuous infusion) on ocular penetration has been characterized in a rabbit model. When animals were given a 40-mg bolus, 13.3 mg every 8 h, or a constant infusion, each administration mode resulted in similar mean concentrations in serum (area under the curve [AUC] of 32.9, 31.9, and 33.8 mg·h/ml, respectively), and peak concentrations in the aqueous humor (30.5, 31.6, and 30.0%) and vitreous humor (6.6, 7.4, and 7.5%). Thus, ocular concentrations were independent of the mode of drug administration (88).

The lipophilicity of quinolones shows an excellent correlation with penetration into and efflux from the vitreous humor following intraocular drug administration (85–87). Carrier-independent penetration into protected compartments such as the eye and central nervous system correlates with protein binding, molecular weight/size, and the physicochemical properties of the compound including lipophilicity (87, 102). Multiple linear regression analysis shows that the logarithm of the penetration of compounds across planar lipid bilayers and tissue membranes correlates with the oil/water partition ratio, the inverse of the square route of the molecular weight (22), and the free fraction of drug (38, 100). Only the unbound fraction of drug diffuses into the eye following systemic administration.

The correlation between lipophilicity and penetration into or elimination from the eye has been recently characterized following systemic and IO quinolone administration (86). Using five quinolones—ciprofloxacin, fleroxacin, ofloxacin, levofloxacin, and sparfloxacin—Liu et al. have shown an excellent correlation ($r^2 > 0.9999$) between lipophilicity and the penetration (Fig. 1). This relationship is expressed as $\log_{10}$ percent penetration = $2.739(p) + 0.58$, where p = the octanol-water partition coefficient. The ability to delineate further the relationship between penetration and protein binding or molecular size/weight was limited by similarities in these independent variables among the quinolones tested.

In vivo and in vitro studies characterizing the rates of ocular and renal elimination of zwitterionic quinolones suggest the presence of separate and distinct carrier-mediated efflux for quinolones (68, 86). As in the cerebrospinal fluid (CSF), there is a directionality to efflux pumps in the eye that is differentially affected by systemic and intracompartmental probenecid administration (11, 86, 98, 125, 145). For quinolone antimicrobials, active efflux from the vitreous humor following intraocular administration is blocked by probenecid or inflammation (86). Quinolone elimination via the posterior route occurs by two independent mechanisms, diffusion and active efflux (86). As with quinolone penetration following systemic administration, an excellent correlation exists with efflux and lipophilicity ($r^2 = 0.9999$). The elimination half-life is expressed as $t_{1/2\beta} = -1.8172)(\log_{10}p) + 2.1239$ (87).

Ocular pharmacokinetics use concentration-versus-time data to model drug absorption, distribution, metabolism, and elimination. The efflux of quinolones from the vitreous humor is rapid following IO administration (87), whereas the elimination rates following systemic drug administration are not rapid and closely mimic those in the serum (44, 87, 88, 96, 118). Quinolones administered by intravitreal and intravenous injections follow one- or two-compartment models, respectively (44, 87, 88, 96, 118). Physiological models based on anatomical eye compartments are of limited use because drug transfer by flow, blood diffusional exchange, and anterior-posterior drainage is nonidentifiable. Ocular pharmacokinetics of quinolones have been measured both in man and animals; most animal studies are done in rabbits.

It is important to understand limitations of these animal and human pharmacological data when reviewing data describing quinolone concentrations and penetration into the eye (Tables 1 to 4). Although rabbits appear to be a valid model to study ocular pharmacokinetics, when possible, human data are preferable. However, obtaining samples from the cornea and aqueous or vitreous humor requires invading the integrity of the eye, a disruption that is not warranted in the absence of disease. As a result, human corneal samples are obtained in conjunction with keratoplasty, aqueous samples in conjunction with cataract surgery, and vitreous samples at the

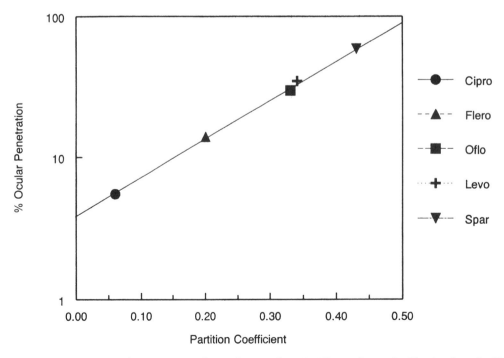

Figure 1. Relationship between the partition coefficient for ciprofloxacin (Cipro), fleroxacin (Flero), ofloxacin (Oflo), levofloxacin (Levo), and sparfloxacin (Spar) and the relative penetration into the vitreous humor.

time of vitrectomy. Following topical drug administration aqueous concentrations should not be affected by breakdown of the blood-aqueous barrier, which should be minimal at the start of surgery. In contrast, pharmacokinetic studies in the vitreous of humans are done in patients with vitrectomies for diseases that often cause a breakdown of the blood-ocular barrier. It should be borne in mind when comparing Tables 2 and 4 that in humans, but not animals, comparisons of penetration into the vitreous humor are generally quantified in the presence of BOB breakdown, whereas in both humans and animals penetration of the aqueous humor is generally done in the absence of BOB breakdown. Aqueous samples have been used as surrogate markers for levels in the corneal stroma following topical application. Following systemic drug administration, aqueous concentrations for most antibiotics are generally much higher than those in the vitreous humor. However, whether this general rule is valid for all quinolone antimicrobials is not known (10).

Another confounding variable is the fact that quinolones bind tightly to pigmented epithelium, and many ocular pharmacokinetic studies are done in albino rabbits. For example, Cochereau-Massin et al. showed that, following the intravitreal administration of pefloxacin into albino and pigmented rabbits, concentrations in the chorioretina were higher and the half-life longer in pigmented than in albino animals (34). However, when Perkins et al. compared the penetration of ofloxacin into, and the efflux from, the vitreous humor of pigmented and albino rabbits, both were similar, with 32 versus 30% penetration and half-lives of 3.21 and 4.32 h, respectively, $P > 0.05$ (118). The risk of iatrogenic complications by using serial needle aspiration has restricted human ocular pharmacokinetic studies to a single sample obtained from different patients. Studies in animals use only one specimen per animal. This approach is based on a concern that serial sampling of individual eyes would introduce artifact due to BOB breakdown.

Generating population data by combining single samples from different subjects has been referred to as the naïve pooled data (NPD) approach. Intrasubject variation using the NPD approach prohibits rigorous determination of pharmacokinetic parameters from small groups of animals or patients, and parameter value estimates cannot address variability in the population being studied, limitations that reduce the value of the information obtained (44, 96).

Penetration data for systemically administered quinolones are often estimated by comparing simultaneous samples in the eye and serum. However,

prior to the pseudoequilibration, this approach does not accurately reflect ocular penetration due to system hysteresis (i.e., the ratio of simultaneous concentrations in ocular humors and serum is not constant). To quantify quinolone penetration in the eye, Barza used an alternative approach (10). Rather than comparing simultaneous drug concentrations, peak concentrations (C_{max}) in aqueous or vitreous humor were compared to peak concentrations in serum. We have used a similar approach to estimate penetration in animals (Table 2) and humans (Table 4). When complete data are presented for concentrations in ocular humors and serum, model-independent methods to estimate the AUC_{ocular} and AUC_{serum} are used to calculate penetration.

For pharmacokinetic analysis in animals it is preferable to obtain complete serum and ocular concentration-time profiles from different subjects. Two methods are available in animals: serial sampling and microdialysis. Multiple samples can be obtained from vitreous humor without altering ocular pharmacokinetics (44, 87, 88, 96, 98, 118). Analysis of pharmacokinetic data using serial ocular and serum data provides more robust data that the NPD approach and decreases the number of animals that are needed (44, 87, 88, 96, 118). The aqueous humor, unlike the vitreous humor, demonstrates breakdown of the blood-aqueous barrier following even a single aspiration from the anterior chamber so that serial sampling is less reliable. Microdialysis provides an important alternative for obtaining serial intraocular pharmacokinetic data (48, 63, 72, 141).

Drusano and colleagues have recently described a third approach, which combines mathematical and statistical tools to determine population pharmacokinetic parameters using a single sample from different patients (e.g., the clinically relevant scenario in humans) and serial plasma samples in the same subjects. This approach has been validated in rabbits receiving systemic ciprofloxacin (44). Derived penetration and pharmacokinetic constants were equivalent when single or complete ocular data sets were used for ciprofloxacin. Although this method has not been used in humans, intensive plasma sampling in conjunction with a single sample from the eye of different subjects holds promise for the analysis of penetration of drugs into privileged spaces such as the eye.

PHARMACODYNAMICS

Pharmacodynamic models characterize the relationship between antimicrobial drug exposure (e.g., pharmacokinetics) and activity, expressed as the

MIC, with efficacy or drug exposure with toxicity. While pharmacodynamics has proven useful in characterizing the relationship between pharmacokinetics in the serum and outcome for quinolones and other antimicrobials (41, 42, 126), this approach has not been used for ocular infections. Ocular pharmacokinetic parameters such as the peak (C_{max}), and mean (AUC) concentrations and elimination-rate half-lives ($t_{1/2\beta}$) differ dramatically from each other (2, 44, 86, 88, 98, 118) and from that in the serum following topical, intraocular, and systemic drug administration. Depending on the dosing schedule and the likelihood of the emergence of resistant mutants, either the C_{max}/MIC ratio or AUC/MIC ratio correlates with outcome for quinolones (42, 43, 119, 126). As a result, pharmacodynamic modeling may be particularly important in optimizing therapy for ocular infections.

Preliminary studies using a human equivalent dose of different quinolones showed that both the AUC/MIC and the C_{max}/MIC ratios correlated with outcome in a *S. epidermidis* endophthalmitis model (85). Because the C_{max} and AUC are linked variables, and because outcome studies that use a single dose in humans do not readily distinguish between AUC/MIC and the C_{max}/MIC ratios (41, 120), dose-fractionation studies are needed to establish the best model for quinolones (43).

OCULAR PHARMACOKINETICS IN ANIMALS FOLLOWING TOPICAL ADMINISTRATION

Table 1 shows the ocular concentrations of fluoroquinolones in rabbits following topical drug administration in the normal eye or those with corneal damage due to penetrating trauma, infection, or alkali burns (12, 51, 111, 115, 116, 133). All studies with ciprofloxacin used eye drops containing 3 mg/ml (0.3%), administered repeatedly from 4 to 14 h prior to sampling. The concentrations of ciprofloxacin in the aqueous humor ranged from 0.14 to 4.8 µg/ml, and in the vitreous humor from 0.65 to 0.77 µg/ml (12, 104, 115, 116). The penetration of ciprofloxacin (or ofloxacin) described by Behrens-Baumann (12) was >10-fold [> 3 standard deviations (SD)] less than that of the other studies; however, fewer doses were given and the interval between administration and sampling was longer than in the other studies.

Concentrations in the vitreous humor were approximately one fourth those in the aqueous. Corneal damage or inflammation increased the mean penetration into both the aqueous and vitreous humors. The coadministration of oral and topical ciprofloxacin (not shown) approximately doubled ciprofloxacin concentrations in aqueous and vitreous humors of rabbits with normal eyes or those with

Table 1. Concentrations of quinolones after topical application in rabbits

Drug	Dosage[a]	Healthy cornea		Corneal damage or inflammation		Reference
		Concn in aqueous humor (µg/g)	Concn in vitreous humor (µg/g)	Concn in aqueous humor (µg/ml)	Concn in vitreous humor (µg/ml)	
Ciprofloxacin	3 mg/ml q1h for					111
Control 7 h	7 or 14 h	1.31	0.65			
Control 14 h		1.85	0.72			
Infected 7 h				2.18	0.67	
Infected 14 h				2.91	1.01	
Ciprofloxacin	3 mg/ml q30min × 8	2.31	0.77	7.36	0.95	112
Ciprofloxacin	3 mg/ml					12
×1		0.1		0.23		
0, 2, 4 h		0.14		0.29		
Ciprofloxacin	3 mg/ml q30min × 6	4.82		12.9		104
Ofloxacin	3 mg/ml					12
× 1		0.04		0.15		
0, 2, 4 h		0.07		0.23		
Ofloxacin	3 mg/ml q30min × 8	3.25	0.17	5.21	0.35	116
Ofloxacin	3 mg/ml q1h × 7	1.45	0.23	2.35	0.29	113
	3 mg/min q1h × 14	2.48	0.27	3.49	0.40	
Enoxacin	3 mg/ml q1h × 4 [b]	0.5		7.1		133
Enoxacin	5 mg/ml × 1			3.7		51
Rosoxacin	10 mg/ml q30min × 6[c]	5.29				64
Rosoxacin	20 mg/ml q30min × 6	5.29				

[a] Abbreviations: concn, concentration; q1h, every hour; q30min, every 30 min.
[b] Concentrations of enoxacin in the healthy or debrided cornea were 12 and 66 µg/ml, respectively.
[c] Concentrations of rosoxacin in the healthy corneal were 6.66 and 15.09 µg/ml following the 10 and 20 µg/ml doses.

surgical trauma plus endophthalmitis (111). In general, the presence of surgery and infection resulted in higher levels particularly in the aqueous humor; however, these differences were not significant (111, 116). Corneal damage due to alkali burns also appeared to modestly increase penetration into the aqueous humor (12), as did more doses (12, 115).

Topical application of 3 mg/ml ofloxacin resulted in concentrations in the aqueous humor of 0.4 to 3.25 µg/ml and concentrations in the vitreous humor ranging from 0.07 to 0.27 µg/ml (12, 115, 116). Corneal damage/inflammation increased aqueous concentrations ~1.5-fold and vitreous humor concentrations ~1.8-fold.

Enoxacin eye drops given as a single 5 mg/ml dose in animals with keratitis or as repeated 3 mg/ml doses in the presence of surgically induced corneal damage resulted in concentrations in aqueous humor of 5 and 3.7 µg/ml, compared with 0.9 µg/ml in normal eyes. Concentrations in corneal tissue were much higher than concentrations in the aqueous humor and were markedly increased with corneal damage (51, 133). A single study by Hulem et al. showed rosoxacin concentrations of ≥5 µg/ml in the aqueous humor following topical application (64).

Reidy and colleagues (122) measured norfloxacin and ciprofloxacin levels in the aqueous humor following topical administration in animals with pseudomonas keratitis. Mean levels were lower for norfloxacin (7.5 µg/ml) than ciprofloxacin (30.5 µg/ml).

Drug-delivery systems are often used to improve the delivery of antimicrobial agents to the eye. Gehlardi examined the utility of tamarin-gum polysaccharide (TGP), a mucoadhesive polymer, on the pharmacokinetics of ofloxacin in the aqueous humor following topical administration (55). Pharmacokinetics in the aqueous humor were determined by pooling data in separate rabbits; ofloxacin-TGP was compared with ofloxacin alone. Topical ofloxacin-TGP approximately tripled the peak and mean aqueous concentrations and doubled the elimination half-lives in rabbits when compared with ofloxacin alone.

OCULAR PHARMACOKINETICS IN ANIMALS FOLLOWING SYSTEMIC ADMINISTRATION

Table 2 shows the penetration of fluoroquinolones into the aqueous and vitreous humor of rabbits following systemic administration. Percent penetration into the aqueous or vitreous humors has been calculated by comparing the AUC_{eye}/AUC_{serum} (32, 87, 88, 98, 103, 118) or the $C_{max,eye}/C_{max,serum}$ (2, 14, 32, 108, 110), as described in the preceding section. It should be noted that data from the different studies shown in Table 2 often were the result of using different dosing schedules and analytical methods. Penetration of ciprofloxacin into the aqueous or vitreous humors ranged from 8.6 to 32.6% and 6.5 to 21%, respectively (5, 14, 87, 88, 110). Excluding the vitreal penetration data of Oosiho et al. (>3 SD

Table 2. Ocular penetration after systemic administration in rabbits

Drug	Dosage and route	% Penetration (concn [µg/ml])[a]			Reference
		Serum	Aqueous humor	Vitreous humor	
Ciprofloxacin	50 mg/kg p.o., 1 dose	(1.5)	21 (0.32)	21 (0.33)	110
Ciprofloxacin	40 mg/kg × 1 i.v.		30.5	6.5	88
	40 mg/kg i.v. infusion		30.0	7.5	
	13.3 mg/kg × 3 i.v. (40 mg/kg)		31.6	7.4	
Ciprofloxacin	30 mg × 1 i.v.			11	5
Ciprofloxacin	12 mg/kg i.v. × 1	(0.7)	8.6(0.06)	4 (0.03)	14
Ofloxacin	40 mg/kg × i.v.		NT	32.6[b]	118
Sparfloxacin	50 mg/kg p.o., 1 dose	(4.0)	18.3 (0.74)		108
Sparfloxacin	40 mg/kg × 1 i.v.		NT	59	86
Trovafloxacin	250 mg/kg p.o. × 1		13	14	103
Trovafloxacin	40 mg/kg i.v. × 1			40	86
Levofloxacin	40 mg/kg i.v. × 1			4.8	86
Fleroxacin	10 mg/kg × 1 i.v.	23.55	27	10	98
Rosoxacin	5 mg/kg i.v., 1 dose	(5.5)	<14 (< 0.75)	<14 (< 0.75)	64
Pefloxacin	50 mg/kg i.m., 1 dose	(33.4)	27 (2.4)	39.5[c]	32
Balofloxacin	20 mg/kg p.o. × 1	(0.27)	66 (0.18)		109

[a] % penetration is based on estimates using highest drug concentrations (concn) in the aqueous or vitreous/serum or AUC_{eye}/AUC_{serum}. All eyes were uninflamed. i.m., intramuscular. Percent penetration is concentration at the site as a percentage of the concentration serum.
[b] Ofloxacin penetration is shown for albino rabbits. Penetration in pigmented rabbits following a single dose and at serum steady state were similar, 30.4 and 30%, respectively.
[c] Pefloxacin concentration is shown for albino rabbits. Penetration into the aqueous and vitreous humor for pigmented rabbits was 24.4 and 45.2%, respectively.

from mean) the mean penetrations into the aqueous and vitreous humor were 24.34 ± 9.76 and 7.28 ± 2.5 µg/ml. A single study by Perkins et al. showed that the penetration of ofloxacin into the vitreous humor was 31% (118). The penetration of the levo isomer of ofloxacin, levofloxacin (35%), was similar to that of ofloxacin (85, 86). Liu et al. found that the vitreal penetration of sparfloxacin, the most lipophilic quinolone, into the vitreous humor was 59% (87), whereas Ooishi found that penetration into the aqueous was 18.3% (108).

Ng and colleagues found that the ocular penetration of trovafloxacin into the aqueous humor and vitreous humor was 13 and 14%, respectively (103), following oral administration. Following intravenous administration Jumbe et al. showed ocular penetration that was almost three times higher, 40% (71). Simultaneous penetration into CSF was 35%; previous studies have shown that penetration into the CSF by several antimicrobials including quinolones is equivalent to that in the vitreous humor (71).

Penetration into the aqueous and vitreous humor for fleroxacin and pefloxacin were 27 versus 19% and 27 versus 29%, respectively (32, 98). Levels of pefloxacin in the lens were 25% of that in serum (32). Aqueous humor penetration of rosoxacin, pefloxacin, and balofloxacin was <14, 29, and 66% , respectively (32, 64, 109).

OCULAR PHARMACOKINETICS IN ANIMALS FOLLOWING INTRAVITREAL ADMINISTRATION

The pharmacokinetics of intravitreal quinolones has been characterized for fleroxacin, ciprofloxacin, ofloxacin, and sparfloxacin (34, 87, 112, 114). Behrens-Baumann and Martell also characterized the pharmacokinetics of ciprofloxacin following subconjunctival administration (14). Liu et al. characterized the elimination rates by obtaining serial samples of vitreous fluids in rabbits that had received ciprofloxacin, fleroxacin, ofloxacin, and sparfloxacin following direct intravitreal injection (87). In each subject one eye received a quinolone and the other both quinolone and probenecid; the effect of inflammation induced by heat-killed bacteria was also studied. The elimination for ciprofloxacin, fleroxacin, ofloxacin, and sparfloxacin was very rapid, with half-lives ranging from 2.8 to 5.2 h. There was an excellent correlation between lipophilicity and the elimination rates ($r^2 > 0.99$). Both probenecid and inflammation induced by heat-killed S. epidermidis decreased quinolone efflux for all quinolones following direct

injection into the vitreous humor (87). These observations suggest that there are two modes of quinolone elimination for the eye, diffusion and carrier-mediated efflux. Ozturk et al. characterized the pharmacokinetics of both ofloxacin (114) and ciprofloxacin (112) following intravitreal injection. In both instances one eye was subjected to surgical trauma and infection with S. aureus. Following a single dose of 200 µg of ciprofloxacin mean concentrations were only slightly higher in the traumatized, infected eyes with elimination half-lives of 6 and 5 h, respectively. Following the intravitreal injection of 200 µg of ofloxacin, there were higher levels at 24 h in the traumatized/infected eye and elimination half-lives of 5.7 and 3 h, respectively.

Cochereau-Massin et al. characterized the elimination rate for pefloxacin in albino and pigmented rabbits following direct ocular injection (34). While concentrations were measured in different subjects at each time point and data combined to calculate elimination rates, the elimination half-life of 3 h was similar to that described for other quinolones (87).

Behrens-Baumann measured the intraocular levels of ciprofloxacin following subconjunctival injection of 1 mg into the perilimbal region or into the lower fornix of rabbits. Aqueous humor levels measured after 1 h were 0.887 and 0.94 mg/ml, and at 10 h were 0.0267 and 0.025 mg/ml, respectively following administration at the two sites of injection (14).

CONCENTRATIONS OF QUINOLONES IN HUMANS AFTER TOPICAL APPLICATION

Table 3 shows aqueous and vitreous concentrations of humans following the topical application of ciprofloxacin, ofloxacin, and norfloxacin. In all cases, drops containing 3 mg/ml were administered repeatedly, at least on an hourly basis. For ciprofloxacin the aqueous concentrations ranged from 0.23 to 2.8; the mean penetration was 0.61 ± 0.84. However, if the data of Akkan et al. are considered an outlier (>3 SD from mean) and excluded from the rest then the mean aqueous concentration of ciprofloxacin is 0.33 ± 0.17 µg/ml (1, 23–25, 27, 29, 45, 140). Concentrations of ofloxacin in the aqueous humor ranged from 0.36 to 2.95 µg/ml with a mean of 1.36 ± 0.84 (1, 24–26, 40, 45, 60, 136, 140). Norfloxacin concentration in the aqueous humor ranged from 0.185 to 1.5 µg/ml. Vitreous humor concentrations for ciprofloxacin were 50% (27) and ofloxacin 25% (26) or 4% (60) of the concentrations in the aqueous humor following topical administration.

Table 3. Concentrations of quinolones after topical application in humans

Drug	Dosage[a]	Procedure	Concn (µg/ml) in: Aqueous humor	Concn (µg/ml) in: Vitreous humor	Reference
Ciprofloxacin	3 mg/ml q30min × 6 then q1h × 3	Cataract surgery	0.33		25
Ciprofloxacin	q1h × 3	Cataract surgery	0.35		24
Ciprofloxacin	q1h × 3	Vitrectomy	0.44	0.22	27
Ciprofloxacin	3 mg/ml q30min × 6/q1h × 3	Vitrectomy	0.23		28
Ciprofloxacin	3 mg/ml q20min × 5	Cataract surgery	0.69		29
Ciprofloxacin	3 mg/ml q15min × 6 h Mode #2 look up	Cataract surgery	0.38		1
Ciprofloxacin	3 mg/ml q15min × 6	Cataract surgery	0.092		140
Ciprofloxacin	3 mg/ml q1h × 6 × 2 at −90 and −30	Cataract surgery	2.80 1.11		45
Ciprofloxacin	3mg/ml q30min × 8	Cataract surgery (prior filtering bleb)	0.21		23
Ofloxacin	3 mg/ml q30min × 6 then qlh × 3	Cataract surgery	1.34		25
Ofloxacin	3 mg/ml q30min × 6/qlh × 3	Cataract surgery	1.43		24
Ofloxacin	3 mg/ml q15min × 8	Cataract surgery	0.56		140
Ofloxacin	3 mg/ml q15min × 6	Cataract surgery	0.964		45
Ofloxacin	3 mg/ml q1h × 6 × 2 at −90 and −30	Cataract surgery	2.95 1.5		1
Ofloxacin	3 mg/ml q30m × 8	Cataract surgery with filtering blebs	0.75		23
Ofloxacin	3 mg/ml q1h × 3	Vitrectomy	1.44	0.37	26
Ofloxacin	3 mg/ml drops q1h × 2 q30min × 6 then 3 mg/ml ointment	Cataract surgery	0.43 0.36		136
Ofloxacin	3 mg/ml q5h × 106	Cataract surgery	2.73		60
Ofloxacin	3 mg/ml q30min × 8	Keratoplasty + vitrectomy[b]	1.34	0.37	40
Norfloxacin	3 mg/ml q15min × 8	Cataract surgery	0.182		140
Norfloxacin	3 mg/ml qlh × 6 × 2 at −90 and −30	Cataract surgery	1.50 1.20		1

[a] Abbreviations: q20min, every 20 min; q15min, every 15 min; q5h, every 5 h.
[b] Ofloxacin concentrations in the cornea were 4.51 µg/ml.

Because of the rapid elimination of quinolones from the vitreous humor after IO injection and their excellent penetration following systemic administration, we and others have questioned the rationale of IO rather than systemic quinolones as adjunctive therapy of endophthalmitis (59, 86). While our studies have focused on the pharmacokinetics and outcome of quinolones following systemic administration, Hainsworth and colleagues (59) have examined the use of implanted devices in prolonging therapeutic concentration of ciprofloxacin in the vitreous humor. These investigators compared ciprofloxacin release from implantable sustained-release devices prepared from polylatic acid and polyvinyl alcohol. In vitro studies showed that there was rapid release of ciprofloxacin from the matrix of dried polylactic acid and polyvinyl alcohol with a release half-life of approximately 2 to 4 h, whereas that from the reservoir device consisting of compressed ciprofloxacin was approximately 3 days. Implantation of the ciprofloxacin reservoir device resulted in prolonged therapeutic intravitreal concentrations that were maintained for at least 2 weeks.

PHARMACOKINETICS IN HUMANS FOLLOWING SYSTEMIC ADMINISTRATION

Table 4 shows human data for the ocular penetration of quinolones following oral (p.o.) or intravenous (i.v.) administration. To simplify this table, only studies for which both serum and ocular drug concentrations were determined are included and all ciprofloxacin studies used a 750-mg dose (47, 70, 75). Penetration of ciprofloxacin into the aqueous humor ranged from 6 to 18% (mean, 13.0 ± 4.89); that in the vitreous humor ranged from 9 to 21% (mean, 16.25 ± 5.51). When doses of ciprofloxacin ranging from 200 to 600 mg i.v. and 500 to 1,000 mg p.o. given as one, two, or three doses were used, penetration was remarkably similar to that following the 750-mg oral dose. Aqueous penetration ranged from 3.3 to 19% (mean, 15.10 ± 7.36) (13, 17, 52, 69, 131, 134) and that in the vitreous 3.2 to 17.7% (mean, 14.38 ± 7.05) (70). Administration p.o. and i.v. of ciprofloxacin in animals shows that the penetration into the aqueous and vitreous

Table 4. Penetration of quinolones other than ciprofloxacin into the human eye following systemic drug administration

Drug	Dosage	Concn, μg/ml (% penetration)				Reference
		Procedure	Serum	Aqueous humor	Vitreous humor	
Ciprofloxacin	750 mg p.o.	Vitreal surgery				75
1× −4 h			1.8		0.17 (9)	
1× −8h			1.0		0.20 (20)	
2×, 12 and −24 h			2.27		0.35 (15)	
Ciprofloxacin	750 mg p.o.	Vitrectomy			(21)	47
Ciprofloxacin	750 mg × 1		2.7	0.15 (6)		70
	750 mg × 2		3.4	0.53 (16)		
	750 mg × 3		3.8	0.69 (18)		
Ofloxacin	200 mg p.o., 1 dose	Cataract extraction	3.0	0.6 (20)		18
Ofloxacin	400 mg p.o., 1 dose	Cataract extraction	5.2	1.14 (22)		83
Ofloxacin	200 mg, −12 h and −2 h	Pars plana vitrectomy	2.23		0.62 (37.8)	139
	400 mg, −12 h and −2 h	Vitrectomy	5.23		1.75 (33.4)	
Sparfloxacin	400 mg, −2 to −24 h	Cataract extraction	1.40	0.40 (29)		21
	1,000 mg total	Pars plana vitrectomy				
Levofloxacin	500 mg, × 1 −12	Vitrectomy	4.34	0.59 (14)	0.32 (7.0)	53
	500 mg × 2 −24 to 12 h		8.02	1.90 (24)	2.39 (30)	
Pefloxacin	400 mg p.o., 1 dose	Cataract extraction	5.0	0.89 (18)		19
	400 mg i.v., 1 dose	Cataract extraction	6.0	1.45 (24)		123
	400 mg p.o., 6 doses	Cataract extraction	15	7.5 (50)		83
	400 mg i.v., 1 dose	Ocular surgery	5.2	0.8 (15)	0.5 (10)	39
	800 mg i.v., 1 dose		13.0	3.3 (25)	4.0 (31)	
Norfloxacin	800 mg p.o., 1 dose	Cataract extraction	3.5	0.56 (16)		20
	1,600 mg, 1 dose		3.3	0.8 (24)		

humors are not affected by the route of systemic drug administration (88).

Three investigators have characterized the penetration of ofloxacin into the aqueous humor following oral doses of 200 or 400 mg given once or twice. Concentrations in the aqueous humor were 20 and 22% (18, 83) and in the vitreous humor were 37.8 and 33.4% (139) of those in the serum.

Ciprofloxacin concentrations in the aqueous and vitreous humors were similar, and ofloxacin concentrations were higher in the vitreous than the aqueous humor. While animal studies show variable results regarding penetration into the aqueous and vitreous humors, studies using serial sampling techniques and optimal pharmacokinetic methods suggest that, for ciprofloxacin at least, in the absence of breakdown of the blood-ocular barrier penetration into the aqueous is greater than that in the vitreous (72, 88) and penetration into vitreous humor increased from 6 to 23% in the presence of BOB breakdown (86). Moreover, in humans vitreal samples are generally obtained from subjects with medical conditions that cause breakdown of the blood-ocular barrier.

Pefloxacin penetration into the aqueous humor ranged from 15 to 50% (mean, 26.4 ± 13.83) (19, 39, 83, 123). Denis et al. showed that following 400 and 800 mg of i.v. pefloxacin the penetration was 10 and

31%, respectively (39). Single studies characterizing sparfloxacin (21) and norfloxacin (17) resulted in penetration into the aqueous humor of 29 and 24%, respectively.

Two investigators characterized the ocular penetration of ofloxacin (23, 40) or ciprofloxacin (23) into the eye following combined topical and oral therapy; neither measured concomitant serum concentrations. Cantor et al. (23) characterized the penetration into the aqueous humor in patients with prior filtering bleb surgery who underwent subsequent cataract surgery. Topical ciprofloxacin or ofloxacin was given as a 3% solution every 30 min for 4 h prior to surgery; oral quinolones were given as a 400-mg dose three times at approximately 24, 12, and 3 h preoperatively. The addition of oral ciprofloxacin to topically administered drug increased aqueous concentrations from 0.21 to 0.35 μg/ml. Oral ofloxacin increased aqueous concentrations from 0.75 to 3.84 μg/ml. Ofloxacin concentrations following both topical therapy and combined topical and oral therapy were significantly higher for ofloxacin than ciprofloxacin. Ofloxacin, but not ciprofloxacin, combined oral and topical therapy resulted in significantly higher aqueous concentrations than topical therapy alone (23). Donnenfeld et al. (40) also compared combined topical and oral ofloxacin in patients undergoing keratoplasty and vitrectomy. Ofloxacin was given topically 3% every 30 min eight times and systemically 400-mg tablets p.o. ~24, 12, and 2 h preoperatively. Combined therapy was compared with topical therapy alone. Combined therapy increased concentrations in the aqueous humor from 1.34 to 2.27 µg/ml and from 0.37 to 2.25 µg/ml in the vitreous humor (40).

In summary, in animal studies the penetration of ciprofloxacin and ofloxacin into the vitreous humor following topical administration appears to be similar, despite the fact that ofloxacin is more lipophilic. On the other hand, in human studies there appeared to be better penetration of ofloxacin than ciprofloxacin following topical drug administration. For all quinolones tested in animals and humans, concentrations in excess of the MIC for most ocular pathogens were achieved in the aqueous humor. The ratio of vitreous to aqueous penetration in humans following topical administration was 0.5 for ciprofloxacin and ~0.25 for ofloxacin (26, 27, 40).

Because of differences in drug administration, study design, analysis, and the likelihood of breakdown of the BOB in human vitreous samples, it is difficult to compare the relative penetration of different quinolones in animals or humans. However, when standardized, validated, and uniform methods were used to characterize penetration following systemic administration in rabbits, the vitreous penetration for ciprofloxacin, fleroxacin, ofloxacin, sparfloxacin, and levofloxacin was 5.5, 13.7, 31.2, 35, and 58.9%, respectively. An excellent correlation also exists between lipophilicity and the penetration of levofloxacin into the vitreous humor (Fig. 1) (71, 87). Overall, the penetration into the aqueous humor of humans was approximately half of that in animals, whereas the penetration into the vitreous humor was double that in animals. Following systemic administration to both animals and man, ofloxacin penetration into the vitreous humor was higher than that of ciprofloxacin, as expected on the basis of their relative lipophilicities. In animals the concomitant use of both topical and oral ciprofloxacin increased the aqueous drug concentrations relative to topical therapy approximately twofold. In humans, relative to topical therapy alone, combined therapy increased the aqueous concentration of both ciprofloxacin and ofloxacin approximately 1.5-fold; and concentrations in the vitreous for both drugs increased approximately sixfold.

Pharmacokinetic studies following direct intravitreal injection have only been performed in rabbits. Unlike other agents that are used for intravitreal therapy of endophthalmitis (e.g., vancomycin, amikacin), for which elimination occurs by the anterior route resulting in therapeutic concentrations that last for days, quinolones are eliminated via the posterior route by both diffusion and active efflux. As with penetration, efflux correlates with lipophilicity. While inflammation slows the elimination somewhat, therapeutic levels nevertheless remain transient.

OUTCOME STUDIES IN ANIMALS WITH EXTERNAL EYE DISEASE

Outcome studies in animals have characterized the use of topical quinolones for the therapy of *P. aeruginosa* and *S. aureus* keratitis (50, 51, 62, 97, 101, 104, 122, 133). A single study has characterized the outcome in rabbits following the injection of *P. aeruginosa* into the anterior chamber treated with topical lomofloxacin (61).

Administration of ciprofloxacin eye drops to rabbits with experimental keratitis due to an aminoglycoside-resistant strain of *P. aeruginosa* resulted in a fall of CFU per milliliter below the levels of detection at the end of therapy. Reidy et al. showed that higher concentrations of ciprofloxacin (7.5 mg/ml) were more effective than fortified tobramycin (13.6 mg/ml) or norfloxacin (10 mg/ml) against an aminoglycoside-resistant *P. aeruginosa*; the MICs of tobramycin, norfloxacin, and ciprofloxacin were 31.25, 0.48, and 0.24 µg/ml. (122). Animals were treated for a total of 4 h. Similar outcomes in rabbits with experimental keratitis due to another aminoglycoside-resistant *P. aeruginosa* strain were described by O'Brien and colleagues (104). Ciprofloxacin (3 mg/ml) drops given every half hour for 12 h also resulted in no viable organisms at the end of therapy (104).

The efficacy of 0.3% ciprofloxacin drops given repeatedly or as a single drop for experimental keratitis due to a susceptible strain of *S. aureus* keratitis was compared clinically and microbiologically against ofloxacin and untreated controls. A sustained release preparation of ciprofloxacin plus polystyrene sulfate (PSS) was also used (101). When treatment was started early, the microbiological outcome for ciprofloxacin was superior to that of ofloxacin or ciprofloxacin plus PSS. When therapy was started later all regimens were roughly equivalent and superior to untreated and vehicle-treated controls. Engle and colleagues also characterized microbiological outcome and the degree of inflammation in animals with *P. aeruginosa* or *S. aureus* keratitis treated with ciprofloxacin plus PSS and ciprofloxacin drops with benzalkonium chloride and EDTA as preservatives (50). Both regimens were highly effective with no difference in microbiological or clinical outcome.

In a study comparing the efficacy of collagen corneal shields hydrated with norfloxacin (40 mg/ml), ciprofloxacin (25 mg/ml), tobramycin (40 mg/ml), or deionized water in animals with tobramycin-resistant *P. aeruginosa* keratitis, ciprofloxacin was the most effective in decreasing colony counts (62).

Using an aminoglycoside-susceptible strain of *P. aeruginosa*, Gritz et al. in a rabbit model of keratitis showed that topical therapy for 12 h with ofloxacin (3 mg/ml) or tobramycin (3 mg/ml) were equally efficacious in decreasing CFU per milliliter at 12 h. At 1 week, eyes were sterile with comparable corneal healing in both treatment groups (56). Melki et al. showed that ofloxacin (3 mg/ml) administered every 30 min for 8 h caused sterilization of the corneas of animals with experimental *S. aureus* keratitis. Povidone-iodine (Betadine, 0.5%) showed less of a fall in CFU per milliliter, however, the differences in CFU per milliliter between povidone-iodine 0.5% therapy and untreated animals were significant (97). Topical enoxacin (3 mg/ml) hourly for 24 h was as effective in the treatment of *P. aeruginosa* keratitis as enoxacin (10 mg/ml) and gentamicin (3 mg/ml) (133).

Topical lomefloxacin (3 mg/ml) given initially every 5 min for 25 min, then twice or thrice daily for 7 days, was also effective in the treatment of *P. aeruginosa* keratitis (90). Outcome was determined clinically and by quantifying CFU per milliliter obtained using conjunctival swabs. By day 3 lomefloxacin showed both significant clinical improvement and sterility in 50% of animals. Whereas most control animals were culture positive on day 6 with continued signs of infection, all swabs from lomefloxacin-treated animals were negative. Kowalski compared the efficacy of lomefloxacin (3 mg/ml) and ciprofloxacin (3 mg/ml) with phosphate-buffered saline control in animals with bacterial keratitis caused by ciprofloxacin-susceptible and resistant strains of *S. aureus*, viridans streptococci, *S. pneumoniae*, *P. aeruginosa*, and *Serratia marcescens* (81). Drug was administered using multiple doses for 4 to 8 h. Either quinolone was significantly more effective than phosphate-buffered saline in decreasing CFU per milliliter. For gram-positive bacteria, the fall in CFU per milliliter was similar for both lomefloxacin and ciprofloxacin, whereas ciprofloxacin was more effective than lomefloxacin in reducing bacterial densities in animals with *P. aeruginosa* and *S. marcescens* keratitis.

OUTCOME STUDIES IN ANIMALS WITH ENDOPHTHALMITIS

Recent studies have characterized the efficacy of quinolones in the therapy of experimental endophthalmitis in animals. Routes of quinolone administration include lomefloxacin eye drops (61), trovafloxacin given systemically (86), and direct injection into the vitreous humor of ciprofloxacin, trovafloxacin, sparfloxacin, or levofloxacin (3, 33, 37, 74, 78) . The outcome of *S. epidermidis* (86, 103) endophthalmitis treated with trovafloxacin has been studied in rabbits. Intravitreal quinolones have been studied for endophthalmitis caused by *P. aeruginosa* (37, 78), streptococci (33), and *Bacillus cereus* (3).

Topical lomefloxcin (3 mg/ml) was compared with gentamicin (3 mg/ml), sulbenicillin (10 mg/ml), or saline in endophthalmitis following *P. aeruginosa* inoculation into the anterior chamber. Outcome was characterized using CFU per milliliter at 6 and 24 h; inflammation of the anterior chamber was monitored for 7 days using a slit lamp. Lomefloxacin appeared to be more effective than gentamicin and sulbenencillin in decreasing CFU per milliliter, with sterility at day 2 in 50% of the animals and decreased anterior chamber inflammation relative to the other treatment groups (61).

Recent studies characterized the outcome of *S. epidermidis* endophthalmitis treated orally (103) or intravenously (87) with trovafloxacin. Both studies characterized clinical inflammation and microbiological and histopathological outcome. Ng et al. (103) used oral trovafloxacin alone, and Liu et al. (87) compared i.v. trovafloxacin with ciprofloxacin. Ng et al. showed that trovafloxacin therapy decreased inflammation of anterior eye structures by day 4 and vitreous inflammation by day 2. The mean CFU per milliliter showed a ~ 1 $\log_{10}$ decrease in trovafloxacin-treated animals compared with controls on days 1 and 2 and a ~ 2 to 3 $\log_{10}$ decrease on days 3 and 4; on day 5, treated eyes showed no growth. Histopathological changes were less marked in treated animals. Liu et al. (86) compared the outcome of a second *S. epidermidis* strain in animals following the administration of intravenous ciprofloxacin or trovafloxacin; the doses used were chosen on the basis of pharmacodynamic data so that serum AUCs and AUC/MIC ratios were identical to those seen in humans. Gross and histopathological changes were less severe in trovafloxacin-treated rabbits. Microbiological outcome studies at day 4 showed that there were no decreases in bacterial densities (CFU/ml) in ciprofloxacin-treated or untreated animals. However, those treated with trovafloxacin had significantly lower bacterial densities in the vitreous humor (86).

Davey et al. (37) and Kim et al. (78) studied the microbiological response in rabbits with *P. aeruginosa* endophthalmitis who received a single intravitreal dose; there were no untreated controls. Outcome was compared in animals receiving ciprofloxacin, gentamicin, or imipenem. When therapy was begun 24 h after infection, ciprofloxacin resulted in a significant decrease in the CFU per milliliter. However, when therapy was begun at 48 h, there was no decrease in bacterial densities. Kim et al. showed that when therapy was started at 6 or 12 h, 300 μg of ciprofloxacin sterilized the vitreous body. However, organisms were present and histopathological abnormalities more marked when therapy was begun at 18 and 24 h. Animals receiving both intravitreal dexamethasone and ciprofloxacin had higher CFU per milliliter when therapy was started at 12 h as compared with animals receiving ciprofloxacin alone.

Cochereau-Massin et al. studied the outcome of streptococcal endophthalmitis following 800-μg intraocular injections of sparfloxacin or pefloxacin. Therapy was started 20 h after infection, and microbiological outcome was measured 24 h thereafter (33). In sparfloxacin-treated animals there was a significant fall in bacterial density when compared with controls or pefloxacin. Karakucuk studied the outcome of *S. epidermidis* endophthalmitis in rabbits receiving 100 μg of intraocular trovafloxacin; therapy was begun at 18 h and outcome determined microbiologically and by clinical scoring. Trovafloxacin was significantly more effective in reducing bacterial density 1 or 2 days after the initiation of therapy than untreated controls (74).

Alfaro and colleagues characterized the natural history of experimental posttraumatic *B. cereus* endophthalmitis and the prevention of disease following the intraocular administration of ciprofloxacin. When given 1 and 6 h after surgical trauma and infection, ciprofloxacin prevented endophthalmitis in rabbits and Yorkshire pigs (5). In a second study of *B. cereus* endophthalmitis, Alfaro compared the natural history of traumatic *B. cereus* endophthalmitis and the efficacy of intravitreal ciprofloxacin, vancomycin, and imipenem therapies in Yorkshire pigs when therapy was begun at 4 h (4). In this study ciprofloxacin proved to be inferior to either vancomycin or imipenem in preventing histopathological changes, which were first noted by 4 h in untreated controls.

OUTCOME STUDIES IN HUMANS

Leibowitz characterized the outcome in 148 patients with culture-positive keratitis treated with 0.3% ciprofloxacin in two concomitant multicenter studies. Outcome was characterized clinically and in some instances microbiologically. In this study >60% of isolates were gram-positive cocci, primarily staphylococci and streptococci. Ciprofloxacin was administered frequently in a decremental fashion with >40 drops on day 0, two drops hourly on day 1, and two drops every 4 h on days 2 through 14; the

frequency thereafter was chosen by the primary ophthalmologist. This study used historical controls or unenrolled patients seen at the time of the study receiving standard regimens consisting of a fortified solution of an aminoglycoside (gentamicin or tobramycin, 14 mg/ml) and cefazolin (14 mg/ml) (84). Approximately 90% of patients responded to ciprofloxacin or fortified drops. There were no serious side effects; corneal precipitates were seen in 17% of ciprofloxacin-treated patients.

Two investigators have used ciprofloxacin to treat bacterial conjunctivitis; one used eye drops (66) and the other used oral therapy (16). In the study by Insler et al. (66) only two patients with keratitis in whom methicillin-resistant *S. aureus* was isolated were evaluated; both responded to therapy with topical applications of 3 mg/ml ciprofloxacin.

In the second study Brennan and Muder treated seven patients with conjunctivitis from whom methicillin-resistant *S. aureus* was isolated with oral ciprofloxacin or topical vancomycin (16). Six of the ciprofloxacin-treated patients also received a second "fortified" antibiotic (i.e., other than a quinolone) eye drops, however, and 7 of 8 patients receiving 50 mg/ml vancomycin drops received other antibiotic eye drops. As a result the role of oral ciprofloxacin as sole therapy is difficult to evaluate. Good outcome was noted in 7 of 8 patients receiving oral ciprofloxacin and all patients receiving topical vancomycin.

Tsai et al. characterized the efficacy of topical ciprofloxacin in 30 Formosan patients whose bacterial keratitis failed to improve with conventional therapy (137). More than 90% had positive cultures. *P. aeruginosa* was the most common pathogen and was isolated in approximately half of the patients. Mycobacteria were next in frequency. Of eleven patients treated with ciprofloxacin, 73% responded with no serious adverse effects. Crystalline deposits were seen in two patients.

In a randomized, masked study Khokhar et al. compared topical ofloxacin (0.3%) with tobramycin 1.5% plus cefazolin 5% in patients with keratitis; the most common isolates were staphylococci (77). Both groups responded equally with comparable time to symptomatic relief and epithelial healing. Posttreatment visual acuity was also comparable. All patients received cycloplegics, vitamins, and antiglaucoma therapy. There were no differences in resolution of ulcers, the mean time to symptomatic relief, or the time for epithelial healing in treated patients.

Oral lomefloxacin in conjunction with topical antimicrobials was used in patients with keratitis and conjunctivitis (89). Forty patients with keratitis, including 10 with ulcers, were treated with twice-daily lomefloxacin in conjunction with topical 0.3%

lomefloxacin, ofloxacin, or tobramycin and anti-inflammatory drugs. Cultures in 29 patients were positive for *S. pneumoniae* in 11, *S. aureus* in 9, and both in 7 patients. *P. aeruginosa* was seen in only two patients. All patients responded with clinical improvement, reepithelialization (in patients with corneal ulcers), and negative cultures by 28 days (many sooner). Twenty-seven patients with conjunctivitis (20 with recalcitrant bacterial conjunctivitis caused primarily by *S. pneumoniae*, 11 with *S. aureus*, and 7 with gonococci) responded as well to oral lomefloxacin in conjunction with topical antimicrobials. In 68 patients with chlamydial conjunctivitis diagnosed clinically, oral lomefloxacin was compared with oral ciprofloxacin or tetracycline. All patients received antibiotic eye ointment as well. Follicles resolved more rapidly in patients receiving either quinolone than in those receiving tetracycline ($P < 0.05$).

Topical or oral norfloxacin (0.3%) has also been used in the therapy of bacterial conjunctivitis (67) and gonococcal keratoconjunctivitis (76). For nongonococcal bacterial conjunctivitis (67) the comparator was tobramycin (0.3%). Treatment consisted of hourly drops the first day and four times daily while awake for at least 6 days; only 50% of patients had pathogens identified. The most common bacterial pathogen was *H. influenzae;* gram-positive isolates included streptococci (*S. pneumoniae*, α-hemolytic streptococci) and staphylococci (*S. aureus* and staphylococcal species). The clinical and bacteriological outcomes were similar in the two groups. No serious side effects of treatment were noted. In the second study, gonococcal keratoconjunctivitis was treated systemically with norfloxacin 1.2 mg daily for 3 days or once (76). In this study 15 men with gonococcal keratoconjunctivitis were treated with oral norfloxacin; all patients responded clinically and microbiologically.

Ooishi and colleagues also reported favorable outcome of infections treated with oral ciprofloxacin (108). Six patients had keratitis or corneal ulcers, and all responded favorably to 200 mg 3 three times daily; two patients with conjunctivitis also responded favorably.

A single study by Kumar and colleagues characterized the efficacy of intraocular quinolones in 20 eyes with suspected endophthalmitis (82). All patients were initially given a single intravitreal injection of pefloxacin (200 μg). Of these 35% had positive cultures. All patients received fortified antibiotics topically (tobramycin and cefazolin) and the majority (60%) received a second intravitreal dose of pefloxacin because of worsening signs of infection after 24 h. On the basis of clinical symptoms, 70%

responded to intraocular pefloxacin alone, and 30% also required vitrectomies. Ninety-five percent of patients had visual acuity of 20/200 after therapy.

OCULAR TOXICITY

Although ocular toxicity involving the cornea, lens, and retina has been reported following the systemic, topical, and direct intraocular administration of quinolones in experimental animals and humans, untoward effects involving the eye are rare in humans treated with conventional doses of topical or systemic quinolones. Following systemic administration of quinolones cataracts have developed in rats and cats treated with pefloxacin and in dogs treated for prolonged periods with rosoxacin (8, 30, 31, 127). However, cataracts have not been seen in other animals given ciprofloxacin or ofloxacin (142) and have not been reported in humans receiving fluoroquinolones (7, 127). Alterations in retinal electrophysiology and histology have been seen in cats given nalidixic acid but were not seen when the animals were given systemic norfloxacin (36) or ciprofloxacin (127).

Flumequine has caused reversible central scotomas due to bulla formation in the maculas of three patients with renal failure (65), but retinal toxicity has not been reported following systemic administration with other fluoroquinolones in humans (95), even when the aqueous and vitreous humors achieved effective antimicrobial levels (35).

When systemic sparfloxacin, enoxacin, and sitafloxacin were given followed by UV-A irradiation, retinal toxicity was induced in mice (128, 129). Of note, similar changes did not occur with levofloxacin.

Using an in vitro model of rabbit corneal epithelial cells stained with ethidium bromide, Matsumoto demonstrated less cell membrane damage by commercially available ofloxacin (Ocuflox) than by ciprofloxacin (Ciloxan) (93). Topical administration of ciprofloxacin (46) and norfloxacin (80) in humans has been associated with corneal deposits associated with corneal epitheliopathy.

In the rabbit, dose-dependent retinal toxicity has been documented following direct injection into the vitreous humor for ciprofloxacin (79, 92, 124, 143), ofloxacin (144), norfloxacin (135), pefloxacin (34), trovafloxacin (57), and levofloxacin (105). Liposomal preparations providing a more sustained release of drug have been formulated at safe yet effective concentrations (143, 144). Injection of ciprofloxacin into the aqueous humor produced dose-dependent corneal toxicity (132). Toxicity was produced when local drug concentrations were substantially higher than those achievable with systemic administration. A retrospective study of corneal ulcers suggested that although the duration of intensive therapy and hospitalization was less in patients treated with topical fluoroquinolones, there appeared to be more serious complications than in the conventionally treated patients (54).

CONCLUSIONS

Pharmacokinetic studies in animals and humans following topical and/or systemic administration of quinolone antimicrobials show that the ocular penetration of quinolones is generally greater than that of other antimicrobials. Following systemic or intraocular injection in rabbits, penetration and efflux show an excellent correlation with lipophilicity. Lipophilic quinolones such as ofloxacin, levofloxacin, and sparfloxacin show good penetration into the vitreous humor following systemic drug administration even in the absence of inflammation. Inflammation increases penetration into the cornea and aqueous humor following topical adminstration and into the vitreous humor following systemic administration. In patients with conjunctivitis or keratitis, quinolone eye drops result in concentrations in tear fluid and in corneal and aqueous humor that generally exceed the MICs for ocular pathogens. Studies in humans show that combined topical and oral quinolones result in higher concentrations in both the aqueous and vitreous humor than results with eye drops alone. These studies also suggest that concentrations following oral therapy alone would be at least equal to or greater than those in the aqueous and vitreous humors, respectively, than the concentrations following topical therapy alone.

Outcome studies in animals with bacterial keratitis due to staphylococci show similar outcomes when compared with fortified antibiotic eye drops. Keratitis in rabbits due to aminoglycoside-susceptible or -resistant *P. aeruginosa* also generally responds to quinolone eye drops. Several studies in rabbits with staphylococcal or streptococcal endophthalitis showed a favorable response following treatment with systemic or IO quinolones. In contrast, animals with *P. aeruginosa* endophthalmits show a poor response to systemic therapy, particularly when therapy is delayed. Quinolones are also less effective than other antibiotics in preventing infection with *B. cereus* in traumatized animals.

Studies in humans with conjunctivitis or keratitis show equivalence but not superiority to fortified antibiotic eye drops. The exception is chlamydial conjunctivitis, for which quinolones appear to be superior to tetracycline. The ability to achieve higher concentrations in the aqueous and vitreous humors when both topical and systemic quinolones are used and the apparent equivalency of aqueous humor concentrations with topical and oral quinolone administration suggest that combination therapy should be considered in patients with bacterial keratitis. Combined oral and topical therapy would help ensure that therapeutic concentration will be maintained when compliance due to frequent drug administration is a problem or the maintenance of therapeutic concentrations during sleep is desirable.

Although quinolones, particularly ciprofloxacin, have been used as adjunctive therapy following IO vancomycin and amikacin administration in humans with bacterial endophthalmits, the potential benefit of combined IO and systemic therapy has not been established. Systemic therapy with antibiotics (vancomycin and ceftazidime) did not improve outcome relative to IO antibiotics in the National Eye Institute's endopthalmitis study. However, unlike lipophilic quinolones, neither antibiotic shows good penetration into the vitreous humor in the absence of inflammation. Pharmacokinetic and pharmacodynamic properties of quinolones include their ability to penetrate the vitreous humor following systemic drug administration and rapid vitreal elimination following IO but not systemic therapy. Pharmacokinetic, toxicity, and outcome studies in animals suggest that if quinolones are used as adjuvant therapy for endophthalmitis, systemic administration may be preferable to IO administration, and it would seem prudent to use quinolones that show both good ocular penetration and antistaphylococcal activity.

REFERENCES

1. Akkan, A. G., I. Mutlu, S. Ozyazgan, A. Gok, U. Yigit, Z. Ozuner, V. Senses, and H. Pekel. 1997. Penetration of topically applied ciprofloxacin, norfloxacin and ofloxacin into the aqueous humor of the uninflamed human eye. *J. Chemother.* 9:257–262.
2. Alexandrakis, G., R. Haimovici, D. Miller, and E. C. Alfonso. 2000. Corneal biopsy in the management of progressive microbial keratitis. *Am. J. Ophthalmol.* 129:571–576.
3. Alfaro, D. V., J. Davis, S. Kim, F. Bia, J. F. Bogard, J. W. Briggs, and P. E. Liggett. 1996. Experimental Bacillus cereus post-traumatic endophthalmitis and treatment with ciprofloxacin. *Br. J. Ophthalmol.* 80:755–758.
4. Alfaro, D. V., III, S. J. Hudson, J. J. Offele, A. A. Bevin, M. Mines, R. M. Laughlin, and R. J. Schoderbek. 1996. Experimental posttraumatic Bacillus cereus endophthalmitis in a swine model. Efficacy of intravitreal ciprofloxacin, vancomycin, and imipenem. *Retina* 16:317–323.
5. Alfaro, D. V., S. J. Hudson, M. M. Rafanan, S. T. Moss, and S. D. Levy. 1996. The effect of trauma on the ocular penetration of intravenous ciprofloxacin. *Am. J. Ophthalmol.* 122:678–683.

6. Assil, K. K., S. R. Zarnegar, B. D. Fouraker, and D. J. Schanzlin. 1992. Efficacy of tobramycin-soaked collagen shields vs tobramycin eyedrop loading dose for sustained treatment of experimental Pseudomonas-aeruginosa-induced keratitis in rabbits. *Am. J. Ophthalmol.* **113:**418–423.

7. Ball, P. 1986. Ciprofloxacin: an overview of adverse experiences. *J. Antimicrob. Chemother.* **18** (Suppl. D):187–193.

8. Ball, P. 1989. Adverse reactions and interactions of fluoroquinolones. *Clin. Investig. Med.* **12:**28–34.

9. Barza, M., J. Baum, W. Taseman, and E. A. Jaeger. 2000. Ocular pharmacology of antibiotics. *In* W. Tasman and E. A. Jaeger (ed.), *Duane's Clinical Ophthalmology on CD ROM.* Lippincott Williams & Wilkins, Philadelphia, Pa.

10. Barza, M. 1993. Treatment of eye infections, p. 423–434. *In* D. C. Hooper and J. S. Wolfson (ed.), *Quinolone Antimicrobial Agents,* 2nd ed. American Society for Microbiology, Washington, D.C.

11. Barza, M., A. Kane, and J. Baum. 1982. The effects of infection and probenecid on the transport of carbenicillin from the rabbit vitreous humor. *Investig. Ophthalmol. Vis. Sci.* **22:**720–726.

12. Behrens-Baumann, W. 1996. Absorption of topically administered ciprofloxacin, ofloxacin and gentamicin in the inflamed rabbit eye. *Ophthalmologica* **210:**119–122.

13. Behrens-Baumann, W., and J. Martell. 1987. Ciprofloxacin concentrations in human aqueous humor following intravenous administration. *Chemotherapy* **33:**328–330.

14. Behrens-Baumann, W., and J. Martell. 1988. Ciprofloxacin concentration in the rabbit aqueous humor and vitreous following intravenous and subconjunctival administration. *Infection* **16:**54–57.

15. Bito, L., and C. DeRousseau. 1980. Transport functions of the blood-retinal barrier system and the micro-environment of the retina, p. 33–163. *In* J. G. Cunha-Vaz (ed.), *NATO Advanced Study Institute Series.* Plenum Press, New York, N. Y.

16. Brennen, C., and R. R. Muder. 1990. Conjunctivitis associated with methicillin-resistant Staphylococcus aureus in a long-term-care facility. *Am. J. Med.* **88:**14N–17N.

17. Bron, A., D. Talon, T. Cellier, J. M. Estavoyer, B. Delbose, and J. Royer. 1989. [Intra aqueous humor penetration of ciprofloxacin in humans]. *Pathol. Biol.* **37:**730–733.

18. Bron, A., D. Talon, B. Delbose, J. M. Estavoyer, G. Kaya, and J. Royer. 1987. [Intracameral penetration of ofloxacin in man]. *J. Fr. Ophtalmol.* **10:**443–446.

19. Bron, A., D. Talon, B. Delbose, J. M. Estavoyer, F. Prost, and M. Montard. 1986. [Intracameral penetration of pefloxacine in man]. *J. Fr. Ophtalmol.* **9:**317–321.

20. Bron, A., D. Talon, J. M. Estavoyer, T. Cellier, B. Delbose, and M. Montard. 1989. Ocular distribution of the new quinolones. *Rev. Infect. Dis.* **11** (Suppl. 5):S1206–S1207.

21. Bron, A. M., A. P. Pechinot, C. P. Garcher, G. A. Guyonnet, A. M. Kazmierczak, D. A. Schott, and H. Lecoeur. 1994. The ocular penetration of oral sparfloxacin in humans. *Am. J. Ophthalmol.* **117:**322–327.

22. Burns-Bellhorn, M. S., R. W. Bellhorn, and J. V. Benjamin. 1978. Anterior segment permeability to fluorescein-labeled dextrans in the rat. *Investig. Ophthalmol. Vis. Sci.* **17:**857–862.

23. Cantor, L. B., E. Donnenfeld, L. J. Katz, W. L. Gee, C. D. Finley, V. K. Lakhani, J. Hoop, and K. Flarty. 2001. Penetration of ofloxacin and ciprofloxacin into the aqueous humor of eyes with functioning filtering blebs: a randomized trial. *Arch. Ophthalmol.* **119:**1254–1257.

24. Cekic, O., C. Batman, Y. Totan, U. Yasar, N. E. Basci, A. Bozkurt, and S. O. Kayaalp. 1999. Penetration of ofloxacin and ciprofloxacin in aqueous humor after topical administration. *Ophthal. Surg. Lasers* **30:**465–468.

25. Cekic, O., C. Batman, Y. Totan, U. Yasar, N. E. Basci, A. Bozkurt, S. O. Kayaalp, and O. Zilelioglu. 1999. Aqueous humour levels of topically applied ciprofloxacin and ofloxacin in the same subjects. *Eye* **13** (Pt. 5):656–659.

26. Cekic, O., C. Batman, U. Yasar, N. E. Basci, A. Bozkurt, and S. O. Kayaalp. 1998. Penetration of ofloxacin in human aqueous and vitreous humors following oral and topical administration. *Retina* **18:**521–525.

27. Cekic, O., C. Batman, U. Yasar, N. E. Basci, A. Bozkurt, and S. O. Kayaalp. 1999. Human aqueous and vitreous humour levels of ciprofloxacin following oral and topical administration. *Eye* **13** (Pt. 4):555–558.

28. Cekic, O., C. Batman, U. Yasar, N. E. Basci, O. Zilelioglu, and A. Bozkurt. 2000. Subretinal fluid levels of topical, oral, and combined administered ciprofloxacin in humans. *Br. J. Ophthalmol.* **84:**1061–1063.

29. Celebi, S., S. Ay, U. Aykan, V. Bulut, G. Alagoz, and U. O. Celiker. 1998. Penetration of oral and topical ciprofloxacin into human aqueous humor. *Acta Ophthalmol. Scand.* **76:**683–685.

30. Christ, W., and T. Lehnert. 1990. Toxicity of the quinolones, p. 165–187. *In* C. Siporin, C. L. Heifetz, and J. M. Domagala (ed.), *The New Generation of Quinolones.* Marcel Dekker, Inc., New York, N. Y.

31. Christ, W., T. Lehnert, and B. Ulbrich. 1988. Specific toxicologic aspects of the quinolones. *Rev. Infect. Dis.* **10** (Suppl. 1):S141–S146.

32. Cochereau-Massin, I., J. Bauchet, F. Faurisson, J. M. Vallois, P. Lacombe, and J. J. Pocidalo. 1991. Ocular kinetics of pefloxacin after intramuscular administration in albino and pigmented rabbits. *Antimicrob. Agents Chemother.* **35:**1112–1115.

33. Cochereau-Massin, I., J. Bauchet, S. Marrakchi-Benjaafar, A. Saleh-Mghir, F. Faurisson, J. M. Vallois, E. Vallee, and J. J. Pocidalo. 1993. Efficacy and ocular penetration of sparfloxacin in experimental streptococcal endophthalmitis. *Antimicrob. Agents Chemother.* **37:**633–636.

34. Cochereau-Massin, I., S. Marrakchi-Benjaafar, J. Bauchet, J. M. Vallois, F. Faurisson, F. D'Hermies, and J. J. Pocidalo. 1994. Kinetics and tolerability of intravitreal pefloxacin in rabbits. *J. Antimicrob. Chemother.* **33:**231–242.

35. Cohen, R. G., M. Raizman, C. Callina, and M. Lahav. 1997. Retinal safety of oral and topical ofloxacin in rabbits. *J. Ocul. Pharmacol. Ther.* **13:**369–379.

36. Corrado, M. L., W. E. Struble, C. Peter, V. Hoagland, and J. Sabbaj. 1987. Norfloxacin: review of safety studies. *Am. J. Med.* **82:**22–26.

37. Davey, P. G., M. Barza, and M. Stuart. 1987. Dose response of experimental Pseudomonas endophthalmitis to ciprofloxacin, gentamicin, and imipenem: evidence for resistance to "late" treatment of infections. *J. Infect. Dis.* **155:**518–523.

38. Davson, H., and M. B. Segal. 1969. Effect of cerebrospinal fluid on volume of distribution of extracellular markers. *Brain* **92:**131–136.

39. Denis, F., M. Mounier, and J. P. Adenis. 1987. [Intraocular penetration of pefloxacin in man and rabbit. The aqueous humor and vitreous body]. *Pathol. Biol.* **35:**772–776.

40. Donnenfeld, E. D., H. D. Perry, R. W. Snyder, R. Moadel, M. Elsky, and H. Jones. 1997. Intracorneal, aqueous humor, and vitreous humor penetration of topical and oral ofloxacin. *Arch. Ophthalmol.* **115:**173–176.

41. Drusano, G. L. 2000. Fluoroquinolone pharmacodynamics: prospective determination of relationships between exposure and outcome. *J. Chemother.* **12** (Suppl. 4):21–26.

42. Drusano, G. L., and W. A. Craig. 1997. Relevance of pharmacokinetics and pharmacodynamics in the selection of

antibiotics for respiratory tract infections. *J. Chemother.* **9**:38–44.

43. **Drusano, G. L., D. E. Johnson, M. Rosen, and H. C. Standiford.** 1993. Pharmacodynamics of a fluoroquinolone antimicrobial agent in a neutropenic rat model of Pseudomonas sepsis. *Antimicrob. Agents Chemother.* **37**:483–490.

44. **Drusano, G. L., W. Liu, R. Perkins, A. Madu, C. Madu, M. Mayers, and M. H. Miller.** 1995. Determination of robust ocular pharmacokinetic parameters in serum and vitreous humor of albino rabbits following systemic administration of ciprofloxacin from sparse data sets by using IT2S, a population pharmacokinetic modeling program. *Antimicrob. Agents Chemother.* **39**:1683–1687.

45. **Durmaz, B., S. Marol, R. Durmaz, O. Oram, I. F. Hepsen, and S. Gunal.** 1997. Aqueous humor penetration of topically applied ciprofloxacin, ofloxacin and tobramycin. *Arzneim.-forsch.* **47**:413–415.

46. **Eiferman, R. A., J. P. Snyder, and R. E. Nordquist.** 2001. Ciprofloxacin microprecipitates and macroprecipitates in the human corneal epithelium. *J. Cataract Refract. Surg.* **27**:1701–1702.

47. **el Baba, F. Z., M. D. Trousdale, W. J. Gauderman, D. G. Wagner, and P. E. Liggett.** 1992. Intravitreal penetration of oral ciprofloxacin in humans. Ophthalmology **99**:483–486.

48. **Elmquist, W. F., and R. J. Sawchuk.** 1997. Application of microdialysis in pharmacokinetic studies. *Pharm. Res. (N. Y.)* **14**:267–288.

49. **Endophthalmitis Vitrectomy Study Group.** 1995. Results of the Endophthalmitis Vitrectomy Study. A randomized trial of immediate vitrectomy and of intravenous antibiotics for the treatment of postoperative bacterial endophthalmitis. *Arch. Ophthalmol.* **113**:1479–1496.

50. **Engel, L. S., M. C. Callegan, J. M. Hill, A. T. Folkens, Y. Shimomura, and R. J. O'Callaghan.** 1996. The effectiveness of two ciprofloxacin formulations for experimental Pseudomonas and Staphylococcus keratitis. *Jpn. J. Ophthalmol.* **40**:212–219.

51. **Esposito, S., H. Thadepalli, H. A. Benler, and S. K. Chuah.** 1991. Enoxacin therapy for experimental pseudomonas keratitis. *J. Chemother.* **3**:147–151.

52. **Fern, A. I., G. Sweeney, M. Doig, and G. Lindsay.** 1986. Penetration of ciprofloxacin into aqueous humor. *Trans. Ophthalmol. Soc. U. K.* **105**(Pt. 6):650–652.

53. **Fiscella, R. G., T. K. Nguyen, M. J. Cwik, B. A. Phillpotts, S. M. Friedlander, D. C. Alter, M. J. Shapiro, N. P. Blair, and J. P. Gieser.** 1999. Aqueous and vitreous penetration of levofloxacin after oral administration. *Ophthalmology* **106**:2286–2290.

54. **Gangopadhyay, N., M. Daniell, L. Weih, and H. R. Taylor.** 2000. Fluoroquinolone and fortified antibiotics for treating bacterial corneal ulcers. *Br. J. Ophthalmol.* **84**:378–384.

55. **Ghelardi, E., A. Tavanti, F. Celandroni, A. Lupetti, C. Blandizzi, E. Boldrini, M. Campa, and S. Senesi.** 2000. Effect of a novel mucoadhesive polysaccharide obtained from tamarind seeds on the intraocular penetration of gentamicin and ofloxacin in rabbits. *J. Antimicrob. Chemother.* **46**:831–834.

56. **Gritz, D. C., P. J. McDonnell, T. Y. Lee, D. Tang-Liu, B. B. Hubbard, and A. Gwon.** 1992. Topical ofloxacin in the treatment of Pseudomonas keratitis in a rabbit model. *Cornea* **11**:143–147.

57. **Gurler, B., Y. Ozkul, M. Bitiren, A. Satici, H. Oguz, and S. Karadede.** 2001. Experimental intravitreal application of trovafloxacin in rabbits. *Ophthalmic Res.* **33**:228–236.

58. **Habgood, M. D., D. J. Begley, and N. J. Abbott.** 2000. Determinants of passive drug entry into the central nervous system. *Cell. Mol. Neurobiol.* **20**:231–253.

59. **Hainsworth, D. P., J. D. Conklin, J. R. Bierly, D. Ax, and P. Ashton.** 1996. Intravitreal delivery of ciprofloxacin. *J. Ocul. Pharmacol. Ther.* **12**:183–191.

60. **Hanioglu-Kargi, S., N. Basci, H. Soysal, A. Bozkurt, E. Gursel, and O. Kayaalp.** 1998. The penetration of ofloxacin into human aqueous humor given by various routes. *Eur. J. Ophthalmol.* **8**:33–36.

61. **Hatano, H., K. Inoue, S. Shia, and W. Liping.** 1993. Application of topical lomefloxacin against experimental Pseudomonas endophthalmitis in rabbits. *Acta Ophthalmol.* **71**:666–670.

62. **Hobden, J. A., J. J. Reidy, R. J. O'Callaghan, M. S. Insler, and J. M. Hill.** 1990. Quinolones in collagen shields to treat aminoglycoside-resistant pseudomonal keratitis. *Investig. Ophthalmol. Vis. Sci.* **31**:2241–2243.

63. **Hughes, P. M., R. Krishnamoorthy, and A. K. Mitra.** 1996. Vitreous disposition of two acycloguanosine antivirals in the albino and pigmented rabbit models: a novel ocular microdialysis technique. *J. Ocul. Pharmacol. Ther.* **12**:209–224.

64. **Hulem, C. D., S. E. Old, L. D. Zeleznick, and I. H. Leopold.** 1982. Intraocular penetration of rosoxacin in rabbits. *Arch. Ophthalmol.* **100**:646–649.

65. **Hurault de Ligny, B., D. Sirbat, M. Kessler, P. Trechot, and J. Chanliau.** 1984. [Ocular side effects of flumequine. 3 cases of macular involvement]. *Therapie* **39**:595–600.

66. **Insler, M. S., L. A. Fish, J. Silbernagel, J. A. Hobden, R. J. O'Callaghan, and J. M. Hill.** 1991. Successful treatment of methicillin-resistant Staphylococcus aureus keratitis with topical ciprofloxacin. *Ophthalmology* **98**:1690–1692.

67. **Jacobson, J. A., N. B. Call, E. M. Kasworm, M. S. Dirks, and R. B. Turner.** 1988. Safety and efficacy of topical norfloxacin versus tobramycin in the treatment of external ocular infections. *Antimicrob. Agents Chemother.* **32**:1820–1824.

68. **Jaehde, U., F. Sorgel, A. Reiter, G. Sigl, K. G. Naber, and W. Schunack.** 1995. Effect of probenecid on the distribution and elimination of ciprofloxacin in humans. *Clin. Pharmacol. Ther.* **58**:532–541.

69. **Janert, B., B. Schull, and H. P. Geisen.** 1989. Concentrations of ciprofloxacin in aqueous humor following intravenous and oral administration. *Rev. Infect. Dis.* **11**(Suppl. 5) S1077.

70. **Joos, B., F. Gassman, and R. Luthy.** 1986. Penetration of ciprofloxacin into the human eye. *In Program and Abstracts of the 26th Interscience Conference on Antimicrobial Agents and Chemotherapy.* American Society for Microbiology, Washington, D.C.

71. **Jumbe, N., W. Liu, G. Drusano, A. Louie, and M. H. Miller.** 1999. Comparison of Quinolone active efflux afer, systemic, intravitreous and intracerebrovascula administration. *In Program and Abstracts of the 39th Interscience Conference on Amtimicrobial Agents and Chemotherapy.* American Society for Microbiology, Washington, D.C.

72. **Jumbe, N., W. Liu, A. Louie, G. Drusano, and M. H. Miller.** 1999. Parametric comparison of microdialysis and direct vitreous sampling techniques at non-steady-state conditions. *In Program and Abstracts of the 39th Interscience Conference of Antimicrobial Agents and Chemotherapy.* American Society for Microbiology, Washington, D. C.

73. **Kalayci, D., N. Basci, S. Kortunay, H. Hasiripa, and A. Bozkurt.** 1999. Penetration of Topical ciprofloxacin by presoaked medicated soft contact lenses. *CLAO J.* **25**:192–184.

74. **Karakucuk, S., E. Mirza, B. Sumerkan, and T. Okten.** 2000. Intravitreal trovafloxacin against experimental Staphylococcus epidermidis endophthalmitis. *Ophthalmic Res.* **32**:126–131.

75. Keren, G., A. Alhalel, E. Bartov, R. Kitzes-Cohen, E. Rubinstein, S. Segev, and G. Treister. 1991. The intravitreal penetration of orally administered ciprofloxacin in humans. *Investig. Ophthalmol. Vis. Sci.* 32:2388–2392.

76. Kestelyn, P., J. Bogaerts, A. M. Stevens, P. Piot, and A. Meheus. 1989. Treatment of adult gonococcal keratoconjunctivitis with oral norfloxacin. *Am. J. Ophthalmol.* 108:516–523.

77. Khokhar, S., N. Sindhu, and B. R. Mirdha. 2000. Comparison of topical 0.3% ofloxacin to fortified tobramycin-cefazolin in the therapy of bacterial keratitis. *Infection* 28:149–152.

78. Kim, I. T., K. H. Chung, and B. S. Koo. 1996. Efficacy of ciprofloxacin and dexamethasone in experimental pseudomonas endophthalmitis. *Korean J. Ophthalmol.* 10:8–17.

79. Kim, S. H., J. H. Kim, K. S. Cho, and J. S. Kwak. 1995. Safety of intravitreally injected ciprofloxacin in phakic rabbit eyes. *Korean J. Ophthalmol.* 9:12–18.

80. Konishi, M., M. Yamada, and Y. Mashima. 1998. Corneal ulcer associated with deposits of norfloxacin. *Am. J. Ophthalmol.* 125:258–260.

81. Kowalski, R. P., E. G. Romanowski, K. A. Yates, and Y. J. Gordon. 2001. Lomefloxacin is an effective treatment of experimental bacterial keratitis. *Cornea* 20:306–308.

82. Kumar, A., M. S. Sridhar, T. Dada, H. K. Tewari, and S. K. Gupta. 2000. Intravitreal pefloxacin therapy in postoperative endophthalmitis. *Clin. Exp. Ophthalmol.* 28:38–40.

83. Lafaix, C., A. Salvanet, A. Fisch, F. Forestier, G. Montay, and A. Meulemans. 1987. [Diffusion of fluoroquinolones in the aqueous humor and crystalline lens]. *Pathol. Biol.* 35:768–771.

84. Leibowitz, H. M. 1991. Clinical evaluation of ciprofloxacin 0.3% ophthalmic solution for treatment of bacterial keratitis. *Am. J. Ophthalmol.* 112:34S–47S.

85. Liu, W., N. Jumbe, P. Kaw, G. Drusano, A. Louie, and M. H. Miller. 1999. Comparison of quinolone pharmacokinetics in the vitreous humor and CSF following IV drug administration in albino rabbits. *Investig. Ophthalmol. Vis. Sci.* 40:S88.

86. Liu, W., P. Kaw, M. Vergara, B. M. Lomaestro, Q. F. Liu, M. Mayers, M. Farber, G. Drusano, A. Louie, and M. H. Miller. 1998. Outcome in rabbits with *S. epidermidis* endophthalmitis treated with a fluoroquinolne and/or rifampin. *Investig. Ophthalmol. Vis. Sci.* 39:S357.

87. Liu, W., Q. F. Liu, R. Perkins, G. Drusano, A. Louie, A. Madu, U. Mian, M. Mayers, and M. H. Miller. 1998. Pharmacokinetics of sparfloxacin in the serum and vitreous humor of rabbits: physicochemical properties that regulate penetration of quinolone antimicrobials. *Antimicrob. Agents Chemother.* 42:1417–1423.

88. Madu, A. A., M. Mayers, R. Perkins, W. Liu, G. L. Drusano, R. Aswani, C. N. Madu, and M. H. Miller. 1996. Aqueous and vitreous penetration of ciprofloxacin following different modes of systemic administration. *Exp. Eye Res.* 63:129–136.

89. Maichuk, I., E. S. Vakhova, and L. A. Kononenko. 1998. [Lomefloxacin in treatment of infectious eye diseases]. *Antibiot. Khimioter.* 43:32–35.

90. Malet, F., J. Colin, A. Jauch, and M. L. Abalain. 1995. Bacterial keratitis therapy in guinea pigs with lomefloxacin by initially high-followed by low-dosage regimen. *Ophthalmic Res.* 27:322–329.

91. Mandell, B. A., T. A. Meredith, E. Aguilar, A. el Massry, A. Sawant, and S. Gardner. 1993. Effects of inflammation and surgery on amikacin levels in the vitreous cavity. *Am. J. Ophthalmol.* 115:770–774.

92. Marchese, A. L., V. S. Slana, E. W. Holmes, and W. M. Jay. 1993. Toxicity and pharmacokinetics of ciprofloxacin. *J. Ocul. Pharmacol.* 9:69–76.

93. Matsumoto, S., and M. E. Stern. 2000. Effect of anti-infective ophthalmic solutions on corneal cells in vitro. *Adv. Ther.* 17:148–151.

94. Maurice, D. M. and S. Mishma. 1984. Ocular pharmacokinetics, p. 19–116. *In* M. Sears (ed.), *Pharmacology of the Eye. Handbook of Experimental Pharmacology*. Springer-Verlag, Berlin, Germany.

95. Mayer, D. G. 1987. Overview of toxicological studies. *Drugs* 34(Suppl. 1):150–153.

96. Mayers, M., D. Rush, A. Madu, M. Motyl, and M. H. Miller. 1991. Pharmacokinetics of amikacin and chloramphenicol in the aqueous humor of rabbits. *Antimicrob. Agents Chemother.* 35:1791–1798.

97. Melki, S. A., A. Safar, F. Yaghouti, P. Scharper, M. Scharper, B. Zeligs, A. L. MacDowell, M. A. Goldberg, and J. Lustbader. 2000. Effect of topical povidone-iodine versus topical ofloxacin on experimental Staphylococcus keratitis. *Graefe's Arch. Clin. Exp. Ophthalmol.* 238:459–462.

98. Miller, M. H., A. Madu, G. Samathanam, D. Rush, C. N. Madu, K. Mathisson, and M. Mayers. 1992. Fleroxacin pharmacokinetics in aqueous and vitreous humors determined by using complete concentration-time data from individual rabbits. *Antimicrob. Agents Chemother.* 36:32–38.

99. Mindel, J. S., W. Tasman, and E. A. Jaeger. 2000. Pharmacokinetics. *In* W. Tasman and E. A. Jaeger (ed.), *Duane's Clinical Ophthalmology on CD Rom.* Lippincott Williams & Wilkins, Philadelphia, Pa.

100. Moog, E., and H. Knothe. 1969. Passage of various tetracyclines into human aqueous humor in dependence of their protien binding in the blood stream. *Ber. Zusammenkunf Dtsch. Ophthalmol. Ges.* 69:536–539.

101. Moreau, J. M., L. C. Green, L. S. Engel, J. M. Hill, and R. J. O'Callaghan. 1998. Effectiveness of ciprofloxacin-polystyrene sulfonate (PSS), ciprofloxacin and ofloxacin in a Staphylococcus keratitis model. *Curr. Eye Res.* 17:808–812.

102. Nau, R., F. Sorgel, and H. W. Prange. 1994. Lipophilicity at Ph 7.4 and molecular-size govern the entry of the free serum fraction of drugs into the cerebrospinal-fluid in humans with uninflamed meninges. *J. Neurol. Sci.* 122:61–65.

103. Ng, E. W., N. Samiy, K. L. Ruoff, F. V. Cousins, D. C. Hooper, S. von Gunten, D. J. D'Amico, and A. S. Baker. 1998. Treatment of experimental Staphylococcus epidermidis endophthalmitis with oral trovafloxacin. *Am. J. Ophthalmol.* 126:278–287.

104. O'Brien, T. P., M. R. Sawusch, J. D. Dick, and J. D. Gottsch. 1988. Topical ciprofloxacin treatment of Pseudomonas keratitis in rabbits. *Arch. Ophthalmol.* 106:1444–1446.

105. Ohkubo, S., K. Mochizuki, M. Torisaki, Y. Yamashita, M. Komatsu, T. Tanahashi, M. Ogata, and T. Kajimura. 1996. [Effects of intravitreal levofloxacin on the rabbit retina]. *Nippon Ganka Gakkai Zasshi* 100:592–598.

106. Okhravi, N., H. M. Towler, P. Hykin, M. Matheson, and S. Lightman. 1997. Assessment of a standard treatment protocol on visual outcome following presumed bacterial endophthalmitis. *Br. J. Ophthalmol.* 81:719–725.

107. Oldendorf, W. H. 1973. Carrier-mediated blood-brain barrier transport of short-chain monocarboxylic organic acids. *Am. J. Physiol* 224:1450–1453.

108. Ooishi, M., and Miyao, M. 1990. Ocular pharmacokinetic studies on AT-4140, abstr. 1258. *In Program and Abstracts of the 30th Interscience Conference on Antimicrobial Agents and Chemotherapy.* American Society for Microbiology, Washington, D.C.

109. Ooishi, M., M. Miyao, T. Abe, T. Sasagawa, M. Motoyama, T. Nakagawa, and T. Okutomi. 1995. [Pharmacokinetics of balofloxacin in the intraocular tissues of pigmented rabbits]. *Jpn. J. Antibiot.* 48:1274–1280.

110. Ooishi, M., F. Sakaue, A. Oonomo, and K. Yoneyama. 1985. Fundamental and clinical studies on Bay o 9867 in ophthalmology. *Chemotherapy* (Tokyo) 33:1014–1021.

111. Ozturk, F., S. Kortunay, E. Kurt, S. S. Ilker, N. E. Basci, and A. Bozkurt. 1999. Penetration of topical and oral ciprofloxacin into the aqueous and vitreous humor in inflamed eyes. *Retina* 19:218–222.

112. Ozturk, F., S. Kortunay, E. Kurt, S. S. Ilker, U. U. Inan, N. E. Basci, A. Bozkurt, and O. Kayaalp. 1999. Effects of trauma and infection on ciprofloxacin levels in the vitreous cavity. *Retina* 19:127–130.

113. Ozturk, F., S. Kortunay, E. Kurt, U. U. Inan, S. S. Ilker, N. Basci, and A. Bozkurt. 1999. The effect of long-term use and inflammation on the ocular penetration of topical ofloxacin. *Curr. Eye Res.* 19:461–464.

114. Ozturk, F., S. Kortunay, E. Kurt, I. U. Ubeyt, I. S. Sami, N. E. Basci, A. Bozkurt, and K. S. Oguz. 1999. Ofloxacin levels after intravitreal injection. Effects of trauma and inflammation. *Ophthalmic Res.* 31:446–451.

115. Ozturk, F., E. Kurt, U. U. Inan, M. C. Kortunay, S. S. Ilker, N. E. Basci, and A. Bozkurt. 2000. Penetration of topical and oral ofloxacin into the aqueous and vitreous humor of inflamed rabbit eyes. *Int. J. Pharm.* 204:91–95.

116. Ozturk, F., E. Kurt, U. U. Inan, S. Kortunay, S. S. Ilker, N. E. Basci, and A. Bozkurt. 2000. The effects of prolonged acute use and inflammation on the ocular penetration of topical ciprofloxacin. *Int. J. Pharm. (Amst.)* 204:97–100.

117. Parkkari, M., H. Paivarinta, and L. Salminen. 1995. The treatment of endophthalmitis after cataract surgery: review of 26 cases. *J. Ocul. Pharmacol. Ther.* 11:349–359.

118. Perkins, R. J., W. Liu, G. Drusano, A. Madu, C. Mayers, C. Madu, and M. H. Miller. 1995. Pharmacokinetics of ofloxacin in serum and vitreous humor of albino and pigmented rabbits. *Antimicrob. Agents Chemother.* 39:1493–1498.

119. Preston, K. E., M. A. Kacica, R. J. Limberger, W. A. Archinal, and R. A. Venezia. 1997. The resistance and integrase genes of pACM1, a conjugative multiple-resistance plasmid, from Klebsiella oxytoca. *Plasmid* 37:105–118.

120. Preston, S. L., G. L. Drusano, A. L. Berman, C. L. Fowler, A. T. Chow, B. Dornseif, V. Reichl, J. Natarajan, and M. Corrado. 1998. Pharmacodynamics of levofloxacin: a new paradigm for early clinical trials. *JAMA* 279:125–129.

121. Rabkin, M. D., M. B. Bellhorn, and R. W. Bellhorn. 1977. Selected molecular weight dextrans for in vivo permeability studies of rat retinal vascular disease. *Exp. Eye Res.* 24:607–612.

122. Reidy, J. J., J. A. Hobden, J. M. Hill, K. Forman, and R. J. O'Callaghan. 1991. The efficacy of topical ciprofloxacin and norfloxacin in the treatment of experimental Pseudomonas keratitis. *Cornea* 10:25–28.

123. Richman, J., H. Zolezio, and D. Tang-Liu. 1990. Comparison of ofloxacin, gentamicin, and tobramycin concentrations in tears and in vitro MICs for 90% of test organisms. *Antimicrob. Agents Chemother.* 34:1602–1604.

124. Rootman, D. S., P. Savage, S. M. Hasany, L. Chisholm, and P. K. Basu. 1992. Toxicity and pharmacokinetics of intravitreally injected ciprofloxacin in rabbit eyes. *Can. J. Ophthalmol.* 27:277–282.

125. Salminen, L. 1978. Cloxacillin distribution in the rabbit eye after intravenous injection. *Acta Ophthalmol.* 56:11–19.

126. Schentag, J. J., L. C. Strenkoski-Nix, D. E. Nix, and A. Forrest. 1998. Pharmacodynamic interactions of antibiotics alone and in combination. *Clin. Infect. Dis.* 27:40–46.

127. Schluter, G. 1987. Ciprofloxacin: review of toxicologic effects. *Am. J. Med.* 82:91–93.

128. Shimoda, K., S. Okawara, and M. Kato. 2001. Phototoxic retinal degeneration and toxicokinetics of sitafloxacin, a quinolone antibacterial agent, in mice. *Arch. Toxicol.* 75:395–399.

129. Shimoda, K., M. Yoshida, N. Wagai, S. Takayama, and M. Kato. 1993. Phototoxic lesions induced by quinolone antibacterial agents in auricular skin and retina of albino mice. *Toxicol. Pathol.* 21:554–561.

130. Silbiger, J., and G. A. Stern. 1992. Evaluation of corneal collagen shields as a drug delivery device for the treatment of experimental pseudomonas keratitis. *Ophthalmology* 99:889–892.

131. Skoutelis, A. T., S. P. Gartaganis, C. J. Chrysanthopoulos, D. Beermann, C. Papachristou, and H. P. Bassaris. 1988. Aqueous humor penetration of ciprofloxacin in the human eye. *Arch. Ophthalmol.* 106:404–405.

132. Stevens, S. X., B. D. Fouraker, and H. G. Jensen. 1991. Intraocular safety of ciprofloxacin. *Arch. Ophthalmol.* 109:1737–1743.

133. Sugar, A., M. A. Cohen, P. A. Bien, T. J. Griffin, C. L. Heifetz, and S. Mehta. 1986. Treatment of experimental Pseudomonas corneal ulcers with enoxacin, a quinolone antibiotic. *Arch. Ophthalmol.* 104:1230–1232.

134. Sweeney, G., A. I. Fern, G. Lindsay, and M. W. Doig. 1990. Penetration of ciprofloxacin into the aqueous humour of the uninflamed human eye after oral administration. *J. Antimicrob. Chemother.* 26:99–105.

135. Tanahashi, T., K. Mochizuki, M. Torisaki, Y. Yamashita, M. Komatsu, T. Higashide, and M. Ogata. 1992. Effect of intravitreal injection of norfloxacin on the retina in pigmented rabbits. *Lens Eye Toxic. Res.* 9:493–503.

136. Tang-Liu, D., J. Lambert, S. Blancaflor, and A. Gwon. 1995. Availability of 0.3% ofloxacin ointment and solution in human conjunctiva and aqueous humor. *J. Ocul. Pharmacol. Ther.* 11:57–63.

137. Tsai, A. C., M. C. Tseng, S. W. Chang, and F. R. Hu. 1995. Clinical evaluation of ciprofloxacin ophthalmic solution in the treatment of refractory bacterial keratitis. *J. Formos. Med. Assoc.* 94:760–764.

138. van de Waterbeemd, H., G. Camenisch, G. Folkers, J. R. Chretien, and O. A. Raevsky. 1998. Estimation of blood-brain barrier crossing of drugs using molecular size and shape, and H-bonding descriptors. *J. Drug Targeting* 6:151–165.

139. Verbraeken, H., A. Verstraete, V. d. Van, and G. Verschraegen. 1996. Penetration of gentamicin and ofloxacin in human vitreous after systemic administration. *Graefe's Arch. Clin. Exp. Ophthalmol.* 234(Suppl. 1):S59–S65.

140. von Keyserlingk, J., R. Beck, U. Fischer, E. M. Hehl, R. Guthoff, and B. Drewelow. 1997. Penetration of ciprofloxacin, norfloxacin and ofloxacin into the aqueous humours of patients by different topical application modes. *Eur. J. Clin. Pharmacol.* 53:251–255.

141. Waga, J., I. Nilsson-Ehle, B. Ljungberg, A. Skarin, L. Stahle, and B. Ehinger. 1999. Microdialysis for pharmacokinetic studies of ceftazidime in rabbit vitreous. *J. Ocul. Pharmacol. Ther.* 15:55–463.

142. Wegener, A., U. D. Kuhn, M. Lorenz, and O. Hockwin. 1990. Evaluation of a possible cocataractogenic potential of ofloxacin. *Lens Eye Toxic. Res.* 7:39–47.

143. Wiechens, B., J. B. Grammer, U. Johannsen, U. Pleyer, J. Hedderich, and G. I. Duncker. 1999. Experimental intravitreal application of ciprofloxacin in rabbits. *Ophthalmologica* 213:120–128.

144. Wiechens, B., D. Neumann, J. B. Grammer, U. Pleyer, J. Hedderich, and G. I. Duncker. 1998. Retinal toxicity of liposome-incorporated and free ofloxacin after intravitreal injection in rabbit eyes. *Int. Ophthalmol.* 22:133–143.

145. Yoshida, A., S. Ishiko, and M. Kojima. 1992. Outward permeability of the blood-retinal barrier. *Graefe's Arch. Clin. Exp. Ophthalmol.* 230:78–83.

Chapter 19

Treatment of Skin and Soft Tissue Infections

ADOLF W. KARCHMER

Bacterial infections of the skin, which often extend to involve adjacent soft tissue, have been classified as primary pyodermas, infectious gangrene and gangrenous cellulitis, and secondary bacterial infections complicating preexisting skin lesions. The primary pyodermas include impetigo, folliculitis, furuncles and carbuncles, ecthyma, erysipelas, and cellulitis with or without associated lymphangitis. Recovery of an etiologic agent from patients with primary pyodermas generally requires culture of a draining portal of entry or drainable abscess or a detectable bacteremia. With a closed cellulitis lesion, culture of material from fine needle aspiration or biopsy of the advancing edge yields a pathogen in only 30% of cases. With the exception of cellulitis associated with unique epidemiologic exposures, e.g., *Erysipelothrix rhusiopathiae* from saltwater fish, *Aeromonas hydrophila* from fresh water, and *Vibrio vulnificus* or *Vibrio alginolyticus* from exposure to saltwater or brackish water, the majority of the primary pyodermas are caused by *Staphylococcus aureus*, *Streptococcus pyogenes*, or occasionally by other beta-hemolytic streptococci (Lancefield group C or G) or group B streptococci, *Streptococcus agalactiae*. Two additional primary pyodermas are defined by characteristic skin lesions, the chancriform lesion and the membranous ulcer of which the prototypic causes are *Bacillus anthracis* and *Corynebacterium diphtheriae*, respectively.

Infection involving skin sites wherein there has been prior injury, often called complicated skin and soft tissue infection, is caused not only by *S. aureus*, *S. pyogenes*, and groups B, C, and G streptococci, but also by an array of facultative gram-negative bacilli and anaerobic bacteria. These infections are often polymicrobial. The infections may involve surgical and traumatic wounds, burns, decubitus ulcers, and foot ulcers in patients with diabetes. In addition, some nonclostridial infections result in cutaneous necrosis and gangrene. Streptococcal gangrene (ecthyma) and

necrotizing fasciitis are caused by group A and occasionally group C or G streptococci. Progressive bacterial synergistic gangrene is a slowly spreading, tissue-destroying infection that typically complicates surgical wounds and is caused by microaerophilic streptococci in combination with *S. aureus*. Synergistic necrotizing cellulitis is a rapidly spreading, often crepitant, skin and subcutaneous tissue polymicrobial infection associated with systemic toxicity and caused by combinations of *Bacteroides* spp., peptostreptococci, and facultative gram-negative bacilli.

The fluoroquinolones have broad antibacterial activity, including activity against many of the bacteria that cause skin and soft tissue infection. In addition, these agents in general have excellent bioavailability after oral administration, favorable pharmacokinetics and penetration into soft tissues, and a good safety profile. As a result, fluoroquinolones have been extensively studied and used to treat these infections, particularly when patients are not severely ill and thus are candidates for initial oral therapy or oral therapy after a brief course of intravenous therapy.

PHARMACOKINETICS AND PHARMACODYNAMICS

Most bacterial infections involving skin and adjacent soft tissues reside in the interstitial spaces of these tissues. Thus, to provide effective therapy, quinolones must reach sufficient concentrations in these spaces to exceed the MIC for the relevant pathogen. In general, quinolones penetrate into these soft tissues well and achieve concentrations that are effective against most susceptible organisms (Table 1). Studies in human volunteers have used cantharides-induced blisters as a source of inflammatory interstitial fluid to assess fluoroquinolone pharmacokinetics (7, 19, 34, 60, 62–66). The time after an oral intravenous dose to reach peak concentration in skin blister fluid generally lags by 2 to

Adolf W. Karchmer • Division of Infectious Diseases, Beth Israel Deaconess Medical Center, 330 Brookline Avenue, Kennedy-6A, Boston, MA 02215.

Table 1. Inflammatory interstitial fluid penetration of selected fluoroquinolones in humans after a single dose

| Drug (reference) | Dose/route[a] | Mean peak concentration | | Penetration[b] (%) | Protein binding % | MIC$_{90}$ for S. aureus[c] |
		Plasma	Skin blister fluid[d]			
Ciprofloxacin (7)	400/i.v.	6.7	2.6	97	20–35	0.5
	750/p.o.	3.9	2.28	105	20–36	0.5
Levofloxacin (60)	500/p.o.	6.92	3.61	124	24–38	0.25
Sparfloxacin (34)	400/p.o.	1.6	1.3	117	45	0.125
Trovafloxacin (66)	200/p.o.	2.9	1.2	64	70–81	0.06
Gatifloxacin (62)	400/p.o.	4.1	3.6	117	20	0.25
Gemifloxacin (60)	320/p.o.	2.33	0.74	61	60	0.06
Moxifloxacin (63)	400/i.v.	5.09	3.23	94	30–45	0.12
	400/p.o.	4.98	2.62	83	30–45	0.12
Clinafloxacin (65)	200/p.o.	1.34	1.13	93	50–60	0.03
Garenoxacin (64)	600/p.o.	10.4	7.2	82	84	0.03

[a]The dose is in milligrams. i.v., intravenous; p.o., oral.
[b]Ratio of AUC extrapolated to infinity for blister fluid to plasma × 100.
[c]Methicillin-susceptible S. aureus.
[d]Blisters induced by application of cantharides-impregnated plasters (1 × 1 cm) to skin.

4 h that required to reach peak concentration in plasma, and the mean peak concentrations in blister fluid are lower than those noted in plasma. Nevertheless, the drug concentration curve over time in blister fluid after reaching peak concentration is nearly superimposable on that of the plasma curve. The percent penetration of fluoroquinolones into skin blister fluid calculated by comparing the area under the concentration-time curve (AUC) for the drug in blister fluid and plasma ranges from approximately 60% of the plasma AUC for gemifloxacin and trovafloxacin to approaching or exceeding 100% for ciprofloxacin, levofloxacin, sparfloxacin, gatifloxacin, moxifloxacin, and garenoxacin. For most of the fluoroquinolones, the free drug in skin blister fluid exceeds the MIC for S. aureus, S. pyogenes, other beta-hemolytic streptococci, and the Enterobacteriaceae, which commonly cause soft tissue infection for the majority of the advised dose-to-dose interval. For quinolones, however, the maximum concentration (C_{max})/MIC ratio is considered the pharmacodynamic marker predictive of bacterial eradication. As can be estimated from Table 1, the C_{max}/MIC at which 90% of the isolates tested are inhibited (MIC$_{90}$) for methicillin-susceptible S. aureus, adjusted for the free drug concentration (non-protein-bound active drug), ranges from 4 to 38, with levofloxacin, trovafloxacin, gatifloxacin, moxifloxacin, clinafloxacin, and garenoxacin. Pharmacokinetic data for moxifloxacin in interstitial spaces suggest the drug would be highly effective for soft tissue infections caused by methicillin-susceptible S. aureus, S. pyogenes, and most Enterobacteriaceae (45). In addition, Trampuz et al. demonstrated that skin blister fluid accumulating for 5 h after intake of a single 500-mg tablet of levofloxacin killed 2.0 log S. aureus at 6 h of incubation (60).

Projected free drug C_{max}/MIC$_{90}$ for methicillin-resistant S. aureus will be marginal, raising questions regarding the efficacy of available fluoroquinolones in the treatment of significant soft tissue infection caused by these organisms. In sum, these data provide a pharmacokinetic-pharmacodynamic rationale for anticipating that fluoroquinolones would be effective in the treatment of skin and soft tissue infections caused by susceptible organisms.

MICROBIOLOGY OF SKIN AND SOFT TISSUE INFECTION

The major pathogens causing primary skin and soft tissue infections among immunocompetent patients, in the absence of unique epidemiologic considerations, are S. aureus and beta-hemolytic streptococci, particularly S. pyogenes. Nosocomial infections of skin and adjacent soft tissue and infections occurring in trauma-induced cutaneous ulcerations and wounds are caused by a broad array of bacteria and are commonly polymicrobial (Table 2). Surveillance programs (SENTRY Antimicrobial Surveillance Program) that have examined the microbiology of nosocomial or community-acquired skin and soft tissue infections occurring in hospitalized patients also indicate differences in the causes of these infections compared with those associated with the primary pyodermas (13, 40). Microbiology laboratories in multiple medical centers from North America, Latin America, and Europe have each submitted the initial 50 consecutive, unique-patient, clinically significant bacterial isolates from hospitalized patients with skin and soft tissue infections during specified time periods

Table 2. Bacterial isolates from skin and soft tissue infections at sites of local injury[a]

Isolates from:	
Foot ulcers in diabetics[b]	Animal and human bite wounds[b]
S. aureus	*Actinobacillus* species
S. agalactiae	*Haemophilus* species
Other streptococci (viridans and beta-hemolytic)	*Capnocytophaga* species
	Eikenella corrodens
Coagulase-negative staphylococci	*Moraxella* species
	Pasteurella multocida subsp. *multocida* and *P. septica*
Enterococci	
Enterobacteriaceae	Other *Pasteurella* species
Pseudomonas aeruginosa	*S. aureus*
Peptostreptococci	Streptococci
Prevotella species	*Weeksella zoohelcum*
Bacteroides fragilis group	*Bacteroides tectum*
Other *Bacteroides* species	*Fusobacterium nucleatum*
	Other *Fusobacterium* species
	Peptostreptococci
	Porphyromonas species
	Prevotella species

[a]Data from references 23, 25, 26, 28, 35, 38, 41, 52.
[b]Multiple isolates from a single infection are noted commonly; the pathogenic role of some isolates is not defined.

to the SENTRY program. These isolates have then been characterized in the central laboratory by reference identification and susceptibility-testing methods advocated by the National Committee for Clinical Laboratory Standards. These extensive data provide a comprehensive view of the microbiology of skin and soft tissue infections among hospitalized patients (Table 3). The potent anti-gram-negative bacillus

Table 3. Bacterial isolates from skin and soft tissue infections in hospitalized patients

Isolate	No. (%) of isolates	
	1997[a] (n = 1,562)	2,000[b] (n = 2,537)
S. aureus	666 (42.6)	1,013 (39.9)
P. aeruginosa	176 (11.3)	307 (12.1)
Enterococci	127 (8.1)	195 (7.7)
Escherichia coli	112 (7.2)	246 (9.7)
Enterobacter spp.	82 (5.2)	141 (5.6)
Beta-hemolytic streptococci	79 (5.1)	47 (1.8)
Other enteric gram-negative bacilli	183 (11.7)	291 (11.4)
Nonenteric gram-negative bacilli	60 (3.8)	55 (2.2)
Coagulase-negative staphylococci	59 (3.8)	107 (4.2)
Non-beta-hemolytic streptococci	18 (1.2)	18 (0.7)
Other		117 (4.6)

[a]Isolates from United States and Canada (13).
[b]Isolates from North America, Latin America, and Europe (40).

activity of the newer fluoroquinolones combined with their enhanced activity against gram-positive cocci (Table 4) makes these agents highly attractive for the treatment of these complex and often more severe skin and soft tissue infections. Of note, however, the two large SENTRY Antimicrobial Surveillance Programs report that 24 and 27% of *S. aureus* isolates are methicillin-resistant (13, 40). Many methicillin-resistant *S. aureus* isolates have acquired high-level resistance to ciprofloxacin and the newer fluoroquinolones. Although the activity of some of the newer quinolones, e.g., trovafloxacin, moxifloxacin, clinafloxacin, and garenoxacin, against ciprofloxacin-resistant methicillin-resistant *S. aureus* appears to have been retained, the efficacy of these drugs in the treatment of serious infections caused by these organisms has not been established (15, 16, 33, 36, 37, 40, 53). There is concern that exposure of these organisms will selectively enrich the infecting bacterial population for decreasing susceptibility and thus predispose patients to treatment failure (67). Similarly, in the SENTRY program, oxacillin resistance was noted in 24% of coagulase-negative staphylococci isolated from skin and soft tissue infections, and many of these were resistant to ciprofloxacin and levofloxacin (40). Also, the activity of the fluoroquinolones against enterococci, particularly against vancomycin-resistant enterococci, many of which are *Enterococcus faecium*, is marginal (33). Thus data from clinical trials are required to define the efficacy of the fluoroquinolones for the treatment of skin and soft tissue infections.

Approximately 5 million Americans are bitten by animals, primarily cats or dogs, or other humans each year, and 5 to 25% of these wounds become infected and require antimicrobial therapy. The soft tissue infections resulting from these bites are caused

Table 4. Activity of fluoroquinolones against the principal staphylococci and streptococci that cause skin and soft tissue infection

Fluoroquinolone	MIC90 (µg/ml)		
	S. aureus[a]	*S. pyogenes*	*S. agalactiae*
Ciprofloxacin	1	1	1
Fleroxacin	1	8	16
Ofloxacin	0.5	2	2
Levofloxacin	0.25	1	2
Sparfloxacin	0.125	0.5	0.5
Tosufloxacin	0.06	0.25	0.25
Trovafloxacin	0.06	0.25	0.5
Clinafloxacin	0.03	0.06	0.12
Moxifloxacin	0.12	0.25	0.5
Gatifloxacin	0.25	0.5	0.5
Gemifloxacin	0.06	0.03	0.03
Garenoxacin	0.03	0.25	0.12

[a]Methicillin-susceptible strains.

not only by *S. aureus* or beta-hemolytic streptococci taking origin from the skin of the bitten person, but more commonly from the oral flora of the biting animal or person. A wide variety of fastidious aerobic and anaerobic bacteria have been recovered from bite-wound infections (Table 2). Aerobic bacteria isolated from bite-related infections are susceptible to fluoroquinolones (Table 5). For *S. aureus*, streptococci, *Eikenella corrodens*, *Capnocytophagia* species, CDC EF₄, *Actinobacillus* and *Haemophilus* spp., and *Moraxella* spp. that were isolated from bite infections, the MIC₉₀s of ciprofloxacin, sparfloxacin, ofloxacin, levofloxacin, moxifloxacin, trovafloxacin, gatifloxacin, and garenoxacin were ≤0.5 μg/ml (25, 26, 28, 29). *Pasturella* species, particularly *Pasteurella multocida* subsp. *multocida* and *P. multocida* subsp. *septica,* which are associated with more serious infections, are highly susceptible to the fluoroquinolones; the MIC₉₀s of ciprofloxacin, sparfloxacin, ofloxacin, levofloxacin, moxifloxacin, trovafloxacin, grepafloxacin, and garenoxacin are ≤0.125 μg/ml and commonly ≤0.03 μg/ml (25, 28, 29). With the exception of *Fusobacterium nucleatum* and other *Fusobacterium* species, for which the MIC₉₀s were commonly ≥8 μg/ml, anaerobes isolated from bite wounds, including *Bacteroides tectum*, *Porphyromonas* species, many *Prevotella* species, and *Peptostreptococcus* species were commonly susceptible to trovafloxacin, gatifloxacin, moxifloxacin, and garenoxacin (24, 25, 27–29). Nevertheless, the

activity of these newer fluoroquinolones against anaerobes is not entirely predictable and clinical experience in treating bite wounds with these drugs is very limited. Because the bacteria causing dog and cat bite infections are often fastidious and difficult to isolate and test for antimicrobial susceptibilty, recommendations for therapy are generally based on published studies of in vitro susceptibility rather than the testing of isolates associated with individual cases. Accordingly, on the basis of in vitro results and general clinical experience, a β-lactam antibiotic such as amoxicillin combined with a β-lactamase inhibitor is recommended. When this combination cannot be used, treatment with a fluoroquinolone in combination with clindamycin has been advised (18, 57).

The activity of earlier quinolones against the *Bacteroides fragilis* group is marginal (32, 49, 61). Thus, older fluoroquinolones, e.g., ciprofloxacin, ofloxacin, and levofloxacin, are not recommended for single agents for treatment of skin and soft tissue infections wherein these anaerobes may play a significant role. Trovafloxacin and garenoxacin, and to a lesser degree moxifloxacin, gemifloxacin, and clinafloxacin, have activity against the *B. fragilis* group and may have a role in the treatment of infections caused by these organisms (8, 9, 31, 39, 43). Nevertheless, activity of these fluoroquinolones against many anaerobic gram-negative bacteria is variable, and many of these organisms, for example, *Bacteroides thetaiotaomicron*, *Bacteroides distaso-*

Table 5. Activity of fluoroquinolones against unusual aerobic and anaerobic bacteria isolated from animal and human bite-wound infections

Organism	MIC range (μg/ml) of:					
	Ciprofloxacin[a]	Levofloxacin[a]	Trovafloxacin[a]	Gatifloxacin[a]	Moxifloxacin[b]	Garenoxacin[c]
Aerobic isolates						
Haemophilus spp.	≤0.001–0.06	≤0.001–0.06	≤0.001–0.03	≤0.001–0.03	0.008–0.06	
Capnocytophaga spp.	0.016–1.0	0.008–1.0			0.004–1.0	
Eikenella corrodens	0.004–0.02	0.008–0.06	0.016–0.06	0.008–0.125	0.008–0.125	≤0.015–0.125
CDC group EF₄	0.004–0.06	0.008–0.06	0.008–0.06	0.004–0.06	0.004–0.5	≤0.015–0.125
Moraxella spp.	0.004–0.06	0.004–0.06	0.008–0.06	≤0.001–0.016	0.004–0.03	≤0.015–0.06
Pasteurella multocida						
Subsp. *multocida*	0.004–0.03	0.008–0.03	0.008–0.03	0.008–0.03	0.008–0.026	≤0.015
Subsp. *septica*	0.004–0.03	0.008–0.03	0.004–0.016	0.008–0.03	0.008–0.016	≤0.015
Pasteurella spp.	0.002–0.03	0.002–0.06	0.002–0.125	0.002–0.03	0.004–0.06	≤0.015
Weeksella zoohelcum	0.002–0.125	0.016–0.125	0.002–0.125	0.004–0.03	0.004–0.016	≤0.015[d]
Anaerobic isolates						
Bacteroides tectum	0.5–4	0.25–1	0.03–0.25	0.06–0.5	0.03–0.25	≤0.015–0.125
Fusobacterium nucleatum	1–>8	0.5–>8	0.25–4	0.25–>8	0.008–8	0.125–>8
Fusobacterium spp. (other)	1–>8	2–>8	0.5–4	0.03–>8	0.03–8	≤0.015–>8
Peptostreptococci	0.25–2	0.25–4	0.06–0.5	0.06–1	0.03–0.5	0.03–0.06
Porphyromonas spp.	0.125–2	0.06–1	0.03–0.5	≤0.03–0.25	0.008–0.5	0.03–0.06
Prevotella spp.	0.125–2	0.25–1	0.06–1	0.06–0.25	0.03–2	0.06–0.25

[a]Data from reference 28.
[b]Data from reference 25.
[c]Data from reference 29.
[d]*Bergeyella zoohelcum.*

nis, and *Bacteroides ovatus*, are relatively resistant. Hence, with the possible exception of trovafloxacin, fluoroquinolones have not been advocated for treatment of infections caused by anaerobic gram-negative bacteria (1, 2, 6, 27, 30, 32, 33, 49).

CLINICAL EVALUATION OF FLUOROQUINOLONE TREATMENT

Ciprofloxacin, one of the earliest developed fluoroquinolones, has been extensively studied as therapy of skin infection. Gentry reviewed 20 open uncontrolled studies that used doses of 500 to 750 mg of ciprofloxacin administered orally every 12 h for 5 to 14 days in the treatment of patients with cellulitis, infected ulcers and wounds, erysipelas, and abscesses. Among the patients in these studies, 60% required hospitalization initially (20). Of 358 patients who were studied, 274 (77%) were treated successfully (complete or substantial resolution of signs and symptoms without need of additional therapy). Cure was achieved in 73% of patients with infection caused by methicillin-resistant *S. aureus*. However, bacterial eradication of methicillin-resistant *S. aureus* was accomplished in only 48% of patients as contrasted with eradication of methicillin-susceptible *S. aureus* in 83% of patients. Infections attributed to *Enterobacteriaceae* and *P. aeruginosa* were cured in 100 and 72% of patients, respectively.

Randomized, open and double-blind clinical trials have been performed to evaluate the safety and efficacy of fluoroquinolones in comparison with other agents considered standards of care. The patients enrolled in these trials were heterogeneous. Thus, the clinical experience is best viewed by categorizing study patients according to the severity of their infection and grouping studies conducted in patients with uncomplicated (less severe) and complicated (more severe) skin and soft tissue infections.

Uncomplicated Skin Infections

In randomized studies, some of which were conducted using a double-blind design, fluoroquinolone treatment of uncomplicated skin and soft tissue infection was highly efficacious. Cure (complete resolution or improvement in multiple clinical parameters without need for additional antibiotic therapy) rates for fluoroquinolones ranged from 85 to 99%, while the cure rates in those patients treated with various comparators ranged from 79 to 97% (Table 6). In each study the outcome of fluoroquinolone treatment did not differ significantly from that achieved with the comparator. The predominant pathogen isolated from patients in each of these studies was *S. aureus*; eradication rates of *S. aureus* by fluoroquinolones in these patients ranged from 92 to 100% with comparable eradication rates by the comparator (46–48, 51, 54). The frequency with which

Table 6. Comparative randomized trials of fluoroquinolone treatment of uncomplicated skin and soft tissue infections

Author (reference)	Fluoroquinolone dose; route (days)[a]	No. cured[b]/ total no. evaluable (%)	Comparative antimicrobial dose; route (days)	No. cured[b]/ total no. evaluable (%)
Neldner (46)	Temafloxacin; 600 mg twice daily, p.o. (7–10)	95/97 (98)	Cefadroxil; 500 mg twice daily, p.o. (7–10)	102/106 (96)
Powers et al. (54)	Ofloxacin; 400 mg twice daily, p.o. (10)	72/73 (99)	Cephalexin; 500 mg 4 times daily, p.o. (10)	63/65 (97)
Nichols et al. (47)	Levofloxacin; 500 mg daily, p.o. (9)	178/182 (98)	Ciprofloxacin; 500 mg twice daily, p.o. (9.6)	187/193 (97)
Tassler et al. (59)	Fleroxacin; 400 mg daily, p.o. (7)	105/114 (92)	Amoxicillin-clavulanate; 500 mg 3 times daily, p.o. (7)	55/57 (96)
Nicodemo et al. (48)[c]	Levofloxacin; 500 mg daily, p.o. (7)	129/136 (95)	Ciprofloxacin; 500 mg twice daily, p.o. (10)	124/130 (91)
Daniel (12)[c]	Trovafloxacin; 100 mg daily, p.o. (7)	106/125 (85)	Flucloxacillin; 500 mg 4 times daily, p.o. (7)	97/123 (79)
Parrish et al. (51)[c]	Moxifloxacin; 400 mg daily, p.o. (7)	162/180 (90)	Cephalexin; 500 mg 3 times daily (7)	156/171 (91)
Tarshis et al. (58)[c]	Gatifloxacin; 400 mg daily, p.o. (7–10)	146/161 (91)	Levofloxacin; 500 mg daily, p.o. (7–10)	145/172 (84)
Dreholb (14)[c]	Ofloxacin; 400 mg twice daily, p.o. (10)	130/157 (83)	Fleroxacin; 400 mg daily, p.o. (10)	122/156 (83)

[a]p.o., oral.
[b]Cure or improved.
[c]Double-blind trial.

patients included in these trials had infections caused by methicillin-resistant, fluoroquinolone-resistant *S. aureus* usually is not reported but presumably was very low. Neldner did note that 11% of *S. aureus* isolated from study patients were methicillin-resistant, but only one isolate was resistant to temafloxacin, the study fluoroquinolone. Although eradication rates for *S. aureus* by temafloxacin and the comparator, cefadroxil, were 87 and 83%, respectively, the methicillin-susceptibility phenotypes of persistent isolates were not identified (46). Tarshis et al. included patients infected by methicillin-resistant *S. aureus* in their trial but did not report their frequency. They did note, however, that no *S. aureus* isolates were gatifloxacin resistant and that only one had intermediate gatifloxacin susceptibility and that one *S. aureus* isolate was resistant to the comparator, levofloxacin. Eradication rates of *S. aureus* for gatifloxacin and levofloxacin in this study were 93 and 92%, respectively (58). Similarly, in the trial comparing moxifloxacin and cephalexin, the frequency of the methicillin-resistant phenotype among *S. aureus* isolates is not noted, but for these *S. aureus* isolates the MIC_{90} for moxifloxacin was 0.125 μg/ml. In this study the eradication rates of *S. aureus* by moxifloxacin and cephalexin were 92 and 93%, respectively, suggesting that the agents may not have been challenged by significant numbers of methicillin-resistant *S. aureus* (51). Although cure rates were comparable in the two arms of the large randomized, blinded trial reported by Drehobl et al., ofloxacin treatment achieved a higher microbiologic eradication rate (153 of 157; 97%) than did fleroxacin (141 of 158; 89%) ($P < 0.05$; treatment difference 8%, 95% confidence interval 2 to 14%) (14). *S. aureus* isolates were eradicated more frequently in the ofloxacin than in the fleroxacin treatment arm (83 of 85; 98% versus 64 of 73; 88%). In general, study drug-related adverse events were relatively infrequent in these trials and few patients discontinued therapy because of drug-related adverse events (12, 46–48, 51, 54, 58, 59). In considering the high cure rates for skin and soft tissue infections attributed to fluoroquinolones in these trials (Table 6) it is important to note that many of the infections studied are milder primary pyodermas (including impetigo, folliculitis, and drained abscesses) and that methicillin-resistant, fluoroquinolone-resistant *S. aureus* strains were encountered infrequently.

Complicated Skin and Soft Tissue Infections

Randomized clinical trials have evaluated fluoroquinolones for the treatment of more severe, so-called complicated skin and soft tissue infections.

Patients treated in these trials are primarily those with surgical or traumatic wound infections, bite-associated infections, complex cellulitis soft tissue abscesses, infected decubitus or diabetic foot ulcers, and occasional patients with necrotizing cellulitis (10, 17, 21, 22, 50, 55). The microbiologic causes of infection in these study patients are similar to those noted in the SENTRY surveillance program (Table 3). In these studies, gram-positive cocci remain the predominant pathogens accounting for 45 to 72% of isolates (10, 21, 55). *S. aureus* is the single most common organism causing infection. Notably, most *S. aureus* isolates are methicillin susceptible, with only rare isolates noted to be methicillin resistant. From 28 to 55% of the pathogens recovered were gram-negative bacilli, and among these, the most common was *Pseudomonas aeruginosa*.

In the randomized trials of treatment for complicated skin and soft tissue infections fluoroquinolones were as effective clinically as the third-generation cephalosporins or β-lactam–β-lactamase inhibitor comparators (Table 7). Clinical cure rates for fluoroquinolones ranged from 69 to 98% but were somewhat clustered around 80%. Cure rates among patients treated with the third-generation cephalosporin or β-lactam–β-lactamase inhibitor comparator were similar (range, 65 to 98%) but tended to cluster in the middle 70% (10, 17, 21, 22, 50, 55). When comparing fluoroquinolones with the comparator in individual studies, cure rates did not differ significantly. Overall, the cure rates are lower than those noted for uncomplicated skin and soft tissue infection, a not surprising reflection of the more severe nature of these complicated infections. While safety of fluoroquinolones in general in these studies was very satisfactory, as anticipated from larger trials and general experience, phototoxicity was noted in 10.5% of clinafloxacin recipients, including two reactions prompting hospitalization for second-degree sunburn (55).

The overall microbiologic eradication rates for initial pathogens in the three largest trials were similar: ciprofloxacin, 200 of 300 (87%) versus cefotaxime, 205 of 246 (83%) (21); clinafloxacin, 97 of 157 (62%) vs. piperacillin-tazobactam, 84 of 151 (56%) (55); trovafloxacin, 88 of 119 (74%) versus amoxicillin-clavulanate 72 of 99 (73%) (10). Of note, in the trial reported by Gentry et al., the rate of persistent plus recurrent original pathogens was significantly lower in ciprofloxacin-treated patients (6%) than in cefotaxime recipients (15%) ($P = 0.012$) (21). This difference was largely the result of persisting *P. aeruginosa* and enteric gram-negative bacilli. In the clinafloxacin trial the overall eradication rate for both study drugs was lower than that in

Table 7. Comparative randomized trials of fluoroquinolone treatment of complicated skin and soft tissue infection

Author (reference)	Fluoroquinolone daily dose; route (mean no. of days)[a]	No. cured[b]/total no. evaluable (%)	Comparative antimicrobial daily dose; route (mean no. of days)	No. cured[b]/total no. evaluable (%)
Gentry (21)[c]	Ciprofloxacin; 1.5 g, p.o. (9.3)	187/230 (81)	Cefotaxime; 6 g, i.v. (8.9)	180/246 (74)
Fass (17)	Ciprofloxacin; 800 mg, i.v./1–1.5 g, p.o.	46/58 (79)	Ceftazidime; 2–4 g, i.v.	28/39 (72)
Gentry (22)	Ofloxacin; 800 mg, p.o. (12)	42/43 (98)	Cefotaxime; 6 g, i.v. (12)	49/50 (98)
Parrish (50)	Fleroxacin; 400 mg, i.v. (7)	74/90 (82)	Ceftazidime; 2–6 g, i.v. (8)	36/49 (73)
Daniel (10)	Trovafloxacin; 200 mg, p.o. (10–14)	111/119 (93)	Amoxicillin-clavulanate; 1.5/375 g, p.o. (10–14)	92/99 (93)
Siami (55)[c]	Clinafloxacin; 400 mg, i.v./400 mg, p.o. (13)	94/144 (69)	Piperacillin-tazobactam[d]; 12/1.5, i.v. Amoxicillin-clavulanate; 1.5/375 g, p.o. (10–14)p.o. (13)	88/135 (65)

[a] p.o., oral; i.v., intravenous.
[b] Cure or improved.
[c] Investigator or double-blind design.
[d] Vancomycin added if methicillin-resistant *S. aureus* recovered from infection site.

the other trials (55). This difference might have related to the decision to classify patients as having "presumed persistent pathogens" if there was no material to culture or if a nonstudy antibiotic had been administered.

In examining treatment of infections caused by *S. aureus*, Gentry et al. noted recurrence or persistence of *S. aureus* in 8 of 107 (7%) of ciprofloxacin-treated patients and emergence of resistance to ciprofloxacin in three *S. aureus* isolates compared with the recurrence or persistence of this organism in 9 of 99 (9%) of cefotaxime recipients. Eradication of methicillin-susceptible and methicillin-resistant *S. aureus*, respectively, was noted in 34 of 54 (63%) and 4 of 7 (51%) patients treated with clinafloxacin and 32 of 54 (59%) and 5 of 14 (35%) treated with piperacillin-tazobactam; one *S. aureus* isolate developed resistance to clinafloxacin (55). Daniel reported that eradication rates of *S. aureus* by trovafloxacin or amoxicillin-clavulanate were 78 and 81%, respectively (10). These modest microbiologic eradication rates by fluoroquinolones and comparator agents for *S. aureus*, unquestionably the premier pathogen for complicated skin and soft tissue infection, should sound a note of caution. This is particularly true when noting that methicillin-resistant *S. aureus*, now a common nosocomial wound infection pathogen, was infrequently encountered in these studies and clinafloxacin and trovafloxacin are among the fluoroquinolones with the greatest potency against *S. aureus* (Table 4).

Diabetic Foot Infection

Polymicrobial infections in the feet of patients with diabetes mellitus (so called "diabetic foot infection") usually arise from neuropathic ulcers and fre-

quently occur in the setting of arterial insufficiency. Although patients with these infections are often included in treatment trials for complicated skin and soft tissue infections, because of the uniqueness of the clinical setting and the frequency of this problem some studies have focused solely on fluoroquinolone treatment of this entity. Ciprofloxacin, ofloxacin, trovafloxacin, and fleroxacin plus clindamycin, often using sequential intravenous to oral routes of administration, have been studied as treatment of diabetic foot infections with encouraging results (4, 11, 41, 44, 52). Lipsky et al. randomly assigned diabetic patients with moderately severe foot infections to sequential intravenous to oral treatment with ofloxacin 400 mg every 12 h or ampicillin-sulbactam 1.5 to 3.0 g intravenously every 6 h followed by amoxicillin-clavulanate 625 mg orally every 8 h (41). The mean duration of the ofloxacin and aminopenicillin treatments were 7.8 and 7.1 days intravenously, respectively, plus 13.2 and 12.0 days orally, respectively. Response rates, cured plus improved including patients with adjacent osteomyelitis (16 in the ofloxacin arm, 5 in the aminopenicillin arm), were 40 of 47 (85%) and 34 of 41 (83%) among evaluable patients receiving ofloxacin or an aminopenicillin, respectively. In an open-label, non-comparative, multicenter study patients with diabetic foot infections of varying degrees of severity (without osteomyelitis) were treated with trovafloxacin, 200 mg orally, administered once daily for 14 days and were observed thereafter for 30 days (11). Of 255 patients enrolled, 214 were clinically evaluable. The spectrum of pathogens was consistent with that encountered in moderately severe diabetic foot infection, and *S. aureus* was the predominant pathogen accounting for 29% of all isolates. The cure rate (complete resolution or incomplete resolution of signs and symptoms but requiring no further antibiotic therapy) at the end of treatment was 93% and the eradication rate of *S. aureus* was 83%. Although a promising agent for treatment of foot infections in patients with diabetes, trovafloxacin was withdrawn from routine clinical use because of infrequent but severe hepatotoxicity.

The necessity to treat anaerobes, at least empirically until excluded, when considering therapy for severe diabetic foot infections involving deeply penetrating neuropathic ulcers requires further elucidation (23, 35). Currently available fluoroquinolones have limited activity against anaerobic gram-negative bacteria. Thus, if a fluoroquinolone is to be used to treat a severe limb-threatening infection wherein gram-negative anaerobes are likely to be present, a second antibiotic with predictable activity against anaerobic gram-negative rods, e.g., clindamycin, should be added (38). Fluoroquinolones alone or in combination with an antianaerobic agent are safe and effective agents for treating more severe diabetic foot infections caused by susceptible pathogens. Alternatively, non-limb-threatening diabetic foot infections, that is those occurring in the absence of a full skin-thickness ulceration and significant ischemia, are often caused by *S. aureus* and streptococci and are most appropriately treated with an antistaphylococcal penicillin or cephalosporin in lieu of a fluoroquinolone (38, 42).

Cutaneous Anthrax

Cutaneous anthrax is the prototype chancriform primary pyoderma. More than 95% of naturally occurring anthrax worldwide is the cutaneous form. This infection arises when spores are introduced at the site of a preexisting skin break. During the bioterrorism cases in the United States in 2001, there were seven definite and four suspected cases of cutaneous anthrax, some of which developed in the absence of a known break in the skin. The clinical evolution of cutaneous anthrax is well described. Following a 1- to 12-day incubation period after exposure to spores of *B. anthracis,* a painless, slightly pruritic papule develops. Over succeeding days the papule vesiculates or becomes surrounded by small vesicles. Thereafter the lesion enlarges, becomes surrounded by gelatinous edema, and subsequently the central papule area becomes necrotic and covered by a black eschar. With control of the infection the eschar dries and is shed over several weeks leaving little or no scar. Although malaise and fever are noted as the lesion progresses in the absence of treatment, bacteremia is a rare complication. In untreated patients gram-positive rods can be seen on smear of vesicle

fluid or ulcer drainage and can be cultured; however, organisms are cleared rapidly with antibiotic treatment. Prior to the bioterrorism episode, penicillin was the therapy of choice for cutaneous anthrax. Subsequently, because β-lactamase genes were discovered in the isolates from the 2001 terrorist outbreak, ciprofloxacin (500 mg orally every 12 h for 7 to 10 days) has been recommended as treatment for mild cutaneous anthrax that is not occurring in natural exposure settings. More severe cases of cutaneous anthrax are treated with parenteral ciprofloxacin. In the setting of suspected bioterrorism, it is advised that ciprofloxacin treatment for cutaneous anthrax be continued for 60 days as prophylaxis against inhalational anthrax (3, 5, 56). Other fluoroquinolones may be effective as treatment for anthrax as well, but they have not been tested in vivo nor approved by the Food and Drug Administration for this use.

CONCLUSION

Data from comparative and noncomparative clinical trials demonstrate that currently available fluoroquinolones are highly effective treatment for mild, uncomplicated as well as for more severe, complicated skin and soft tissue infections. The fluoroquinolones, however, with their exceptional, broad antimicrobial spectrum, usually bring excessive potency and spectrum of activity to the treatment of uncomplicated primary pyoderma. Thus, these agents should not be used routinely for treatment of uncomplicated skin infections wherein *S. aureus* and beta-hemolytic streptococci are overwhelmingly the likely pathogens. Indiscriminate use may help to select increasingly fluoroquinolone-resistant pathogens. Furthermore, resistance to fluoroquinolones is increasing among *S. aureus* isolates, in particular those that are methicillin resistant; this may limit the utility of these agents. Appropriate treatment for these uncomplicated primary skin infections should use regimens focused on *S. aureus.* In contrast, when treating complex, complicated, and more severe skin and soft tissue infections, which are more likely polymicrobial and caused by gram-negative bacilli and gram-positive cocci, fluoroquinolones with their broad antimicrobial activity and good safety profile may be appropriate choices. The available fluoroquinolones, however, should not be used alone to treat skin infections wherein anaerobic gram-negative bacilli combined with other bacteria are anticipated, for example, synergistic necrotizing cellulitis, Fournier's gangrene, and severe crepitant fetid diabetic foot infections. If fluoroquinolones are to be used in these patients, a second drug with predictable antianaerobic activity should be included in the regimen. Similarly, fluoroquinolones should be used with caution when infections are known or likely to be caused by methicillin-resistant *S. aureus*. Thus, with judicious use these broad-spectrum, relatively nontoxic, orally bioavailable antimicrobials can be a major resource in the treatment of skin and soft tissue infections.

REFERENCES

1. Aldridge, K. E., D. Ashcraft, and K. A. Bowman. 1997. Comparative in vitro activities of trovafloxacin (CP 99,219) and other antimicrobials against clinically significant anaerobes. *Antimicrob. Agents Chemother.* 41:484–487.

2. Appelbaum, P. C. 1999. Quinolone activity against anaerobes. *Drugs* 58(Suppl. 2):60–64.

3. Bartlett, J. G., T. V. Inglesby, and L. Borio. 2002. Management of anthrax. *Clin. Infect. Dis.* 35:851–858.

4. Beam, T. R., Jr., I. Gutierrez, S. Powell, R. Hewitt, M. Hocko, M. Brackett, and M. Craver. 1989. Prospective study of the efficacy and safety of oral and intravenous ciprofloxacin in the treatment of diabetic foot infections. *Rev. Infect. Dis.* 11(Suppl. 5):S1163–S1163

5. Bell, D. M., P. E. Kozarsky, and D. S. Stephens. 2002. Clinical issues in the prophylaxis, diagnosis, and treatment of anthrax. *Emerg. Infect. Dis.* 8:222–225.

6. Betriu, C., M. Gomez, L. Palau, A. Sanchez, and J. J. Picazo. 1999. Activities of new antimicrobial agents (trovafloxacin, moxifloxacin, sanfetrinem, and quinupristin-dalfopristin) against *Bacteroides fragilis* group: comparison with the activities of 14 other agents. *Antimicrob. Agents Chemother.* 43:2320–2322.

7. Catchpole, C., J. M. Andrews, J. Woodcock, and R. Wise. 1994. The comparative pharmacokinetics and tissue penetration of single-dose ciprofloxacin 400 mg IV and 750 mg PO. *J. Antimicrob. Chemother.* 33:103–110.

8. Citron, D. M., and M. D. Appleman. 1997. Comparative in vitro activities of trovafloxacin (CP-99,219) against 221 aerogic and 217 anaerobic bacteria isolated from patients with intra-abdominal infections. *Antimicrob. Agents Chemother.* 41:2312–2316.

9. Credito, K. L., M. R. Jacobs, and P. C. Appelbaum. 2003. Time-kill studies of the antianaerobe activity of garenoxacin compared with those of nine other agents. *Antimicrob. Agents Chemother.* 47:1399–1402.

10. Daniel, R., for The Trovafloxacin Study Group. 1999. Comparison of the efficacy and safety of once-daily oral trovafloxacin and 3-times-daily amoxicillin/clavulanic acid for the treatment of complicated skin and soft-tissue infections. *Drugs* 58(Suppl. 2):288–290.

11. Daniel, R., for The Trovafloxacin Study Group. 1999. Once-daily oral trovafloxacin in the treatment of diabetic foot infections. *Drugs* 58(Suppl. 2):291–292.

12. Daniel, R., for The Trovafloxacin Study Group. 1999. Trovafloxacin once daily vs. flucloxacillin four times daily in the treatment of uncomplicated skin and skin-structure infections. *Drugs* 58(Suppl. 2):293–294.

13. Doern, G. V., R. N. Jones, M. A. Pfaller, K. C. Kugler, and M. L. Beach, for the SENTRY Study Group (North America). 1999. Bacterial pathogens isolated from patients with skin and soft tissue infections: frequency of occurrence and antimicrobial susceptibility patterns from the SENTRY antimicrobial surveillance program (United States and Canada, 1997). *Diagn. Microbiol. Infect. Dis.* 34:65–72.

14. Drehobl, M., L. Koenig, M. Barker, P. St Clair, and D. Maladorno. 1997. Fleroxacin 400 mg once daily versus ofloxacin 400 mg twice daily in skin and soft tissue infections. *Chemotherapy* 43:378–384.

15. Eliopoulos, G. M. 1999. Activity of newer fluoroquinolones *in vitro* against gram-positive bacteria. *Drugs* 58(Suppl. 2):23–28.

16. Endtz, H. P., J. W. Mouton, and J. G. den Hollander. 1997. Comparative in vitro activities of trovafloxacin (CP 99,219) against 445 gram-positive isolates from patients with endocarditis and those with other blood stream infections. *Antimicrob. Agents Chemother.* 41:1146–1149.

17. Fass, R. L., J. F. Plouffe, and J. A. Russell. 1989. Intravenous/oral ciprofloxacin versus ceftazidime in the treatment of serious infections. *Am. J. Med.* 18(Suppl. D):153–157.

18. Fleisher, G. R. 1999. The management of bite wounds. *N. Engl. J. Med.* 340:138–140.

19. Gee, T., J. M. Andrews, J. P. Ashby, G. Marshall, and R. Wise. 2001. Pharmacokinetics and tissue penetration of gemifloxacin following a single oral dose. *J. Antimicrob. Chemother.* 47:431–434.

20. Gentry, L. O. 1991. Review of quinolones in the treatment of infections of skin and skin structure. *J. Antimicrob. Chemother.* 28(Suppl. C):97–110.

21. Gentry, L. O., C. H. Ramirez-Ronda, E. Rodriguez-Noreiga, H. Thadepalli, P. L. del Rosal, and C. Ramirez. 1989. Oral ciprofloxacin vs. parenteral cefotaxime in treatment of difficult skin and skin structure infections: a multicenter trial. *Arch. Intern. Med.* 149:2579–2583.

22. Gentry, L. O., G. Rodriguez-Gomez, B. J. Zeluff, A. Koshdel, and M. Price. 1989. A comparative evaluation of oral ofloxacin versus intravenous cefotaxime therapy for serious skin and skin structure infections. *Am. J. Med.* 87(Suppl. 6C):57S–60S.

23. Gerding, D. N. 1995. Foot infections in diabetic patients: the role of anaerobes. *Clin. Infect. Dis.* 20(Suppl. 2):S283–S288

24. Goldstein, E. J., D. M. Citron, Y. Warren, K. Tyrrell, and C. V. Merriam. 1999. In vitro activity of gemifloxacin (SB265805) against anaerobes. *Antimicrob. Agents Chemother.* 43:2231–2235.

25. Goldstein, E. J. C., D. M. Citron, M. Hudspeth, S. H. Gerardo, and C. V. Merriam. 1997. In vitro activity of Bay 12-8039, a new 8-methoxyquinolone, compared to the activities of 11 other oral antimicrobial agents against 390 aerobic and anaerobic bacteria isolated from human and animal bite wound skin and soft tissue infections in humans. *Antimicrob. Agents Chemother.* 41:1552–1557.

26. Goldstein, E. J. C., D. M. Citron, S. Hunt-Gerardo, M. Hudspeth, and C. V. Merriam. 1997. Comparative in vitro activities of DU-6859a, levofloxacin, ofloxacin, sparfloxacin, and ciprofloxacin against 387 aerobic and anaerobic bite wound isolates. *Antimicrob. Agents Chemother.* 41:1193–1195.

27. Goldstein, E. J. C., D. M. Citron, C. V. Merriam, K. Tyrrell, and Y. Warren. 1999. Activities of gemifloxacin (SB 265805, LB20304) compared to those of other oral antimicrobial agents against unusual anaerobes. *Antimicrob. Agents Chemother.* 43:2726–2730.

28. Goldstein, E. J. C., D. M. Citron, C. V. Merriam, K. Tyrrell, and Y. Warren. 1999. Activity of gatifloxacin compared to those of five other quinolones versus aerobic and anaerobic isolates from skin and soft tissue samples of human and animal

bite wound infections. *Antimicrob. Agents Chemother.* **43**:1475–1479.

29. **Goldstein, E. J. C., D. M. Citron, C. V. Merriam, Y. A. Warren, K. L. Tyrrell, and H. Fernandez.** 2002. In vitro activities of the des-fluoro(6) quinolone BMS-284756 against aerobic and anaerobic pathogens isolated from skin and soft tissue animal and human bite wound infections. *Antimicrob. Agents Chemother.* **46**:866–870.

30. **Goldstein, E. J. C.** 1996. Possible role for the new fluoroquinolones (levofloxacin, grepafloxacin, trovafloxacin, clinafloxacin, sparfloxacin, and DU-6859a) in the treatment of anaerobic infections: review of current information on efficacy and safety. *Clin. Infect. Dis.* **23**(Suppl. 1):S25–S30.

31. **Hecht, D. W., and J. R. Osmolski.** 2003. Activities of garenoxacin (BMS-284756) and other agents against anaerobic clinical isolates. *Antimicrob. Agents Chemother.* **47**:910–916.

32. **Hecht, D. W., and H. M. Wexler.** 1996. In vitro susceptibility of anaerobes to quinolones in the United States. *Clin. Infect. Dis.* **23**(Suppl. 1):S2–S8

33. **Hooper, D. C.** 2000. New uses for new and old quinolones and the challenge of resistance. *Clin. Infect. Dis.* **30**:243–254.

34. **Johnson, J. H., M. A. Cooper, J. M. Andrews, and R. Wise.** 1992. Pharmacokinetics and inflammatory fluid penetration of sparfloxacin. *Antimicrob. Agents Chemother.* **36**:2444–2446.

35. **Johnson, S., F. Lebahn, L. P. Peterson, and D. N. Gerding.** 1995. Use of an anaerobic collection and transport swab device to recover anaerobic bacteria from infected foot ulcers in diabetics. *Clin. Infect. Dis.* **20**(Suppl. 2):S289–S290.

36. **Jones, M. E., M. R. Visser, M. Klootwijk, P. Heisig, J. Verhoef, and F. J. Schmitz.** 1999. Comparative activities of clinafloxacin, grepafloxacin, levofloxacin, moxifloxacin, ofloxacin, sparfloxacin, and trovafloxacin and nonquinolones linozelid, quinupristin-dalfopristin, gentamicin, and vancomycin against clinical isolates of ciprofloxacin-resistant and -susceptible *Staphylococcus aureus* strains. *Antimicrob. Agents Chemother.* **43**:421–423.

37. **Jones, R. N., M. L. Beach, M. A. Pfaller, and G. V. Doern.** 1998. Antimicrobial activity of gatifloxacin tested against 1676 strains of ciprofloxacin-resistant gram-positive cocci isolated from patient infections in North and South America. *Diagn. Microbiol. Infect. Dis.* **32**:247–252.

38. **Karchmer, A. W., and G. W. Gibbons.** 1994. Foot infections in diabetes: evaluation and management, p. 1–22. *In* J. S. Remington and M. N. Swartz (ed.), *Current Clinical Topics in Infectious Diseases.* Blackwell Scientific Publications, Boston, Mass.

39. **King, A., J. May, G. French, and I. Phillips.** 2000. Comparative *in vitro* activity of gemifloxacin. *J. Antimicrob. Chemother.* **45**(Suppl. S1):1–12.

40. **Kirby, J. T., A. H. Mutnick, R. N. Jones, D. J. Biedenbach, and M. A. Pfaller, for the SENTRY Participants Group.** 2002. Geographic variations in garenoxacin (BMS284756) activity tested against pathogens associated with skin and soft tissue infections: report from the SENTRY Antimicrobial Surveillance Program (2000). *Diagn. Microbiol. Infect. Dis.* **43**:303–309.

41. **Lipsky, B. A., P. D. Baker, G. C. Landon, and R. Fernau.** 1997. Antibiotic therapy for diabetic foot infections: Comparison of two parenteral-to-oral regimens. *Clin. Infect. Dis.* **24**:643–648.

42. **Lipsky, B. A., R. E. Pecoraro, S. A. Larson, M. E. Hanley, and J. H. Ahroni.** 1990. Outpatient management of uncomplicated lower-extremity infections in diabetic patients. *Arch. Intern. Med.* **150**:790–797.

43. **Lowe, M. N., and H. M. Lamb.** 2000. Gemifloxacin. *Drugs* **59**:1137–1147.

44. **Malanoski, G. J., G. W. Gibbons, J. S. Chrzan, E. Levin, and A. W. Karchmer.** 1995. Fleroxacin plus clindamycin in the treatment of limb-threatening foot infections in diabetic patients. *Clin. Drug Invest.* **9**(Suppl. 1):30–35.

45. **Muller, M., H. Stab, M. Brunner, J. G. Moller, E. Lackner, and H. G. Eichler.** 1999. Penetration of moxifloxacin into peripheral compartments in humans. *Antimicrob. Agents Chemother.* **43**:2345–2349.

46. **Neldner, K. H.** 1991. Double-blind randomized study of oral temafloxacin and cefadroxil in patients with mild to moderately severe bacterial skin infections. *Am. J. Med.* **91**(Suppl. 6A):111S–114S.

47. **Nichols, R. L., J. W. Smith, L. O. Gentry, J. Gezon, T. Campbell, and R. R. Williams.** 1997. Multicenter, randomized study comparing levofloxacin and ciprofloxacin for uncomplicated skin and skin structure infections. *South. Med. J.* **90**:1193–1200.

48. **Nicodemo, A. C., J. A. Robledo, A. Jasovich, and W. Neto.** 1998. A multicenter, double-blind, randomised study comparing the efficacy and safety of oral levofloxacin versus ciprofloxacin in the treatment of uncomplicated skin and skin structure infections. *Int. J. Clin. Pract.* **52**:69–74.

49. **Nord, C. E.** 1996. In vitro activity of quinolones and other antimicrobial agents against anaerobic bacteria. *Clin. Infect. Dis.* **23**(Suppl. 1):S15–S18

50. **Parrish, L. C., and D. L. Jungkind.** 1993. Systemic antimicrobial therapy for skin and skin structure infections: comparison of fleroxacin and ceftazidime. *Am. J. Med.* **94**(Suppl. 3A):166S–173S.

51. **Parrish, L. C., H. B. Routh, B. Miskin, J. Fidelholtz, P. Werschler, A. Heyd, D. Haverstock, and D. Church.** 2000. Moxifloxacin versus cephalexin in the treatment of uncomplicated skin infections. *Int. J. Clin. Pract.* **54**:497–503.

52. **Peterson, L. R., L. M. Lissack, K. Canter, C. E. Fasching, C. Clabots, and D. N. Gerding.** 1989. Therapy of lower extremity infections with ciprofloxacin in patients with diabetes mellitus, peripheral vascular disease, or both. *Am. J. Med.* **86**:801–808.

53. **Pong, A., K. S. Thomson, E. S. Moland, S. A. Chartrand, and C. C. Sanders.** 1999. Activity of moxifloxacin against pathogens with decreased susceptibility to ciprofloxacin. *J. Antimicrob. Chemother.* **44**:621–627.

54. **Powers, R. D., R. Schwartz, R. M. Snow, and D. R. Yarbrough, III.** 1991. Ofloxacin versus cephalexin in the treatment of skin, skin structure, and soft-tissue infections in adults. *Clin. Ther.* **13**:727–736.

55. **Siami, G., N. Christou, I. Eiseman, and K. J. Tack, for The Clinafloxacin Severe Skin and Soft Tissue Infections Study Group.** 2001. Clinafloxacin versus piperacillin-tazobactam in treatment of patients with severe skin and soft tissue infections. *Antimicrob. Agents Chemother.* **45**:525–531.

56. **Swartz, M. N.** 2001. Recognition and management of anthrax: an update. *N. Engl. J. Med.* **345**:1621–1626.

57. **Talan, D. A., D. M. Citron, F. M. Abrahamian, G. J. Moran, and E. J. C. Goldstein, for The Emergency Medicine Animal Bite Infection Study Group.** 1999. Bacteriologic analysis of infected dog and cat bites. *N. Engl. J. Med.* **340**:85–92.

58. **Tarshis, G. A., B. M. Miskin, T. M. Jones, J. Champlin, K. J. Wingert, J. D. Breen, and M. J. Brown.** 2001. Once-daily oral gatifloxacin versus oral levofloxacin in treatment of uncomplicated skin and soft tissue infections: double-blind, multicenter, randomized study. *Antimicrob. Agents Chemother.* **45**:2358–2362.

59. **Tassler, H.** 1993. Comparative efficacy and safety of oral fleroxacin and amoxicillin/clavulanate potassium in skin and soft tissue infection. *Am. J. Med.* **94**(Suppl. 3A):159S–165S.

60. Trampuz, A., M. Wenk, Z. Rajacic, and W. Zimmerli. 2000. Pharmacokinetics and pharmacodynamics of levofloxacin against *Streptococcus pneumoniae* and *Staphylococcus aureus* in human skin blister fluid. *Antimicrob. Agents Chemother.* 44:1352–1355.

61. Wexler, H. M., E. Molitoris, D. Molitoris, and S. M. Finegold. 1998. In vitro activity of levofloxacin against a selected group of anaerobic bacteria isolated from skin and soft tissue infections. *Antimicrob. Agents Chemother.* 42:984–986.

62. Wise, R., J. M. Andrews, J. P. Ashby, and J. Marshall. 1999. A study to determine the pharmacokinetics and inflammatory fluid penetration of gatifloxacin following a single oral dose. *J. Antimicrob. Chemother.* 44:701–704.

63. Wise, R., J. M. Andrews, G. Marshall, and G. Hartman. 1999. Pharmacokinetics and inflammatory-fluid penetration of moxifloxacin following oral or intravenous administration. *Antimicrob. Agents Chemother.* 43:1508–1510.

64. Wise, R., T. Gee, G. Marshall, and J. M. Andrews. 2002. Single-dose pharmacokinetics and penetration of BMS 284756 into an inflammatory exudate. *Antimicrob. Agents Chemother.* 46:242–244.

65. Wise, R., J. Jones, I. Das, and J. M. Andrews. 1998. Pharmacokinetics and inflammatory fluid penetration of clinafloxacin. *Antimicrob. Agents Chemother.* 42: 428–430.

66. Wise, R., D. Mortiboy, J. Child, and J. M. Andrews. 1996. Pharmacokinetics and penetration into inflammatory fluid of trovafloxacin (CP-99,219). *Antimicrob. Agents Chemother.* 40:47–49.

67. Zhao, X., W. Eisner, N. Perl-Rosenthal, B. Kreiswirth, and K. Drlica. 2003. Mutant prevention concentration of garenoxacin (BMS-284756) for ciprofloxacin-susceptible or -resistant *Staphylococcus aureus. Antimicrob. Agents Chemother.* 47:1023–1027.

Chapter 20

Treatment of Intracellular Infections

JEAN-MARC ROLAIN AND DIDIER RAOULT

INTRACELLULAR BEHAVIOR OF PATHOGENS

The intracellular location of some bacteria remains a critical point to explain failures of antibiotic treatment from infected hosts. Parasites that multiply only within eukaryotic cells are obligate intracellular pathogens, whereas facultative intracellular pathogens may multiply in cell-free models (Table 1). Bacteria can reside in phagocytic cells including neutrophils, macrophages, and monocytes or in nonphagocytic cells such as endothelial cells or in erythrocytes (Table 1). Bacteria can survive with or without multiplication in such cells by resistance to the intracellular bactericidal phagolysosomal pathway with various strategies (Fig. 1). Engulfment of parasites inside phagocytic cells leads to the formation of a phagosome that fuses with lysosomes within 20 min. An intracellular parasite can be killed either by an oxygen-dependent killing mechanism (oxidative burst) or by an oxygen-independent mechanism due to the acidity of the phagolysosomal medium (pH = 4.5) and the acidic activation of lysosomes enzymes. Intracellular microorganisms that survive inside eukaryotic cells have elaborated various mechanisms to resist the phagolysosomal pathway. Some of them can infect lysosome-free cells such as erythrocytes, e.g., *Plasmodium* spp. and *Babesia* spp. among protozoa or *Bartonella bacilliformis* (the agent of Carrion's disease) among bacteria. Microorganisms can infect nonphagocytic cells such as endothelial cells (*Rickettsia* spp., *Bartonella* spp.), fibroblasts and epithelial cells (*Chlamydia*), which display lower microbicidal activity than polymorphonuclear leukocytes (PMNs) and macrophages. Only a few bacteria, such as the agent of the human granulocytic ehrlichiosis, can survive in polymorphonuclear cells because of the strong microbicidal activity. Monocytes and macrophages possess lower microbicidal properties than PMNs and can support the survival and multiplication of various microorganisms (*Legionella* spp., *Salmonella* spp., *Brucella* spp., *Yersinia*, *Shigella*,

Coxiella burnetii). Bacteria ingested in these cells lead to the formation of early endosomes, late endosomes, and finally to phagolysosomes in which most organisms are killed due to the presence of local acidity (i.e., pH < 5) and enzymes. Four categories of mechanisms exist to explain the survival of bacteria in such cells (Fig. 1): (i) surviving in cytoplasm after exit from the endosomal compartment with or without fusion of the phagosomal vacuole with lysosomes (*Rickettsia*, *Shigella*, *Listeria*); (ii) surviving in nonfused phagosomes (*Legionella*); (iii) surviving in fused phagosomes (*Chlamydia*, *Salmonella*); and (iv) surviving in lysosomes (*C. burnetii*).

INTRACELLULAR ACTIVITY OF ANTIBIOTICS

Intracellular Uptake and Subcellular Localization of Antibiotics

Activity of antibiotics against intracellular bacteria depends on several factors, including pharmacodynamic and pharmacokinetic properties of drugs (Fig. 2). First, to be active, antibiotics need to reach the cells in tissue compartments by the systemic route. Second, antibiotics need to reach and concentrate in the intracellular compartments. Mechanisms of uptake and subcellular localization of antibiotics are presented in Table 2. The intracellular-to-extracellular ratio (*C/E* ratio) is the most important factor and can be determined by several methods including radiometric, fluorometric, or chemical techniques. Intracellular uptake of antibiotics has been studied by using cell models to determine the intracellular concentration and location in mouse cell lines or human phagocytic cell lines such as PMNs or monocytes. The fluoroquinolones accumulate within phagocytes to give a *C/E* ratio of 6:7 for granulocytes, 3:4 for macrophages, and about 2 in epithelial cells (36–40, 75–80). Accumulation is

Jean-Marc Rolain and Didier Raoult • Unité des Rickettsies CNRS UMR 6020, Faculté de Médecine, Université de la Méditerranée, 27, Boulevard Jean Moulin, 13385 Marseille Cedex 05, France.

Table 1. Target cells and subcellular localization of intracellular bacteria

Type of intracellular bacteria	Target cells	Subcellular localization
Obligate		
Rickettsia	Endothelial cells	Cytosol
Ehrlichia	Macrophages, PMN	Phagosome
Coxiella burnetii	Macrophages	Phagolysosome
Chlamydia	Macrophages, epithelial cells	Phagosome
Tropheryma whipplei	Macrophages	Phagolysosome
Facultative		
Bartonella	Endothelial cells	Phagosome
Brucella	Macrophages	Phagosome
Francisella	Macrophages	Phagolysosome
Legionella	Macrophages	Phagosome
Salmonella	Macrophages	Phagosome
Shigella	Epithelial cells	Cytosol
Yersinia	Macrophages, epithelial cells	Phagosome
Mycobacterium	Macrophages	Phagolysosome
Listeria	Macrophages	Cytosol

temperature dependent and is inhibited at 4°C. Uptake is passive and does not require energy because it persists even when using dead cells. Third, antibiotic should remain active in the intracellular compartment without inactivation by cell metabolism and/or by deleterious effect of the pH (66, 68). Antibiotics can be more effective at neutral or basic pH values (especially the fluoroquinolone compounds), and conversely, antibiotics such as rifampin and pyrazinamide are more effective at acidic pH values. Subcellular localization of antibiotics is also an important factor because bacteria can be concentrated either in cytosol or in lysosome or phagolysosome (Table 2). Fluoroquinolone compounds in cells may be located both in the cytosol and lysosomes, whereas weak base antibiotics such as the aminoglycosides and the macrolides are concentrated within lysosomes. These properties may confer the activity of quinolones on various intracellular pathogens, but acidic pH within phagosomes and phagolysosomes may reduce their antimicrobial activity.

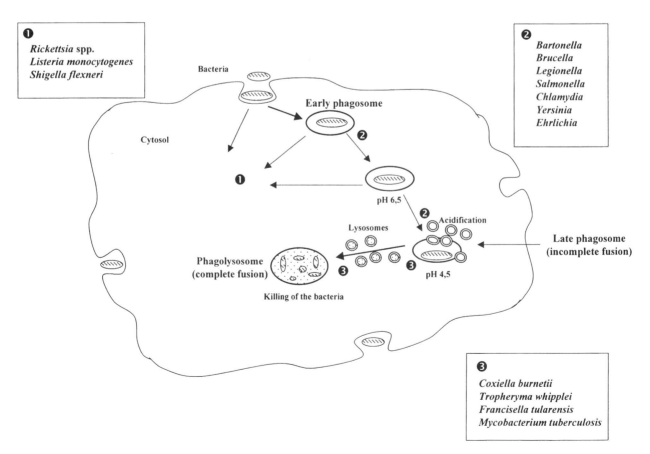

Figure 1. Strategy for survival of intracellular bacteria in cells.

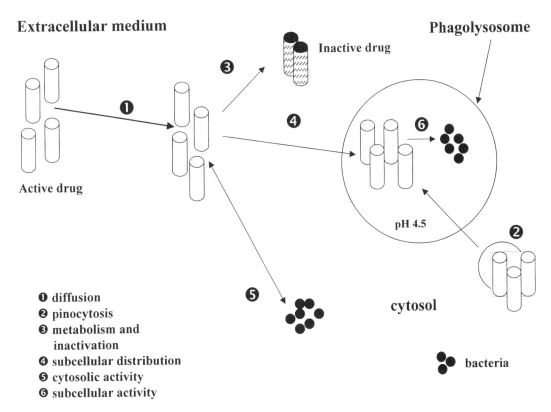

Figure 2. Intracellular uptake and subcellular localization of antibiotics.

Intracellular Antibiotic Activity

Methods

Cell culture models. Although antibiotic susceptibility of facultative intracellular bacteria can be assessed in cell-free systems using classic MIC determination methods, the antibiotic susceptibility of obligate intracellular bacteria should be determined only in infected cell models. In vitro models have been established for determination of the intracellular activity of antibiotics against strict intracellular pathogens (25). These cell

systems may also be useful for facultative intracellular pathogens because of the poor ability of MICs as determined in axenic medium to predict in vivo efficacy of antibiotics. The choice of the cell system depends on each pathogen, but usually the methods used involve cell lines that are easy to obtain and grow, such as Vero, Hel, and MRC5 cells. These models share common features, including infection of cells with the pathogen for a sufficient time to allow penetration of the bacteria, removal of nonphagocytized microorganisms from the extracellular medium, addition of the antibiotic to the culture medium, and evaluation of antibiotic activity using several methods adapted to each bacterium. For some pathogens such as *Chlamydia, Rickettsia,* and *C. burnetii,* centrifugation of the inoculum onto the cell monolayer increases the ratio of infected cells and facilitates the intracellular penetration of pathogens (107). The method of evaluation of antibiotic may vary according to the pathogen considered (69) and the most accurate technique is enumeration of viable intracellular microorganisms (CFU or plaque forming unit counts) after various times of antibiotic exposure as compared with drug-free controls (*Rickettsia, Coxiella*). Measurement of viable bacteria can be done directly after staining the bacteria or indirectly by the formation of plaque due to a cytopathic effect (*Rickettsia*). Other methods of eval-

Table 2. Antibiotic uptake, subcellular localization, and pH of optimum activity of antibiotics[a]

Antibiotic	Mode of entry	Cytosol	Lysosomes	PH of optimum activity
Aminoglycosides	Pinocytosis		+++	7
β-Lactams	Diffusion	+		7
Chloramphenicol	Diffusion	++	Unknown	7
Erythromycin	Transport	+	+++	7.8
Fluoroquinolones	Unknown	++	++	8
Rifampin	Diffusion	++	++	<5
Tetracyclines	Diffusion	++	Unknown	6.6

[a]Symbols: +, low concentration; ++, medium concentration; +++, high concentration.

uation have been used, including determination of the percentage of infected cells (*Ehrlichia, Chlamydia*), flow cytometry (*Chlamydia, Rickettsia*) (35, 56), and the luciferase technique (Mycobacteria) (2).

A bacteriostatic activity corresponds to the inhibition of growth of viable bacteria titer after antibiotic exposure as compared with the same inoculum not treated with antibiotics. A bactericidal effect corresponds to reduction of viable bacteria after antibiotic exposure as compared with the inoculum. The determination of the bactericidal activity of antibiotics is crucial because only such antibiotics would allow eradication of the pathogen from the infected cells, especially in the immunocompromised host. Nevertheless, in vitro models, although very useful to assess the antibiotic susceptibility to antibiotics of the intracellular form of the pathogen, do not reflect the clinical situation.

Animal models. Animal models have been used to assess antibiotic therapeutic efficacy against intracellular pathogens. The design of an animal model should consider the choice of the animal species, the dose of the inoculum, the route of inoculation and of treatment, and the timing between inoculation and treatment (25). The choice of an animal model should be based on a model that reproduces some clinical and most pathological features of the human disease. The route of inoculation must be carefully chosen. In most cases, the pathogen is inoculated intravenously or intraperitoneally even when such routes do not mimic the natural route of infection. For pathogens that naturally invade via the respiratory tract (*Legionella, Coxiella*), experimental inhalation can be performed. However, animal models are not available for most intracellular pathogens, including rickettsial or chlamydial agents, and diseases induced in animals may not reflect accurately the pathophysiological manifestations of human diseases. The difficulty in extrapolating experimental data obtained both in in vitro and animal models to

the clinical situation emphasizes that only clinical data obtained from infected humans are reliable indicators of the utility of an antibiotic regimen.

Results

Many studies have compared the efficacy of quinolones in vitro and in vivo against intracellular pathogens. Indeed, because of their high uptake in cells, fluoroquinolone compounds are of current interest in treating infections due to intracellular pathogens. Antibiotic susceptibility of obligate intracellular bacteria as determined by using in vitro cell models are summarized in Table 3.

Rickettsia are naturally resistant to β-lactams, aminoglycosides, and co-trimoxazole. The typhus group is susceptible to erythromycin, whereas the spotted fever group is not (92). Fluoroquinolones are very effective against *Rickettsia* with similar activity for pefloxacin, ciprofloxacin, sparfloxacin, ofloxacin, and levofloxacin (70, 82, 92). *C. burnetii* is also susceptible to some quinolones to varying degrees (88, 89, 91), and strains resistent in vitro have been found to have mutations in the *gyrA* gene (72). For *Ehrlichia* spp. a wide heterogeneity of susceptibility to fluoroquinolones exists between various *Ehrlichia* species. This variation is due to a natural gyrase-mediated resistance to quinolones in the *Ehrlichia canis* subgroup (65).

Chlamydia are naturally resistant to β-lactams, aminoglycosides, glycopeptides, and imidazoles. *Chlamydia pneumoniae* is naturally resistant to sulfonamides, whereas *Chlamydia trachomatis* is not resistant. In vitro, tetracyclines, macrolides (azithromycin and clarithromycin are more effective than erythromycin), rifampin, and fluoroquinolones (ofloxacin and sparfloxacin) are the most active antibiotics against bacteria of the genus *Chlamydia* (18, 23, 73).

Bacteria of the genus *Salmonella* are usually extremely sensitive to the fluoroquinolone antibiotics

Table 3. Antibiotic susceptibility of obligate intracellular bacteria, as determined using in vitro cell models[a]

Organism	Blm	Amg	Tet	Chm	Sxt	Qui	Rif	Ery	Rox	Azm	Cla
Rickettsia conorii	R	R	S	S	R	S	S	R	S	R	S
Rickettsia rickettsii	R	R	S	S	R	S	S	R	S	R	S
Rickettsia prowazekii	R	R	S	S	R	S	S	S	ND	S	S
Ehrlichia chaffeensis	R	R	S	R	R	R	S	R	ND	ND	ND
Coxiella burnetii	R	R	S	R	S	S	S	S	S	R	S
Chlamydia trachomatis	R	R	S	R	R	S	S	S	S	S	S
Chlamydia psittaci	R	R	S	R	R	S	S	S	S	S	S
Chlamydia pneumoniae	R	R	S	R	R	S	S	S	S	S	S

[a]Abbreviations: Amg, aminoglycosides; Azm, azithromycin; Blm, betalactams; Chm, chloramphenicol; Cla, clarithromycin; Ery, erythromycin; ND, not determined; Qui, quinolones; R, resistant; Rif, rifampin; Rox, roxithromycin; S, susceptible; Sxt, co-trimoxazole; Tet, tetracyclines.

(MICs from 0.03 to 0.125 µg/ml) (108). In time-kill studies, the fluoroquinolones are more rapidly bactericidal than the third-generation cephalosporins. Nevertheless, fluoroquinolone resistance has now been reported in association with single-point mutations in the quinolone resistance-determining region of the *gyrA* gene (13, 104) of *Salmonella enterica* serovar Paratyphi (14) and *Senterica* serovar Typhi (20, 93)

For *Legionella*, fluoroquinolones are more active than all macrolides in vitro and in vivo. Ciprofloxacin, enoxacin, grepafloxacin, levofloxacin, ofloxacin, pefloxacin, sparfloxacin, and trovafloxacin were all active by in vitro dilution methods (103). The quinolones were more active than erythromycin in irreversibly inhibiting the growth of *Legionella pneumophila* within guinea pig alveolar macrophages, peripheral blood monocytes, guinea pig peritoneal macrophages, and HL60 cells (30, 31, 59, 98). Ciprofloxacin, levofloxacin, pefloxacin, sparfloxacin, and trovafloxacin were more active than erythromycin or no therapy in guinea pig models for pneumonia and peritonitis (103).

Studies on the in vitro activity of fluoroquinolones against *Francisella tularensis* are scarce. Only two studies report the in vitro antibiotic sus-

ceptibility of quinolones, including ciprofloxacin, levofloxacin, grepafloxacin, and trovafloxacin (MICs ranging from 0.016 to 0.047 µg/ml) (52, 99). These studies, which show the bactericidal effect of quinolones against *F. tularensis* in an in vitro cell model, were confirmed by Maurin et al. (67).

CLINICAL RELEVANCE OF QUINOLONES FOR THE TREATMENT OF INTRACELLULAR PATHOGENS

Antibiotic treatment recommendations for intracellular pathogens are given in Table 4.

Obligate Intracellular Bacteria

Rickettsia

The genus *Rickettsia* includes spotted fever group rickettsiae, typhus group rickettsiae, and scrub typhus (due to *Orientia tsutsugamushi*). The spotted fever group comprises 14 known species that are responsible for diseases in humans and includes *R. conorii*, the agent of Mediterranean spotted fever (MSF), and

Table 4. Antibiotic treatment recommendations for intracellular pathogens[a]

Disease/causative organism	Treatment recommendation(s) for:	
	Adult	Children
Spotted fever group rickettsiae	Doxycycline 200 mg b.i.d., 1 day	Doxycycline 5 mg/kg b.i.d., 1 day
	Or ofloxacin 200 mg b.i.d., 7 days	Or josamycin 50 mg/kg/day, 14 days
Typhus	Doxycycline 200 mg b.i.d., 1 day	Doxycycline 5 mg/kg b.i.d., 1 day
Acute Q fever	Doxycycline 100 mg b.i.d., 21 days	Co-trimoxazole (trimethoprim-sulfamethoxazole)
	Or ofloxacin 200 mg b.i.d., 14 days	16/80 mg/5 kg b.i.d., 14 days
Chlamydia trachomatis	Doxycycline 100 mg b.i.d., 7 days	Erythromycin 10 mg/kg q.i.d., 14 days
	Or azithromycin 1 g orally, single dose	
Chlamydia psittaci	Doxycycline 100 mg b.i.d., 14 days	Erythromycin 50 mg/kg/day, 14 days
	Or erythromycin 500 mg q.i.d., 14 days	
	Or ofloxacin 200 mg b.i.d., 14 days	
Chlamydia pneumoniae	Doxycycline 100 mg b.i.d., 14 days	Erythromycin 50 mg/kg/day, 14 days
	Or erythromycin 500 mg q.i.d., 14 days	
	Or ofloxacin 250 mg q.i.d., 21 days	
Legionellosis	Azithromycin 500 mg, 7 to 10 days	Erythromycin 50 mg/kg/day, 14 days
	Or ofloxacin 400 mg b.i.d., 10 days	
Typhoid	Ofloxacin (200 mg b.i.d.)	Ceftriaxone 100 mg/kg once a day
	Or ciprofloxacin (500 mg b.i.d.), 7 days	Or cotrimoxazole 16/80 mg/5 kg b.i.d., 14 days
	Or ceftriaxone 2 g once a day	
Salmonella enteritis	Ciprofloxacin 500 mg b.i.d., 7 days	Ceftriaxone 100 mg/kg once a day
	Or Ceftriaxone 2 g once a day	Or cotrimoxazole 16/80 mg/5 kg b.i.d., 14 days
Yersiniosis	Ofloxacin 400 mg/day, 7 to 14 days	Gentamicin 3 mg/kg/day, 7 to 14 days
	Or gentamicin 3 mg/kg/day, 7 to 14 days	
	Or doxycycline 200 mg/day, 7 to 14 days	
Shigellosis	Ciprofloxacin 500 mg b.i.d., 5 days	Ceftriaxone 50 mg/kg/day single dose
Tularemia	Streptomycin 10 mg/kg b.i.d., i.m., 7 to 10 days	Streptomycin 10 mg/kg b.i.d., i.m., 7 to 10 days
	Or doxycycline 200 mg/day, 14 days	
	Or ciprofloxacin 750 mg b.i.d., 14 days	

[a]Abbreviations: i.m., intramuscular; q.i.d., 4 times daily.

Rickettsia rickettsii, the agent of Rocky Mountain spotted fever (RMSF) (85). The typhus group includes *Rickettsia typhi*, the agent of murine typhus, and *Rickettsia prowazekii*, the agent of epidemic typhus (85). The tetracyclines [mainly doxycycline 100 mg twice a day (b.i.d.) orally or intravenously in severe cases] remain the first-line antibiotic regimen to treat rickettsial diseases. A single-day regimen of doxycycline orally (200 mg b.i.d.) is currently used for Mediterranean spotted fever, epidemic typhus, murine typhus, and scrub typhus (5, 12, 51, 81, 84). Pefloxacin (400 mg/b.i.d. for 11 days), either alone or in combination with rifampin in severe cases, was used successfully to treat patients with MSF, including two patients with neuromeningeal complications (54). Ciprofloxacin was used also in five patients with MSF, including a human immunodeficiency virus (HIV)-infected patient (83). Ciprofloxacin has been compared with doxycycline in the treatment of MSF in a randomized double-blind evaluation (46). Although doxycycline yielded a more rapid defervescence than ciprofloxacin, and clinical manifestations such as headache, arthralgia, and myalgia resolved more rapidly, ciprofloxacin was considered as an effective alternative. Apyrexia was obtained with ofloxacin (200 mg b.i.d. for 7 days) in 15 patients with MSF and is currently the recommended alternative to doxycycline (8).

Coxiella

C. burnetii is the etiological agent of Q fever (71). The disease may present acutely with a self-limited febrile illness, pneumonitis, or hepatitis. Chronic Q fever is typically due to endocarditis. Although acute infections respond to antibiotic therapy, chronic infections are difficult to cure. Tetracyclines remain the first-line antibiotics to treat acute Q fever. Oral doxycycline (100 mg b.i.d. for 21 days) allows reduction of the febrile period. Fluoroquinolones are effective against *C. burnetii* in vitro (44, 57, 70, 87, 91, 110) and have been used as an alternative to tetracyclines in vivo to treat patients suffering from acute Q fever (9, 71). Ofloxacin (200 mg b.i.d.) is considered the best alternative to doxycycline to treat acute Q fever in adults. For chronic Q fever, mainly endocarditis, the treatment combination currently used is a combination of doxycycline and hydroxychloroquine for 18 months, a combination that is more effective with fewer relapses than the combination of ofloxacin and doxycycline (86).

Ehrlichia

Ehrlichia chaffeensis is the etiological agent of human monocytic ehrlichiosis in the United States (21). The disease is most often diagnosed in spring and summer in patients with a history of tick bite. Clinical manifestations of the disease may vary from asymptomatic to severe, and symptoms are similar to those of RMSF: patients typically present with high fever, headache, chills, malaise, and myalgia. Rash occurs in only one-third, and the lack of rash may help to distinguish ehrlichiosis from RMSF. The etiological agent of human granulocytic ehrlichiosis (HGE) is closely related to the veterinary pathogens *Ehrlichia phagocytohila* and *Ehrlichia equi* and has recently been described in a patient who was bitten by ticks. Clinical manifestations of HGE are similar to those of ehrlichiosis due to *E. chaffeensis* but in general are more severe. Sennetsu fever is a mononucleosis-like illness caused by *Erhlichia sennetsu*, which was discovered in Japan. Patients have a self-limited febrile illness with malaise, anorexia, and lymphadenopathy. No fatalities or severe complications have been reported.

Tetracyclines are highly active in vitro against *E. sennetsu*, *E. chaffeensis*, and the HGE agent (10, 11, 60), and doxycycline is currently the first-line antibiotic in treating ehrlichial diseases (3, 26, 106). However, these antibiotics are contraindicated in children younger than 8 years old because of tooth discoloration and in pregnant women because of bone toxicity to the fetus. Failures have been reported with chloramphenicol in patients with monocytic ehrlichiosis or human granulocytic ehrlichiosis, and the agents of these conditions are not susceptible to chloramphenicol in vitro (26). Rifampin is active against ehrlichia in vitro and may represent a safe alternative in these situations. Its clinical use has been suggested for pregnant women with HGE (15). In vitro susceptibility to fluoroquinolones depends on *Ehrlichia* species, with *E. sennetsu* and the HGE agent being susceptible (10, 60) and *E. chaffeensis* being resistant (11). This difference in susceptibility to fluoroquinolones has been related recently to a natural DNA gyrase-mediated resistance in the latter group (65). Fluoroquinolones have not been used extensively in ehrlichial diseases.

Chlamydial diseases

The genus *Chlamydia* comprises three species responsible for human infections: *C. trachomatis*, the agent of trachoma (a chronic keratoconjunctivitis leading to blindness) in developing countries and sexually transmitted diseases (urethritis in men; cervicitis, salpingitis, and uretritis in women) and neonatal infections (conjunctivitis and pneumonia) worldwide; *Chlamydia psittaci*, the etiological agent of psittacosis; and *C. pneumoniae*, an etiological agent of atypical pneumonia.

Doxycycline and azithromycin are the antibiotics of choice for the treatment of infections due to *C. trachomatis*. The currently recommended regimens are doxycycline 200 mg/day for 7 days for urethritis in men and 10 to 14 days for cervicitis, or azithromycin 250 mg b.i.d. (100). Azithromycin can be used as the first single-dose therapy (1 g) for *C. trachomatis* infections (69). Ciprofloxacin was effective in chlamydial infections of the urogenital tracts of women treated with a dosage regimen of 500 mg orally b.i.d. for 7 days (1) or 1.5 g/day (55). Ofloxacin may be an effective drug for the treatment of lower genital tract infections with *C. trachomatis* in men and women, and there are indications that ofloxacin may also be of value in the treatment of chlamydial epididymitis and salpingitis (74). Salpingitis is often associated with other pathogens such as enterobacteria and anaerobic bacteria, and the treatment of choice is amoxicillin-clavulanic acid plus doxycycline or ofloxacin for 14 days. For neonatal pulmonary infections due to *C. trachomatis*, the treatment of choice is erythromycin (40 mg/kg of body weight/day), since tetracyclines and fluoroquinolones are contraindicated.

C. pneumoniae can cause acute atypical pneumonia. Transmission occurred from human to human by the airborne route, via infected respiratory secretions. The proportion of community-acquired pneumonias associated with *C. pneumoniae* has been estimated to be 6 to 22%, depending on geographical location, age group, and then diagnostic methods used (49). *C. psittaci* is the agent of psittacosis, a zoonosis transmitted by birds (especially *Psittacides*). The disease is usually an acute pneumonia with various extrapulmonary clinical manifestations, including meningitis or meningoencephalitis, endocarditis or myocarditis, and hepatitis. The drugs of choice for the treatment of acute respiratory infections due to *C. pneumoniae* or *C. psittaci* include doxycycline (100 mg b.i.d. for 14 days) or erythromycin (500 mg four times daily for 14 days) (53). Psittacosis has a high mortality rate and must be treated with tetracyclines immediately on clinical suspicion (96). For children, only erythromycin should be used at 30 to 50 mg/kg/day every 6 h. More recently it has been demonstrated that clarithromycin and azithromycin are likely to be at least as effective as doxycycline or erythromycin for *C. pneumoniae* infections (53). Although the newer fluoroquinolones are two- to tenfold more potent in vitro than the older agents against *C. pneumoniae*, they are still less potent than the macrolides and tetracyclines. Considering the enhanced pharmacokinetic properties and tissue penetration of the newer quinolones, these agents might be expected to be as effective as the macrolides in the treatment of pneumonias due to *C. pneumoniae*. Successful treatment of patients with pneumonia and bronchitis caused by *C. pneumoniae* has been reported with ofloxacin (400 mg b.i.d. for 14 days) (48, 64), sparfloxacin (200 mg b.i.d. for 14 days) (22), and levofloxacin (33). In these studies diagnosis of the disease was only based on serology, and improvment of clinical manifestations was the criterion for cure. Only one anecdotal report exists of the use of quinolones in *C. pneumoniae* infection in which cultures were performed (90). Three patients with *C. pneumoniae*-positive cultures were treated with grepafloxacin (600 mg p.o. orally daily for 10 to 14 days). Two of the three patients remained culture positive and symptomatic despite 2 weeks of treatment. In conclusion, new quinolones might be useful in the treatment of chlamydial respiratory infections, but more clinical trials are needed.

Facultative Intracellular Bacteria

Bartonella and Brucella

Bartonella and *Brucella* species belong to the α2 subgroup of *Proteobacteria*. The genus *Bartonella* includes 14 validated species, five of which have been associated with human infections: *B. henselae*, *B. quintana*, *B. elizabethae*, *B. clarridgeiae*, and *B. bacilliformis*. The spectrum of diseases caused by *Bartonella* species includes cat scratch disease, bacillary angiomatosis, peliosis hepatitis, endocarditis, trench fever, bacteremia in homeless persons, and Carrion's disease, which manifests as Oroya fever or verruga peruana. Infections due to *Brucella* spp. are common zoonoses in many parts of the world and may present with a broad spectrum of clinical manifestations. The most frequent complications involve the gastrointestinal tract (hepatitis, splenitis), the skeletal (arthritis, spondylitis, osteomyelitis), the central nervous system (meningitis, meningoencephalitis), and the cardiovascular system (endocarditis). Two combination antibiotic regimens are recommended for human brucellosis, including doxycycline 100 mg b.i.d. with streptomycin 500 mg b.i.d., and doxycycline 100 mg b.i.d. with rifampin 300 mg b.i.d. or three times daily for 6 weeks (47). Prolonged therapy for at least 3 months is recommended when complications occur. Available clinical trials using fluoroquinolones do not support clinical efficacy despite the promising in vitro activity of these compounds (62).

Current knowledge indicates that brucellosis and *Bartonella*-related infections share comparable microbiological, pathophysiological, and clinical findings. Brucellosis and *Bartonella* infections are mainly characterized by two clinical forms: acute and chronic stages. A broad spectrum of chronic infections are caused by *Bartonella* species: endocarditis, cutaneous tumor (verruga peruana due to *B. bacilliformis* and bacillary angiomatosis due to *B. henselae* and *B. quintana*), and osteoarticular damages. Streptomycin is considered regularly effective to treat verruga peruana (16). Aminoglycosides, especially gentamicin, are also used to treat patients with *Bartonella*-related endocarditis (34). In our experience (unpublished results) and in experience reported in the literature, all patients treated with a combination of tetracycline for 6 weeks and an aminoglycoside for 2 weeks fully recovered without any relapse, although valve replacement was required for most of the patients because of extensive valvular damage.

Salmonella, Shigella, and *Yersinia*

Salmonellosis is a relatively common infection in humans, most often as a food-borne gastrointestinal illness and less often as a nonintestinal illness. Salmonellosis can be divided in two subgroups of clinical entities: (i) gastroenteritis and associated complications and (ii) typhoid or enteric fever. Enteritis due to *Salmonella* consists of a diarrheal illness with abdominal pain and fever, but clinical symptomatology is quite variable. The diarrhea is watery and mild or prolonged and associated with blood and mucus. Disease onset occurs most often in 48 to 72 h after ingestion. Complications from intestinal salmonellosis may occur simultaneously with the acute diarrheal disease or at least within a short time thereafter (45). The more common complications concern bone and joint, hepatobiliary and spleen, pulmonary, genital, central nervous system, and vascular. The clinical features of enteric fever may vary considerably between different geographic regions. Symptoms of typhoid and paratyphoid are similar, although paratyphoid tends to be a milder infection. Untreated, typhoid fever will often resolve after several weeks, but patients may die during the course of the illness from circulatory collapse. Chloramphenicol has long been considered the antibiotic of choice to treat typhoid fever but has now been abandoned because of a high rate of relapses and possible bone marrow toxicity. Currently recommended regimen of typhoid fever include a broad-spectrum cephalosporin (ceftriaxone, 2 g once daily for 7 to 10 days), or a quinolone (ciprofloxacin, 500 mg b.i.d. intravenously for 7 to 14 days) (97). Indeed, the newer fluoroquinolones have proved to be the most effective drugs for treatment of enteric fever (28, 105). Clinical trials have been performed with several quinolones, including ofloxacin, ciprofloxacin, norfloxacin, and fleroxacin (108) and for a total of 19 randomized trials (corresponding to 788 patients with culture-confirmed enteric fever due to *S. enterica* serovar Typhi), the overall pooled cure rate was of 97.3%. Conversely, randomized trials involving third-generation cephalosporins display a cure rate of 79%. Thus, the fluoroquinolones were clearly superior to oral or parenteral third-generation cephalosporins in typhoid (108). Moreover, treatment plays an important role in the eradication of biliary and urinary foci of bacteria. Treatment of nontyphoidal salmonellosis primarily involves rehydration and does not require administration of antibiotics. Antibiotic therapy using either a quinolone or a third-generation cephalosporin for 7 days should be recommended to prevent bacteremia in some patient groups, including immunocompromised patients, the elderly, especially those with atherosclerosis or cardiovascular abnormalities, and neonates (third-generation cephalosporin only).

The clinical manifestation of shigellosis, like salmonelloses, is mainly diarrhea, but the spectrum of intestinal illness is variable. The incubation period ranges from 48 to 96 h. Nevertheless, shigellosis is often more severe than salmonellosis, with fever, abdominal pain, and severe diarrhea. Trimethoprim-sulfamethoxazole and ampicillin have long been considered the treatment of choice for shigellosis and severe travelers' diarrhea (29, 94), but quinolones represent the optimal agent for therapy of bacterial diarrhea in adults in areas where trimethoprim and ampicillin-resistant enteric pathogens are common (27). Ciprofloxacin (500 mg every 12 h for 5 days) is the currently recommended antibiotic regimen in treating patients with shigellosis (6, 7, 58). A short-course therapy with norfloxacin can be used effectively to treat shigellosis in adults in developing countries (4). Nevertheless, quinolone resistance among *Shigella* has been reported recently (43) but is rare (109) and should be investigated to better define the optimum treatment in such situations.

Gastrointestinal infection due to *Yersinia enterocolitica* is the most common form of the yersinioses. Patients often have prominent abdominal pain with or without fever. In its severe enteric form the diarrheal illness is a dysentery. During the enteritis the bacteria can become invasive, and complications may occur in certain patients. As a consequence of the bacteremia various sites may become involved with secondary infection including large blood vessels, bone, joint, liver, and central nervous system. Untreated, the morbidity and mortality of such complications are high. Although *Y. enterocolitica* is susceptible to several antibiotics in vitro, only a few antibiotics display in vivo activity, including chloramphenicol, doxycycline, cotrimoxazole, and ciprofloxacin (41, 50). The most advisable antibiotic regimen is an aminoglycoside (gentamicin 3 mg/kg/day in two or three doses intravenously), either alone or combined with doxycycline or ofloxacin (400 mg/day for 10 to 14 days). Ofloxacin should be preferred for invasive infections due to *Y. enterocolitica*, especially for bone and joint infections (19)

Legionella

L. pneumophila is the agent of Legionnaires' disease, which manifests typically by bilateral pneumonia, or Pontiac fever, a febrile, self-limited, flu-like illness without apparent lung involvment. Infection occurs via the respiratory tract by inhalation of contaminated aerosols. Erythromycin was historically considered the antibiotic of choice (500 mg 4 times daily orally for 10 to 14 days) for the treatment of Legionnaires' disease. The new macrolides, especially azithromycin (500 mg daily for 7 to 10 days), are promising (103).

Promising results have been obtained with the newer fluoroquinolones. Monotherapy with ciprofloxacin was described as clinically effective in 80% (8 of 10) of critically ill immunocompromised patients with community and nosocomially acquired Legionnaires' disease (102). In this same study, 40% (4 of 10) of the patients were initially unresponsive to treatment with erythromycin and rifampin, but treatment with ciprofloxacin resulted in clinical cure in 75% (3 of 4) of these nonresponders. Clinical failures of ciprofloxacin treatment have been reported in three cases in which a low dosage of 400 mg daily was given (61, 102).

Ofloxacin (400 mg b.i.d. for 10 days) has been used successfully in the treatment of Legionnaires' disease (42). Clinical failure of ofloxacin treatment was reported in a HIV-infected patient receiving a low dosage of 200 mg b.i.d. (103).

In four prospective, randomized trials, oral sparfloxacin (400 mg on day 1 followed by 200 mg daily for 10 to 14 days) resulted in 75% (3 of 4) cure in patients with serologically confirmed Legionnaires' disease (103). In a prospective, randomized trial, oral sparfloxacin (400 mg on day 1 followed by 200 mg daily for up to 10 days) yielded a bacteriological response in two patients with Legionnaires' disease, diagnosed by a positive sputum culture in one patient and by a positive urinary antigen in the other (24).

In two prospective, randomized trials of intravenous alatrofloxacin (the prodrug of trovafloxacin) followed by oral trovafloxacin (200 mg daily to complete a total of 7 to 14 days of therapy), there was a 77% (10 of 13) cure of patients with serologically confirmed Legionnaires' disease (103).

Successful treatment of Legionnaires' disease has also been reported with levofloxacin (500 mg daily for 7 to 14 days) (33) and grepafloxacin (600 mg daily for 10 days) (101).

For nosocomal pneumonias, nursing home pneumonias, and transplant recipients in whom *L. pneumophila* is considered a potential pathogen, the quinolones (especially ciprofloxacin, levofloxacin, and trovafloxacin) may be the empirical drugs of choice.

Francisella

The drug of choice for the treatment of tularemia is streptomycin, with tetracycline and chloramphenicol being used as alternatives (52). Gentamicin has recently been suggested as an acceptable alternative to streptomycin (32). In Europe, *F. tularensis* causes mild infections, while ulceroglandular tularemia with primary ulceration and regional lymphadenopathy is the most common form of the disease. These infections are not usually severe enough to require hospitalization of the patients, and oral antibiotic treatment at home would be ideal. In vitro and in vivo studies have shown that quinolones are promising alternatives for such treatment of tularemia. Three patients with pneumonic tularemia and one with ulceroglandular tularemia were successfully treated with ciprofloxacin (750 mg b.i.d.), and one patient has been successfully cured with norfloxacin (400 mg b.i.d. for 10 days) (99). All five patients responded to treatment within 48 h, and no relapses occurred within 6 months. Scheel reported in 1992 the case of a veterinarian with ulceroglandular tularemia cured with ciprofloxacin (750 mg b.i.d. for 2 weeks without relapse at a follow-up examination 2 months later) (95). In 1999 Limaye and Hooper discussed two patients with tularemia successfully treated with levofloxacin and reviewed eight cases of tularemia treated with quinolones with a favorable clinical response in all cases (63). Recently, Chocarro et al. reported 14 cases of an outbreak of tularemia treated with quinolones, and seven patients relapsed after treatment with ciprofloxacin (17). In conclusion, quinolone compounds should be considered as alternative agents for tularemia therapy.

CONCLUSIONS

Fluoroquinolones are extremely effective against intracellular pathogens in vitro and in vivo due to their ability to penetrate eukaryotic cells and to concentrate in subcellular compartments. Thus, these compounds represent valuable therapeutic alternatives or drugs of choice for infections caused by intracellular pathogens, including Q fever, spotted fever group rickettsiosis, tularemia, *Salmonella* enteritis and typhoid, yersiniosis and shigellosis, *Chlamydia* infections, and legionellosis. The newer fluoroquinolones are promising antimicrobial agents for these diseases, but multicenter clinical trials may be necessary to confirm their effectiveness, especially when the disease is rare.

REFERENCES

1. Ahmed-Jushuf, I. H., O. P. Arya, D. Hobson, B. C. Pratt, C. A. Hart, S. J. How, I. A. Tait, and P. M. Rao. 1988. Ciprofloxacin treatment of chlamydial infections of urogenital tracts of women. *Genitourin. Med.* 64:14–17.

2. Arain, T. M., A. E. Resconi, D. C. Singh, and C. K. Stover. 1996. Reporter gene technology to assess activity of antimycobacterial agents in macrophages. *Antimicrob. Agents Chemother.* 40:1542–1544.

3. Bakken, J. S., J. Krueth, C. Wilsonnordskog, R. L. Tilden, K. Asanovich, and J. S. Dumler. 1996. Clinical and laboratory characteristics of human granulocytic ehrlichiosis. *JAMA* 275:199–205.

4. Bassily, S., K. C. Hyams, N. A. el Masry, Z. Farid, E. Cross, A. L. Bourgeois, E. Ayad, and R. G. Hibbs. 1994. Short-course norfloxacin and trimethoprim-sulfamethoxazole treatment of shigellosis and salmonellosis in Egypt. *Am. J. Trop. Med. Hyg.* 51:219–223.

5. Bella-Cueto, F., B. Font-Creus, F. Segura-Porta, E. Espejo-Arenas, P. Lopez-Parez, and T. Munoz-Espin. 1987. Comparative, randomized trial of one-day doxycycline versus 10-day tetracycline therapy for Mediterranean spotted fever. *J. Infect. Dis.* 155:1056–1058.

6. Bennish, M. L., M. A. Salam, R. Haider, and M. Barza. 1990. Therapy for shigellosis. II. Randomized, double-blind comparison of ciprofloxacin and ampicillin. *J. Infect. Dis.* 162:711–716.

7. Bennish, M. L., M. A. Salam, W. A. Khan, and A. M. Khan. 1992. Treatment of shigellosis: III. Comparison of one- or two-dose ciprofloxacin with standard 5-day therapy. A randomized, blinded trial. *Ann. Intern. Med.* 117:727–734.

8. Bernard, E., M. Carles, S. Politano, C. Laffont, and P. Dellamonica. 1989. Rickettsiosis caused by *Rickettsia conorii*: treatment with ofloxacin. *Rev. Infect. Dis.* 11:S989–S991.

9. Bertrand, A., F. Janbon, O. Jonquet, and J. Reynes. 1988. Infections par les rickettsiales et fluoroquinolones. *Pathol. Biol.* 36:493–495.

10. Brouqui, P., and D. Raoult. 1990. In vitro susceptibility of *Ehrlichia sennetsu* to antibiotics. *Antimicrob. Agents Chemother.* 34:1593–1596.

11. Brouqui, P., and D. Raoult. 1992. In vitro antibiotic susceptibility of the newly recognized agent of ehrhlichiosis in humans, *Ehrlichia chaffeensis*. *Antimicrob. Agents Chemother.* 36:2799–2803.

12. Brown, G. W., J. P. Saunders, S. Singh, D. L. Huxsoll, and A. Shirai. 1978. Single dose doxycycline therapy for scrub typhus. *Trans. R. Soc. Trop. Med. Hyg.* 72:412–416.

13. Brown, J. C., C. J. Thomson, and S. G. Amyes. 1996. Mutations of the gyrA gene of clinical isolates of Salmonella typhimurium and three other Salmonella species leading to decreased susceptibilities to 4-quinolone drugs. *J. Antimicrob. Chemother.* 37:351–356.

14. Brown, N. M., M. R. Millar, J. A. Frost, and B. Rowe. 1994. Ciprofloxacin resistance in *Salmonella* paratyphi A. *J. Antimicrob. Chemother.* 33:1258–1259.

15. Buitrago, M. I., J. W. Ijdo, P. Rinaudo, H. Simon, J. Copel, J. Gadbaw, R. Heimer, E. Fikrig, and F. J. Bia. 1998. Human granulocytic ehrlichiosis during pregnancy treated successfully with rifampin. *Clin. Infect. Dis.* 27:213–215.

16. Caceres-Rios, H., J. Rodriguez-Tafur, F. Bravo-Puccio, C. Maguin-Avargas, C. S. Diaz, D. C. Ramos, and R. Patarca. 1995. Verruga peruana: an infectious endemic angiomatosis. *Crit. Rev. Oncog.* 6:47–56.

17. Chocarro, A., A. Gonzalez, and I. Garcia. 2000. Treatment of tularemia with ciprofloxacin. *Clin. Infect. Dis.* 31:623.

18. Cooper, M. A., J. M. Andrews, J. P. Ashby, R. S. Matthews, and R. Wise. 1990. In-vitro activity of sparfloxacin, a new quinolone antimicrobial agent. *J. Antimicrob. Chemother.* 26:667–676.

19. Crowe, M., K. Ashford, and P. Ispahani. 1996. Clinical features and antibiotic treatment of septic arthritis and osteomyelitis due to *Yersinia enterocolitica*. *J. Med. Microbiol.* 45:302–309.

20. Daga, M. K., K. Sarin, and R. Sarkar. 1994. A study of culture positive multidrug resistant enteric fever—changing pattern and emerging resistance to ciprofloxacin. *J. Assoc. Physicians India* 42:599–600.

21. Dawson, J. E., B. E. Anderson, D. B. Fishbein, J. L. Sanchez, C. S. Goldsmith, K. H. Wilson, and C. W. Duntley. 1991. Isolation and characterization of an *Ehrlichia* sp. from a patient diagnosed with human Ehrlichiosis. *J. Clin. Microbiol.* 29:2741–2745.

22. DeAbate, C. A., D. Henry, G. Bensch, A. Jubran, S. Chodosh, L. Harper, D. Tipping, and G. H. Talbot. 1998. Sparfloxacin vs ofloxacin in the treatment of acute bacterial exacerbations of chronic bronchitis: a multicenter, double-blind, randomized, comparative study. Sparfloxacin Multicenter ABECB Study Group. *Chest* 114:120–130.

23. Donati, M., F. M. Rodriguez, A. Olmo, L. D'Apote, and R. Cevenini. 1999. Comparative in-vitro activity of moxifloxacin, minocycline and azithromycin against *Chlamydia* spp. *J. Antimicrob. Chemother.* 43:825–827.

24. Donowitz, G. R., M. L. Brandon, J. P. Salisbury, C. P. Harman, D. M. Tipping, A. E. Urick, and G. H. Talbot. 1997. Sparfloxacin versus cefaclor in the treatment of patients with community-acquired pneumonia: a randomized, double-masked, comparative, multicenter study. *Clin. Ther.* 19:936–953.

25. Drancourt, M., and D. Raoult. 1993. Methodology of antibiotics testing for intracellular pathogens, p. 71–85. *In* D. Raoult (ed.), *Antimicrobial Agents and Intracellular Pathogens*. CRC Press, Boca Raton, Fla.

26. Dumler, J. S., and J. S. Bakken. 1995. Ehrlichial diseases of humans: emerging tick-borne infections. *Clin. Infect. Dis.* 20:1102–1110.

27. DuPont, H. L. 1991. Use of quinolones in the treatment of gastrointestinal infections. *Eur. J. Clin. Microbiol. Infect. Dis.* 10:325–329.

28. DuPont, H. L. 1993. Quinolones in *Salmonella* typhi infection. *Drugs* 45(Suppl. 3):119–124.

29. DuPont, H. L., C. D. Ericsson, A. Robinson, and P. C. Johnson. 1987. Current problems in antimicrobial therapy for bacterial enteric infection. *Am. J. Med.* 82:324–328.

30. Edelstein, P. H., M. A. Edelstein, and B. Holzknecht. 1992. In vitro activities of fleroxacin against clinical isolates of *Legionella* spp., its pharmacokinetics in guinea pigs, and use to treat guinea pigs with L. pneumophila pneumonia. *Antimicrob. Agents Chemother.* 36:2387–2391.

31. Edelstein, P. H., M. A. Edelstein, J. Weidenfeld, and M. B. Dorr. 1990. In vitro activity of sparfloxacin (CI-978; AT-4140) for clinical Legionella isolates, pharmacokinetics in guinea pigs, and use to treat guinea pigs with L. pneumophila pneumonia. *Antimicrob. Agents Chemother.* **34:**2122–2127.

32. Enderlin, G., L. Morales, R. F. Jacobs, and J. T. Cross. 1994. Streptomycin and alternative agents for the treatment of tularemia: review of the literature. *Clin. Infect. Dis.* **19:**42–47.

33. File, T. M., Jr. 1999. Levofloxacin in the treatment of community acquired pneumonia. *Can. Respir. J.* **6**(Suppl. A):35A–39A.

34. Fournier, P. E., H. Lelievre, S. J. Eykyn, J. L. Mainardi, T. J. Marrie, F. Bruneel, C. Roure, J. Nash, D. Clave, E. James, C. Benoit-Lemercier, L. Deforges, H. Tissot-Dupont, and D. Raoult. 2001. Epidemiologic and clinical characteristics of *Bartonella quintana* and *Bartonellahenselae* endocarditis: a study of 48 patients. *Medicine (Baltimore)* **80:**245–251.

35. Gant, V. A., G. Warnes, I. Philips, and G. F. Savidge. 1993. The application of flow cytometry to the study of bacterial responses to antibiotics. *J. Med. Microbiol.* **39:**147–154.

36. Garcia, I., A. Pascual, S. Ballesta, and E. J. Perea. 2000. Uptake and intracellular activity of ofloxacin isomers in human phagocytic and non-phagocytic cells. *Int. J. Antimicrob. Agents* **15:**201–205.

37. Garcia, I., A. Pascual, M. C. Conejo, and E. J. Perea. 1996. [Intracellular penetration of 5 quinolones into non-phagocytic cells]. *Enferm. Infecc. Microbiol. Clin.* **14:**167–170.

38. Garcia, I., A. Pascual, M. C. Guzman, and E. J. Perea. 1992. Uptake and intracellular activity of sparfloxacin in human polymorphonuclear leukocytes and tissue culture cells. *Antimicrob. Agents Chemother.* **36:**1053–1056.

39. Garcia, I., A. Pascual, and E. J. Perea. 1994. Intracellular penetration and activity of BAY Y 3118 in human polymorphonuclear leukocytes. *Antimicrob. Agents Chemother.* **38:**2426–2429.

40. Garraffo, R., D. Jambou, R. M. Chichmanian, S. Ravoire, and P. Lapalus. 1991. In vitro and in vivo ciprofloxacin pharmacokinetics in human neutrophils. *Antimicrob. Agents Chemother.* **35:**2215–2218.

41. Gayraud, M., M. R. Scavizzi, H. H. Mollaret, L. Guillevin, and M. J. Hornstein. 1993. Antibiotic treatment of *Yersinia enterocolitica* septicemia: a retrospective review of 43 cases. *Clin. Infect. Dis.* **17:**405–410.

42. Gentry, L. O. 1991. Review of quinolones in the treatment of infections of the skin and skin structure. *J. Antimicrob. Chemother.* **28**(Suppl. C):97–110.

43. Ghosh, A. S., J. Ahamed, K. K. Chauhan, and M. Kundu. 1998. Involvement of an efflux system in high-level fluoroquinolone resistance of *Shigella dysenteriae*. *Biochem. Biophys. Res. Commun.* **242:**54–56.

44. Gikas, A., I. Spyridaki, A. Psaroulaki, D. Kofterithis, and Y. Tselentis. 1999. In vitro susceptibility of *Coxiella burnetii* to trovafloxacin in comparison with susceptibilities to pefloxacin, ciprofloxacin, ofloxacin, doxycycline, and clarithromycin. *Antimicrob. Agents Chemother.* **42:**2747–2748.

45. Goldberg, M. B., and R. H. Rubin. 1988. The spectrum of *Salmonella* infection. *Infect. Dis. Clin. N. Am.* **2:**571–598.

46. Gudiol, F., R. Pallares, J. Carratala, F. Bolao, J. Ariza, G. Rufi, and P. F. Viladrich. 1989. Randomized double-blind evaluation of ciprofloxacin and doxycycline for Mediterranean spotted fever. *Antimicrob. Agents Chemother.* **33:**987–988.

47. Hall, W. H. 1990. Modern chemotherapy for brucellosis in humans. *Rev. Infect. Dis.* **12:**1060–1099.

48. Hammerschlag, M. R. 1999. Activity of quinolones against *Chlamydia pneumoniae*. *Drugs* **58**(Suppl. 2):78–81.

49. Hammerschlag, M. R. 2000. Activity of gemifloxacin and other new quinolones against *Chlamydia pneumoniae:* a review. *J. Antimicrob. Chemother.* **45**(Suppl. 1):35–39.

50. Hoogkamp-Korstanje, J. A. 1987. Antibiotics in *Yersinia enterocolitica* infections. *J. Antimicrob. Chemother.* **20:**123–131.

51. Huys, J., J. Kayhigi, P. Freyens, and G. V. Berghe. 1973. Single-dose treatment of epidemic typhus with doxycycline. *Chemotherapy* **18:**314–317.

52. Ikaheimo, I., H. Syrjala, J. Karhukorpi, R. Schildt, and M. Koskela. 2000. In vitro antibiotic susceptibility of *Francisella tularensis* isolated from humans and animals. *J. Antimicrob. Chemother.* **46:**287–290.

53. Jackson, L. A., and J. T. Grayston. 1998. *Chlamydia pneumoniae*. p. 583–586. In V. L. Yu, T. C. Merigan, Jr., and S. L. Barriere. (ed.), *Antimicrobial Therapy and Vaccines.* Williams and Wilkins, Baltimore, Md.

54. Janbon, F., O. Jonquet, J. Reynes, and A. Bertrand. 1989. Use of pefloxacin in the treatment of Rickettsiosis and Coxiellosis. *Rev. Infect. Dis.* **11:**990–991.

55. Jeskanen, L., L. Karppinen, L. Ingervo, S. Reitamo, H. P. Happonen, and A. Lassus. 1989. Ciprofloxacin versus doxycycline in the treatment of uncomplicated urogenital *Chlamydia trachomatis* infections. A double-blind comparative study. *Scand. J. Infect. Dis. Suppl.* **60:**62–65.

56. Kelly, D. J., K. F. Salata, D. Strickman, and J. N. Hershey. 1995. *Rickettsia tsutsugamushi* infection in cell culture: antibiotic susceptibility determined by flow cytometry. *Am. J. Trop. Med. Hyg.* **53:**602–606.

57. Keren, G., A. Keysary, R. Goldwasser, and E. Rubinstein. 1994. The inhibitory effect of fluoroquinolones on *Coxiella burnetii* growth in in-vitro systems. *J. Antimicrob. Chemother.* **33:**1254–1255.

58. Khan, W. A., C. Seas, U. Dhar, M. A. Salam, and M. L. Bennish. 1997. Treatment of shigellosis: V. Comparison of azithromycin and ciprofloxacin. A double-blind, randomized, controlled trial. *Ann. Intern. Med.* **126:**697–703.

59. Kitsukawa, K., J. Hara, and A. Saito. 1991. Inhibition of *Legionella pneumophila* in Guinea pig peritoneal macrophages by new quinolones, macrolides and other antimicrobial agents. *J. Antimicrob. Chemother.* **27:**343–353.

60. Klein, M. B., C. M. Nelson, and J. L. Goodman. 1997. Antibiotic susceptibility of the newly cultivated agent of human granulocytic ehrlichiosis: promising activity of quinolones and rifamycins. *Antimicrob. Agents Chemother.* **41:**76–79.

61. Kurz, R. W., W. Graninger, T. P. Egger, H. Pichler, and K. H. Tragl. 1988. Failure of treatment of *Legionella pneumonophila* with ciprofloxacin. *J. Antimicrob. Chemother.* **22:**389–391.

62. Lang, R., and E. Rubinstein. 1992. Quinolones for the treatment of brucellosis. *J. Antimicrob. Chemother.* **29:**357–360.

63. Limaye, A. P., and C. J. Hooper. 1999. Treatment of tularemia with fluoroquinolones: two cases and review. *Clin. Infect. Dis.* **29:**922–924.

64. Lipsky, P. E. 1994. Rheumatoïd arthritis, p. 1648–1653. In K. J. Isselbacher, E. Braunwald, J. D. Wilson, J. B. Martin, A. S. Fauci, and D. L. Kasper (ed.), *Harrisson's Principles of Internal Medicine.* Mc Graw-Hill, Inc., New York, N.Y.

65. Maurin, M., C. Abergel, and D. Raoult. 2001. DNA gyrase-mediated natural resistance to fluoroquinolones in *Ehrlichia* spp. *Antimicrob. Agents Chemother.* **45:**2098–2105.

66. Maurin, M., A. M. Benoliel, P. Bongrand, and D. Raoult. 1992. Phagolysosomal alkalinization and the bactericidal effect of antibiotics: the *Coxiella burnetii* paradigm. *J. Infect. Dis.* **166:**1097–1102.

67. **Maurin, M., N. F. Mersali, and D. Raoult.** 2000. Bactericidal activities of antibiotics against intracellular *Francisella tularensis*. *Antimicrob. Agents Chemother.* **44:**3428–3431.

68. **Maurin, M., and D. Raoult.** 1994. Phagolysosomal alkalinization and intracellular killing of *Staphylococcus aureus* by amikacin. *J. Infect. Dis.* **169:**330–336.

69. **Maurin, M., and D. Raoult.** 1996. Optimum treatment of intracellular infection. *Drugs* **52:**45–59.

70. **Maurin, M., and D. Raoult.** 1997. Bacteriostatic and bactericidal activity of levofloxacin against *Rickettsia rickettsii*, *Rickettsia conorii*, "Israeli spotted fever group rickettsia" and *Coxiella burnetii*. *J. Antimicrob. Chemother.* **39:**725–730.

71. **Maurin, M., and D. Raoult.** 1999. Q fever. *Clin. Microbiol. Rev.* **12:**518–553.

72. **Musso, D., M. Drancourt, S. Osscini, and D. Raoult.** 1996. Sequence of quinolone resistance-determining region of gyrA gene for clinical isolates and for an in vitro-selected quinolone-resistant strain of *Coxiella burnetii*. *Antimicrob. Agents Chemother.* **40:**870–873.

73. **Nagayama, A., T. Nakao, and H. Taen.** 1988. In vitro activities of ofloxacin and four other new quinoline- carboxylic acids against *Chlamydia trachomatis*. *Antimicrob. Agents Chemother.* **32:**1735–1737.

74. **Oriel, J. D.** 1989. Use of quinolones in chlamydial infection. *Rev. Infect. Dis.* **11**(Suppl. 5):S1273–S1276

75. **Ozaki, M., K. Komori, M. Matsuda, R. Yamaguchi, T. Honmura, Y. Tomii, I. Nishimura, and T. Nishino.** 1996. Uptake and intracellular activity of NM394, a new quinolone, in human polymorphonuclear leukocytes. *Antimicrob. Agents Chemother.* **40:**739–742.

76. **Pascual, A., I. Garcia, S. Ballesta, and E. J. Perea.** 1997. Uptake and intracellular activity of trovafloxacin in human phagocytes and tissue-cultured epithelial cells. *Antimicrob. Agents Chemother.* **41:**274–277.

77. **Pascual, A., I. Garcia, S. Ballesta, and E. J. Perea.** 1999. Uptake and intracellular activity of moxifloxacin in human neutrophils and tissue-cultured epithelial cells. *Antimicrob. Agents Chemother.* **43:**12–15.

78. **Pascual, A., I. Garcia, M. C. Conejo, and E. J. Perea.** 1991. Fluorometric and high-performance liquid chromatographic measurement of quinolone uptake by human neutrophils. *Eur. J. Clin. Microbiol. Infect. Dis.* **10:**969–971.

79. **Pascual, A., I. Garcia, and E. J. Perea.** 1992. Entry of lomefloxacin and temafloxacin into human neutrophils, peritoneal macrophages, and tissue culture cells. *Diagn. Microbiol. Infect. Dis.* **15:**393–398.

80. **Perea, E. J., I. Garcia, and A. Pascual.** 1992. Comparative penetration of lomefloxacin and other quinolones into human phagocytes. *Am. J. Med.* **92:**48S–51S.

81. **Perine, P. L., D. W. Krause, S. Awoke, and J. E. McDade.** 1974. Single-dose doxycycline treatment of louse-borne relapsing fever and epidemic typhus. *Lancet* **ii:**742–744.

82. **Raoult, D., P. Bres, M. Drancourt, and G. Vestris.** 1991. In vitro susceptibilities of *Coxiella burnetii*, *Rickettsia rickettsii*, and *Rickettsia conorii* to the fluoroquinolone sparfloxacin. *Antimicrob. Agents Chemother.* **35:**88–91.

83. **Raoult, D., H. Gallais, P. De Micco, and P. Casanova.** 1986. Ciprofloxacin therapy for Mediterranean spotted fever. *Antimicrob. Agents Chemother.* **30:**606–607.

84. **Raoult, D., J. B. Ndihokubwayo, H. Tissot-Dupont, V. Roux, B. Faugere, R. Abegbinni, and R. J. Birtles.** 1998. Outbreak of epidemic typhus associated with trench fever in Burundi. *Lancet* **352:**353–358.

85. **Raoult, D., and J. G. Olson.** 1999. Emerging rickettsioses, p. 17–35. *In* W. M. Scheld, W. A. Craig, and J. M. Hughes

(ed.), *Emerging Infections 3*. ASM Press, Washington, D.C.

86. **Raoult, D., H. Tissot-Dupont, C. Foucault, J. Gouvernet, P. E. Fournier, E. Bernit, A. Stein, M. Nesri, J. R. Harle, and P. J. Weiller.** 2000. Q fever 1985–1998: clinical and epidemiologic features of 1,383 infections. *Medicine* **79:**109–123.

87. **Raoult, D., H. Torres, and M. Drancourt.** 1991. Shell-vial assay: evaluation of a new technique for determining antibiotic susceptibility, tested in 13 isolates of *Coxiella burnetii*. *Antimicrob. Agents Chemother.* **35:**2070–2077.

88. **Raoult, D., M. Yeaman, and O. Baca.** 1989. Susceptibility of *Rickettsia* and *Coxiella burnetii* to quinolones. *Rev. Infect. Dis.* **11:**986

89. **Raoult, D., M. R. Yeaman, and O. G. Baca.** 1989. Susceptibility of *Coxiella burnetii* to pefloxacin and ofloxacin in ovo and persistently infected L929 cells. *Antimicrob. Agents Chemother.* **33:**621–623.

90. **Roblin, P. M., G. Montalban, and M. R. Hammerschlag.** 1994. In vitro activities of OPC-17116, a new quinolone; ofloxacin; and sparfloxacin against *Chlamydia pneumoniae*. *Antimicrob. Agents Chemother.* **38:**1402–1403.

91. **Rolain, J. M., M. Maurin, and D. Raoult.** 2001. Bacteriostatic and bactericidal activities of moxifloxacin against *Coxiella burnetii*. *Antimicrob. Agents Chemother.* **45:**301–302.

92. **Rolain, J. M., M. Maurin, G. Vestris, and D. Raoult.** 1998. In vitro susceptibilities of 27 Rickettsiae to 13 antimicrobials. *Antimicrob. Agents Chemother.* **42:**1537–1541.

93. **Rowe, B., L. R. Ward, and E. J. Threlfall.** 1995. Ciprofloxacin-resistant *Salmonella typhi* in the UK. *Lancet* **346:**1302.

94. **Salam, M. A., and M. L. Bennish.** 1991. Antimicrobial therapy for shigellosis. *Rev. Infect. Dis.* **13**(Suppl. 4):S332–S341.

95. **Scheel, O., R. Reiersen, and T. Hoel.** 1992. Treatment of tularemia with ciprofloxacin. *Eur. J. Clin. Microbiol. Infect. Dis.* **11:**447–448.

96. **Schlick, W.** 1993. The problems of treating atypical pneumonia. *J. Antimicrob. Chemother.* **31**(Suppl. C):111–120.

97. **Stanley, P. J., P. J. Flegg, B. K. Mandal, and A. M. Geddes.** 1989. Open study of ciprofloxacin in enteric fever. *J. Antimicrob. Chemother.* **23:**789–791.

98. **Stout, J. E., B. Arnold, and V. L. Yu.** 1998. Comparative activity of ciprofloxacin, ofloxacin, levofloxacin, and erythromycin against *Legionella* species by broth microdilution and intracellular susceptibility testing in HL-60 cells. *Diagn. Microbiol. Infect. Dis.* **30:**37–43.

99. **Syrjala, H., R. Schildt, and S. Raisainen.** 1991. In vitro susceptibility of *Francisella tularensis* to fluoroquinolones and treatment of tularemia with norfloxacin and ciprofloxacin. *Eur. J. Clin. Microbiol. Infect. Dis.* **10:**68–70.

100. **Toomey, K. E., and R. C. Barnes.** 1990. Treatment of *Chlamydia trachomatis* genital infection. *Rev. Infect. Dis.* **12**(Suppl. 6):S645–S655.

101. **Topkis, S., H. Swarz, S. A. Breisch, and A. N. Maroli.** 1997. Efficacy and safety of grepafloxacin 600 mg daily for 10 days in patients with community-acquired pneumonia. *Clin. Ther.* **19:**975–988.

102. **Unertl, K. E., F. P. Lenhart, H. Forst, G. Vogler, V. Wilm, W. Ehret, and G. Ruckdeschel.** 1989. Ciprofloxacin in the treatment of legionellosis in critically ill patients including those cases unresponsive to erythromycin. *Am. J. Med.* **87:**128S–131S.

103. **Vergis, E. N., and V. L. Yu.** 1998. *Legionella* species, p. 257–272. *In* V. L. Yu, T. C. Merigan, Jr., and S. L. Barriere (ed.), *Antimicrobial Therapy and Vaccines*. Williams and Wilkins, Baltimore, Md.

104. **Wain, J., N. T. Hoa, N. T. Chinh, H. Vinh, M. J. Everett, T. S. Diep, N. P. Day, T. Solomon, N. J. White, L. J. Piddock,**

and C. M. Parry. 1997. Quinolone-resistant *Salmonella typhi* in Viet Nam: molecular basis of resistance and clinical response to treatment. *Clin. Infect. Dis.* **25:**1404–1410.

105. **Waiz, A.** 1995. The new quinolones in the treatment of diarrhea and typhoid fever. *Drugs* **49**(Suppl. 2):132–135.

106. **Walker, D. H., and J. S. Dumler.** 1996. Emergence of the ehrlichioses as human health problems. *Emerg. Infect. Dis.* **2:**1–15.

107. **Weiss, E., and H. R. Dressler.** 1960. Centrifugation of rickettsiae and viruses into cells and its effect on infection. *Proc. Soc. Exp. Biol. Med.* **103:**691–695.

108. **White, N. J.** 1998. *Salmonella typhi* and *paratyphi*, p. 361–376. *In* V. L. Yu, T. C. Merigan, Jr., and S. L. Barriere (ed.), *Antimicrobial Therapy and Vaccines*, Williams and Wilkins, Baltimore, Md.

109. **Willke, A.** 2000. Low-level resistance to fluoroquinolones among *Salmonella* and *Shigella. Clin. Microbiol. Infect.* **6:**687.

110. **Yeaman, M. R., L. A. Mitscher, and O. G. Baca.** 1987. In vitro susceptibility of *Coxiella burnetii* to antibiotics, including several quinolones. *Antimicrob. Agents Chemother.* **31:**1079–1084.

Chapter 21

Fluoroquinolones in Intensive Care Unit Infections

ETHAN RUBINSTEIN

Patients with life-threatening severe community-acquired infections or infections that compromise vital organ functions are often treated in intensive care units (ICUs). In recent years, a rise has also occurred in the number of severe and complex non-infectious diseases that are treated in ICUs with more aggressive therapies than previously, which has led to an increase in the prevalence and severity of nosocomial infections. Thus, the ICU is the "meeting point" for severe community-acquired infections and nosocomial infections.

These problems are further complicated by the emergence and spread of multiple resistant bacterial strains in a hospital setting that is under intense antibacterial pressure. Antimicrobial resistance in the ICU has been recognized as an important variable, influencing patient outcome and overall resource utilization. While bacterial resistance is accelerating, the available tools to combat such infections are decreasing in efficacy and in variety, leaving the clinician with few choices (16).

In some ICUs, at times, 100% of patients staying more than 48 h receive antibacterial therapy or prophylaxis. The relative shortage of manpower, along with the present invasive monitoring techniques, only aggravates this situation. Thus, for example, in an ICU in Israel, during a 12-month survey there were 20 ventilator-associated pneumonias/1,000 ventilator days, 12 bloodstream infections/1,000 central vascular catheter days, and 14 urinary tract infections/1,000 indwelling urinary catheter days (6). In another European study, 1,589 patients (16,970 patient days) were included, and the infection rate was 21.6% (13.1% of patients). The rates of infection were as follows: ventilator-associated pneumonia, 9.6%; sinusitis, 1.5%; central venous catheter-associated infection, 3.5%; central venous catheter-associated bacteremia, 4.8%; urinary catheter-associated urinary tract infection, 7.8%; and primary bacteremia, 4.5%. The total incidence of ICU-acquired infections was 20.3% (22). In

another study conducted in ICUs in 17 countries in Western Europe, all patients (>10 years of age) occupying an ICU bed over a 24-h period were included. A total of 1,417 ICUs provided 10,038 patient case reports. A total of 4,501 patients (44.8%) were infected, and 2,064 (20.6%) had ICU-acquired infections. Pneumonia (46.9%), lower respiratory tract infections (17.8%), urinary tract infections (17.6%), and bloodstream infections (12%) were the most frequent types of ICU infections reported, all increasing the risk of death 1.71- to 3.5-fold (34). Taken together, it is reasonable to assume that presently the rate of nosocomial infections in ICUs is about 20%, with infections of the respiratory tract, urinary tract, and bloodstream being the most common.

The most frequently reported microorganisms identified in ICU nosocomial infections were *Enterobacteriaceae* (34.4%), *Staphylococcus aureus* (30.1%; 60% resistant to methicillin [MRSA]), *Pseudomonas aeruginosa* (28.7%), coagulase-negative staphylococci (19.1%), and fungi (17.1%) (34).

In a study evaluating the susceptibility of ICU pathogens, 118 European hospitals in five countries were screened. A total of 9,166 gram-negative strains were initially isolated from 7,308 patients between June 1994 and June 1995. Decreased antibiotic susceptibility across all species and drugs was highest in the Portuguese ICU. The highest incidence of resistance was seen in all countries for *P. aeruginosa* (up to 37% resistant to ciprofloxacin in Portuguese ICUs and 46% resistant to gentamicin in French ICUs). Among the gram-negative pathogens, decreased susceptibility to ciprofloxacin ranged from 7 (Sweden) to 25% (Portugal) compared with ~10% decreased susceptibility to imipenem, 7 to 21% to ceftazidime, 20 to 30% to ceftriaxone, 20 to 40% to piperacillin, 11 to 25% to piperacillin-tazobactam, 6 to 29% to gentamicin, and 4 to 11% to amikacin. Among the specific gram-negative pathogens, *Acinetobacter* spp. were the most resistant with decreased susceptibility to ciprofloxacin ranging from 18 (Belgium) to 81%

Ethan Rubinstein • Unit of Infectious Diseases, Sheba Medical Center, University of Tel Aviv, Tel Aviv, Israel.

(Spain). Among *Enterobacter* spp. decreased ciprofloxacin susceptibility ranged from 0 (Sweden) to 31% (Belgium). Among *Escherichia coli* it ranged from 1 to 2% (Sweden and France) to 14% (Spain), and among *Klebsiella* sp. it ranged from 1 to 2 (Belgium and Spain) to 18% (France) (17). Another study demonstrated that among 890 strains from ICU and hematology units in Switzerland, 100% of *Enterococcus* sp., *Streptococcus agalactiae*, *Streptococcus pneumoniae*, and other gram-positive cocci were susceptible to levofloxacin; 94% of 95 *S. aureus* strains and 65% of 85 coagulase-negative staphylococci strains were also susceptible to levofloxacin. Of 510 gram-negative strains only *P. aeruginosa* exhibited 87% susceptibility. Ninety-seven percent of 111 *E. coli* strains and 98% of 45 strains of *Klebsiella pneumoniae* strains were susceptible to levofloxacin. All other strains were 99 to 100% susceptible to levofloxacin (30). A recent study from Taiwan, however, demonstrated an alarming situation in which 17.5% of *E. coli* strains from ICU patients showed resistance to ciprofloxacin, and an additional 30.9% of the strains demonstrated reduced susceptibility to fluoroquinolones (23). There is a consensus that antimicrobial resistance in the ICU setting is an important factor influencing patient outcome, particularly if the involved pathogen is multiresistant (12, 17, 20, 31).

Among resistant gram-negative pathogens, the most common sources in the ICU are infections of the respiratory tract and urinary tract. Pneumonia occurs in 9 to 20% of patients requiring mechanical ventilation, with an associated mortality of 20 to 80% (10). These infections are commonly caused by gram-negative organisms (75 to 90%), such as *Acinetobacter baumanii*, *P. aeruginosa*, *K. pneumoniae* carrying extended spectrum β-lactamases (ESBLs), and *Stenotrophomonas maltophilia*, among others, which are frequently resistant to many antibiotics. Thus, fluoroquinolone resistance patterns among ICU isolates can vary greatly. Treatment recommendations, therefore, have to be developed locally according to the ICU resistance pattern and updated periodically.

As therapy is started in the ICU, infected patients frequently require initial empiric antibacterials that have high efficacy against all possible pathogens until culture results and antibacterial susceptibilities become known. Attempts to cycle empiric antibacterial therapy to overcome resistance have been made. In one such study (20), 6-month periods of ceftazidime use were followed by 6-month periods of ciprofloxacin use followed by 6 months of cefepime for the treatment of suspected gram-negative bacterial infections. The authors found that inadequate therapy of nosocomial infections decreased from one period to the other,

although this change was not reflected in overall hospital mortality. In another study by the same authors that was initiated because of a high rate of resistance to ceftazidime in gram-negative ICU pathogens, ciprofloxacin was selected for empirical therapy of gram-negative infections. This change resulted in a reduced occurrence of ventilator-associated pneumonia and bloodstream infections primarily due to a reduction of ceftazidime-resistant pathogens causing these infections (18).

In a study that compared "blind" therapy for suspected nosocomial infections in the ICU, three periods were chosen. A baseline period in which ceftazidime was prescribed to 1,323 patients, a second period in which ciprofloxacin was administered to 1,243 patients, and a third period in which cefepime was administered to 1,102 patients. The overall administration of inadequate antimicrobial treatment for nosocomial infections decreased during the course of the study (6.1, 4.7, and 4.5%; $P = 0.15$). This difference was primarily because of a significant decrease in the administration of inadequate treatment for gram-negative bacterial infections (4.4, 2.1, and 1.6; $P < 0.001$). There were no significant differences in the overall hospital mortality rate among the three periods and the three antimicrobials used (15.6, 16.4, and 16.2% of patients; $P = 0.828$). The data suggest that scheduled changes of antibiotic classes for the empirical treatment of gram-negative bacterial infections, with the inclusion of a fluoroquinolone between two broad-spectrum cephalosporin periods, can reduce the occurrence of "blinded" inadequate antibiotic treatment for nosocomial infections, possibly improving the outcome of critically ill patients (20).

Nevertheless, extensive use of fluoroquinolones in the ICU certainly has its drawbacks. A recent article found an association in an ICU setting between the amount of intravenous fluoroquinolones prescribed and the incidence of endemic infection with *A. baumanii* and *E. coli* strains resistant to fluoroquinolones (33). However, the extensive use of ciprofloxacin in ICUs in recent years has been followed by an increase in resistance to ciprofloxacin occurring among nosocomial pathogens, especially *P. aeruginosa* and *S. aureus*. From 1989 to 1992, ciprofloxacin susceptibility results from 8,517 *P. aeruginosa* and 9,021 *S. aureus* isolates associated with nosocomial infections were reported to the National Nosocomial Infections Surveillance System in the United States; 27.1% of *S. aureus* isolates and 4.7% of *P. aeruginosa* isolates were resistant to ciprofloxacin. Ciprofloxacin resistance was highest (80%) among MRSA strains and was more common among *S. aureus* isolated from the urinary and respiratory tracts than from other sites of isolation. The model showed a 123% increase in the odds of ciprofloxacin resistance from 1989 to 1990 to 1991 to 1992. For *P. aeruginosa* resistance varied by site of infection and rose most for respiratory-tract isolates from 2.0% in 1989 to 1990 to 5.3% in 1991 to 1992 (2, 5).

It seems, therefore, that in centers in which fluoroquinolones are heavily used, and in which rates of fluoroquinolone resistance are high, fluoroquinolone efficacy against nosocomial ICU isolates is rather limited, and other options are to be sought. On the other hand, a low resistance level in *P. aeruginosa*, *Acinetobacter* spp., *K. pneumoniae*, and *S. aureus* toward the fluoroquinolones justifies their consideration for use as empiric therapy for suspected nosocomial infections in the ICU.

PHARMACOKINETICS/ PHARMACODYNAMICS OF FLUOROQUINOLONES IN ICU INFECTIONS

Many patients in the ICU are in a critical condition, are frequently intubated, and need hemodynamic assistance, hemodialysis, and hemofiltration. Thus, the pharmacokinetics of many antibacterial agents may be different from those in patients with less severe diseases and certainly different from volunteers from whom most pharmacokinetic data are derived. Pharmacokinetic factors that are likely to differ in ICU patients include the following.

1. Volume of distribution may vary due to anasarca, low serum albumin levels, fluid overload, different tissue binding of drugs, and change in the intra- and extracellular volumes. Thus, for example, patients with extensive burns or septic shock may have larger distribution volumes leading to reduced serum drug concentrations. In such patients who are near or below their ideal body weight, the actual weight should be used for dose calculation. In those who are >25% above ideal weight (because of obesity, edema, or third-space fluid) a reasonable approach is to add 43% of the "nonlean" weight to the ideal body weight (32).

   Fluoroquinolone antibacterial efficacy correlates best with either their maximum concentration of drug in serum (C_{max}) divided by the MIC or by their area under the time concentration curve (AUC) divided by the MIC (AUIC). C_{max}/MIC is the best predictor for the rapidity of bacterial kill, at least when *S. pneumoniae* and gram-negative bacteria are considered (24, 36). With this property in mind, it is reasonable to assume that fluoroquinolones should preferentially be adminis-

tered at high doses at infrequent intervals, rather than low doses given more frequently. The achievement of minimally effective antibiotic action consisting of an AUIC of at least 125 is associated with bacterial eradication, in particular, for gram-negative bacterial infections. When AUIC is increased to 250, ciprofloxacin (which displays concentration-dependent bacterial killing in vivo) is able to eliminate the bacterial pathogen within 1 to 2 days. β-Lactams, even when dosed to an AUIC of 250, require longer treatment duration to eliminate the bacterial pathogen, because their in vivo bacterial killing rate is slower than that of the quinolones. The AUIC value of >250 is also highly predictive of the lack of development of bacterial resistance. Antimicrobial regimens that do not achieve an AUIC of at least 125 cannot prevent the selective pressure, so pronounced in the ICU, that leads to overgrowth of resistant bacterial subpopulations. Indeed, there is considerable belief among experts that conventional management strategies that prescribe fluoroquinolone doses that fail to attain AUIC values of at least 125 are contributing to the rise in fluoroquinolone resistance levels in bacteria (28).

2. Altered drug clearance occurs because of reduced renal perfusion, decreased liver clearance function due to diminished liver perfusion (e.g, occurring in severe cirrhosis, the initial phase of severe hepatic trauma, shock states, use of vasopressors), and altered metabolism.

3. Altered absorption and bioavailability can be due to intestinal edema, delayed gastric emptying, alteration in intestinal peristalsis, or reduction in splanchnic perfusion, all of which impede drug absorption and may decrease intestinal drug secretion. Altered intestinal flora and use of sedatives and H_2 receptor blocking agents may also change intestinal motility and intraluminal pH affecting drug absorption.

4. Because most agents are administered intravenously to patients in the ICU, knowledge of drug incompatibilities is essential to prevent drug interactions. In depth charts of allowed admixtures are available and should be consulted (9). In addition, the relatively large number of administered agents may cause displacement from serum protein of one drug by the other. An example is displacement of warfarin by highly bound compounds that may lead to bleeding complications.

THERAPY

Fluoroquinolones have been used frequently to treat nosocomial infections in the ICU because of their pronounced activity against resistant gram-negative bacteria, their lack of association with *Clostridium difficile* colitis, and their lack of promotion of vancomycin-resistant enterococci (29).

Bacteremia

Bacteremia is commonly associated with intravascular catheters. Approximately 10% of patients in an ICU with an intravascular catheter of more than 72 h duration will develop bacteremia. *Staphylococcus epidermidis*, which is usually methicillin-resistant, and MRSA are common pathogens, but gram-negative pathogens, as mentioned before, are also frequent (25).

During 1997, a total of 4,267 nosocomial and community-acquired bloodstream infections due to gram-negative organisms were reported from SENTRY hospitals in Canada (8), the United States (19), and Latin America (10). *E. coli* was the most common isolate (41% of all gram-negative isolates), followed by *Klebsiella* species (17.9%), *P. aeruginosa* (10.6%), and *Enterobacter* species (9.4%). For all gram-negative isolates combined, the most active antimicrobials tested were meropenem, imipenem, and cefepime. Levofloxacin [MIC at which 90% of the isolates tested are inhibited (MIC_{90}, 2 mg/liter], ciprofloxacin (MIC_{90}, 1 mg/liter), gatifloxacin (MIC_{90}, 2 mg/liter), sparfloxacin (MIC_{90}, 2 mg/liter), and trovafloxacin (MIC_{90}, 2 mg/liter) were also active against most isolates. Bloodstream infection isolates from Latin America were uniformly more resistant to all classes of antimicrobial agents tested than were isolates from Canada or the United States (18). In another prospective study (26) of 452 episodes of bacteremia, 25 (5.5%) were caused by *K. pneumoniae* resistant to ciprofloxacin in vitro. ESBL production was detected in 15 (60%) of 25 ciprofloxacin-resistant isolates, compared with 68 (16%) of 427 ciprofloxacin-susceptible strains ($P = 0.0001$). Multivariate analysis revealed that risk factors for ciprofloxacin resistance in *K. pneumoniae* included prior receipt of a quinolone ($P = 0.0065$) and an ESBL-producing strain ($P = 0.012$). Pulsed-field gel electrophoresis suggested that patient-to-patient transmission occurred. The close relationship between ESBL production and ciprofloxacin resistance is particularly worrisome because the first reported instance of plasmid-mediated ciprofloxacin resistance was in an isolate of *K. pneumoniae* also possessing an ESBL.

In a clinical study evaluating ciprofloxacin in the therapy of various severe infections, the response rate of patients with bacteremia treated with ciprofloxacin monotherapy was 92% at the end of therapy and similar (92%) to the rate obtained by a combination of aminoglycoside/β-lactam regimens. For patients receiving ciprofloxacin in combination with another antibacterial agent, the success rate was 83%, while the rate was 67% (confidence interval, −0.41 to 0.74) with standard therapy. Similar success rates were also noted 7 to 14 days after the end of therapy (21).

In an open, randomized, multinational, multicenter study, the efficacy, safety, and tolerability of levofloxacin 500 mg twice daily was compared with imipenem/cilastatin 1 g intravenously three times daily in the treatment of hospitalized adult patients with clinically suspected bacteremia/sepsis. A total of 503 patients were randomly selected, and 499 patients were included in the intent-to-treat population. Clinical cure rates in the intent-to-treat population and per-protocol population were not significantly different between the two treatment arms; these were 77% (184 of 239) and 89% (125 of 140), respectively, for levofloxacin and 68% (178 of 260) and 85% (125 of 147), respectively, for imipenem/cilastatin. At follow-up, the cure rates were 84% for levofloxacin and 69% for imipenem/cilastatin. The authors concluded that levofloxacin was as effective as imipenem/cilastatin. A satisfactory bacteriological response was obtained in 87% (96 of 110) of levofloxacin patients and 84% (97 of 116) of imipenem/cilastatin patients (8).

In some countries, increasing resistance of pathogens to ciprofloxacin and ofloxacin has resulted in an increased therapeutic failure rate in patients with bacteremia; e.g, from 1993 to 1998, 40 cases of fluoroquinolone-resistant *E. coli* bacteremia were observed in a teaching hospital in South Korea; 25 episodes (63.5%) were community acquired. The incidence of quinolone-resistant *E. coli* bacteremia increased steadily, from 6.7 to 24.6% during the 5 years of the study, and correlated with the significantly increased use of fluoroquinolones ($P = 0.003$, $r = 0.98$). When the 40 fluoroquinolone-resistant *E. coli* bacteremic patients were compared with 80 patients with bacteremia due to quinolone-susceptible *E. coli*, prior fluoroquinolone use was the only independent risk factor for fluoroquinolone-resistant bacteremia ($P = 0.001$). The rate of multidrug resistance of fluoroquinolone-resistant pathogens was much higher (60%) than that of quinolone-susceptible isolates (13.8%). The isolates revealed little evidence of clonal spread and may have emerged in direct response to the selective pressure exerted by prior fluoroquinolone use (3).

In contrast to these observations, other centers have reported the long-standing efficacy of ciprofloxacin therapy against *P. aeruginosa* and other pathogens originating in the ICU. Antimicrobial susceptibilities of blood culture isolates obtained before and after the introduction of ciprofloxacin were similar (14, 27). On the other hand, other centers reported rising incidence of resistance to fluoroquinolones, frequently associated with the density of the use of the agent in the particular unit (13, 19).

Streptococcus viridans is a "new pathogen" in ICUs, infecting neutropenic patients and causing severe sepsis. The MIC_{90} for these isolates were as follows: penicillin, 0.5 μg/ml; amoxicillin, 0.5 μg/ml; cefotaxime, 0.25 μg/ml; ciprofloxacin, 4 μg/ml; sparfloxacin, 0.5 μg/ml; vancomycin, 0.5 μg/ml; teicoplanin, 0.25 μg/ml; and quinupristin-dalfopristin, 1 μg/ml. The rate of susceptibility of penicillin-resistant *S. viridans* to ciprofloxacin was only 23%, and no resistance to sparfloxacin, vancomycin, teicoplanin, and quinupristin-dalfopristin was demonstrable (32). Among the fluoroquinolones, clinafloxacin was most active (MIC_{90}, 0.19 μg/ml), whereas ciprofloxacin and fleroxacin were the least active (both MIC_{90}, 16 μg/ml) (15). Because many of the pathogens causing bacteremia are gram-positive pathogens, the activity of fluoroquinolones against these pathogens is of particular interest.

The in vitro spectrum of a novel des-fluoro(6) quinolone, BMS-284756 (garenoxacin), was compared with those of five fluoroquinolones (trovafloxacin, moxifloxacin, levofloxacin, ofloxacin, and ciprofloxacin). Garenoxacin was among the most active and often was the most active quinolone against staphylococci (including MRSA), streptococci, pneumococci (including ciprofloxacin-nonsusceptible and penicillin-resistant strains), and *Enterococcus faecalis*. Garenoxacin inhibited approximately 60 to 70% of the *Enterococcus faecium* (including vancomycin-resistant) at the anticipated MIC susceptible breakpoint (≤4 μg/ml) (35).

Sinusitis

Sinusitis occurring in intubated patients, patients with nasogastric tubes, or those with facial trauma is also a relatively common infection in the ICU. Surgical drainage is usually required, and antibiotic therapy, including that with fluoroquinolones, is of secondary importance (11).

Wound Infections

Wound infections, while common in surgical ICUs, play a small role in medical ICUs (12).

Urinary Tract Infections

Hospital-acquired urinary tract infections occur in approximately 3.0% of hospitalized patients with a 1% rate of associated bacteremia. These infections are most commonly caused by resistant gram-negative bacteria, enterococci, and fungi.

Pseudomembranous Colitis

Antibiotic-associated pseudomembranous colitis is a common nosocomial infection caused by the toxin producing *C. difficile* in ICU patients who receive antibiotics, in particular, third-generation cephalosporins. Fluoroquinolones, however, have been considered only rarely as being responsible for this infection (6a). On the other hand, most fluoroquinolones have activity against this organism that is insufficient to allow their use in therapy of *C. difficile* colitis (1, 22).

At present, the newer fluoroquinolones (levofloxacin, moxifloxacin, and gatifloxacin) with their improved activity against gram-positive pathogens do not seem to add much to present therapeutic options for nosocomial infections. However, in vitro data of some of the more advanced fluoroquinolones, like gemifloxacin, garenoxacin and clinafloxacin, might make them useful alternatives for treatment of nosocomial gram-positive infections in ICUs (7).

REFERENCES

1. **Alonso, R., T. Pelaez, M. J. Gonzalez-Abad, L. Alcala, P. Munoz, M. Rodriguez-Creixems, and E. Bouza.** 2001. In vitro activity of new quinolones against Clostridium difficile. *J. Antimicrob. Chemother.* **47:**195–197.
2. **Carmeli, Y., N. Troillet, G. M. Eliopoulos, and M. H. Samore.** 1999. Emergence of antibiotic-resistant Pseudomonas aeruginosa: comparison of risks associated with different antipseudomonal agents. *Antimicrob. Agents Chemother.* **43:**1379–1382.
3. **Cheong, H. J., C. W. Yoo, J. W. Sohn, W. J. Kim, M. J. Kim, and S. C. Park.** 2001. Bacteremia due to quinolone-resistant Escherichia coli in a teaching hospital in South Korea. *Clin. Infect. Dis.* **33:**48–53.
4. **Civetta, J. M., R. W. Taylor, and R. R. Kirby (ed.).** 1997. *Critical Care*, 3rd ed. Lippincott-Raven, Philadelphia, Pa.
5. **Coronado, V. G., J. R. Edwards, D. H. Culver, and R. P. Gaynes, for the National Nosocomial Infections Surveillance (NNIS) System.** 1995. Ciprofloxacin resistance among nosocomial Pseudomonas aeruginosa and Staphylococcus aureus in the United States. *Infect. Control. Hosp. Epidemiol.* **16:**71.
6. **Finkelstein, R., G. Rabino, I. Kassis, and I. Macmid.** 2000. Device-associated, device-day infection rates in an Israeli adult general intensive care unit. *J. Hosp. Infect.* **44:**200–205.
6a. **Fraisse, A., C. Croix, D. Maniere, and P. Pfitzenmeyer.** 1999. Diarrhee a Clostridium difficile chez le sujet tres age. Particularites cliniques et evolutives de 21 cases. [Clostridium difficile diarrhea in the very old. Clinical features and course in 21 cases] *Presse. Med.* **28:**1748–1752.

7. Fung-Tomc, J.-C., B. Minassian, B. Kolek, E. Huczko, L. Aleksunes, T. Stickle, T. Washo, E. Gradelski, L. Valera, and D. P. Bonner. 2000. Antibacterial spectrum of a novel desfluoro(6) quinolone, BMS-284756. *Antimicrob. Agents Chemother.* **44**:3351–3356.

8. Geddes, A., M. Thaler, S. Schonwald, M. Harkonen, F. Jacobs, and I. Nowotny. 1999. Levofloxacin in the empirical treatment of patients with suspected bacteraemia/sepsis: comparison with imipenem/cilastatin in an open, randomized trial. *J. Antimicrob. Chemother.* **44**:799–810.

9. Gilman, A. G., L. S. Goodman, T. W. Rall, et al. (ed.). 2000. *The Pharmacologic Basis of Therapeutics.* Macmillan Publishing Co., New York, N.Y.

10. Hanberger, H., J. A. Garcia-Rodriguez, M. Gobernado, H. Goossens, L. E. Nilsson, and M. J. Struelens. 1999. Antibiotic susceptibility among aerobic gram-negative bacilli in intensive care units in 5 European countries. French and Portuguese ICU Study Groups. *JAMA* **281**:67–71.

11. Hansen, M., M. R. Poulsen, D. K. Bendixen, and F. Hartmann-Andersen. 1988. Incidence of sinusitis in patients with nasotracheal intubation. *Br. J. Anaesth.* **61**:231.

12. Heyland, D. K., D. J. Cook, L. Griffith, S. P. Keenan, and C. Bruin-Buisson. 1999. The attributable morbidity and mortality of ventilator-associated pneumonia in critically ill patients. *Am. J. Respir. Crit. Care Med.* **159**:1249–1256.

13. Hsueh, P.-R., L. J. Teng, P. C. Yang, Y. C. Chen, S. W. Ho, and K. T. Luh. 1998. Persistence of a multidrug-resistant Pseudomonas aeruginosa clone in an intensive care burn unit. *J. Clin. Microbiol.* **36**:1347–1351.

14. Jamal, W.-Y., K. El-Din, V. O. Rotimi, and T. D. Chugh. 1999. An analysis of hospital-acquired bacteraemia in intensive care unit patients in a university hospital in Kuwait. *J. Hosp. Infect.* **43**:49–56.

15. Kerr, K.-G., H. T. Armitage, and P. H. McWhinney. 1999. Activity of quinolones against viridans group streptococci isolated from blood cultures of patients with haematological malignancy. *Support. Care Cancer* **7**:28–30.

16. Koleff, M., and M. Niederman. 2001. Antimicrobial resistance in the ICU. The time for action is now. *Crit. Care Med.* **29**(Suppl.):N63.

17. Kollef, M. H., G. Sherman, S. Ward, and V. J. Fraser. 1999. Inadequate antimicrobial treatment of infections: a risk factor for hospital mortality among critically ill patients. *Chest* **115**:462–474.

18. Kollef, M.H., J. Vlasnik, L. Sharpless, C. Pasque, D. Murphy, and V. J. Fraser. 1997. Scheduled rotation of antibiotic classes. A strategy to decrease the incidence of ventilator-associated pneumonia due to antibiotic-resistant gram-negative bacteria. *Am. J. Respir. Crit. Care Med.* **156**:1040–1048.

19. Kollef, M.-H., J. Vlasnik, L. Sharpless, C. Pasque, D. Murphy, and V. Fraser. 1997. Scheduled change of antibiotic classes: a strategy to decrease the incidence of ventilator-associated pneumonia. *Am. J. Respir. Crit. Care Med.* **156**:1040–1048.

20. Koleff, M. H., S. Ward, G. Sherman, D. Prentice, R. Schaiff, W. Huey, and V. J. Fraser. 2000. Inadequate treatment of nosocomial infections is associated with certain empiric antibiotic choices. *Crit. Care Med.* **28**:3456–3464.

21. Krumpe, P.-E., S. Cohn, J. Garreltes, J. Ramirez, H. Coulter, D. Haverstock, and R. Echols. 1999. Intravenous and oral mono- or combination-therapy in the treatment of severe infections: ciprofloxacin versus standard antibiotic therapy. Ciprofloxacin Study Group. *J. Antimicrob. Chemother.* **43**(Suppl. A):117–128.

22. Legras, A., D. Malvy, A. I. Quinioux, D. Villers, G. Bouachour, R. Robert, and R. Thomas. 1998. Nosocomial infections: prospective survey of incidence in five French intensive care units. *Intensive Care Med.* **24**:1040–1046.

23. McDonald, L. C., F. J. Chen, H. J. Lo, H. C. Yin, P. L. Lu, C. H. Huang, P. Chen, T. L. Lauderdale, and M. Ho. 2001. Emergence of reduced susceptibility and resistance to fluoroquinolones in Escherichia coli in Taiwan and contributions of distinctive selective pressures. *Antimicrob. Agents Chemother.* **45**:3084–3091.

24. MacGowan, A. P., C. A. Rogers, A. Holt, M. Wooton, and K. E. Bowker. 2001. Pharmacodynamics of Gemifloxacin against Streptococcus pneumoniae in an in vitro pharmacokinetic model of infection. *Antimicrob. Agents Chemother.* **45**:2916–2921.

25. Mermel, L. A., B. M. R. J. Farr, Sheretz, I. I. Raad, N. O'Grady, J. A. Harris, and D. E. Craven. 2001. Guidelines for the management of intravascular related infections. *Clin. Infect. Dis.* **32**:1249–1272.

26. Paterson, D. L., L. Mulazimoglu, J. M. Casssellas, W. C. Ko, H. Goossens, A. Von-Gottberg, S. Mohapatra, G. N. Trenholme, K. P. Klugman, J. G. McCormack, and V. L. Yu. 2000. Epidemiology of ciprofloxacin resistance to extended-spectrum beta-lactamase production I Klebsiella pneumoniae isolates causing bactermia. *Clin. Infect. Dis.* **30**:473–478.

27. Pieroni, P., J. Goodfellow, L. Reesor, M. Louie, and A. E. Simor. 1997. Antimicrobial susceptibilities of blood culture isolates obtained before and after the introduction of ciprofloxacin. *J. Antimicrob. Chemother.* **39**:419–422.

28. Puzniak, L. A., J. Mayfield, T. Leet, M. Kollef, and L. M. Mundy. 2001. Acquisition of vancomycin-resistant enterococci during scheduled antimicrobial rotation in an intensive care unit. *Clin. Infect. Dis.* **33**:151–157.

29. Schentag, J. J. 1999. Antimicrobial action and pharmacokinetics/pharmacodynamics: the use of AUIC to improve efficacy and avoid resistance. *J. Chemother.* **11**:426–439.

30. Siegrist, H. H, M. C. Nepa, and A. Jacquet. 1999. Susceptibility to levofloxacin of clinical isolates of bacteria from intensive care and haematology/oncology patients in Switzerland: a multicentre study. *J. Antimicrob. Chemother.* **43**(Suppl. C):51–54.

31. Solomkin, J.S. 1996. Antimicrobial resistance: an overview. *New Horiz.* **4**:319–320.

32. Traynor, A. M., A. N. Nafziger, and J. S. Bertino. 1995. Aminoglycoside dosing weight correction factors for patients of various body sizes. *Antimicrob. Agents Chemother.* **39**:545–551.

33. Villers, D., E. Espaze, M. F. Coste-Burel, F. Giauffret, E. Ninin, F. Nicolas, and H. Richet. 1998. Nosocomial Acinetobacter baumanii infections: microbiological and clinical epidemiology. *Ann. Intern. Med.* **129**:182–189.

34. Vincent, J. L., D. J. Bihari, P. M. Suter, H. A. Bruining, J. White, M. H. Nicolas-Chanoin, M. Wolff, R. C. Spencer, and M. Hemmer. 1995. The prevalence of nosocomial infection in intensive care units in Europe. Results of the European Prevalence of Infection in Intensive Care (EPIC) Study. EPIC International Advisory Committee. *JAMA* **274**:639–644.

35. Wisplinghoff, H., R. R. Reinert, O. Cornely, and H. Seifert. 1999. Molecular relationships and antimicrobial susceptibilities of viridans group streptococci isolated from blood of neutropenic cancer patients. *J. Clin. Microbiol.* **37**:1876–1880.

36. Wright, D.H., L. B. Horde, M. Peterson, A. D. Hoang, and J. C. Rotscafer. 1998. *Program and Abstracts of the 98th General Meeting of the American Society for Microbiology, 1998,* abstr. A-86, p. 53. American Society for Microbiology, Washington, D.C.

Chapter 22

Quinolones in Pediatrics

FARYAL GHAFFAR AND GEORGE H. MCCRACKEN, JR.

SPECTRUM OF ACTION

Quinolones are bactericidal and active against a wide range of gram-positive and gram-negative bacterial pathogens relevant to pediatric infections. These include *Pseudomonas aeruginosa*, nosocomially acquired *Enterobacteriaceae*, methicillin-sensitive and methicillin-resistant *Staphylococcus aureus* and *Staphylococcus epidermidis*. They also show excellent activity against other gram-negative pathogens, including β-lactamase-producing strains of *Haemophilus influenzae*, *Moraxella catarrhalis*, *Shigella* and *Salmonella* species, *Neisseria meningitides*, and *Neisseria gonorrhoeae*. The activity against streptococci, such as group A and B streptococci, pneumococci, and enterococci, varies with the more recent compounds having excellent activity. These agents have very poor activity against anaerobes and *Nocardia* organisms. Quinolones have in vitro activity against *Chlamydia*, *Mycoplasma*, *Mycobacterium*, *Plasmodium*, and *Rickettsia* species as well as *Bartonella henselae*, but their clinical efficacy in treating such infections in children is unknown.

Compared with ciprofloxacin (the prototypical agent of the original fluoroquinolones), the newest fluoroquinolones (levofloxacin, sparfloxacin, grepafloxacin, clinafloxacin, gatifloxacin, and moxifloxacin) all have increased potency against gram-positive bacteria. This activity along with anaerobic coverage and substantial retention of the gram-negative activity of these new fluoroquinolones results in compounds of exceptional broad antimicrobial activity, similar to that of the carbapenems (6, 19, 104). Although ciprofloxacin is not as active against *S. aureus* or *S. pneumoniae* as the newer quinolones, it remains the most active quinolone against *P. aeruginosa*.

Ciprofloxacin, ofloxacin, levofloxacin, sparfloxacin, grepafloxacin, moxifloxacin, gatifloxacin, and gemifloxacin all have activity against *Chlamydia pneu-moniae*, *Chlamydia trachomatis*, *Ureaplasma urealyticum*, *Mycoplasma pneumoniae*, *Mycoplasma hominis*, and *Legionella pneumophila*. Ciprofloxacin, sparfloxacin, levofloxacin, ofloxacin, gatifloxacin, and moxifloxacin have demonstrated activity against *Mycobacterium tuberculosis*, *Mycobacterium fortuitum*, *Mycobacterium kansasii*, and some strains of *Mycobacterium chelonae*, but have only fair or poor activity against *Mycobacterium avium-M. intracellulare*. Ofloxacin and pefloxacin have activity against *Mycobacterium leprae* in animal models. Quinolones also inhibit *Rickettsia* species and *Coxiella burnetii*, and they have some activity against *Plasmodium* species.

RESISTANCE

Widespread use of fluoroquinolones has resulted in emergence of resistance; therefore, it is important to give careful thought to the site of infection and pathogens in each patient (34, 52, 54, 56, 57, 76, 92, 108, 110).

Widely varying rates of resistance have been reported worldwide, according to the bacterial species, clinical setting, and country (1, 2, 13, 25, 26, 59, 82, 91). Several reports have described resistance developing in staphylococcal species in hospitals with frequent quinolone use and, more disturbingly, among susceptible organisms during therapy (59). There have been rapid increases in resistance among *Serratia marcescens*, *Citrobacter freundii*, *Providentia* spp., *Klebsiella pneumoniae*, *Streptococcus pneumoniae*, and methicillin-resistant *S. aureus*. The emergence of fluoroquinolone resistance among adults worldwide is of major concern if these agents are used in pediatrics. Selection and expansion of resistant clones in daycare and other facilities could result in limiting the use of fluoroquinolones in pediatric patients. Preliminary data from an ongoing prospective study at our center

---

Faryal Ghaffar and George H. McCracken, Jr. • Southwestern Medical School, 5323 Harry Hines Boulevard, Dallas, TX 75235-9063.

in Dallas, Tex., assessing the effect of gatifloxacin on nasopharyngeal colonization in children with recurrent or persistent acute otitis media showed decreased carriage of *S. pneumoniae* directly after treatment without induction of fluoroquinolone resistance. Similarly, Dagan et al. studied the dynamics of nasopharyngeal pneumococcal carriage in children with recurrent and nonresponsive acute otitis media treated with gatifloxacin. The results of the study showed decreased pneumococcal carriage during treatment followed by a colonization rate 2 to 3 weeks later higher than that at pretreatment. The treated patients became colonized with new serotypes that were susceptible to penicillin. There was no selection of gatifloxacin resistance among pneumococcal isolates (32).

Use of fluoroquinolones in children should be strictly limited to those specific infections complicated by special conditions for which the benefit of these drugs is clear and for which no alternative safe and effective antibiotic therapy is available. Avoidance of their routine administration may play a significant role in limiting the spread of bacterial resistance to these drugs. Surveillance is necessary to detect the emergence of, or increase in, fluoroquinolone resistance among various bacterial species.

PHARMACOLOGY

All commercially available fluoroquinolones as well as those under development are rapidly absorbed after oral administration. In addition, some drugs of this class (e.g., ciprofloxacin, ofloxacin, levofloxacin, gatifloxacin) are available for intravenous infusion. Quinolones penetrate well into tissues, especially into infected tissues, and are accumulated within macrophages and the polymorphonuclear leukocytes.

Clearance mechanisms differ between the quinolones (95). In renal failure doses of ciprofloxacin, ofloxacin, levofloxacin, lomefloxacin, sparfloxacin, and gatifloxacin should be adjusted in accordance with the decrease in glomerular filtration rate. Pefloxacin (not available in the United States) and moxifloxacin are entirely metabolized and should be used cautiously in case of liver impairment.

PHARMACOKINETIC STUDIES

Pharmacokinetic data of fluoroquinolones in pediatric patients are limited as a consequence of their restricted use. Peltola et al. (87) studied the pharmacokinetics of oral ciprofloxacin (15 mg/kg of body weight) administered to seven infants and nine children. The elimination half-life of ciprofloxacin was longer in infants than it was in children (2.73 ± 0.28 versus 1.28 ± 0.52 h, respectively; $P < 0.001$). Ciprofloxacin elimination half-life in children is shorter than in adults (3 to 5 h). The mean ± SD peak concentration (C_{max}) values in infants and children were 3.3 ± 1.3 and 2.1 ± 1.4 mg/liter, respectively; times to reach C_{max} (t_{max}) were 1.18 ± 0.46 and 1.0 ± 0.25 h, respectively. There was no significant difference in the C_{max} in the serum and t_{max} in the infants compared with children. On the basis of these data, children between 1 and 5 years of age should receive ciprofloxacin at more frequent intervals than infants or older children. On the basis of that limited study, an oral dose of 10 to 15 mg of ciprofloxacin per kg three times daily may be appropriate for children 1 to 5 years of age.

In another study, the pharmacokinetic properties of sequential intravenous/oral ciprofloxacin were studied in children with cystic fibrosis. Eighteen children (age, 5 to 17 years) were given intravenous ciprofloxacin 10 mg/kg every 8 h and 20 mg/kg orally every 12 h. The mean steady-state C_{max} after intravenous infusion and oral doses were 5.0 ± 1.5 and 3.7 ± 1.4 mg/liter, respectively, the t_{max} was 2.5 ± 1.8 h following oral doses. The mean oral bioavailability of ciprofloxacin in younger children was less than that in older children (68 versus 95%, respectively); oral bioavailability in adults was 75%. The mean half-life ranged from 2.6 to 3.4 h. The authors recommended higher doses of ciprofloxacin (30 mg/kg/day intravenously and 40 mg/kg/day orally) in patients with cystic fibrosis (97).

Capparelli et al. reported the single-dose pharmacokinetics of oral gatifloxacin in 88 pediatric patients <2 to 16 years of age. The pharmacokinetics of gatifloxacin were not significantly different among the four age groups (<2, 2 to 6, 6 to 12, and 12 to 16 years old). A single oral 10 mg/kg dose resulted in drug exposure values (serum area under the curve, 36.0 ± 12.0 µg·h/ml) in pediatric patients similar to those in adults given a 400-mg-daily dose (24).

In another study, pharmacokinetics of intravenous gatifloxacin was studied in 43 children (3 months to 16 years). Subjects received gatifloxacin in a dosage of 2.5, 5, 7.5, 10, or 12.5 mg/kg (maximum, 600 mg). The results indicated that the drug exposure (serum area under the curve from zero to infinity) in children increased in a dose-related manner and was similar across different age groups. A 10 mg/kg dose of gatifloxacin in children resulted in drug exposure similar to that in adults given 400 mg intravenously and in children given 10 mg/kg as oral suspension (10).

Chen et al. studied the pharmacokinetics of intravenous levofloxacin in 40 pediatric patients in five different age groups (6 months to 2 years, 2 to 5 years, 5 to 10 years, 10 to 12 years, and 12 to 16 years). Each subject received a single 7 mg/kg intravenous dose of levofloxacin. The levofloxacin C_{max} was similar across all age groups. Age-related decreases in clearance of levofloxacin were observed. As compared with adult data, higher or more frequent doses appear necessary in infants and young children to maintain effective drug exposure (27).

ADVERSE EFFECTS AND TOXICITIES IN CHILDREN

Extraarticular Effects

Fluoroquinolones are relatively safe and well tolerated. Adverse effects occur in 5 to 10% of adults and necessitate discontinuation of treatment in 1 to 2% of cases. Similar experiences have been found in children. The restriction of fluoroquinolone use in children has limited the safety data in this population. Safety data are currently available from compassionate use of ciprofloxacin. Chysky et al. (29) reported on the follow-up of 634 children, aged 3 days to 17 years, who received ciprofloxacin. The data were compiled from information submitted by physicians who treated patients with ciprofloxacin on a compassionate basis. Eighty percent of the patients were 10 to 17 years of age. Eighty (12.6%) patients reported adverse effects. The most frequently reported side effects were gastrointestinal (31 patients), skin (21 patients), and central nervous system (CNS) complaints such as dizziness, headache, hallucinations, anxiety, tinnitus, and taste perversion (14 patients). Nine children had genitourinary problems such as dysuria, nephritis, and increased serum creatinine values. Arthralgia was reported by eight (1.3%) children; all were girls with cystic fibrosis and all had transient joint symptoms.

Photosensitivity occurs most often with agents containing a halogen substituent at the 8 position, such as lomefloxacin, clinafloxacin, and sparfloxacin (39). In adults, photosensitivity reactions were reported in 10% of patients taking lomefloxacin, 7.9% taking sparfloxacin, and <1% taking ciprofloxacin, ofloxacin, and levofloxacin. It is unclear whether the incidence of photosensitivity would be different in children compared with that in adults (77).

Reversible intracranial hypertension (15), interstitial nephritis, crystalluria, and anaphylaxis have been associated with fluoroquinolones, as has hemolytic anemia in patients with glucose-6-phos-

phate dehydrogenase deficiency who received nalidixic acid. The staining of teeth reported in infants from Thailand has not been observed elsewhere (72). Trovafloxacin, grepafloxacin, and temafloxacin were withdrawn from the market because of unexpected toxicity problems. In 1999, two recently released fluoroquinolones (trovafloxacin and grepafloxacin) were withdrawn from the market because trovafloxacin resulted in possible acute liver failure (73) and grepafloxacin resulted in prolongation of QT intervals and sudden death. Temafloxacin was removed from sale in 1992 because it resulted occasionally in a fatal syndrome of hemolysis, renal failure, thrombocytopenia, and hypoglycemia (18). Sparfloxacin is also no longer marketed in the United States.

Cartilage Toxicity (Preclinical and Clinical Data)

When administered to immature animals (dogs, rabbits, rats, guinea pigs, pigs, marmosets, monkeys, ferrets), all of the quinolones studied, older and new derivatives, cause arthropathic effects in major, usually weight-bearing synovial joints. This arthropathy evolves in days to weeks, and the typical histopathologic lesions (fluid-filled blisters, fissures, erosions, clusters of chondrocytes) are accompanied by noninflammmatory joint effusion (65, 103). The quinolone-induced joint lesion in animals can manifest as acute arthritis, evident by limping and swelling. Cartilage damage in animals has been shown to be dose-dependent, occurring at different doses in different species (47, 60, 66, 70). Despite these early descriptions, case-controlled retrospective studies with nalidixic acid and controlled clinical and radiographic studies with ciprofloxacin raise doubts concerning the applicability of these animal studies to humans. The exact mechanism of quinolone induced arthropathy is still unknown. It is hypothesized that it could be related to one or more of the following: (i) inhibition of the mitochondrial DNA synthesis in immature chondrocytes (5, 66); (ii) direct toxicity to cartilage from the fluorine substituent (however, this latter possibility seems unlikely since quinolones without a fluorine induce cartilage toxicity in experimental animals; in addition, fluorinated agents other than fluoroquinolones do not cause cartilage toxicity); (iii) compromised mitochondrial integrity; (iv) quinolone-induced oxidative injury to chondrocytes; (v) the chelating properties of the quinolones for magnesium (recent data indicate that they might play an important role because magnesium-deficient juvenile rats showed cartilage lesions that were identical to quinolone-induced lesions [41]).

Studies in Children

Experience with the use of quinolones in children has increased, particularly in children with cystic fibrosis who are given ciprofloxacin. These children, and others receiving nalidixic acid, norfloxacin, and ciprofloxacin, have only had joint symptoms (i.e., arthralgias) that have been reversible occasionally (3, 4). This raises the possibility that humans may have a higher threshold for arthropathy than other species. Moreover, since some children have received the older quinolones for several years (for chronic urinary tract infections), it is likely that arthropathy would have been detected if humans are prone to this complication.

Several case reports of successful quinolone treatment in children without significant adverse side effects have been published (11, 12, 33, 58). Schaad et al. evaluated the effects of orally administered ciprofloxacin (30 mg/kg per day) on cartilage at baseline and after receiving ciprofloxacin for 3 months in 13 prepubertal and 5 postpubertal children with cystic fibrosis. The children were reevaluated at 4 to 6 months later. The investigators used magnetic resonance imaging, growth velocity, bone metabolic studies, and roentgenograms to examine the children for skeletal deformity. Toxic effects on cartilage were not noted in any child enrolled in the study (101). In a subsequent report, Schaad et al. (100) provided data from the autopsies of two children who died of bronchopulmonary disease associated with cystic fibrosis. These children had received oral ciprofloxacin (30 mg/kg per day) for 9 to 10 months during their last 3 years of life. Both children had normal cartilage of the knee at autopsy. Another study of 463 infants and children from 3 to 17 years of age showed that the safety profile of ciprofloxacin did not differ substantially from that in adults; specifically, no arthropathy was reported (64).

Studies to identify subclinical cartilage damage by roentgenogram and nuclear magnetic resonance imaging revealed no abnormalities in children given ciprofloxacin and norfloxacin (7, 100). In patients with cystic fibrosis, reversible arthralgia, sometimes accompanied by discrete synovial effusion with possible or probable relation to quinolone therapy, occurred in 8 of 634 (1.3%) pediatric patients treated with ciprofloxacin (28) and in 9 of 63 (14%) treated with pefloxacin (88). In addition to patients with cystic fibrosis, studies on the use of quinolones (including norfloxacin, ciprofloxacin, and trovafloxacin) in children with other conditions, such as shigellosis, salmonellosis, and meningococcal meningitis, reported no cases of arthropathy (7, 16, 29, 68, 88).

Results of a retrospective cohort study from 1992 to 1998 of more than 6,000 fluoroquinolone-treated children showed that the incidence of tendon-joint disorders 2 months posttherapy was <1% and was comparable with that of the reference group, children treated with azithromycin (111).

In summary, data from studies of ciprofloxacin in children have failed to demonstrate an irreversible drug-induced arthropathy with the morphologic or histologic features consistent with those observed in animal toxicology studies. On the basis of this limited experience and of the potential usefulness of the fluoroquinolones in pediatric infections, the Food and Drug Administration signaled its willingness to consider protocols to study these agents in selected infectious diseases of infants and children.

CLINICAL USES IN PEDIATRICS

The available data about fluoroquinolones suggest that (i) they do not (or, at worst, very rarely) cause arthropathy or bone abnormality in children, (ii) they are well tolerated, and (iii) they are effective. Therefore, the Committee on Infectious Diseases of the American Academy of Pediatrics recommended that these antibiotics should be considered after careful assessment of the risks and benefits for the individual for the following conditions (8): (i) bronchopulmonary exacerbation in patients with cystic fibrosis, (ii) complicated urinary tract infections, (iii) multiresistant gram-negative infection in an immunocompromised host for whom prolonged oral therapy is desired, (iv) chronic osteomyelitis, (v) chronic suppurative otitis media, (vi) infections with multiresistant mycobacteria, and (vii) gastrointestinal infections caused by multiresistant *Salmonella* or *Shigella* species.

CYSTIC FIBROSIS

Chronic relapsing bronchopulmonary infection by *P. aeruginosa* is a major cause of morbidity and mortality for patients with cystic fibrosis. Antibiotic therapy has been shown to be a major factor in improving survival in patients with cystic fibrosis (106). Combination therapy with β-lactam antibiotics and an aminoglycoside have shown the best results. However, parenteral therapy often requires hospitalization, and relapse after treatment may necessitate maintenance therapy. Fluoroquinolones, in particular ciprofloxacin, are the principal drugs for long-term ambulatory treatment of this infection because they are currently the only orally administered agents available for treatment of *P. aeruginosa* infection.

Ciprofloxacin as monotherapy has been shown to be as effective as the standard combination therapy with a β-lactam and an aminoglycoside in pediatric patients (20, 28, 46, 94). However, a major concern of using ciprofloxacin alone in these patients is the emergence of resistance (46), which is particularly an issue when prolonged maintenance or prophylactic therapy is used. To reduce the risk of resistance, intravenous fluoroquinolones should be reserved for the treatment of acute exacerbations when standard therapy has failed or cannot be used because of microbial resistance or adverse effects, or when prolonged oral therapy is required.

FEBRILE NEUTROPENIA

Bacterial infections are a common cause of morbidity and mortality in neutropenic cancer patients. Empiric antibiotic therapy has become a standard of care for these patients during febrile episodes. Many clinical trials during the past three decades have demonstrated that a variety of antibiotic combinations and, more recently, potent antibiotic monotherapies are effective for management of febrile, neutropenic children with cancer (42). The predominant pathogens are gram-negative bacteria, including *Escherichia coli*, *Klebsiella*, *Enterobacter*, and *P. aeruginosa*, and gram-positive bacteria, including coagulase-negative staphylococci, *S. aureus* (including methicillin-resistant *S. aureus*), viridans streptococci, and enterococci. These drugs are potentially useful for preventing infections with gram-negative bacteria, but infections with gram-positive bacteria can occur during use of these drugs (21, 37, 85).

Intravenous ciprofloxacin has been used alone in treating sepsis in the neutropenic host but is less effective than combination therapy of ceftazidime or piperacillin plus amikacin (44).

A prospective evaluation of ciprofloxacin compared with piperacillin and amikacin treatment showed that it performed poorly. Overall success was 47% among those randomized to receive ciprofloxacin compared with 88% for combination therapy. Of greatest concern in this study was the poor response of children with gram-positive bacteremias to ciprofloxacin monotherapy, with only 25% of the children being treated successfully (78).

In contrast, when fluoroquinolones have been used to treat "low-risk" febrile neutropenic patients, they have shown potential benefits (30, 42). Because these agents do not have reliable gram-positive coverage, they are unsuitable for empiric therapy in high-risk febrile neutropenic children especially in conditions that are prone to infections caused by staphylococci.

The improved gram-positive and excellent gram-negative activity of agents like gatifloxacin and moxifloxacin should make these agents excellent candidates for use in high-risk children with febrile neutropenia. As yet, however, data are lacking.

URINARY TRACT INFECTIONS

The fluoroquinolones can be considered as potential candidates for use in pediatric urinary tract infections (UTIs) because (i) more than 90% of all UTI pathogens are gram-negative organisms; (ii) the organisms in complicated UTI are often multiply resistant; and (iii) fluoroquinolones can be given orally, which can avoid hospitalization and allow resumption of normal activity more quickly. Because most of the UTIs are caused by gram-negative bacilli, many of which are multidrug resistant in complicated cases, the fluoroquinolones are a logical choice for treatment, especially when an oral agent is preferred. Resistance can occur after prolonged use, and therefore, they may not be the best choice for prophylaxis (107). Urinary tract infections are one of the principal indications of the fluoroquinolones in adults; however, clinical experience with these antibiotics in children is limited. Two studies (43, 107) reported uniformly excellent success in eradicating the infecting bacteria in 148 patients treated with norfloxacin (6 to 16 mg/kg/day). Ciprofloxacin, norfloxacin, and gatifloxacin are primarily excreted in the urine, making them excellent agents to treat urinary tract infections (53, 81, 102).

GASTROINTESTINAL INFECTIONS

Gastrointestinal infections are a major health problem in infants and children worldwide, causing severe morbidity and mortality. Fluoroquinolones offer an advantage over other classes of antibiotics for gastrointestinal infections because they exhibit excellent activity in vitro against all major enteric bacterial pathogens except *Clostriduim difficile*. Other advantages of using quinolones in the treatment of gastrointestinal infections include the following. Gastrointestinal pathogens, especially *Shigella* and *Salmonella* spp., are becoming increasingly resistant to many antibacterials, including ampicillin, amoxicillin, trimethoprim-sulfamethoxazole, and nalidixic acid (62, 96). High concentrations of these drugs are achieved in feces and are maintained at therapeutic values for several days, permitting a short course of therapy (86). The fluoroquinolones achieve high biliary and intraphagocytic concentrations, which may help in eradicating or preventing the development of the *Salmonella* carrier state after oral treatment. Oral administration of fluoroquinolones eliminates major components of gram-negative aerobic microflora with little effect on the anaerobic flora, and gastrointestinal absorption of fluoroquinolones is not affected by diarrhea (69). These features and the increasing antibiotic resistance of some pathogens causing gastroenteritis (e.g., *Salmonella* and *Shigella*) suggest that the use of these drugs for gastrointestinal infections in children will be successful.

Increasing numbers of studies have documented the efficacy of the fluoroquinolones in the treatment of *Salmonella* or *Shigella*. Lolekha et al. (71) treated 73 children who had shigellosis with trimethoprim-sulfamethoxazole, nalidixic acid, or norfloxacin. The clinical cure rate among patients receiving quinolones was significantly better than that in the trimethoprim-sulfamethoxazole-treated group. In Madagascar 38 children with shigellosis, ranging from 8 months to 13 years of age, were treated with one to three doses of pefloxacin. Sixty-eight percent of the isolates were multidrug resistant. The clinical response and the elimination of *Shigella* from stools were achieved for 84 and 89% of patients after one to two doses of pefloxacin (51). Another study demonstrated that norfloxacin is a safe and effective alternative to nalidixic acid for the treatment of shigellosis and is effective in shigellosis cases infected by nalidixic acid-resistant *Shigella* (16).

In a study in Zaire, 53 children with extraintestinal salmonellosis were treated with oral ciprofloxacin for 5 days or until resolution of fever (up to 6 weeks in bone, joint, or CNS infections). Fifty-one children (96%) were bacteremic. Therapy was judged to be effective in 96% of patients (50). In 21 children with multidrug-resistant typhoid fever with diarrhea, ciprofloxacin was as successful as furazolidone (36).

However, it is necessary to distinguish severe forms (typhoid fever and extraintestinal *Salmonella* infections), in which fluoroquinolone treatment is often necessary, from the nontyphoid *Salmonella* infections, in which the indication of fluoroquinolones is more limited.

In extraintestinal *Salmonella* infections in children, fluoroquinolones can be used effectively because of excellent intracellular penetration, including excellent concentrations in the cerebrospinal fluid (50).

Another problem, particularly in children with sickle cell anemia, is that of *Salmonella* infection of the bones. It is often necessary to use fluoro-

quinolones to facilitate oral treatment if the strain is multidrug resistant.

In addition, therapy with ciprofloxacin has been reported to reduce significantly the duration of diarrhea caused by enteropathogenic *E. coli*, an important cause of diarrhea in developing countries, and of traveler's diarrhea (38, 105).

Reports from Southeast Asia and Spain tell of quinolone resistance among *Salmonella* and *Shigella* strains, which poses a problem for future treatment of these infections (17, 23, 55). High rates of quinolone resistance among *Campylobacter* spp. have been reported as well (80, 90).

BONE AND JOINT INFECTIONS

Ciprofloxacin has been shown to be an effective agent in the treatment of osteomyelitis, especially when the pathogen is a gram-negative organism. Infections of bone and joints have typically required prolonged therapy for cure, most often 4 to 6 weeks and sometimes longer. The prolonged antimicrobial therapy usually used for bone and joint infections is facilitated by effective oral agents, and quinolones may fill this role in some cases. The ease and lower cost of administration of oral agents is important in this context. The most common pathogens are staphylococci, but mixed infections including gram-negative bacilli are often seen in patients with infections of bone developing after open trauma, or in patients with deep ulcers of overlying skin and soft tissues that provide a source of contiguous spread of infection. In addition, *Pseudomonas* is the principal pathogen in osteochondritis of the foot after penetration of a nail through a sneaker tread. Fluoroquinolones offer several advantages over traditional compounds for treatment of osteomyelitis. They inhibit a broad spectrum of gram-negative and gram-positive bacteria, they penetrate into bone at sufficient concentrations, and they can be administered orally. These are important features because osteomyelitis is caused by a variety of organisms and the treatment period is long. Ciprofloxacin, gatifloxacin, and moxifloxacin exhibit good activity against methicillin-susceptible *S. aureus* and *Streptococcus pyogenes*, the two leading organisms in acute osteomyelitis and suppurative arthritis in immunocompetent children. Ciprofloxacin has excellent activity against *P. aeruginosa* and *Salmonella* spp. but lacks reliable activity against pneumococci. By contrast, gatifloxacin and moxifloxacin exhibit excellent activity against penicillin-resistant pneumococci (104). Twelve children with septic arthritis (one with concomitant osteomyelitis) caused by

Salmonella spp. were completely cured by 4 to 6 weeks of treatment with ciprofloxacin (with joint aspiration and irrigation at the start of treatment). There were no adverse effects (48). Raz and Miron (93) documented the efficacy of surgery followed by oral ciprofloxacin therapy for up to 14 days in patients with pseudomonal osteochondritis.

RECURRENT AND PERSISTENT ACUTE OTITIS MEDIA

Fluoroquinolones should not be used for routine treatment of acute otitis media because other antibiotics have adequate efficacy but should be considered for recurrent and nonresponsive acute otitis media. Gatifloxacin, given as 10 mg/kg for 10 days for children between 6 months and 7 years of age with recurrent or nonresponsive acute otitis media, had an overall cure rate of 87% (150 of 173); among evaluable patients with *S. pneumoniae*, the cure rate was 91% (30 of 33). The most frequent drug-related adverse events were vomiting (15%) and diarrhea (5%). There have been no reports of arthropathy (9).

CHRONIC SUPPURATIVE OTITIS MEDIA

Fluoroquinolones should not be used for routine treatment of acute otitis media because other conventionally used antibiotics are satisfactory. However, when *P. aeruginosa* is the causative agent, which often is the case in chronic suppurative otitis media and malignant otitis externa, fluoroquinolones are a logical choice because of their activity against *P. aeruginosa*, good penetration into bone and cartilage, and clinical success in the management of ear and sinus infections in adults (79, 89). Lang et al. published the results of ciprofloxacin treatment in 21 patients between 22 months and 14 years of age with chronic suppurative otitis without cholesteatoma. All patients had previously been treated unsuccessfully with conventional oral agents for otitis, and *P. aeruginosa* was isolated from 86%. Ciprofloxacin for 2 to 3 weeks was successful in 18 of the 21 patients. Resistance developed in three patients, and there was recurrence in 7 of 18 patients during a 16-month follow-up visit (67). The results of this study illustrate that children with chronic suppurative otitis without cholesteatoma can be effectively treated with oral ciprofloxacin. This novel approach may avoid hospitalization. Ciprofloxacin ear drops three times daily for 14 days was also successful in 10 of 11 children (aged 3 to 8 years) with chronic otitic disease and persistent otorrhea for many months. There were no adverse effects (40). Ofloxacin otic solution has been approved by the U.S. Food and Drug Administration for acute otorrhea associated with tympanostomy tubes and otitis externa caused by *S. aureus* and *P. aeruginosa* in children one year of age or older, and for chronic suppurative otitis media with perforated tympanic membranes in children ≥12 years of age (35).

CNS INFECTION

Fluoroquinolones penetrate well into the cerebrospinal fluid (CSF) in the presence of even mildly inflamed meninges, and the concentrations in CSF exceed the MICs for susceptible organisms (49). The increasing prevalence of multidrug-resistant *S. pneumoniae* isolates is a concern worldwide. Although ciprofloxacin does not have good activity against *S. pneumoniae*, the new generation of fluoroquinolones, especially gatifloxacin and moxifloxacin, has excellent activity against even highly penicillin- and cephalosporin-resistant pneumococci, thereby allowing effective bactericidal activity in the central nervous system (14, 74, 83, 84). Data from the rabbit meningitis model demonstrated excellent bacteriologic effectiveness of trovafloxacin, gatifloxacin, and moxifloxacin in meningitis by resistant pneumococci (74, 83, 84). Trovafloxacin was shown in a multicentered, prospective controlled study to be as efffective as conventional treatment (ceftriaxone with or without vancomycin) of infants and children with bacterial meningitis (98). In that study, bacteriologic eradication in CSF at 24 to 36 h after the start of therapy occurred in 95% or more of the patients. Adverse effects were minimal and joint symptoms occurred more often in patients receiving ceftriaxone. Besides *S. pneumoniae*, another potential indication for fluoroquinolones is multidrug-resistant gram-negative meningitis in neonates and in immunocompromised children. Thus, fluoroquinolones may be particularly useful in areas where bacterial resistance is a problem and prolonged parenteral therapy is not feasible. Published case reports demonstrate the successful treatment of infants and children with gram-negative CNS infections (45, 61). Gatifloxacin looks promising for this indication, having shown activity in an animal model of bacterial meningitis caused by gram-negative organisms (74).

In neonates, besides gram-negative organisms, pathogens such as *Listeria monocytogenes*, group B streptococci, and *Mycoplasma hominis* are also susceptible to gatifloxacin, moxifloxacin, and clinafloxacin (14, 109).

RESISTANT PNEUMOCOCCAL INFECTIONS

Increasing resistance of pneumococcal isolates to the penicillins, macrolides, and cephalosporins is a universal concern, especially when empiric use of vancomycin is limited in most centers to avoid selection for vancomycin-resistant enterococci and intermediately resistant *S. aureus* strains. Because new fluoroquinolones such as gatifloxacin and moxifloxacin are highly active against multidrug-resistant strains of *S. pneumoniae* (18, 74, 83, 84), assessment of these agents is indicated in selected pediatric patients with recurrent or persistent acute otitis media and sinusitis, especially those who have failed repeated courses of appropriate antibiotics.

MYCOBACTERIAL INFECTIONS

The fluoroquinlones have good bactericidal activity against many mycobacteria and achieve adequate serum and tissue concentrations. The new methoxyquinolone, moxifloxacin, has bactericidal activity against *M. tuberculosis* similar to that of isoniazid in vitro and in mice (63). Atypical mycobacterial infections in children have been satisfactorily treated with ciprofloxacin as part of combination therapy (75), and gatifloxacin has been shown in vitro to be active against *M. leprae* (99). Fluoroquinolones should not be used alone or as first-line therapy, and they should be reserved for treatment of *M. tuberculosis*, which is resistant to both rifampin and isoniazid. The Centers for Disease Control and Prevention recommend that in areas with multidrug-resistant tuberculosis (i.e., resistance to both isoniazid and rifampin), administration of a fluoroquinolone in combination with pyrazinamide for 6 to 12 months should be considered when prophylaxis is indicated.

PREVENTION OF MENINGOCOCCAL CARRIAGE

Close contacts of patients infected with meningococci are at greater risk of developing the disease than is the general population. chemoprophylaxis is used to eradicate nasopharyngeal carriage of meningococci from such high-risk individuals. Rifampin is used generally, but four doses are required. Ciprofloxacin is effective as a single dose. In Malawi, 469 children were treated effectively with ciprofloxacin, with eradication in more than 90% and no hospitalizations for meningococcal disease in the ensuing 12 months. The rate of adverse effects was similar to that after treatment with rifampin (31).

CONCLUSION

Some fluoroquinolones have been used safely and effectively in selected pediatric patients. As the experience with these agents increases they will become part of the pediatrician's armamentarium for treatment of nosocomial pneumonia, meningitis caused by resistant pneumococci and gram-negative enteric organisms, febrile neutropenic patients managed on an ambulatory basis, chronic *Pseudomonas* infections, acute exacerbation of chronic pulmonary disease in children with cystic fibrosis-selected enteric pathogens caused by *Shigella*, *Salmonella*, and *Campylobacter* species, and possibly in those with persistent or recurrent acute otitis media. Use of these agents in pediatrics must be tempered by the realization that overuse is likely to result in resistance in a fashion similar to that observed with β-lactam antibiotics among pneumococci in infants and young children.

REFERENCES

1. Acar, J. F., and F. W. Goldstein. 1997. Trends in bacterial resistance to fluoroquinolones. *Clin. Infect. Dis.* 24:S67–S73.
2. Acar J. F., T. F. O'Brien, F. W. Goldstein, and R. N. Jones. 1993. The epidemiology of bacterial resistance to quinolones. *Drugs* 45(Suppl. 3):S24–S28.
3. Adam D. Use of quinolones in pediatric patients. 1989. *Rev. Infect. Dis.* 11(Suppl. 5):S1113–S1116.
4. Alghasham, A. A., and M. C. Nahata. 2000. Clinical use of fluoroquinolones in children. *Ann. Pharmacother.* 34:347–359.
5. Amacher, D. E., S. J. Schomaker, T. D. Gootz, and P. R. McGuirk. 1989. Proteoglycan and procollagen synthesis in rat embryo limb bud cultures treated with quinolone antibacterials. *Altern. Methods Toxicol.* 7:307–312.
6. Ambrose, P. G., R. C. Owens, R. Quintiliani, and C. H. Nightingale. 1997. New generations of quinolones: with particular attention to levofloxacin. *Conn. Med.* 61:269–272.
7. Anco, M., G. Bossi, D. Gaselli, G. Cosi, A. Villa, and G. Beluffi. 1995. Long term magnetic resonance survey of cartilage damage in leukemic children treated with fluoroquinolones. *Pediatr. Infect. Dis. J.* 14:713–714.
8. Aradottir, E., and R. Yogev. 1999. The use of fluoroquinolones in pediatrics: a reassessment. *Semin. Pediatr. Infect. Dis.* 10:31–37.
9. Arguedas, A., L. Sher, E. Lopez, X. Saez-Llorens, K. Skuba, and P. Pierce. 2001. Gatifloxacin treatment of recurrent/nonresponsive acute otitis media, abstr. G-1534. *In Program and Abstracts of the 41st Interscience Conference on Antimicrobial Agents and Chemotherapy.* American Society for Microbiology, Washington, D.C.
10. Avila-Aguero, M., J. Blumer, J. Bradley, X. Saez-Llorens, M. O'Ryan, D. Grasela, F. Lacreta, M. Swingle, G. H.

McCracken, and H. Jafri. 2001. Single dose safety and pharmacokinetics of intravenous gatifloxacin in pediatric patients, abstr. A-39. *In Program and Abstr 41st Intersci Conf Antimicrob. Agents Chemother.* American Society for Microbiology, Washington, D.C.

11. Ball, P. 1989. Long term use of quinolones and their safety. *Rev. Infect. Dis.* **11:**S1365–S1370.

12. Bannon, M. J., P. R. Stutchfield, A. M. Weindling, and Damjanovic. 1989. Ciprofloxacin in neonatal *Enterobacter cloacae* septicemia. *Arch. Dis. Child.* **64:**1388–1391.

13. Bast, D. J., D. E. Low, C. L. Duncan, L. Kilburn, L. A. Mandell, R. J. Davidson, J. C. S. De Azavedo. 2000. Fluoroquinolone resistance in clinical isolates of *Streptococcus pneumoniae*: contributions of type II topoisomerase mutations and efflux to levels of resistance. *Antimicrob. Agents Chemother.* **44:**3049–3054.

14. Bauernfeind, A. 1997. Comparison of the antibacterial activities of the quinolones Bay 12–8039, gatifloxacin (AM 1155), trovafloxacin, clinafloxacin, levofloxacin and ciprofloxacin. *J. Antimicrob. Chemother.* **40:**639–651.

15. Bedu, A., I. Naar, and C. Farnoux. 1998. Hypertension intracraienne chez un nouveau-ne traite par quinolones. *Presse Med.* **27:**1140–1142.

16. Bhattacharya, S. K., M. K. Bhattacharya, P. Dutta, D. Sen, R. Raisaily, A. Moitra, and S. C. Pal. 1991. Randomized clinical trial of norfloxacin for shigellosis. *Am. J. Trop. Med. Hyg.* **45:**683–687.

17. Bhutta, Z. A. 1997. Quinolone-resistant Salmonella paratyphi B meningitis in newborn: a case report. *J. Infect.* **35:**308–310.

18. M. D. Blum, D. J. Graham, and C. A. McCloskey. 1994. Temafloxacin syndrome: review of 95 cases. *Clin. Infect. Dis.* **18:**946–950.

19. Borcherding, S. M., R. Stevens, R. A. Nicholas, C. R. Corley, and T. Self. 1996. Quinolones: a practical review of clinical uses, dosing considerations, and drug interactions. *J. Fam. Pract.* **42:**69–78.

20. Bosso, J. A. 1989. Use of ciprofloxacin in cystic fibrosis patients. *Am. J. Med.* **87**(Suppl. 5A):120S–127S.

21. Bow, E. J., E. Rayner, and T. J. Louie. 1988. Comparison of norfloxacin with co-trimoxazole for infection prophylaxis in acute leukemia: the trade-off for reduced gram-negative sepsis. *Am. J. Med.* **84:**847–854.

22. Burkhardt, J. E., J. N. Walterspiel, and U. B. Schhad. 1997. Quinolone arthropathy in animals versus children. *Clin. Infect. Dis.* **25:**1196–1204.

23. Campo, P., A. Gutierrez, and C. Landron de Guevera. 1997. Evolution of susceptibility of non-typhi Salmonella in a Spanish hospital (1992–1994) and report of a Salmonella ser. Typhimurium isolate resistant to quinolones. *Eur. J. Epidemiol.* **13:**239–241.

24. Capparelli, E., F. Lecreta, J. Blumer, J. Bradley, T. Wells, G. Kearns, M. Swingle, G. Duncan, and D. Graela. 2000. Single dose safety and pharmacokinetics of oral gatifloxacin in pediatric patients, abstr. A-15. *In Program and Abstr 40th Intersci Conf Antimicrob Agents Chemother.* American Society for Microbiology, Washington, D.C.

25. Carratala, J., A. Fernandez-Sevilla, F. Tubau, M. Callis, and F. Gudiol. 1995. Emergence of quinolone-resistant Escherichia coli bacteremia in neutropenic patients with cancer who have received prophylactic norfloxacin. *Clin. Infect. Dis.* **20:**557–560.

26. Chen, D. K., A. McGeer, J. C. de Azavedo, and D. E. Low. 1999. Decreased susceptibility of *Streptococcus pneumoniae* to fluoroquinolones in Canada. *N. Engl. J. Med.* **341:**233–239.

27. Chen, S., R. Abels, J. Blumer, A. Chow, H. Goldstein, G. Kearns, S. Maldonado, G. Noel, T. Wells, and S. Spielberg. 2001. Single-dose pharmacokinetics and tolerability of intravenous levofloxacin in pediatric patients, abstr. A-42. *In Program and Abstracts of the 41st Interscience Conference on Antimicrobial Agents and Chemotherapy.* American Society of Microbiology, Washington, D.C.

28. Church, D. A., J. F. Kanga, R. J. Kuhn, T. T. Rubio, W. A. Spohn, J. C. Stevens, P. G. Painter, B. E. Thurberg, D. C. Haverstock, R. Y. Perroncel, and R. M. Echols. 1997. Sequential ciprofloxacin therapy in pediatric cystic fibrosis: comparative study vs. ceftazidime/tobramycin in the treatment of acute pulmonary exacerbations. *Pediatr. Infect. Dis. J.* **16:**97–105.

29. Chysky, V., K. Kapila, R. Hullmann, G. Arcieri, P. Schacht, and R. Echols. 1991. Safety of ciprofloxacin in children. World-wide clinical experience based on compassionate use. Emphasis on joint evaluation. *Infection* **19:**289–296.

30. Cruciani, M., E. Concia, A. Nevarra, L. Pervers, F. Bonetti, M. Arico, and L. Nespoli. 1989. Prophylactic co-trimoxazole vs norfloxacin in neutropenic children-perspective randomized study. *Infection* **17:**65–69.

31. Cuevas, L. E., P. Kazembe, G. K. Mughogho, G. S. Tillotson, and C. A. Hart. 1995. Eradication of nasopharyngeal carriage of *Neisseria meningitidis* in children and adults in rural Africa: a comparison of ciprofloxacin and rifampicin. *J. Infect. Dis.* **171:**728–731.

32. Dagan, R., L. Piglansky, D. Greenberg, A. Leiberman, P. Pierce, L. Wilhelm, and E. Libovitz. 2001. Dynamics of nasopharyngeal pneumococcal carriage in children with recurrent and non-responsive acute otitis media treated with gatifloxacin, abstr. G-1825. *In Program and Abstracts of the 41st Interscience Conference on Antimicrobial Agents and Chemotherapy.* American Society for Microbiology, Washington, D.C.

33. Dagan, R., F. Schlaeffer, and M. Einhorn. 1989. Parenteral fluoroquinolones for the treatment of children with life-threatening infections. *Infection* **18:**237–238.

34. Drlica, K., and X. L. Zhao. 1997. DNA gyrase, topoisomerase IV, and the 4-quinolones. *Microbial. Rev.* **61:**377–392.

35. Daiichi Pharmaceutical. Product information. February 1998. Floxacin otic (ofloxacin otic solution). Fort Lee, N.J.

36. Dutta, P., U. Mitra, R. Rasaily, M. R. Saha, B. Manna, M. K. Chatterjee, T. Garai, M. Sengupta, and S. K. Bhattacharya. 1997. Multi-drug resistant typhoid fever with diarrhea. *Indian Pediatr.* **34:**891–899.

37. Elting, L. S., G. P. Bodey, and B. H. Keefe. 1992. Septicemia and shock syndrome due to viridans streptococci: a case-control study of predisposing factors. *Clin. Infect. Dis.* **14:**1201–1207.

38. Ericsson, C. D., P. C. Johnson, H. L. Dupont, D. Morgan, J. A. M. Bitsura, and F. J. Cabada. 1987. Ciprofloxacin or trimethoprim-sulfamethoxazole as initial therapy for travellers' diarrhea: a placebo-controlled, randomized trial. *Ann. Intern. Med.* **106:**216–220.

39. Ferguson, J., and R. Dawe. 1997. Phototoxicity in quinolones: comparison of ciprofloxacin and grepafloxacin. *J. Antimicrob. Chemother.* **40**(Suppl. A):93–98.

40. Force R. W., M. C. Hart, S. A. Plummer, D. A. Powell, and M. C. Nahata. 1995. Topical ciprofloxacin for otorrhoea after tympanostomy tube placement. *Arch. Otolaryngol. Head Neck Surg.* **121:**880–884.

41. Forster, C., R. Schwabe, E. Lozo, U. Zippel, J. Vormann, T. Gunther, H. J. Merker, and R. Stahlmann. 1997. Quinolone-induced arthropathy: exposure of magnesium-deficient aged

rats or immature rats, mineral concentrations in the target tissues and pharmacokinetics. *Arch. Toxicol.* 72:26–32.

42. Freifeld, A., and P. Pizzo. 1997. Use of fluoroquinolones for empirical management of febrile neutropenia in pediatric cancer patients. *Pediatr. Infect. Dis. J.* 16:140–146.

43. Fuji, R., H. Meguro, O. Arimasu, K. Ushijima, T. Abe, S. Nakazawa, H. Sato, A. Narita, K. Niino, and H. Ichihashi. 1990. Evaluation of norfloxacin in the pediatric field Pediatric Study Group for Norfloxacin. *Jpn. J. Antibiot.* 43:181–215.

44. Gendrel, D., and F. Moulin. 2001. Fluoroquinolones in paediatrics. *Drugs.* 3:365–377.

45. Goepp, J. G., C. K. Lee, T. Anderson, J. D. Dick, J. M. Stokoe, and J. Eiden. 1992. Use of ciprofloxacin in an infant with ventriculitis. *J. Pediatr.* 121:303–305.

46. Goldbarb, J., R. C. Stern, M. D. Reed, T. S. Yamashita, C. M. Myers, and J. L. Blumer. 1987. Ciprofloxacin monotherapy for acute pulmonary exacerbation of cystic fibrosis. *Am. J. Med.* 82(Suppl. 4A):174–179.

47. Gough, A. W., O. B. Kasali, R. E. Sigler, and V. Baragi. 1992. Quinolones arthropathy-acute toxicity to immature articular cartilage. *Toxicol. Pathol.* 20:436–449.

48. Green, S. D. R. 1996. Management of typhoid fever and multi-resistant salmonellosis in children. Presented at First European Congress of Chemotherapy, Glasgow.

49. Green S. D. R., S. M. Ilunga, J. S. Cheesburgh, G. S. Tillotson, M. Hitchens, and D. Felmingham. 1993. The treatment of neonatal meningitis due to gram-negative bacilli with ciprofloxacin: evidence of satisfactory penetration into the CSF. *J. Infect.* 26:253–256.

50. Green S. D. R., and F. Mewa Ilunga. 1992. An open study of ciprofloxacin for the treatment of proven or suspected extraintestinal salmonellosis in African children: a preliminary report. *Adv. Antimicrob. Antineoplast. Chemother.* 11:181–187.

51. Guyon, P., A. M. Cassel-Beraud, G. Rakotonirine, and D. Gendrel. 1994. Short-term pefloxacin therapy in Madagascan children with shigellosis due to multiresistant organisms. *Clin. Infect. Dis.* 19:1172–1173.

52. Hawkey, P. M. 2000. Resistance to ciprofloxacin and the new quinolones. *J. Chemother.* 12:12–14.

53. Hendershot, E. F. 1995. Fluoroquinolones. *Infect. Dis. Clin. N. Am.* 3:715–730.

54. Hoban, D. J., R. N. Jones, L. J. Harrell, M. Knudson, and D. Sewell. 1993. The North American component (the United States and Canada) of an international comparative MIC trial monitoring ofloxacin resistance. *Diagn. Microbiol. Infect. Dis.* 17:157–161.

55. Hoge, C. W., L. Bodhidatta, and C. Tungaem. 1995. Emergence of nalidixic acid resistant *Shigella* dysenteriae type 1 in dessert. *Int. J. Epidemiol.* 24:1228–1232.

56. Hooper, D. C. 1998. Bacterial topoisomerases, anti-topoisomerases, and antitopoisomerase resistance. *Clin. Infect. Dis.* 27(Suppl. 1):S54–S63.

57. Hooper, D. C. 1995. Quinolones, p. 364–376. *In* G. L. Mandell, J. E. Benett, and R. Dolin (ed.). *Principles and Practice of Pediatric Infectious Diseases*, 4th ed. Churchill Livingstone, New York, N.Y.

58. Houwen, R. H., C. M. Bijleveld, and H. G. de Vries-Hospers. 1987. Ciprofloxacin for cholangitis after hepatic portoenterostomy. *Lancet.* i:1367.

59. Iqbal, J., M. Rahman, and M. S. Kabir. 1999. Ciprofloxacin resistance among community-derived methicillin-resistant Staphylococcus aureus (MRSA) strains. *Southeast Asian J. Trop. Med. Public Health.* 30:779–780.

60. Ingham, B., D. W. Brentuall, E. A. Dale, and V. A. McFadzean. 1977. Arthropathy induced by antibacterial fused N-alkyl-pyridone-3-carboxylic acid. *Toxicol. Lett.* 1:21–26.

61. Isaacs, D., M. P. E. Slack, A. R. Wilkinson, and A. W. Westwood. 1986. Successful treatment of *pseudomonas* ventriculitis with ciprofloxacin. *J. Antimicrob Chemother.* 17:535–538.

62. Jahan, Y., and A. Hossain. 1997. Multiple drug-resistant *Shigella dysenteriae* type 1 in Rajban district. Bangladesh. *J. Diarrhoeal Dis. Res.* 15:17–20.

63. Ji, B., N. Lounis, C. Maslo, C. Truffot-Pernot, P. Bonnafous, and J. Grosset. 1998. In vitro and in vivo activities of moxifloxacin and clinafloxacin against *Mycobacterium tuberculosis*. *Antimicrob. Agents Chemother.* 42:2066–2069.

64. Reference deleted.

65. Kato, M., S. Takada, Y. Kashida, and M. Nomura. 1995. Histologic examination on Achilles tendon lesions induced by quinolone antibacterial agents in juvenile rats. *Toxicol. Pathol.* 23:385–392.

66. Kubin, R. 1993. Safety and efficacy of ciprofloxacin in paediatric patients: review. *Infection* 21:413–421.

67. Lang, R., S. Goshen, and A. Raas-Rothschild. 1992. Oral ciprofloxacin in the management of chronic suppurative otitis media without cholesteatoma in children: preliminary experience in 21 children. *Pediatr. Infect. Dis. J.* 11:925–929.

68. Leibovitz, E., J. Janco, L. Piglansky, J. Press, P. Yagupsky, H. Reinhart, I. Yaniv, and R. Dagan. 2000. Oral ciprofloxacin vs IM ceftriaxone as empiric treatment of acute invasive diarrhea in children. *Pediatr. Infect. Dis. J.* 19:1060–1067.

69. Leigh, D. A., B. Walsh, K. Harris, P. Hankok, and G. Travers. Pharmacokinetics of ofloxacin and the effect of the fecal flora of healthy volunteers. *J. Antimicrob. Chemother.* 22(Suppl. C):115–125.

70. Linseman, D. A., L. A. Hampton, and D. G. Branstetter. 1995. Quinolone-induced arthropathy in neonatal mouse. Morphological analysis of articular lesions produced by pipemidic acid and ciprofloxacin. *Fundam. Appl. Toxicol.* 28:59–64.

71. Lolekha, S. S., P. Vivulbanhitkit, and P. Poonyarit. 1991. Response to antomicrobial therapy for shigellosis in Thailand. *Rev. Infect. Dis.* 13(Suppl. 4):342–346.

72. Lumbiganon, P., K. Pengsaa, and T. Sookpranee. 1991. Ciprofloxacin in neonates and its possible adverse effects on the teeth. *Pediatr. Infect. Dis. J.* 10:619–620.

73. Lumpkin, M. M. June 9 1999. Public health advisory. Trovan (trovafloxacin/ alatrofloxacin mesylate). U.S. Food and Drug Administration, Washington, D.C. http://www.fda.gov/cder/news/trovan/trovan-advisory.htm. Accessed March 22, 2000.

74. Lutsar, I., I. R. Friedland, L. Wubbel, C. C. McCoig, H. S. Jafri, W. Ng, F. Ghaffar, and G. H. McCracken. Pharmacodynamics of gatifloxacin in cerebrospinal fluid in experimental cephalsporin-resistant pneumococcal meningitis. 1998. *Antimicrob. Agents Chemother.* 42:2650–2655.

75. Makhani, S., K. R. Postlethwaite, N. M. Renny, C. J. Kerawala, and A. T. Carton. 1998. Atypical cervico-facial mycobacterial infections in childhood. *Br. J. Oral Maxillofac. Surg.* 36:119–122.

76. Martinez-Martinez, L., A. Pascual, and G. A. Jacoby. 1998. Quinolone resistance from a transferable plasmid. *Lancet* 351:797–799.

77. Ma run, S. J., J. M. Meyer, S. J. Chuck, R. Jung, C. R. Messick, and S. L. Pendland. 1998. Levofloxacin and sparfloxacin: new quinolone antibiotics. *Ann. Pharmacother.* 32:320–326.

78. Meunier, F., S. H. Zinner, H. Gaya, T. Calandra, C. Viscoli,

J. Klastersky, and M. Glauser. 1991. Prospective randomized evaluation of ciprofloxacin versus piperacillin plus amikacin for empiric antibiotic therapy of febrile granulocytopenic cancer patients with lymphomas and solid tumors. *Antimicrob. Agents Chemother.* **35**:873–878.

79. Morrison, G. A., and C. M. Baiy. 1988. Relapsing malignant otitis externa successfully treated with ciprofloxacin. *J. Laryngol. Otol.* **102**:872–876.

80. Murphy, G. S., Jr., P. Echeverria, L. R. Jackson, M. K. Arness, C. LeBron, and C. Pitarangsi. 1996. Ciprofloxacin- and azithromycin-resistant Campylobacter causing traveler's diarrhea in U.S. troops deployed to Thailand in 1994. Clin. Infect. Dis. **22**:868–869.

81. Naber, K. G. 2001. Which fluoroquinolones are suitable for the treatment of urinary tract infections?. *Int. J. Antimicrob. Agents.* **17**:331–341.

82. Okusu, H., D. Ma, and H. Nikaido. 1996. AcrAB efflux pump plays a major role in the antibiotic resistance phenotype of *Escherichia coli* multiple-antibiotic-resistance (Mar) mutants. *J. Bacteriol.* **178**:306–308.

83. Ostergaard, C., T. K. Sorensen, J. D. Knudsen, and N. Frimodt-Moller. 1998. Evaluation of moxifloxacin, a new 8-methoxyquinolone, for treatment of meningitis caused by a penicillin-resistant pneumococcus in rabbits. *Antimicrob. Agents Chemother.* **42**:1706–1712.

84. Paris, M. M., S. M. Hickey, M. Trujillo, S. Shelton, and G. H. McCracken, Jr. 1995. Evaluation of CP-99, 219, a new fluoroquinolone, for treatment of experimental penicillin- and cephalosporin-resistant pneumococcal meningitis. *Antimicrob. Agents Chemother.* **39**:1243–1246.

85. Patrick, C. C. 1997. Use of fluoroquinolones as prophylactic agents in patients with neutropenia. *Pediatr. Infect. Dis. J.* **16**:135–139.

86. Pecquet, S., S. Ravoire, and A. Andremont. 1990. Fecal excretion of ciprofloxacin after a single oral dose and its effect on fecal bacteria in healthy volunteers. *J. Antimicrob. Chemother.* **26**:145–150.

87. Peltola, H., M. Vaarala, O. V. Renkonen, and P. J. Neuvonen. 1992. Pharmacokinetics of single-dose oral ciprofloxacin in infants and small children. *Antimicrob. Agents Chemother.* **36**:1086–1090.

88. Pertuiset, E., G. Lenoir, M. Jehanne, F. Douchain, M. Guillot, and C. J. Menkes. 1989. Tolérance articulaire de la péfloxacine et de l'ofloxacine chez les enfants et adolescents atteints de mucoviscidose. *Rev. Rhum. Mal. Osteoartic.* **56**:735–740.

89. Piccirillo, J. F., and S. M. Parnes. 1989. Ciprofloxacin for the treatment of chronic ear disease. *Laryngoscope* **99**:510–513.

90. Pigaru, C., R. Bartolome, B. Almirante, A. M. Planes, J. Gavalda, and A. Pahissa. 1997. Bacteremia due to *Campylobacter* species: clinical findings and antimicrobial susceptibility patterns. *Clin. Infect. Dis.* **25**:1414–1420.

91. Poole, K., K. Tetro, Q. Zhao, S. Neshat, D. E. Heinrichs, and N. Bianco. 1996. Expression of the multidrug resistance operon mexA-mexB-oprM in *Pseudomonas aeruginosa*: mexR encodes a regulator of operon expression. *Antimicrob. Agents Chemother.* **40**:2021–2028.

92. Rattan, A. 1999. Mechanisms of resistance to fluoroquinolones. *Natl. Med. J. India.* **12**:162–164.

93. Raz, R., and D. Miron. 1994. Oral ciprofloxacin for treatment of infection following nail puncture wounds of the foot. *Clin. Infect. Dis.* **21**:194–195.

94. Richard, D. A., S. Nousia-Arvanitakis, V. Sollich, B. J. Hampel, B. Sommerauer, and U. B. Schaad. 1997. Oral ciprofloxacin vs. intravenous ceftazidime plus tobramycin in pediatric cystic fibrosis patients: comparison of antipseudomonas efficacy and assessment of safety with

ultrasonography and magnetic resonance imaging. *Pediatr. Infect. Dis. J.* **16**:572–578.

95. Robson, R. A. 1992. Quinolone pharmacokinetics. *Int. J. Antimicrob. Agents* **2**:3–10.

96. Rowe, B., L. R. Ward, and E. J. Threlfall. 1997. Multidrug resistant *Salmonella typhi*: a worldwide epidemic. *Clin. Infect. Dis.* **24**(Suppl. 1):S106–S109.

97. Rubio, T. T., M. V. Miles, J. T. Lettieri, R. J. Kuhn, R. M. Echols, and D. A. Church. 1997. Pharmacokinetic disposition of sequential intravenous/oral ciprofloxacin in pediatric cystic fibrosis patients with acute pulmonary exacerbation. *Pediatr. Infect. Dis. J.* **16**:112–117.

98. Saez-Llorens, X., C. McCoig, J. M. Feris, S. L. Vargas, K. P. Klugman, G. D. Hussey, R. W. Frenk, L. H. Falleiros-Carvalho, A. G. Arguedas, J. Bradley, A. C. Arrieta, E. R. Wald, S. Pancorbo, G. H. McCracken, Jr., and the Trovan Meningitis Study Group. 2002. Quinolone treatment for pediatric bacterial meningitis. A comparative study of trovafloxacin and ceftriaxone with or without vancomycin. *Pediatr. Infect. Dis. J.* **21**:14–22.

99. Saito, H., M. Gidoh, and K. Kobayashi. 1998. *In vitro* activity of gatifloxacin (AM-1155) against *Mycobacterium leprae*, abstr. E-185. *In Program and Abstracts of the 38th Interscience Conference on Antimicrobial Agents and Chemother.* American Society for Microbiology. Washington, D.C.

100. Schaad, U. B., E. Sander, J. Wedgwood, and T. Schaffner. 1992. Morphologic studies for skeletal toxicity after prolonged ciprofloxacin therapy in two juvenile cystic fibrosis patients. *Pediatr. Infect. Dis. J.* **11**:1047–1049.

101. Schaad, U. B., C. Stoupis, J. Wedgwood, H. Tschaeppeler, and P. Vock. 1991. Clinical, radiologic and magnetic resonance monitoring for skeletal toxicity in pediatric patients with cystic fibrosis receiving a three-month course of ciprofloxacin. *Pedatr. Infect. Dis. J.* **10**:723–729.

102. Stahlberg, H. J., K. Goehler, and M. Guillaume. 1998. Pharmacokinetics of the R- and S-enantiomers of gatifloxacin (GTX), a new fluoroquinolone antibiotic, following single oral doses to healthy caucasian volunteers, abstr. A-25. *In Programs and Abstracts of the 38th Interscience Conference on Antimicrobial Agents and Chemotherapy.* American Society for Microbiology, Washington, D.C.

103. Stahlmann, R., H. J. Merker, N. Hinz, I. Chahoud, J. Webb, W. Herger, and D. Neubert. 1990. Ofloxacin in juvenile non-human primates and rats. Arthropathia and drug plasma concentrations. *Arch. Toxicol.* **64**:193–204.

104. Stein, G. E. 1996. Pharmacokinetics and pharmacodynamics of newer fluoroquinolones. *Clin. Infect. Dis.* **23**(Suppl. 1):S19–S24.

105. Taylor, D. N., J. L. Sanchez, W. Candler, S. Thornton, C. McQueen, and P. Echeverria. 1991. Treatment of travellers' diarrhea: ciprofloxacin plus loperamide compared with ciprofloxacin alone: a placebo controlled, randomized trial. *Ann. Intern. Med.* **114**:731–734.

106. Thomassen, M. J., C. A. Demko, and C. F. Doershuk. 1987. Cystic fibrosis: a review of pulmonary infections and interventions. *Pediatr. Pulmonol.* **3**:334–351.

107. Van Wijk, A. E., T. P. V. M. Dejong, and J. D. Van Gool. 1992. Using quinolones in urinary tract infections in children. *Antimicrob. Agents Chemother.* **11**:157S–161S.

108. Vila, J., J. Ruiz, P. Goni, and T. Jimenez de Anta. 1997. Quinolone-resistance mutations in the topoisomerase IV parC gene of *Acinetobacter baumannii*. *J Antimicrob. Chemother.* **39**:757–762.

109. Waites, K. B., K. C. Canupp, and G. E. Kenny. 1998. Quantitative determination of in vitro susceptibilities of Mycoplasma hominis to fluoroquinolones and quinopristin-

dalfopristin, using E-tests and commercially prepared media, abstr. E-31. *In Program and Abstracts of the 38th Interscience Conference on Antimicrobial Agents and Chemotherapy.* American Society for Microbiology, Washington, D.C.

110. **Wolfson, J. S., and D. C. Hooper.** 1989. Bacterial resistance to quinolones: mechanisms and clinical importance. *Rev. Infect. Dis.* **11:**S960–S968.

111. **Yee, C. L., C. Duffy, P. G. Gerbino, S. Stryker, and G. J. Noel.** 2002. Tendon or joint disorders in children after treatment with fluoroquinolones or azithromycin. *Pediatr. Infect. Dis. J.* **21:**525–529.

Quinolone Antimicrobial Agents, 3rd ed.
Edited by David C. Hooper and Ethan Rubinstein
© 2003 ASM Press, Washington, D.C.

Chapter 23

Quinolone Resistance and Its Clinical Relevance

DONALD E. LOW

Although the introduction of the quinolones proved to be a major therapeutic advance, shortly after their introduction resistance in both gram-negative and gram-positive bacteria was reported and in some circumstances was dramatic (168, 220, 224). New knowledge about the pharmacokinetic/pharmacodynamic (PK/PD) parameters of these agents and how resistance emerges and disseminates may have prevented or at least delayed it (60, 141, 293). The adoption of clinical rather than microbiologic susceptibility interpretive breakpoints has allowed the emergence of resistant subpopulations to go undetected (12, 212). In addition, such resistant subpopulations may have a greater propensity to acquire subsequent mutations that could result in the development of resistance to therapy and lead to clinical failures (103, 180, 236, 262, 291). This chapter focuses on important examples of where resistance has emerged to the fluoroquinolones, the factors responsible, and how this resistance has affected patient management.

RESPIRATORY TRACT PATHOGENS

Streptococcus pneumoniae

The emergence of *S. pneumoniae* resistance to the β-lactam and macrolide antimicrobials has raised concerns regarding the use of these agents for the treatment of suspected or proven pneumococcal infections (17). As a result, fluoroquinolones with increased activity against *S. pneumoniae*, such as levofloxacin, moxifloxacin, and gatifloxacin, are now being recommended and used for the treatment of patients who are at risk for infection due to multidrug-resistant strains (17, 89, 128, 194, 221, 238). However, there has been relatively little experience with the use of these agents as monotherapy for large biomass pneumococcal infections such as community-

acquired pneumonia, as compared with the β-lactam and macrolide antibiotics, especially regarding the potential for the emergence of resistance during therapy.

Drivers of resistance

One possible driver of fluoroquinolone resistance in pneumococci may have been the use of fluoroquinolones, with marginal pneumococcal activity, for respiratory tract infections. When first introduced in 1987, ciprofloxacin was promoted for the treatment of respiratory tract infections, including those caused by *S. pneumoniae*. Results from early preliminary trials supported their use for such an indication (11, 86). However, subsequent studies found that the use of ciprofloxacin for pneumococcal infections was associated with poor eradication rates in both acute exacerbations of chronic bronchitis (AECB) and pneumonia (67, 140, 192, 301). Reports of the development of resistance soon followed (58, 113, 172, 232, 301). PK/PD parameters allow us to understand now why this occurred. In general, the area under the curve (AUC)/MIC ratio now accepted to be most predictive of bacterial eradication and clinical success in gram-positive bacteria is >35 (6, 59, 190, 323). The maximum concentration of drug in serum (C_{max})/MIC ratio accepted to be most predictive for prevention of resistance selection is >4 (191, 295). Following a 750-mg oral dose of ciprofloxacin, the C_{max} is only 3 μg/l and the AUC is 31 μg/ml (111). The MIC at which 90% of the isolates tested are inhibited (MIC_{90}) of *S. pneumoniae* is 1 μg/ml. Therefore, for pneumococci, the C_{max}/MIC ratio is typically only 3 and the AUC/MIC ratio is only 31 (198).

Once clinical failures were recognized to occur when ciprofloxacin was used for the treatment of pneumococcal infections, it was no longer promoted or widely used for the treatment of pneumococcal

Donald E. Low • Department of Microbiology, Toronto Medical Laboratories and Mount Sinai Hospital, and University of Toronto, Ontario, Canada M5G 1X5.

infections, including community-acquired pneumonia. However, it continued to be used for the treatment of AECB at a dose of 500 mg twice daily (319). Eradication rates of *S. pneumoniae* in AECB varied from 63 to 90% (7, 52). Failure to eradicate was associated with the development of resistance during therapy in some patients (7, 53). Surveillance studies conducted in Canada, where ~30% of ciprofloxacin use was for the treatment of AECB, documented the emergence of pneumococci resistant to ciprofloxacin, especially in respiratory isolates from older patients (47).

Another possible cause for the emergence of fluoroquinolone resistance in pneumococci was the acquisition of genes encoding altered target sites for the fluoroquinolones from the less susceptible viridans group streptococci (VGS), analogous to the exchange of chromosomal DNA between VGS and pneumococci that gave rise to penicillin-binding proteins with decreased affinity for penicillin (78). The VGS, which are closely related to pneumococci, are frequently fluoroquinolone resistant (70, 98, 123). Janoir and colleagues (151) investigated the possibility of reciprocal interspecies exchange in vitro of topoisomerase genes between *S. pneumoniae* and VGS. Transformants were obtained with DNA from resistant strains of *Streptococcus oralis, Streptococcus mitis, Streptococcus sanguis,* and *Streptococcus constellatus.* When a double *parC-gyrA* high-level resistant mutant of *S. mitis* was used as a DNA donor, high-level fluoroquinolone-resistant transformants of *S. pneumoniae* were obtained. Ferrándiz et al. (88) analyzed three clinical isolates of *S. pneumoniae* with high-level ciprofloxacin resistance. The structure of the *gyrA* and *parC* genes from two of the isolates was organized in such a way as to suggest genetic transformation with DNA from VGS, supporting the notion that genetically related VGS could act as a reservoir for fluoroquinolone resistance genes. However, Bast et al. (18) analyzed 71 ciprofloxacin-resistant *S. pneumoniae* clinical isolates and found only one for which the quinolone resistance-determining regions (QRDR) of the *parC, parE,* and *gyrB* genes were genetically related to those of VGS. Although their findings support the occurrence of interspecies recombination of type II topoisomerase genes, its contribution to the emergence of quinolone resistance among pneumococci appears to be minimal. This contribution could become more important in certain patient groups or clinical situations where the prevalence of fluoroquinolone resistance in VGS is high enough to increase the likelihood of such exchange.

Another possible driver of resistance may be the increasing unrecognized pool of first-step mutants in the community. Effective surveillance depends on the ability to detect and predict trends in low-level resistance prior to the development of clinically relevant resistance (12). However, this objective may not be realized if the agents in the class, such as levofloxacin or more active fluoroquinolones, are used as the measure of the prevalence of pneumococcal resistance (44, 154). Lim et al. (182) found that 59% of isolates with first-step mutations had a levofloxacin MIC of 2 µg/ml, a level that is considered susceptible according to National Committee for Clinical Laboratory Standards (NCCLS) criteria. Davies et al. (68) found that of 14 strains for which levofloxacin MICs were 2 µg/ml, 10 (71%) had a *parC* mutation. As with gram-negative organisms, first-step mutations in *S. pneumoniae* were more likely to develop second-step mutations when compared with those not having mutations (103, 180, 236, 262, 291). Therefore, because first-step mutants are likely to go unrecognized, physicians may treat infections, such as pneumococcal pneumonia, in which the infecting strain has a first-step mutation and the antimicrobial agent has only marginal activity. In such a setting fluoroquinolone resistance may develop and clinical failures could occur (65).

Finally, preliminary evidence suggests that the fitness cost of pneumococci developing resistance to the fluoroquinolones is not substantial, and in fact, in some cases may be neutral. Gillespie and colleagues (104) selected resistance to these agents in a wild-type strain and measured their fitness in comparative growth experiments. They found that mutation in the *parC* and *gyrA* genes, on some occasions, were not be associated with a physiological deficit.

Prevalence of resistance

Emergence of resistance in *S. pneumoniae* to the fluoroquinolones has been described in Canada, Spain, Hong Kong, Eastern and Central Europe, and to a lesser extent, the United States (Fig. 1). In Canada, Chen et al. (47) found that the prevalence of ciprofloxacin-resistant pneumococci (MIC, ≥4 µg/ml) increased overall from 0% in 1993 to 1.7% in 1997 to 1998 ($P = 0.01$) and in adults to 3.7% (Fig. 2). In addition, the degree of resistance also increased (Fig. 3). From 1994 to 1998, a statistically significant increase occurred in the proportion of isolates with a MIC for ciprofloxacin of ≥32 µg/ml ($P = 0.04$). Linares et al. (183) found in Spain an increase of ciprofloxacin-resistant pneumococci from 0.9% in 1991 to 1992 to 3% in 1997 to 1998. A similar study performed by Perez-Trallero et al. (231) between November 1998 and October 1999 found 7% of *S. pneumoniae* were resistant to ciprofloxacin. Ho and colleagues (133, 135) documented a marked increase

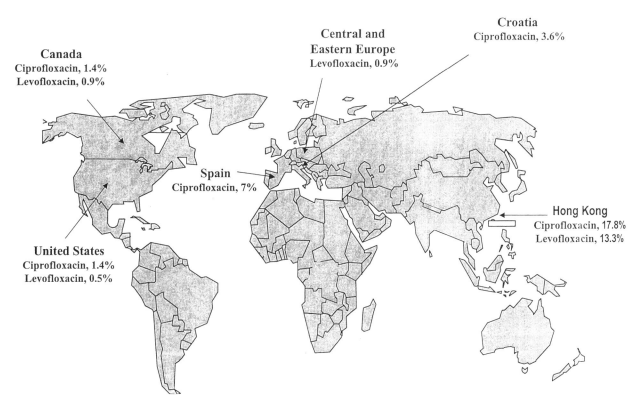

Figure 1. The prevalence of ciprofloxacin-resistant (MIC, ≥4 µg/ml) and levofloxacin-nonsusceptible (MIC, ≥4 µg/ml) *S. pneumoniae* worldwide. Adapted from references 77, 135, 188, 217, 228, 231, and 296.

in the overall prevalence of nonsusceptibility to the fluoroquinolones when comparing results of surveillance studies conducted in 1998 and 2000. Over a two-year period, the prevalence of levofloxacin nonsusceptibility (MIC, ≥4 µg/ml) increased from 5.5 to 13.3% among all isolates and from 9.2 to 28.4% among the penicillin-resistant strains. Nagai and col-

leagues (217) performed surveillance in 10 Central and Eastern European countries between 1999 and 2000. Overall levofloxacin resistance was 0.9%. Pankuch et al. (228) conducted a surveillance study in Croatia where they studied a total of 585 pneumococcus strains isolated from adults in 22 hospitals from 15 Croatian cities between November 2000 and April

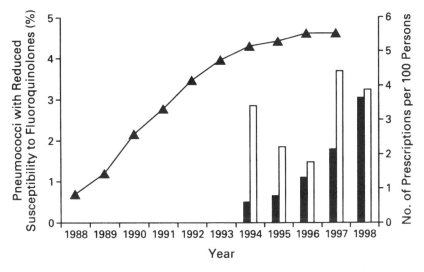

Figure 2. Fluoroquinolone prescriptions per capita (curve) and frequency of pneumococci with ciprofloxacin MICs of ≥4 µg/ml in Canada according to the patient's age (bars). Reprinted from reference 47 with permission. © 1999 Massachusetts Medical Society. All rights reserved.

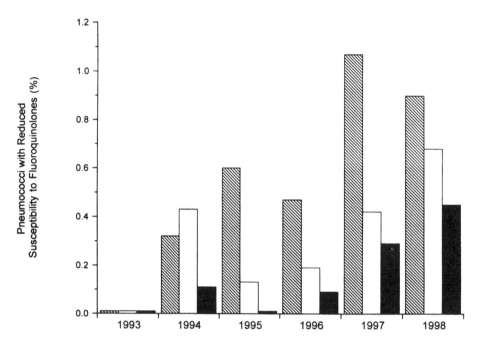

Figure 3. The increasing prevalence and MICs of *S. pneumoniae* resistant to ciprofloxacin (MIC, ≥4 μg/ml) in Canada. The hatched, white, and black bars represent isolates for which the MICs were 4, 8 and 16, and >16 μg/ml, respectively. Reprinted from Clinical Infectious Diseases (187) with permission from University of Chicago Press.

2001. Twenty-one strains (3.6%) were quinolone nonsusceptible. MICs of all quinolones were high for seven strains tested with the same serotype (23F), and mutations were found in *gyrA, parC*, and *parE*. The remaining 14 strains were more heterogeneous and had mutations only in *parC* and/or *parE*. In Northern Ireland, ciprofloxacin resistance was linked to penicillin resistance. Eighteen (42.9%) of 42 penicillin-resistant pneumococci were resistant to ciprofloxacin (110). Rates of resistance in the United States have been found to be <2% (44, 77, 265, 266). Doern et al. (77) reported ciprofloxacin resistance rates of 1.4%. The Centers for Disease Control and Prevention's Active Bacterial Core Surveillance program conducted between 1995 and 1999 reported levofloxacin-nonsusceptible rates of 0.2% (44). They did not include ciprofloxacin as one of the agents tested.

In most countries, reporting increasing ciprofloxacin resistance has been the result of the emergence of de novo resistance in many different serotypes (5, 47, 231). However, in Hong Kong the emergence of resistance has been due to the dissemination of a multiply resistant clone that shares an identical multilocus sequence-typing allelic profile with the globally distributed strain Spain[23F]-1. This fluoroquinolone-resistant variant, designated Hong Kong[23F]-1, was found to have serotype 14 and 19F variants (135). As noted, in Croatia one third of quinolone-resistant strains were serotype 23F (228). McGee et al. (203) characterized a collection of strains that were obtained from a study in Northern

Ireland and from the Alexander Project, an international network that was established in 1992 to monitor the development of antimicrobial resistance to major lower respiratory tract bacterial pathogens. Twenty-nine fluoroquinolone-resistant (ofloxacin MIC, ≥4 mg/liter) isolates of *S. pneumoniae* were selected from the collection of clinical isolates from the Alexander Project and strains from Northern Ireland. Of the 29 fluoroquinolone-resistant strains, eight (28%) belonged to serotype 23F, eight (28%) to serotype 9V, and five (17%) to serogroup 6. Serotypes 35, 22, 34, 14, and 20 accounted for the remaining eight isolates.

Clinical relevance

Although treatment failures due to β-lactams, macrolides, and cotrimoxazole resistance in pneumococci have been reported with meningitis and otitis media, the relation between drug resistance and treatment failures among patients with pneumococcal pneumonia is less clear (71, 283). However, fluoroquinolone resistance in pneumococci causing pneumonia in association with clinical failures, although anecdotal, has been well described (65, 67, 81, 140, 159, 169, 192, 258, 301, 318). Reports of the development of resistance and clinical failures appeared shortly after the introduction of the ciprofloxacin in 1987 (58, 113, 172, 232, 301). Weiss and colleagues (318) described a nosocomial outbreak of fluoroquinolone-resistant pneumococci. Over the course of a 20-month period, in a hospital respiratory ward where ciprofloxacin was often used as empirical antimicrobial therapy for lower respiratory tract infections, 16 patients with chronic bronchitis developed lower respiratory tract infections caused by a strain of penicillin- and ciprofloxacin-resistant *S. pneumoniae* (serotype 23 F). The MIC of ciprofloxacin for all isolates was ≥4 µg/ml. All five patients with AECB treated with ciprofloxacin failed therapy. Davidson et al. (65) reported four cases of pneumococcal pneumonia, treated empirically with oral levofloxacin, that failed therapy. All cases were associated with the isolation of an organism that was either resistant to levofloxacin prior to therapy or that acquired resistance during therapy. Two patients had previously received ciprofloxacin. One of the four patients died after 6 days of monotherapy with levofloxacin.

From these and other studies a number of risk factors have been recognized that identify patients who are likely to be colonized or infected with a fluoroquinolone-resistant pneumococci: patients who are >64 years of age, have a history of chronic obstructive lung disease, and/or prior fluoroquinolone exposure (44, 47, 134, 135, 266). None of the community-acquired pneumonia position papers published since the introduction of the "respiratory" fluoroquinolones has suggested that a history of previous fluoroquinolone use should be a reason for caution when using one of these antimicrobials empirically (17, 128, 194, 221).

Haemophilus influenzae and *Moraxella catarrhalis*

The fluoroquinolones have excellent activity against both *H. influenzae* and *M. catarrhalis*, with ciprofloxacin MIC$_{90}$s of <0.06 µg/ml (316). Resistance rates to ciprofloxacin remain <0.2% for both respiratory pathogens, despite the use of the fluoroquinolones for the treatment of AECB for more than a decade (26, 27, 36, 62, 137, 195). Resistance, when described, is usually associated with prolonged continuous or intermittent therapy and clinical failures (13, 62, 75, 115, 311). The AUC/MIC ratio when treating infections due to *H. influenzae* and *M. catarrhalis* is >300, a value well above the 125 that is predictive of clinical cures and microbiological eradication when treating infections due to gram-negative pathogens (92, 186). The rarity of fluoroquinolone resistance in *H. influenzae* and *M. catarrhalis* may provide support for the strategy of using a fluoroquinolone that has the greatest likelihood of resulting in eradication of the infecting pathogen.

Nazir et al. (219) provided a cautionary note, however, regarding the potential for the emergence of fluoroquinolone resistance in *H. influenzae* and its dissemination. During routine microbiologic surveillance of antibiotic susceptibility, they noted 36% levofloxacin resistance among *H. influenzae* isolates in 2001. Review of surveillance data since 1996 revealed the following proportions of levofloxacin-resistant *H. influenzae*: 0% in 1996, 1% in 1997, 5% in 1998, and 15% in 1999. Thirty-seven of 101 *H. influenzae* isolates in 2001 were resistant. Twenty-eight were recovered from sputum submitted from patients from a long-term care facility, and nine were submitted from patients in hospital (eight from sputum, one from blood). Eight of these hospital patients had been in the long-term care facility previously. The levofloxacin, moxifloxacin, trovafloxacin and ciprofloxacin MICs for all of the long-term care facility isolates was 32 µg/ml.

Streptococcus pyogenes

Although ciprofloxacin and levofloxacin have only moderate activity against group A streptococci, with MIC$_{90}$s of 0.5 µg/ml, previous reports of resistance have been rare (14, 325). However, in a nationwide multicenter susceptibility surveillance study in Spain by Pérez-Trallero et al. (231), 70 (3.4%) of 2,039 isolates of *S. pyogenes* had a ciprofloxacin MIC of ≥4 µg/ml and were found equally in children and adults. Ciprofloxacin resistance was more prevalent among erythromycin-nonsusceptible group A streptococci than among erythromycin-susceptible ones.

Other Respiratory Pathogens

Although fluoroquinolone resistance has been described in clinical isolates of *Mycoplasma hominis*, it has yet to be described in *Mycoplasma pneumoniae* (20, 21). Similarly, fluoroquinolone resistance has been described in *Chlamydia trachomatis*, but not yet in *Chlamydia pneumoniae* (281). Morrissey et al. (211) investigated the in vitro development of fluoroquinolone resistance in *C. trachomatis* and *C. pneumoniae* after exposure to subinhibitory concentrations of fluoroquinolones for numerous passages. Although they were able to select for strains of *C. trachomatis* that were highly resistant, they could not sustain reduced fluoroquinolone susceptibility with *C. pneumoniae*. Finally, although fluoroquinolone resistance has not been described in clinical isolates of *Legionella* spp., resistance has been obtained in vitro (222). A concern is that these agents are not routinely isolated from patients with clinical infections and susceptibility testing is problematic. Therefore resistance may well emerge and go undetected.

SEXUALLY TRANSMITTED DISEASES

Fluoroquinolones are highly active in vitro against *Neisseria gonorrhoeae* (ciprofloxacin MIC, ≤0.03 µg/ml) and are effective in treating gonococcal infections. As a result of the emergence of penicillin-, tetracycline-, and spectinomycin-resistant strains of *N. gonorrhoeae* in the 1980s in the United States, the Centers for Disease Control and Prevention (CDC) included fluoroquinolones for the treatment of uncomplicated gonorrhea (40, 41). In 1993, the CDC recommended single-dose, oral therapy with ciprofloxacin (500 mg) or ofloxacin (400 mg) as two of the primary regimens for the treatment of uncomplicated gonorrhea (41).

Drivers of Resistance

In some countries, gonococcal infections have been treated with a single, orally administered dose of 250 mg of ciprofloxacin as opposed to the 500 mg recommended by the CDC (116). This may be one of the factors that explain the emergence of resistance in Asia and the failure of resistance to emerge in the United States, and when it has been recognized, it has often been imported (42, 165). Once fluoroquinolone resistance emerged, its dissemination was facilitated by the failure of treatment to eradicate the organism, resulting in an increased likelihood for person-to-person transmission, locally, nationally, and internationally (8, 21, 25, 247, 288, 290, 302).

Prevalence of Resistance

Current NCCLS guidelines now define isolates with intermediate susceptibility (low-level resistance) to ciprofloxacin and ofloxacin when the MIC is 0.125 to 0.5 µg/ml and 0.5 to 1.0 µg/ml, respectively. Resistance is defined as when the ciprofloxacin and ofloxacin MIC is ≥1 and ≥2 µg/ml, respectively. Quinolone-nonsusceptible *N. gonorrhoeae* strains first appeared in Southeast Asia in the early 1980s. They were initially only low-level resistant. This pattern remained unchanged until 1991, when resistant strains were first identified (164).

Low-level resistant strains have now been reported from many countries worldwide (164). Resistant strains have been reported most frequently from the Philippines, Hong Kong, and Japan, and less frequently from Australia, Canada, Spain, Thailand, United Kingdom, and the United States (164). The frequency of fluoroquinolone-nonsusceptible strains has increased dramatically since the early 1990s. For example, in Hong Kong, fluoroquinolone-nonsusceptible strains were isolated inter-

mittently from 1990 to 1992 (157) but increased from an estimated 0.5% in late 1992 to 10.4% in late 1994 (156).

From 1994 to 1995, strains with low-level resistance to ciprofloxacin and ofloxacin accounted for approximately 36, 54, and 22% of strains in Hong Kong, the Philippines, and Thailand, respectively (164). During the same period, resistant strains accounted for approximately 10, 12, and 1% of all strains in Hong Kong, the Philippines, and Thailand, respectively (164).

In other geographic areas, fluoroquinolone-nonsusceptible strains have been isolated only sporadically, although with increasing frequency. Ison et al. (149) presented results from a surveillance study that included 10 hospitals in the London area that was conducted in 1997. They found that only 0.4% of isolates were ciprofloxacin resistant (MIC, ≥1 µg/ml). Rahman et al. (248) tested a total of 343 gonococcal strains isolated from persons in Bangladesh from 1997 to 1999. Of the isolates from 1997, 9% were resistant (MIC, ≥1.0 µg/ml) to ciprofloxacin, whereas 41 and 49% of the isolates from 1998 and 1999, respectively, were resistant to ciprofloxacin. In Sweden, they compared epidemiological data with antibiotic susceptibility patterns of strains isolated from February 1998 through January 1999, so as to characterize the risk of infection with a highly resistant *N. gonorrhoeae* strain (23). Epidemiological data were received from each clinician reporting a case of gonorrhea, and these data were linked to the *N. gonorrhoeae* strains. Of a total of 348 *N. gonorrhoeae* isolates, representing 89% of all Swedish cases diagnosed during the 12-month period, 18% had decreased susceptibility to ciprofloxacin (MIC, >0.064 mg/liter). The antibiotic susceptibility varied with the places where patients were exposed to infection. When exposed in Asia, 63% of the isolates showed reduced susceptibility to ciprofloxacin, compared with 0 to 8.5% of the isolates from patients exposed in other places (relative risk, 8.5; $P < 0.001$). In Sydney, Australia, fluoroquinolone-nonsusceptible strains were isolated infrequently in 1991 to 1994 (289). In 1999, 17% of gonococcal isolates displayed reduced susceptibilities to the quinolones, three times the number seen in 1998 (287). In Israel, at the end of 1999, ciprofloxacin-resistant strains of *N. gonorrhoeae* (MICs, ≥32 µg/ml) were isolated for the first time in southern Israel, as well as in other regions of the country (64, 324). The incidence of male gonococcal urethritis in the South increased in a 1.5-year period from 3 of 100,000 to 12 of 100,000 ($P < 0.05$) in correlation with increased isolation of ciprofloxacin-resistant organisms (324). A marked increase in the incidence of gonorrhea was also encountered in Jerusalem, where 54.5% of the isolates in 2000 were ciprofloxacin resistant. Pulsed-field gel electrophoresis typing of gonococci from different areas of Israel indicated that all of the ciprofloxacin-resistant isolates belonged to identical or related strains. In China resistance rates to ciprofloxacin were reported to be 34% (326). The CDC-sponsored Gonococcal Isolate Surveillance Project in the United States reported that the frequency of strains with low-level resistance increased from 0.3% (17 of 5,238) in 1991 to 1.3% (65 of 4,996) in 1994 ($P < 001$); however, resistant strains accounted for only 0.04% (2 of 4,996) of strains in 1994. In the United States, the increase in strains with low-level resistance was associated largely, but not exclusively, with the persistence of such strains in Cleveland, Ohio. First detected in 1992, these strains accounted for ~16% of isolates in Cleveland in 1994 (114, 166). In addition, a sustained outbreak caused by ciprofloxacin-resistant isolates has been reported from Seattle, Wash., in 1995; these strains had MICs of 8.0 μg/ml of ciprofloxacin and ofloxacin (42). The percentage of gonococcal isolates in Hawaii that were ciprofloxacin resistant increased from 1.4% (4 of 290) in 1997 to 9.5% (22 of 231) in 1999 (43). Otherwise, fluoroquinolone-resistant *N. gonorrhoeae* occurs rarely in the United States: less than 0.05% of 4,639 isolates collected by CDC's Gonococcal Isolate Surveillance Project during 1996 had MICs of ≥1.0 μg/ml to ciprofloxacin. There are, however, areas where rates of fluoroquinolone resistance have required changes in first-line therapy.

Clinical Relevance

Rahman and colleagues (247) performed a prospective study of 217 female sex workers in Dhaka, Bangladesh. Overall, 37.8% of the gonococcal isolates recovered from female sex workers were resistant to ciprofloxacin. For 95% of the isolates from patients who had treatment success, the MICs were 0.008 to 0.06 μg/ml. On the other hand, for 96% of the isolates from patients who had treatment failure, the MICs were 1 to 32 μg/ml. Aplasca de los Reyes and colleagues (8) performed a study whereby 105 female sex workers with gonorrhea were prospectively randomly selected to receive treatment with oral ciprofloxacin (500 mg) or cefixime (400 mg) and followed up for test of cure. *N. gonorrhoeae* was reisolated within 28 days after treatment from 1 (3.8%) of 26 women given cefixime (to which all strains were susceptible) versus 24 (32.3%) of 72 women given ciprofloxacin ($P < 0.01$). Treatment failure (reisolation of pretreatment auxotype/serovar) occurred in 14

(46.7%) of 30 women infected with strains with ciprofloxacin MICs of ≥4.0 μg/ml versus 1 (3.6%) of 28 infected by strains with MICs <4.0 μg/ml ($P < 0.01$).

Chlamydia trachomatis

A well documented feature of chlamydial infection has been its high rate of recurrence among sexually active populations. However, determining whether recurrent disease is due to reinfection or to persistent infection with the same organism has been difficult. Of particular concern is whether some persistent infections are a consequence of resistance to standard antimicrobial agents. Although *C. trachomatis* historically has been sensitive to the tetracyclines, macrolides, and fluoroquinolones, recent reports have noted increasing in vitro resistance to tetracycline and erythromycin. Somani et al. (281) conducted in vitro susceptibility testing and genotyping on urogenital isolates of *C. trachomatis* from three patients, two of whom showed evidence of clinical treatment failure with azithromycin and one of whom was the wife of a patient. All three isolates demonstrated multidrug resistance to doxycycline, and azithromycin, and had an ofloxacin MIC of >4.0 μg/ml. Recurrent disease due to relapsing infection with the same resistant isolate was documented on the basis of identical genotypes of both organisms. Fluoroquinolone resistance will emerge in *C. trachomatis* (72). Morrissey and colleagues (211) were readily able to select for resistant mutants by several passages in subinhibitory concentrations of fluoroquinolones. In addition, because of the technical expertise and time required to determine antimicrobial susceptibilities for *C. trachomatis*, resistance may go unrecognized.

ENTERIC PATHOGENS

Food-borne infections are an important cause of illness and hospitalization in developing and developed countries. Although antimicrobial agents are not essential for the treatment of most of these infections, they can be lifesaving in cases of severe infection. The use of ampicillin, chloramphenicol, and cotrimoxazole is limited because of increasing antimicrobial resistance to these agents. Fluoroquinolones such as ciprofloxacin are commonly used for adult patients with *Salmonella* and *Campylobacter* infections and for the treatment of acute gastroenteritis. However, their use has become threatened by the emergence of isolates with reduced susceptibility to the fluoroquinolones during the past decade.

Before fluoroquinolones were introduced in agriculture, nontyphoidal *Salmonella* and *Campylobacter* resistance to quinolones was rare. However, quinolone resistance in humans appeared shortly after their approval for use in animal husbandry (85). Accordingly, the alarming increase in quinolone resistance observed during the past few years among nontyphoidal *Salmonella* and *Campylobacter* has aroused speculation that this might be an effect of the use of quinolones in animal husbandry (51, 176, 200, 208). In Asia, several quinolones, including three fluoroquinolones licensed for humans (ciprofloxacin, ofloxacin, and norfloxacin), have been approved for animal use (121). In Taiwan, enrofloxacin has been used as a growth promoter (202). In Europe, none of the fluoroquinolones licensed for humans are approved for animal use, although many other quinolone preparations are allowed for the treatment of livestock, poultry, and fish. In the United States, enrofloxacin is allowed for treatment of poultry and cattle respiratory infections (204). In Canada, enrofloxacin was only approved for egg dipping for a brief period of time. The manufacturer voluntarily withdrew the drug in 1997 because of extensive extra label use in food-producing animals (2).

Salmonella

Typhoid fever is a life-threatening illness caused by the bacterium *Salmonella enterica* serovar Typhi. In the United States about 400 cases occur each year, and 70% of these are acquired while traveling internationally. Typhoid fever is still common in the developing world, where it affects about 12.5 million persons each year. *S. enterica* serovar Typhi lives only in humans and would therefore not be affected by the use of fluoroquinolones in agriculture. Nontyphoidal *Salmonella* spp. are associated with animals, and salmonellosis is usually linked to foods of animal origin.

Fluoroquinolones have excellent in vitro and clinical activity against isolates of the *Salmonella* with MIC_{90}s of ≤ 0.06 μg/ml (9). *Salmonella* isolates with reduced susceptibilities to the quinolones typically have single amino acid substitutions in the QRDR. Although the mutations that have been reported are clustered between Ala67 and Tyr122, it is Ser83 and Asp87 that are most commonly substituted (Table 1). In contrast, GyrB substitutions are rare, and no substitutions in ParC or ParE have been described to the best of my knowledge (Table 1). Although it is unclear as to the absence of ParC and ParE mutations, it is possible that such alterations may have a prohibitive cost to the fitness of *Salmonella* spp. (105). Decreased susceptibility to ciprofloxacin due to active efflux may also contribute to a reduction in activity of the fluoroquinolones (106, 241).

The NCCLS guidelines use the MICs of ≤ 1 and ≥ 4 μg/ml and ≤ 16 and ≥ 32 μg/ml as respective breakpoints for susceptibility and resistance for ciprofloxacin and nalidixic acid, respectively (218). First-step mutations of the *gyrA* gene result in ciprofloxacin MICs that are ≥ 0.125 but ≤ 1 μg/ml (105, 106, 122). Typically *Salmonella* that have MICs of ≥ 4 μg/ml have two amino acid substitutions in GyrA or a combination of amino acid substitutions in GyrA and GyrB (105, 129). However, isolates have been identified with MICs of ≥ 4 μg/ml that only have a single mutation in *gyrA*, suggesting some other additional mechanism (105). Single-point mutation in the QRDR of the *gyrA* gene in salmonellas usually leads simultaneously to resistance to nalidixic acid (122).

Table 1. The frequency of mechanisms responsible for a reduction of fluoroquinolone activity in *Salmonella* isolated from humans and animals[a]

| Amino acid substitution (mutation) in | | Efflux | Frequency | Frequency of occurrence of the following MIC (μg/ml) | | | |
GyrA	GyrB			0.12 to 0.5	1	2	≥4
Ser83→Phe			+++	+++	+	+	+
Ser83→Phe	Asp87→Asn		−/+				+
Ser83→Phe	Asp87→Gly		−/+				+
Ser83→Tyr			++	+	+	+	+
Ser83→Ala	Asp→78Asn						+
Asp87→Asn			+++	+++			
Asp87→Gly			++	++	+	+	
Asp87→Tyr			++	+++			
Asp87→Tyr	Ser83→Phe		−/+	+			
Ala119→Glu			−/+	+			
	Ser463→Tyr		−/+	+			
		Yes		+			

[a] Clonal isolates were counted as one. Table adapted from references 35, 105, 118, 122, 171, 181, 208, 225, 240, 256, 314.

Hakanen et al. (122) evaluated 1,010 *Salmonella* isolates for susceptibility to nalidixic acid and ciprofloxacin. These isolates were divided into two distinct subpopulations, with the great majority (*n* = 960) being fully ciprofloxacin susceptible and a minority (*n* = 50) exhibiting reduced ciprofloxacin susceptibility (MICs ranging between ≥0.125 and ≤1 µg/ml). The less ciprofloxacin-susceptible isolates were uniformly resistant to nalidixic acid, whereas only 12 (1.3%) of the fully susceptible isolates were nalidixic acid resistant. A mutation of the *gyrA* gene could be demonstrated in all isolates for which the ciprofloxacin MICs were ≥0.125 µg/ml and in 94% of the nalidixic acid-resistant isolates, but in none of the nalidixic acid-susceptible isolates analyzed. Identification of nalidixic acid resistance by the disk diffusion method provided a sensitivity of 100% and a specificity of 87.3% as tools to screen for isolates for which the MICs of ciprofloxacin were ≥0.125 µg/ml.

Liebana et al. (181) characterized 100 veterinary isolates of *Salmonella* isolates selected on the basis of nalidixic acid resistance. All but a single isolate showed at least decreased susceptibility to ciprofloxacin (MICs of ≥0.25 µg/ml). All but one isolate had a mutation in *gyrA*.

Drivers of resistance

As noted above the major reasons for the rapid increase in nontyphoidal *Salmonella* spp. with reduced susceptibility to the fluoroquinolones has been the use of the fluoroquinolones in agriculture, especially in pigs and poultry (101, 139, 143, 241). Fluoroquinolone-resistant *Salmonella* is then transferred to humans by eating colonized meat. Chiu and colleagues (51) documented the dramatic rise of fluoroquinolone resistance in clinical isolates (70% from blood cultures) of *S. enterica* serovar Choleraesuis in Taiwan, where fluoroquinolones have been added to animal feed as a growth promoter for several years (202). They first observed ciprofloxacin resistance in 2000. By the third quarter of 2001, 60% of clinical isolates of serovar Choleraesuis were resistant to ciprofloxacin (Fig. 4). Antibiograms, plasmid-profiling, and molecular-typing results all implicated swine as the source of the resistant strains. Another source of resistance is the selection of spontaneous mutants with reduced susceptibilities to the fluoroquinolones in patients during therapy (234).

Once established, a resistant clone can then spread from person to person (208, 225). An example of the clonal spread of a resistant clone is *S. enterica* serovar Typhimurium DT104. Since the 1990s, infections with DT104 have been recognized in several countries; DT104 is the second most prevalent salmonella in humans in England and Wales (108, 208, 297, 299). Since 1994, the incidence of multiresistant DT104, with additional resistance phenotypes, has increased including the presence of reduced susceptibility to the fluoroquinolones (8, 66, 108, 208, 256).

An additional source of strains of *Salmonella* with reduced susceptibility to the fluoroquinolones is

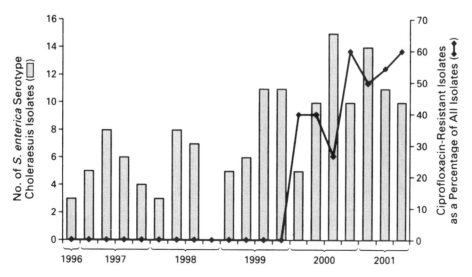

Figure 4. Emergence of fluoroquinolone resistance among *S. enterica* serovar Choleraesuis isolates in Taiwan. Shown here are the total quarterly numbers of serovar Choleraesuis isolates from Chang Gung Memorial Hospital and Chang Gung Children's Hospital from the fourth quarter of 1996 through the third quarter of 2001 (bars) and the percentage of these isolates that were resistant to ciprofloxacin (curve). Ciprofloxacin was not available in these hospitals before October 1996. Reprinted from reference 51 with permission. © 2002 Massachusetts Medical Society. All rights reserved.

the return traveler or visitor from an endemic area of resistance (94, 121). Hakanen et al. (121) in Finland collected 1,210 *Salmonella* isolates; 629 were from Finnish travelers returning from abroad. From 1995 to 1999, the annual proportion of travelers' isolates with reduced ciprofloxacin susceptibility (MIC, ≥0.125 μg/ml) increased from 3.9 to 23.5% (*P* < 0.001). The increasing trend was particularly striking among the isolates from Southeast Asia; isolates with reduced ciprofloxacin susceptibility from Thailand alone increased from 5.6 to 50.0% (*P* < 0.001).

Prevalence of resistance

Salmonella isolates with reduced susceptibility to the fluoroquinolones have increased in both humans and animals, especially in Europe, Southeast Asia, and the Indian subcontinent (Fig. 5) (28, 45, 51, 63, 94, 108, 136, 208, 242, 297).

Nontyphoidal *Salmonella* spp. Between 1991 and 1994, *Salmonella* with reduced fluoroquinolone susceptibility isolated from humans in England and Wales increased from 0.3 to 2.1% (94, 297). Among the most prevalent serotypes, the highest incidence was seen in *S. enterica* serovar Hadar, where isolates with reduced fluoroquinolone susceptibility increased from

2.0% in 1991 to 39.6% in 1994. In 1994, 5.1% of *S. enterica* serovar Virchow and *S. enterica* serovar Newport were resistant compared with 1.4% of *S. enterica* serovar Typhimurium and 0.4% of *S. enterica* serovar Enteritidis. This trend continues (317).

In Belgium, Van Looveren and colleagues (306) studied a random sample of 378 *Salmonella* strains of human origin that were collected during 1998. In total, 38 serotypes were represented, of which *S. enterica* serovar Enteritidis (20.4%), serovar Typhimurium (20.4%), serovar Hadar (9.0%), serovar Brandenburg (7.9%), serovar Infantis (7.7%), and serovar Virchow (5.3%) were the most common. All strains were susceptible to ceftriaxone and ciprofloxacin. For nalidixic acid the rate of resistance was 19.0%. Of the 72 strains resistant to nalidixic acid, 31 were serovar Hadar. Most of the serovar Hadar strains were also resistant to ampicillin, tetracycline, and sulfamethoxazole, and had elevated ciprofloxacin MICs at which 50% of the isolates tested are inhibited (MIC_{50}s) (0.25 μg/ml) and MIC_{90}s (1 μg/ml). In Spain, Prats et al. (246) studied the trends of resistance in enteropathogenic bacteria from between 1985 and 1987 and 1995 and 1998. Although ciprofloxacin resistance remained <1, nalidixic acid resistance increased from <1 to 11%. Eighty-six percent of serovar Hadar was nalidixic acid resistant in 1995 to 1999.

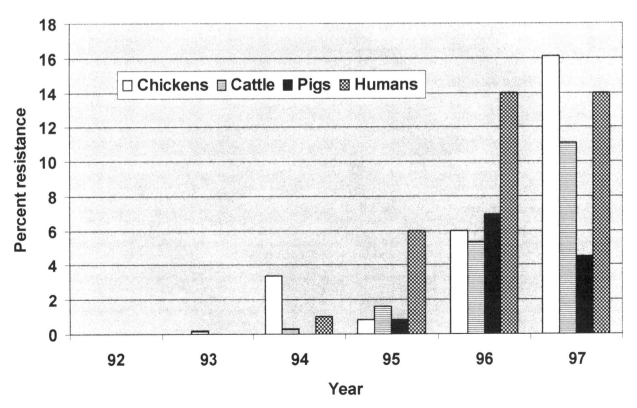

Figure 5. Prevalence of *Salmonella* with decreased susceptibility to ciprofloxacin (MIC, >0.06 μg/ml). Adapted from references 51, 94, 121, 136, 138, 298.

In the United States fluoroquinolone-resistant *Salmonella* is rare. Only 21 (0.5%) of the 4,008 *Salmonella* isolates collected and analyzed from 1994 to 1995 were resistant to nalidixic acid (132). Even in multidrug-resistant *S. enterica* serovar Typhimurium DT104, quinolone resistance in the United States has remained rare (108,253). Olsen and colleagues (225) reported a nosocomial outbreak of *Salmonella* infection in Oregon. Eleven patients with fluoroquinolone-resistant salmonellosis were identified at two nursing homes. The index patient had been hospitalized in the Philippines and had probably acquired the infection there. The isolates from the outbreak were also similar to the only previous isolate of fluoroquinolone-resistant salmonella, which came from a patient in New York who had been transferred from a hospital in the Philippines. Rossiter et al. (259) reported the emergence of fluoroquinolone resistance among nontyphoidal *Salmonella* detected by the National Antimicrobial Resistance Monitoring System. After serotyping, public health laboratories in the 17 National Antimicrobial Resistance Monitoring System participating sites forwarded every tenth nontyphoidal *Salmonella* isolate to the CDC for susceptibility testing to ciprofloxacin. Patients with isolates exhibiting decreased susceptibility (MIC, >0.25 μg/ml) to ciprofloxacin, including ciprofloxacin resistance (MIC, >4 μg/ml), were interviewed. The percent of isolates that demonstrate decreased susceptibility to fluoroquinolones was 0.4% (5 of 1,326) in 1996 and 1.4% (20 of 1,378) in 2000. Seven (0.1%) of these isolates were ciprofloxacin-resistant (MIC, ≥4 μg/ml). All seven infections were associated with international travel. Of 28 of the 50 patients with ciprofloxacin MICs of >0.25 and <4 μg/ml, 20 (71%) did not travel internationally in the week before illness onset.

Isenbarger and colleagues (148) characterized bacterial isolates from studies of community-acquired diarrhea conducted in Thailand and Vietnam from 1996 to 1999. From Thailand there were 696 salmonella isolates, of which 20% were nalidixic acid resistant and <1% were ciprofloxacin resistant. There were only 30 isolates from Vietnam, all of which were susceptible to both antimicrobials. In Ontario, Canada, nontyphoidal *Salmonella* resistance rates to ciprofloxacin and nalidixic acid are <1%. However, up to a third of all *S. enterica* serovar Typhi isolates are resistant to nalidixic acid (150).

Typhoidal *Salmonella*. *S. enterica* serovar Typhi is endemic in developing countries in Africa, South and Central America, and the Indian subcontinent,

with an estimated incidence of 33 million cases each year. By contrast, in developed countries such as the United Kingdom or the United States, incidence is much lower, and most cases are in travelers returning from endemic areas. Serovar Typhi with decreased susceptibility to ciprofloxacin (MIC, ≥0.125 μg/ml) increased to 23% in the United Kingdom in 1999 (298). All strains with decreased sensitivity to ciprofloxacin were also resistant to nalidixic acid. Most patients had recently returned from India or Pakistan. However, in 1998 and 1999, strains with decreased susceptibility to ciprofloxacin were also isolated from travelers returning from Sri Lanka, Nepal, Bangladesh, and Thailand.

Since 1993, strains of serovar Typhi with decreased susceptibility to ciprofloxacin have been isolated in Vietnam, although they still remain rare (148, 260).

In Mumbai, India, nalidixic acid resistance in serovar Typhi increased from zero in 1990 to 82% in 2000 (257). In 1997, an outbreak of nalidixic acid-resistant serovar Typhi with decreased susceptibility to ciprofloxacin involved more than 6,000 people in Tajikistan (214). The epidemic strain had a pulsed-field gel electrophoresis profile indistinguishable from that of isolates of multidrug-resistant Vi-phage type E1 from patients infected in India (125).

Clinical relevance

Although case reports of infections caused by salmonella with reduced susceptibility to the fluoroquinolones are rare, there is increasing evidence that such infections may be associated with a less than satisfactory outcome when infections due to such organisms are treated with a fluoroquinolone (132, 234, 241, 304, 308). In most cases, the isolates have had ciprofloxacin MICs of ≥0.125 μg/ml but ≤1 μg/ml and have included both systemic and enteric infections (94, 153, 208, 234, 244, 298, 304, 314). This includes situations where either the original strain had reduced susceptibility to the fluoroquinolones (208, 298, 314) or resistance developed during therapy (94, 101, 143, 234, 244, 308).

Typhoidal *Salmonella*. To reduce the cost and possible toxicity, courses of fluoroquinolones shorter than one week have been evaluated in patients with mild-to-moderate typhoid fever. Studies conducted in Vietnam have shown that courses of treatment as short as 2 days are >90% effective (279, 313). Wain et al. (314) reported their findings in a trial of short-course ofloxacin therapy in adults and children with blood-culture-confirmed, uncomplicated typhoid fever. Adults received ofloxacin either at a dosage of

10 mg/kg body weight in two daily divided doses for 3 days or 15 mg /kg of body weight in two daily divided doses for 2 days. Children were given ofloxacin at a dosage of 15 mg/kg body weight in two daily divided doses for either 2 or 3 days. Clinical failure was defined as failure to resolve fever 7 days after the start of treatment in association with persistence of symptoms and signs or the development of severe or complicated enteric fever. The MIC of ofloxacin for the nalidixic acid-resistant *S. enterica* serovar Typhi was 0.125 to 1.0 μg/ml. The MIC of ofloxacin for the nalidixic acid susceptible serovar Typhi was 0.03 to 0.25 μg/ml. There were 132 nalidixic acid-susceptible isolates and 18 resistant isolates. The median time to fever clearance was 156 h (range, 30 to 366 h) for patients infected with nalidixic acid-resistant serovar Typhi and 84 h (range, 12 to 378 h) for those infected with nalidixic acid-susceptible strains (*P* < 0.001). Six (33.3%) of 18 nalidixic acid-resistant serovar Typhi infections required retreatment, whereas 1 (0.8%) of 132 infections due to susceptible strains required retreatment (relative risk, 44; 95% confidence interval, 5.6 to 345; *P* < 0.0001).

Threlfall and Ward (298) reported two patients infected with a serovar Typhi with reduced susceptibility to ciprofloxacin. In 1991, a strain of serovar Typhi resistant to nalidixic acid (MIC, 512 μg/ml) was isolated from a 1-year-old child who had recently returned from India. The ciprofloxacin MIC was 0.6 μg/ml. The patient did not respond to treatment with ciprofloxacin despite serum levels of 1.5 mg/liter. A 65-year-old woman who returned from India infected with a strain of phage-type E1 (MIC to ciprofloxacin of 1.0 mg/liter) did not respond to twice-a-day treatment with ciprofloxacin, 400 mg intravenously. After 5 days, treatment was changed to amoxicillin and ceftriaxone. Within 3 days, the patient's condition improved, and after a further 5 days she was afebrile.

John (153) reported the experience with the use of ciprofloxacin monotherapy in India for the treatment of enteric fever. Since 1991, isolates of serovar Typhi with reduced susceptibility have been reported and continue to increase. In 1993, the recommended therapy became ciprofloxacin 750 mg twice daily for 7 days. However, since 1997 an increase has been noted in the number of patients failing ciprofloxacin monotherapy as defined by failure of patients to respond after 72 h of monotherapy.

Nontyphoidal *Salmonella*. Helms and colleagues (130) from Denmark performed a matched cohort study to determine death rates associated with drug resistance in *S. enterica* serovar Typhimurium. They linked data from the Danish Surveillance Registry for Enteric Pathogens with the Civil Registration System and the Danish National Discharge Registry. By survival analysis, the 2-year death rates were compared with a matched sample of the general Danish population, after the data were adjusted for differences in comorbidity. Of 4,075 cases of serovar Typhimurium infections reported in Denmark from January 1995 to October 1999, the antimicrobial-drug susceptibility was determined in isolates from 2,059 cases, and a successful link to the Civil Registry System was obtained for 2,047 (99.4%). In 2,047 patients with serovar Typhimurium, 59 deaths were identified. Patients with susceptible strains of serovar Typhimurium were 2.3 times more likely to die 2 years after infection than persons in the general Danish population. Patients infected with strains resistant to ampicillin, chloramphenicol, streptomycin, sulfonamide, and tetracycline were 4.8 times (95% confidence interval 2.2 to 10.2) more likely to die, whereas quinolone resistance, as defined by resistance to nalidixic acid, was associated with a mortality rate 10.3 times higher than the general population. No ciprofloxacin-resistant strains were found. The MIC of ciprofloxacin for the nalidixic acid-resistant isolates ranged from 0.06 to 0.38 μg/ml (median, 0.09 μg/ml).

Molbak et al. (208) reported an outbreak of DT104 causing enteric disease consisting of 25 culture-confirmed cases in which the strain was resistant to nalidixic acid and had reduced susceptibility to the fluoroquinolones. Five patients were treated with a fluoroquinolone, of which four failed therapy. Patients 10, 12, and 19 had persistent diarrhea despite treatment with ciprofloxacin or fleroxacin; they recovered after treatment with mecillinam (patient 19) or discontinuation of treatment (patients 10 and 12). From patient 19, three strains isolated after treatment had a ciprofloxacin MIC of 0.09 μg/ml. The fourth patient (patient 14) was a 62-year-old woman without chronic or malignant disease. She was admitted to the hospital after 9 days with gastrointestinal symptoms. During 5 days of treatment with ciprofloxacin (250 mg twice daily), an intestinal perforation developed.

Pers et al. (234) described an 82-year-old man with pneumonia from whom *S. enterica* serovar Enteritidis was isolated from the pleural fluid. He was treated with ciprofloxacin 500 mg orally twice daily for 3 weeks. He was readmitted a month after discharge because of fever and was treated with ciprofloxacin, but only 250 mg orally twice daily because of impaired renal function. He was found to have a splenic abscess also due to serovar Enteritidis. The ciprofloxacin MIC of the original isolate was 0.032 μg/ml, and the splenic abscess isolate was 1 μg/ml.

Piddock and colleagues (240, 244) reported two patients that failed therapy with ciprofloxacin. The first patient (patient A), who had a history of renal disease and recurrence, was treated with ciprofloxacin 500 mg orally twice daily for 14 days for a urinary tract infection due to *S. enterica* serovar Typhimurium. One month later the infection recurred. The ciprofloxacin MIC of the original isolate was 0.03 µg/ml and of the posttherapy isolate was 2 µg/ml. A second patient (patient B) was a 52-year-old male that had a serovar Typhimurium infection of a hematoma that was a complication of a ruptured aortic aneurysm. He was treated with 200 mg of ciprofloxacin twice daily intravenously for at least 10 days. The ciprofloxacin MIC of the original isolate was 0.03 µg/ml, whereas the posttherapy isolates had MICs that ranged from 0.12 to 0.5 µg/ml.

These findings would argue that, although the clinical importance of the reduced fluoroquinolone susceptibility of salmonella is anecdotal, it might be valuable for laboratories to be able to identify such isolates if identified from patients who are failing clinically.

Campylobacter spp.

Identifying *Campylobacter* with reduced susceptibilities to the fluoroquinolones does not suffer the same problems as *Salmonella*. Fluoroquinolones are not as active against *Campylobacter* as they are against *Salmonella*. The MIC_{90}s are 0.25 µg/ml, as compared with the MIC_{90}s of ciprofloxacin for *Salmonella* of $\leq$ 0.06 µg/ml (9,205). A single-point mutation in the QRDR of the *gyrA* gene of *Campylobacter* will result in an MIC of $\geq$2 µg/ml, nonsusceptible according to NCCLS guidelines (218). Mutations in the *gyrA* gene have been implicated in fluoroquinolone resistance of *Campylobacter* in numerous studies (102, 246, 278, 286). High-level resistance is associated with two mutations in *gyrA* (10).

Drivers of resistance

The major source of fluoroquinolone-resistant isolates has been from animals (124). Published epidemiologic and laboratory data from several countries provide evidence that the use of fluoroquinolones in poultry has had a primary role in increasing resistance to quinolones among *Campylobacter jejuni* isolates from humans (84, 97, 177, 210, 233, 246, 249, 251, 268, 278, 286, 307, 310). Treatment with fluoroquinolones of broiler chickens infected with quinolone-sensitive *C. jejuni* does not eradicate the organism; rather, it selects for quinolone-resistant mutants (200). Enrofloxacin was introduced in The Netherlands for veterinary use in 1987 and has been used extensively as a therapeutic agent in poultry since that time (84). Ciprofloxacin-resistant human *Campylobacter* isolates increased from 0% in 1985 to 11% in 1989, closely associated with an increase in ciprofloxacin-resistant *Campylobacter* isolates from retail poultry products (84). In Spain, the percentage of ciprofloxacin-resistant human campylobacter isolates increased from 0 to 3% in 1989 to 30 to 50% in 1991. This coincided with the licensure of enrofloxacin for veterinary use in 1990 (251, 268, 310). Ciprofloxacin-resistant *Campylobacter* spp. have also been isolated from retail poultry products in Spain (233), Taiwan (177), the United Kingdom (97), and the United States (277).

Another source of fluoroquinolone resistance is the traveler returning from areas where quinolone resistance is endemic (34, 97, 215, 249, 275, 276, 278). Smith and colleagues (278) conducted a study of patients with ciprofloxacin-resistant *C. jejuni* isolated during 1996 and 1998 in Minnesota. The proportion of quinolone-resistant *C. jejuni* isolates from humans increased from 1.3% in 1992 to 10.2% in 1998 ($P < 0.001$). During 1996 and 1997, infection with quinolone-resistant *C. jejuni* was associated with foreign travel and with the use of a quinolone before the collection of stool specimens. However, they were also able to show that the number of quinolone-resistant infections that were acquired domestically increased during the study period. Ciprofloxacin-resistant *C. jejuni* was isolated from 14% of 91 domestic chicken products obtained from retail markets in 1997. Molecular subtyping showed an association between resistant *C. jejuni* strains from chicken products and domestically acquired infections in Minnesota residents.

Prevalence of resistance

Resistance to fluoroquinolones in *Campylobacter* has increased dramatically during the past decade in many parts of the world (Fig. 6). Before 1989, resistance was rare. Talsma et al. (286) studied resistance trends in The Netherlands between 1994 and 1997. The ofloxacin-resistance rates among *Campylobacter* isolates increased from 11 to 29%. In Spain, resistance rates up to 88% have been reported (246, 264, 268, 310). In Taiwan, rates of fluoroquinolone resistance in *Campylobacter* spp. were 57% (177). Isenbarger and colleagues (148), when comparing rates of ciprofloxacin resistance between Thailand and Vietnam, found 77 versus 7%, respectively ($P < 0.05$). Since quinolones were

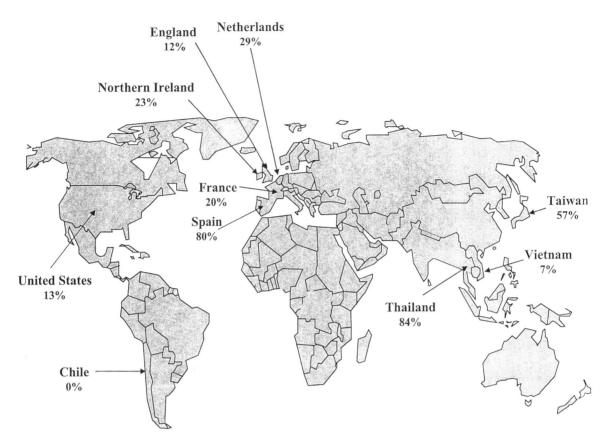

Figure 6. Prevalence of fluoroquinolone resistance in *Campylobacter*. Adapted from references 85, 87, 138, 148, 178, 210, 246, 286, 300, 329.

approved for veterinary use in the United Kingdom and the United States in late 1993 and 1995, respectively, reports have shown increasing quinolone resistance in both animal and human isolates (243, 278). In Northern Ireland the percentage of ciprofloxacin-resistant isolates increased from 9% in 1996 to 23% in 1999 (210).

Clinical relevance

Most cases of *Campylobacter* enteritis do not require antimicrobial treatment, because it is usually a brief, clinically mild, and self-limiting illness. However, some patients will require treatment. These patients include severe and prolonged cases of enteritis, septicemia, and other extraintestinal infections. In immunosuppressed patients, including those with AIDS, *Campylobacter* enteritis can be prolonged, severe, and relapsing. Early clinical trials of both community-acquired acute diarrhea and travelers' diarrhea caused by *Campylobacter* spp. demonstrated that patients treated with a fluoroquinolone had a good clinical response (112, 239, 321). However, it soon became apparent that resistance in *Campylobacter* spp. could arise in vivo, sometimes

after only one or two administrations of fluoroquinolones, in association with bacteriologic and clinical failures (3, 112, 170, 322). Eight of the 15 subjects in a placebo-controlled randomized trial received norfloxacin for acute enteritis due to norfloxacin-sensitive strains of *C. jejuni*. In three of these eight subjects, high-level quinolone-resistant *Campylobacter* strains, of the same serotype as in pre-treatment samples, were isolated 4 to 90 days after the initiation of treatment (322). Goodman et al. (112) described two patients infected with *C. jejuni* who received ciprofloxacin that failed bacteriologically, and one of whom also failed clinically. Smith and colleagues (278) found that patients infected with resistant *C. jejuni* who were treated with fluoroquinolones were found to have a longer duration of diarrhea than were patients with fluoroquinolone-sensitive isolates (an average of 10 days versus 7 days). Kuschner et al. (170) evaluated the use of azithromycin (500 mg) or ciprofloxacin (500 mg) daily for 3 days for the treatment of acute diarrhea among United States military personnel in Thailand. *Campylobacter* spp. were the most common pathogens isolated (44 isolates from 42 patients). All *Campylobacter* isolates were susceptible to azithromycin; 22 were resistant to ciprofloxacin. Among the 42 patients with *Campylobacter* infection, there were two clinical and six bacteriologic treatment failures in the ciprofloxacin group and no treatment failures in the azithromycin group (*P* = 0.021 for bacteriologic failures). Tee et al. (292) reported the emergence of multidrug resistance in *C. jejuni* isolates from three patients with AIDS. Each patient was infected with a single strain that progressively acquired resistance to the antibiotics used during treatment, including ciprofloxacin. In these patients the development of resistance was associated with bacteriologic and clinical failure.

Shigella spp.

Shigellosis is principally a disease of humans and rarely occurs in animals. The organism is frequently found in water polluted with human feces. In general, *Shigella dysenteriae*, *Shigella flexneri*, and *Shigella boydii* account for most isolates in developing countries. Conversely, *Shigella sonnei* is most common and *S. dysenteriae* is least common in developed countries. *S. sonnei*, also known as "Group D" *Shigella*, accounts for more than two-thirds of the cases of shigellosis in the United States. A second type, *S. flexneri*, or "group B" *Shigella*, accounts for almost all of the rest. Nalidixic acid is recommended for the treatment of shigellosis caused by strains of *Shigella* that are resistant to ampicillin and cotrimoxazole. Ciprofloxacin resistance is still relatively uncommon, but nalidixic acid resistance is increasing, a harbinger for fluoroquinolone resistance. For example, in 1990, >50% of *S. dysenteriae* type I isolates in Bangladesh were resistant to nalidixic acid, but ciprofloxacin remained susceptible according to current breakpoints (22, 193). In China up to 50% of *S. dysenteriae*, *S. sonnei*, and *S. boydii* are resistant to nalidixic acid (1). Antimicrobial resistance trends were examined for enteric isolates from Thailand between 1981 and 1995. Although resistance to *S. dysenteriae* type 1 to nalidixic acid was >97% and 1 to 2% in Shigella other than *S. dysenteriae* type 1, fluoroquinolone resistance was not found (138). Isenbarger and colleagues compared resistance rates in *Shigella* spp., other than *S. dysenteriae* type 1, between Thailand and Vietnam between 1996 and 1999 and found nalidixic acid resistance rates to be <1% in Thailand and 0% in Vietnam.

Despite increasing resistance to other antimicrobials, in many developed countries *Shigella* spp. have remained susceptible to nalidixic acid with resistance rates <5%, especially when examining indigenous strains (*S. flexneri* and *S. sonnei*) (46, 173, 246, 252).

However, as resistance to ampicillin and co-trimoxazole develops, fluoroquinolones are being recommended and used as first-line empiric therapy, which could lead to the emergence of resistance (46, 173, 252).

Quinolone resistance in *Shigella* has been shown to be caused by mutations in the *gyrA* and by efflux (99, 142). Clinical failures in association with reduced susceptibility to quinolones or resistance to nalidixic acid are few (142, 312). The development of resistance to nalidixic acid during therapy, which resulted in clinical failure, has been reported (312). Khan et al. (163) found that resistance to nalidixic acid was a predictor of reduced susceptibility and clinical failures. Seventeen percent (3 of 18) of patients infected by *S. dysenteriae* type 1, of which 97% were nalidixic acid-resistant, failed ciprofloxacin therapy (500 mg every 12 h for 5 days), whereas only 6% (1 of 18) with nalidixic acid-susceptible isolator failed therapy. For ciprofloxacin, the median MIC was 0.125 µg/ml for *S. dysenteriae* type 1 isolates and 0.016 µg/ml for isolates of other species. This suggests that, as is the case with *Salmonella* spp., strains resistant to nalidixic acid and with reduced susceptibility to ciprofloxacin (MIC, ≥0.125 µg/ml) may be associated with a worse clinical outcome and failure of bacterial eradication when treated with ciprofloxacin.

OTHER GRAM-NEGATIVE BACTERIA

Escherichia coli and *Klebsiella* spp.

The emergence of fluoroquinolone resistance in highly susceptible *E. coli* and *Klebsiella* spp. was unexpected because multiple mutations are required for clinically important levels of resistance to emerge. Before 1990, resistance of these organisms to the fluoroquinolones was extremely rare (15, 167). However, since then high rates of resistance have been reported in some regions of the world (Fig. 7). As with *Salmonella*, emerging resistance in *E. coli* and *Klebsiella* spp. may not be detected using current NCCLS breakpoints of ≤1, 2, and ≥4 µg/ml for susceptible, intermediate, and resistant, respectively (218). Chen et al. (48) characterized isolates of *E. coli* from a national surveillance program in Taiwan. They chose 20 *E. coli*-resistant isolates, 44 isolates with reduced susceptibility (≥0.125 but ≤1 µg/ml), and 17 susceptible isolates, and assessed them for point mutations in the QRDRs of *gyrA* and *parC*. They found that all resistant isolates had two mutations in *gyrA* and at least one additional mutation in *parC*, and all isolates with reduced susceptibility had

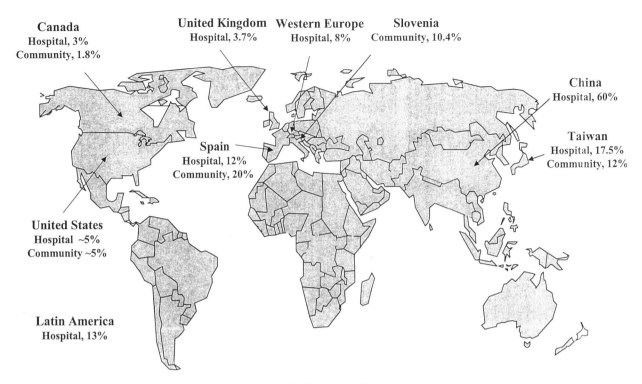

Figure 7. Prevalence of fluoroquinolone-resistant *E. coli* (MIC, ≥4 µg/ml) in the hospital and community. Adapted from references 54, 69, 74, 91, 96, 158, 185, 196, 197, 201, 309, 315.

at least one mutation in *gyrA*. As with *Salmonella*, a surrogate marker for the detection of first-step mutants of *E. coli* and *Klebsiella* spp. is the presence of nalidixic acid resistance. Ruiz and colleagues (262) studied the prevalence of the nalidixic acid-resistant, ciprofloxacin-susceptible phenotype in *Enterobacteriaceae*. The results showed that 113 of 151 (74.8%) strains of the *Enterobacteriaceae* with diminished susceptibility to ciprofloxacin (MICs, 0.06 to 1 µg/ml) were resistant to nalidixic acid (MICs > 32 µg/ml). Of the 89 *E. coli* strains with this phenotype 83 already had a mutation in the amino acid codon Ser-83 of the *gyrA* gene, whereas none of the nalidixic acid-susceptible strains did. It may not only be of epidemiological significance to identify such isolates, but it may be of clinical importance. As with pneumococci and other gram-negative organisms, using a fluoroquinolone to treat infections caused by strains with first-step mutations may lead to failure as a result of the selection of a second-step mutation that renders the organism resistant (103, 180, 236, 262, 291).

Drivers of resistance

The origin of quinolone resistance has been from both human and animal reservoirs. In humans, although possible, the emergence of resistance to *E. coli* and *Klebsiella* spp. de novo in a wild-type strain

while receiving treatment with a quinolone is unlikely because multiple mutations are required for clinically important levels of resistance to emerge. Rather resistance is more likely to emerge in a step-wise fashion as the result of multiple exposures or prolonged therapy.

Fluoroquinolones have been widely accepted and used for the prevention of bacterial infections in neutropenic patients as well as other patients at risk for gram-negative infections, including those with cirrhosis and liver transplantation (61, 82, 144). However, in those institutions using fluoroquinolone prophylaxis resistance in gram-negative organisms has emerged as compared with those institutions that do not (19, 39, 57, 216, 305). Cometta et al. (57) reported the occurrence of fluoroquinolone-resistant *E. coli* bacteremia in patients with cancer and neutropenia. They compared the susceptibilities of blood culture isolates from patients before the widespread use of fluoroquinolone prophylaxis in 1993 and after. All 92 strains of *E. coli* isolated from blood specimens between 1983 and 1990 were fluoroquinolone-susceptible (MIC, <1 µg/ml). But 11 of 40 strains of *E. coli* isolated between 1991 and 1993 were highly fluoroquinolone resistant (MIC, ≥16 µg/ml). These strains were recovered from 10 patients, all of whom had received fluoroquinolones as prophylaxis. In contrast, only 1 of 29 patients infected with fluoroquinolone-sensitive *E. coli* strains had been given quinolone prophylaxis ($P < 0.001$). The resistant strains were isolated from patients hospitalized in six institutions and were therefore thought likely to have emerged independently.

Increasing fluoroquinolone consumption has also been associated with increasing cases of fluoroquinolone-resistant *E. coli* infections in nonneutropenic hospitalized patients and patients in the community and colonization with *E. coli* in the hospital and community setting (54, 83, 96, 109, 230, 230, 255). Goettsch and colleagues (109) studied resistance to the antibiotics most commonly prescribed for urinary tract infections in The Netherlands from 1989 to 1998 in >90,000 *E. coli* isolates. Resistance to norfloxacin increased from 1.3% in 1989 to 5.8% in 1998. A comparison of the trend in norfloxacin resistance and the rates of prescription for fluoroquinolones showed that increasing fluoroquinolone resistance was associated with increasing fluoroquinolone consumption in the community.

Another reason for the increase in fluoroquinolone-resistant *E. coli* and *Klebsiella* spp. has been the increased prevalence of extended spectrum β-lactamases (ESBL). In many regions of the world, ESBLs are present in ~25% of all *Klebsiella pneumoniae* isolates from intensive care units (229). For reasons that are unknown, there is a high association with fluoroquinolone resistance in strains that produce ESBLs (229). Paterson and colleagues (229) reported a prospective study of *K. pneumoniae* bacteremia in 12 hospitals in seven countries. Of 452 episodes of bacteremia, 25 (5.5%) were caused by *K. pneumoniae* that was resistant in vitro to ciprofloxacin. ESBL production was detected in 15 (60%) of 25 ciprofloxacin-resistant isolates, compared with 68 (16%) of 427 ciprofloxacin-susceptible strains ($P = 0.0001$). Multivariate analysis revealed that risk factors for ciprofloxacin resistance in *K. pneumoniae* included prior receipt of a quinolone ($P = 0.0065$) and an ESBL-producing strain ($P = 0.012$). In all, 18% of ESBL-producing isolates were also ciprofloxacin resistant. Pulsed-field gel electrophoresis showed that 11 of the 15 ciprofloxacin-resistant ESBL-producing strains belonged to just four genotypes, suggesting that patient-to-patient transmission of such strains had occurred. Winokur et al. (320) evaluated the prevalence of ESBL-producing strains among strains of *K. pneumoniae*, *E. coli*, *Proteus mirabilis*, and *Salmonella* spp. that were isolated as part of the worldwide antimicrobial resistance surveillance project. The highest percentage of ESBL phenotype was detected among *K. pneumoniae* strains from Latin America (45%) followed by those from the Western

Pacific region (25%), Europe (23%), the United States (8%), and Canada (5%). ESBL-producing strains of *P. mirabilis* and *E. coli* were more prominent in Latin America. Rates of coresistance to ciprofloxacin ranged from 14 to 80%, with particularly high levels of quinolone resistance noted among the *P. mirabilis* isolates. At the National Taiwan University Hospital in 1999 46% of *E. coli* and 18% of *K. pneumoniae* resistant to extended-spectrum cephalosporins were also resistant to ciprofloxacin (152). As with the close linkage of fluoroquinolone resistance with methicillin-resistant *S. aureus* (MRSA), the reasons for the association of fluoroquinolone resistance with ESBLs are unknown.

Finally, as noted previously, another important reservoir for fluoroquinolone resistance in *E. coli*, *Klebsiella* spp., and other gram-negatives organisms is the use of fluoroquinolones in agriculture. Several investigators have described increases in the levels of resistance to the fluoroquinolones among *E. coli* strains isolated from animals (29, 107, 226). Garau et al. (96) studied the evolution of resistance to quinolones in *E. coli* from 1992 to 1997 in Barcelona, Spain. In addition to the emergence of fluoroquinolone resistance as a cause of nosocomial and community-acquired infections the prevalence of fluoroquinolone-resistant *E. coli* in the feces of healthy people was found to be unexpectedly high (24% in adults and 26% in children). They postulated that the source for the fluoroquinolone resistance in children was from food animals. Among the 56 samples from 56 different pigs, fluoroquinolone resistance was found in isolates from 25 (44.6%). Among the 105 *E. coli* isolates from poultry, 95 (90.4%) were resistant to ciprofloxacin. Linton (184) demonstrated that antibiotic-resistant *E. coli* could be transferred from poultry to a food handler's hands during food preparation and, finally, to food. Finally, Cherifi and colleagues (49) demonstrated a clonal relationships among *E. coli* isolates from human and animal infections, indicating that animals are a source of *E. coli* infections in humans.

Prevalence of resistance

In Beijing from 1997 to 1999, approximately 60% of *E. coli* strains isolated from hospital-acquired infections and 50% of the *E. coli* strains isolated from the community were resistant to ciprofloxacin (315). Of those fluoroquinolone-resistant strains, 80% exhibited ciprofloxacin MICs of >32 µg/ml. In Taiwan, 11.3% of *E. coli* were resistant to fluoroquinolones, and 21.7% had reduced susceptibility (201). Resistance was more common in isolates from patients in the intensive care unit

(17.5%) than in other adult inpatient (11.4%; $P =$ 0.08) and outpatient isolates (11.9%; $P > 0.1$). Sheng and colleges (274) demonstrated the rapid increase in fluoroquinolone resistance in a major teaching hospital in Taiwan. Resistance was uncommon in the early 1990s, but by 1996 20% of isolates were resistant. Resistance has also been reported from various other countries of East Asia (179, 227, 327). In Spain fluoroquinolone-resistant *E. coli* has emerged during the past decade. Garau and colleagues (96) found that resistant strains were more common in patients with nosocomial infections but also increased in patients with community-acquired infections (9% in 1992 to 17% in 1996). Twelve percent of the episodes of *E. coli* bacteremia were due to fluoroquinolone-resistant strains. Resistance is increasing in other parts of Spain (69, 230), and other European countries (54, 91, 109, 174, 223, 305). Although there are a few reports of resistance in gram-negative organisms in North America (37), overall rates remain low (74, 79, 267, 328). The rates of fluoroquinolone resistance in *K. pneumoniae* show marked geographic differences, but now exceed 5% in many centers in North America, Europe, and Asia (30, 74, 79, 91, 155, 263, 294, 303). Edmond and colleagues (79) performed concurrent surveillance for nosocomial bloodstream infections at 49 hospitals over a 3-year period, during which they detected >10,000 infections. The most common gram-negative organisms were *E. coli* (5.7%) and *Klebsiella* spp. (5.4%). Ciprofloxacin resistance rates were 1 and 8%, respectively. Diekema et al. (74) during 1997 investigated nosocomial and community-acquired bloodstream infections due to gram-negative organisms involving hospitals in Canada, the United States, and Latin America. *E. coli* was the most common isolate (41% of all gram-negative isolates), followed by *Klebsiella* spp. (17.9%). Ciprofloxacin resistance rates among *E. coli* from Canada, the United States, and Latin America were 3, 2.6, and 13.2%, respectively. For *Klebsiella* spp. the resistance rates were 1.6, 4.4, and 16, respectively. Fridkin and colleagues (93) examined changes in resistance prevalence in 23 hospitals in the United States from 1996 to 1999 and found significant increases in ciprofloxacin-resistant *E. coli* in isolates from patients outside of the intensive care unit setting. Using NCCLS criteria, in 1998 to 1999, they found 2.5 and 1.4% of *E. coli* were ciprofloxacin resistant when isolated from patients on the clinical ward and in outpatient settings, respectively. Livermore et al. (185) reported resistance trends to ciprofloxacin, the most widely used fluoroquinolone in the United Kingdom, in the prevalent *Enterobacteriaceae* species (*E. coli*,

Klebsiella spp., *Enterobacter* spp., and *P. mirabilis*) from bacteremias in England and Wales during the 1990s. Significant increases in resistance were observed for all four species groups. For *E. coli*, ciprofloxacin resistance rose from 0.8% in 1990 to 3.7% in 1999 and became widely scattered among reporting hospitals. The prevalence of resistance in *Klebsiella* spp. rose from 3.5% in 1990, to 9.5% in 1996 and 7.1% in 1999, while that in *Enterobacter* spp. rose from 2.1% in 1990 to 10.5% in 1996 and 10.9% in 1999. For both *Klebsiella* and *Enterobacter* spp., most resistance was localized in a few centers. Resistance was infrequent and scattered in *P. mirabilis* but reached a prevalence of 3.3% in 1999.

Clinical relevance

Only anecdotal case reports describe clinical failures in patients being treated for a fluoroquinolone-resistant *E. coli* or *Klebsiella* spp. infection with a fluoroquinolone. Paterson and colleagues (229) in their prospective study of *K. pneumoniae* bacteremia described two patients with ciprofloxacin-resistant strains who were treated empirically with ciprofloxacin and one patient who was treated empirically with ofloxacin. Two of the three patients failed therapy, one of whom died.

Fluoroquinolones have been advocated for both the prevention and treatment of infections in the febrile neutropenic patient (61, 100, 147). However, the emergence of quinolone-resistant gram-negative bacilli has been demonstrated in both groups of patients (39, 57, 96, 162, 282, 305, 327). Giamarello et al. (100) used monotherapy with intravenous, followed by oral high-dose ciprofloxacin as initial empiric therapy for granulocytopenic patients with fever. Thirteen patients with bacteremia caused by ciprofloxacin-resistant microorganisms were clinical failures, an unspecified number of which were due to either *E. coli*, *Klebsiella* spp., and/or *Enterobacter* spp. Of all the risk factors identified in numerous studies of various patient populations, the constant risk factor for infection or colonization with a fluoroquinolone-resistant strain was prior receipt of a fluoroquinolone (39, 96, 229, 230, 254, 255).

Pseudomonas aeruginosa

Although ciprofloxacin was approved for the treatment of infections caused by *P. aeruginosa*, its in vitro activity was marginal. Early studies found that the MIC$_{90}$s were 0.5 µg/ml (269). In hindsight, one could have predicted that selection of fluoroquinolone-resistant strains would occur readily, knowing that a single mutation causes the MIC of ciprofloxacin to approach or exceed achievable concentrations in serum.

Drivers of resistance

Although clonal spread of a multiresistant strain of *P. aeruginosa* in the hospital setting can account for the high prevalence of resistance, the emergence of resistance worldwide is primarily accounted for by the development of resistance in an individual stain either associated with prior therapy or arising during therapy (38, 80, 126, 175).

Le Thomas et al. (175) reported the emergence, after 4 days of ciprofloxacin monotherapy, of a double mutant of *P. aeruginosa* overexpressing the multidrug efflux system MexAB-OprM and harboring a mutation in the *gyrB* gene. Compared with its initial susceptible counterpart, this mutant exhibited a significant increase in resistance to most of the β-lactam antibiotics tested and to ciprofloxacin.

Prevalence of resistance

Rates of resistance of *P. aeruginosa* to ciprofloxacin vary from 0 to 40% depending on the site of isolation (community versus hospital), ward in hospital, age of patient, underlying illness, and prior antimicrobial use (1, 31, 91, 93, 131, 145, 146, 152, 284). Huang et al. (146) examined the susceptibilities of all blood-culture isolates identified from microbiology laboratories in all 13 hospitals in San Francisco County from 1996 to 1999. *P. aeruginosa* isolates showed increasing annual countywide resistance to ciprofloxacin (7 to 21%, $P = 0.005$). Ciprofloxacin resistance approached 20% in adult intensive care unit and adult medical and surgical wards countywide. No isolates resistant to ciprofloxacin were cultured from pediatric wards. Karlowsky et al. (158) prospectively collected from 26 hospital laboratories across the United States clinical isolates of nonfermentative gram-negatives organisms from January to May 2000, as part of the Tracking Resistance in the United States Today (TRUST) surveillance initiative. Twenty-seven percent of the isolates of *P. aeruginosa* were resistant to ciprofloxacin. As part of the Global SENTRY Antimicrobial Surveillance Program (1997 to 1999), SENTRY participants reported a total of 70,067 strains from 1997 to 1999, of which 6,631 were *P. aeruginosa* (95). Resistance rates to ciprofloxacin in 1999 were 16% in the Asia-Pacific region, 19% in Canada, 25% in the United Sates, 32% in Europe, and 39% in Latin America. Similar surveillance results were reported by facilities participating in Project Intensive Care Antimicrobial

Resistance Epidemiology (ICARE) and the (Meropenem Yearly Susceptibility Test Information Collection (MYSTIC) program in the United States during 1999 and 2000 (93, 155). In the United Kingdom, 25 hospitals in 1999 participated in a country surveillance program by providing clinically significant isolates of *P. aeruginosa* for susceptibility testing (131). The results found resistance rates to ciprofloxacin of 8%. These rates were mostly unchanged since a previous survey conducted in 1993. High resistance rates were nevertheless reported for isolates from patients with cystic fibrosis. In Taiwan, drug resistance data were collected from a nationwide resistance survey of clinical isolates from 12 major hospitals located in different parts of the country (145). The prevalence of ciprofloxacin-resistant *P. aeruginosa* ranged from 10 to 36%. In Taipei, Jean and colleagues (152) evaluated the in vitro susceptibilities of isolates of extended-spectrum cephalosporin-resistant gram-negative bacteria recovered between January 1999 and December 1999 in a major teaching hospital. Forty-eight percent of ceftazidime-resistant *P. aeruginosa* were resistant to ciprofloxacin. Sheng et al. (274) found 13% of *P. aeruginosa* isolated from patients in a large teaching hospital during 1996 and 1997 in Taiwan were ciprofloxacin resistant.

Clinical relevance

Early studies, especially for the treatment of patients with cystic fibrosis, found that *P. aeruginosa* was not being eradicated during fluoroquinolone therapy, despite clinical improvement (120, 261). In subsequent studies it was noted that resistance was developing while patients were receiving therapy and, in some cases, resulting in clinical failures (38, 50, 90, 127, 175, 272, 273). Harris et al. (127) conducted a case-series study of multiresistant *P. aeruginosa* in patients who did not have cystic fibrosis. Twenty-two patients were identified from whom *P. aeruginosa* resistant to ciprofloxacin, imipenem, ceftazidime, and piperacillin was isolated. In 16 of 22 cases, isolation of susceptible *P. aeruginosa* preceded the culture of multiresistant isolates. All 16 patients were exposed to antibiotics prior to the development of resistance, seven of which received ciprofloxacin. Of three patients with pneumonia treated with ciprofloxacin, one died and another failed therapy. As with pneumococci, clinicians should avoid readministering previously prescribed antibiotics when initiating empiric therapies for possible *P. aeruginosa* bacteremia, especially when the previous antibiotics have been given as monotherapy (80). In addition, physicians must recognize that resistance can develop while giving therapy and be associated with clinical failure (127).

OTHER GRAM-POSITIVE COCCI

Staphylococcus spp.

The early investigations with the new fluoroquinolones, in particular, ciprofloxacin, demonstrated in vitro activity against both methicillin-susceptible and -resistant staphylococci, although marginal with MIC_{90}s of 0.5 μg/ml (16, 280). A single mutation in the primary target would increase the MIC of ciprofloxacin 4- to 16-fold, a level of resistance at or above peak drug concentrations achievable in serum, providing an opportunity for such first-step mutants to survive and emerge when a patient was exposed to fluoroquinolones (141).

Drivers of resistance

An association between methicillin and fluoroquinolone resistance has been recognized since fluoroquinolone resistance was first described in staphylococci. Blumberg et al. (32) reported their experience following the introduction of ciprofloxacin onto their hospital formulary. Prior to the introduction of ciprofloxacin in 1988, 159 methicillin-susceptible *S. aureus* (MSSA) and 131 MRSA were found to be susceptible to ciprofoxacin. One year after introduction, 79% of MRSA and 13.6% of MSSA were ciprofloxacin resistant. Phage typing revealed both clonal dissemination as well as the development of resistance in genetically diverse backgrounds.

The reason for the differences in the ease of acquisition of fluoroquinolone resistance in MRSA, as compared with MSSA, has not yet been elucidated. This difference may be explained in part by the dissemination of clonal strains, coselection of MRSA with other antimicrobial agents, the more frequent use of fluoroquinolones to treat patients colonized/infected with MRSA, as opposed to MSSA, and/or as yet unrecognized genetic traits (270, 271).

Prevalence of resistance

Fluoroquinolone resistance in MRSA and coagulase-negative staphylococci is now >50% worldwide (1, 270, 285). Fluoroquinolone resistance in methicillin-susceptible staphylococci vary from <5 to 22%, depending on the location of the study (199, 209). Santos and colleagues (270) conducted an international study with isolates being provided from countries in Europe, Asia, and Latin America.

Ciprofloxacin resistance in MRSA, MSSA, methicillin-resistant and -susceptible coagulase-negative staphylococci was 90, 21, 50, and 22%, respectively. Susceptibility testing was performed on 602 geographically and genetically diverse *S. aureus* from across North America by Low and colleagues (189). A total of 70% of MRSA and 3.5% of MSSA were found to be ciprofloxacin resistant.

Clinical relevance

Initial investigations reported the successful use of oral ciprofloxacin in the eradication of MRSA colonization and in the treatment of MRSA and MSSA infections (117, 213, 245). However, it was soon recognized that when a fluoroquinolone, such as ciprofloxacin, was used alone that resistance frequently developed and was often associated with clinical failures (32, 213, 237, 245). Piercy et al. (245) reported that 6 (16%) of 37 patients treated for MRSA colonization developed resistance during therapy, while Mulligan et al. (213) noted that ciprofloxacin resistance developed in 7 (32%) of 22 patients treated for MRSA colonization.

Viridans Group Streptococci

Although the earlier fluoroquinolones were not promoted for the prevention or treatment of infections caused by VGS, they were accepted for prophylaxis and treatment of febrile neutropenia, a condition that is associated with infections due to VGS (56, 79, 147). In fact, VGS infections have been associated with a number of risk factors, including fluoroquinolones prophylaxis (33, 55, 56, 161, 207, 235). The earlier fluoroquinolones have borderline activity against the VGS, being inhibited by 0.5 to 4 μg/ml of ciprofloxacin (160, 269). Surveillance performed by Doern et al. (76) during 1993 and 1994 found <1% of blood-culture isolates of VGS were resistant to ofloxacin (MIC, ≥8 μg/ml). Two cross-Canada surveillance studies of the susceptibility of VGS blood-culture isolates conducted between 1995 and 1997 and again in 2000 found that 8% of isolates were ciprofloxacin resistant (MIC, ≥4 μg/ml) (70, 98). In both studies, there were no differences in the rates of resistance, whether from community or tertiary care hospitals. Diekema et al. (73) investigated the antimicrobial susceptibility of VGS among patients with and without the diagnosis of cancer in the United States, Canada, and Latin America. These were bloodstream isolates of VGS collected between January 1997 and December 1999. Only 44% of isolates were susceptible to ciprofloxacin (MIC, ≤1 μg/ml). Guerin and colleagues (119) isolated VGS from oropharyngeal samples of hospitalized patients and nonhospitalized healthy control subjects. One-third of the hospitalized patients, whether treated with fluoroquinolones or not, carried ciprofloxacin-resistant (MIC, ≥4 μg/ml) VGS, while only 3 of 13 healthy control subjects were colonized with such strains.

Of concern is that patients receiving fluoro-quinolone prophylaxis will not only be at higher risk for VGS bacteremia, but that fluoroquinolone resistance will emerge and result in clinical failures (206, 207, 250). Razonable et al. (250) reported that VGS bacteremia developed in 6 of 37 (16.2%) patients who were on levofloxacin prophylaxis following autologous peripheral blood stem cell transplantation during an eight month period in 2001. All isolates were genetically unrelated and were nonsusceptible to levofloxacin (MIC, ≥4 μg/ml). Three patients developed septic shock.

CONCLUSION

There are very few examples in which such widespread resistance has emerged to an antimicrobial class in such a short period of time. Had we known then, when the quinolones were first introduced, what we know now regarding the ease with which resistance can arise and disseminate, we might have been able to prevent or at least to delay this problem. From this past experience there are several important lessons learned. First, isolates with decreased susceptibility to fluoroquinolones can occur as the result of a spontaneous point mutation. Such isolates are more likely to survive the effect of the treating fluoroquinolone if that agent has less than optimal PK/PD parameters. Second, resistance is also more likely to occur when using fluoroquinolones to treat large bacterial population infections such as pneumonia, in which the presence of spontaneous first- and/or second-step mutants is high. Third, infections caused by an organism that already has a first-step mutant are more likely to give rise to a subsequent mutation than the wild-type strain. Such a secondary mutation may result in resistance and clinical failure. Therefore, physicians must recognize risk factors associated with an organism causing the infection that is likely to be fluoroquinolone resistant, the most important of which is prior therapy with a quinolone. Finally, there are several examples in which the use of clinical rather than microbiological breakpoints fails to identify those strains with reduced susceptibility to the fluoroquinolones as a result of mutations in the target sites. Such a circumstance not only may result in the inad-

vertent treatment of a patient with a less-than-optimal fluoroquinolone, but may also mask the emergence of resistance. This information could preserve this important class of antimicrobials if applied appropriately.

REFERENCES

1. Acar, J. F., and F. W. Goldstein. 1997. Trends in bacterial resistance to fluoroquinolones. *Clin. Infect. Dis.* **24**(Suppl. 1):S67–S73.
2. Adewoye, L. 2002. Personal communication.
3. Adler-Mosca, H., J. Luthy-Hottenstein, L. G. Martinetti, A. Burnens, and M. Altwegg. 1991. Development of resistance to quinolones in five patients with campylobacteriosis treated with norfloxacin or ciprofloxacin. *Eur. J. Clin. Microbiol. Infect. Dis.* **10**:953–957.
4. Akkina, J. E., A. T. Hogue, F. J. Angulo, R. Johnson, K. E. Petersen, P. K. Saini, P. J. Fedorka-Cray, and W. D. Schlosser. 1999. Epidemiologic aspects, control, and importance of multiple-drug resistant *Salmonella* Typhimurium DT104 in the United States. *J. Am. Vet. Med. Assoc.* **214**:790–798.
5. Alou, L., M. Ramirez, C. Garcia-Rey, J. Prieto, and H. de Lencastre. 2001. *Streptococcus pneumoniae* isolates with reduced susceptibility to ciprofloxacin in Spain: clonal diversity and appearance of ciprofloxacin-resistant epidemic clones. *Antimicrob. Agents Chemother.* **45**:2955–2957.
6. Ambrose, P. G., D. M. Grasela, T. H. Grasela, J. Passarell, H. B. Mayer, and P. F. Pierce. 2001. Pharmacodynamics of fluoroquinolones against *Streptococcus pneumoniae* in patients with community-acquired respiratory tract infections. *Antimicrob. Agents Chemother.* **45**:2793–2797.
7. Anzueto, A., M. S. Niederman, and G. S. Tillotson, for the Bronchitis Study Group. 1998. Etiology, susceptibility, and treatment of acute bacterial exacerbations of complicated chronic bronchitis in the primary care setting: ciprofloxacin 750 mg b.i.d. versus clarithromycin 500 mg b.i.d. *Clin. Ther.* **20**:885–900.
8. Aplasca De Los Reyes, M. R., V. Pato-Mesola, J. D. Klausner, R. Manalastas, T. Wi, C. U. Tuazon, G. Dallabetta, W. L. Whittington, and K. K. Holmes. 2001. A randomized trial of ciprofloxacin versus cefixime for treatment of gonorrhea after rapid emergence of gonococcal ciprofloxacin resistance in The Philippines. *Clin. Infect. Dis.* **32**:1313–1318.
9. Asperilla, M. O., R. A. Smego, Jr., and L. K. Scott. 1990. Quinolone antibiotics in the treatment of *Salmonella* infections. *Rev. Infect. Dis.* **12**:873–889.
10. Bachoual, R., S. Ouabdesselam, F. Mory, C. Lascols, C. J. Soussy, and J. Tankovic. 2001. Single or double mutational alterations of *gyrA* associated with fluoroquinolone resistance in *Campylobacter jejuni* and *Campylobacter coli*. *Microb. Drug Resist.* **7**:257–261.
11. Ball, A. P. 1986. Overview of clinical experience with ciprofloxacin. *Eur. J. Clin. Microbiol.* **5**:214–219.
12. Baquero, F. 2001. Low-level antibacterial resistance: a gateway to clinical resistance. *Drug Resist. Update* **4**:93–105.
13. Barriere, S. L., and J. A. Hindler. 1993. Ciprofloxacin-resistant *Haemophilus influenzae* infection in a patient with chronic lung disease. *Ann. Pharmacother.* **27**:309–310.
14. Barry, A. L., P. C. Fuchs, and S. D. Brown. 2001. In vitro activities of three nonfluorinated quinolones against representative bacterial isolates. *Antimicrob. Agents Chemother.* **45**:1923–1927.

15. Barry, A. L., P. C. Fuchs, M. A. Pfaller, S. D. Allen, and E. H. Gerlach. 1990. Prevalence of fluoroquinolone-resistant bacterial isolates in four medical centers during the first quarter of 1990. *Eur. J. Clin. Microbiol. Infect. Dis.* **9:**906–908.

16. Barry, A. L., and R. N. Jones. 1987. In vitro activity of ciprofloxacin against gram-positive cocci. *Am. J. Med.* **82:**27–32.

17. Bartlett, J. G., S. F. Dowell, L. A. Mandell, T. M. File, Jr., D. M. Musher, and A. Fine. 2000. Practice guidelines for the management of community-acquired pneumonia in adults. *Clin. Infect. Dis.* **31:**347–382.

18. Bast, D. J., J. C. de Azavedo, T. Y. Tam, L. Kilburn, C. Duncan, L. A. Mandell, R. J. Davidson, and D. E. Low. 2001. Interspecies recombination contributes minimally to fluoroquinolone resistance in *Streptococcus pneumoniae*. *Antimicrob. Agents Chemother.* **45:**2631–2634.

19. Baum, H. V., U. Franz, and H. K. Geiss. 2000. Prevalence of ciprofloxacin-resistant *Escherichia coli* in hematologic-oncologic patients. *Infection* **28:**278–281.

20. Bebear, C. M., H. Renaudin, A. Bryskier, and C. Bebear. 2000. Comparative activities of telithromycin (HMR 3647), levofloxacin, and other antimicrobial agents against human mycoplasmas. *Antimicrob. Agents Chemother.* **44:**1980–1982.

21. Bebear, C. M., J. Renaudin, A. Charron, H. Renaudin, B. de Barbeyrac, T. Schaeverbeke, and C. Bebear. 1999. Mutations in the *gyrA*, *parC*, and *parE* genes associated with fluoroquinolone resistance in clinical isolates of *Mycoplasma hominis*. *Antimicrob. Agents Chemother.* **43:**954–956.

22. Bennish, M. L., M. A. Salam, M. A. Hossain, J. Myaux, E. H. Khan, J. Chakraborty, F. Henry, and C. Ronsmans. 1992. Antimicrobial resistance of *Shigella* isolates in Bangladesh, 1983–1990: increasing frequency of strains multiply resistant to ampicillin, trimethoprim-sulfamethoxazole, and nalidixic acid. *Clin. Infect. Dis.* **14:**1055–1060.

23. Berglund, T., M. Unemo, P. Olcen, J. Giesecke, and H. Fredlund. 2002. One year of *Neisseria gonorrhoeae* isolates in Sweden: the prevalence study of antibiotic susceptibility shows relation to the geographic area of exposure. *Int. J. STD AIDS* **13:**109–114.

24. Bhuiyan, B. U., R. A. Miah, M. Rahman, K. M. Rahman, and M. J. Albert. 1998. High prevalence of ciprofloxacin resistance amongst strains of *Neisseria gonorrhoeae* isolated from commercial sex workers in Bangladesh. *J Antimicrob. Chemother.* **42:**675–676.

25. Bhuiyan, B. U., M. Rahman, M. R. Miah, S. Nahar, N. Islam, M. Ahmed, K. M. Rahman, and M. J. Albert. 1999. Antimicrobial susceptibilities and plasmid contents of *Neisseria gonorrhoeae* isolates from commercial sex workers in Dhaka, Bangladesh: emergence of high-level resistance to ciprofloxacin. *J. Clin. Microbiol.* **37:**1130–1136.

26. Biedenbach, D. J., and R. N. Jones. 2000. Fluoroquinolone-resistant *Haemophilus influenzae*: frequency of occurrence and analysis of confirmed strains in the SENTRY antimicrobial surveillance program (North and Latin America). *Diagn. Microbiol. Infect. Dis.* **36:**255–259.

27. Biedenbach, D. J., R. N. Jones, and M. A. Pfaller. 2001. Activity of BMS284756 against 2,681 recent clinical isolates of *Haemophilus influenzae* and *Moraxella catarrhalis*: report from The SENTRY Antimicrobial Surveillance Program (2000) in Europe, Canada and the United States. *Diagn. Microbiol. Infect. Dis.* **39:**245–250.

28. Biswal, N., B. Mathai, B. D. Bhatia, S. Srinivasan, and P. Nalini. 1994. Enteric fever: a changing perspective. *Indian Pediatr.* **31:**813–819.

29. Blanco, J. E., M. Blanco, A. Mora, and J. Blanco. 1997. Prevalence of bacterial resistance to quinolones and other antimicrobials among avian *Escherichia coli* strains isolated from septicemic and healthy chickens in Spain. *J. Clin. Microbiol.* **35:**2184–2185.

30. Blondeau, J. M., Y. Yaschuk, M. Suter, and D. Vaughan, for the Canadian Antimicrobial Study Group. 1999. In-vitro susceptibility of 1982 respiratory tract pathogens and 1921 urinary tract pathogens against 19 antimicrobial agents: a Canadian multicentre study. *J. Antimicrob. Chemother.* **43**(Suppl. A):3–23.

31. Blondeau, J. M., Y. Yaschuk, and The Canadian Ciprofloxacin Study Group. 1996. Canadian ciprofloxacin susceptibility study: comparative study from 15 medical centers. *Antimicrob. Agents Chemother.* **40:**1729–1732.

32. Blumberg, H. M., D. Rimland, D. J. Carroll, P. Terry, and I. K. Wachsmuth. 1991. Rapid development of ciprofloxacin resistance in methicillin-susceptible and -resistant *Staphylococcus aureus*. *J. Infect. Dis.* **163:**1279–1285.

33. Bochud, P. Y., P. Eggiman, T. Calandra, G. Van Melle, L. Saghafi, and P. Francioli. 1994. Bacteremia due to viridans streptococcus in neutropenic patients with cancer: clinical spectrum and risk factors. *Clin. Infect. Dis.* **18:**25–31.

34. Bowler, I., and D. Day. 1992. Emerging quinolone resistance in campylobacters. *Lancet* **340:**245.

35. Brown, J. C., P. M. Shanahan, M. V. Jesudason, C. J. Thomson, and S. G. Amyes. 1996. Mutations responsible for reduced susceptibility to 4-quinolones in clinical isolates of multi-resistant *Salmonella typhi* in India. *J. Antimicrob. Chemother.* **37:**891–900.

36. Campos, J., F. Roman, M. Georgiou, C. Garcia, R. Gomez-Lus, R. Canton, H. Escobar, and F. Baquero. 1996. Long-term persistence of ciprofloxacin-resistant *Haemophilus influenzae* in patients with cystic fibrosis. *J. Infect. Dis.* **174:**1345–1347.

37. Canawati, H. N., R. el Farra, J. Seymour, J. Shimashita, D. Dunn, and J. Z. Montgomerie. 1997. Ciprofloxacin-resistant *Escherichia coli* emerging in a rehabilitation medical center. *Diagn. Microbiol. Infect. Dis.* **29:**133–138.

38. Carmeli, Y., N. Troillet, G. M. Eliopoulos, and M. H. Samore. 1999. Emergence of antibiotic-resistant *Pseudomonas aeruginosa*: comparison of risks associated with different antipseudomonal agents. *Antimicrob. Agents Chemother.* **43:**1379–1382.

39. Carratala, J., A. Fernandez-Sevilla, F. Tubau, M. Callis, and F. Gudiol. 1995. Emergence of quinolone-resistant *Escherichia coli* bacteremia in neutropenic patients with cancer who have received prophylactic norfloxacin. *Clin. Infect. Dis.* **20:**557–560.

40. Centers for Disease Control and Prevention. 1989. Sexually transmitted diseases treatment guidelines. *Morb. Mortal. Wkly. Rep.* **38**(Suppl. 8):1–43.

41. Centers for Disease Control and Prevention. 1993. Sexually transmitted diseases treatment guidelines. *Morb. Mortal. Wkly. Rep.* **42:**1–102.

42. Centers for Disease Control and Prevention. 1995. Fluoroquinolone resistance in *Neisseria gonorrhoeae* Colorado and Washington. *Morb. Mortal. Wkly. Rep.* **44:**761–764.

43. Centers for Disease Control and Prevention. 2000. Fluoroquinolone-resistance in *Neisseria gonorrhoeae*, Hawaii, 1999, and decreased susceptibility to azithromycin in *N. gonorrhoeae*, Missouri. *Morb. Mortal. Wkly. Rep.* **49:**833–837.

44. Centers for Disease Control and Prevention. 2001. Resistance of *Streptococcus pneumoniae* to fluoro-

quinolones, United States, 1995–1999. *Morb. Mortal. Wkly. Rep.* **50**:800–804.

45. Chandel, D. S., R. Chaudhry, B. Dhawan, A. Pandey, and A. B. Dey. 2000. Drug-resistant *Salmonella enterica* serotype paratyphi A in India. *Emerg. Infect. Dis.* **6**:420–421.

46. Cheasty, T., J. A. Skinner, B. Rowe, and E. J. Threlfall. 1998. Increasing incidence of antibiotic resistance in shigellas from humans in England and Wales: recommendations for therapy. *Microb. Drug Resist.* **4**:57–60.

47. Chen, D., A. McGeer, J. C. de Azavedo, and D. E. Low, for The Canadian Bacterial Surveillance Network. 1999. Decreased susceptibility of *Streptococcus pneumoniae* to fluoroquinolones in Canada. *N. Engl. J. Med.* **341**:233–239.

48. Chen, F. J., L. C. McDonald, M. Ho, and H. J. Lo. 2001. Identification of reduced fluoroquinolone susceptibility in *Escherichia coli*: a herald for emerging resistance. *J. Antimicrob. Chemother.* **48**:936–938.

49. Cherifi, A., M. Contrepois, B. Picard, P. Goullet, I. Orskov, and F. Orskov. 1994. Clonal relationships among *Escherichia coli* serogroup O78 isolates from human and animal infections. *J. Clin. Microbiol.* **32**:1197–1202.

50. Chin, N. X., N. Clynes, and H. C. Neu. 1989. Resistance to ciprofloxacin appearing during therapy. *Am. J. Med.* **87**:28S–31S.

51. Chiu, C. H., T. L. Wu, L. H. Su, C. Chu, J. H. Chia, A. J. Kuo, M. S. Chien, and T. Y. Lin. 2002. The emergence in Taiwan of fluoroquinolone resistance in *Salmonella enterica* serotype choleraesuis. *N. Engl. J. Med.* **346**:413–419.

52. Chodosh, S., A. Schreurs, G. Siami, H. W. Barkman, A. Anzueto, M. Shan, H. Moesker, T. Stack, and S. Kowalsky, for the Bronchitis Study Group. 1998. Efficacy of oral ciprofloxacin vs. clarithromycin for treatment of acute bacterial exacerbations of chronic bronchitis. *Clin. Infect. Dis.* **27**:730–738.

53. Chodosh, S., A. Schreurs, G. Siami, H. W. J. Barkman, A. Anzueto, M. Shan, H. Moesker, T. Stack, and S. Kowalsky, for the Bronchitis Study Group. 1998. Efficacy of oral ciprofloxacin vs. clarithromycin for treatment of acute bacterial exacerbations of chronic bronchitis. *Clin. Infect. Dis.* **27**:730–738.

54. Cizman, M., A. Orazem, V. Krizan-Hergouth, and J. Kolman. 2001. Correlation between increased consumption of fluoroquinolones in outpatients and resistance of *Escherichia coli* from urinary tract infections. *J. Antimicrob. Chemother.* **47**:502.

55. Classen, D. C., J. P. Burke, C. D. Ford, S. Evershed, M. R. Aloia, J. K. Wilfahrt, and J. A. Elliott. 1990. *Streptococcus mitis* sepsis in bone marrow transplant patients receiving oral antimicrobial prophylaxis. *Am. J. Med.* **89**:441–446.

56. Collin, B. A., H. L. Leather, J. R. Wingard, and R. Ramphal. 2001. Evolution, incidence, and susceptibility of bacterial bloodstream isolates from 519 bone marrow transplant patients. *Clin. Infect. Dis.* **33**:947–953.

57. Cometta, A., T. Calandra, J. Bille, and M. P. Glauser. 1994. *Escherichia coli* resistant to fluoroquinolones in patients with cancer and neutropenia. *N. Engl. J. Med.* **330**:1240–1241.

58. Cooper, B., and M. Lawlor. 1989. Pneumococcal bacteremia during ciprofloxacin therapy for pneumococcal pneumonia. *Am. J. Med.* **87**:475.

59. Craig, W. A. 1998. Pharmacokinetic/pharmacodynamic parameters: rationale for antibacterial dosing of mice and men. *Clin. Infect. Dis.* **26**:1–12.

60. Craig, W. A. 2001. Does the dose matter? *Clin. Infect. Dis.* **33**(Suppl. 3):S233–S237.

61. Cruciani, M., R. Rampazzo, M. Malena, L. Lazzarini, G. Todeschini, A. Messori, and E. Concia. 1996. Prophylaxis with fluoroquinolones for bacterial infections in neutropenic patients: a meta-analysis. *Clin. Infect. Dis.* **23**:795–805.

62. Cunliffe, N. A., F. X. Emmanuel, and C. J. Thomson. 1995. Lower respiratory tract infection due to ciprofloxacin resistant *Moraxella catarrhalis*. *J. Antimicrob. Chemother.* **36**:273–274. (Letter.)

63. Daga, M. K., K. Sarin, and R. Sarkar. 1994. A study of culture positive multidrug resistant enteric fever—changing pattern and emerging resistance to ciprofloxacin. *J. Assoc. Physicians India* **42**:599–600.

64. Dan, M., F. Poch, and B. Sheinberg. 2002. High prevalence of high-level ciprofloxacin resistance in *Neisseria gonorrhoeae* in Tel Aviv, Israel: correlation with response to therapy. *Antimicrob. Agents Chemother.* **46**:1671–1673.

65. Davidson, R., R. Cavalcanti, J. L. Brunton, D. J. Bast, J. C. de Azavedo, P. Kibsey, C. Fleming, and D. E. Low. 2002. Resistance to levofloxacin and failure of treatment of pneumococcal pneumonia. *N. Engl. J. Med.* **346**:747–750.

66. Davies, A., P. O'Neill, L. Towers, and M. Cooke. 1996. An outbreak of *Salmonella* typhimurium DT104 food poisoning associated with eating beef. *Commun. Dis. Rep. CDR Rev.* **6**:R159-R162.

67. Davies, B. I., F. P. Maesen, and C. Baur. 1986. Ciprofloxacin in the treatment of acute exacerbations of chronic bronchitis. *Eur. J. Clin. Microbiol.* **5**:226–231.

68. Davies, T. A., A. Evangelista, S. Pfleger, K. Bush, D. F. Sahm, and R. Goldschmidt. 2002. Prevalence of single mutations in topoisomerase type II genes among levofloxacin-susceptible clinical strains of *Streptococcus pneumoniae* isolated in the United States in 1992 to 1996 and 1999 to 2000. *Antimicrob. Agents Chemother.* **46**:119–124.

69. Daza, R., J. Gutierrez, and G. Piedrola. 2001. Antibiotic susceptibility of bacterial strains isolated from patients with community-acquired urinary tract infections. *Int. J. Antimicrob. Agents* **18**:211–215.

70. de Azavedo, J. C., L. Trpeski, S. Pong-Porter, S. Matsumura, and D. E. Low. 1999. In vitro activities of fluoroquinolones against antibiotic-resistant blood culture isolates of viridans group streptococci from across Canada. *Antimicrob. Agents Chemother.* **43**:2299–2301.

71. Deeks, S. L., R. Palacio, R. Ruvinsky, D. A. Kertesz, M. Hortal, A. Rossi, J. S. Spika, and J. L. Di Fabio, for The *Streptococcus pneumoniae* Working Group. 1999. Risk factors and course of illness among children with invasive penicillin-resistant *Streptococcus pneumoniae*. *Pediatrics* **103**:409–413.

72. Dessus-Babus, S., C. M. Bebear, A. Charron, C. Bebear, and B. de Barbeyrac. 1998. Sequencing of gyrase and topoisomerase IV quinolone-resistance-determining regions of *Chlamydia trachomatis* and characterization of quinolone-resistant mutants obtained in vitro. *Antimicrob. Agents Chemother.* **42**:2474–2481.

73. Diekema, D. J., M. L. Beach, M. A. Pfaller, and R. N. Jones. 2001. Antimicrobial resistance in viridans group streptococci among patients with and without the diagnosis of cancer in the USA, Canada and Latin America. *Clin. Microbiol. Infect.* **7**:152–157.

74. Diekema, D. J., M. A. Pfaller, R. N. Jones, G. V. Doern, P. L. Winokur, A. C. Gales, H. S. Sader, K. Kugler, and M. Beach. 1999. Survey of bloodstream infections due to gram-negative bacilli: frequency of occurrence and antimicrobial susceptibility of isolates collected in the United States, Canada, and Latin America for the SENTRY Antimicrobial Surveillance Program, 1997. *Clin. Infect. Dis.* **29**:595–607.

75. DiPersio, J. R., R. N. Jones, T. Barrett, G. V. Doern, and M. A. Pfaller. 1998. Fluoroquinolone-resistant *Moraxella*

catarrhalis in a patient with pneumonia: report from the SENTRY Antimicrobial Surveillance Program (1998). *Diagn. Microbiol. Infect. Dis.* 32:131–135.

76. Doern, G. V., M. J. Ferraro, A. B. Brueggemann, and K. L. Ruoff. 1996. Emergence of high rates of antimicrobial resistance among viridans group streptococci in the United States. *Antimicrob. Agents Chemother.* 40:891–894.

77. Doern, G. V., K. P. Heilmann, H. K. Huynh, P. R. Rhomberg, S. L. Coffman, and A. B. Brueggemann. 2001. Antimicrobial resistance among clinical isolates of *Streptococcus pneumoniae* in the United States during 1999–2000, including a comparison of resistance rates since 1994–1995. *Antimicrob. Agents Chemother.* 45:1721–1729.

78. Dowson, C. G., T. J. Coffey, and B. G. Spratt. 1994. Origin and molecular epidemiology of penicillin-binding-protein-mediated resistance to beta-lactam antibiotics. *Trends Microbiol.* 2:361–366.

79. Edmond, M. B., S. E. Wallace, D. K. McClish, M. A. Pfaller, R. N. Jones, and R. P. Wenzel. 1999. Nosocomial bloodstream infections in United States hospitals: a three- year analysis. *Clin. Infect. Dis.* 29:239–244.

80. El Amari, E. B., E. Chamot, R. Auckenthaler, J. C. Pechere, and C. Van Delden. 2001. Influence of previous exposure to antibiotic therapy on the susceptibility pattern of *Pseudomonas aeruginosa* bacteremic isolates. *Clin. Infect. Dis.* 33:1859–1864.

81. Empey, P. E., H. R. Jennings, A. C. Thornton, R. P. Rapp, and M. E. Evans. 2001. Levofloxacin failure in a patient with pneumococcal pneumonia. *Ann. Pharmacother.* 35:687–690.

82. Emre, S., A. Sebastian, L. Chodoff, P. Boccagni, B. Meyers, P. A. Sheiner, E. Mor, S. R. Guy, E. Atillasoy, M. E. Schwartz, and C. M. Miller. 1999. Selective decontamination of the digestive tract helps prevent bacterial infections in the early postoperative period after liver transplant. *Mt. Sinai J. Med.* 66:310–313.

83. Ena, J., M. M. Lopez-Perezagua, C. Martinez-Peinado, M. A. Cia-Barrio, and I. Ruiz-Lopez. 1998. Emergence of ciprofloxacin resistance in *Escherichia coli* isolates after widespread use of fluoroquinolones. *Diagn. Microbiol. Infect. Dis.* 30:103–107.

84. Endtz, H. P., G. J. Ruijs, B. van Klingeren, W. H. Jansen, R. T. van der, and R. P. Mouton. 1991. Quinolone resistance in campylobacter isolated from man and poultry following the introduction of fluoroquinolones in veterinary medicine. *J. Antimicrob. Chemother.* 27:199–208.

85. Engberg, J., F. M. Aarestrup, D. E. Taylor, P. Gerner-Smidt, and I. Nachamkin. 2001. Quinolone and macrolide resistance in *Campylobacter jejuni* and *C. coli*: resistance mechanisms and trends in human isolates. *Emerg. Infect. Dis.* 7:24–34.

86. Fass, R. J. 1987. Efficacy and safety of oral ciprofloxacin in the treatment of serious respiratory infections. *Am. J. Med.* 82:202–207.

87. Fernandez, H., M. Mansilla, and V. Gonzalez. 2000. Antimicrobial susceptibility of *Campylobacter jejuni* subsp. *jejuni* assessed by E-test and double dilution agar method in Southern Chile. *Mem. Inst. Oswaldo Cruz* 95:247–249.

88. Ferrándiz, M. J., A. Fenoll, J. Linares, and A. G. De La Campa. 2000. Horizontal transfer of *parC* and *gyrA* in fluoroquinolone-resistant clinical isolates of *Streptococcus pneumoniae*. *Antimicrob. Agents Chemother.* 44:840–847.

89. File, T. M., Jr., J. Segreti, L. Dunbar, R. Player, R. Kohler, R. R. Williams, C. Kojak, and A. Rubin. 1997. A multicenter, radomized study comparing the efficacy and safety of intravenous and/or oral levofloxacin versus ceftriaxone and/or cefuroxime axetil in treatment of adults with community-acquired pneumonia. *Antimicrob. Agents Chemother.* 41:1965–1972.

90. Fink, M. P., D. R. Snydman, M. S. Niederman, K. V. Leeper, Jr., R. H. Johnson, S. O. Heard, R. G. Wunderink, J. W. Caldwell, J. J. Schentag, and G. A. Siami, for The Severe Pneumonia Study Group. 1994. Treatment of severe pneumonia in hospitalized patients: results of a multicenter, randomized, double-blind trial comparing intravenous ciprofloxacin with imipenem-cilastatin. *Antimicrob. Agents Chemother.* 38:547–557.

91. Fluit, A. C., M. E. Jones, F. J. Schmitz, J. Acar, R. Gupta, and J. Verhoef. 2000. Antimicrobial susceptibility and frequency of occurrence of clinical blood isolates in Europe from the SENTRY antimicrobial surveillance program, 1997 and 1998. *Clin. Infect. Dis.* 30:454–460.

92. Forrest, A., D. E. Nix, C. H. Ballow, T. F. Goss, M. C. Birmingham, and J. J. Schentag. 1993. Pharmacodynamics of intravenous ciprofloxacin in seriously ill patients. *Antimicrob. Agents Chemother.* 37:1073–1081.

93. Fridkin, S. K., H. A. Hill, N. V. Volkova, J. R. Edwards, R. M. Lawton, R. P. Gaynes, and J. E. McGowan, Jr. 2002. Temporal changes in prevalence of antimicrobial resistance in 23 US hospitals. *Emerg. Infect. Dis.* 8:697–701.

94. Frost, J. A., A. Kelleher, and B. Rowe. 1996. Increasing ciprofloxacin resistance in salmonellas in England and Wales 1991–1994. *J. Antimicrob. Chemother.* 37:85–91.

95. Gales, A. C., R. N. Jones, J. Turnidge, R. Rennie, and R. Ramphal. 2001. Characterization of *Pseudomonas aeruginosa* isolates: occurrence rates, antimicrobial susceptibility patterns, and molecular typing in the global SENTRY Antimicrobial Surveillance Program, 1997–1999. *Clin. Infect. Dis.* 32(Suppl.2):S146–S155.

96. Garau, J., M. Xercavins, M. Rodriguez-Carballeira, J. R. Gomez-Vera, I. Coll, D. Vidal, T. Llovet, and A. Ruiz-Bremon. 1999. Emergence and dissemination of quinolone-resistant *Escherichia coli* in the community. *Antimicrob. Agents Chemother.* 43:2736–2741.

97. Gaunt, P. N., and L. J. Piddock. 1996. Ciprofloxacin resistant *Campylobacter* spp. in humans: an epidemiological and laboratory study. *J. Antimicrob. Chemother.* 37:747–757.

98. Gershon, A. S., J. C. de Azavedo, A. McGeer, K. I. Ostrowska, D. Church, D. J. Hoban, G. K. Harding, K. Weiss, L. Abbott, F. Smaill, M. Gourdeau, G. Murray, and D. E. Low. 2002. Activities of new fluoroquinolones, ketolides, and other antimicrobials against blood culture isolates of viridans group streptococci from across Canada, 2000. *Antimicrob. Agents Chemother.* 46:1553–1556.

99. Ghosh, A. S., J. Ahamed, K. K. Chauhan, and M. Kundu. 1998. Involvement of an efflux system in high-level fluoroquinolone resistance of *Shigella dysenteriae*. *Biochem. Biophys. Res. Commun.* 242:54–56.

100. Giamarellou, H., H. P. Bassaris, G. Petrikkos, W. Busch, M. Voulgarelis, A. Antoniadou, E. Grouzi, and N. Zoumbos. 2000. Monotherapy with intravenous followed by oral high-dose ciprofloxacin versus combination therapy with ceftazidime plus amikacin as initial empiric therapy for granulocytopenic patients with fever. *Antimicrob. Agents Chemother.* 44:3264–3271.

101. Gibb, A. P., C. S. Lewin, and O. J. Garden. 1991. Development of quinolone resistance and multiple antibiotic resistance in *Salmonella bovismorbificans* in a pancreatic abscess. *J. Antimicrob. Chemother.* 28:318–321.

102. Gibreel, A., E. Sjogren, B. Kaijser, B. Wretlind, and O. Skold. 1998. Rapid emergence of high-level resistance to quinolones in *Campylobacter jejuni* associated with muta-

tional changes in *gyrA* and *parC*. *Antimicrob. Agents Chemother.* **42**:3276–3278.

103. **Gillespie, S. H., and A. Dickens.** 2002. Variation in mutation rate of quinolone resistance in *Streptococcus pneumoniae*. *3rd International Symposium on Pneumococci and Pneumococcal Disease.* Centers for Disease Control and Prevention, Atlanta, Ga.

104. **Gillespie, S. H., L. L. Voelker, and A. Dickens.** 2002. Evolutionary barriers to quinolone resistance in *Streptococcus pneumoniae. Microb. Drug Resist.* **8**:79–84.

105. **Giraud, E., A. Brisabois, J. L. Martel, and E. Chaslus-Dancla.** 1999. Comparative studies of mutations in animal isolates and experimental in vitro- and in vivo-selected mutants of *Salmonella* spp. suggest a counterselection of highly fluoroquinolone-resistant strains in the field. *Antimicrob. Agents Chemother.* **43**:2131–2137.

106. **Giraud, E., A. Cloeckaert, D. Kerboeuf, and E. Chaslus-Dancla.** 2000. Evidence for active efflux as the primary mechanism of resistance to ciprofloxacin in *Salmonella enterica* serovar typhimurium. *Antimicrob. Agents Chemother.* **44**:1223–1228.

107. **Giraud, E., S. Leroy-Setrin, G. Flaujac, A. Cloeckaert, M. Dho-Moulin, and E. Chaslus-Dancla.** 2001. Characterization of high-level fluoroquinolone resistance in *Escherichia coli* O78:K80 isolated from turkeys. *J. Antimicrob. Chemother.* **47**:341–343.

108. **Glynn, M. K., C. Bopp, W. Dewitt, P. Dabney, M. Mokhtar, and F. J. Angulo.** 1998. Emergence of multidrug-resistant *Salmonella enterica* serotype typhimurium DT104 infections in the United States. *N. Engl. J. Med.* **338**:1333–1338.

109. **Goettsch, W., W. van Pelt, N. Nagelkerke, M. G. Hendrix, A. G. Buiting, P. L. Petit, L. J. Sabbe, A. J. van Griethuysen, and A. J. de Neeling.** 2000. Increasing resistance to fluoroquinolones in *Escherichia coli* from urinary tract infections in the Netherlands. *J. Antimicrob. Chemother.* **46**:223–228.

110. **Goldsmith, C. E., J. E. Moore, P. G. Murphy, and J. E. Ambler.** 1998. Increased incidence of ciprofloxacin resistance in penicillin-resistant pneumococci in Northern Ireland. *J. Antimicrob. Chemother.* **41**:420–421. (Letter.)

111. **Gonzalez, M. A., F. Uribe, S. D. Moisen, A. P. Fuster, A. Selen, P. G. Welling, and B. Painter.** 1984. Multiple-dose pharmacokinetics and safety of ciprofloxacin in normal volunteers. *Antimicrob. Agents Chemother.* **26**:741–744.

112. **Goodman, L. J., G. M. Trenholme, R. L. Kaplan, J. Segreti, D. Hines, R. Petrak, J. A. Nelson, K. W. Mayer, W. Landau, G. W. Parkhurst, and S. Levin.** 1990. Empiric antimicrobial therapy of domestically acquired acute diarrhea in urban adults. *Arch. Intern. Med* **150**:541–546.

113. **Gordon, J. J., and C. A. Kauffman.** 1990. Superinfection with *Streptococcus pneumoniae* during therapy with ciprofloxacin. *Am. J. Med.* **89**:383–384.

114. **Gordon, S. M., C. J. Carlyn, L. J. Doyle, C. C. Knapp, D. L. Longworth, G. S. Hall, and J. A. Washington.** 1996. The emergence of *Neisseria gonorrhoeae* with decreased susceptibility to ciprofloxacin in Cleveland, Ohio: epidemiology and risk factors. *Ann. Intern. Med.* **125**:465–470.

115. **Gould, I. M., K. J. Forbes, and G. S. Gordon.** 1994. Quinolone resistant *Haemophilus influenzae. J. Antimicrob. Chemother.* **33**:187–188.

116. **Gransden, W. R., C. A. Warren, I. Phillips, M. Hodges, and D. Barlow.** 1990. Decreased susceptibility of *Neisseria gonorrhoeae* to ciprofloxacin. *Lancet* **335**:51.

117. **Greenberg, R. N., D. J. Kennedy, P. M. Reilly, K. L. Luppen, W. J. Weinandt, M. R. Bollinger, F. Aguirre, F. Kodesch, and A. M. Saeed.** 1987. Treatment of bone, joint, and soft-tissue infections with oral ciprofloxacin. *Antimicrob. Agents Chemother.* **31**:151–155.

118. **Griggs, D. J., K. Gensberg, and L. J. Piddock.** 1996. Mutations in gyrA gene of quinolone-resistant Salmonella serotypes isolated from humans and animals. *Antimicrob. Agents Chemother.* **40**:1009–1013.

119. **Guerin, F., E. Varon, A. B. Hoi, L. Gutmann, and I. Podglajen.** 2000. Fluoroquinolone resistance associated with target mutations and active efflux in oropharyngeal colonizing isolates of viridans group streptococci. *Antimicrob. Agents Chemother.* **44**:2197–2200.

120. **Haddow, A., S. Greene, G. Heinz, and D. Wantuck.** 1989. Ciprofloxacin (intravenous/oral) versus ceftazidime in lower respiratory tract infections. *Am. J. Med.* **87**:113S–115S.

121. **Hakanen, A., P. Kotilainen, P. Huovinen, H. Helenius, and A. Siitonen.** 2001. Reduced fluoroquinolone susceptibility in *Salmonella enterica* serotypes in travelers returning from southeast Asia. *Emerg. Infect. Dis.* **7**:996–1003.

122. **Hakanen, A., P. Kotilainen, J. Jalava, A. Siitonen, and P. Huovinen.** 1999. Detection of decreased fluoroquinolone susceptibility in salmonellas and validation of nalidixic acid screening test. *J. Clin. Microbiol.* **37**:3572–3577.

123. **Hakenbeck, R., N. Balmelle, B. Weber, C. Gardes, W. Keck, and A. de Saizieu.** 2001. Mosaic genes and mosaic chromosomes: intra- and interspecies genomic variation of *Streptococcus pneumoniae. Infect. Immun.* **69**:2477–2486.

124. **Hamer, D. H., and C. J. Gill.** 2002. From the farm to the kitchen table: the negative impact of antimicrobial use in animals on humans. *Nutr. Rev.* **60**:261–264.

125. **Hampton, M. D., L. R. Ward, B. Rowe, and E. J. Threlfall.** 1998. Molecular fingerprinting of multidrug-resistant *Salmonella enterica* serotype Typhi. *Emerg. Infect. Dis.* **4**:317–320.

126. **Harbarth, S., A. D. Harris, Y. Carmeli, and M. H. Samore.** 2001. Parallel analysis of individual and aggregated data on antibiotic exposure and resistance in gram-negative bacilli. *Clin. Infect. Dis.* **33**:1462–1468.

127. **Harris, A., C. Torres-Viera, L. Venkataraman, P. DeGirolami, M. Samore, and Y. Carmeli.** 1999. Epidemiology and clinical outcomes of patients with multiresistant *Pseudomonas aeruginosa. Clin. Infect. Dis.* **28**:1128–1133.

128. **Heffelfinger, J. D., S. F. Dowell, J. H. Jorgensen, K. P. Klugman, L. R. Mabry, D. M. Musher, J. F. Plouffe, A. Rakowsky, A. Schuchat, and C. G. Whitney.** 2000. Management of community-acquired pneumonia in the era of pneumococcal resistance: a report from the Drug-Resistant *Streptococcus pneumoniae* Therapeutic Working Group. *Arch. Intern. Med.* **160**:1399–1408.

129. **Heisig, P.** 1993. High-level fluoroquinolone resistance in a *Salmonella typhimurium* isolate due to alterations in both *gyrA* and *gyrB* genes. *J. Antimicrob. Chemother.* **32**: 367–377.

130. **Helms, M., P. Vastrup, P. Gerner-Smidt, and M. lbak.** 2002. Excess mortality associated with antimicrobial drug-resistant *Salmonella* Typhimurium. *Emerg. Infect. Dis.* **8**:490–495.

131. **Henwood, C. J., D. M. Livermore, A. P. Johnson, D. James, M. Warner, and A. Gardiner.** 2000. Susceptibility of gram-positive cocci from 25 UK hospitals to antimicrobial agents including linezolid. The Linezolid Study Group. *J. Antimicrob. Chemother.* **46**:931–940.

132. **Herikstad, H., P. Hayes, M. Mokhtar, M. L. Fracaro, E. J. Threlfall, and F. J. Angulo.** 1997. Emerging quinolone-resistant *Salmonella* in the United States. *Emerg. Infect. Dis.* **3**:371–372.

133. **Ho, P. L., T. L. Que, D. N. Tsang, T. K. Ng, K. H. Chow, and W. H. Seto.** 1999. Emergence of fluoroquinolone resistance among multiply resistant strains of *Streptococcus pneu-*

moniae in Hong Kong. *Antimicrob. Agents Chemother.* 43:1310–1313.

134. Ho, P. L., W. S. Tse, K. W. Tsang, T. K. Kwok, T. K. Ng, V. C. Cheng, and R. M. Chan. 2001. Risk factors for acquisition of levofloxacin-resistant *Streptococcus pneumoniae*: a case-control study. *Clin. Infect. Dis.* 32:701–707.

135. Ho, P. L., R. W. Yung, D. N. Tsang, T. L. Que, M. Ho, W. H. Seto, T. K. Ng, W. C. Yam, and W. W. Ng. 2001. Increasing resistance of *Streptococcus pneumoniae* to fluoroquinolones: results of a Hong Kong multicentre study in 2000. *J. Antimicrob. Chemother.* 48:659–665.

136. Hoa, N. T., T. S. Diep, J. Wain, C. M. Parry, T. T. Hien, M. D. Smith, A. L. Walsh, and N. J. White. 1998. Community-acquired septicaemia in southern Viet Nam: the importance of multidrug-resistant *Salmonella typhi*. *Trans. R. Soc. Trop. Med. Hyg.* 92:503–508.

137. Hoban, D. J., G. V. Doern, A. C. Fluit, M. Roussel-Delvallez, and R. N. Jones. 2001. Worldwide prevalence of antimicrobial resistance in *Streptococcus pneumoniae*, *Haemophilus influenzae*, and *Moraxella catarrhalis* in the SENTRY Antimicrobial Surveillance Program, 1997–1999. *Clin. Infect. Dis.* 32(Suppl. 2):S81–S93.

138. Hoge, C. W., J. M. Gambel, A. Srijan, C. Pitarangsi, and P. Echeverria. 1998. Trends in antibiotic resistance among diarrheal pathogens isolated in Thailand over 15 years. *Clin. Infect. Dis.* 26:341–345.

139. Hohmann, E. L. 2001. Nontyphoidal salmonellosis. *Clin. Infect. Dis.* 32:263–269.

140. Hoogkamp-Korstanje, J. A., and S. J. Klein. 1986. Ciprofloxacin in acute exacerbations of chronic bronchitis. *J. Antimicrob. Chemother.* 18:407–413.

141. Hooper, D. C. 2001. Emerging mechanisms of fluoroquinolone resistance. *Emerg. Infect. Dis.* 7:337–341.

142. Horiuchi, S., Y. Inagaki, N. Yamamoto, N. Okamura, Y. Imagawa, and R. Nakaya. 1993. Reduced susceptibilities of *Shigella sonnei* strains isolated from patients with dysentery to fluoroquinolones. *Antimicrob. Agents Chemother.* 37:2486–2489.

143. Howard, A. J., T. D. Joseph, L. L. Bloodworth, J. A. Frost, H. Chart, and B. Rowe. 1990. The emergence of ciprofloxacin resistance in *Salmonella typhimurium*. *J. Antimicrob. Chemother.* 26:296–298.

144. Hsieh, W. J., H. C. Lin, S. J. Hwang, M. C. Hou, F. Y. Lee, F. Y. Chang, and S. D. Lee. 1998. The effect of ciprofloxacin in the prevention of bacterial infection in patients with cirrhosis after upper gastrointestinal bleeding. *Am. J. Gastroenterol.* 93:962–966.

145. Hsueh, P. R., C. Y. Liu, and K. T. Luh. 2002. Current status of antimicrobial resistance in Taiwan. *Emerg. Infect. Dis.* 8:132–137.

146. Huang, S. S., B. J. Labus, M. C. Samuel, D. T. Wan, and A. L. Reingold. 2002. Antibiotic resistance patterns of bacterial isolates from blood in San Francisco County, California, 1996–1999. *Emerg. Infect. Dis.* 8:195–201.

147. Hughes, W. T., D. Armstrong, G. P. Bodey, E. J. Bow, A. E. Brown, T. Calandra, R. Feld, P. A. Pizzo, K. V. Rolston, J. L. Shenep, and L. S. Young. 2002. 2002 guidelines for the use of antimicrobial agents in neutropenic patients with cancer. *Clin. Infect. Dis.* 34:730–751.

148. Isenbarger, D. W., C. W. Hoge, A. Srijan, C. Pitarangsi, N. Vithayasai, L. Bodhidatta, K. W. Hickey, and P. Dac Cam. 2002. Comparative antibiotic resistance of diarrheal pathogens from Vietnam and Thailand, 1996–1999. *Emerg. Infect. Dis.* 8:175–180.

149. Ison, C. A., and I. M. Martin, for the London Gonococcal Working Group. 1999. Susceptibility of gonococci isolated in London to therapeutic antibiotics: establishment of a London surveillance programme. *Sex. Transm. Infect.* 75:107–111.

150. Jamieson, F. 2002. Personal communication.

151. Janoir, C., I. Podglajen, M. D. Kitzis, C. Poyart, and L. Gutmann. 1999. In vitro exchange of fluoroquinolone resistance determinants between *Streptococcus pneumoniae* and viridans streptococci and genomic organization of the *parE*-*parC* region in *S. mitis*. *J. Infect. Dis.* 180:555–558.

152. Jean, S. S., L. J. Teng, P. R. Hsueh, S. W. Ho, and K. T. Luh. 2002. Antimicrobial susceptibilities among clinical isolates of extended- spectrum cephalosporin-resistant Gram-negative bacteria in a Taiwanese University Hospital. *J. Antimicrob. Chemother.* 49:69–76.

153. John, M. 2001. Decreasing clinical response of quinolones in the treatment of enteric fever. *Indian J. Med. Sci.* 55:189–194.

154. Jones, M. E., J. A. Karlowsky, R. Blosser-Middleton, I. A. Critchley, E. Karginova, C. Thornsberry, and D. F. Sahm. 2002. Longitudinal assessment of antipneumococcal susceptibility in the United States. *Antimicrob. Agents Chemother.* 46:2651–2655.

155. Jones, R. N., and M. A. Pfaller. 2002. Ciprofloxacin as broad-spectrum empiric therapy-are fluoroquinolones still viable monotherapeutic agents compared with beta-lactams? Data from the MYSTIC Program (US). *Diagn. Microbiol. Infect. Dis.* 42:213–215.

156. Kam, K. M., K. K. Lo, N. K. Ho, and M. M. Cheung. 1995. Rapid decline in penicillinase-producing *Neisseria gonorrhoeae* in Hong Kong associated with emerging 4-fluoroquinolone resistance. *Genitourin. Med.* 71:141–144.

157. Kam, K. M., K. K. Lo, C. F. Lai, Y. S. Lee, and C. B. Chan. 1993. Ofloxacin susceptibilities of 5,667 *Neisseria gonorrhoeae* strains isolated in Hong Kong. *Antimicrob. Agents Chemother.* 37:2007–2008.

158. Karlowsky, J. A., L. J. Kelly, C. Thornsberry, M. E. Jones, A. T. Evangelista, I. A. Critchley, and D. F. Sahm. 2002. Susceptibility to fluoroquinolones among commonly isolated Gram- negative bacilli in 2000: TRUST and TSN data for the United States. *Int. J. Antimicrob. Agents* 19:21–31.

159. Kays, M. B., D. W. Smith, M. E. Wack, and G. A. Denys. 2002. Levofloxacin treatment failure in a patient with fluoroquinolone-resistant *Streptococcus pneumoniae* pneumonia. *Pharmacotherapy* 22:395–399.

160. Kayser, F. H., and J. Novak. 1987. In vitro activity of ciprofloxacin against gram-positive bacteria. An overview. *Am. J. Med.* 82:33–39.

161. Kern, W., E. Kurrle, and T. Schmeiser. 1990. Streptococcal bacteremia in adult patients with leukemia undergoing aggressive chemotherapy. A review of 55 cases. *Infection* 18:138–145.

162. Kern, W. V., E. Andriof, M. Oethinger, P. Kern, J. Hacker, and R. Marre. 1994. Emergence of fluoroquinolone-resistant *Escherichia coli* at a cancer center. *Antimicrob. Agents Chemother.* 38:681–687.

163. Khan, W. A., C. Seas, U. Dhar, M. A. Salam, and M. L. Bennish. 1997. Treatment of shigellosis: V. Comparison of azithromycin and ciprofloxacin. A double-blind, randomized, controlled trial. *Ann. Intern. Med.* 126:697–703.

164. Knapp, J. S., K. K. Fox, D. L. Trees, and W. L. Whittington. 1997. Fluoroquinolone resistance in *Neisseria gonorrhoeae*. *Emerg. Infect. Dis.* 3:33–39.

165. Knapp, J. S., R. Ohye, S. W. Neal, M. C. Parekh, H. Higa, and R. J. Rice. 1994. Emerging in vitro resistance to quinolones in penicillinase-producing *Neisseria gonorrhoeae* strains in Hawaii. *Antimicrob. Agents Chemother.* 38:2200–2203.

166. Knapp, J. S., J. A. Washington, L. J. Doyle, S. W. Neal, M. C. Parekh, and R. J. Rice. 1994. Persistence of *Neisseria gonorrhoeae* strains with decreased susceptibilities to ciprofloxacin and ofloxacin in Cleveland, Ohio, from 1992 through 1993. *Antimicrob. Agents Chemother.* **38:**2194–2196.

167. Kresken, M., A. Jansen, and B. Wiedemann. 1990. Prevalence of resistance of aerobic gram-negative bacilli to broad-spectrum antibacterial agents: results of a multicentre study. *J. Antimicrob. Chemother.* **25:**1022–1024.

168. Kresken, M., and B. Wiedemann. 1988. Development of resistance to nalidixic acid and the fluoroquinolones after the introduction of norfloxacin and ofloxacin. *Antimicrob. Agents Chemother.* **32:**1285–1288.

169. Kuehnert, M. J., F. S. Nolte, and C. A. Perlino. 1999. Fluoroquinolone resistance in *Streptococcus pneumoniae*. *Ann. Intern. Med.* **131:**312–313. (Letter.)

170. Kuschner, R. A., A. F. Trofa, R. J. Thomas, C. W. Hoge, C. Pitarangsi, S. Amato, R. P. Olafson, P. Echeverria, J. C. Sadoff, and D. N. Taylor. 1995. Use of azithromycin for the treatment of *Campylobacter enteritis* in travelers to Thailand, an area where ciprofloxacin resistance is prevalent. *Clin. Infect. Dis.* **21:**536–541.

171. Launay, O., V. J. Nguyen, A. Buu-Hoi, and J. F. Acar. 1997. Typhoid fever due to a *Salmonella typhi* strain of reduced susceptibility to fluoroquinolones. *Clin. Microbiol. Infect.* **3:**541–544.

172. Lee, B. L., R. C. Kimbrough, S. R. Jones, J. Mills, and M. A. Sande. 1991. Infectious complications with respiratory pathogens despite ciprofloxacin therapy. *N. Engl. J. Med.* **325:**520–521.

173. Lee, J. C., J. Y. Oh, K. S. Kim, Y. W. Jeong, J. W. Cho, J. C. Park, S. Y. Seol, and D. T. Cho. 2001. Antimicrobial resistance of *Shigella sonnei* in Korea during the last two decades. *APMIS* **109:**228–234.

174. Lehn, N., J. Stower-Hoffmann, T. Kott, C. Strassner, H. Wagner, M. Kronke, and W. Schneider-Brachert. 1996. Characterization of clinical isolates of *Escherichia coli* showing high levels of fluoroquinolone resistance. *J. Clin. Microbiol.* **34:**597–602.

175. LeThomas, I., G. Couetdic, O. Clermont, N. Brahimi, P. Plesiat, and E. Bingen. 2001. In vivo selection of a target/efflux double mutant of *Pseudomonas aeruginosa* by ciprofloxacin therapy. *J. Antimicrob. Chemother.* **48:**553–555.

176. Levy, S. B. 1998. Multidrug resistance—a sign of the times. *N. Engl. J. Med.* **338:**1376–1378.

177. Li, C. C., C. H. Chiu, J. L. Wu, Y. C. Huang, and T. Y. Lin. 1998. Antimicrobial susceptibilities of *Campylobacter jejuni* and coli by using E-test in Taiwan. *Scand. J. Infect. Dis.* **30:**39–42.

178. Reference deleted.

179. Li, J. B., Y. S. Yu, Y. L. Ma, W. L. Zhou, and X. Z. Yu. 2001. Prevalence and analysis of risk factors for infections caused by resistant *Escherichia coli* strains in Anhui, China. *Infection* **29:**228–231.

180. Li, X., X. Zhao, and K. Drlica. 2002. Selection of *Streptococcus pneumoniae* mutants having reduced susceptibility to moxifloxacin and levofloxacin. *Antimicrob. Agents Chemother.* **46:**522–524.

181. Liebana, E., C. Clouting, C. A. Cassar, L. P. Randall, R. A. Walker, E. J. Threlfall, F. A. Clifton-Hadley, A. M. Ridley, and R. H. Davies. 2002. Comparison of gyrA Mutations, Cyclohexane Resistance, and the Presence of Class I Integrons in *Salmonella enterica* from Farm Animals in England and Wales. *J. Clin. Microbiol.* **40:**1481–1486.

182. Lim, S., Bast, D., de Azavedo, J., McGeer, A., and Low, D. E. 2002. Failure of current susceptibility testing methodologies to detect first-step *Streptococcus pneumoniae* mutants, abstr. 2388. *In Program and Abstracts of the 42nd Interscience Conference on Antimicrobial Agents Chemotherapy.* American Society for Microbiology, Washington, D.C.

183. Linares, J., A. G. De La Campa, and R. Pallares. 1999. Fluoroquinolone resistance in *Streptococcus pneumoniae*. *N. Engl. J. Med.* **341:**1546–1547. (Letter.)

184. Linton, A. H. 1977. Animal to man transmission of *Enterobacteriaceae*. *R. Soc. Health J.* **97:**115–118.

185. Livermore, D. M., D. James, M. Reacher, C. Graham, T. Nichols, P. Stephens, A. P. Johnson, and R. C. George. 2002. Trends in fluoroquinolone (ciprofloxacin) resistance in *Enterobacteriaceae* from bacteremias, England and Wales, 1990–1999. *Emerg. Infect. Dis.* **8:**473–478.

186. Lode, H., K. Borner, and P. Koeppe. 1998. Pharmacodynamics of fluoroquinolones. *Clin. Infect. Dis.* **27:**33–39.

187. Low, D. E. 2001. Antimicrobial drug use and resistance among respiratory pathogens in the community. *Clin. Infect. Dis.* **33**(Suppl. 3):S206–S213.

188. Low, D. E., J. de Azavedo, K. Weiss, T. Mazzulli, M. Kuhn, D. Church, K. Forward, G. Zhanel, A. E. Simor, Canadian Bacterial Surveillance Network, and A. McGeer. 2002. Antimicrobial resistance among clinical isolates of *Streptococcus pneumoniae* in Canada during 2000. *Antimicrob. Agents Chemother.* **46:**1295–1301.

189. Low, D. E., B. N. Kreiswirth, K. Weiss, and B. M. Willey. 2002. Activity of GAR-936 and other antimicrobial agents against North American isolates of *Staphylococcus aureus*. *Int. J. Antimicrob. Agents* **20:**220.

190. MacGowan, A., C. Rogers, and K. Bowker. 2000. The use of in vitro pharmacodynamic models of infection to optimize fluoroquinolone dosing regimens. *J. Antimicrob. Chemother.* **46:**163–170.

191. Madaras-Kelly, K. J., and T. A. Demasters. 2000. In vitro characterization of fluoroquinolone concentration/MIC antimicrobial activity and resistance while simulating clinical pharmacokinetics of levofloxacin, ofloxacin, or ciprofloxacin against *Streptococcus pneumoniae*. *Diagn. Microbiol. Infect. Dis.* **37:**253–260.

192. Maesen, F. P., B. I. Davies, W. H. Geraedts, and C. Baur. 1987. The use of quinolones in respiratory tract infections. *Drugs* **34**(Suppl. 1):74–79.

193. Mamun, K. Z., S. Tabassum, M. A. Hussain, and P. Shears. 1997. Antimicrobial susceptibility of *Shigella* from a rural community in Bangladesh. *Ann. Trop. Med. Parasitol.* **91:**643–647.

194. Mandell, L. A., T. J. Marrie, R. F. Grossman, A. W. Chow, and R. H. Hyland. 2000. Canadian guidelines for the initial management of community-acquired pneumonia: an evidence-based update by the Canadian Infectious Diseases Society and the Canadian Thoracic Society. *Clin. Infect. Dis.* **31:**383–421.

195. Marco, F., J. Garcia-de-Lomas, C. Garcia-Rey, E. Bouza, L. Aguilar, and C. Fernandez-Mazarrasa. 2001. Antimicrobial susceptibilities of 1,730 *Haemophilus influenzae* respiratory tract isolates in Spain in 1998–1999. *Antimicrob. Agents Chemother.* **45:**3226–3228.

196. Mathai, D., R. N. Jones, and M. A. Pfaller. 2001. Epidemiology and frequency of resistance among pathogens causing urinary tract infections in 1,510 hospitalized patients: a report from the SENTRY Antimicrobial Surveillance Program (North America). *Diagn. Microbiol. Infect. Dis.* **40:**129–136.

197. Mazzulli, T. 2001. Antimicrobial resistance trends in common urinary pathogens. *Can. J. Urol.* **8**(Suppl. 1):2–5.

198. Mazzulli, T., A. E. Simor, R. Jaeger, S. Fuller, and D. E. Low. 1990. Comparative in vitro activities of several new fluoroquinolones and *B*-lactam antimicrobial agents against community isolates of *Streptococcus pneumoniae*. *Antimicrob. Agents Chemother.* **34**:467–469.

199. McCloskey, L., T. Moore, N. Niconovich, B. Donald, J. Broskey, C. Jakielaszek, S. Rittenhouse, and K. Coleman. 2000. In vitro activity of gemifloxacin against a broad range of recent clinical isolates from the USA. *J. Antimicrob. Chemother.* **45**(Suppl. 1):13–21.

200. McDermott, P. F., S. M. Bodeis, L. L. English, D. G. White, R. D. Walker, S. Zhao, S. Simjee, and D. D. Wagner. 2002. Ciprofloxacin resistance in *Campylobacter jejuni* evolves rapidly in chickens treated with fluoroquinolones. *J. Infect. Dis.* **185**:837–840.

201. McDonald, L. C., F. J. Chen, H. J. Lo, H. C. Yin, P. L. Lu, C. H. Huang, P. Chen, T. L. Lauderdale, and M. Ho. 2001. Emergence of reduced susceptibility and resistance to fluoroquinolones in *Escherichia coli* in Taiwan and contributions of distinct selective pressures. *Antimicrob. Agents Chemother.* **45**:3084–3091.

202. McDonald, L. C., M. T. Chen, T. L. Lauderdale, and M. Ho. 2001. The use of antibiotics critical to human medicine in food-producing animals in Taiwan. *J. Microbiol. Immunol. Infect.* **34**:97–102.

203. McGee, L., C. E. Goldsmith, and K. P. Klugman. 2002. Fluoroquinolone resistance among clinical isolates of *Streptococcus pneumoniae* belonging to international multiresistant clones. *J. Antimicrob. Chemother.* **49**:173–176.

204. McKellar, Q., I. Gibson, A. Monteiro, and M. Bregante. 1999. Pharmacokinetics of enrofloxacin and danofloxacin in plasma, inflammatory exudate, and bronchial secretions of calves following subcutaneous administration. *Antimicrob. Agents Chemother.* **43**:1988–1992.

205. McNulty, C. A., J. Dent, and R. Wise. 1985. Susceptibility of clinical isolates of *Campylobacter pyloridis* to 11 antimicrobial agents. *Antimicrob. Agents Chemother.* **28**:837–838.

206. McWhinney, P. H., S. Patel, R. A. Whiley, J. M. Hardie, S. H. Gillespie, and C. C. Kibbler. 1993. Activities of potential therapeutic and prophylactic antibiotics against blood culture isolates of viridans group streptococci from neutropenic patients receiving ciprofloxacin. *Antimicrob. Agents Chemother.* **37**:2493–2495.

207. Menichetti, F., R. Felicini, G. Bucaneve, F. Aversa, M. Greco, C. Pasquarella, M. V. Moretti, A. Del Favero, and M. F. Martelli. 1989. Norfloxacin prophylaxis for neutropenic patients undergoing bone marrow transplantation. *Bone Marrow Transplant.* **4**:489–492.

208. Molbak, K., D. L. Baggesen, F. M. Aarestrup, J. M. Ebbesen, J. Engberg, K. Frydendahl, P. Gerner-Smidt, A. M. Petersen, and H. C. Wegener. 1999. An outbreak of multidrug-resistant, quinolone-resistant *Salmonella enterica* serotype typhimurium DT104. *N. Engl. J. Med.* **341**:1420–1425.

209. Monsen, T., M. Ronnmark, C. Olofsson, and J. Wistrom. 1999. Antibiotic susceptibility of staphylococci isolated in blood cultures in relation to antibiotic consumption in hospital wards. *Scand. J. Infect. Dis.* **31**:399–404.

210. Moore, J. E., M. Crowe, N. Heaney, and E. Crothers. 2001. Antibiotic resistance in *Campylobacter* spp. isolated from human faeces (1980–2000) and foods (1997–2000) in Northern Ireland: an update. *J. Antimicrob. Chemother.* **48**:455–457.

211. Morrissey, I., H. Salman, S. Bakker, D. Farrell, C. M. Bebear, and G. Ridgway. 2002. Serial passage of *Chlamydia* spp. in sub-inhibitory fluoroquinolone concentrations. *J. Antimicrob. Chemother.* **49**:757–761.

212. Mouton, J. W. 2002. Breakpoints: current practice and future perspectives. *Int. J. Antimicrob. Agents* **19**:323–331.

213. Mulligan, M. E., P. J. Ruane, L. Johnston, P. Wong, J. P. Wheelock, K. MacDonald, J. F. Reinhardt, C. C. Johnson, B. Statner, I. Blomquist, J. McCarthy, W. O'Brien, S. Gardner, L. Hammer, and D. M. Citron. 1987. Ciprofloxacin for eradication of methicillin-resistant *Staphylococcus aureus* colonization. *Am. J. Med.* **82**:215–219.

214. Murdoch, D. A., N. Banatvaia, A. Bone, B. I. Shoismatulloev, L. R. Ward, E. J. Threlfall, and N. A. Banatvala. 1998. Epidemic ciprofloxacin-resistant *Salmonella typhi* in Tajikistan. *Lancet* **351**:339.

215. Murphy, G. S., Jr., P. Echeverria, L. R. Jackson, M. K. Arness, C. LeBron, and C. Pitarangsi. 1996. Ciprofloxacin- and azithromycin-resistant *Campylobacter* causing traveler's diarrhea in U.S. troops deployed to Thailand in 1994. *Clin. Infect. Dis.* **22**:868–869.

216. Murphy, M., A. E. Brown, K. A. Sepkowitz, E. M. Bernard, T. E. Kiehn, and D. Armstrong. 1997. Fluoroquinolone prophylaxis for the prevention of bacterial infections in patients with cancer—is it justified? *Clin. Infect. Dis.* **25**:346–348.

217. Nagai, K., P. C. Appelbaum, T. A. Davies, L. M. Kelly, D. B. Hoellman, A. T. Andrasevic, L. Drukalska, W. Hryniewicz, M. R. Jacobs, J. Kolman, J. Miciuleviciene, M. Pana, L. Setchanova, M. K. Thege, H. Hupkova, J. Trupl, and P. Urbaskova. 2002. Susceptibilities to telithromycin and six other agents and prevalence of macrolide resistance due to L4 ribosomal protein mutation among 992 pneumococci from 10 Central and Eastern European countries. *Antimicrob. Agents Chemother.* **46**:371–377.

218. **National Committee for Clinical Laboratory Standards.** 2002. Performance standards for antimicrobial susceptibility testing. Twelfth informational supplement, M100-S12. National Committee for Clinical Laboratory Standards, Wayne, Pa.

219. Nazir, J., C. Urban, N. Mariano, J. Burns, S. Segal-Maurer, and J. J. Rahal. 2002. Levofloxacin resistant *Haemophilus influenzae* in a long term care facility, abstr. 647. *Program and Abstracts of the 42nd Interscience Conference on Antimicrobial Agents and Chemotherapy.* American Society for Microbiology, Washington, D.C.

220. Neu, H. C. 1988. Bacterial resistance to fluoroquinolones. *Rev. Infect. Dis.* **10**(Suppl. 1):S57–S63.

221. Niederman, M. S., L. A. Mandell, A. Anzueto, J. B. Bass, W. A. Broughton, G. D. Campbell, N. Dean, T. File, M. J. Fine, P. A. Gross, F. Martinez, T. J. Marrie, J. F. Plouffe, J. Ramirez, G. A. Sarosi, A. Torres, R. Wilson, and V. L. Yu. 2001. Guidelines for the management of adults with community-acquired pneumonia. Diagnosis, assessment of severity, antimicrobial therapy, and prevention. *Am. J. Respir. Crit. Care Med.* **163**:1730–1754.

222. Nielsen, K., J. M. Bangsborg, and N. Hoiby. 2000. Susceptibility of *Legionella* species to five antibiotics and development of resistance by exposure to erythromycin, ciprofloxacin, and rifampicin. *Diagn. Microbiol. Infect. Dis.* **36**:43–48.

223. Oethinger, M., S. Conrad, K. Kaifel, A. Cometta, J. Bille, G. Klotz, M. P. Glauser, R. Marre, and W. V. Kern. 1996. Molecular epidemiology of fluoroquinolone-resistant *Escherichia coli* bloodstream isolates from patients admitted to European cancer centers. *Antimicrob. Agents Chemother.* **40**:387–392.

224. Ogle, J. W., L. B. Reller, and M. L. Vasil. 1988. Development of resistance in *Pseudomonas aeruginosa* to imipenem, norfloxacin, and ciprofloxacin during therapy:

proof provided by typing with a DNA probe. *J. Infect. Dis.* **157:**743–748.

225. Olsen, S. J., E. E. DeBess, T. E. McGivern, N. Marano, T. Eby, S. Mauvais, V. K. Balan, G. Zirnstein, P. R. Cieslak, and F. J. Angulo. 2001. A nosocomial outbreak of fluoro-quinolone-resistant salmonella infection. *N. Engl. J. Med.* **344:**1572–1579.

226. Orden, J. A., J. A. Ruiz-Santa-Quiteria, D. Cid, R. Diez, S. Martinez, and F. R. de La. 2001. Quinolone resistance in potentially pathogenic and non-pathogenic *Escherichia coli* strains isolated from healthy ruminants. *J. Antimicrob. Chemother.* **48:**421–424.

227. Ozeki, S., T. Deguchi, M. Yasuda, M. Nakano, T. Kawamura, Y. Nishino, and Y. Kawada. 1997. Development of a rapid assay for detecting *gyrA* mutations in *Escherichia coli* and determination of incidence of *gyrA* mutations in clinical strains isolated from patients with complicated urinary tract infections. *J. Clin. Microbiol.* **35:**2315–2319.

228. Pankuch, G. A., B. Bozdogan, K. Nagai, A. Tambic-Andrasevic, A. Schoenwald, T. Tambic, S. Kalenic, S. Plesko, N. K. Tepes, Z. Kotarski, M. Payerl-Pal, and P. C. Appelbaum. 2002. Incidence, epidemiology, and characteristics of quinolone-nonsusceptible *Streptococcus pneumoniae* in Croatia. *Antimicrob. Agents Chemother.* **46:**2671–2675.

229. Paterson, D. L., L. Mulazimoglu, J. M. Casellas, W. C. Ko, H. Goossens, A. von Gottberg, S. Mohapatra, G. M. Trenholme, K. P. Klugman, J. G. McCormack, and V. L. Yu. 2000. Epidemiology of ciprofloxacin resistance and its relationship to extended-spectrum beta-lactamase production in *Klebsiella pneumoniae* isolates causing bacteremia. *Clin. Infect. Dis.* **30:**473–478.

230. Pena, C., J. M. Albareda, R. Pallares, M. Pujol, F. Tubau, and J. Ariza. 1995. Relationship between quinolone use and emergence of ciprofloxacin-resistant *Escherichia coli* in bloodstream infections. *Antimicrob. Agents Chemother.* **39:**520–524.

231. Perez-Trallero, E., C. Fernandez-Mazarrasa, C. Garcia-Rey, E. Bouza, L. Aguilar, J. Garcia-de-Lomas, and F. Baquero. 2001. Antimicrobial susceptibilities of 1,684 *Streptococcus pneumoniae* and 2,039 *Streptococcus pyogenes* isolates and their ecological relationships: results of a 1-year (1998–1999) multicenter surveillance study in Spain. *Antimicrob. Agents Chemother.* **45:**3334–3340.

232. Perez-Trallero, E., J. M. Garcia-Arenzana, J. A. Jimenez, and A. Peris. 1990. Therapeutic failure and selection of resistance to quinolones in a case of pneumococcal pneumonia treated with ciprofloxacin. *Eur. J. Clin. Microbiol. Infect. Dis.* **9:**905–906.

233. Perez-Trallero, E., M. Urbieta, C. L. Lopategui, C. Zigorraga, and I. Ayestaran. 1993. Antibiotics in veterinary medicine and public health. *Lancet* **342:**1371–1372.

234. Pers, C., P. Sogaard, and L. Pallesen. 1996. Selection of multiple resistance in *Salmonella enteritidis* during treatment with ciprofloxacin. *Scand. J. Infect. Dis.* **28:**529–531.

235. Persson, L., T. Vikerfors, L. Sjoberg, P. Engervall, and U. Tidefelt. 2000. Increased incidence of bacteraemia due to viridans streptococci in an unselected population of patients with acute myeloid leukaemia. *Scand. J. Infect. Dis.* **32:**615–621.

236. Pestova, E., J. J. Millichap, G. A. Noskin, and L. R. Peterson. 2000. Intracellular targets of moxifloxacin: a comparison with other fluoroquinolones. *J. Antimicrob. Chemother.* **45:**583–590.

237. Peterson, L. R., J. N. Quick, B. Jensen, S. Homann, S. Johnson, J. Tenquist, C. Shanholtzer, R. A. Petzel, L. Sinn, and D. N. Gerding. 1990. Emergence of ciprofloxacin resist-

ance in nosocomial methicillin-resistant *Staphylococcus aureus* isolates. Resistance during ciprofloxacin plus rifampin therapy for methicillin-resistant *S aureus* colonization. *Arch. Intern. Med.* **150:**2151–2155.

238. Petitpretz, P., P. Arvis, M. Marel, J. Moita, and J. Urueta. 2001. Oral moxifloxacin vs high-dosage amoxicillin in the treatment of mild- to-moderate, community-acquired, suspected pneumococcal pneumonia in adults. *Chest* **119:**185–195.

239. Piddock, L. J. 1995. Quinolone resistance and *Campylobacter* spp. *J. Antimicrob. Chemother.* **36:**891–898.

240. Piddock, L. J. 2002. Fluoroquinolone resistance in *Salmonella* serovars isolated from humans and food animals. *FEMS Microbiol. Rev.* **26:**3–16.

241. Piddock, L. J., D. J. Griggs, M. C. Hall, and Y. F. Jin. 1993. Ciprofloxacin resistance in clinical isolates of *Salmonella typhimurium* obtained from two patients. *Antimicrob. Agents Chemother.* **37:**662–666.

242. Piddock, L. J., V. Ricci, I. McLaren, and D. J. Griggs. 1998. Role of mutation in the *gyrA* and *parC* genes of nalidixic-acid-resistant salmonella serotypes isolated from animals in the United Kingdom. *J. Antimicrob. Chemother.* **41:**635–641.

243. Piddock, L. J., V. Ricci, K. Stanley, and K. Jones. 2000. Activity of antibiotics used in human medicine for *Campylobacter jejuni* isolated from farm animals and their environment in Lancashire, UK. *J. Antimicrob. Chemother.* **46:**303–306.

244. Piddock, L. J., K. Whale, and R. Wise. 1990. Quinolone resistance in salmonella: clinical experience. *Lancet* **335:**1459.

245. Piercy, E. A., D. Barbaro, J. P. Luby, and P. A. Mackowiak. 1989. Ciprofloxacin for methicillin-resistant *Staphylococcus aureus* infections. *Antimicrob. Agents Chemother.* **33:**128–130.

246. Prats, G., B. Mirelis, T. Llovet, C. Munoz, E. Miro, and F. Navarro. 2000. Antibiotic resistance trends in enteropathogenic bacteria isolated in 1985–1987 and 1995–1998 in Barcelona. *Antimicrob. Agents Chemother.* **44:**1140–1145.

247. Rahman, M., A. Alam, K. Nessa, S. Nahar, D. K. Dutta, L. Yasmin, S. Monira, Z. Sultan, S. A. Khan, and M. J. Albert. 2001. Treatment failure with the use of ciprofloxacin for gonorrhea correlates with the prevalence of fluoroquinolone-resistant *Neisseria gonorrhoeae* strains in Bangladesh. *Clin. Infect. Dis.* **32:**884–889.

248. Rahman, M., Z. Sultan, S. Monira, A. Alam, K. Nessa, S. Islam, S. Nahar, A. W. Shama, K. S. Alam, J. Bogaerts, N. Islam, and J. Albert. 2002. Antimicrobial susceptibility of *Neisseria gonorrhoeae* isolated in Bangladesh (1997 to 1999): rapid shift to fluoroquinolone resistance. *J. Clin. Microbiol.* **40:**2037–2040.

249. Rautelin, H., O. V. Renkonen, and T. U. Kosunen. 1991. Emergence of fluoroquinolone resistance in *Campylobacter jejuni* and *Campylobacter coli* in subjects from Finland. *Antimicrob. Agents Chemother.* **35:**2065–2069.

250. Razonable, R. R., M. R. Litzow, Y. Khaliq, K. E. Piper, M. S. Rouse, and R. Patel. 2002. Bacteremia due to viridans group streptococci with diminished susceptibility to levofloxacin among neutropenic patients receiving levofloxacin prophylaxis. *Clin. Infect. Dis.* **34:**1469–1474.

251. Reina, J., N. Borrell, and A. Serra. 1992. Emergence of resistance to erythromycin and fluoroquinolones in thermotolerant *Campylobacter* strains isolated from feces 1987–1991. *Eur. J. Clin. Microbiol. Infect. Dis.* **11:**1163–1166.

252. Replogle, M. L., D. W. Fleming, and P. R. Cieslak. 2000. Emergence of antimicrobial-resistant shigellosis in Oregon. *Clin. Infect. Dis.* **30:**515–519.

253. Ribot, E. M., R. K. Wierzba, F. J. Angulo, and T. J. Barrett. 2002. *Salmonella enterica* serotype Typhimurium DT104 isolated from humans, United States, 1985, 1990, and 1995. *Emerg. Infect. Dis.* 8:387–391.

254. Richard, P., M. H. Delangle, D. Merrien, S. Barille, A. Reynaud, C. Minozzi, and H. Richet. 1994. Fluoroquinolone use and fluoroquinolone resistance: is there an association? *Clin. Infect. Dis.* 19:54–59.

255. Richard, P., M. H. Delangle, F. Raffi, E. Espaze, and H. Richet. 2001. Impact of fluoroquinolone administration on the emergence of fluoroquinolone-resistant gram-negative bacilli from gastrointestinal flora. *Clin. Infect. Dis.* 32:162–166.

256. Ridley, A., and E. J. Threlfall. 1998. Molecular epidemiology of antibiotic resistance genes in multiresistant epidemic *Salmonella typhimurium* DT 104. *Microb. Drug Resist.* 4:113–118.

257. Rodrigues, C., A. Mehta, and V. R. Joshi. 2002. *Salmonella typhi* in the past decade: learning to live with resistance. *Clin. Infect. Dis.* 34:126.

258. Ross, J. J., M. G. Worthington, S. L. Gorbach, G. S. Tillotson, X. Zhao, K. Drlica, G. G. Zhanel, D. J. Hoban, C. K. Chan, J. Hutchinson, D. E. Low, J. de Azavedo, and D. Bast. 2002. Resistance to levofloxacin and failure of treatment of pneumococcal pneumonia. *N. Engl. J. Med.* 347:65–67.

259. Rossiter, S., J. McClellan, T. Barrett, K. Joyce, and A. D. Anderson, for the NARMS Working Group. 2002. Emerging fluoroquinolone resistance among non-typhoidal *Salmonella* in the United States: NARMS 1996–2000. *Program Abstracts International Conference on Emerging Infectious Diseases.* 2002. Centers for Disease Control and Prevention, Atlanta, Ga.

260. Rowe, B., L. R. Ward, and E. J. Threlfall. 1990. Spread of multiresistant *Salmonella typhi. Lancet* 336:1065–1066.

261. Rubio, T. T. 1990. Ciprofloxacin in the treatment of Pseudomonas infection in children with cystic fibrosis. *Diagn. Microbiol. Infect. Dis.* 13:153–155.

262. Ruiz, J., J. Gomez, M. M. Navia, A. Ribera, J. M. Sierra, F. Marco, J. Mensa, and J. Vila. 2002. High prevalence of nalidixic acid resistant, ciprofloxacin susceptible phenotype among clinical isolates of *Escherichia coli* and other *Enterobacteriaceae. Diagn. Microbiol. Infect. Dis.* 42:257–261.

263. Rydberg, J., C. Larsson, and H. Miorner. 1994. Resistance to fluoroquinolones in *Pseudomonas aeruginosa* and *Klebsiella pneumoniae. Scand. J. Infect. Dis.* 26:317–320.

264. Saenz, Y., M. Zarazaga, M. Lantero, M. J. Gastanares, F. Baquero, and C. Torres. 2000. Antibiotic resistance in *Campylobacter* strains isolated from animals, foods, and humans in Spain in 1997–1998. *Antimicrob. Agents Chemother.* 44:267–271.

265. Sahm, D. F., J. A. Karlowsky, L. J. Kelly, I. A. Critchley, M. E. Jones, C. Thornsberry, Y. Mauriz, and J. Kahn. 2001. Need for annual surveillance of antimicrobial resistance in *Streptococcus pneumoniae* in the United States: 2-year longitudinal analysis. *Antimicrob. Agents Chemother.* 45:1037–1042.

266. Sahm, D. F., D. E. Peterson, I. A. Critchley, and C. Thornsberry. 2000. Analysis of ciprofloxacin activity against *Streptococcus pneumoniae* after 10 years of use in the United States. *Antimicrob. Agents Chemother.* 44:2521–2524.

267. Sahm, D. F., C. Thornsberry, D. C. Mayfield, M. E. Jones, and J. A. Karlowsky. 2001. Multidrug-resistant urinary tract isolates of *Escherichia coli*: prevalence and patient demographics in the United States in 2000. *Antimicrob. Agents Chemother.* 45:1402–1406.

268. Sanchez, R., V. Fernandez-Baca, M. D. Diaz, P. Munoz, M. Rodriguez-Creixems, and E. Bouza. 1994. Evolution of susceptibilities of *Campylobacter* spp. to quinolones and macrolides. *Antimicrob. Agents Chemother.* 38:1879–1882.

269. Sanders, C. C. 1988. Ciprofloxacin: in vitro activity, mechanism of action, and resistance. *Rev. Infect. Dis.* 10:516–527.

270. Santos, S., I, R. Mato, H. de Lencastre, and A. Tomasz. 2000. Patterns of multidrug resistance among methicillin-resistant hospital isolates of coagulase-positive and coagulase-negative staphylococci collected in the international multicenter study RESIST in 1997 and 1998. *Microb. Drug Resist.* 6:199–211.

271. Schmitz, F. J., A. C. Fluit, D. Hafner, A. Beeck, M. Perdikouli, M. Boos, S. Scheuring, J. Verhoef, K. Kohrer, and C. Von Eiff. 2000. Development of resistance to ciprofloxacin, rifampin, and mupirocin in methicillin-susceptible and -resistant *Staphylococcus aureus* isolates. *Antimicrob. Agents Chemother.* 44:3229–3231.

272. Scully, B. E., H. C. Neu, M. F. Parry, and W. Mandell. 1986. Oral ciprofloxacin therapy of infections due to *Pseudomonas aeruginosa. Lancet* i:819–822.

273. Shalit, I., H. R. Stutman, M. I. Marks, S. A. Chartrand, and B. C. Hilman. 1987. Randomized study of two dosage regimens of ciprofloxacin for treating chronic bronchopulmonary infection in patients with cystic fibrosis. *Am. J. Med.* 82:189–195.

274. Sheng, W. H., Y. C. Chen, J. T. Wang, S. C. Chang, K. T. Luh, and W. C. Hsieh. 2002. Emerging fluoroquinolone-resistance for common clinically important gram-negative bacteria in Taiwan. *Diagn. Microbiol. Infect. Dis.* 43:141–147.

275. Sjogren, E., G. B. Lindblom, and B. Kaijser. 1997. Norfloxacin resistance in *Campylobacter jejuni* and *Campylobacter coli* isolates from Swedish patients. *J. Antimicrob. Chemother.* 40:257–261.

276. Slavin, M. A., I. Jennens, and W. Tee. 1996. Infection with ciprofloxacin-resistant *Campylobacter jejuni* in travellers returning from Asia. *Eur. J. Clin. Microbiol. Infect. Dis.* 15:348–350.

277. Smith, K. E., J. M. Besser, C. W. Hedberg, F. T. Leano, J. B. Bender, J. H. Wicklund, B. P. Johnson, K. A. Moore, and M. T. Osterholm, for the Investigation Team. 1999. Quinolone-resistant *Campylobacter jejuni* infections in Minnesota, 1992–1998. *N. Engl. J. Med.* 340:1525–1532.

278. Reference deleted.

279. Smith, M. D., N. M. Duong, N. T. Hoa, J. Wain, H. D. Ha, T. S. Diep, N. P. Day, T. T. Hien, and N. J. White. 1994. Comparison of ofloxacin and ceftriaxone for short-course treatment of enteric fever. *Antimicrob. Agents Chemother.* 38:1716–1720.

280. Smith, S. M. 1986. In vitro comparison of A-56619, A-56620, amifloxacin, ciprofloxacin, enoxacin, norfloxacin, and ofloxacin against methicillin-resistant *Staphylococcus aureus. Antimicrob. Agents Chemother.* 29:325–326.

281. Somani, J., V. B. Bhullar, K. A. Workowski, C. E. Farshy, and C. M. Black. 2000. Multiple drug-resistant *Chlamydia trachomatis* associated with clinical treatment failure. *J. Infect. Dis.* 181:1421–1427.

282. Somolinos, N., R. Arranz, M. C. Del Rey, and M. L. Jimenez. 1992. Superinfections by *Escherichia coli* resistant to fluoroquinolones in immunocompromised patients. *J. Antimicrob. Chemother.* 30:730–731.

283. Straus, W. L., S. A. Qazi, Z. Kundi, N. K. Nomani, and B. Schwartz for the Pakistan Co-trimoxazole Study Group. 1998. Antimicrobial resistance and clinical effectiveness of

co-trimoxazole versus amoxycillin for pneumonia among children in Pakistan: randomised controlled trial. *Lancet* 352:270–274.

284. Tacconelli, E., M. Tumbarello, S. Bertagnolio, R. Citton, T. Spanu, G. Fadda, and R. Cauda. 2002. Multidrug-resistant *Pseudomonas aeruginosa* bloodstream infections: analysis of trends in prevalence and epidemiology. *Emerg. Infect. Dis.* 8:218–220.

285. Tacconelli, E., M. Tumbarello, K. G. Donati, M. Bettio, T. Spanu, F. Leone, L. A. Sechi, S. Zanetti, G. Fadda, and R. Cauda. 2001. Glycopeptide resistance among coagulase-negative staphylococci that cause bacteremia: epidemiological and clinical findings from a case-control study. *Clin. Infect. Dis.* 33:1628–1635.

286. Talsma, E., W. G. Goettsch, H. L. Nieste, P. M. Schrijnemakers, and M. J. Sprenger. 1999. Resistance in *Campylobacter* species: increased resistance to fluoroquinolones and seasonal variation. *Clin. Infect. Dis.* 29:845–848.

287. Tapsall, J. 2000. Annual report of the Australian Gonococcal Surveillance Programme, 1999. *Commun. Dis. Intell.* 24:113–117.

288. Tapsall, J. W., E. A. Limnios, C. Thacker, B. Donovan, S. D. Lynch, L. J. Kirby, K. A. Wise, and C. J. Carmody. 1995. High-level quinolone resistance in *Neisseria gonorrhoeae*: a report of two cases. *Sex. Transm. Dis.* 22:310–311.

289. Tapsall, J. W., E. A. Phillips, T. R. Shultz, and C. Thacker. 1996. Quinolone-resistant *Neisseria gonorrhoeae* isolated in Sydney, Australia, 1991 to 1995. *Sex. Transm. Dis.* 23:425–428.

290. Tapsall, J. W., T. R. Shultz, R. Lovett, and R. Munro. 1992. Failure of 500 mg ciprofloxacin therapy in male urethral gonorrhoea. *Med. J. Aust.* 156:143.

291. Tavio, M. M., J. Vila, J. Ruiz, J. Ruiz, A. M. Martin-Sanchez, and M. T. Jimenez de Anta. 1999. Mechanisms involved in the development of resistance to fluoroquinolones in *Escherichia coli* isolates. *J. Antimicrob. Chemother.* 44:735–742.

292. Tee, W., A. Mijch, E. Wright, and A. Yung. 1995. Emergence of multidrug resistance in *Campylobacter jejuni* isolates from three patients infected with human immunodeficiency virus. *Clin. Infect. Dis.* 21:634–638.

293. Thomas, J. K., A. Forrest, S. M. Bhavnani, J. M. Hyatt, A. Cheng, C. H. Ballow, and J. J. Schentag. 1998. Pharmacodynamic evaluation of factors associated with the development of bacterial resistance in acutely ill patients during therapy. *Antimicrob. Agents Chemother.* 42:521–527.

294. Thomson, C. J. 1999. The global epidemiology of resistance to ciprofloxacin and the changing nature of antibiotic resistance: a 10 year perspective. *J. Antimicrob. Chemother.* 43(Suppl. A):31–40.

295. Thorburn, C. E., and D. I. Edwards. 2001. The effect of pharmacokinetics on the bactericidal activity of ciprofloxacin and sparfloxacin against *Streptococcus pneumoniae* and the emergence of resistance. *J. Antimicrob. Chemother.* 48:15–22.

296. Thornsberry, C., D. F. Sahm, L. J. Kelly, I. A. Critchley, M. E. Jones, A. T. Evangelista, and J. A. Karlowsky. 2002. Regional trends in antimicrobial resistance among clinical isolates of *Streptococcus pneumoniae, Haemophilus influenzae,* and *Moraxella catarrhalis* in the United States: results from the TRUST Surveillance Program, 1999–2000. *Clin. Infect. Dis.* 34(Suppl. 1):S4–S16.

297. Threlfall, E. J., J. A. Frost, L. R. Ward, and B. Rowe. 1996. Increasing spectrum of resistance in multiresistant *Salmonella typhimurium. Lancet* 347:1053–1054.

298. Threlfall, E. J., and L. R. Ward. 2001. Decreased susceptibility to ciprofloxacin in *Salmonella enterica* serotype Typhi, United Kingdom. *Emerg. Infect. Dis.* 7:448–450.

299. Threlfall, E. J., L. R. Ward, J. A. Skinner, and B. Rowe. 1997. Increase in multiple antibiotic resistance in nontyphoidal salmonellas from humans in England and Wales: a comparison of data for 1994 and 1996. *Microb. Drug Resist.* 3:263–266.

300. Thwaites, R. T., and J. A. Frost. 1999. Drug resistance in *Campylobacter jejuni, C coli,* and *C lari* isolated from humans in north west England and Wales, 1997. *J. Clin. Pathol.* 52:812–814.

301. Thys, J. P. 1988. Quinolones in the treatment of bronchopulmonary infections. *Rev. Infect. Dis.* 10(Suppl. 1):S212–S217.

302. Turner, A., K. R. Gough, A. E. Jephcott, and A. N. McClean. 1995. Importation into the UK of a strain of *Neisseria gonorrhoeae* resistant to penicillin, ciprofloxacin and tetracycline. *Genitourin. Med.* 71:265–266.

303. Turnidge, J. 1995. Epidemiology of quinolone resistance. Eastern hemisphere. *Drugs* 49(Suppl. 2):43–47.

304. Umasankar, S., R. A. Wall, and J. Berger. 1992. A case of ciprofloxacin-resistant typhoid fever. *Commun. Dis. Rep. CDR Rev.* 2:R139–R140.

305. Van Belkum, A., W. Goessens, S. C. van Der, N. Lemmens-Den Toom, M. C. Vos, J. Cornelissen, E. Lugtenburg, S. de Marie, H. Verbrugh, B. Lowenberg, and H. Endtz. 2001. Rapid emergence of ciprofloxacin-resistant *Enterobacteriaceae* containing multiple gentamicin resistance-associated integrons, the Netherlands. *Emerg. Infect. Dis.* 7:862–871.

306. Van Looveren, M., M. L. Chasseur-Libotte, C. Godard, C. Lammens, M. Wijdooghe, L. Peeters, and H. Goossens. 2001. Antimicrobial susceptibility of nontyphoidal *Salmonella* isolated from humans in Belgium. *Acta Clin. Belg.* 56:180–186.

307. Van Looveren, M., G. Daube, L. De Zutter, J. M. Dumont, C. Lammens, M. Wijdooghe, P. Vandamme, M. Jouret, M. Cornelis, and H. Goossens. 2001. Antimicrobial susceptibilities of *Campylobacter* strains isolated from food animals in Belgium. *J. Antimicrob. Chemother.* 48:235–240.

308. Vasallo, F. J., P. Martin-Rabadan, L. Alcala, J. M. Garcia-Lechuz, M. Rodriguez-Creixems, and E. Bouza. 1998. Failure of ciprofloxacin therapy for invasive nontyphoidal salmonellosis. *Clin. Infect. Dis.* 26:535–536.

309. Velasco, M., J. P. Horcajada, J. Mensa, A. Moreno-Martinez, J. Vila, J. A. Martinez, J. Ruiz, M. Barranco, G. Roig, and E. Soriano. 2001. Decreased invasive capacity of quinolone-resistant *Escherichia coli* in patients with urinary tract infections. *Clin. Infect. Dis.* 33:1682–1686.

310. Velazquez, J. B., A. Jimenez, B. Chomon, and T. G. Villa. 1995. Incidence and transmission of antibiotic resistance in *Campylobacter jejuni* and *Campylobacter coli. J. Antimicrob. Chemother.* 35:173–178.

311. Vila, J., J. Ruiz, F. Sanchez, F. Navarro, B. Mirelis, M. T. de Anta, and G. Prats. 1999. Increase in quinolone resistance in a *Haemophilus influenzae* strain isolated from a patient with recurrent respiratory infections treated with ofloxacin. *Antimicrob. Agents Chemother.* 43:161–162.

312. Vinh, H., J. Wain, M. T. Chinh, C. T. Tam, P. T. Trang, D. Nga, P. Echeverria, T. S. Diep, N. J. White, and C. M. Parry. 2000. Treatment of bacillary dysentery in Vietnamese children: two doses of ofloxacin versus 5-days nalidixic acid. *Trans. R. Soc. Trop. Med. Hyg.* 94:323–326.

313. Vinh, H., J. Wain, T. N. Vo, N. N. Cao, T. C. Mai, D. Bethell, T. T. Nguyen, S. D. Tu, M. D. Nguyen, and N. J. White. 1996. Two or three days of ofloxacin treatment for

uncomplicated multidrug-resistant typhoid fever in children. *Antimicrob. Agents Chemother.* 40:958–961.

314. Wain, J., N. T. Hoa, N. T. Chinh, H. Vinh, M. J. Everett, T. S. Diep, N. P. Day, T. Solomon, N. J. White, L. J. Piddock, and C. M. Parry. 1997. Quinolone-resistant *Salmonella typhi* in Viet Nam: molecular basis of resistance and clinical response to treatment. *Clin. Infect. Dis.* 25:1404–1410.

315. Wang, H., J. L. Dzink-Fox, M. Chen, and S. B. Levy. 2001. Genetic characterization of highly fluoroquinolone-resistant clinical *Escherichia coli* strains from China: role of *acrR* mutations. *Antimicrob. Agents Chemother.* 45:1515–1521.

316. Wannamaker, L. W., and P. M. Schlievert. 1988. Exotoxins of group A streptococci, p. 267–296. *In* M. C. Hardegree and A. T. Tu (ed.), *Bacterial Toxins*. Marcel Dekker, New York, N.Y.

317. Ward, L. R., and B. Rowe. 1999. Resistance to ciprofloxacin in non-typhoidal salmonellas from humans in England and Wales—the current situation. *Clin. Microbiol. Infect.* 5:130–134.

318. Weiss, K., C. Restieri, M. Laverdiere, A. McGeer, R. J. Davidson, L. Kilburn, D. J. Bast, J. de Azavedo, and D. E. Low. 2001. A nosocomial outbreak of fluoroquinolone-resistant *Streptococcus pneumoniae*. *Clin. Infect. Dis.* 33: 517–522.

319. Wilson, R. 1999. Ten years of ciprofloxacin: the past, present and future. Acute exacerbations of chronic bronchitis. *J. Antimicrob. Chemother.* 43(Suppl. A):95–96.

320. Winokur, P. L., R. Canton, J. M. Casellas, and N. Legakis. 2001. Variations in the prevalence of strains expressing an extended-spectrum beta-lactamase phenotype and characterization of isolates from Europe, the Americas, and the Western Pacific region. *Clin. Infect. Dis.* 32(Suppl. 2):S94–S103.

321. Wistrom, J., and S. R. Norrby. 1995. Fluoroquinolones and bacterial enteritis, when and for whom? *J. Antimicrob. Chemother.* 36:23–39.

322. Wretlind, B., A. Stromberg, L. Ostlund, E. Sjogren, and B. Kaijser. 1992. Rapid emergence of quinolone resistance in

323. Wright, D. H., G. H. Brown, M. L. Peterson, and J. C. Rotschafer. 2000. Application of fluoroquinolone pharmacodynamics. *J. Antimicrob. Chemother.* 46:669–683.

324. Yagupsky, P., A. Schahar, N. Peled, N. Porat, R. Trefler, M. Dan, Y. Keness, and C. Block. 2002. Increasing incidence of gonorrhea in Israel associated with countrywide dissemination of a ciprofloxacin-resistant strain. *Eur. J. Clin. Microbiol. Infect. Dis.* 21:368–372.

325. Yan, S. S., M. L. Fox, S. M. Holland, F. Stock, V. J. Gill, and D. P. Fedorko. 2000. Resistance to multiple fluoroquinolones in a clinical isolate of *Streptococcus pyogenes*: identification of *gyrA* and *parC* and specification of point mutations associated with resistance. *Antimicrob. Agents Chemother.* 44:3196–3198.

326. Ye, S., X. Su, Q. Wang, Y. Yin, X. Dai, and H. Sun. 2002. Surveillance of antibiotic resistance of *Neisseria gonorrhoeae* isolates in China, 1993–1998. *Sex. Transm. Dis.* 29:242–245.

327. Yoo, J. H., D. H. Huh, J. H. Choi, W. S. Shin, M. W. Kang, C. C. Kim, and D. J. Kim. 1997. Molecular epidemiological analysis of quinolone-resistant *Escherichia coli* causing bacteremia in neutropenic patients with leukemia in Korea. *Clin. Infect. Dis.* 25:1385–1391.

328. Zhanel, G. G., J. A. Karlowsky, G. K. Harding, A. Carrie, T. Mazzulli, D. E. Low, and D. J. Hoban for The Canadian Urinary Isolate Study Group. 2000. A Canadian national surveillance study of urinary tract isolates from outpatients: comparison of the activities of trimethoprim-sulfamethoxazole, ampicillin, mecillinam, nitrofurantoin, and ciprofloxacin. *Antimicrob. Agents Chemother.* 44:1089–1092.

329. Zirnstein, G., Y. Li, B. Swaminathan, and F. Angulo. 1999. Ciprofloxacin resistance in *Campylobacter jejuni* isolates: detection of gyrA resistance mutations by mismatch amplification mutation assay PCR and DNA sequence analysis. *J. Clin. Microbiol.* 37:3276–3280.

Campylobacter jejuni in patients treated with norfloxacin. *Scand. J. Infect. Dis.* 24:685–686.

Chapter 24

Veterinary Use of Quinolones and Impact on Human Infections

HENRIK C. WEGENER AND JØRGEN ENGBERG

USE OF ANTIMICROBIALS IN ANIMALS

Antimicrobials are used primarily in domesticated animals and much less frequently in wild animals. The domesticated animals consist of two very different entities, companion animals and food animals. Companion animals have population patterns like humans and receive close veterinary attention, and treatment is not highly dependent on economics. The patterns of disease and antimicrobial usage reflect this circumstance. Food animals, in contrast, are kept in large groups and often housed with high animal densities for the entire rearing period. Meat-producing animals are rapidly raised to slaughter weight, which is usually before they reach physical maturity. The youth of the animals and their housing in large groups facilitate the development and spread of infectious disease. Treatment of entire groups of animals as soon as clinical symptoms appear in a few members of the group is common practice (therapeutic usage). Furthermore, in many production systems treatment of groups of animals in advance of clinical symptoms is practiced regularly, for instance, in connection with movement of animals, mingling of animals from different litters, or other factors that predispose to outbreaks of disease (prophylactic usage). The most common syndromes that require antimicrobial therapy are diarrhea and pneumonia. Finally, antimicrobials are also used to enhance growth rates and increase feed efficiency in food animals (growth promotion).

Quinolones are primarily used for treatment and prevention of animal diseases. They are not used for growth promotion, according to the available information. Quinolones are primarily available for animals on prescription in most countries.

Nalidixic acid was the first quinolone used clinically in animals. This drug is no longer used, according to the available information. Subsequent quinolones, synthesized in the 1960s and 1970s (oxolinic acid, flumequine), are still used in animals in some countries. The modern fluoroquinolones were introduced into the animal market in the late 1980s and early 1990s. In 1987 and 1989 they were introduced into veterinary medicine in The Netherlands and Germany, respectively, and then in France in 1991 and the United Kingdom in 1993; they are now licensed in all European Union (EU) countries. In the United States (USA), sarafloxacin was licensed for use in poultry in 1995 as was enrofloxacin in 1996 (10). Recently, the U.S. Food and Drug Administration (FDA) banned the extra-label use of fluoroquinolones for food animals (25). The FDA has furthermore taken steps to withdraw the approval of sarafloxacin and enrofloxacin for poultry (26). Several types of fluoroquinolones are available for animals in other regions of the world. However, the usage of fluoroquinolones differs greatly regarding animal species, label indications, and geographic spread. Tables 1 through 3 show the pattern of fluoroquinolone usage in food animals worldwide (98).

Quinolone production and usage in animals has been estimated to amount to about 50 tons for proprietary products (mainly EU, USA, Japan, South Korea) and, because of the lower prices, 70 tons of generic quinolone are used for the same purposes. However, usage data, particularly for nonproprietary products, are grossly incomplete. For instance, data from China estimated annual quinolone consumption for animals in China alone to be approximately 470 tons in 1997. The consumption of quinolones in human medicine was estimated to be 800 tons in the same year (98).

MODE OF QUINOLONE USE IN DIFFERENT ANIMAL SPECIES

The fluoroquinolones approved for use in food animals can be administered by injection or given

Henrik C. Wegener • Danish Zoonosis Centre, Danish Veterinary Institute, Bülowsvej 27, DK-1790 Copenhagen V, Denmark.
Jørgen Engberg • Department of Gastrointestinal and Parasitic Infections, Division of Diagnostics, Statens Serum Institut, Artillerivej 5, DK-2300 Copenhagen S, Denmark.

Table 1. Proprietary quinolones licensed for use in animals (92)[a]

Generic name	Trade name	Licensed for use in:						
		Cattle	Swine	Chicken	Turkeys	Dogs	Cats	Fish
Enrofloxacin	Baytril	X	X	X	X	X	X	X[b]
Danofloxacin	Advocin	X	X	X				
	Advocid							
Norfloxacin	Quinabic			X	X			
Ofloxacin	Oxaldin			X	X			
Ciprofloxacin	Generic		X	X				
Sarafloxacin	Floxasol			X	X			X
	Saraflox							
	Sarafin							
Orbifloxacin	Victas	X	X			X	X	
	Orbax							
Marbofloxacin	Marbocyl	X	X			X	X	
Flumequine	Many	X	X	X				X
Oxolinic acid	Many	X	X	X				X
Difloxacin	Vetequinon		X	X	X	X		
	Dicural							

[a] Table reproduced from reference 98 with permission.
[b] Baytril is not licensed for this use, but generic products are available in some countries.

Table 2. Quinolones licensed for use in food animals by region of the world[a]

Region	Quinolones licensed for use in the following animals[b]			
	Livestock	Poultry	Pet animals	Fish
Europe	Enrofloxacin	Enrofloxacin	Enrofloxacin	Sarafloxacin
	Flumequine	Difloxacin	Difloxacin	(Oxolinic acid)
	Marbofloxacin	Flumequine	Marbofloxacin	
	Danofloxacin	Oxolinic acid		
USA	Enrofloxacin	Enrofloxacin	Enrofloxacin	None
		Sarafloxacin[c]	Difloxacin	
			Orbifloxacin	
Japan	Enrofloxacin	Enrofloxacin	Enrofloxacin	Oxolinic acid
	Danofloxacin	Danofloxacin	Orbifloxacin	
	Orbifloxacin	Ofloxacin		
	Difloxacin	Vebufloxacin		
	Oxolinic acid	Oxolinic acid		
Asia	Enrofloxacin	Enrofloxacin	Enrofloxacin	Oxolinic acid
	Danofloxacin	Danofloxacin		Enrofloxacin
	Ciprofloxacin	Ciprofloxacin		Flumequine
		Ofloxacin		
		Flumequine		
		Norfloxacin		
		Oxolinic acid		
Latin America	Enrofloxacin	Enrofloxacin	Enrofloxacin	Oxolinic acid
	Ciprofloxacin	Ciprofloxacin		
	Danofloxacin	Danofloxacin		
	Norfloxacin	Norfloxacin		
	(Flumequine)	(Flumequine,		
		oxolinic acid)[d]		
Canada		Enrofloxacin	Enrofloxacin	
Australia	None	None	Enrofloxacin	None
South Africa	Danofloxacin	Danofloxacin	Enrofloxacin	
		Norfloxacin		

[a] Table reproduced from reference 98 with permission.
[b] Substances in parentheses are in limited use.
[c] Voluntarily withdrawn from the market in 2001.
[d] Voluntarily withdrawn from the market in 1998.

Table 3. Indications of use and formulation of quinolones for treatment of infection in animals[a]

Animal species	Licensed use	Major bacteria	Formulation
Cattle	Respiratory, enteric	*Pasteurella* spp., *Haemophilus somnus*, *Mycoplasma bovis*	Injectable, bolus
Swine	Respiratory, enteric, mastitis/metritis	*Pasteurella* spp., *Actinobacillus pleuropneumoniae*, *Mycoplasma hyosynoviae*, *E. coli*	Injectable, oral solution, feed medication
Broilers	Respiratory, enteric	*E. coli*, *Mycoplasma* spp., *Pasteurella* spp., *Salmonella* spp.	Oral (water medication)
Turkeys	Respiratory, enteric	*E. coli*, *Mycoplasma* spp., *Pasteurella* spp., *Salmonella* spp.	Oral (water medication)
Fish	Generalized conditions (septicemia), skin/ulcers	*Aeromonas hydrophila*, *Vibrio* spp.	Oral (feed medication)
Dogs	Skins/wounds, urinary tract, respiratory	*S. intermedius*, *E. coli*, *Pasteurella* spp.	Oral (tablets), injectables
Cats	Skins/wounds, urinary tract, respiratory	*S. intermedius*, *E. coli*, *Pasteurella* spp.	Oral (tablets), injectables

[a] Table reproduced from reference 98 with permission.

orally in feed or water. The fluoroquinolones are often used for group or flock treatment of animals that are sick or at risk of becoming sick. Because the intake of feed and water varies between animals, in particular when some are sick, underdosing of animals is inevitable. Underdosing is probably an important risk factor for the selection of quinolone-resistant bacteria in animals (10).

Cattle

Antimicrobial therapies differ in dairy and beef units. Treatment may be oral or parenteral or occasionally by water medication. Fluoroquinolones are potentially useful for treatment of diarrhea caused by *Escherichia coli* and *Salmonella enterica* in calves and for treatment of pneumonia caused by *Pasteurella multocida*, *Pasteurella haemolytica*, *Haemophilus somnus*, *Actinomyces pyogenes*, and *Mycoplasma bovis* in calves and older animals. Mastitis is the most common infection in dairy herds. Fluoroquinolones are generally not used for intramammary treatment of mastitis and are not the drugs of choice for systemic treatment of mastitis. In the USA enrofloxacin was approved in 1998 for use in bovine respiratory disease associated with *P. haemolytica*, *P. multocida*, and *H. somnus* (25).

Swine

Piglets primarily receive antimicrobial treatment for enteritis, pneumonia, and septicemia. At weaning (usually 3 to 4 weeks) all piglets are gathered, mixed, and then reared to finishing weight. The first stage "weaners" are highly prone to develop postweaning diarrhea caused by a limited range of *E. coli* serotypes. In later stages of weaning and early finish-

ing *Lawsonia intracellularis* is recognized as an important cause of diarrhea, and meningitis caused by *Streptococcus suis* is a cause of mortality in this age group. From 8 to 10 weeks (25 to 30 kg) until slaughter, pigs are called "finishers." In this age group pneumonia caused by *Mycoplasma hyopneumoniae* and *Actinobacillus pleuropneumoniae* and dysentery caused by *Brachyspira pilosicoli* are common indications for antimicrobial therapy. Pigs are moved and mixed with other pigs several times during production. At every move there is increased risk of infection due to stress and exposure to pathogens. This risk is reflected in the extensive use of medicated feed for swine. Dewey et al. (19) found, in a survey of 712 American swine farms, that 77% of farms provided weaners with antimicrobials in feed on a continuous basis. The lowest continuous use was in late finishers, in which medicated feed was used continuously in "only" 55% of herds. Fluoroquinolones are primarily used to treat or prevent postweaning diarrhea, especially in cases in which alternative, less expensive therapies may be found to be ineffective because of multiresistant pathogens. No fluoroquinolones are currently approved for use in swine in the USA, but they are widely used in swine production in Central and South America as well as in Europe (80).

Poultry

The poultry industry is divided into two sectors: egg producers and slaughter poultry producers. Treatment is required for outbreaks of necrotic enteritis (*Clostridium perfringens* type A), coli-septicemia (*E. coli*), salmonellosis, mycoplasma infections (*Mycoplasma synoviae*), and necrotic dermatitis caused by *Staphylococcus aureus*. Fluoroquinolones are used primarily for the treatment and prevention of coli-septicemia by injection into eggs before hatching and by administration to chickens through medicated water. According to Smith et al. (79) poultry producers in Mexico used 326 million medicated liters for poultry in 1997 (equal to approximately half a liter of fluoroquinolone-medicated water per head produced in the country in 1997).

Fish

Second-generation quinolones (oxolinic acid and flumequine) have been used in freshwater and marine aquaculture in several regions of the world. Recently, effective vaccines against infections with *Aeromonas salmonicida* (furunculosis) have reduced the use of antimicrobials in aquaculture in some developed countries (31). Nearly 90% of the global aquaculture production (22.8 million tons in 1996) is estimated to take place in Asia (99). Only limited data are available on the extent and pattern of antimicrobial usage in aquaculture worldwide.

Companion Animals

A wider range of fluoroquinolones, including several formulations for humans, is used in companion animals. Fluoroquinolones are used for a wide range of indications. In the USA they have been approved for urinary tract infections and soft tissue infections in dogs and cats. Only limited information exists on the extent of quinolone usage in companion animals, but label and extra-label use of fluoroquinolones is common practice.

RESISTANCE TO QUINOLONES IN ANIMAL PATHOGENS

Resistance in pathogenic bacteria from food animals is monitored less intensively than that in bacteria causing human infections. The major reasons for this lack of data are the cost and limited availability of veterinary diagnostic laboratory services. Few countries have active centralized surveillance of resistance in animal pathogens, and there are problems of data comparability between existing systems (13, 105).

Occurrence of antimicrobial resistance in animal pathogenic and zoonotic bacteria depends on the use of antimicrobials for treatment and prevention of disease, as well as for growth promotion, in the particular animal host species (88).

Fluoroquinolones are active against several of the major causes of enteric and respiratory tract infec-

tions and generalized infections in food animals. Consequently, they constitute a treatment option for the veterinary practitioner. The higher cost of these drugs has hitherto limited the extent of their use in animals (48).

Antimicrobial resistance has emerged in several animal pathogens with the introduction of fluoroquinolones for use in animals. Figure 1 shows the emergence of quinolone resistance in different animal pathogens following the licensing of enrofloxacin for treatment of infections in swine, cattle, and poultry in Denmark in 1993. Resistance has emerged rapidly despite low relative levels of consumption representing less than 1/100th of the total volume of antimicrobials used in food animals in Denmark in the same period (17).

Escherichia coli

E. coli is a major animal pathogen. It causes septicemia, mastitis, neonatal and postweaning diarrhea in most species, and a range of specialized syndromes such as "watery mouth" in lambs and edema disease in pigs. In poultry, coli-septicemia (colibacillosis) is one of the most important bacterial infections. Fluoroquinolones are often active against animal-pathogenic *E. coli* and are widely used for treatment and prevention of this disease (82). Despite the limited amounts of fluoroquinolones used, a correlation was observed between the volumes used and the levels of resistance in animal pathogenic serotypes of *E. coli* in Denmark (Fig. 2) (17). In a study from Spain, where fluoroquinolones are widely used to prevent colibacillosis, Blanco et al. (12) found that 17% of *E. coli* isolates, collected during 1992 and 1993, were resistant to fluoroquinolones, and 48% of the same isolates were resistant to nalidixic acid. In Saudi Arabia, another country with widespread use of fluoroquinolones in poultry production, it was reported that more than 50% of clinical *E. coli* isolates from poultry were resistant to fluoroquinolones (6, 11). It appears that indiscriminate use of fluoroquinolones in poultry production could rapidly mean the end of these important drugs for treatment of colibacillosis.

Salmonella

S. enterica causes enteric infections, as well as a range of other infections in food animals. Most animals colonized with zoonotic salmonella, however, show no clinical signs of infection. Enteric infections are primarily treated with ampicillin, amoxicillin-clavulanic acid, oxytetracycline, and other non-quinolone antimicrobials.

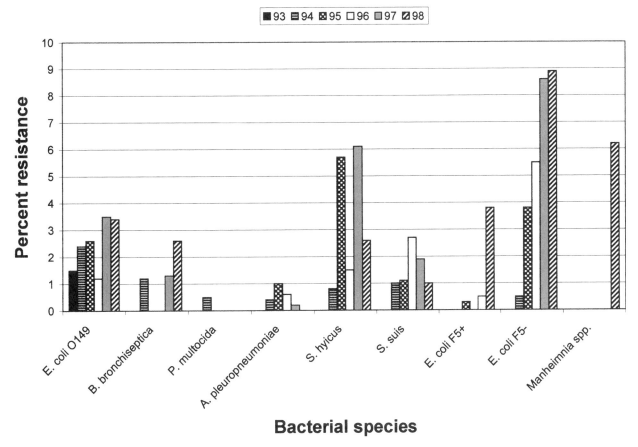

Figure 1. Percentage of fluoroquinolone-resistant isolates among bacteria from clinical infections in pigs and cattle in Denmark from 1993 to 1998. (Reproduced from the Veterinary Record [3] with permission.)

Campylobacter

Campylobacter species found in food animals (*C. jejuni, C. coli, C. lari, C. fetus, C. upsaliensis,* and *C. hyointestinalis*) only rarely cause infections, with the exception of *C. fetus,* which causes infections of the reproductive tract of cattle and sheep.

Staphylococci

Major staphylococcal infections in animals are mastitis in cattle and other food animal species (*S. aureus* and coagulase-negative staphylococci), exudative epidermitis in pigs (*Staphylococcus hyicus*), as well as a large number of individual wound

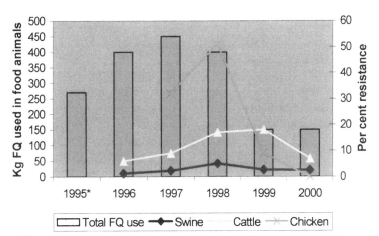

Figure 2. Consumption of fluoroquinolones in food animals and occurrence of fluoroquinolone resistance in animal-pathogenic *E. coli* in Denmark. (Reproduced from DANMAP [17] with permission.)

infections in all food animal species. Infections are often treated with β-lactam antibiotics and streptomycin (alone or in combination). Quinolones are used infrequently for the treatment of staphylococcal infections. Nevertheless, a survey from Denmark found that 30% of *S. aureus* and 8.5% of coagulase-negative staphylococci, isolated from infections in poultry, were resistant to fluoroquinolones (4).

Streptococci

Streptococci cause mastitis in bovine and other species (*S. agalactiae*, *S. dysgalactiae*, and *S. uberis*), as well as joint infections in young animals of most species. A major use of antimicrobials against streptococcal infections is *S. suis* infections in pigs. The same antimicrobials that are used against staphylococci are also commonly used against streptococcal infections in food animals. Quinolones are used less frequently.

Pasteurellaceae

This diverse group of bacteria is one of the major causes of infections in food animals. The family is composed of three genera, *Haemophilus*, *Actinobacillus*, and *Pasteurella* (the HAP group). Major pathogens include *P. multocida*, a cause of respiratory tract infections in most species, and *P. parahaemolyticus* and *H. somnus*, a major cause of pneumonia in cattle and sheep, and *A. pleuropneumoniae* and *H. parasuis*, a cause of pneumonia in pigs. Fluoroquinolones are active against all members of the HAP group and are useful for the treatment of pneumonia in most animal species. Human infections with *P. multocida* can occur after dog or cat bites. Fluoroquinolones can be used to treat human infections with β-lactamase producing *P. multocida* (8).

Mycoplasmas

Mycoplasmas are important pathogens of poultry and pigs and are also causes of pneumonia in calves and mastitis in cattle. Pneumonia in pigs caused by *M. hyopneumonia* is a major reason for the use of significant amounts of antibiotics in that species, including fluoroquinolones. A survey of different animal pathogenic *Mycoplasma* spp. from the USA indicated that enrofloxacin was active against all clinical isolates (32, 33). A survey from Denmark of *M. hyosynoviae* showed that all clinical isolates from swine were sensitive to enrofloxacin after 4 years of enrofloxacin use in swine production (2). Nevertheless, another drug unrelated to human ther-

apeutics, tiamulin, has superior in vitro activity to enrofloxacin and remains the drug of choice for these infections in pigs.

MECHANISM OF QUINOLONE RESISTANCE

Quinolones act by directly inhibiting bacterial DNA synthesis. Inhibition appears to occur by interaction of the drug with complexes composed of DNA and either of the two target enzymes, DNA gyrase and topoisomerase IV. Resistance to quinolones largely depends on chromosomal mutations.

Resistance to quinolones in *Salmonella* is associated with mutations in the molecular target: the DNA gyrase subunits A and B. Mutations are located in the highly conserved regions of the *gyrA* and *gyrB*. Resistance to first-generation quinolones, such as nalidixic acid, is primarily associated with single-point mutations in *gyrA* (97). *Salmonella* strains with single mutations in *gyrA* also have reduced susceptibility to fluoroquinolones (low-level resistance). High-level resistance to fluoroquinolones in *Salmonella* is associated with two mutations in *gyrA* and *gyrB*, respectively (34).

Resistance to quinolones in *Campylobacter* also appears to be due most often to mutations in the genes encoding subunits of DNA gyrase (*gyrA*). In the *gyrA* gene, mutations are located at positions Thr-86, Asp-90, and Ala-70 (72, 95). The most common mechanism of resistance among wild-type isolates is a single mutation at position Thr-86. Mutations at Thr-86 are associated with higher-level resistance to nalidixic acid (MIC, 64 to 128 µg/ml) and ciprofloxacin (MIC, 16 to 64 µg/ml) than mutations at Asp-90 or Ala-70. *C. jejuni* isolates resistant to even higher levels of quinolones (ciprofloxacin MIC of 125 µg/ml) carry two mutations, one in *gyrA* Thr-86 and the other in the topoisomerase IV subunit *parC* at Arg-139 (30). Evidence of efflux of fluoroquinolones in *C. jejuni* (15) also exists but has not yet been shown to be clinically relevant.

OCCURRENCE OF QUINOLONE RESISTANCE IN ZOONOTIC BACTERIA

Most data on resistance in zoonotic bacteria come from testing of clinical isolates from humans. Testing of animal isolates is primarily determined to guide the veterinarian's choice of appropriate therapy. Consequently, resistance to quinolones is determined infrequently in zoonotic bacteria from food animals because they rarely cause clinical disease. An even greater paucity of data exists for zoonotic bacterial isolates from food. Data on resistance primarily stem from surveys of limited size and duration. In a few countries active surveillance programs of antimicrobial resistance in bacteria from food animals and food have been initiated in recent years, e.g., the National Antimicrobial Resistance Monitoring System program in the USA (47) and the DANMAP program in Denmark (9, 17). Such programs have greatly enhanced the availability of high-quality data on trends in antimicrobial resistance in food-borne zoonoses. In Denmark, surveillance of resistance is linked to surveillance of use of antimicrobials in food animals and humans (9, 17).

The two most common food-borne zoonoses worldwide are campylobacteriosis and salmonellosis (101). Both infections most often present as an acute gastroenteritis characterized by diarrhea, fever, nausea, vomiting, headache, and occasionally other symptoms. The infections are often self-limiting, but in vulnerable patients, or in complicated infections such as infection of the bloodstream, treatment is required. Fluoroquinolones are standard empirical treatment for acute gastrointestinal tract infections in humans in most parts of the world. Resistance to quinolones in *Campylobacter* and *Salmonella* has been shown to reduce the efficacy of treatment as described below.

Salmonella enterica subsp. *enterica*

Resistance to fluoroquinolones and earlier-generation quinolones has emerged in salmonella in food animals and food of animal origin following the licensing of fluoroquinolones for veterinary use in animals (10, 40, 79, 97, 98). A parallel increase in quinolone resistance in human clinical isolates has been reported in some countries (Fig. 3) (69, 85, 98).

The epidemiology of resistant bacteria is complex, and many factors, other than the use of antimicrobials, affect their spread. This complexity is particularly true for *Salmonella*. *Salmonella* serotypes vary in their host specificity and in their ability to survive and multiply under different environmental conditions (39, 104). Consequently, the use of antimicrobials is only one of several factors that may affect the introduction, establishment, and spread of a particular salmonella clone in food animal and food production. This phenomenon has been reflected in the periodic introduction, rapid establishment and spread, and subsequent disappearance of different *Salmonella* clones in food animals locally as well as globally. Quinolone-sensitive clones may replace quinolone-resistant clones of *Salmonella* in the absence of apparent changes in quinolone selective pressure. This phenomenon has

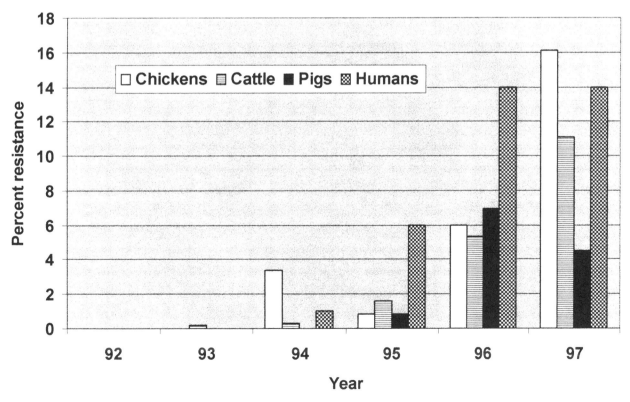

Figure 3. Percentage of *S. enterica* serovar Typhimurium DT104 isolates with low-level resistance to ciprofloxacin in United Kingdom 1993 to 1997. Enrofloxacin was licensed for animals in 1993. (Reproduced from Drug Resistance Updates [81] with permission.)

been observed in United Kingdom, Germany, and Belgium (40, 46, 69, 103).

Quinolone resistance, due to the mechanisms of resistance, is usually only spread clonally in *Salmonella*. The occurrences of resistance reported in the literature vary with animal and food sources, countries, and serotypes. Table 4 shows data on quinolone resistance in common *Salmonella* serovars from a number of recent publications. The comparability of data is hampered by the differences in sampling schemes, isolation methods, and susceptibility-testing methods used in the different studies. Nonetheless, the data confirm an association between licensing of fluoroquinolones for animals in some countries and emergence of resistance in *Salmonella* and furthermore that resistance remains at low levels in *Salmonella* isolated from animals in countries in which fluoroquinolones are not used or are used restrictively (USA and Australia). Because fluoroquinolones have been used widely for

treatment of acute diarrhea in humans in the USA and Australia in the same period (7, 42), this observation indirectly supports that human use of fluoroquinolones is not a major factor in the selection and spread of quinolone-resistant nontyphoidal *Salmonella*.

A recent cause of concern is that resistance to quinolones is now rapidly emerging in *S. enterica* serovar Enteritidis in some regions. *S. enterica* serovar Enteritidis is the most common serovar in human infections. This serovar has hitherto remained remarkably sensitive to antimicrobials when compared with other salmonella serovars such as Typhimurium, Virchow, and Hadar. However, this pattern of antibiotic susceptibility is not reflected with the quinolones, potentially due to the mutational nature of the resistance and the practice of injecting fluoroquinolones into eggs, the predilection site for *S. enterica* serovar Enteritidis, to prevent colisepticemia in chickens (54).

Table 4. Low-level (FQR_l) and high-level (FQR_h) resistance to fluoroquinolones in nontyphoidal *Salmonella* isolated from humans and food animals in different countries

Country	Origin	Year	Serovar	No. of isolates with:		Reference
				FQR_l (%)	FQR_h (%)	
UK	Human	1999	Enteritidis	8	0	82
	Human	1999	Typhimurium	8	0	
	Human	1999	Virchow	39	0	
	Human	1999	Hadar	70	0	
Denmark	Human	2000	Typhimurium	2	0	13
	Human	2000	Enteritidis	5	0	
	Cattle[a]	1995–99	Typhimurium	1.5	0	100
	Cattle[a]	1995–99	Dublin	3.5	0	
	Broiler	1997–99	Enteritidis	27	0	
	Broiler	1997–99	Typhimurium	0.8	0	
	Swine	1997–99	Typhimurium	1.3	0	
Poland	Human	1998–99	Typhimurium	41	0	79
	Human	1998–99	Enteritidis	7.3	0	
	Human	1998–99	Virchow	45	0	
	Human	1998–99	Hadar	91	0	
Belgium	Cattle	1991–98	Typhimurium	NA	4.5[b]	36
Germany	Non-human	1994–98	Multiple types	5.2	0.35	32
	Human	1996–97	Multiple types	NA	0.15	
USA	Cattle	1997	Multiple types	0	0	23
	Swine	1997	Multiple types	0	0	
	Chicken	1997	Multiple types	0.3	0	
	Turkey	1997	Multiple types	8.3	0	
Australia	Non-human	1994–98	Multiple types	0.1	0	41
	Human	1994–98	Multiple types	0.7	0	
UK	Non-human	1999	Typhimurium	11.3	NA	43
	Non-human		Multiple types	5.3	NA	
Greece	Human	1996–97	Enteritidis	NA	0	88
			Typhimurium	NA	0	
Belgium	Human	1998	Multiple types	19	0	85
			Hadar	91	0	

[a] A total of 580 bovine salmonella isolates from 1986 to 1992 (before licensing of enrofloxacin in Denmark) all tested sensitive to nalidixic acid and to ciprofloxacin.
[b] An epidemic of fluoroquinolone-resistant *S. enterica* serovar Typhimurium DT204C peaked in 1993 (25%). In 1998 the level of FQR_h-resistant *S. enterica* serovar Typhimurium in cattle was 0.5%.

C. jejuni and C. coli

As for *Salmonella*, veterinary data on resistance to fluoroquinolones in *Campylobacter* isolated from food animals is incomplete. *C. jejuni* is predominant in broilers and cattle but is infrequent in pigs in which *C. coli* predominates. The reported levels of resistance vary with reference to *Campylobacter* species and animal origin. Increased rates of resistance to fluoroquinolones was first reported for *Campylobacter* from chickens (21). In vitro susceptibility of *Campylobacter* and *Salmonella* isolates from broilers to quinolones, ampicillin, tetracycline, and erythromycin, reported by Jacobs-Reitsma et al. in 1994, indicated almost 30% fluoroquinolone resistance among *Campylobacter* isolates from broilers in The Netherlands (41). In Denmark, in year 2000, 15% of *C. jejuni* from cattle and 8% of *C. jejuni* from broilers were resistant to ciprofloxacin (17). In the same year ciprofloxacin resistance was detected in 8 and 10% of *C. coli* from swine and broilers, respectively (17). Ciprofloxacin-resistant *C. jejuni* was isolated from 14 % of 91 domes-

tic chicken products obtained from retail markets in United States in 1997 (38). In recent reports from Belgium and Spain, the rate of quinolone resistance is very high, e.g., 62.1% in *C. coli* from Belgian broilers (90) and 100% in *C. coli* from Spanish pigs (73).

Emerging resistance to fluoroquinolones in *Campylobacter* isolated from humans has clearly been documented in numerous countries during the past decade (Fig. 4) (23). In some countries the rise in resistance has been remarkably rapid and extensive, whereas in other countries the resistance rates have risen more slowly but steadily. Before 1989, resistance was rare, but with the introduction of enrofloxacin in veterinary medicine and (probably less important) fluoroquinolones in human medicine in mainland Europe (The Netherlands, Finland, France, and Spain), a rapid emergence of quinolone resistance in *Campylobacter* isolates from patients was noted (5, 16, 21, 50, 70, 71, 77).

Surveillance data on resistance rates in human isolates from Asia soon indicated a similar increase (43, 84). Quinolones were approved for veterinary use in

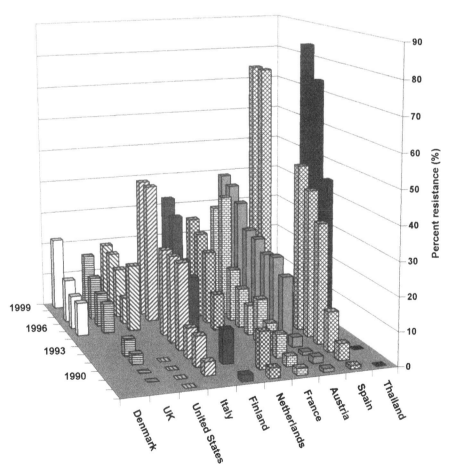

Figure 4. Trends for quinolone resistance rates (in percentages) among *C. coli* and *C. jejuni* combined from human sources around the world. The bars represent both nalidixic acid and fluoroquinolone resistance and are based on mean values of resistance from numerous reports. (Reproduced from Emerging Infectious Diseases [23] with permission.)

the United Kingdom and the USA in late 1993 and 1995, respectively; reports from these areas now show increasing quinolone resistance profiles (67, 74, 79).

In newer data from Taiwan, Thailand, and Spain, rates of fluoroquinolone resistance in *C. jejuni*, or *C. jejuni* and *C. coli* combined, were 56.9, 84, and 75 to 88%, respectively. Although lower frequencies are reported from other regions, recent trends show a clear tendency of emerging quinolone resistance in many countries. Quinolone resistance in human isolates often coincides with or follows the approval of fluoroquinolones for use in animal husbandry, although some differences in resistance rates between countries may be explained by differences in association with foreign travel, commerce, methods of testing, and surveillance activity.

E. coli

E. coli is one of the most common causes of infection in humans and animals worldwide. *E. coli* is associated with a wide variety of diseases, but a large degree of host and disease specificity exists for the different serotypes. Thus, certain pathogenic *E. coli* serovars predominate as causes of intestinal infections in humans and different animal species. Even though many different *E. coli* serovars might be zoonotic, the only *E. coli* clearly documented to have a reservoir in food animals and to infect humans through the food chain is enterohemorrhagic *E. coli* of serotype O157. Currently, reduced susceptibility to quinolones has not been reported in this *E. coli* serotype, but their emergence would be a concern with increasing use of fluoroquinolones in ruminants (2).

TRANSFER OF QUINOLONE-RESISTANT ZOONOTIC BACTERIA FROM ANIMALS TO HUMANS AND ITS PUBLIC HEALTH IMPACT

Resistance to quinolones depends largely on chromosomal mutations. Resistance, however, has recently been found on transferable genetic elements in *Klebsiella* and *E. coli*. The dissemination of quinolone resistance from animals to humans has been thought to be mediated exclusively by the dissemination of resistant strains, but the potential for plasmid spread has now emerged. Thus, the epidemiology of quinolone-resistant zoonoses is complex and multifactorial.

Salmonella enterica subsp. *enterica*

Food animals are the major reservoir for zoonotic *Salmonella* infections in humans, and food (untreated, insufficiently cooked, or recontaminated)

serves as the main vehicle for the infection. In the USA it is estimated that 95% of nontyphoidal salmonella infections are food borne (49). Other sources of infection, such as human and animal contacts, water, and other factors, also contribute but, in developed countries, only in a minor way. The routes of transmission of the resistant *Salmonella* infections do not differ from those of *Salmonella* infections in general (7).

Quinolone resistance in veterinary *Salmonella* isolates was first observed in 1988 in Germany. Strains of multidrug-resistant *S. enterica* serovar Typhimurium phage type 204c (DT204c) highly resistant to fluoroquinolones were isolated from cattle in an area near the Dutch border with Germany (69). Resistance was caused by mutations in the *gyrA* and *gyrB* genes (34). Hof et al. (37) reported on a nonfatal case of salmonellosis in an 11-year-old girl who was infected with such a strain presumably by ingestion of contaminated meat. In 1990 the number of *S. enterica* serovar Typhimurium DT204c isolates decreased in Germany. However, in parallel, the number of pentadrug-resistant isolates (resistant to ampicillin, chloramphenicol, streptomycin, sulfonamides, and tetracyclines) of *S. enterica* serovar Typhimurium DT104 increased, and the strains soon became the most prevalent *Salmonella* serovar and phage type among veterinary isolates (69). A similar emergence and disappearance of fluoroquinolone-resistant *S. enterica* serovar Typhimurium DT204 in cattle was detected in Belgium in 1991 to 1995. This clone was substituted by *S. enterica* serovar Typhimurium DT104, originally sensitive to fluoroquinolones, but now showing increasing levels of low-level resistance to fluoroquinolones (40). In England and Wales a decrease in susceptibility to fluoroquinolones in isolates of *S. enterica* serovar Typhimurium DT 104 was observed following the licensing of enrofloxacin for veterinary use in 1993 (18, 68, 86).

In humans most infections caused by nontyphoidal salmonellae are self-limiting, and antibiotic therapy is not indicated. However, in severe cases of *Salmonella* enteritis and in life-threatening situations, such as invasive salmonellosis, treatment is recommended, and this is particularly applicable for infections caused by multidrug-resistant salmonellae (7, 89). Treatment may eradicate the infection, but in some patients relapses occur, and it may prolong shedding. Resistance can emerge during the course of therapy (54, 66, 93).

Recently, in Denmark, a fatal case of quinolone-resistant *S. enterica* serovar Typhimurium DT104 was reported in an outbreak associated with the consumption of contaminated pork (53). The outbreak included 25 culture-confirmed cases, and the outbreak strain was resistant to nalidixic acid and had reduced susceptibility to ciprofloxacin (MICs ranging from 0.064 to 0.128 μg/ml). The median age of patients was 45 years, and at least seven had a history of antibiotic usage prior to the infection. Eleven patients were admitted to the hospital because of gastroenteritis or septicemia. Fluoroquinolone treatment was reported to lack clinical effect in at least four patients. One previously healthy patient died of complications of intestinal perforation, which developed during ciprofloxacin treatment. Another patient with severe underlying disease died of complications of intestinal perforation caused by the *Salmonella* infection. The molecular epidemiology and data from patients indicated that the primary source of the outbreak was a Danish swine herd colonized with quinolone-resistant *S. enterica* serovar Typhimurium DT104. The outbreak highlighted the transfer of quinolone-resistant strains from animals to humans and the potential problems associated with the treatment of patients infected with such clones.

Reduced treatment effect has also been reported in other studies of human infections with nalidixic acid-resistant nontyphoidal and typhoidal salmonellae (91, 94). However, others have reported that treatment failure does not always correlate with higher MICs of nalidixic acid and ciprofloxacin (14).

In a recent study, Helms and colleagues (35) investigated the survival rates (at 2-year follow-up) associated with *S. enterica* serovar Typhimurium infections in Denmark. The study included data on 2,047 patients. For every patient, data on 10 matched referents were included. The study found that *S. enterica* serovar Typhimurium patients had a 2.3 times higher mortality than comparators (95% confidence interval 1.7 to 3.2), when adjusted for comorbidity. The case-fatality rate was 0.9%, and the majority of deaths occurred within 30 days from the date that the sample was received in the diagnostic laboratory. When patients infected with low-level resistant strains (MICs of ciprofloxacin ranged from 0.06 to 0.38 μg/liter) were compared with patients infected with sensitive strains, the patients infected with quinolone-resistant strains had a fivefold higher mortality rate (10.2) than patients infected with sensitive strains. More studies are needed to address this issue.

Several investigations have found that treatment of humans with antimicrobials predisposes the patient to infections with resistant *Salmonella*. This risk has also been documented for quinolone-resistant *Salmonella* (59). Antimicrobial therapy can also predispose patients to infections with sensitive *Salmonella* strains (63). Considering that patients receiving antimicrobial therapy may already have one infection, acquiring an additional *Salmonella*

infection may seriously worsen the patient's condition. There is concern that with increasing levels of resistance in *Salmonella* the risk of nosocomial *Salmonella* outbreaks could increase.

C. jejuni and *C. coli*

C. jejuni, first identified as a human diarrheal pathogen in 1973, is the most frequently diagnosed bacterial cause of human gastroenteritis in the USA and throughout the world. Contaminated food is the usual source of human infections; therefore, the presence of fluoroquinolone-resistant strains in the food chain has raised concerns that the treatment of human infections will be compromised. As for *Salmonella* enteritis, most cases of *Campylobacter* infections do not require antimicrobial treatment, being brief, clinically mild, and self-limiting. However, a substantial proportion of these infections require treatment. Infections requiring treatment include severe and prolonged cases of enteritis, septicemia, and other extraintestinal infections. Erythromycin has been the most commonly used agent for treating *Campylobacter* enteritis. In the 1980s, the introduction of fluoroquinolones, which are effective against most major pathogens causing bacterial enteritis, offered a new approach to antibiotic intervention. Fluoroquinolones initially had good in vitro activity for thermophilic *Campylobacter* species, as well as for members of the family of *Enterobacteriaceae*.

Early clinical trials of both community-acquired acute diarrhea and traveler's diarrhea caused by *Campylobacter* demonstrated that patients treated with a fluoroquinolone had good clinical response. It soon became apparent, however, that resistance in *Campylobacter* spp. could arise in vivo, sometimes after only one or two administrations of fluoroquinolones (1). Moreover, Endtz and colleagues (21) reported as early as 1991 that the emergence of quinolone-resistant *C. jejuni* and *C. coli* isolated from humans in The Netherlands coincided with the introduction of fluoroquinolones in veterinary medicine.

Fluoroquinolone resistance in *Campylobacter* from food animals is now recognized as an emerging public health problem. In Minnesota Smith et al. (79) found that patients who were treated with a fluoroquinolone after the collection of stool specimens, the duration of diarrhea was longer for the patients with quinolone-resistant *C. jejuni* infections (median, 10 days) than for the patients with quinolone-sensitive *C. jejuni* infections (median, 7 days; *P* = 0.03). Because *Campylobacter* infections can be serious in immunocompromised patients, the identified treatment failure raises the concern that fluoroquinolone-resistant strains may increase *Campylobacter*-associated deaths in this group of patients.

Campylobacteriosis is primarily a zoonosis. Evidence to indicate that fresh raw meat, especially poultry, is a major source of infection is ample, even though other sources such as raw milk, water, and pets may contribute to human infection (22, 28, 60, 78). In contrast to *Salmonella* infections, food-borne *Campylobacter* enteritis rarely takes the form of explosive outbreaks. This difference may be because *Campylobacter* spp. do not multiply in food, as salmonellae do. A frequent route of infection with *Campylobacter* is cross-contamination of odd food items from raw meats by means of hands and utensils resulting in sporadic or small family outbreaks. This mode of transmission is difficult to substantiate, possibly accounting for the difficulty in identifying the source of many sporadic infections. Studying the transmission of antimicrobial resistance from animals (especially poultry to humans) has been difficult because the chain of transmission is often complex. Several studies, however, have shown that food animals can be a substantial source of infection in humans and that the same sero- and genotypes can be isolated from food animals, food of animal origin, and humans (56, 57, 58, 60, 61, 62, 64). In addition, fluoroquinolone-resistant *C. jejuni* and *C. coli* have been isolated from retail chicken products in several countries including Denmark, The Netherlands, Spain, Taiwan, the United Kingdom, and the USA.

Typing data on resistant isolates are sparse, but Smith and colleagues (79) found DNA fingerprints of quinolone-resistant *C. jejuni* from U.S.-produced poultry identical to those of resistant *C. jejuni* from domestically acquired infections in humans. Therefore, the susceptibility of human strains originating in animals to antibiotics can be related to the exposure of animal strains to antibiotic agents used in farming. A summary of these data strongly adds to the cumulative evidence that the veterinary usage of fluoroquinolones, especially in poultry, is a major contributor to human infections with quinolone-resistant *Campylobacter*.

Multidrug resistance to macrolides and fluoroquinolones must be considered highly undesirable in *Campylobacter* because, in general, these two classes are advocated as first- and second-line drugs for antimicrobial treatment of *Campylobacter* enteritis. Additional resistance to other relevant therapeutic agents poses a risk when there is no effective antimicrobial regimen for *Campylobacter* infections. Recently, Hoge et al. (38) found 100% coresistance between Thai isolates resistant to azithromycin and ciprofloxacin in the last 2 years of surveillance. In addition, the level of tetracycline and ampicillin resistance in Thailand is so high that these agents now have

no role in the treatment of *Campylobacter* or non-cholera diarrhea. Li et al. (44) reported that concomitant resistance rates among nalidixic acid-resistant *C. jejuni* isolates from their patients (exclusively children) were as follows: gentamicin, 2%; erythromycin, 12%; clindamycin, 12%; tetracycline, 97%; and ciprofloxacin, 66%. All the human erythromycin-resistant *C. jejuni* isolates and 90% of the *C. coli* isolates were concomitantly resistant to clindamycin.

Consequences of Resistance for the Clinical Decision-Making Process

It is seldom possible to establish the causative agent of an acute case of diarrhea in a patient prior to treatment onset, so the decision of antimicrobial drug use in the clinical setting is of empiric treatment of acute diarrhea in general. Fluoroquinolones are the drug of choice in this situation. Increasing rates of quinolone resistance in *Campylobacter* and *Salmonella*, the predominating causes of community-acquired diarrhea, in most developed countries therefore constitutes a major problem for public health.

THE CONTRIBUTION OF FLUOROQUINOLONE USE IN HUMANS TO RESISTANT INFECTIONS

S. enterica subsp. enterica

The emergence of resistance in salmonella due to treatment with fluoroquinolones in humans has been documented in several reports (66). But humans themselves are not a major source of *Salmonella* infections (49). Quinolones were used in humans before they were approved for use in animals. Early quinolone usage in humans was not followed by emergence of resistance in community-acquired salmonellosis (7). In contrast, quinolone resistance has emerged in *Salmonella* from food animals, and simultaneously in human infections, following the introduction of quinolones for veterinary use. Underdosing is a major risk factor for the development of quinolone resistance. Underdosing is much more likely to occur in food animals than in humans, as explained previously (10). Thus, the majority of quinolone resistance in human *Salmonella* infections is most likely to have an animal origin and to be caused by the use of quinolones in food animals and not in humans.

C. jejuni and C. coli

Some investigators suggest that resistance in *C. jejuni* and *C. coli* is driven by use of antibiotics for treating human infections rather than by veterinary use. Selection of fluoroquinolone resistance during treatment is well recognized and often reported (5, 20, 76, 84). A predicted 10% of patients treated with a fluoroquinolone for *Campylobacter* enteritis harbor quinolone-resistant *Campylobacter* strains (96). Recently, in their prospective trial, Ellis-Pegler et al. (20) found that fluoroquinolone resistance developed in 18 to 28% of patients during therapy.

Smith et al. (79) showed in their study that prior use of a quinolone accounted for a maximum of 15% of resistant isolates from 1996 to 1998. In addition, an increasing number of reports claim that fluoroquinolone-resistant strains have been isolated from patients who had not received medical treatment, suggesting that strains were already fluoroquinolone-resistant before causing the infection (16, 29, 44, 67, 71, 75). Because human-to-human transmission of *C. jejuni* and *C. coli* is rare (21), patients infected with resistant *Campylobacter* strains are not an important source of resistant *Campylobacter* infection for other humans.

CONTROL MEASURES

Surveillance of quinolone resistance in *Campylobacter* and *Salmonella* is of paramount importance when fluoroquinolones are used to treat human and animal infections. Systematic surveillance and timely reporting of antibiotic resistance patterns in *Campylobacter, Salmonella*, and other enteric pathogens should be given a high priority. The main purpose of monitoring antimicrobial resistance trends in enteric pathogens is to provide clinicians and veterinarians with data that can be used to select appropriate treatment regimens, as well as to provide regulatory authorities with an early warning system to enable preventive action to be taken when resistance exceeds acceptable levels. Surveillance should emphasize antibiotics that are being used routinely to treat humans and animals. For quinolones, quantitative nalidixic acid susceptibility data are more sensitive than fluoroquinolone susceptibility data for detecting common first-step mutations causing clinically relevant reduced susceptibility.

To circumvent the development of resistance, a two-tiered control strategy should be used. Improved infection control strategies along the chain "stable to the table" and guidelines for prudent use of antimicrobial agents in food animal production should be developed promptly (96, 100). To prevent further development of resistance in *Campylobacter* and *Salmonella,* limiting the use of fluoroquinolones for food animals as much as possible is recommended. In

the USA authorities have been restrictive in the licensing of fluoroquinolones for food animals, and recently the regulatory authority has initiated a process to withdraw the approval of fluoroquinolones for use in poultry (26) as well as banning the extralabel use of fluoroquinolones (24). In Europe, the approval of fluoroquinolones for animals is broader and covers a wide range of animals and infections. Guidelines for practicing veterinarians, aiming at avoiding unnecessary use of important human drugs such as fluoroquinolones in animals, have been developed in many countries (65, 87, 100). In Denmark, fluoroquinolones are not essential for treatment of the vast majority of infections in food animals, according to surveillance performed by the Danish Veterinary Institute, and their use is only recommended for the rare occasion when no other therapeutic options are available. Veterinary prescription guidelines, consumer pressure, and public health officials' attention have kept the use of fluoroquinolones in food animals at a minimum in Denmark (Fig. 2).

SUMMARY AND FUTURE PERSPECTIVES

Fluoroquinolones are effective for treatment and prevention of a wide range of bacterial infections in food and companion animals. Resistance is emerging, and limited alternatives make it important to preserve the effect of fluoroquinolones. Resistance in zoonotic bacteria, caused by use of quinolones in animals, is a concern for public health, because fluoroquinolones are important drugs in the treatment of human infections. Low-level resistance to fluoroquinolones in *Salmonella* and high-level resistance in *Campylobacter* causing human infections have emerged, in part, as a result of the use of fluoroquinolones in food animals. There are reports of increased human morbidity and even mortality due to this resistance. Thus, a need exists to preserve the effect of quinolones for humans, and their use in animals should be avoided when therapeutic alternatives exist. Fluoroquinolone resistance may decrease in bacteria from food animals following reductions in selective pressure.

REFERENCES

1. **Aarestrup, F. M., and N. F. Friis.** 1998. Antimicrobial susceptibility testing of *Mycoplasma hyosynoviae* isolated from pigs during 1968 to 1971 and during 1995 and 1996. *Vet. Microbiol.* 61:33–39.
2. **Aarestrup, F. M., and H. C. Wegener.** 1999. The effects of antibiotic usage in food animals on the development of antimicrobial resistance of importance for humans in

Campylobacter and *Escherichia coli. Microbes Infect.* 1:639–644.

3. **Aarestrup, F. M., N. E. Jensen, S. E. Jorsal, and T. K. Nielsen.** 2000. Emergence of resistance to fluoroquinolones among bacteria causing infections in food animals in Denmark. *Vet. Rec.* **146:**76–78.

4. **Aarestrup, F. M., Y. Agersø, P. Ahrens, J. C. Jørgensen, M. Madsen, and L. B. Jensen.** 2000. Antimicrobial susceptibility and presence of resistance genes in staphylococci from poultry. *Vet. Microbiol.* **74:**353–364.

5. **Adler-Mosca, H., J. Lüthy-Hottenstein, G. Martinetti Lucchini, A. Burnens, and M. Altwegg.** 1991. Development of resistance to quinolones in five patients with campylobacteriosis treated with norfloxacin or ciprofloxacin. *Eur. J. Clin. Microbiol. Infect. Dis.* **10:**953–957.

6. **Al-Mustafa, Z.H., and M.S. Al-Ghamdi.** 2000. Use of norfloxacin in poultry production in the eastern province of Saudi Arabia and its possible impact on public health. *Int. J. Environ. Health Res.* **10:**291–299.

7. **Angulo, F. J., K. R. Johnson, R. V. Tauxe, and M. L. Cohen.** 2000. Origins and consequences of antimicrobials-resistant nontyphoidal salmonella: implications for the use of fluoroquinolones in food animals. *Microb. Drug Resist.* **6:**77–83.

8. **Avril, J. L., and P. Y. Donnio.** 1995. Pasteurelloses. *Presse Med.* **24:**516–518.

9. **Bager, F.** 2000. DANMAP: monitoring antimicrobial resistance in Denmark. *Int. J. Antimicrob. Agents* **14:**271–274.

10. **Bager, F., and R. Helmuth.** 2001. Epidemiology of resistance to quinolones in Salmonella. *Vet. Res.* **32:**285–290.

11. **Bazile-Pham-Khac, S., Q. C. Truong, J. P. Lafont, L. Gutmann, X. Y. Zhou, M. Osman, and N. J. Moreau.** 1996. Resistance to fluoroquinolones in *Escherichia coli* isolated from poultry. *Antimicrob. Agents Chemother.* **40:**1504–1507.

12. **Blanco, J. E., M. Blanco, A. Mora, and J. Blanco.** 1997. Prevalence of bacterial resistance to quinolones and other antimicrobials among avian *Escherichia coli* strains isolated from septicemic and healthy chickens in Spain. *J. Clin. Microbiol.* **35:**2184–2185.

13. **Caprioli, A., L. Busani, J. L. Martel, and R. Helmuth.** 2000. Monitoring of antibiotic resistance in bacteria of animal origin: epidemiological and microbiological methodologies. *Int. J. Antimicrob. Agents* **14:**295–301.

14. **Chandel, D. S., and R. Chaudhry.** 2001. Enteric fever treatment failures: a global concern. *Emerg. Infect. Dis.* **7:**762–763.

15. **Charvalos, E., Y. Tselentis, M. M. Hamzehpour, T. Köhler, and J-C. Pechere.** 1995. Evidence for an efflux pump im multidrug-resistant *Campylobacter jejuni. Antimicrob. Agents Chemother.* **39:**2019–2022.

16. **Chatzipanagiotou, S., E. Papavasiliou, and E. Malamou Lada.** 1993. Isolation of *Campylobacter jejuni* strains resistant to nalidixic acid and fluoroquinolones from children with diarrhea in Athens, Greece. *Eur. J. Clin. Microbiol. Infect. Dis.* **12:**566–568. (Letter.)

17. **DANMAP.** 2000. DANMAP 2000 - Consumption of antimicrobial agents and occurrence of antimicrobial resistance in bacteria from food animals and humans in Denmark. Statens Serum Institut, Danish Veterinary and Food Administration, Danish Medicines Agency, Danish Veterinary Laboratory. Available at: www.vetinst.dk and www.dzc.dk.

18. **Davies, R. H. A., C. J. Teale, C. Wray, I. H. McLaren, Y. E. Jones, S. Chappell, and S. Kidd.** 1999. Nalidixic acid resistance in *Salmonellae* isolated from turkeys and other livestock in Great Britain. *Vet. Rec.* **144:**320–322.

19. **Dewey, C. E, B. D. Cox, B. E. Straw, E. J. Bush, and S. Hurd.** 1999. Use of antimicrobials in swine feed in the United States. *Swine Health Prod.* **7:**19–25.

20. **Ellis-Pegler, R. B., L. K. Hyman, R. J. Ingram, and M. McCarthy.** 1995. A placebo controlled evaluation of lomefloxacin in the treatment of bacterial diarrhoea in the community. *J. Antimicrob. Chemother.* **36:**259–263.

21. **Endtz, H. P., G. J. Ruijs, B. van Klingeren, W. H. Jansen, T. van der Reyden, and R. P. Mouton.** 1991. Quinolone resistance in *Campylobacter* isolated from man and poultry following the introduction of fluoroquinolones in veterinary medicine. *J. Antimicrob. Chemother.* **27:**199–208.

22. **Engberg, J., P. Gerner-Smidt, F. Scheutz, E. M. Nielsen, S. L. W. On, and K. Mølbak.** 1998. Water-borne *Campylobacter jejuni* infection in a Danish town: a 6-week continuous source outbreak. *Clin. Microbiol. Infect.* **4:**648–656.

23. **Engberg, J., F. M. Aarestrup, D. E. Taylor, P. Gerner-Smidt, and I. Nachamkin.** 2001. Quinolone and macrolide resistance in *Campylobacter jejuni* and *C. coli*: resistance mechanisms and trends in human isolates. *Emerg. Infect. Dis.* **7:**24–34.

24. **FDA.** 1997. Extralabel animal drug use; fluoroquinolones and glycopeptides; order of prohibition. *Fed. Regist.* **62:**27944–27947.

25. **FDA.** 1998. New animal drug approvals. *Vet. Newsl.* **13:**1.

26. **FDA.** 2001. Sarafloxacin for poultry; withdrawal of approval of NADAs. *Fed. Regist.* **66:**21282.

27. **Fedorka-Cray, P. J., M. A. Miller, D. A. Dargatz, N. E. Wineland, and L. Tollefson.** 1998. Prevalence/trends of quinolone resistace in *Salmonella* isolates from animals in the USA, p. 221–228. *In Use of Quinolones in Food Animals and Potential Impact on Public Health. Report and Proceedings of a WHO Meeting, Geneva, Switzerland, 2–5 June 1998* (WHO/EMC/ZDI/98.12). World Health Organization, Geneva, Switzerland.

28. **Friedman, C. R., J. Neimann, H. C. Wegener, and R. V. Tauxe.** 2000. Epidemiology of *Campylobacter jejuni* infections in the United States and other industrialized nations, p. 121–138. *In* I. Nachamkin and M. J. Blaser (ed.), *Campylobacter*, 2nd ed. ASM Press, Washington, D.C.

29. **Gaunt, P. N., and L. J. Piddock.** 1996. Ciprofloxacin resistant *Campylobacter* spp. in humans: an epidemiological and laboratory study. *J. Antimicrob. Chemother.* **37:**47–57.

30. **Gibreel, A., E. Sjögren, B. Kaijser, B. Wretlind, and O. Sköld.** 1998. Rapid emergence of high-level resistance to quinolones in *Campylobacter jejuni* associated with mutational changes in *gyrA* and *parC. Antimicrob. Agents Chemother.* **42:**3276–3278.

31. **Grave, K., E. Lingaas, M. Bangen, and M. Ronning.** 1999. Surveillance of the overall consumption of antibacterial drugs in humans, domestic animals and farmed fish in Norway in 1992 and 1996. *J. Antimicrob. Chemother.* **43:**243–252.

32. **Hannan, P. C., H. M. Windsor, and P. H. Ripley.** 1997. In vitro susceptibilities of recent field isolates of *Mycoplasma hyopneumoniae* and *Mycoplasma hyosynoviae* to valnemulin (Econor), tiamulin and enrofloxacin and the in vitro development of resistance to certain antimicrobial agents in *Mycoplasma hyopneumoniae. Res. Vet. Sci.* **63:**157–160.

33. **Hannan, P. C., G. D. Windsor, A. de Jong, N. Schmeer, and M. Stegemann.** 1997. Comparative susceptibilities of various animal-pathogenic mycoplasmas to fluoroquinolones. *Antimicrob. Agents Chemother.* **41:**2037–2040.

34. **Heisig, P.** 1993. High-level fluoroquinolone resistance in *Salmonella typhimurium* is due to alterations in both *gyrA* and *gyrB* genes. *J. Antimicrob. Chemother.* **32:**367–377.

35. **Helms, M., P. Vastrup, P. Gerner-Smidt, and K. Mølbak.** 2002. Excess mortality associated with antimicrobial drug resistance in *Salmonella enterica* serovar Typhimurium. *Emerg. Infect. Dis.* **8:**490–495.

36. Helmuth, R., A. Schroeter, H. Trolldenier, and H. Tschäpe. 1998. Examples of *in vitro* quinolone resistance prevalence/trends in foodborne *Salmonella* and other enterics in Germany, p. 175–178. *In Use of Quinolones in Food Animals and Potential Impact on Public Health. Report and Proceedings of a WHO Meeting. Geneva, Switzerland, 2–5 June 1998* (WHO/EMC/ZDI/98.12). World Health Organization, Geneva, Switzerland.

37. Hof, H., I. Ehrhard, and H. Tscäpe. 1991. Presence of quinolone resistance in a strain of *Salmonella typhimurium*. *Eur. J. Clin. Microbiol. Infect. Dis.* 10:747–749.

38. Hoge, C. W., J. M. Gambel, A. Srijan, C. Pitarangsi, and P. Echeverria. 1998. Trends in antibiotic resistance among diarrheal pathogens isolated in Thailand over 15 years. *Clin. Infect. Dis.* 26:341–345.

39. Humphrey, T. 2000. Public-health aspects of Salmonella infections, p. 245–263. *In* C. Wray and A. Wray (ed.), *Salmonella in Domestic Animals.* C.A.B. (Commonwealth Agricultural Bureaux) International Institute of Entomology, London, England.

40. Imberechts, H., I. D'hooghe, H. Bouchet, C. Godard, and P. Pohl. 2000. Apparent loss of enrofloxacin resistance in bovine *Salmonella typhimurium* strains isolated in Belgium, 1991 to 1998. *Vet. Rec.* 147:76–77.

41. Jacobs-Reitsma, W. F., P. M. Koenraad, N. M. Bolder, and R. W. Mulder. 1994. In vitro susceptibility of *Campylobacter* and *Salmonella* isolates from broilers to quinolones, ampicillin, tetracycline, and erythromycin. *Vet. Q.* 16:206–208.

42. JETACAR. 1999. The use of antimicrobials in food-producing animals: antibiotic resistant bacteria in animals and humans. Commonwealth Department of Health and Aged Care and Commonwealth Department of Agriculture, Fisheries and Forestry, Australia.

43. Kuschner, R. A., A. F. Trofa, R. J. Thomas, C. W. Hoge, C. Pitarangsi, S. Amato, R. P. Olafson, P. Echeverria, J. C. Sadoff, and D. N. Taylor. 1995. Use of azithromycin for the treatment of *Campylobacter* enteritis in travelers to Thailand, an area where ciprofloxacin resistance is prevalent. *Clin. Infect. Dis.* 21:536–541.

44. Li, C. C., C. H. Chiu, J. L. Wu, Y. C. Huang, and T. Y. Lin. 1998. Antimicrobial susceptibilities of *Campylobacter jejuni* and *coli* by using E-test in Taiwan. *Scand. J. Infect. Dis.* 30:39–42.

45. Lightfood, D., M. Hubbard, and M. Valcanis. Examples of *in vitro* quinolone resistance prevalence/trends in human and animal isolates of foodborne *Salmonella* in Australia, p. 163–167. *In Use of Quinolones in Food Animals and Potential Impact on Public Health. Report and Proceedings of a WHO Meeting, Geneva, Switzerland, 2–5 June 1998* (WHO/EMC/ZDI/98.12). World Health Organization, Geneva, Switzerland.

46. Malorny, B., A. Schroeter, and R. Helmuth. 1999. Incidence of quinolone resistance over the period 1986 to 1998 in veterinary *Salmonella* isolates from Germany. *Antimicrob. Agents Chemother.* 43:2278–2282.

49. Marano, N. N., S. Rossiter, K. Stamey, K. Joyce, T. J. Barrett, L. K. Tollefson, and F. J. Angulo. 2000. The National Antimicrobial Resistance Monitoring System (NARMS) for enteric bacteria, 1996–1999: surveillance for action. *J. Am. Vet. Med. Assoc.* 217:1829–1830.

48. McMullin, P. F. 1998. Quinolone usage in poultry medication in Europe, p. 123–129. *In Use of Quinolones in Food Animals and Potential Impact on Public Health. Report and Proceedings of a WHO Meeting, Geneva, Switzerland, 2–5 June 1998* (WHO/EMC/ZDI/98.12). World Health Organization, Geneva, Switzerland.

49. Mead, P. S., L. Slutsker, V. Dietz, L. F. McCaig, J. S. Bresee, C. Shapiro, P. M. Griffin, and R. V. Tauxe. 1999. Food-related illness and death in the United States. *Emerg. Infect. Dis.* 5:607–625.

50. Megraud, F. 1998. Les infections à *Campylobacter* en France (1986–1997). *Bull. Epidémiol. Ann.* 2:83–84.

51. Ministry of Agriculture, Fisheries and Food. 1998. A review of antimicrobial resistance in the food chain. A technical report for MAFF. Ministry of Agriculture, Fisheries and Food, United Kingdom.

52. Ministry of Agriculture, Fisheries and Food. 1999. Salmonella in Livestock Production 1999. Veterinary Laboratories Agency. Ministry of Agriculture, Fisheries and Food. United Kingdom.

53. Mølbak, K., D. L. Baggesen, F. M. Aarestrup, J. M. Ebbesen, J. Engberg, K. Frydendahl, P. Gerner-Smidt, A. M. Petersen, and H. C. Wegener. 1999. An outbreak of multidrug-resistant, quinolone-resistant *Salmonella enterica* serotype Typhimurium DT104. *N. Engl. J. Med.* 341:1420–1425.

54. Mølbak, K., P. Gerner-Smidt, and H. C. Wegener. 2002. Increasing quinolone resistance in *Salmonella enterica* serotype Enteritidis. *Emerg. Infect. Dis.* 8:514–515.

55. Neill, M. A., S. M. Opal, J. Heelan, R. Giusti, J. E. Cassidy, R. White, and K. H. Mayer. 1991. Failure of ciprofloxacin to eradicate convalescent fecal excretion after acute salmonellosis: experience during an outbreak in health care workers. *Ann. Intern. Med.* 114:195–199.

56. Nielsen, E. M., J. Engberg, and M. Madsen. 1997. Distribution of serotypes of *Campylobacter jejuni* and *C. coli* from Danish patients, poultry, cattle and swine. *FEMS Immunol. Med. Microbiol.* 19:47–56.

57. Nielsen, E. M., and N. L. Nielsen. 1999. Serotypes and typability of *Campylobacter jejuni* and *Campylobacter coli* isolated from poultry products. *Int. J. Food Microbiol.* 46:199–205.

58. Nielsen, E. M., J. Engberg, V. Fussing, L. Petersen, C. H. Brogren, and S. L. W. On. 2000. Evaluation of phenotypic and genotypic methods for subtyping *Campylobacter jejuni* isolates from humans, poultry, and cattle. *J. Clin. Microbiol.* 38:3800–3810.

59. Olsen, S. J., E. E. DeBess, T. E. McGivern, N. Marano, T. Eby, S. Mauvais, V. K. Balan, G. Zirnstein, P. R. Cieslak, and F. J. Angulo. 2001. A nosocomial outbreak of fluoroquinolone-resistant salmonella infection. *N. Engl. J. Med.* 344:1572–1579.

60. On, S. L. W., E. M. Nielsen, J. Engberg, and M. Madsen. 1998. Validity of *Sma*I-defined genotypes of *Campylobacter jejuni* examined by *Sal*I, *Kpn*I, and *Bam*HI polymorphisms: evidence of identical clones infecting humans, poultry, and cattle. *Epidemiol. Infect.* 120:231–237.

61. Orr, K. E., N. F. Lightfoot, P. R. Sisson, B. A. Harkis, J. L. Tveddle, P. Boyd, A. Carroll, C. J. Jackson, D. R. Wareing, and R. Freeman. 1995. Direct milk excretion of *Campylobacter jejuni* an a dairy cow causing cases of human enteritis. *Epidemiol. Infect.* 114:15–24.

62. Owen, R. J., and S. Leeton. 1999. Restriction fragment length polymorphism analysis of the flaA gene of *Campylobacter jejuni* for subtyping human, animal and poultry isolates. *FEMS Microbiol. Lett.* 176:345–350.

63. Pavia, A. T., L. D. Shipman, J. G. Wells, N. D. Puhr, J. D. Smith, T. W. McKinley, and R. V. Tauxe. 1990. Epidemiologic evidence that prior antimicrobial exposure decreases resistance to infection by antimicrobial-sensitive Salmonella. *J. Infect. Dis.* 161:255–260.

64. Pearson, A. D., M. H. Greenwood, J. Donaldson, T. D. Healing, D. M. Jones, M. Shahamat, R. K. Feltham, and R.

R. Colwell. 2000. Continuous source outbreak of campylobacteriosis traced to chicken. *J. Food Prot.* **63**:309–314.

65. Pedersen, K. B., F. M. Aarestrup, N. E. Jensen, F. Bager, L. B. Jensen, S. E. Jorsal, T. K. Nielsen, H. C. Hansen, A. Meyling, and H. C. Wegener. 1999. The need for a veterinary antibiotic policy. *Vet. Rec.* **145**:50–53.

66. Pers, C., P. Søgaard, and L. Pallesen. 1996. Selection of multiple resistance in *Salmonella enteritidis* during treatment with ciprofloxacin. *Scand. J. Infect. Dis.* **28**:529–531.

67. Piddock, L. J. 1995. Quinolone resistance and *Campylobacter* spp. *J. Antimicrob. Chemother.* **36**:891–898.

68. Piddock, L. J., and A. de Jong. 1999. Implications of quinolone resistance in veterinary isolates of *Salmonella*. *Vet. Rec.* **145**:380.

69. Rabsch, W., H. Tschäpe, and A. J. Bäumler. 2001. Nontyphoidal salmonellosis: emerging problems. *Microbes Infect.* **3**:237–247.

70. Rautelin, H., O. V. Renkonen, and T. U. Kosunen. 1991. Emergence of fluoroquinolone resistance in *Campylobacter jejuni* and *Campylobacter coli* in subjects from Finland. *Antimicrob. Agents Chemother.* **35**:2065–2069.

71. Reina, J., N. Borrell, and A. Serra. 1992. Emergence of resistance to erythromycin and fluoroquinolones in thermotolerant *Campylobacter* strains isolated from feces 1987–1991. *Eur. J. Clin. Microbiol. Infect. Dis.* **11**:1163–1166.

72. Ruiz, J., P. Goni, F. Marco, F. Gallardo, B. Mirelis, T. Jimenez De Anta, and J Vila. 1998. Increased resistance to quinolones in *Campylobacter jejuni*: a genetic analysis of *gyr*A gene mutations in quinolone-resistant clinical isolates. *Microbiol. Immunol.* **42**:223–226.

73. Saenz Y., M. Zarazaga, M. Lantero, M. J. Gastanares, F. Baquero, and C. Torres. 2000. Antibiotic resistance in *Campylobacter* strains isolated from animals, foods, and humans in Spain in 1997–1998. *Antimicrob. Agents Chemother.* **44**:267–271.

74. Sam, W. I. C., M. M. Lyons, and D. J. Waghorn. 1999. Increasing rates of ciprofloxacin resistant *Campylobacter*. *J. Clin. Pathol.* **52**:709. (Letter.)

75. Sanchez, R., V. Fernandez Baca, M. D. Diaz, P. Munoz, M. Rodriguez Creixems, and E. Bouza. 1994. Evolution of susceptibilities of *Campylobacter* spp. to quinolones and macrolides. *Antimicrob. Agents Chemother.* **38**:1879–1882.

76. Segreti, J., T. D. Gootz, L. J Goodman, G. W. Parkhurst, J. P. Quinn, B. A. Martin, and G. M. Trenholme. 1992. High-level quinolone resistance in clinical isolates of *Campylobacter jejuni*. *J. Infect. Dis.* **165**:667–770.

77. Shah, P. M., V. Schafer, and H. Knothe. 1993. Medical and veterinary use of antimicrobial agents: implications for public health. A clinician's view on antimicrobial resistance. *Vet. Microbiol.* **35**:269–274.

78. Skirrow, M. B., M. J. Blaser, P. D. Smith, J. I. Ravdin, and H. B. Greenberg (ed.). 1995. *Infections of Gastrointestinal Tract*, p. 825–848. Raven Press, New York, N.Y.

79. Smith, K. E., J. M. Besser, C. W. Hedberg, F. T. Leano, J. B. Bender, J. H. Wicklund, B. P. Johnson. K. A. More, and M. T. Osterholm. 1999. Quinolone-resistant *Campylobacter jejuni* infections in Minnesota, 1992–1998. *N. Engl. J. Med.* **340**:1525–1532

80. Stephano, A. 1998. Examples of fluoroquinolone usage in pig production in Latin America, p. 139–144. *In Use of Quinolones in Food Animals and Potential Impact on Public Health. Report and Proceedings of a WHO Meeting, Geneva, Switzerland, 2–5 June 1998* (WHO/EMC/ZDI/98.12). World Health Organization, Geneva, Switzerland.

81. Stöhr, K., and H. C. Wegener. 2000. Animal use of antimicrobials: impact on resistance. *Drug Resist. Updates* **3**:207–209.

82. Sumano, L. H., C. L. Ocampo, G. W. Brumbaugh, and R. E. Lizarraga. 1998. Effectiveness of two fluoroquinolones for the treatment of chronic respiratory disease outbreak in broilers. *Br. Poult. Sci.* **139**:42–46.

83. Szych, J., A. Cieslik, J. Paciorek, and S. Kaluzewski. 2001. Antibiotic resistance in *Salmonella enterica* subsp. *enterica* strains isolated in Poland from 1998 to 1999. *Int. J. Antimicrob. Agents.* **18**:37–42

84. Tee, W., A. Mijch, E. Wright, and A. Yung. 1995. Emergence of multidrug resistance in *Campylobacter jejuni* isolates from three patients infected with human immunodeficiency virus. *Clin. Infect. Dis.* **21**:634–638.

85. Threlfall, E. J., L. R. Ward, A. M. Ridley, and B. Rowe. 1998. Resistance to fluoroquinolone antibiotics in salmonellas from humans in England and Wales: the current situation, p. 199–204. *In Use of Quinolones in Food Animals and Potential Impact on Public Health. Report and Proceedings of a WHO Meeting, Geneva, Switzerland, 2–5 June 1998* (WHO/EMC/ZDI/98.12). World Health Organization, Geneva, Switzerland.

86. Threlfall, E. J., L. Ward, J. A. Skinner, and A. Graham. 2000. Antimicrobial drug resistance in non-typhoidal salmonellas from humans in England and Wales in 1999; decrease in multiple resistance in *Salmonella enterica* serotypes Typhimurium, Virchow, and Hadar. *Microb. Drug Resist.* **6**:319–325.

87. van den Bogaard, A. E. 1993. A veterinary antibiotic policy: a personal view on the perspectives in The Netherlands. *Vet. Microbiol.* **35**:303–312.

88. van den Bogaard, A. E., and E. E. Stobberingh. 2000. Epidemiology of resistance to antibiotics. Links between animals and humans. *Int. J. Antimicrob. Agents* **14**:327–325.

89. van Looveren, M., M. L. Chasseur-Libotte, C. Godard, C. Lammens, M. Wijdooghe, L. Peeters, and H. Goossens. 2001. Antimicrobial susceptibility of nontyphoidal *Salmonella* isolated from humans in Belgium. *Acta Clin. Belg.* **56**:180–186.

90. van Looveren, M., G. Daube, L. De Zutter, J. M. Dumont, C. Lammens, M. Wijdooghe, P. Vandamme, M. Jouret, M. Cornelis, and H. Goossens. 2001. Antimicrobial susceptibilities of *Campylobacter* strains isolated from food animals in Belgium. *J. Antimicrob. Chemother.* **48**:235–240.

91. Vasallo, F. J., P. Martin-Rabadan, L. Alcala, J. M. Garcia-Lechuz, M. Rodriguez-Creixems, and E. Bouza. 1998. Failure of ciprofloxacin therapy for invasive nontyphoidal salmonellosis. *Clin. Infect. Dis.* **26**:535–536.

92. Velonakis, E. N., A. Markogiannakis, L. Kondili, E. Varjioti, Z. Mahera, E. Dedouli, A. Karaitianou, N. Vakalis, and Bethimouti. 2001. Evolution of antibiotic resistance of non-typhoidal salmonellae in Greece during 1990–97. *Eur. Surveill.* **6**:117–120.

93. Voltersvik, P., A. Halstensen, N. Langeland, A. Digranes, L. E. Peterson, T. Rolstad, and S. O. Solberg. 2000. Eradication of non-typhoid salmonellae in acute enteritis after therapy with ofloxacin for 5 or 10 days. *J. Antimicrob. Chemother.* **46**:457–459.

94. Wain, J., N. T. Hoa, N. T. Chinh, H. Vinh, M. J. Everett, T. S. Diep, N. P. Day, T. Solomon, N. J. White, L. J. Piddock, and C. M. Parry. 1997. Quinolone-resistant *Salmonella typhi* in Viet Nam: molecular basis of resistance and clinical response to treatment. *Clin. Infect. Dis.* **25**:1404–1410.

95. Wang, Y., W. M. Huang, and D. E. Taylor. 1993. Cloning

and nucleotide sequence of the *Campylobacter jejuni gyrA* gene and characterization of quinolone resistance mutations. *Antimicrob. Agents Chemother.* **37:**457–463.

96. **Wistrom, J., and S. R. Norrby.** 1995. Fluoroquinolones and bacterial enteritis, when and for whom? *J. Antimicrob. Chemother.* **36:**23–39.

97. **Wiuff, C., M. Madsen, D. L. Baggesen, and F. M. Aarestrup.** 2000. Quinolone resistance among Salmonella enterica from cattle, broilers, and swine in Denmark. *Microb. Drug Resist.* **6:**11–17.

98. **World Health Organization.** 1998. *Use of Quinolones in Food Animals and Potential Impact on Public Health. Report and Proceedings of a WHO Meeting, Geneva, Switzerland, 2–5 June 1998* (WHO/EMC/ZDI 98.12). World Health Organization, Geneva, Switzerland.

99. **World Health Organization.** 1999. *Food Safety Issues Associated with Products from Aquaculture. Report from a Joint FAO/NACA/WHO study group.* WHO Technical Report Series, No. 883. World Health Organization, Geneva, Switzerland.

100. **World Health Organization.** 2000. *WHO Global Principles for the Containment of Antimicrobial Resistance in Animals Intended for Food.* Report of a WHO Consultation 5–9 June 2000 (WHO/CDS/CSR/APH/2000.4). World Health Organization, Geneva, Switzerland.

101. **World Health Organization.** 2001. *The Increasing Incidence of Human Campylobacteriosis. Report and Proceedings from a WHO Consultation of Experts, Copenhagen, Denmark, 21–25 November 2001* (WHO/CDS/CSR/APH 2001.7). World Health Organization, Geneva, Switzerland.

102. **World Health Organization.** 2001. *WHO Global Strategy for Containment of Antimicrobial Resistance* (WHO/CDS/CSR/DSR/2001.2). World Health Organization, Geneva, Switzerland.

103. **Wray, C., I. M. McLaren, and Y. E. Beedell.** 1993. Bacterial resistance monitoring of salmonellas isolated from animals, national experience of surveillance schemes in the United Kingdom. *Vet. Microbiol.* **35:**313–319.

104. **Wray, C., and R. H. Davies.** 2000. Salmonella infections in cattle, p. 169–190. *In* C. Wray and A. Wray (ed.), *Salmonella in Domestic Animals.* C.A.B. (Commonwealth Agricultural Bureaux) International Institute of Entomology, London, England.

105. **Wray, C., and J. C. Gnanou.** 2000. Antibiotic resistance monitoring in bacteria of animal origin: analysis of national monitoring programmes. *Int. J. Antimicrob. Agents* **14:**291–294.

IV. ADVERSE AND OTHER EFFECTS

Quinolone Antimicrobial Agents, 3rd ed.
Edited by David C. Hooper and Ethan Rubinstein
© 2003 ASM Press, Washington, D.C.

Chapter 25

Adverse Effects

HARTMUT LODE AND ETHAN RUBINSTEIN

The fluoroquinolone class of agents has been plagued by a number of compounds that have undergone an extensive clinical evaluation and have achieved distinctive clinical results but were not introduced into the market because of unacceptable safety and tolerability. Examples of such compounds are Bay 3118 and clinafloxacin. On the other hand, several fluoroquinolones introduced into the market were withdrawn early because of safety issues. Temafloxacin was removed from the market a few months after its introduction because of the hemolytic-uremic syndrome it caused. The pathophysiology of this adverse event was never adequately explored. Trovafloxacin was also removed from the market a short while after its introduction because of unacceptable liver toxicity causing hepatic necrosis and acute hepatic failure in six patients. Sparfloxacin use was severely curtailed because of associated phototoxic effects and cardiotoxicity. Grepafloxacin was also removed from the market shortly after its introduction because of cardiotoxicity (Table 1).

Because the basic structure of the fluoroquinolones is the same, some adverse events can be assigned to distinct parts of the basic molecule (Fig. 1). Core nuclear structure differences, such as a nitrogen atom at the nuclear 8 position (instead of carbon as in the fluoroquinolone core structure) in the related fluoronaphthyridones, such as trovafloxacin, and tosufloxacin, have been associated with organ-targeted toxicity. A cyclopropyl at the R1 position increases clastogenicity and interactions with theophylline. The (2,4) difluorophenyl substitution at position 1 that is common to trovafloxacin, temafloxacin, and tosufloxacin caused immunologically mediated toxicity. No such adverse events were reported with gemifloxacin, a fluoronaphthypyridone with a 1-cyclopropyl substituent. The substituents at positions 3 and 4 are linked to chelation of metals. The moiety at position 5 can contribute not only to phototoxicity and genetic toxicity

but also to QTc prolongation on the electrocardiogram. Substituents at position 7 are involved in central nervous system toxicity, as this position has the greatest influence on γ-aminobutyric acid-binding inhibition as well as on the interaction of quinolones with theophylline and nonsteroidal anti-inflammatory agents (33, 68). A halogen (usually a fluorine atom) at position 8 is generally associated with increased phototoxicity. Examples of such compounds are sparfloxacin, Bay 3118, fleroxacin, lomefloxacin, sitafloxacin, and clinafloxacin.

Fluoroquinolones presently marketed, or those that are in the final stage of clinical trials, seem to be well tolerated, with average adverse event rates of 20 to 30% for most compounds that are not significantly different from those of cephalosporins (5, 6, 63, 76) (Tables 2 and 3). Many prospective randomized, double-blind, placebo- or comparator-controlled clinical trials revealed that the fluoroquinolones (except for fleroxacin) were not significantly different from nonfluoroquinolone comparator agents in terms of proportion of patients experiencing a range of adverse events (48, 63). Such studies are the most reliable source of information and reveal the highest rate of adverse events (105). Because the severity of adverse events is difficult to assess, antibiotic discontinuation due to adverse events has been used as a marker of those with greater severity (6). The rates for drug discontinuation due to adverse events of some of the newer fluoroquinolones are shown in Table 4 (6). An estimate of the frequency of adverse events can also be drawn from the number of such events reported to monitoring agencies following the launch of the product (Table 5).

The most frequently reported adverse events associated with fluoroquinolones are as follows (8, 63):

- Gastrointestinal, including nausea, dyspepsia, vomiting, abdominal pain, flatulence, diarrhea, constipation, and anorexia.

Hartmut Lode • Department of Pulmonary Infectious Diseases, City Hospital Zehlendorf/Heckeshorn, Freie Universität Berlin, Zum Heckeshorn 33, D-14109 Berlin, Germany. **Ethan Rubinstein** • Unit of Infectious Diseases, Sheba Medical Center, University of Tel Aviv, Tel Aviv, Israel.

Table 1. Serious fluoroquinolone-associated adverse events leading to drug withdrawals, severe restrictions, or suspensions from the market

Compound	Year	Toxicity	Outcome
Temafloxacin	1992	Hemolytic-uremic syndrome	Withdrawn after launch
Bay 3118	1993	Phototoxicity	Withdrawn pre-launch
Sparfloxacin	1994	Phototoxicity, QTc prolongation	Warning
Tosufloxacin	1996	Thrombocytopenia, nephritis	Warning
Trovafloxacin	1999	Liver toxicity	Restricted use/suspension
Grepafloxacin	1999	QTc prolongation, TdP[a]	Withdrawn after launch
Clinafloxacin	1999	Phototoxicity, hypoglycemia	Withdrawn pre-launch

[a] TdP, torsades de pointes.

- Central nervous system, including headache, dizziness, lightheadedness, drowsiness, sleep disorder(s), somnolence, mood changes, confusion, agitation, tremor, delirium, psychosis, and seizures.
- Hepatic, including transient rise in liver enzymes, cholestatic jaundice, hepatitis, and hepatic failure.
- Renal, including azotemia, crystalluria, hematuria, interstitial nephritis, nephropathy, renal failure, and the hemolytic-uremic syndrome.
- Dermatologic, including rash, pruritus, photosensitivity, phototoxicity, hemorrhagic bullae, pigmentation, excessive sweating, flushing, and urticaria.
- Musculoskeletal, including arthropathy, tendinitis, and tendon rupture.

- Cardiovascular, including hypotension, ventricular tachycardia (torsade de pointes), QTc interval prolongation.
- Sensory organs, including tinnitus, blurred vision, colored vision disturbances, and taste perversion.
- Other, including drug fever, chills, serum sickness-like reactions, anaphylactoid reactions, anaphylaxis, angioedema, bronchospasm, and vasculitis (63).

In general, the elderly are considered more at risk for drug-induced adverse events than younger individuals. In a summary of clinical data on oral ciprofloxacin, nearly one fourth of the 1,652 patients were >70 years old. There was a tendency for all adverse events to occur more frequently in the elderly

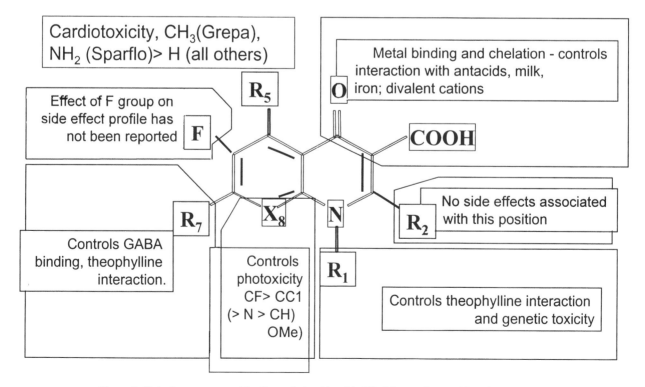

Figure 1. Quinolone structure-side effect relationships. Modified from reference 33 with permission.

Table 2. Overall incidence of
fluoroquinolone-associated adverse events

Drug/phase	Adverse event rate (%)
Levofloxacin phase III (USA)	9.9
Levofloxacin phase III (Japan)	3.8
Trovafloxacin (all doses)	27
Grepafloxacin (600 mg)	47
Gatifloxacin (phase III)	28.9
Moxifloxacin (phase III)	27.5

rather than in young persons; thus three of four episodes of hallucinations were reported by the elderly (33, 93). All these changes are dealt with in greater detail in this chapter.

EFFECTS ON THE BONE MARROW AND IMMUNE SYSTEM

Bone marrow cells are the most rapidly dividing eukaryotic cells, and therefore, considered most susceptible to agents affecting DNA synthesis. Because fluoroquinolones affect bacterial DNA synthesis, the effects of these agents on the bone marrow were carefully studied from the early period of fluoroquinolone development. In addition, fluoroquinolones are often administered to patients with leukemia and to bone marrow transplant patients; thus their effect on the bone marrow is of particular importance. The effect of several fluoroquinolones on granulocyte-macrophage colonies was studied in the soft agar system by several authors. Significant inhibition was found by rufloxacin in a concentration of 50 μg/ml and by ofloxacin in a concentration of 100 μg/ml, concentrations that exceed therapeutic serum drug concentrations by a factor of ~12. Therapeutic concentrations (10 μg/ml) had no effect on murine cell proliferation (81). The addition of clinically attainable

concentrations of ciprofloxacin, sparfloxacin, or clinafloxacin with pokeweed mitogen to murine spleen cells resulted in a significant enhancement in colony-stimulating activity, resulting in a 1.5- to 1.8-fold increase in the number of myeloid progenitors compared with control cultures. Other quinolones showed either no stimulatory effect (fleroxacin, norfloxacin) or had an inhibitory effect (ofloxacin) on myeloid progenitor cell growth. The stimulatory quinolones have in common a cyclopropyl moiety at position N1 of the quinolone ring (61). Similar results were also observed with human bone marrow myeloid precursors exposed to high and therapeutic concentrations of pefloxacin, ofloxacin, and ciprofloxacin (17, 46, 79). Ciprofloxacin at high doses (100 mg/kg of body weight/24 h) also suppressed bone marrow engraftment of murine bone marrow when donor and recipient mice were treated, whereas pefloxacin and lower doses of ciprofloxacin (25 and 50 mg/kg/24 h) had no such effect (100). The suppressive effect was short lived and lasted only for 3 days after the discontinuation of the treatment in recipient mice (98). With ciprofloxacin administered at therapeutic dosages, repopulation of hematopoietic organs in addition to the spleen was also observed, suggesting enhanced production of colony-stimulating factors (CSFs), an effect that could be abolished with anti-CSF antibodies (61, 97). In the same model of sublethally irradiated mice, the number of myeloid progenitors in the bone marrow and the number of peripheral white blood cells 8 days after irradiation was significantly enhanced in mice treated with ciprofloxacin (45 mg/kg/day), sparfloxacin (22.5 mg/kg/day), and clinafloxacin (11.25 mg/kg/day) compared with saline-treated animals ($P \leq 0.05$). Clinafloxacin at a higher dosage (45 mg/kg/day) resulted in a decrease in myeloid progenitors in the bone marrow. A similar increase in myeloid progenitors and white blood cell count was observed in animals treated with high doses

Table 3. Overall incidence of adverse events associated with fluoroquinolones (U.S./European data)

Agent	Incidence (%) of adverse events				References
	Total	Gastrointestinal	CNS[a]	Skin	
Ciprofloxacin	5.8	3.4	1.1	0.7	7, 47, 48, 63, 68, 72, 76, 93, 102
Norfloxacin	9.1	3.9	4.4	0.5	23, 26, 47, 48, 76, 102, 110, 113
Pefloxaxcin	8.0	5.6	0.9	2.2	23, 45, 47, 48, 68, 76, 113
Ofloxacin	4.2	2.6	0.89	0.53	23, 48, 55, 68, 72, 76, 102
Levofloxacin	2.0–9.9	5.1	0.2–1.1	0.2	48, 63, 76, 102
Sparfloxacin	32	10	>3	1.9(7.4[b])	63, 89, 102
Grepafloxacin	47	15	5	2.0	63, 102, 104, 109
Moxifloxacin	27	8.0	5.4	2.0	5, 9, 52, 68, 72
Trovafloxacin	27	4–7		1.0	5, 63, 102, 108

[a] CNS, central nervous system.
[b] Phototoxicity.

Table 4. Drug discontinuation rate of new fluoroquinolones
due to adverse events

Fluoroquinolone, dose[a]	% discontinuation due to adverse event
Levofloxacin, 500 mg (U.S. data)	3.7
Sparfloxacin, 400/200 mg (RTI)	3.0
Gatifloxacin	2.9
Moxifloxacin	3.3
Trovafloxacin, i.v.-p.o.	7.0
Grepafloxacin, 600 mg	6.4

[a] RTI, respiratory tract infection; i.v., intravenously; p.o., orally.

(greater than those of clinical relevance) of ofloxacin, and norfloxacin (90 mg/kg/day) and fleroxacin (45 and 90 mg/kg/day). Quinolone-treated animals, at the above-cited doses, showed enhanced survival compared with saline-treated animals. The only exception was the higher mortality of clinafloxacin-treated mice (61). Similar results were obtained in cyclophosphamide-treated animals that were dosed with both moxifloxacin and ciprofloxacin, suggesting stimulated hematopoiesis (97). Corresponding clinical studies in humans, however, have not yet borne out a salutary effect of fluoroquinolones on hematopoietic cell recovery in patients undergoing transplantation (37).

With levofloxacin, no mutagenic effects on the bone marrow were observed in lacZ transgenic mice (Muta Mouse) with doses of 300 or 600 mg/kg (50% lethal dose in ddY starin mice), suggesting the safety of this agent in this respect (54).

Ciprofloxacin, enoxacin, levofloxacin, nalidixic acid, ofloxacin, pipemidic acid, and N1-cyclopropyl quinolones were capable of inducing micronuclei in in vitro assays of mouse bone marrow cells. Levofloxacin and other quinolones induced neither micronuclei in mouse bone marrow nor unscheduled DNA synthesis in rat hepatocytes when administered to intact live animals, stressing the lack of effect of these compounds on eukaryotic DNA (98). With trovafloxacin, a single human case of associated leukopenia was reported without an appropriate investigation (70).

Fluoroquinolones have been used extensively for prophylaxis in febrile neutropenia and also as therapy in low-risk neutropenic patients; in some instances fluoroquinolones have been administered for prolonged periods and in relatively high doses.

No bone marrow-associated ill effects caused by the quinolones on the recovery of WBC were reported in any of the studies conducted (including those using ofloxacin, ciprofloxacin, and norfloxacin) (36, 38, 50, 57, 58, 90).

It is reasonable to conclude that the older fluoroquinolones have no bone marrow toxicity in humans when administered in conventional dosages, even for prolonged periods. For the fluoroquinolones of the newer generation, no such information is yet available.

At clinically achievable concentrations fluoroquinolones do not affect phagocytosis and chemotaxis, whereas preincubation of bacteria with fluoroquinolones facilitates the phagocytosis of bacteria (84).

It has been repeatedly shown that fluoroquinolones in supertherapeutic concentrations inhibit mammalian cell growth and block cell cycle progression due to inhibition of mammalian topoisomerase II (37). Paradoxically, a two- to threefold increase in thymidine accumulation is observed in phytohemagglutinin-stimulated cells treated with quinolones, possibly because of increased interleukin-2 (IL-2) synthesis produced early after exposure to quinolones and before cell division ensues (87). Most fluoroquinolones (including cipro-floxacin, enoxacin, levofloxacin, ofloxacin, norfloxacin, pefloxacin, and nalidixic acid) in therapeutic and supertherapeutic concentrations have been reported to induce IL-2 synthesis. IL-2 upregulation occurs through the action of ciprofloxacin and presumably other fluoroquinolones on the transcription process (86). Concomitantly, IL-2 receptor density increases as well (summarized in reference 37). Ciprofloxacin in various concentrations, as well as norfloxacin and ofloxacin, was reported to induce interferon γ (IFN-γ) production in stimulated blood cells (4, 31, 86). In contrast to the enhanced

Table 5. Post-launch adverse reaction spontaneous reporting to the
FDA[a] (levofloxacin/trovafloxacin)

Drug	Period (mo.)	No. of prescriptions	ADR[b] reports/ 100,000	Serious ADR reports/100,000
Ciprofloxacin	4	196,000	13	6
Ofloxacin	4	267,000	25	3
Levofloxacin	17	3,000,000	16.4	3
Trovafloxacin	5	392,000	98	17
Temafloxacin	4	174,000	108	28

[a] Data from references 5 and 6.
[b] ADR, adverse reaction.

production of IL-2 by ciprofloxacin, the production of IL-1β and tumor necrosis factor α (TNF-α) is inhibited by stimulated human monocytes under the influence of ciprofloxacin. A contradictory observation is that in human volunteers treated for 7 days with ciprofloxacin, monocytes obtained from the peripheral blood had an enhanced production of IL-1α, IL-1β, IL-6, and TNF-α (4). The synthesis of other inflammatory cytokines, such as E-selectin and IL-8, is stimulated in human endothelial cells by trovafloxacin and ciprofloxacin (40, 85).

Ciprofloxacin, in addition to its stimulatory activity on IL-2 and IFN-γ synthesis, induces in lymphocyte up-regulation of the early immediate genes, c-*myc*, c-*jun*, JunB, and Fra-1, a reaction similar to the SOS response seen in bacteria exposed to ciprofloxacin. This upregulation results in inhibition of cell division and in enhanced cell repair (12). Concomitantly, ciprofloxacin upregulates mRNA of IL-1α, TNF-α, IL-2, IL-2R, IL-3, IL-4, and granulocyte-macrophage colony-stimulating factor (GM-CSF) in mitogen-stimulated lymphocytes (85).

Ciprofloxacin has also been shown to upregulate IL-3 and GM-CSF synthesis, thereby preventing experimental antiphospholipid syndrome and the associated fetal loss in the mouse model of antiphospholipid syndrome (12, 94).

Because ciprofloxacin was shown to inhibit TNF-α and IL-1, the known inflammatory cytokines, the effect of ciprofloxacin was investigated further in type II collagen-induced arthritis in the rat, a model that simulates human rheumatoid arthritis. Ciprofloxacin prevented the development of arthritis in this model without affecting the level of anticollagen antibodies (15). In mice challenged with lethal doses of lipopolysaccharide there is a sharp rise in levels of IL-6 and TNF-α in serum; in animals treated with ciprofloxacin (250 mg/kg), trovafloxacin (100 mg/kg), and tosufloxacin (100 mg/kg), serum IL-6 and TNF-α concentrations were significantly reduced and were associated with improved animal survival (59). A similar beneficial effect on animal survival and cytokine serum levels was observed in the *Bacteroides fragilis* intra-abdominal abscess model in mice (44).

In summary, the immunomodulatory effects of the fluoroquinolones in suppressing TNF-α and IL-1 seen in vitro and in animal models might potentially be beneficial in infectious processes but have not yet been documented to be beneficial in humans. Likewise, the stimulatory effect of fluoroquinolones on IL-2, IL-3, and GM-CSF production might be beneficial to patients with bone marrow grafts, but a beneficial effect awaits proof in clinical trials.

RENAL EFFECTS

Antimicrobials often concentrate in the kidney and can potentially damage the organ by a variety of mechanisms, including direct tubular injury, interstitial inflammation (allergic interstitial nephritis), changes in renal electrolyte levels, or damage to the glomerular apparatus (56).

Acute renal failure was a rare adverse event associated with the older quinolone antibacterials, e.g., piromidic acid (43). Early review of ciprofloxacin also noted hematuria, minor transient elevations in the levels of serum creatinine or blood urea nitrogen, and hyaline and amorphous casts in the urine (7).

In general, nephrotoxic reactions to newer fluoroquinolones appear to be unusual but potentially serious. Because of its extensive usage, ciprofloxacin has been the quinolone most often reported in association with nephrotoxicity.

Allergic Interstitial Nephritis

Allergic interstitial nephritis (AIN) is thought to be the most common form of fluoroquinolone nephrotoxicity and is attributed to a type III hypersensitivity reaction. The identification of fluoroquinolone-induced AIN is usually based on the clinical presentation, which includes acute arthralgia, eosinophilia, eosinophiluria, fever, skin rashes, proteinuria, hematuria, pyuria, loin pain, and renal failure (49). The onset of symptoms and azotemia occur most often within 3 to 10 days after initiation of the fluoroquinolone. A history of recent exposure to potential nephrotoxins and improvement after the drug is discontinued are also typical. The clinical course and laboratory findings in AIN are nonspecific, not dose related, and often complicated by other concurrently administered agents. Nonoliguric renal failure is more common than oliguric renal failure.

Interstitial Nephritis

Acute renal toxicity typically developed within hours to weeks in patients who had preexisting underlying renal pathology. Other than elevation of serum creatinine levels, clinical manifestations and abnormal laboratory findings are often not characteristic. Urinalysis results include pyuria (white cells), granular casts, microscopic hematuria, and proteinuria (49).

Granulomatous Interstitial Nephritis

Another possible mechanism of fluoroquinolone nephrotoxicity centers on a cell-mediated immunologic process, suggested by the findings of granulomatous interstitial nephritis (GIN). GIN is characterized by granulomas formed by nodular infiltrates similar in size to a glomerulus. The cellular infiltrate consists predominantly of histiocytes and T lymphocytes. Drug-induced GIN can occur with or without vasculitits or glomerulonephritis. Renal biopsy is useful in guiding therapy because patients with GIN may benefit from a prolonged course of corticosteroid therapy. The prognosis of GIN is generally good (62).

Acute Renal Failure

Acute renal failure is probably not dose related and has occurred with doses of ciprofloxacin as low as 200 to 250 mg twice daily. Resolution of the acute renal failure has usually occurred within 1 to 8 weeks following drug discontinuation, with or without the administration of a short course of corticosteroid therapy. Treatment with corticosteroids is controversial, however. Most cases resolve over time with normalization or near normalization of renal function, further supporting the diagnosis of drug-induced disease (65).

Acute Tubular Necrosis

Acute tubular necrosis has also been reported in association with ciprofloxacin overdose (32). In this case a 15-year-old girl ingested 7.5 to 10.0 g of ciprofloxacin with 100 mg of trazodone 24 h before admission. The creatinine reached a maximum of 6.2 mg/dl on day 6, when the patient became anuric. One week after ingestion, her creatinine level began to decrease with a concomitant rise in urine output. The distal nephron can also be involved in acute renal failure, and electron microscopy or plastic-embedded sections may be necessary to define its involvement.

Crystalluria

Another postulated mechanism of fluoroquinolone nephrotoxicity is renal damage due to a foreign body reaction caused by crystallization of the antimicrobial (62, 67). In mild forms, tubular acidification defects are associated at an early stage. Such defects may lead to precipitation of fluoroquinolones that is more likely to occur in a neutral to alkaline environment. Animal studies suggested the relative insolubility of ciprofloxacin at alkaline pH leads to crystalluria and resultant tubular damage due to a foreign body reaction. Ciprofloxacin is associated with crystalluria mainly when the urine pH is >7.0 (65). However, adequate hydration appears to prevent acute renal failure induced by ciprofloxacin in neutropenic patients given ciprofloxacin 750 mg every 8 h (32).

Temafloxacin Syndrome

A multisystem syndrome consisting of hemolysis often combined with renal failure, coagulopathy, and hepatic dysfunction known as the temafloxacin syndrome has been estimated to occur in 1 of 3,500 patients treated with temafloxacin. In a review of 114 cases of the syndrome, a new onset of renal toxicity was observed in 54 cases with dialysis required in 34 cases (13). Renal dysfunction was associated with the onset of hemolysis on the first day of temafloxacin use and with the presence of disseminated intravascular coagulation. On the basis of this severe side effect, temafloxacin was removed from the market. This syndrome has not been reported with other quinolones, although some features overlap with the syndrome of severe hepatotoxicity seen with trovafloxacin.

Conclusion

Fluoroquinolones are usually well tolerated with a minimum of serious adverse effects, and renal toxicity is uncommon. Nearly all reported cases of acute renal failure associated with fluoroquinolones have involved patients older than 50 years of age. The incidence of elevated serum creatinine levels related to therapy with ciprofloxacin, norfloxacin, ofloxacin, or pefloxacin is estimated to range from 0.25 to 0.3%. Crystalluria, interstitial nephritis, and acute renal failure have not been causally associated with levofloxacin, sparfloxacin, grepafloxacin, or trovafloxacin (63). However, the possibility of "silent" acute renal failure makes routine and close follow-up of renal function parameters and clinical course in patients prescribed fluoroquinolones mandatory, especially in transplant patients or others who may be receiving nephrotoxic immunosuppressive or chemotherapeutic agents.

HEPATIC EFFECTS

In general, the quinolones are well tolerated by the liver. However, in human pharmacology, intrahepatic quinolone concentrations have been found to be as high as eight times the corresponding concentrations in serum (71). Also, in quinolone-uptake studies in rat hepatocytes, pefloxacin at a concentration of 400 µg/ml and ciprofloxacin at 200 µg/ml were found to be hepatotoxic (71). The rise of the intracellular enzymes released into the culture medium in these studies suggested a change in the hepatocyte membrane permeability or/and cellular lysis (75). Because the release of intracellular enzymes was associated with morphological hepatocyte alteration, it was suggested that high concentrations of pefloxacin or ciprofloxacin might lead to hepatocyte injury. However, this cellular damage was only observed when concentrations of ciprofloxacin or pefloxacin were 20-fold the average concentrations in human serum.

The largest safety database available for any fluoroquinolone is that for ciprofloxacin, which has been administered for nearly 8,000 patients in clinical trials and until 2000 had been prescribed to more than 200 million patients. Spontaneous reports showed that only few ciprofloxacin-treated patients had serious abnormalities in liver function test values; small numbers of patients also developed hepatitis, liver necrosis, or hepatic insufficiency or failure. Two cases of cholestatic jaundice, possibly induced by ciprofloxacin, have been reported, and hepatotoxicity has also been observed during therapy with enoxacin, norfloxacin, and ofloxacin (63).

In general, liver enzyme abnormalities have been noted in 2 to 3% of patients receiving fluoroquinolone therapy (113). Elevations in serum transaminases and alkaline phosphatase levels are most common. These are usually mild and reversible on discontinuation of the therapy. On the basis of crude pooled estimates of data supplied by manufacturers, elevated levels of serum aspartate aminotransferase, alanine aminotransferase, or alkaline phosphatase occurred in 24.9, 24.0, and 17.8 of 1,000 patients treated with ciprofloxacin, ofloxacin, and pefloxacin, respectively (47). These liver enzyme abnormalities rarely led to discontinuation of therapy.

Clinical trial data for levofloxacin indicate the very low frequency (0.3%) of abnormal liver function test values, none of which necessitated discontinuation of therapy (63). Elevated transaminase levels were found in 2% of patients treated with sparfloxacin in North American trials (112, 113). Clinical trials with data for 2,500 patients treated with grepafloxacin demonstrated increased levels of hepatic transaminases, gamma-glutamyltranspeptidase, and alkaline phosphatase in a few patients (<1%) (104). Some reports on gatifloxacin-induced hepatotoxicty have also appeared recently (25, 73)

With trovafloxacin administerd both orally and intravenously, a specific and severe hepatic side effect was seen after the treatment of nearly 2.5 million patients worldwide. A severe eosinophilic hepatitis was reported in a frequency of 1 in 17,000 courses of therapy and finally led to the removal of this drug from the market in Europe and to severe limitation of

trovafloxacin use in the United States (108). In the United States a year following the introduction of trovafloxacin into the market, more than 140 reports of cases with severe clinically symptomatic liver diseases were registered in patients receiving trovafloxacin. There were 14 cases of acute liver failure, and four of these required liver transplantation. In six patients the liver damage was fatal (21, 108). This liver toxicity appears to be an idiosynchratic hypersensitivity reaction leading to hepatic cell necrosis that at times was not reversible following discontinuation of trovafloxacin therapy. The hepatotoxicity was unpredictable and could occur even after a single dose, although it was more common after 14 days of therapy. Tovafloxacin-induced hepatotoxicity is initially manifested as elevations of the transaminases that may reach extreme levels.

The recently approved quinolones moxifloxacin and gatifloxacin are usually well tolerated with liver enzyme abnormalities noted in the usual range of 2 to 3% of patients receiving these antimicrobials (16, 52).

OTHER LABORATORY ABNORMALITIES

Laboratory test abnormalities associated with older quinolones (norfloxacin, ciprofloxacin, ofloxacin, pefloxacin) include mild reversible elevations of liver enzymes, usually transaminases, in 1.8 to 4.5% of patients. Hematopoetic abnormalities are also uncommon and typically mild and reversible, with 0.2 to 2.1% of patients having leukopenia or eosinophilia. Abnormalities of renal function are uncommon. Occasional mild elevations of blood urea nitrogen or creatinine have been reported (112). No effect of fluoroquinolones on serum creatinine measurements by the picric acid and enzymatic methods was seen in a carefully performed study (69).

In a recent study, the cross-reaction of 13 different quinolone antimicrobials in five common opiate-screening assays was investigated (3). Nine of the quinolones caused positive assay results (above the threshold) in at least one of the assays. Four of the assay systems caused false-positive results for at least one quinolone. Eleven of the 13 compounds caused some opiate activity by at least one assay system. At least one compound caused opiate assay activity in all five assay systems. Levofloxacin, ofloxacin, and pefloxacin were most likely to lead to a false-positive opiate result. Positive opiate results were obtained in urine from all six volunteers.

Clinically relevant changes in laboratory values were reported in only a small proportion of patients (<1%) receiving oral gatifloxacin 400 mg once daily: bilirubin levels increased from baseline in 10 of 2,624 patients; neutropenia was reported in 4 of 2,584 patients; and chloride levels decreased in 6 of 2,649 patients. There were no reports of hyperglycemia, hypernatriemia, anemia, or leukopenia (80).

In a recent report on the safety profile of moxifloxacin covering 6,178 patients from the clinical trial database and 5,805 patients from postmarketing observational studies, the same low figures as with gatifloxacin were reported (52), except for the rare cases of hepatitis (25, 73).

In general, quinolone trials are connected with no unusual laboratory abnormalities.

ALLERGIC REACTIONS

Anaphylactic or anaphylactoid reactions to fluoroquinolones are estimated to occur in 0.46 to 1.2 of 100,000 patients (12 cases in a population of 972,000) (30), and allergic dermatologic reactions have also been reported infrequently, occurring in 0.4 to 2.2% of patients. In several trials involving fluoroquinolones, the rate of hypersensitivity reactions, often manifested on the skin, has occurred at a frequency of 0.6 to 1.4% (5, 72). In a recent survey in Italy in an area of approximately 20 million people, on the basis of the Critical Term List of the World Health Organization, skin reactions were voluntarily reported and classified by a panel of dermatologists as either serious or nonserious events. A total of 2,224 adverse skin reaction reports (44.7% of all of the reported adverse reactions) were identified, yielding a reporting rate of about 5.5 per 100,000 inhabitants per year. The female-to-male ratio was 1.58, and the reporting rate increased progressively with age. The drug categories with the highest number of cutaneous reactions were antimicrobials. A total of 372 (16.9%) serious reactions were reported, the most frequent being angioedema (171 cases), erythema multiforme (68 cases), and photosensitivity (37 cases). Co-trimoxazole, followed by cephalosporins and fluoroquinolones, were associated with the highest rate among the antimicrobials (72). In comparative trials, the rate of skin allergy in patients who received a fluoroquinolone or a comparator was usually equal or smaller in the fluoroquinolone arm. The dermatologic adverse events of most fluoroquinolones are shown in Table 6.

Anaphylaxis (recurrent) has been described with pefloxacin (1), levofloxacin (99), and ciprofloxacin (18). Recently, because of meningococcal infection among university students, ciprofloxacin 500 mg orally was administered to about 3,200 persons. Three cases of anaphylactoid reaction occurred, a rate of about 1:1,000, much higher than the

Table 6. Skin rashes (%) associated with fluoroquinolones[a]

Fluoroquinolone	Skin effects (%)
Norfloxacin	0.5
Pefloxacin	2.2
Lomefloxacin	2.4
Fleroxacin	3.0
Ciprofloxacin	0.7
Ofloxacin	0.53
Levofloxacin	0.2
Sparfloxacin	1.9
Grepafloxacin	2.0
Moxifloxacin	2.0
Gatifloxacin	0.65
Trovafloxacin	0.2–1.0
Pazufloxacin	0.4
Tosufloxacin	0.4
Prulifloxacin	0.5
Deasquin	?
Balofloxacin	0.85
Sitafloxacin	1.15

[a] Modified from reference 5 with permission.

1:100,000 quoted above (2). Some of the skin manifestations may be caused by a histamine-release phenomenon (83). Vasculitis in the skin and kidneys has been rarely described with ciprofloxacin, even in infants (82). Bullous pemphigoid (60) as well as toxic epidermolysis (64, 114) has been associated with ciprofloxacin, and fixed drug eruption has been associated with norfloxacin (35) and tosufloxacin (74, 92). A rash similar to an ampicillin-induced rash was also described in a patient with infectious mononucleosis who received levofloxacin (78).

Desensitization to ciprofloxacin in a patient with a prior history of maculopapular rash was attempted successfully (11). Some patients with prior anaphylaxis have also been desensitized successfully with an oral regimen (28, 41). There seems to be cross-reactivity among various fluoroquinolones in their capacity to produce allergic reactions, and therefore a hypersensitivity to one fluoroquinolone precludes the use of another (8, 23, 28). Although most allergic adverse events subside when therapy is withdrawn, fatal vasculitis has been described with ciprofloxacin and ofloxacin (23, 63, 77).

Eosinophilic meningitis associated with quinolone therapy has also been described in an isolated case report (2).

EFFECTS IN PREGNANCY

In animals, norfloxacin failed to produce malformations in the offspring of mice, rats, rabbits, and monkeys, although it produced some fetal loss in monkeys when administered in very high doses (26, 27, 48). Ciprofloxacin and ofloxacin also produced no teratogenic effects in rats, mice, and rabbits. Both agents, however, were associated with an increased incidence of abortion in rabbits because of gastrointestinal toxicity (23, 106). Pefloxacin, enoxacin, and fleroxacin produced no teratogenic effects in rats (23, 51). In macaques, temafloxacin in high doses produced fetal waste but no fetal malformations (107). Administered to pregnant rats at doses of up to 810 mg/kg, levofloxacin produced decreased body weight, retardation of ossification, and increases in mortality and skeletal variations in fetuses (23, 111) No adverse effects were observed in perinatal and postnatal toxicity studies in rats at doses of up to 360 mg/kg (51). Levofloxacin administered at a dose of 50 mg/kg to rabbits showed no adverse effects on fertility or teratogenicity (23); however, decreases in maternal body weight and food intake were observed.

In the cynomolgus macaque (*Macaca fascicularis*), oral administration of fleroxacin (35 and 70 mg/kg/day) during gestational days 20 to 34 or 35 to 49 increased maternal toxicity (weight loss, anorexia, emesis), and embryo lethality was observed at 70 mg/kg/day. No malformations or growth retardation were observed. Fleroxacin levels in embryonic tissues were similar to maternal plasma levels. A correlation between exposure and embryo toxicity for ciprofloxacin, temafloxacin, and norfloxacin resulted in embryo lethality except for norfloxacin (51).

The use of fluoroquinolones in pregnant humans has increased over the years because many of the pregnancies are unplanned and because this class of agents has been widely used for the treatment of urinary tract infections, a condition common in young females and in pregnant women. In 1988, Jungst et al. (55) reported on 39 women who received ofloxacin during pregnancy. In 33 cases (15 exposed before day 17 of pregnancy, 9 exposed after day 17, and 9 with an unspecified time of exposure) babies were born healthy. One miscarriage and four congenital malformations were reported in this cohort, with no clear relationship to ofloxacin treatment. Another study reported a rate of congenital abnormalities of 9.5% among 63 infants whose mothers were exposed to ciprofloxacin during the first trimester of their pregnancy and reported to the manufacturer before the outcome of the pregnancy was known (66). In another prospective study, 549 pregnancies were collected by the European Network of Teratology Information Services (ENTIS) between 1986 and 1994, in addition to 116 previously documented pregnancies with prenatal quinolone expo-

sure. The live newborn babies malformation rate in the ENTIS group was 4.8%, and no specific pattern of congenital abnormalities was found (95). A higher rate of fetal distress and delivery by cesarian section but no malformations were also reported for a cohort of 38 women exposed to quinolones compared with a rate of controls not exposed to teratogenic agents (14).

In an additional definitive prospective study, 200 women with a mean age of 30.8 years exposed to fluoroquinolones (norfloxacin, 93 women; ciprofloxacin, 105 women; and ofloxacin, 2 women) during gestation were studied. Pregnancy outcome was compared with 200 controls matched for age, smoking, and alcohol consumption habits, who were exposed to nonteratogenic, nonembryotoxic antimicrobials matched for the indication and length of therapy with the women who received the fluoroquinolones (10). Rates for major congenital malformations were similar between the two groups in those with exposures in the first trimester (2.2 and 2.6% for the quinolone and control group, respectively; relative risk, 0.85; 95% confidence interval, 0.21 to 3.49). Women treated with quinolones had an increased risk for unnecessary therapeutic abortions compared with the control group (relative risk, 4.50; confidence interval, 0.908 to 20.57) resulting in a lower rate of live births (86 versus 94%, $P = 0.02$). More importantly, the rates of spontaneous abortions, fetal distress, prematurity rate, and birth weight did not differ between the children born to the mothers of the two treatment groups. Neither did gross motor development differ between the two groups. No clinically significant musculoskeletal abnormalities occurred in the children exposed to fluoroquinolones (66). Recently, recommendations for therapy of inhalational anthrax, as well as postexposure prophylaxis in pregnant women, which have included ciprofloxacin in doses of 400 mg intravenously every 12 h or 500 mg by mouth every 12 h, respectively, for up to 60 days, have been published in the United States and adopted by many other countries as well (20, 53). Nevertheless, other authorities believe that the data on ciprofloxacin use during pregnancy are insufficient to determine that there is no risk (39).

In summary, the available data suggest that short therapy periods with ciprofloxacin and norfloxacin are probably safe in pregnant women. The situation with ofloxacin is unclear, but the available reports call for caution in the use of this fluoroquinolone during pregnancy. There are no data regarding the use of the newer agents during pregnancy, and they should best be avoided until more data on their safety in pregnancy become available.

CANDIDIASIS

The reason for the emergence of candidal organisms as frequent and important pathogens is probably related to the ability of *Candida* spp. to colonize individuals who are treated with multiple antibiotics. It is thought that candida competes with bacteria for an ecological niche. When antibiotics suppress the normal bacterial flora, candidal organisms can proliferate and then disseminate to the deep organs. Antibiotic use is frequently complicated with candidal vaginal overgrowth, and this side effect is usually tracked as vaginitis in the monitoring system during clinical trials with antibiotics.

With the old quinolones vaginitis was reported infrequently, e.g., in the spontaneous reporting system for serious adverse reactions associated with ciprofloxacin from a patient population of approximately eight million, no vaginitis was mentioned (76). In 1,609 patients treated with 400 mg of grepafloxacin daily, vaginitis was observed in 3% (103); less than 1% of patients had vaginitis in a trovafloxacin trial including 875 patients (103). In analysis of data from 3,021 recipients of oral gatifloxacin 400 mg once daily, the most frequently reported adverse event besides nausea (incidence 8%) was vaginitis (6%) (103). In several studies with moxifloxacin the incidence of vaginitis was very low (< 1%) (9, 22). Also, in a review addressing the comparative tolerability of newer fluoroquinolones (levofloxacin, lomefloxacin, fleroxacin, sparfloxacin, grepafloxacin, trovafloxacin, moxifloxacin) vaginitis as a reported event was not mentioned (5).

In summary, antibiotic treatment, in general, can lead to vaginitis induced by candida in a frequency varying between 0.5 and 8%. The class of fluoroquinolones falls also in this category, but major differences among the different fluoroquinolones are not apparent.

REFERENCES

1. **Al-Hedaithy, M. A., and A. M., Noreddin.** 1996. Hypersensitivity an aphylactoid reaction to pefloxacin in a patient with AIDS. *Ann. Pharmacother.* 30:612–614.

2. **Asperilla, M. O., and R. A. Smego, Jr.** 1989. Eosinophilic meningitis associated with ciprofloxacin. *Am. J. Med.* 87:589–590.

3. **Baden, L. R., G. Horowitz, H. Jacoby, and G. M. Eliopoulos.** 2001. Quinolones and false-positive urine screening for opiates by immunoassay technology. *JAMA* 286:3115–3119.

4. **Bailly, S., M. Fay, B. Ferrua, and M. A. Gougerot-Pocidalo.** 1991. Ciprofloxacin treatnment in vivo increases the ex-vivo capacity of lipopolysaccharide-stimulated human monocytes to produce IL-1, IL-6 and tumor necrosis factor-alpha. *Clin. Exp. Immunol.* 85:331–334.

5. **Ball, P., L. Mandell, Y. Niki, and G. Tillotson.** 1999. Comparative tolerability of the newer fluoroquinolones antibacterials. *Drug Saf.* 21:407–421.

6. **Ball, P.** 2001. Future of the quinolones. *Semin. Respir. Infect.* 16:215–224.

7. **Ball, P.** 1986. Ciprofloxacin: an overview of adverse experiences. *J. Antimicrob. Chemother.* 18(Suppl. D):187–193.

8. **Ball, P., and G. S. Tillotson.** 1995. Tolerability of fluoroquinolone antibiotics: past, present and future. *Drug Saf.* 13:343–358.

9. **Barman Balfour, J. A., and H. M. Lamb.** 2000. Moxifloxacin. *Drugs* 59:115–139.

10. **Berkovitch, M., A. Pastuszak, M. Gazarian, M. Lewis, and G. Koren.** 1994. Safety of new quinolones in pregnancy. *Obst. Gynecol.* 84:535–538.

11. **Bircher A. J., and M. Rutishauser.** 1997. Oral "desensitization" of maculopapular exanthema from ciprofloxacin. *Allergy* 52:1246–1248.

12. **Blank, M., J. George, P. Fishman Y. Levy, V. Toder, S. Savyon, V. Barak, T. Koike, and Y. Schoenfeld.** 1998. Ciprofloxacin immunomodulation of experimental antiphospholipid syndrome associated with elevation of interleukin-3 and granulocyte-macrophage-colony-stimulating factor expression. *Arthritis Rheum.* 41:224–232.

13. **Blum, M. D., D. J. Graham, and C. A McCloskey.** 1994. Temafloxacin syndrome: review of 95 cases. *Clin. Infect. Dis.* 18:946–950.

14. **Bomford, J. A. L, J. C. Ledger, B. J. O'Keefe, and C. Reiter.** 1993. Ciprofloxacin use during pregnancy. *Drugs* 45(Suppl. 3):461–462.

15. **Breban, M., C. Fournier, M. A. Gougerot-Pocidalo, M. Muffat-Joly, and J. J. Pocidalo.** 1992. Protective effects of ciprofloxacin against type II collagen induced arthritis in rats. *J. Rheumatol.* 19:216–222.

16. **Breen, J., K. Skuba, and D. Grasela.** 1999. Safety and tolerability of gatifloxacin, an advanced-generation 8-methoxy fluoroquinolone. *J. Respir. Dis.* 20:70–76.

17. **Broide, E., B. Douer, N. Shaked, A. Yellin, Y. Liberman, N. Rosen, S. Segev, and E. Rubinstein.** 1992. Effect of short term therapy with ciprofloxacin, ceftriaxone and placebo on human peripheral WBC and marrow derived granulocytes, macrophages progenitor cells (CFU-GM). *Eur. J. Haematol.* 48:276–277.

18. **Burke, P., and S. R. Burne.** 2000. Allergy associated with ciprofloxacin *Br. Med. J.* 320:679.

19. **Campoli-Richards, D. M., J. P. Monk, A. Price, P. Benfield, P. A. Todd, and A. Ward.** 1988. Ciprofloxacin. A review of its antibacterial activity, pharmacokinetic properties and therapeutic use. *Drugs* 35:373–447.

20. **Centers for Disease Control and Prevention Update.** 2001. Investigation of bioterrorism-related anthrax and interim guidelines for exposure management and antimicrobial therapy. *Morb. Mortal. Wkly. Rep.* 50:909–919.

21. **Chen, H. J. L., K. J. Bloch, and J. A. Mclean.** 2000. Acute eosinophilic hepatitis from trovafloxacin. *N. Engl. J. Med.* 342:359–360.

22. **Chodosh, S., C.A. De Abate, D. Havestode, L. Aneiro, and D. Church.** 2000. Short-course moxifloxacin therapy for treatment of acute bacterial exacerbations of chronic bronchitis. *Respir. Med.* 94:18–27.

23. **Christ, W., T. Lehnert, and B. Ulbrich.** 1988. Specific toxicologic aspects of the quinolones. *Rev. Infect. Dis.* 10(Suppl.):S141–S146.

24. **Clutterbuck, D. J., and A. McMillan.** 1997. Anaphylactoid reaction to ciprofloxacin. *Int. J. STD AIDS* 8:707–708.

25. **Coleman, C. I., J. V. Spencer, J. O Chung, and P. Reddy.**

2002. Possible gatifloxacin induced fulminant hepatic failure. *Ann. Pharmacother* **36**:1162–1167.

26. Corrado, M. L., W. E. Struble, C. Peter, V. Hoagland, and J. Sabbaj. 1987. Norfloxacin: review of safety studies. *Am. J. Med.* **82**(Suppl. 6A):129S–133S.

27. Cukierski, M. A., S. Prahalada, A. G. Zacchei, C. P. Peter, J. D. Todgers, D. L. Hess, M. J. Cukierski, A. F. Trantal, T. Nyland, and R. T. Robertson. 1989. Embryotoxicity studies of norfloxacin in cynomolgus monkeys. I. Teratology studies and norfloxacin plasma concentration in pregnant and non-pregnant monkeys. *Teratology* **39**:39–52.

28. Davila, I., M. L. Diez, S. Quirce, J. Fraj, B. De La Hoz, and M. Lazaro. 1993. Cross reactivity between quinolones. Report of three cases. *Allergy* **48**:388–390.

29. Davis, R., and H. M. Bryson. 1994. Levofloxacin: a review of its antibacterial activity, pharmacokinetics and therapeutic efficacy. *Drugs* **47**:677–700.

30. Davis, H., E. McGoodwin, T. Greene, and T. Reed. 1989. Anaphylactoid reactions reported after treatment with ciprofloxacin. *Ann. Intern. Med.* **111**:1041.

31. De Simone, C., L. Baldinelli, M. Ferrazzi, S. De Santis, L. Pugnaloni, and F. Sorice. 1986. Influence of ofloxacin, norfloxacin, nalidixic acid, pyromidic acid and pipemidic acid on human gamma-interferon production and blastogenesis. *J. Antimicrob. Agents Chemother.* **17**:811–814.

32. Dharnidharka, V. R., K. Nadeau., C. L. Cannon., H. W. Harris., and S. Rosen. 1995. Ciprofloxacin overdose: acute renal failure with prominent apoptotic changes. *Am. J. Kidney Dis.* **26**:516–519.

33. Domagala, J. M. 1994. Structure-activity and structure-side-effect relationships for the quinolone antibacterials. *J. Antimicrob. Chemother.* **33**:685–706.

34. Erdem, G., M. A. Staat, B. L. Connelly, and A. Assa'ad. 1999. Anaphylactic reaction to ciprofloxacin in a toddler: successful desensitization. *Pediatr. Infect. Dis. J.* **18**:563–564.

35. Fernandez-Rivas, M. 1997. Fixed drug eruption (FDE) caused by norfloxacin. *Allergy* **52**:477–478.

36. Ford, C. D., W. Reiley, J. Wood, D. C. Classen, and J. P. Burke. 1998. Oral antimicrobial prophylaxis in bone marrow transplant recipients: randomized trial of ciprofloxacin versus ciprofloxacin-vancomycin. *Antimicrob. Agents Chemother.* **42**:1402–1408.

37. Forsgren, A., S. F. Sclossman, and T. F. Tedder. 1987. 4-Quinolone drugs affect cell cycle progression and function of human lymphocytes in vitro. *Antimicrob. Agents Chemother.* **31**:768–773.

38. Freifield, A., D. Marchigiani, T. Walsh, S. Chanock, L. Lewis, J. Hiemenz, S. Hiemenz, J. E,. Hicks, C. Gill, S. M. Steinberg, and P. A. Pizzo. 1999. A double blind comparison of empirical oral and intravenous antibiotic therapy for low-risk febrile patients with neutropenia during cancer chemotherapy. *N. Engl. J. Med.* **341**:305–311.

39. Friedman, J. M., and J.E. Polifka. *Teratogenic Effects of Drugs: a Resource for Clinicians (TERIS)*, p. 149–195. Johns Hopkins University Press, Baltimore, Md.

40. Galley, H. F, J. K. Dhillon, R. L. Patterson, and N. R. Webster. 2000. Effect of ciprofloxacin on the activation of the transcription factors, nuclear factor kappaB, activator protein-1 and nuclear-factor-IL-6 and interleukin-6 and interleukin-8 mRNA expression in human endothelial cell line. *Clin. Sci. (Lond.)* **99**:405–410.

41. Gea-Banacloche, J. C., and D. D. Metcalfe. 1996. Ciprofloxacin desensitization. *J. Allergy Clin. Immunol.* **97**:1426–1427.

42. Geddes, A., M. Thaler, S. Schonwald, M. Harkonen, F.

Jacobs, and I. Nowotny. 1999. Levofloxacin in the empirical treatment of patients with suspected bacteraemia/sepsis: comparison with imipenem/cilastatin in an open, randomized trial. *J. Antimicrob. Chemother.* **44**:799–810.

43. Godin, M., T. Ducastelle., E. Bercoff, D. Dubois, J. P. Fillastre, and J. Bouneille. 1984. Renal failure and quinolone. *Nephron* **37**:70.

44. Gollapudi, S. V., S. K. Chuah, T. Harvey, H. D. Thadepalli, and H. Thadepalli. 1993. In vivo effects of rufloxacin and ciprofloxacin on T-cell subsets and tumor necrosis factor production in mice infected with Bacteroides fragilis. *Antimicrob. Agents Chemother.* **37**:1711–1712.

45. Gonzalez, J.P., and J. M. Henwood. 1989. Pefloxacin: a review of its antibacterial activity, pharmacokinetic properties, and therapeutic uses. *Drugs* **37**:628–686.

46. Hahn, T., Y. Barak, E. Leibovitch, L. Malach, O. Dagan, and E. Rubinstein. 1991. Ciprofloxacin inhibits human hematopoietic cell growth synergism with tumor necrosis factor and interferon. *Exp. Hematol.* **19**:157–160.

47. Halkin, H. 1988. Adverse effects of the fluoroquinolones. *Rev. Infect. Dis.* **10**(Suppl. 1):258–261.

48. Hooper, D. C., and J. S. Wolfson. 1993. Adverse effects, p. 489–512. In D. C. Hooper and J. S. Wolfson (ed.), *Quinolone Antimicrobial Agents*, 2nd ed. American Society for Microbiology, Washington, D.C.

49. Hootkins, R., A. Z. Fenves, and M. K. Stephens. 1989 Acute renal failure secondary to oral ciprofloxacin therapy: a presentation of three cases and a review of the literature. *Clin. Nephrol.* **32**:75–78.

50. Hughes, W. T., D. Armstrong, G. P. Bodey, A. E. Brown, J. E., Edwards, R. Feld, P. Pizzo, K. V. I. Rolston, J. L. Shenep, and L. S. Young. 1997. Guidelines for the use of antimicrobial agents in neutropenic patients with unexplained fevers. *Clin. Infect. Dis.* **25**:551–573.

51. Hummler, H., W. F. Richter, and A. G. Hendrickx. 1993. Developmental toxicity of fleroxacin and comparative pharmacokinetics of four fluoroquinolones in the cynomolgus macaque (Macaca fascicularis). *Toxicol. Appl. Pharmacol.* **122**:34–45.

52. Iannini, P. B., R. Rubin, C. Reiter, and G. Tillotson. 2001. Reassuring safety profile of moxifloxacin. *Clin. Infect. Dis.* **32**:1112–1114.

53. Inglesby, T. V., D. A. Henderson, J. G. Bartlett, M. S. Ascher, E. Eitzen, A. M. Friedlander, J. Hauer, J. McDade, M. T. Osterholm, T. O'Toole, G. Parker, T. M. Perl, P. K. Russell, and K. Tonat for the Working Group on Civilian Biodefense. 1999. Anthrax as a biological weapon: medical and public health management. *JAMA* **281**:1735–1745.

54. Itoh, S., M. Miura, and H. Shimada. 1998. Lack of mutagenicity of levofloxacin in lacZ transgenic mice. *Mutagenesis***13**:51–55.

55. Jungst, G., and R. Mohr. 1988. Overview of post-marketing experience with ofloxacin in Germany. *J. Antimicrob. Chemother.* **22**:(Suppl. C):167–175.

56. Kaloyanides, G. J. 1994. Antibiotic-related nephrotoxicity. *Nephrol. Dial. Transplant.* **9**(Suppl. 4):130–134.

57. Kern, W., and E. Kurrle. 1991. Ofloxacin versus trimethoprim-sulfamethoxazole for prevention of infection in patients with acute leukemia and granulocytopenia. *Infection* **19**:73–80.

58. Kern, W. V., A. Cometta, R. De Bock, J. Lamgenakken, M. Paesmans, H. Gaya. 1999. Oral versus intravenous empirical therapy for fever in patients with granulocytopenia who are receiving cancer chemotherapy. *N. Engl. J. Med.* **341**:312–318.

59. Khan, A. A., T. R. Slifer, F. G. Araujo, Y. Suzuki, and J. S.

Remington. 2000. Protection against lipopolysaccharide-induced death by fluoroquinolones. *Antimicrob. Agents Chemother.* **44**:3169–3173.

60. Kimyai-Asadi, A., A. Usman, and H. C. Noiusari. 2000. Ciprofloxacin-induced bullous pemphigoid. *J. Am. Acad. Dermatol.* **42**(5 Pt 1):847.

61. Kletter, Y., I. Riklis, and I. Shalit, I. Fabian. 1991 Enhanced repopulation of murine hematopoietic organs in sublethally irradiated mice after treatment with ciprofloxacin. *Blood* **78**:1685–1691.

62. Lien, Y. H., R. Hansen, W. F. Kern, J. Bagert, R. B. Nagle, and M. Ko, and M. S. Siskind. 1993. Ciprofloxacin-induced granulomatous interstitial nephritis and localized elastolysis. *Am. J. Kidney Dis.* **22**:598–602.

63. Lipsky, B. A., and C. A. Baker. 1999. Fluoroquinolone toxicity profiles: a review focusing on newer agents *Clin. Infect. Dis.* **28**:352–364.

64. Livasy, C. A., and A. M. Kaplan. 1997. Ciprofloxacin-induced toxic epidermal necrolysis: a case report and a review. *Dermatology* **195**:173–175.

65. Lo, W. K., K. V. I. Rolston, E. B. Rubenstein, and G. P. Bodey. 1993. Ciprofloxacin induced nephrotoxicity in patients with cancer. *Arch. Intern. Med.* **153**:1258–1262.

66. Loebstein, R., A. Addis, E. Ho, R. Andreou, S. Sage, A. E. Donnenfeld, B. Schick, M. Bonati, M. Moretti, A. Lalkin, A. Pastuszak, and G. Keren. 1998. Pregnancy outcome following gestational exposure to fluoroquinolones: a multicenter prospective controlled study. *Antimicrob. Agents Chemother.* **42**:1336–1339.

67. Lomaestro, B. M. 2000. Fluoroquinolone-induced renal failure. *Drug Saf.* **22**:479–485.

68. Mandell, L. A., P. Ball, and G. Tillotson. 2001. Antimicrobial safety and tolerability: differences and dilemmas. *Clin. Infect. Dis.* **32**(Suppl. 1):S72–S79.

69. Massoomi, T., H. G Mathews, and C. J. Destache. 1993. Effect of seven fluoroquinolones on the detemination of serum creatinine by the picric acid and enzymatic methods. *Ann. Pharmacother.* **27**:586–588.

70. Mitropoulos, F. A, P. B. Angood, and R. Rabinovici. 2001. Trovafloxacin-associated leukopenia. *Ann. Pharmacother.* **35**:41–44.

71. Montey, G., Y. Goueffon, and F. Roquet. 1984. Absorption, distribution, metabolic fate, and elimination of pefloxacin mesylate in mice, rats, dogs, monkeys, and humans. *Antimicrob. Agents Chemother.* **25**:463–472.

72. Naldi, L., A. Conforti, M. Venegoni, M. G. Troncon, A. Caputi, E. Ghiotto, A. Cocci, U. Moretti, G. Velo, and R. Leone. 1999. Cutaneous reactions to drugs. An analysis of spontaneous reports in four Italian regions. *Br. J. Clin. Pharmacol.* **48**:839–846.

73. Nicholson, S. C., C. D. Webb, and R. C. Moellering. 2002. Antimicrobial-associated acute hepatitis. *Pharmacotherapy* **22**:794–796.

74. Nishijima, S., and M. Nakagawa. 1997. Fixed drug eruption caused by tosufloxacin tosillate. *J. Int. Med. Res.* **25**:359–363.

75. Nordmann, P., M. Diez-Ibanez, M. Chessebeuf-Padieu, B. Luu, G. Mack, and M. Mersel. 1999. Toxic effects of 7 β-hydroxycholesterol on rat liver cells primary cultures, epithelial lines, and co-cultures. *Cell Biol. Toxicol.* **5**:261–270.

76. Norrby, S. R., and P. S. Lietman. 1993. Safety and tolerability of fluoroquinolones. *Drugs* **45**(Suppl. 3):59–64.

77. Pace, J. L., and P. Gatt. 1989. Fatal vasculitis associated with ofloxacin. *Br. Med. J.* **299**:658.

78. Paily, R. 2000. Quinolone drug rash in a patient with infectious mononucleosis. *J. Dermatol.* **27**:405–406.

79. Pallavacini, F., A. Antinori, G. Frederico, M. Funtoni, and P. Neruo. 1989. Influence of two quinolones, ofloxacin and pefloxacin, on human myelopoesis in vitro. *Antimicrob. Agents Chemother.* **33**:122–123.

80. Perry, C. M., D. Ormrod, M. Hurst, and S. V. Onrust. 2001. Gatifloxacin: a review of its use in the management of bacterial infections. *Drugs* **61**:1–37.

81. Pessina, A., M. G. Neri, E. Muschiato, E. Mineo, and G. Cocuzza. 1989. Effect of fluoroquinolones on the in-vitro proliferation of myeloid precursor cells. *J. Antimicrob. Chemother.* **24**:203–208.

82. Reano, M., R. Vives, J. Rodriguez, P. Daroca, G. Canto, and J. Fernandez. 1997. Ciprofloxacin-induced vasculitis. *Allergy* **52**:599–600.

83. Remuzon, P., D. Bouzard, C. Guiol, and J. Jacquet. 1992. Fluoronaphtypyridines as antibacterial agents. 6. Synthesis and structure activity relationship of new chiral 7-(1-,3-,4-, and 6-methyl-2,5-diazabicyclo[2.2.1]-heptan-2-yl]-1-(1,1 dimethyl)-6-fluoro-1,4-dihydro-oxo-1,8-naphthyridine-3-carboxylix acid. Influence of the configuration on blood pressure in dogs: a quinolone-class effect. *J. Med. Chem.* **35**:2898–2899.

84. Riesbeck, K. 2002. Immunomodulating activity of quinolones. *Rev. J. Chemother.* **14**:3–12.

85. Riesbeck, K., A. Forsgren, A. Henriksson, and A. Bredberg. 1998. Ciprofloxacin induces an immunomodulatory stress response in human T lymphocytes. *Antimicrob. Agents Chemother.* **42**:1923–1930.

86. Riesbeck, K., and A. Forsgren. 1994. Increased Il-2 transcription in murine lymphocyte by ciprofloxacin. *Immunopharmacology* **27**:155–164.

87. Riesbeck, K., and A. Forsgren. 1998. Commentary on ciprofloxacin superinduction of Il-2 synthesis and thymidine uptake. *Transplantation* **65**:1282–1283.

88. Riesbeck, K., H. Schatz, Ö. Östraat, G. Tufveson, and H. Ekberg. 1995. Enhancement of the immuno-suppressive effect of cyclosporin A by ciprofloxacin in a rat cardiac transplantation model. *Transplant. Int.* **8**:96–102.

89. Rubinstein, E. 1996. Safety profile of sparfloxacin in the treatment of respiratory tract infections. *J. Antimicrob. Chemother.* **37**:(Suppl. A):145–160.

90. Rubinstein, E., P. Potgieter, P. Davey, and S. R. Norrby. 1994. The use of fluoroquinolones in neutropenic patients—analysis of adverse effects. *J. Antimicrob. Chemother.* **34**:7–19.

91. Salon, E. J., M. A. Newbrough, C. A. Albarracin, and J. E. Hernandez. 1997. Anaphylactoid reaction to ciprofloxacin versus toxic shock syndrome. *Ann. Pharmacother.* **1**:119–120.

92. Sangen, Y., A. Kawada, M. Asai, Y. Aragane, T. Yudate, and T. Tezuka. 2000. Fixed drug eruption induced by tosufloxacin tosilate. *Contact Dermatitis* **42**:285.

93. Sanders, W. E., Jr. 1988. Efficacy, safety and potential economic benefits of oral ciprofloxacin in the treatment of infections. *Rev. Infect. Dis.* **10**:528–543.

94. Savion, S, M. Lank, J. Shepshelovich, P. Fishman, Y. Schoenfeld, and V. Toder. 2000. Ciprofloxacin affects pregnancy loss in CBA/JxDBA/2J mice possibly via elevation of interleukin-3 and granulocyte-macrophage-colony-stimulating factor production. *Am. J. Reprod. Immunol.* **44**:293–298.

95. Schaefer, C., E. Amoura-Elefant, T. Vial, A. Ornoy, H. Garbis, E. Robert, E. Rodriguez-Pinilla, T. Pexeider, N. Prapas, and P. Merlob. 1996. Pregnancy outcome after prenatal quinolone exposure. Evaluation of a case registry of the European Network of Teratology Information Services (ENTIS). *Eur. J. Obst. Gynecol.* **69**:83–89.

96. Shalit, I., Y. Kletter, K. Weiss, T. Gruss, and I. Fabian. 1997. Enhanced hematopoiesis in sublethally irradiated mice treated with various quinolones. *Eur. J. Haematol.* **58**:92–98.

97. Shalit, I., Y. Kletter, D. Halperin, D. Waldman, E. Vasserman, A. Nagler, and I. Fabian. 2001. Immunomo-dulatory effects of moxifloxacin in comparison to ciprofloxacin and G-CSF in a murine model of cyclophosphamide-induced leukopenia. *Eur. J. Haematol.* **66:**287–296.

98. Shimada, H., and S. Itoh. 1996. Effects of new quinolone antibacterial agents on mammalian chromosomes. *J. Toxicol. Environ. Health* **47:**115–123.

99. Smythe, M. A., and D. M. Cappelletty. 2000. Anaphylactoid reaction to levofloxacin. *Pharmacotherapy* **20:**1520–1523.

100. Somekh, E., B. Lew, E. Schwartz, A. Barzilai, and E. Rubinstein. 1989. The effect of ciprofloxacin and pefloxacin on bone marrow engraftment in the spleen of mice. *J. Antimicrob. Chemother.* **19:**781–790.

101. Somekh, E., S. West, A. Barzilai, and E. Rubinstein. 1989. The lack of long term suppressive effect of ciprofloxacin on murine bone marrow. *J. Antimicrob. Chemother.* **24:**209–213.

102. Stahlmann, R. 1990. Safety profile of the quinolones. *J. Antimicrob. Chemother.* **26**(Suppl. D):31–34.

103. Stahlmann R., and H. Lode. 2000. Safety overview: Toxicity, adverse effects, and drug interactions, p. 370–416. *In* V. T. Andriole (ed.), *The Quinolones*, 2nd ed. Academic Press, Inc., New York. N.Y.

104. Stahlmann, R., and R. Schwabe. 1997. Safety profile of grepafloxacin compared with other fluoroquinolones. *J. Antimicrob. Chemother.* **40**(Suppl. A):83–92.

105. Takayama, S., M. Hirohashi, M. Kato, and H. Shimada. 1995. Toxicity of quinolone antimicrobial agents. *J. Toxicol. Environ. Health* **45:**1–45.

106. Takayama, S., T. Watanabe, Y. Akiyama, K. Ohura, S. Harada, K. Matsuhashi, K. Mochida, and N. Yamashita. 1986. Reproductive toxicity of ofloxacin. *Arzneim.-Forsch.* **36:**1244–1248.

107. Tarantal, A. F., S. B. Lehrer, B. L. Lasley, and A. G. Hendrickx. 1990. Developmental toxicity of temafloxacin hydrochloride in the long-tailed macquaque (Maccaca fascicularis). *Teratology* **42:**233–242.

108. U.S. Food and Drug Administration. 1999. *Public Health Advisory. Trovan (Trovafloxacin/Alatrofloxacin Mesylate. 9 June 1999)*. U.S. Food and Drug Administration, Washington, D.C.

109. Wagstaff, A. J., and J. A. Balfour. 1997. Grepafloxacin. *Drugs* **53:**817–824.

110. Wang, C. X., J. Sabbaj, M. Corrado, and J. Hoagland. 1986. Worldwide clinical experience with norfloxacin: efficacy and safety. *Scand. J. Infect. Dis. Suppl.* **28:**81–89.

111. Watanabe, T., K. Fujikawa, S. Harada, K. Ohura, T. Sasaki, and S. Takayama. 1992. Reproductive toxicity of the new quinolone antibacterial agent levofloxacin in rats and rabbits. *Arzneim.-Forsch.* **43:**374–377.

112. Wolfson, J. S. 1989. Quinolone antimicrobial agents: adverse effects and bacterial resistance. *Eur. J. Clin. Microb. Infect. Dis.* **8:**1080–1092.

113. Wolfson, J. S., and D. C. Hooper. 1991. Overview of fluoroquinolone safety. *Am. J. Med.* **91**(Suppl. 6A):153–161.

114. Yerasi, A. B., and M. D. Oertal. 1996. Ciprofloxacin-induced toxic epidermal necrolysis. *Ann. Pharmacother.* **30:**297.

115. Zakari, S. M., H. Meyer, G. Meinhardt, W. Reinisch, K. Scrattbauer, M. Knoefler, and L. H. Block. 2000. Effects of trovafloxacin on the IL-1 dependent activation of E-selection in human endothelial cells in vitro. *Immunopharmacology* **48:**27–34.

Quinolone Antimicrobial Agents, 3rd ed.
Edited by David C. Hooper and Ethan Rubinstein
© 2003 ASM Press, Washington, D.C.

Chapter 26

QT Prolongation with Quinolone Antimicrobial Agents

YEE GUAN YAP AND A. JOHN CAMM

The QT interval is defined as the duration between the beginning of the QRS complex and the end of the T wave on the electrocardiogram (ECG). It represents the time interval between the beginning of ventricular depolarization and the end of ventricular repolarization. It is well recognized that a prolonged QT interval may herald or facilitate the occurrence of a specific form of polymorphic ventricular tachyarrhythmia, namely, torsades de pointes (TdP). If rapid or prolonged, this arrhythmia can sometimes lead to ventricular fibrillation and sudden cardiac death (Fig. 1A and B).

Since the original description of TdP by Dessertenne, it has been recognized that many clinical conditions can cause prolonged or abnormal repolarization (i.e., QT interval prolongation or abnormal T or T/U wave morphology) and/or TdP. TdP may be associated with congenital or acquired QT interval prolongation. Medication is the most common cause of acquired long QT syndrome. Many drugs are known to prolong the QT interval, with antiarrhythmic medications being implicated most often. However, a spectrum of noncardiac drugs, such as nonsedating antihistamines, macrolide antibiotics, quinolone antimicrobials, antipsychotics, etc., can cause QT prolongation and induce TdP (127). Several of these drugs have now been withdrawn from the market or have had their sale restricted. Many investigational drugs have also been implicated. Of concern is that the pro-arrhythmic risk of many of these drugs is difficult to detect during the developmental phase of the drug and may not be recognized until some years after being marketed.

The number of drugs associated with QT prolongation and TdP may increase. This issue has been identified as a considerable public health problem and has attracted attention from the drug regulatory authorities. In a survey in both the United Kingdom (U.K.) and Italy, noncardiac drugs that have proarrhythmic potential (i.e., official warnings on QT pro-

longation or TdP or with published data on QT prolongation, ventricular tachycardia, or a class III effect) alone represented 3 and 2% of total prescriptions in both countries, respectively (28). Drug-induced proarrhythmia may be a highly prevalent issue, and it is prudent that all prescribing physicians and their patients should be aware of this risk and take the precautions to minimize proarrhythmia.

MECHANISM OF DRUG-INDUCED QT PROLONGATION AND TdP

The cardiac action potential is generated by the transmembrane movement of several ions, including Na^+, Ca^{2+}, and K^+. The intracellular potential of myocytes is negative compared with the extracellular space (resting transmembrane potential = -80 to -90 mV). However, cardiac cells are excitable and, when appropriately stimulated, membrane ionic channels in the cell open and close sequentially. Depending on their voltage and time dependencies, the movement of ions back and forth leads to changes of the transmembrane potential, and hence generation of action potentials. The initial depolarization (phase 0) is triggered by a rapid influx of sodium ions (I_{Na}) which changes the cell potential from -90 to mV to $+30$ mV (110, 129). The transient outward I_{to} potassium current is subsequently responsible for the slight immediate repolarization (phase 1). During the following plateau phase (phase 2), the cell potential is maintained by the influx of calcium ions (I_{ca}). Cellular depolarization leads to generation of the QRS complex on the surface ECG. The repolarization phase (phase 3) of the myocytes is driven predominantly by outward movement of the potassium currents, carried by the rapid (I_{Kr}) and slow (I_{Ks}) components of the delayed rectifier potassium channel. This ionic movement gives rise to the T wave on the ECG, as the cellular potentials return

Yee Guan Yap and A. John Camm • Department of Cardiological Sciences, St. George's Hospital Medical School, London, United Kingdom.

A

B

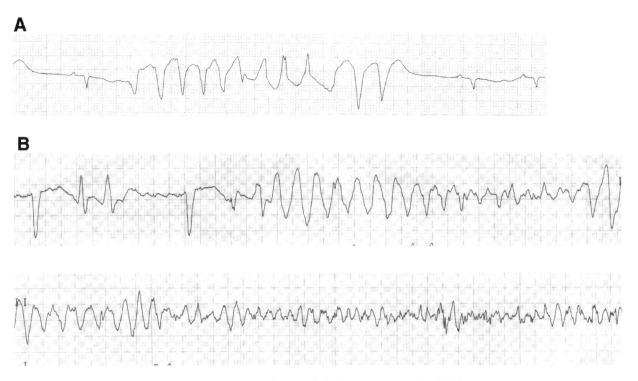

Figure 1. (A) Self-limiting TdP. (B) TdP leading onto ventricular fibrillation.

in sequence to their resting states. The diastolic depolarization (phase 4) results from a combination of the decay of the outward delayed rectifier I_{Kr} and I_{Ks} currents, which maintains the resting potential at approximately −90 mV, and the activation of a specific inward pacemaker current (I_f) and the inward sodium background leak current ($I_{Na\text{-}B}$). A variety of other different potassium channel subtypes are also present in the heart (88) (Fig. 2), and blockade of

each of these potassium channels has a different effect on the action potential (Fig. 3).

MECHANISM OF ACQUIRED QT PROLONGATION AND TdP

Disturbances in any of these ionic movements, in particular the potassium ions, may cause arrhythmias.

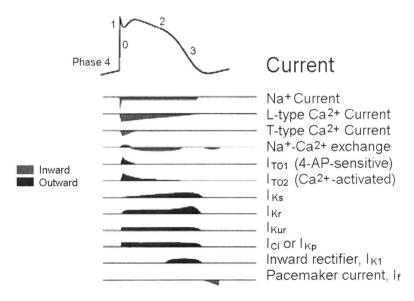

Figure 2. Cardiac ionic currents and their relationship to action potential. Modified from reference 88.

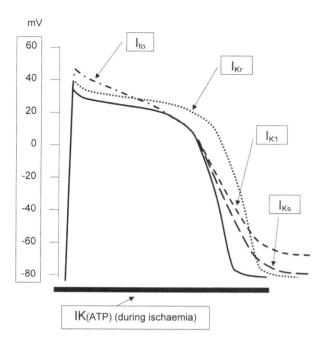

Figure 3. Alteration in action potential with individual blockade of some potassium channels.

There are at least eight different potassium channel subtypes in the heart (24). The individual potassium channels differ in their voltage-, rate-, and time-dependent opening and closing characteristics and by their regulation and response to drugs. Each of them may be a target for drug effect. Each potassium channel has a different effect on the action potential (Fig. 2 and 3), and various potassium channels may not be expressed equally in all species, individuals, or tissues. The principal K^+ currents participating in the repolarization of the action potential in the human ventricular myocardium under normal conditions are the delayed rectifier K^+ current (I_{Kr} and I_{Ks}) (98), the inward rectifier I_{K1} (96), and the transient outward K^+ current I_{to} (92). I_{Kr} seems to play the most important role in determining the duration of the action potential.

The evidence suggests that the drug-induced proarrhythmias are mostly mediated by drugs that suppress the I_{K1} and I_{Kr} channels that govern the rapid repolarization phase (98). I_{K1} is an outward current that is time independent but voltage dependent. I_{K1} determines and stabilizes the resting membrane potential near the equilibrium potential for potassium and also contributes to the final phase of repolarization of the action potential. I_{K1} is also termed the inward rectifying current because it allows current to flow more easily in the inward direction (96).

The evidence is now clear that the blockade of I_{Kr} is reponsible for quinolone-induced TdP (17, 34, 103). The blockade of the I_{Kr} current results in the prolongation of the action potential duration and the slowing of

repolarization. It manifests clinically as a prolonged QT interval and a lower-amplitude T wave on the surface ECG. Prolongation of repolarization often results in a bifid T wave. Prolongation of repolarization may also lead to activation of an inward depolarization current, known as an early after-depolarization (8), which is responsible for the increased amplitude of the U wave on the ECG and may promote repetitive triggered activity. When accompanied by the presence of markedly increased dispersion of repolarization, often induced by the same drug, this may induce re-entry and provoke TdP, which is then sustained by further re-entry or spiral-wave activity (37) (Fig. 4). Such phenomena are more readily induced in the His-Purkinje network and also from a subset of myocardial cells from the midventricular myocardium, known as M cells (71). One reason for this cell selectivity may be that the resting membrane potential in Purkinje fibers is more positive than that in the ventricle, and the blockade of I_{Kr} channel is voltage dependent, with more block in depolarized tissue (7). This property may then lead to dispersion of refractoriness between the two tissue types, which is a potentially arrhythmogenic effect. M cells are a subset of myocardial cells located deep in the subepicardium, which are electrophysiologically different from those of epicardium and endocardium but intermediate between those of epi- and endomyocardial cells and Purkinje fibers. Compared with subendocardial or subepicardial cells, M cells show more pronounced action potential prolongation and easier induction of early after-depolarizations and triggered activity in response to I_{Kr} blockade (37, 71).

MEASUREMENT OF QT INTERVAL

When measuring the QT interval, the ECG is best recorded at a paper speed of 50 mm/s and at an amplitude of 0.5 mV/cm using a multichannel recorder capable of simultaneous recording of all 12 leads. The end of T wave is defined by the intercept of a tangent to the steepest part of the descending portion of the T wave and the isoelectric line. The QT interval is measured from the beginning of the QRS complex to the end of the T wave on a standard ECG, traditionally from lead II.

The QT interval is influenced by heart rate. At least 3 or 4 RR intervals preceding the QT interval should be measured for rate correction. Several formulas may be used to correct the QT interval for the biophysical effect of heart rate (QTc). The most commonly used formulas are Fridericia's cube-root formula (QTc = $QT/RR^{1/3}$) and Bazett's square-root formula (QTc = $QT/RR^{1/2}$). Between the two, Bazett's formula is more popular, but Fridericia's

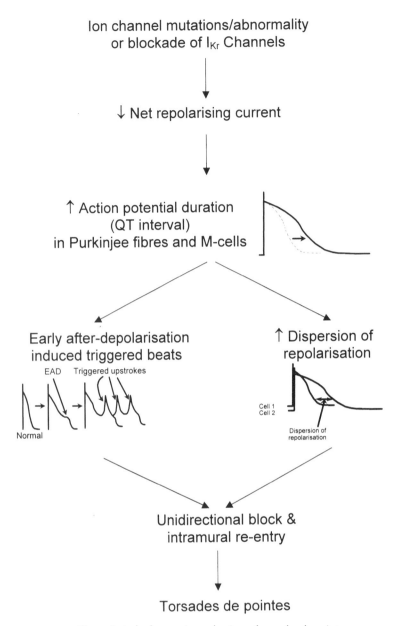

Figure 4. Arrhythmogenic mechanism of torsades de pointes.

correction is preferred because it is more accurate at the extremes of physiological heart rate.

Newer repolarization parameters such as QT dispersion (maximum − minimum QT intervals) on the 12-lead surface ECG, which is considered to be an indirect measure of spatial heterogeneity of repolarization, may be useful in assessing drug efficacy and safety. In one important study patients in whom a class 1a antiarrhythmic drug provoked QT prolongation and TdP had significantly increased precordial QT interval dispersion (51). In contrast, patients receiving amiodarone or class 1a antiarrhythmics without developing TdP did not have increased QT dispersion although the QT interval was similarly prolonged (51). Thus, spatial heterogeneity/dispersion of ventricular repolarization may be required in addition to QT prolongation for the genesis of TdP. Although the use of QT dispersion in the assessment of drugs that prolong the QT interval needs further confirmation, it may provide information about the clinical significance of QT prolongation.

QUINOLONES AND THE RISK OF QT PROLONGATION AND TdP

The risk of QT prolongation and potentially fatal ventricular arrhythmias associated with quinolones was highlighted following the withdrawal of grepafloxacin due to several cases of sudden death and TdP, which were not anticipated during initial drug development. However, the cardiotoxicity of quinolones as a group is not clear. While it has been suggested that the QT prolonging effect of quinolone is a class effect (12), others have stated that the cardiotoxic potential of grepafloxacin and sparfloxacin are higher than those of other quinolones (103). The data on the cardiotoxicity of quinolones, in general, are still sparse.

Grepafloxacin has been marketed in the U.K. since 1998 and in the United States since 1997, until recently due to its cardiotoxicity. During animal studies on both rabbit and dog models, grepafloxacin prolonged the QT interval after intravenous dosage of 10 to 30 mg/kg of body weight (104). In the phase I study on healthy volunteers, grepafloxacin was noted to mildly prolong the QT interval with a mean QTc prolongation of only 10 ms (108). However, it was withdrawn voluntarily in the U.K. and the United States in 1999 by its manufacturer due to seven possibly associated sudden deaths and several cases of TdP (13). Another fluoroquinolone, temafloxacin, introduced in the United States in 1992, was also withdrawn from the market less than 4 months after its introduction, but primarily because of numerous reports (approximately 50 cases) of serious noncardiac adverse events, including three deaths (http://www.fda.gov/ohrms/dockets /ac/99/slides/3558s1/index.htm). The major noncardiac side effects included hypoglycemia in elderly patients as well as a constellation of multisystem organ involvement characterized by anaphylaxis, severe hemolytic anemia, renal failure, abnormal liver function tests, hypoglycemia, and coagulopathy. The cardiotoxicity of temafloxacin is unclear.

Most data on the cardiac adverse effect of quinolones centered on a new fluoroquinolone, sparfloxacin, because it was the original fluoroquinolone described to be associated with proarrhythmia. Sparfloxacin was observed to prolong the QT interval in dogs during preclinical development of the drug (55). The Sparfloxacin Safety Group has confirmed that sparfloxacin prolonged the QTc interval by an average of 3% in healthy volunteers (phase I study) as well as in patients with renal or hepatic impairment (phase III study) (55). Since the drug was marketed in 1994, there have been some cases of ventricular arrhythmia (three reversible ventricular tachycardia) reported during the European postmarketing surveillance of sparfloxacin, all of which occurred in patients with underlying cardiac conditions (55). An integrated analysis of the safety data of sparfloxacin from six multicenter phase III

trials, consisting of five double-masked, randomized, comparative trials of sparfloxacin (a 400-mg oral loading dose followed by 200 mg/day for 10 days) versus standard comparative therapies (erythromycin, cefaclor, ofloxacin, clarithromycin, and ciprofloxacin), confirmed that the mean change from the QTc interval baseline was significantly greater in sparfloxacin-treated patients (10 ms) than in patients given comparator drugs (3 ms), although no associated ventricular arrhythmias were detected (70).

In a separate small double-blind, randomized, placebo-controlled, crossover study of 15 healthy volunteers, sparfloxacin at two different doses of 200 and 400 mg prolonged the QT interval to the same extent (by 4%) compared with placebo (30). No significant reverse rate dependence of QT interval was observed. However, another clinical study on 90 healthy male volunteers showed that the increases in the placebo-adjusted mean change and mean maximum change in QT interval were dose related. The placebo-adjusted increases in QTc interval on day 1 loading dose were 9, 16, and 28 ms after the subjects received 200, 400, and 800 mg of sparfloxacin, respectively. The corresponding increases on day 4 steady state were 7, 12, and 26 ms, respectively. In an in vitro study on rabbit Purkinje fibers, the effect of sparfloxacin on cardiac action potential was compared with that of ofloxacin and levofloxacin (1). Sparfloxacin prolonged the duration of action potential in a concentration-dependent manner. In contrast, ofloxacin and levofloxacin did not alter the action potential duration at various concentrations (1 to 100 μM). At low stimulation rates, the sparfloxacin-induced prolongation of the action potential was greater and early after-depolarizations occurred in a concentration-dependent manner. Thus, sparfloxacin exerts a pure class III electrophysiological effect, whereas levofloxacin and ofloxacin apparently do not. Sparfloxacin was metabolized by the kidney, and its clearance was reduced and concentrations in plasma were raised in patients with moderate [creatinine clearance (CL_{CR}) 30 to 49 ml/min per 1.73 m^2] or severe (CL_{CL} 10 to 29 ml/min per 1.73 m^2) renal insufficiency, but increases did not appear to augment drug effects on the QT interval or enhance the risk for adverse events compared with patients with normal renal function (31). It is yet uncertain whether sparfloxacin will cause an unacceptable incidence of spontaneous TdP, in particular in low-risk patients, but an anecdotal case has been reported (34).

Moxifloxacin in a preclinical study on anesthetized rabbit models produced no ventricular arrhythmia at doses up to 120 mg/kg, whereas sparfloxacin induced ventricular tachycardia, including TdP in 50% (3 of 6 animals) at similar dosage.

Data from the worldwide phase III clinical trials showed that the degree of QTc prolongation measured at baseline and 2 h postdose on days 3 to 5 of 400-mg-daily of oral moxifloxacin was slightly greater at 6 ± 26 ms ($n = 787$) than at 2 ± 23 ms with clarithromycin ($n = 136$), with 0.4% of patients having QTc > 500 ms and 1.3% with ΔQTc > 60 ms while receiving moxifloxacin (15). No cardiovascular morbidity or mortality attributable to QT prolongation has occurred so far, with moxifloxacin treatment in more than 4,000 patients (http:// www.fda.gov/cder/foi/label/1999/210851bl.pdf). There are, as yet, no data concerning the possible clinical sequelae of this effect in patients at risk of QT interval prolongation during the early phase of clinical trials (11). Moxifloxacin is an I_{Kr} blocker and prolonged the QT interval in a dose-dependent manner but did not exert reverse rate dependency (http://www.fda.gov/ohrms/dockets/ac/99/transcpt/3558t2b.pdf). Moxifloxacin is about one third as potent as sparfloxacin in blocking the I_{Kr} channel in mouse atrial cells. Moxifloxacin also showed some blockage of the I_{Ks} channel, and the action potential duration was prolonged by moxifloxacin at a concentration much higher than by sparfloxacin (50 versus 3 μM) (http://www.fda.gov/ohrms/dockets/ac/99 /transcpt/3558t2b.pdf).

Gatifloxacin is an advanced-generation, 8-methoxyfluoroquinolone that is active against a broad spectrum of pathogens. Clinical studies have shown that gatifloxacin has limited potential to prolong the QT interval (45). In a study on 55 volunteers using oral and intravenous doses of gatifloxacin ranging from 200 to 800 mg, the prolongation of the QTc interval was 2.9 ± 16.5 ms, and no subject had a QTc interval >450 ms in this study (http:// www.fda.gov/cder/foi/label/1999/210621bl.pdf). No cardiovascular morbidity or mortality attributable to QT prolongation has occurred with gatifloxacin treatment in more than 4,000 patients, including 118 patients concurrently receiving drugs known to prolong the QT interval and 139 patients with uncorrected hypokalemia (although ECG monitoring was not performed). However, the likelihood of QT prolongation may increase with increasing concentrations of the drug and may potentially lead to TdP. Therefore, the recommended dose should not be exceeded. Pharmacokinetic studies between gatifloxacin and drugs that prolong the QT interval such as cisapride, erythromycin, antipsychotics, and tricyclic antidepressants have not been performed. Therefore, similar to other QT-prolonging drugs, gatifloxacin should be used with caution when given concurrently with these drugs, as well as in patients with ongoing proarrhythmic conditions, such as clinically significant bradycardia or acute myocardial ischemia.

Levofloxacin has been implicated in the etiology of QT prolongation and TdP (http://www.bmj.com /cgi/eletters/320/7243/1158#EL5;), although it did not alter the action potential duration in an experimental study on rabbit Purkinje fibers (1). In a retrospective study of 23 patients who received a standard dose of 500 mg of levofloxacin daily and had ECGs during treatment, levofloxacin prolonged the QTc interval >30 ms in 17% of patients and >60 ms in 9% of patients. Absolute QT interval prolongation greater than 500 ms was present in 17% of patients, one of whom developed TdP, although this patient was also receiving amiodarone (http://www.bmj .com/cgi/eletters/320/7243/1158#EL5). During the postmarketing surveillance, a case of QT prolongation and polymorphic ventricular tachycardia was reported in association with levofloxacin use (97). The U.S. Food and Drug Administration's spontaneous reporting system documented 11 other cases of TdP in 3 million treatments with levofloxacin (12). These reports generally involve patients who had concurrent medical conditions; the relationship to levofloxacin has not been established. The manufacturer is now required to conduct further electrophysiological studies to investigate the in vitro effect of levofloxacin and similar agents on the I_{Kr} channel and its dose response to QT intervals in male and female healthy volunteers over a broad age range, including subjects >65 years of age and placebo and active control arms using other antimicrobials with all the recommended doses.

ARRHYTHMOGENIC RISK OF QUINOLONES: A CLASS EFFECT?

The cardiotoxicity of quinolones as a class remains unclear, in part because of a lack of data, especially on the newer quinolones that are yet to be marketed. What is probably clear now is that fluoroquinolones prolong the QT interval or action potential duration to different degrees, at least in animal models, although some controversy remains whether QT prolongation with quinolones is a class effect. For instance, as discussed earlier, Adamantidis demonstrated that sparfloxacin, but not levofloxacin or ofloxacin, prolonged the cardiac repolarization in rabbit Purkinje fibers (1). Anderson and colleagues also showed that in a rabbit model sparfloxacin had a far greater effect on the potassium channel than did grepafloxacin and gatifloxacin, although all three agents could cause ventricular arrhythmia (5). Sparfloxacin had the greatest effect for blocking the

I_{Kr} channel with a 50% inhibitory concentration (IC_{50}) of 0.23 μM compared with IC_{50} of 26.5 μM for gatifloxacin and IC_{50} of 27.2 μM for grepafloxacin (5). In a comparative study using patch-clamp electrophysiology, it was shown that quinolones inhibited the human HERG potassium currents, but with widely differing potencies. Among the quinolones tested, sparfloxacin was the most potent compound, displaying an IC_{50} of 18 μM, whereas ofloxacin was the least potent compound, with an IC_{50} value of 1,420 μM. Other IC_{50} were as follows: grepafloxacin, 50 μM; moxifloxacin, 129 μM; gatifloxacin, 130 μM; levofloxacin, 915 μM; and ciprofloxacin, 966 μM. Blockade of HERG channel by sparfloxacin displayed a positive voltage dependence. In contrast to HERG, the KvLQT1/minK potassium channel was not a target for blockade by the fluoroquinolones. These results provided a mechanism for the QT prolongation observed clinically with administration of sparfloxacin and certain other fluoroquinolones because free plasma levels of these drugs after therapeutic doses approximate those concentrations that inhibit HERG channel current. In levofloxacin, ciprofloxacin, and ofloxacin, inhibition of HERG

occurs at concentrations much greater than those observed clinically. The data indicate that clinically relevant HERG channel inhibition by the fluoroquinolones is not a class effect but is highly dependent on specific substitutions within the chemical structure of this series of compounds. Furthermore, there may be significant differences between quinolones, as shown by the large difference in the arrhythmogenic doses, for instance, between grepafloxacin (10 to 30 mg/kg) and ciprofloxacin (300 mg/kg) (103).

In a recent study on an in vivo rabbit arrhythmia model, sparfloxacin, moxifloxacin, gatifloxacin, and grepafloxacin were all shown to block I_{Kr} channel with descending order. Similarly, sparfloxacin prolonged the QT interval by 370 ± 30 ms, followed by moxifloxacin (270 ± 30 ms), grepafloxacin (280 ± 25 ms), and gatifloxacin(255 ± 23 ms) Fig. 5 and 6) (42). In isolated canine Purkinje fibers, sparfloxacin, grepafloxacin, moxifloxacin, and ciprofloxacin prolonged action potential in a descending order. The prolongation was inverse frequency dependent with larger increases in action potential duration occurring when the stimulation frequency was reduced to 0.5 Hz (43). The most comprehensive study was by

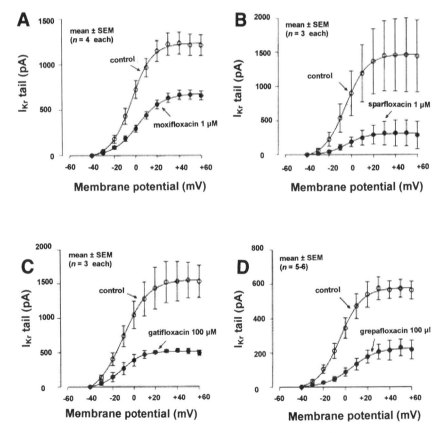

Figure 5. I_{Kr} blockade by quinolones (voltage-clamp study) showing voltage dependence of I_{Kr} blockade with sparfloxacin being the most potent I_{Kr} blocker, followed by grepafloxacin (equipotency as gatifloxacin) and moxifloxacin. Adapted from reference 85.

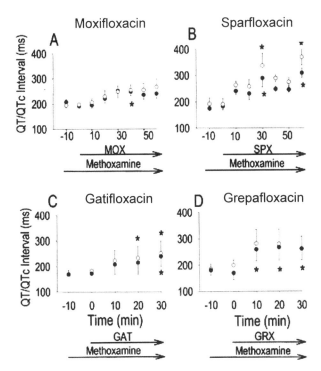

Figure 6. QT prolongation with quinolones (rabbit arrhythmia model) showing sparfloxacin is the most potent in prolonging the QT interval, followed by grepafloxacin (equipotency as gatifloxacin) and moxifloxacin. ○, QT; ●, QTc. *, $P < 0.05$ of baseline (both QT and QTc). Adapted and modified from reference 85.

Hagiwara et al. (49). They examined the effects of 10 fluoroquinolone antibacterial agents, namely, levofloxacin, sitafloxacin, trovafloxacin, ciprofloxacin, gemifloxacin, tosufloxacin, gatifloxacin, grepa-

floxacin, moxifloxacin, and sparfloxacin, on action potentials recorded from guinea pig ventricular myocardia. Sparfloxacin prolonged action potential duration (APD) by about 8% at 10 μM and by about 41% at 100 μM. Gatifloxacin, grepafloxacin, and moxifloxacin also prolonged APD at 100 μM by about 13, 24, and 25%, respectively. In contrast, levofloxacin, sitafloxacin, trovafloxacin, ciprofloxacin, gemifloxacin, and tosufloxacin had little or no APD-prolonging effect at concentrations as high as 100 μM (Fig. 7). Thus, the evidence from all these studies suggested that differences exist in the potency to prolong QT interval among the various fluoroquinolones, and the risk of arrhythmias is probably not a class effect. However, there is still a paucity of information and lack of objective data on the cardiac safety of other old and new quinolones, including norfloxacin, pefloxacin, fleroxacin, clinafloxacin, lomefloxacin, sitafloxacin, trovafloxacin, and tosufloxacin. Figure 8 summarizes the effect of the few most commonly investigated quinolones on I_{Kr} blockade, action potential prolongation, QT prolongation, and TdP.

EFFECTS OF QUINOLONES ON HEPATIC CYTOCHROME P450 ENZYMIC SYSTEM

Quinolones have varying effects on the hepatic cytochrome P450 system. For instance, enoxacin and ciprofloxacin inhibit the hepatic cytochrome P450 enzyme system; others, such as ofloxacin and lome-

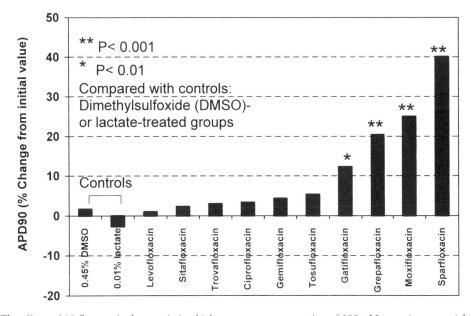

Figure 7. The effects of 10 fluoroquinolone antimicrobial agents at a concentration of 100 μM on action potential duration at 90% repolarization (ADP$_{90}$) of action potentials recorded from isolated guinea pig right ventricular myocardia (n = 4 to 6; mean ADP$_{90}$ in each group shown). This study showed the difference in the potency to prolong QT intervals among various fluoroquinolones. Modified from reference 49 with permission.

I_{Kr} Blockade (Descending order)	$\uparrow APD_{90}$* (Descending order)	$\uparrow$ QT (ms)	TdP
Sparfloxacin		9-28 (200-800mg)	+ (rabbit/dog)
Grepafloxacin		10	+ (human)
Moxifloxacin		6±26	?
Gatifloxacin	?	2.9±16.5	?
Levofloxacin	-	>60ms (9% of pts)	+ (human)
Ciprofloxacin		?	+ (human)
Ofloxacin	-	?	?

*Canine or rabbit Purkinje fibres

Figure 8. The effects of various quinolones on the I_{Kr} blockade, action potential prolongation, QT prolongation, and TdP.

floxacin have minimal effects on the system, whereas levofloxacin, gatifloxacin, and moxifloxacin have no effect at all on the system. Quinolones that inhibit hepatic cytochrome P450 enzyme should not be administered with other drugs that are metabolized by this enzymic system, especially other QT-prolonging drugs that are metabolized by the hepatic cytochrome P450 CYP3A4 (terfenadine, astemizole, ziprasidone, haloperidol, desipramine, and clomipramine). The coadministration of quinolones that inhibit hepatic cytochrome P450 enzyme and such drugs exacerbates the risk of TdP and must be avoided.

OTHER ANTIMICROBIALS AND ANTIMALARIALS THAT MAY PROLONG QT INTERVAL AND CAUSE TdP

Apart from quinolones, several other antimicrobials and antimalarials also have the propensity to cause QT prolongation and TdP. It is vital that physicians who prescribe multiple antimicrobials are aware of the potential synergistic proarrhythmia effect between different classes of antimicrobials.

Macrolides

Several recent anecdotal reports have identified that erythromycin, apart from inhibiting the hepatic

cytochrome P450 3A4 isoenzyme and increasing the concentration in serum of QT-prolonging drugs that are metabolized by hepatic enzymes such as terfenadine, can in itself cause QT prolongation (ranging from 0.56 to 0.70 s) and TdP (19, 40, 42, 46, 60, 93). Most of the patients who developed TdP were critically ill in the intensive care unit, but others had ischemic heart disease, congenital heart disease, or congenital long QT syndrome. Some patients were otherwise healthy, except for the chest infection for which erythromycin was prescribed. Most cases of proarrhythmia with erythromycin have occurred with intravenous infusion. However, oral erythromycin did prolong QT intervals by 13.8 ± 31 ms (3.7% ± 7.9%) as a comparator drug in one study, although the actual dosage and duration was unclear (55).

Erythromycin prolonged the action potential by inhibiting the delayed rectifier potassium current, I_{Kr} (95), preferentially on M cells compared with the epicardial or endocardial cells (9), and at high concentration (100 to 200 mg/liter), inducing phase 2 and phase 3 early after-depolarizations (95), which is the basis of its proarrhythmic tendency.

In a prospective evaluation of critically ill patients, erythromycin significantly prolonged the QTc interval from a baseline of 524 ± 105 ms to 555 ± 134 ms after slow infusion of the drug (mean rate, 8.9 ± 3.5 mg/min) compared with controls who received cephalosporins and had no change in their QTc interval (from 423 ± 96 to 419 ± 96 after infusion) (33,

118). The extent of QT prolongation correlated strongly with the erythromycin infusion rate (48) and the QT-prolonging effect is rapid (75). Therefore, intravenous erythromycin should always be administered as a slow infusion, and ECG monitoring should accompany erythromycin therapy, particularly in critically ill patients. Erythromycin should never be rapidly administered intravenously because it can lead to TdP, circulatory arrest, and death (14, 20). While QT prolongation with erythromycin is quite common, particularly in patients with heart disease, the incidence of TdP is rare despite the anecdotal cases reported (81). Erythromycin has also been reported to prolong QT further and/or TdP when it is coadministered with quinidine (68), cisapride (74), terfenadine (53), or ebastine (79), all of which are known to prolong QT intervals themselves.

Oral clarithromycin has also been reported to cause QT prolongation, TdP, or ventricular tachycardia in several cases (57, 63, 66, 91, 100, 119). In contrast, azithromycin and dirithromycin do not cause any further increase in QT interval compared with placebo when given to healthy men receiving terfenadine (10, 50). The risk of QT prolongation and TdP with other less commonly used macrolide antibiotics such as troleandomycin, josamycin, flurythromycin, and ponsinomycin is less clear (39). All macrolides (except azithromycin) are hepatic cytochrome P450 3A4 inhibitors and should therefore not be given concomitantly with any QT-prolonging drugs that are metabolized by hepatic cytochrome P450 3A4 isoenzyme, such as terfenadine and cisapride (74).

Azole Antifungals

The azole antifungal agents including imidazoles (ketoconazoles and miconazoles) and triazoles (itraconazole and fluconazole) have been reported to cause QT prolongation, either when given alone or concomitantly with other drugs such as nonsedating antihistamines (primarily terfenadine and astemizole) and tricyclic antidepressants (32, 87, 117, 121, 130). Ketoconazole prolongs the QT interval by the blocking the I_{Kr} channel (125). Although the blocking effect on the I_{Kr} channel by other azoles is less clear, it is probably a class effect.

Similar to macrolide antibiotics, ketoconazole and itraconazole also inhibit the hepatic cytochrome P450 CYP3A4 isoenzyme. Therefore, coadministration of ketoconazole, fluconazole, or itraconazole with other QT-prolonging drugs that are metabolized by the cytochrome P450 CYP3A4 isoenzyme will result in a markedly prolonged QT interval and increase the risk of TdP (4, 32, 87, 117, 130).

Antimalarials

Antimalarials deserve some attention because they are commonly prescribed worldwide. Quinine is the diastereomer of quinidine (59), and both drugs produce prolongation of the QT interval. The threshold for the quinidine effect was lower than that for quinine, but the change in QTc interval for a given change in free drug concentration was similar between the two drugs (59), although other workers have shown contrary results (124). The change in QT interval is not predictive of the plasma quinine concentration because the concentration within the therapeutic range produced only minor and unpredictable abnormalities. The effect of QT prolongation (as well as QRS interval prolongation) with intravenous quinine infusion (given at 5 mg/kg over 5 min) was greatest between 1 and 4 min after completion of the quinine infusion (123). The proarrhythmic risk of quinine is of particular concern in patients with acute renal failure, especially after 3 days of therapy (107).

The proarrhythmic risk of chloroquine is unclear despite two cases of TdP or ventricular fibrillation in the literature with a halofantrine overdose (25, 29). Of note, both chloroquine and halofantrine caused significant inhibition of hepatic cytochrome CYP2D6 enzymic activity at therapeutic loading doses. Therefore, the combination of these drugs with other drugs known to prolong the QT interval should be avoided, especially those that are metabolized significantly by CYP2D6 (101).

Halofantrine induced a dose-related PR and QT prolongation as well as syncope in adults with no preexisting QT prolongation (47, 65, 80) and in children who received therapeutic doses of halofantrine (88). Halofantrine also induced TdP and/or ventricular fibrillation in patients with congenital long QT syndrome (78, 114). At a standard dose of 24 mg/kg/day, halofantrine lengthened the QT interval duration from a mean QTc of 400 ms to 440 ms, and the maximum QT interval with halofantrine treatment was observed at 12 h after administration (73). The QTc interval significantly correlated with the plasma level of the parent drug halofantrine, but not with its plasma metabolite, N-desbutyl-halofantrine, level (77, 116). Like all QT-prolonging drugs, halofantrine is a potent inhibitor of the I_{Kr} channel with an IC_{50} value of 196.9 nM (113). Blockade of the I_{Kr} channel by halofantrine is predominantly caused by high-affinity binding to the open and inactivated channel states, with only a small contribution from lower-affinity binding to closed channels. Halofantrine is very highly bound in whole blood (83% to proteins in serum, 17% to erythrocytes), which may contribute partly to its potent cardiotoxicity (22).

Pentamidine

Since 1987, pentamidine has been reported to cause QT prolongation and TdP when given in intravenous form (16, 26, 43, 69, 76, 84, 89, 106, 111, 115, 122). In addition, pentamidine can also induce tachycardia, hypotension, T wave inversion, ST segment depression (56, 86, 122), and U wave alternans (16). Stein et al. estimated that the cumulative incidence of QT prolongation (defined as QTc > 480 ms) was 27% after 7 days and 50% during 14 of 21 days of intravenous pentamidine therapy (105). In another study, Eisenhauer et al. found that, among the patients receiving intravenous pentamidine therapy with QT prolongation, the risk of TdP was 75% (3 of 4 patients) if QTc prolongation was >480 ms or 60% (3 of 5 patients) if ΔQTc was 80 ms (36). However, the overall evidence suggested that the proarrhythmic risk of intravenous pentamidine appeared to be an idiosyncratic phenomenon rather than the outcome of cumulative dose-related effects (36, 41).

There is a lack of study on the electrophysiological properties of pentamidine. However, it is known that pentamidine is structurally similar to procainamide (122), and it is therefore reasonable to postulate that pentamidine shares the same proarrhythmic properties as procainamide. Despite the cardiotoxicity of intravenous pentamidine (84), inhalatory pentamidine is safe and did not prolong the QT interval, even when given at high dose (300 mg biweekly) for a prolonged period (>1 month) (21, 112).

Pentavalent Antimonial Meglumine

Pentavalent antimony is used to treat leishmaniasis and has been noted to cause abnormal repolarization, including QT prolongation, flattened and/or T wave, TdP, and syncope (23, 83, 94, 99). Repolarization abnormalities were related to the total daily dose of antimony and duration of treatment. Repolarization abnormalities are common when pentavalent antimony is used at doses above 20 mg/kg/day for more than 15 days, and life-threatening arrhythmias may occur if very high doses are used (23), but QTc prolongation of >500 ms has been reported in 11% of patients receiving short-term, low-dose pentavalent antimony (94).

FACTORS THAT MAY FURTHER PROLONG VENTRICULAR REPOLARIZATION OR PREDICT TdP

There are many causes of QT interval prolongation, although, by far, the most common is drug administration. The medications that can cause QT prolongation and TdP are listed in Table 1. It is important that those patients who receive multiple drugs have their medications cross-checked so that those drugs that have the propensity to prolong the QT interval and/or to cause TdP are not prescribed together. Apart from drugs, other conditions that are likely to cause QT prolongation include:

- Organic heart disease (e.g., congenital long QT syndrome [Fig. 9]; ischemic heart disease, congestive heart failure, dilated cardiomyopathy, hypertrophic cardiomyopathy, myocarditis, and Kawasaki syndrome) (2, 44, 72, 90; http://www.fda.gov/ohrms/dockets/ac/99/slides/3558s1/index.htm).
- Metabolic abnormalities, e.g., hypokalemia (by far the most common, Fig. 10), hypocalcemia, hypomagnesemia (3, 27, 61).
- Bradycardia, atrioventricular and sinoatrial blocks (18, 64).
- Drug-related factors (e.g., narrow therapeutic window, a multiplicity of pharmacological actions, and inhibition and induction of cytochrome P450 enzymes, polypharmacy) (109, 129, 130).
- Female gender because of reduced ion channel density differences (35, 67).
- Hepatic impairment (126).

PREVENTION AND TREATMENT OF DRUG-INDUCED QT PROLONGATION

In clinical practice, adverse proarrhythmic effects of quinolones may be prevented by not exceeding the recommended dose and by avoiding use in patients with preexisting heart disease or other risk factors, previous ventricular arrhythmias, and/or electrolyte imbalance such as hypokalemia. Concomitant administration of drugs that inhibit the cytochrome P450 (e.g., imidazole antifungals, macrolide antibiotics) (Table 2) or those that can prolong the QT interval or cause electrolyte disturbance should also be avoided. The serum potassium level should be checked regularly as a matter of routine care when the patient is taking potassium-depleting diuretics. Drugs that can prolong the QT interval should ideally be listed and regularly updated in a national drug formulary, which is not the case at present. Any adverse event suggestive of cardiac arrhythmias should be reported to drug safety authorities and/or drug manufacturers. In our institution, we routinely give out an advice leaflet regarding the risk of QT prolongation and TdP to at-risk

Table 1. Drugs that can prolong QT interval and TdP[a]

Drug type	Example
Antiarrhythmic drugs	Type 1A (TdP reported in all)
	Ajmaline (TdP reported)
	Aprindine
	Disopyramide (TdP reported)
	Procainamide (TdP reported)
	Quinidine (TdP reported)
	Type 1C (increase QT by prolonging QRS interval)
	Encainide
	Flecainide
	Moracizine
	Propafenone
	Type 3 (TdP reported in all)
	Amiodarone
	Dronedarone
	Sotalol
	d-Sotalol
	Bretylium
	Azimlijde
	Dofetilide
	Ersentilide
	Ibutilide
	Semantilide
	Trecetilide
	Tedisamil
	Almokalant
Calcium channel blocker	Prenylamine (TdP reported, withdrawn)
	Bepridil (TdP reported, withdrawn)
	Terodiline (TdP reported, withdrawn)
Psychiatric drugs	Chlorpromazine (TdP reported)
	Thioridazine (TdP reported)
	Droperidol (TdP reported)
	Haloperidol (TdP reported)
	Amitriptyline
	Nortriptyline
	Clomipramine
	Desipramine (TdP reported)
	Imipramine (TdP reported)
	Maprotiline (TdP reported)
	Chloral hydrate
	Doxepin (TdP reported)
	Lithium (TdP reported)
	Pimozide (TdP reported)
	Sertindole (TdP reported, withdrawn in the U.K.)
	Ziprasidone
Antihistamines	Astemizole (TdP reported)
	Diphenhydramine (TdP reported)
	Ebastine
	Hydroxyzine
	Loratadine
	Mizolastine
	Terfenadine (TdP reported, withdrawn in the U.S.)
Antimicrobial and antimalarial drugs . . .	Clarithromycin (TdP reported)
	Erythromycin (TdP reported)
	Fluconazole
	Itraconazole
	Ketoconazole
	Miconazoles
	Grepafloxacin (TdP reported, withdrawn worldwide)
	Levofloxacin (TdP reported)
	Moxifloxacin
	Sparfloxacin

Continued on following page

Table 1. (*Continued*)

Drug type	Example
	Chloroquine (TdP reported)Halofantrine (TdP reported)
	Quinine
	Pentamidine (TdP reported)
	Pentavalent antimonial meglumine
Prokinetics (serotonin agonists)	Cisapride (TdP reported, withdrawn in the U.S. and U.K.)
5HT$_2$ serotonin antagonist	Ketanserin (TdP reported, withdrawn in the U.S. and U.K.)
Immunosuppressant	Tacrolimus (TdP reported)
Antidiuretic hormone	Vasopressin (TdP reported)
Other agents	Adenosine (TdP reported)
	Organophosphates (TdP reported)
	Papaverine (TdP reported)
	Probucol (TdP reported)
	Cocaine

^{a}This list is not comprehensive.

groups such as patients who are prescribed multiple QT-prolonging drugs, have underlying heart disease, or have congenital long QT syndrome (Table 3). Several websites are available for the public to check out the risk of QT prolongation with a particular drug, although none is comprehensive (Table 3).

TdP is often self-limiting and associated with recurrent dizziness and syncope but may progress to ventricular fibrillation and sudden death. The management of patients with drug-induced TdP includes identifying and withdrawing the offending drug(s) and correcting any potassium and/or magnesium abnormalities. The potassium level should be replenished to 4.5 to 5 mmol/liter. The choices of treatment include intravenous infusion of magnesium sulfate (1 to 2 g), and, in resistant cases, isoproterenol or temporary atrial or ventricular cardiac pacing may be needed to increase the heart rate and shorten the QT

interval (102). Magnesium has no direct effect on the QT interval but reduces the I_{Ca-L} current and acts on the sodium/potassium-activated adenosine triphosphate system, which facilitates potassium influx into the cardiac cell and corrects abnormal repolarization (120).

REGULATORY PERSPECTIVE IN DRUG DEVELOPMENT

Apart from antiarrhythmics, many drugs capable of inducing TdP are noncardiac and are used for relatively benign conditions. Regulatory authorities are concerned that the risk should be identified and, if possible, quantified during the preclinical and clinical development of a drug. Currently, there are recommendations from the Committee for Proprietary

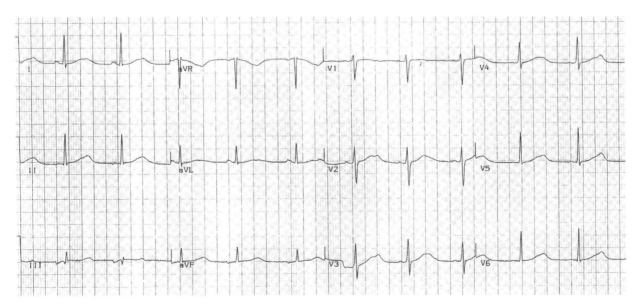

Figure 9. The electrocardiogram of a female patient with congenital long QT syndrome with a QTc interval of 573 ms.

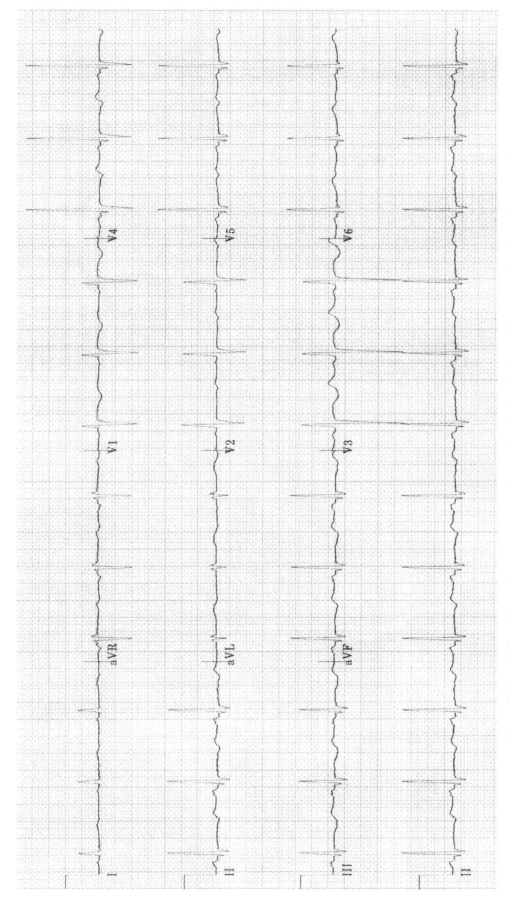

Figure 10. Acquired long QT syndrome in a patient with severe hypokalemia (2.6 mmol/liter). Note the prolonged QT interval of 639 ms and abnormal bizarre T/U wave.

REFERENCES

1. Adamantidis, M. M., B. M. Dumotier, J. P. Caron, and R. Bordet. 1998. Sparfloxacin but not levofloxacin or ofloxacin prolongs cardiac repolarization in rabbit Purkinje fibres. *Fund. Clin. Pharmacol.* **12:**70–76.

2. Ahnve, S. 1985. QT interval prolongation in acute myocardial infarction. *Eur. Heart J.* **6:**D85–D95.

3. Akiyama, T., J. Batchelder, J. Worsman, H. W. Moses, and M. Jedlinski. 1989. Hypocalcemic torsades de pointes. *J. Electrocardiol.* **22:**89–92.

4. Albengres, E., H. Le Louet, and J. P. Tillement, 1998. Systemic antifungal agents. Drug interactions of clinical significance. *Drug Safety* **18:**83–97.

5. Anderson, M. E., A. Mazur, T. Yang, and D. M. Roden. Comparison of K current antagonistic properties and proarrhythmic consequences of gatifloxacin, grepafloxacin and sparfloxacin, abstr. M161. *Spanish J. Chemother.*, in press.

6. Anderson, M. E., A. Mazur, T. Yang, and D. M. Roden. 2001. Potassium current antagonist properties and proarrhythmic consequences of quinolone antibiotics. *J. Pharmacol. Exp. Ther.* **296:**806–810.

7. Antzelevitch, C., J. M. Davidenko, S. Sicouri, et al. 1989. Quinidine-induced early afterdepolarization and triggered activity. *J. Electrophysiol.* **3:**323–338.

8. Antzelevitch, C., and S. Sicouri. 1994. Clinical relevance of cardiac arrhythmias generated by afterdepolarization: role of M cells in the generation of U wave, triggered activity, and torsades de pointes. *J. Am. Coll. Cardiol.* **23:**259–277.

9. Antzelevitch, C., Z. Q. Sun, Z. Q. Zhang, and G. X. Yan. 1996. Cellular and ionic mechanisms underlying erythromycin-induced long QT intervals and torsade de pointes. *J. Am. Coll. Cardiol.* **28:**1836–1848.

10. Bachmann, K., T. J. Sullivan, J. H. Reese, L. Jauregui, K. Miller, M. J. Scott, J. Stotka, and J. Harris. 1997. A study of the interaction between dirithromycin and astemizole in healthy adults. *Am. J. Ther.* **4:**73–79.

11. Balfour, J. A., and H. M. Lamb. 2000. Moxifloxacin: a review of its clinical potential in the management of community-acquired respiratory tract infections. *Drugs* **59:**115–139.

12. Ball, P., L. Mandell, Y. Niki, and G. Tillotson. 1999. Comparative tolerability of the newer fluoroquinolone antibacterials. *Drug Safety* **21:**407–421.

13. Ball, P. 2000. Quinolone-induced QT interval prolongation: a not-so-unexpected class effect. *J. Antimicrob. Chemother.* **45:**557–559.

14. Benoit, A., C. Bodiou, E. Villain, F. Bavoux, A. Checoury, and J. Badoual. 1991. QT prolongation and circulatory arrest after an injection of erythromycin in a newborn infant. *Arch. Fr. Pediatr.* **48:**39–41.

15. Bertino, J., Jr., and D. Fish. 2000. The safety profile of the fluoroquinolones. *Clin. Ther.* **22:**798–817.

16. Bibler, M. R., T. C. Chou, R. J. Toltzis, and P. A. Wade. 1988. Recurrent ventricular tachycardia due to pentamidine-induced cardiotoxicity. *Chest* **94:**1303–1306.

17. Bischoff, U., C. Schmidt, R. Netzer, and O. Pongs. 2000. Effects of fluoroquinolones on HERG currents. *Eur. J. Pharmacol.* **406:**341–343.

18. Brachmann, J., B. J. Scherlag, L. V. Rosenshtraukh, and R. Lazzara. 1983. Bradycardia-dependent triggered activity: relevance to drug-induced multiform ventricular tachycardia. *Circulation* **68:**846–856.

19. Brandriss, M. W., W. S. Richardson, and S. S. Barold. 1994. Erythromycin-induced QT prolongation and polymorphic ventricular tachycardia (torsades de pointes): case report and review. *Clin. Infect. Dis.* **18:**995–998.

20. Camilleri, J. F., J. C. Deharo, D. Panagides, P. Broin, T. Mesana, D. Blin, A. Mouly-Bandini, C. Dubouloz, A. Goudard, and J. R. Monties. 1989. Jet intravenous injection of erythromycin lactobionate. A possible cause of the occurrence of crisis in torsade de pointe. *Ann. Cardiol. Angelol.* **38:**657–659.

21. Cardoso, J. S., A. Mota-Miranda, C. Condo, B. Moura, F. Rocha-Goncalves, and H. Lecour. 1997. Inhalatory pentamidine therapy and the duration of the QT interval in HIV-infected patients. *Int. J. Cardiol.* **59:**285–289.

22. Cenni, B., J. Meyer, R. Brandt, and B. Betschart. 1995. The antimalarial drug halofantrine is bound mainly to low and high density lipoprotein in human serum. *Br. J. Clin. Pharmacol.* **39:**519–526.

23. Chulay, J. D., H. C. Spencer, and M. Mugambi. 1985. Electrocardiographic changes during treatment of leishmaniasis with pentavalent antimony (sodium stibogluconate). *Am. J. Trop. Med. Hyg.* **34:**702–709.

24. Colatsky, T. J. p. 304–340. *In* A. H. Weston and T. C. Hamilton (ed.), *Potassium Channel Modulators.* Blackwell Scientific Publications, Oxford, United Kingdom.

25. Collee, G. G., G. S. Samra, and G. C. Hanson. 1992. Chloroquine poisoning: ventricular fibrillation following 'trivial' overdose in a child. *Intensive Care Med.* **18:**170–171.

26. Cortess, L. M., R. A. Gasser, Jr., D. C. Bjornson, M. J. Dacey, and C. N. Oster. 1992. Prolonged recurrence of pentamidine-induced torsades de pointes. *Ann. Pharmacother.* **26:**1365–1369.

27. Curry, P., D. Fitchett, W. Stubb, and D. Krikler. 1976. Ventricular arrhythmias and hypokalaemia. *Lancet* ii:231–233.

28. De Ponti, F., E. Poluzzi, N. Montanaro, and J. Ferguson. 2000. QTc and psychotropic drugs. *Lancet* **356:**75–76.

29. Demaziere, J., J. M. Fourcade, O. T. Busseuil, P. Adeleine, S. M. Meyer, and J. M. Saissy. 1995. The hazards of chloroquine self prescription in west Africa. *J. Toxicol. Clin. Toxicol.* **33:**369–370.

30. Demolis, J. L., A. Charransol, C. Funck-Brentano, and P. Jaillon. 1996. Effects of a single oral dose of sparfloxacin on ventricular repolarization in healthy volunteers. *Br. J. Clin. Pharmacol.* **41:**499–503.

31. Dorr, M. B., R. D. Johnson, B. Jensen, D. Magner, T. Marbury, and G. H. Talbot. 1999. Pharmacokinetics of sparfloxacin in patients with renal impairment. *Clin. Ther.* **21:**1202–1215.

32. Dorsey, S. T., and L. A. Biblo. 2000. Prolonged QT interval and torsades de pointes caused by the combination of fluconazole and amitriptyline. *Am. J. Emerg. Med.* **18:**227–229.

33. Drici, M. D., B. C. Knollmann, W. X. Wang, and R. L. Woosley. 1998. Cardiac action of erythromycin: influence of female sex. *JAMA* **280:**1774–1776.

34. Dupont, H., J. F. Timsit, B. Souweine, B. Gachot, M. Wolff, and B. Regnier. 1996. Torsades de pointes probably related to sparfloxacin. *Eur. J. Clin. Microbiol. Infect. Dis.* **15:**350–351.

35. Ebert, S. N., X. K. Liu, and R. L. Woosley. 1998. Female gender as a risk for drug-induced cardiac arrhythmias: evaluation of clinical experimental evidence. *J. Womens Health* **7:**547–557.

36. Eisenhauer, M. D., A. H. Eliasson, A. J. Taylor, P. E. Coyne, Jr., and D. C. Wortham. 1994. Incidence of cardiac arrhythmias during intravenous pentamidine therapy in HIV-infected patients. *Chest* **105:**389–394.

37. El-Sherif, N., M. Chinushi, E. B. Caret, and M. Restivo. 1997. Electrophysiological mechanism of the characteristic electrocardiographic morphology of torsade de pointes tachyarrhythmias in the long-QT syndrome: detailed analysis of ventricular tridimensional activation patterns. *Circulation* 96:4392–4399.

38. **European Agency for the Evaluation of Medicinal Products. Human Medicines Evaluation Unit. Committee from Proprietary Medicinal Products (CPMP).** Points to consider: the assessment of the potential for QT interval prolongation by non-cardiovascular medicinal products. March 1997 (CPMP/986/96).

39. Fournier, P., G. Pacouret, and B. Charbonnier. 1993. A new cause of torsades de pointes: combination of terfenadine and troleandomycin. *Ann. Cardiol. Angeiol.* 42:249–252.

40. Freedman, R. A., K. P. Anderson, L. S. Green, and J. W. Mason. 1987. Effect of erythromycin on ventricular arrhythmias and ventricular repolarization in idiopathic long QT syndrome. *Am. J. Cardiol.* 59:168–169.

41. Girgis, I., J. Gualberti, L. Langan, S. Malek, V. Mustaciuolo, T. Costantino, and T. G. McGinn. 1997. A prospective study of the effect of IV pentamidine therapy on ventricular arrhythmias and QTc prolongation in HIV-infected patients. *Chest* 112:646–653.

42. Gitler, B., L. S. Berger, and S. D. Buffa. 1994. Torsades de pointes induced by erythromycin. *Chest* 105:368–372.

42a. **Glaxo Wellcome UK Ltd.** *Raxar Tablets. Summary of Product Characteristics.* Glaxo Wellcome.

43. Gonzalez, A., P. T. Sager, B. Akil, S. H. Rahimtoola, A. K. Bhandari. 1991. Pentamidine-induced torsades de pointes. *Am. Heart J.* 122:1489–1492.

44. Gottlieb, S. S., M. Cines, and J. Marshall. 1997. Torsades de pointes with administration of high-dose intravenous d-sotalol to a patient with congestive heart failure. *Pharmacotherapy* 17:830–831.

45. Grasela, D. M. 2000. Clinical pharmacology of gatifloxacin, a new fluoroquinolone. *Clin. Infect. Dis.* 31(Suppl. 2):S51–S58.

46. Guelon, D., B. Bedock, C. Chartier, and J. Harberer. 1986. QT prolongation and recurrent torsades de pointes during erythromycin lactobionate infusion. *Am. J. Cardiol.* 58:666.

47. Gundersen, S. G., M. Rostrup, E. von der Lippe, E. S. Platou, B. Myrvang, and G. Edwards. 1997. Halofantrine-associated ventricular fibrillation in a young woman with no predisposing QTc prolongation. *Scand. J. Infect. Dis.* 29:207–208.

48. Haefeli, W. E., R. A. Schoenenberger, Ph. Weiss, and R. Ritz. 1992. Possible risk for cardiac arrhythmia related to intravenous erythromycin. *Intensive Care Med.* 18:469–473.

49. Hagiwara, T., S. Satoh, Y. Kasai, and K. Takasuna. 2001. A comparative study of the various fluoroquinolones antibacterial agents on the cardiac action potential in guinea pig right ventricular myocardium. *Jpn. J. Pharmacol.* 87:231–234.

50. Harris, S., D. M. Hilligoss, P. M. Colangelo, M. Eller, and R. Okerholm. 1995. Azithromycin and terfenadine: lack of drug interaction. *Clin. Pharmacol. Ther.* 58:310–315.

51. Hii, J. T. Y., D. G. Wyse, A. M. Gillis, H. J. Duff, M. A. Solylo, and L. B. Mitchell. 1992. Precordial QT interval dispersion as a marker of torsade de pointes. *Circulation* 86:1376–1382.

52. Honig, P. K., D. C. Wortham, K. Zamani, D. P. Connor, J. C. Mulin, and L. R. Cantilena. 1993. Terfenadine-ketoconazole interaction. *JAMA* 269:1513–1518.

53. Honig, P. K., D. C. Wortham, K. Zamani, J. C. Mullin, D. P. Conner, and L. R. Cantilena. 1993. The effect of fluconazole on the steady-state pharmacokinetics and electrocardiographic pharmacodynamics of terfenadine in humans. *Clin. Pharmacol. Ther.* 53:630–636.

54. Ichida, F., N. S. Fatica, J. E. O'Loughlin, M. S. Snyder, K. H. Ehlers, and M. A. Engle. 1988. Correlation of electrocardiographic and echocardiographic changes in Kawasaki syndrome. *Am. Heart J.* 116:812–819.

55. Jaillon, P., J. Morganroth, I. Brumpt, and G. Talbot, for the Sparfloxacin Safety Group. 1996. Overview of electrocardiographic and cardiovascular safety data for sparfloxacin. *J. Antimicrob. Chemother.* 37(Suppl. A):161–167.

56. Jha, T.K. 1983. Evaluation of diamidine compound (pentamidine isethionate) in the treatment of resistant cases of kala-azar occurring in North Bihar, India. *Trans. R. Soc. Trop. Med. Hyg.* 77:167–170.

57. Kamochi, H., T. Nii, K. Eguchi, T. Mori, A. Yamamoto, K. Shimoda, and K. Ibaraki. 1999. Clarithromycin associated with torsades de pointes. *Jpn. Circ. J.* 63:421–422.

58. Kang, J., L. Wang, X. L. Chen, D. J. Triggle, and D. Rampe. 2001. Interactions of a series of fluoroquinolone antibacterial drugs with the human cardiac K(+) channel HERG. *Mol. Pharmacol.* 59:122–126.

59. Karbwang, J., T. M. Davis, S. Looareesuwan, P. Molunto, D. Bunnag, and N. J. White. 1993. A comparison of the pharmacokinetic and pharmacodynamic properties of quinine and quinidine in healthy Thai males. *Br. J. Clin. Pharmacol.* 35:265–271.

60. Katapadi, K., G. Kostandy, M. Katapadi, K. M. Hussain, and D. Schifter. 1997. A review of erythromycin-induced malignant tachyarrhythmia—torsade de pointes. A case report. *Angiology* 48:821–826.

61. Kay, G. N., V. J. Plumb, J. G. Arciniegas, R. W. Henthorn, and A. L. Waldo. 1983. Torsades de pointes: the long-short initiating sequence and other clinical features; observation in 32 patients. *J. Am. Coll. Cardiol.* 2:806–817.

62. King, D. E., R. Malone, and S. H. Lilley. 2000. New classification and update on the quinolone antibiotics. *Am. Fam. Physician* 61:2741–2748.

63. Kundu, S., S. R. Williams, S. P. Nordt, and R. F. Clark. 1997. Clarithromycin-induced ventricular tachycardia. *Ann. Emerg. Med.* 30:542–544.

64. Kurita, T., T. Ohe, N. Marui, N. Aihara, H. Takaki, S. Kamakura, M. Matsuhisa, and K. Shimomura. 1992. Bradycardia-induced abnormal QT prolongation in patients with complete heart block with torsades de pointes. *Am. J. Cardiol.* 69:628–633.

65. Laothavorn, P., J. Karbwang, K. Na Bangchang, D. Bunnag, and T. Harinasuta. 1992. Effect of mefloquine on electrocardiographic changes in uncomplicated falciparum malaria patients. *Southeast Asian J. Trop. Med. Public Health* 23:51–54.

66. Lee, K. L., M. H. Jim, S. C. Tang, and Y. T. Tai. 1998. QT prolongation and torsades de pointes associated with clarithromycin. *Am. J. Med.* 104:395–396.

67. Lehmann, M. H., S. Hardy, D. Archibald, B. Quart, and D. J. MacNeil. 1996. Sex difference in risk of torsades de pointes with d,l-sotalol. *Circulation* 94:2534–2541.

68. Lin, J. C., and H. A. Quasny. 1997. QT prolongation and development of torsades de pointes with the concomitant administration of oral erythromycin base and quinidine. *Pharmacotherapy* 17:626–630.

69. Lindsay, J., Jr. M. A. Smith, and J. A. Light. 1990. Torsades de pointes associated with antimicrobial therapy pneumonia. *Chest* 98:222–223.

70. Lipsky, B. A., M. B. Dorr, D. J. Magner, and G. H. Talbot. 1999. Safety profile of sparfloxacin, a new fluoroquinolone antibiotic. *Clin. Ther.* 21:148–159.

71. Liu, D. W., and C. Antzelevitch. 1995. Characteristics of the delayed rectifier current (IKr and IKs) in canine ventricular

epicardial, midmyocardial, and endocardial myocytes. A weaker IKs contributes to the longer action potential of the M cell. *Circ. Res.* **76:**351–365.

72. Martin, A. B., A. Garson Jr., and J. C. Perry. 1994. Prolonged QT interval in hypertrophic and dilated cardiomyoapthy. *Am. Heart J.* **127:**64–70.

73. Matson, P. A., S. P. Luby, S. C. Redd, H. R. Rolka, and R. A. Meriwether. 1996. Cardiac effects of standard-dose halofantrine therapy. *Am. J. Trop. Med. Hyg.* **54:**229–231.

74. Michalets, E. L., and C. R. Williams. 2000. Drug interactions with cisapride: clinical implications. *Clin. Pharmacokinet.* **39:**49–75.

75. Mishra, A., H. S. Friedman, and A. K. Sinha. 1999. The effects of erythromycin on the electrocardiogram. *Chest* **115:**983–986.

76. Mitchell, P., P. Dodek, L. Lawson, M. Kiess, and J. Russell. 1989. Torsades de pointes during intravenous pentamidine isethionate therapy. *Can. Med. Assoc. J.* **140:**173–174.

77. Monlun, E. P. Le Metayer, S. Szwandt, D. Neau, M. Longy-Boursier, J. Horton, and M. Le Bras. 1995. Cardiac complications of halofantrine: a prospective study of 20 patients. *Trans. R. Soc. Trop. Med. Hyg.* **89:**430–433.

78. Monlun, E., A. Leehardt, O. Pillet, M. C. Gaston Receveur, K. Bouabdallah, M. Longy-Boursier, J. C. Favarel-Garrigues, and M. Le Bras. 1993. Ventricular arrhythmia and halofantrine intake. Probable deleterious effect. Apropos of 3 cases. *Bull. Soc. Pathol. Exot Fil.* **86:**365–367.

79. Moss, A. J., P. Chaikin, J. D. Garcia, M. Gillen, D. J. Roberts, and J. Morganroth. 1999. A review of the cardiac systemic side-effects of antihistamines: ebastine. *Clin. Exp. Allergy* **29**(Suppl. 3):200–205.

80. Nosten, F., F. O. ter Kuile, C. Luxemburger, C. Woodrow, D. E. Kyle, T. Chongsuphajaisiddhi, N. J. White. 1993. Cardiac effects of antimalarial treatment with halofantrine. *Lancet* **341:**1054–1056.

81. Oberg, K. C., and J. L. Bauman. 1995. QT interval prolongation and torsades de pointes due to erythromycin lactobionate. *Pharmacotheraphy* **15:**687–692.

82. Olivier, C., C. Rizk, D. Zhang, and E. Jacqz-Aigrain. 1999. Long QTc interval complicating halofantrine therapy in 2 children with plasmodium falciparum malaria. *Arch. Pediatr.* **6:**966–970.

83. Ortega-Carnicer, J., R. Alcazar, M. De la Torre, and J. Benezet. 1997. Pentavalent antimonial-induced torsade de pointes. *J. Electrocardiol.* **30:**143–145.

84. Otsuka, M., H. Kanamori, S. Sasaki, J. Taguchi, H. Harano, K. Ogawa, M. Matsuzaki, H. Mohri, T. Okubo, S. Sumita, and H. Ochiai. 1997. Torsades de pointes complicating pentamidine therapy of Pneumocystis carinii pneumonia in acute myelogenous leukemia. *Intern. Med.* **36:**705–708.

85. Patmore, L., S. Fraser, D. Mair, and A. Templeton. 2000. Effects of sparfloxacin, grepafloxacin, moxifloxacin, and ciprofloxacin on cardiac action potential duration. *Eur. J. Pharmacol.* **406:**449–452.

86. Pearson, R. D., and E. L. Hewlett. 1985. Pentamidine for the treatment of Pneumocystis Carinii pneumonia and other protozoal diseases. *Ann. Intern. Med.* **103:**782–786.

87. Pohjola-Sintonen, S., M. Viitasalo, L. Toivonen, and P. Neuvonen. 1993. Itraconazole prevents terfenadine metabolism and increases risk of torsades de pointes ventricular tachycardia. *Eur. J. Clin Pharmacol.* **45:**191–193.

88. Priori, S. G., J. Barhanin, R. N. Hauer, W. Haverkamp, H. J. Jongsma, A. G. Kleber, W. J. McKenna, D. M. Roden, Y. Rudy, K. Schwartz, P. J. Schwartz, J. A. Towbin, and A. M. Wilde. 1999. Genetic and molecular basis of cardiac arrhythmias: impact on clinical management part III. *Circulation* **99:**674–681.

89. Pujol, M., J. Carratala, J. Mauri, and P. F. Viladrich. 1988. Ventricular tachycardia due to pentamidine isethionate. *Am. J. Med.* **84:**980.

90. Ramamurthy, S., K. K. Talwar, K. C. Goswami, S. Shrivastava, P. Chopra, S. Broor, and A. Malhotra. 1993. Clinical profile of proven idiopathic myocarditis. *Int. J. Cardiol.* **41:**225–232.

91. Ramirez, J., J. Jnowsky, G. H. Talbot, H. Zhang, and L. Townsend. 1999. Sparfloxacin versus clarithromycin in the treatment of community-acquired pneumonia. *Clin. Ther.* **21:**103–117.

92. Rees, S., and M. J. Curtis. 1996. Which cardiac potassium channel subtype is the preferable target for suppression of ventricular arrhythmia? *Pharmacol. Ther.* **69:**199–217.

93. Rezkalla, M. A., and C. Pochop. 1994. Erythromycin induced Torsades de Pointes: case report and review of the literature. *S. D. J. Med.* **47:**161–164.

94. Ribeiro, A. L., J. B. Drummond, A. C. Volpini, A. C. Andrade, and V. M. Passos. 1999. Electrocardiographic changes during low-dose, short-term therapy of cutaneous leishmaniasis with the pentavalent antimonial meglumine. *Braz. J. Med. Biol. Res.* **32:**297–301.

95. Rubart, M., M. L. Pressler, H. P. Pride, and D. P. Zipes. 1993. Electrophysiological mechanisms in a canine model of erythromycin-associated long QT syndrome. *Circulation* **88:**1832–1844.

96. Sakmann, B., and G. Trube. 1984. Conductance properties of single inwardly rectifying potassium channels in ventricular cells from guinea pig heart. *J. Physiol.* **347:**641–657.

97. Samaha, F. F. 1999. QTc interval prolongation and polymorphic ventricular tachycardia in association with levofloxacin. *Am. J. Med.* **107:**528–529.

98. Sanguinetti, M. C. and N. K. Jurkiewicz. 1990. Two components of cardiac delayed rectifier current: differential sensitivity to block by class III antiarrhythmic agents. *J. Gen. Physiol.* **96:**195–215.

99. Segura, I., and I. Garcia-Bolao. 1999. Meglumine antimoniate, amiodarone and torsades de pointes: a case report. *Resuscitation* **42:**65–68.

100. Sekkarie, M. A. 1997. Torsades de pointes in two chronic renal failure patients treated with cisapride and clarithromycin. *Am. J. Kidney Dis.* **30:**437–439.

101. Simooya, O. O., G. Sijumbil, M. S. Lennard, and G. T. Tucker. 1998. Halofantrine and chloroquine inhibit CYP2D6 activity in healthy Zambians. *Br. J. Clin. Pharmacol.* **45:**315–317.

102. Smith, S. J. 1994. Cardiovascular toxicity of antihistamines. *Otolaryngol. Head Neck Surg.* **111:**348–354.

103. Stahlmann, R., and H. Lode. 1999. Toxicity of quinolones. *Drugs* **58**(Suppl. 2):37–42.

104. Stahlmann, R., and R. Schwabe. 1997. Safety profile of grepafloxacin compared with other fluoroquinolones. *J. Antimicrob. Chemother.* **40**(Suppl. A):83–92.

105. Stein, K. M., C. Fenton, A. M. Lehany, P. M. Okin, and P. Kligfield. 1991. Incidence of QT interval prolongation during pentamidine therapy of pneucocytis carinil pneumonia. *Am. J. Cardiol.* **68:**1091–1094.

106. Stein, K. M., H. Haronian, G. A. Mensah, A. Acosta, J. Jacobs, and P. Kligfield. 1990. Ventricular tachycardia and torsades de pointes complicating pentamidine therapy of Pneucocytis carinii pneumonia in the acquired immunodeficiency syndrome. *Am. J. Cardiol.* **66:**888–889.

107. Sukontason, K., J. Karbwang, W. Rimchala, T. Tin, K. Na-Bangchang, V. Banmairuroi, and D. Bunnag. 1996. Plasma quinine concentrations in falciparum malaria with acute renal failure. *Trop. Med. Int. Health* **1:**236–242.

108. Reference deleted.

109. **Surawicz, B.** 1989. Electrophysiologic substrate of torsades de pointes: dispersion of repolarization or early afterdepolarization. *J. Am. Coll. Cardiol.* **14:**172–184.

110. **Tan, H. L., C. J. Y. Hou, M. R. Lauer, and R. J. Sung.** 1995. Electrophysiologic mechanism of the long QT interval syndrome and torsades de pointes. *Ann. Intern. Med.* **122:** 701–714.

111. **Taylor, A. J., R. W. Hull, P. E. Coyne, R. L. Woosley, and A. H. Eliasson.** 1991. Pentamidine-induced torsades de pointes: safe completion of therapy with inhaled pentamidine. *Clin. Pharmacol. Ther.* **49:**698–700.

112. **Thalhammer, C., J. R. Bogner, and G. Lohmoller.** 1993. Chronic pentamidine aerosol prophylaxis does not induce QT prolongation. *Clin. Investig.* **71:**319–322.

113. **Tie, H., B. D. Walker, C. B. Singleton, S. M. Valenzuela, J. A. Bursill, K. R. Wyse, S. N. Breit, and T. J. Campbell.** 2000. Inhibition of HERG potassium channels by the antimalarial agent halofantrine. *Br. J. Pharmacol.* **130:**1967–1975.

114. **Toivonen, L., M. Viitasalo, H. Siikamaki, M. Raatikka, and S. Pohjola-Sintonen.** 1994. Provocation of ventricular tachycardia by antimalarial drug halofantrine in congenital long QT syndrome. *Clin. Cardiol.* **17:**403–404.

115. **Topol, E. J., and B. B. Lerman.** 1988. Hypomagnesemic torsades de pointes. *Am. J. Cardiol.* **52:**1367–1368.

116. **Touze, J. E., J. Bernard, A. Keundjian, P. Imbert, A. Viguier, H. Chaudet, and J. C. Doury.** 1996. Electrocardiographic changes and halofantrine plasma level during acute falciparum malaria. *Am. J. Trop. Med. Hyg.* **54:**225–228.

117. **Tsai, W. C., L. M. Tsai, and J. H. Chen.** 1997. Combined use of astemizole and ketoconazole resulting in torsades de pointes. *J. Formos. Med. Assoc.* **96:**144–146.

118. **Tschida, S. J., D. R. Guay, R. J. Straka, L. L. Hoey, R. Johanning, and K. Vance-Bryan.** 1996. QTc-interval prolongation associated with slow intravenous erythromycin lactobionate infusions in critically ill patients: a prospective evaluation and review of the literature. *Pharmacotherapy* **16:**663–674.

119. **Van Haarst, A. D., G. A. van't Klooster, J. M. van Gerven, R. C. Schoemaker, J. C. van Oene, J. Burggraaf, M. C. Coene, and R. F. Cohen.** 1998. The influence of cisapride and clarithromycin on QT intervals in healthy volunteers. *Clin. Pharmacol. Ther.* **64:**542–546.

120. **Vukmir, R. B.** 1991. Torsades de pointes: a review. *Am. J. Emerg. Med.* **9:**250–255.

121. **Wassmann, S., G. Nickenig, and M. Bohm.** 1999. Long QT syndrome and torsades de pointes in a patient receiving fluconazole. *Ann. Intern. Med.* **131:**797.

122. **Wharton, J. M., P. A. Demopulos, and N. Goldschlager.** 1987. Torsades de pointes during administration of pentamidine isethionate. *Am. J. Med.* **83:**571–575.

123. **White, N. J., P. Chanthavanich, S. Krishna, C. Bunch, and K. Silamut.** 1983. Quinine disposition kinetics. *Br. J. Clin. Pharmacol.* **16:**399–403.

124. **White, N. J., S. Looareesuwan, and D. A. Warrell.** 1983. Quinine and quinidine: a comparison of ECG effects during the treatment of malaria. *J. Cardiovasc. Pharmacol.* **5:**173–175.

125. **Woosley, R. L., Y. Chen, J. P. Freiman, R. A. Gillis.** 1993. Mechanism of the cardiotoxic actions of terfenadine. *JAMA* **269:**1532–1536.

126. **Woosley, R. L.** 1996. Cardiac actions of antihistamines. *Annu. Rev. Pharmacol. Toxicol.* **36:**233–252.

127. **Yap, Y. G., and A. J. Camm.** 2000. Risk of torsades de pointes with non-cardiac drugs. *Br. Med. J.* **320:**1158–1159.

128. **Zechnich, A. D., J. R. Hedges, D. Eiselt-Proteau, D. Haxby.** 1994. Possible interactions with terfenadine or astemizole. *West. J. Med.* **160:**321–325.

129. **Zhang, M.-Q.** 1997. Chemistry underlying the cardiotoxicity of antihistamines. *Curr. Med. Chem.* **4:**171–184.

130. **Zimmermann, M., H. Duruz, O. Guinand, O. Broccard, P. Levy, D. Locatis, and A. Bloch.** 1992. Torsades de pointes after treatment with terfenadine and ketoconazole. *Eur. Heart J.* **13:**1002–1003.

Quinolone Antimicrobial Agents, 3rd ed.
Edited by David C. Hooper and Ethan Rubinstein
© 2003 ASM Press, Washington, D.C.

Chapter 27

Effects on Connective Tissue Structures

RALF STAHLMANN

Quinolones have the potential to damage cartilage as well as tendons, thus being able to cause unusual forms of adverse drug reactions. Arthropathy in juvenile animals is the best known of these effects and has been observed in all animal species and with all quinolones tested so far. Because of this chondrotoxic potential quinolones are contraindicated in children and adolescents in the growing phase and during pregnancy and lactation, although the significance of the findings for humans is still unclear (see below).

Less is known about the effects on the epiphyseal growth plate, tendons, and other connective tissue structures, than about quinolone-induced lesions of the immature articular cartilage in animals. Some limited data show that very young animals react more sensitively than animals at later developmental stages with respect to changes in the epiphyseal growth plate, but systematic studies defining the vulnerable window for this toxic effect are missing. Also, immature animals seem to be more sensitive than adults to toxic effects on tendons. The current knowledge about the various target tissues is summarized in this section, but first, some brief general remarks about pharmacokinetics in experimental animals and humans and about the hypothetical mechanism of the toxic effects on connective tissue structures are given.

EXPERIMENTAL DATA

General Aspects

Mechanism

The exact mechanism of quinolone-induced arthropathy or tendopathy is still unknown. Several proposals have been made over the years, but definitive data are still missing. Some results from our laboratory indicate that the affinity of the drugs for magnesium could be the crucial initial step (Table 1). When immature rats were fed a magnesium-deficient diet they developed cartilage lesions that could not be distinguished from lesions induced by quinolone treatment. Possibly, integrins, which mediate interaction between the cells and the extracellular matrix, are affected, since their function is critically regulated by divalent cations, such as magnesium (7, 31, 41). It has been shown before in rats that magnesium deficiency induces oxygen radicals and NO production in plasma and some tissues (26), although it is unknown if this induction also occurs in cartilage. However, a further consequence of the depletion of functionally available magnesium in joint cartilage could be the production of oxygen-derived reactive species, as observed in chondrocytes from quinolone-treated juvenile rabbits (11). In agreement with these results Simonin and co-workers demonstrated by Western blot analysis of mouse articular cartilage proteins oxidative damage to collagen in addition to a decrease in proteoglycan synthesis after treatment with pefloxacin (38).

Probably because of the disturbance of the cell-matrix interaction and oxidative stress, chondrocytes and/or cartilage matrix are finally irreversibly damaged, and characteristic blisters and clefts in the immature cartilage are formed. The finding that supplementation with magnesium and tocopherol diminishes quinolone-induced chondrotoxicity in immature rats supports this hypothesis (44). Furthermore, a pronounced synergistic toxicity exists between fluoroquinolone treatment and magnesium deficiency. Juvenile rats treated with low doses of a fluoroquinolone that induced no chondrotoxicity when given to rats with a normal magnesium status caused joint cartilage lesions when they were given to rats which had been kept on a magnesium-deficient diet for one week.

Interestingly, magnesium concentrations in joint cartilage from 28-day-old rats are significantly lower than those in younger or older rats. This difference

---

Ralf Stahlmann • Institute of Clinical Pharmacology and Toxicology, Freie Universität Berlin, Garystrasse 5, 14195 Berlin, Germany.

Table 1. Toxic effects of quinolones on connective tissue structures[a]

1. High concentrations in cartilage (tendon?)
2. Chelate complexes with Mg^{2+} (other cations?)
3. Reduction of functionally available Mg^{2+}
4. Reduction cannot be counterbalanced (not or poorly vascularized tissues!)
5. Reduction of Mg^{2+} concentration below a critical threshold
6. Mg^{2+} deficiency induces radical formation
7. Cartilage and tendon damage

[a] Effects are listed in sequence of events leading to tissue daamge.

might explain the "phase specificity" of quinolone-induced arthropathy, i.e., the pronounced sensitivity of immature animals during a certain developmental stage (55).

Similarities between the symptoms of a dietarily induced magnesium deficiency and those of quinolone-induced arthropathy have also been described in a second species. Lameness and gait alterations closely resembling those associated with quinolone-induced arthropathy were observed in magnesium-deficient beagles, but no histology was performed with cartilage samples from these dogs (48). More recent comparative studies showed that ultrastructural changes in canine cartilage are similar after ciprofloxacin treatment or in magnesium deficiency (45, 46).

Pharmacokinetics

Because the pharmacokinetics of fluoro-quinolones differ considerably between rodents and humans, data on bioavailability and on drug concentrations in plasma or target tissues in animals have to be taken into account if results from experiments in rats are compared with the human clinical situation. For example, the bioavailability of sparfloxacin in rats after gastric intubation is poor, with a high dose of 1,800 mg of sparfloxacin per kg of body weight, producing peak concentrations of drug in plasma that were less than 20 μg/ml (43).

Similarly, in immature rats a single dose of 600 mg of ofloxacin/kg of body weight (representing 100 times the therapeutic dose) results in a mean concentration in plasma of 33 μg/ml, which is only 5 to 10 times higher than those measured in patients during therapy with ofloxacin. Oral treatment of juvenile rats with 100 mg ofloxacin/kg of body weight b.i.d for 5 days corresponds to an exposure that is roughly equivalent to normal human exposure during therapy with high doses of the drug. Concentrations in joint cartilage are three times higher than the corresponding concentrations in plasma under these conditions (30).

In addition to the species differences, major differences exist between the pharmacokinetics of individual quinolones in rats. For example, concentrations of ciprofloxacin in plasma were significantly lower than those of ofloxacin after the same doses (6, 42). Peak concentrations measured after a single, oral dose of 1,200 mg of ciprofloxacin or ofloxacin per kg in juvenile rats were 5.1 ± 2.3 and 45.4 ± 12.4 mg/liter, respectively.

Effects on Immature Joint Cartilage (Articular-Epiphyseal Cartilage Complex)

Quinolone-induced arthropathy has been observed almost exclusively in animals during defined postnatal periods of rapid growth. Therefore, the drugs are restrictively used in children and adolescents. Elderly persons who are prone to cartilage diseases might be considered another possible population at risk, but no clinical data and only a few animal experiments are available addressing this topic. Pefloxacin is the only drug that has been reported to induce arthropathies in adult dogs after 12 months of oral treatment. However, no details of these experiments, such as age of dogs at start of treatment, are available (8). When 15-month-old rats were treated for 4 weeks with daily doses of ofloxacin that were high enough to induce chondrotoxicity in juvenile rats and were given simultaneously a magnesium-deficient diet, no cartilage defects were found histologically in the knee joints of these animals. However, cartilage defects in adult rats were detectable when the animals had been treated several months before during the sensitive period of postnatal development (6, 8).

The reasons for the special vulnerability of immature animals is unknown, but the fact that the juvenile cartilage layer is thicker than adult joint cartilage might be *one* possible explanation why, in the nonvascularized tissue, a lack of functionally available magnesium (or other cations) is not readily counterbalanced. Dogs are more sensitive than other species to cartilage defects inducible with rather low doses of quinolones (10 to 50 mg/kg of body weight). Initially, arthropathy was described in dogs more than 20 years ago after oral administration of the nonfluorinated quinolones nalidixic acid, oxolinic acid, and pipemidic acid. Blisters and erosions in articular cartilage were detected at autopsy; clinical recovery usually occurred within 2 or 3 weeks, but the cartilage lesions were present several months after withdrawal of the drug (13, 49).

Corresponding results have been found with all of the newer fluoroquinolones developed so far (e.g., ciprofloxacin, ofloxacin, levofloxacin, fleroxacin, sparfloxacin, moxifloxacin, gatifloxacin, gemifloxacin, etc.), but only a few comparative studies have been published. In two such studies in immature dogs and rats, grepafloxacin was described as having a relatively low potential for joint toxicity, but pharmacokinetic differences between grepafloxacin and the comparative quinolones probably are the main reason for these differences (50, 51).

Garenoxacin is a non-6-fluorinated quinolone that seems to be less chondrotoxic than other quinolones. It was selected for clinical development from a series of related quinolones because it exhibited less cytotoxicity in a screening in vitro test relative to other quinolones, e.g., the corresponding 6-fluoro-derivative (20). Kawamura and coworkers performed a comparative study with garenoxacin, norfloxacin, and ciprofloxacin. The drugs were given orally to 3-month-old dogs at a daily dose of 50 mg/kg for 1 week. Blister formation was less pronounced with garenoxacin than with the other two agents. The results were confirmed under similar conditions but with intravenous injection (19).

The chondrotoxic potential was also relatively low in juvenile rats, which can be used as a model for quinolone-induced chondrotoxicity (6, 7, 17, 40, 41, 43). When given orally for 1 or 3 months, garenoxacin at daily doses of 400 mg/kg or more induced erosions, blisters, and chondrocyte degeneration in joint cartilage from rats that were 6 weeks of age at the start of the treatment. However, histological changes in knee joints from 4-week-old rats were not detectable when treated with daily doses of 600 mg/kg for a period of 5 days only, resembling more closely the length of a possible treatment period. Similarly, ciprofloxacin was not chondrotoxic under these conditions, but ofloxacin induced lesions in knee joint cartilage (47).

Peak concentrations of garenoxacin in plasma in 4-week-old rats following repeated daily administration of 600 mg/kg were 25 μg/ml. Data on the kinetic behavior of the drug in pediatric patients are not available, but first results in adults show that after an oral dose of 400 mg, peak concentrations in plasma reach approximately 5 to 6 μg/ml and thus are considerably lower than those reached in the toxicological experiment (9). In a further study starting treatment with garenoxacin in 4-day-old rats, peak concentrations in plasma of more than 75 μg/ml were measured. Also under these conditions no histological changes were noted, but on an ultrastructural level effects of the drug on chondrocytes and tenocytes were demonstrated (5, 36).

Taken together, available information indicates that all quinolones (fluorinated or nonfluorinated) induce joint cartilage lesions in immature animals

from multiple species. Minimal doses producing an effect are low in dogs (10 to 50 mg/kg of body weight), which represent the most sensitive species, but the immature rat is a suitable model to study the effects more systematically if the pharmacokinetic differences between rodents and humans are considered. Very little is known about the effects of fluoroquinolones during the neonatal period, but in early developmental phases the epiphyseal growth plate in addition to the articular cartilage appears to be a sensitive target.

Effects on Epiphyseal Growth Plates

The effects of trovafloxacin mesylate at daily doses of 75 mg/kg were studied by the manufacturer of the drug in immature Sprague-Dawley rats from postnatal day 4 to postnatal day 55. The peak concentration of trovafloxacin was 11.3 μg/ml on study day 1. This treatment induced an apparent interruption of normal growth, which was evident in reduced body size and lower body weights when compared with control animals. The gait alterations observed were the result of morphological changes in the cartilage of growth plates that included changes in the shape and lengths of the long bones in the fore- and hindlimbs of young adult rats (24). Clefts in the epiphyseal growth plate were also observed when trovafloxacin was given to rats from day 8 to 35 at doses of 50 or 100 mg/kg of body weight or at one single dose of 200 mg/kg on day 4 postnatally, a dose that was also associated with signs of general toxicity (25).

Effects on the epiphyseal growth plate have also been reported after treatment with moxifloxacin in immature dogs. When beagles aged 10 to 12 weeks were treated with moxifloxacin, degeneration of the matrix as well as the chondrocytes was observed in the epiphyseal growth plates; however, no such effects were found in 18- to 22-week-old dogs under otherwise identical conditions. Chondrotoxic effects on immature articular cartilage were seen in beagles at both developmental stages at lower doses of moxifloxacin (54).

A 3-week treatment period with garenoxacin starting during the first week postnatally (days 4 to 24 postnatally) did not induce defects in articular or epiphyseal cartilage, but ultrastructural findings showed that this quinolone also has the potential to damage chondrocytes (5).

Effects on Tendons

In addition to the clinical experience many toxicological studies have been published confirming that quinolone-induced tendinopathy is a drug-induced, dose-dependent toxic effect of these agents. Kato and coworkers described edema with mononuclear cell infiltration in the inner sheath of the Achilles tendon after single oral administration of pefloxacin or ofloxacin. The tendon lesions were induced in juvenile rats (4 weeks of age) but not in 12-week-old rats (18). Tendon lesions were inhibited by coadministration with dexamethasone and N-nitro-L-arginine methyl ester. Phenidone (1-phenyl-3-pyrazolidinone) and 2-(12-hydroxydodeca-5,10-diynyl)3,5,6-trimethyl-1,4-benzoquinone (AA861) also decreased the incidence of tendon lesions. In contrast, several other agents did not modify these tendon lesions. Overall, the results suggest that nitric oxide and 5-lipoxigenase products partly mediate fluoroquinolone-induced tendon lesions (16).

A group of French toxicologists investigated the effect of pefloxacin on Achilles tendon proteoglycans and collagen in rodents and showed convincingly that quinolone-induced oxidative stress on the Achilles tendon altered proteoglycan anabolism and oxidized collagen. Biphasic changes in proteoglycan synthesis were observed after single administration of pefloxacin, consisting of an early inhibition followed by a repair-like phase. Pefloxacin treatment for several days induced oxidative damage of collagen type I, with the alterations being identical with those observed in the experimental tendinous ischemia and reperfusion model. Oxidative damage was prevented by coadministration of N-acetylcysteine (39).

Ultrastructural alterations in tenocytes can be observed in juvenile and adult rats after treatment with quinolones. Effects were more pronounced when the animals were simultaneously given a magnesium-deficient diet, suggesting that the pathophysiology of tendopathy resembles that of arthropathy (32). In Achilles tendons from quinolone-treated adult rats, specific pathological alterations were demonstrated at the lowest dose level (30 mg/kg) and increased in severity with increasing doses. Tenocytes detached from the extracellular matrix and exhibited degenerative changes, such as multiple vacuoles and large vesicles in the cytoplasm that resulted from swellings and dilatations of cell organelles (mitochondria, endoplasmic reticulum). Other findings were a general decrease of the fibril diameter and an increase in the distance between the collagenous fibrils (33, 34).

Figure 1 provides an example of a tenocyte from a juvenile rat after treatment with ciprofloxacin in comparison to a cell from a control rat. Similar changes were observed after treatment with ofloxacin or garenoxacin (36).

The effects of ciprofloxacin or a magnesium-deficient diet on cellular or matrix proteins of Achilles tendons in immature dogs were studied quantitatively by Western blot analysis. Densitometric analysis of the immunoblots with anticollagen type I, antielastin, antifibronectin, and antiintegrin antibodies showed a

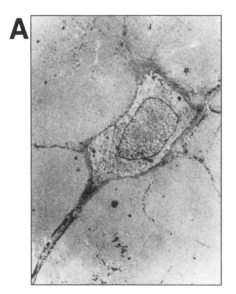
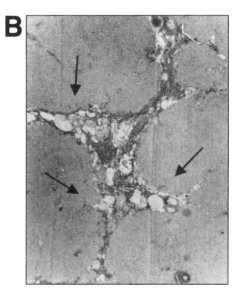

Figure 1. Tenocytes from rat achilles tendons. (A) Rat was treated orally with the vehicle from day 32 to day 36 postnatally. (B) Rat was treated orally with 600 mg ciprofloxacin/kg of body weight from day 32 to day 36 postnatally. In comparison with the controls, cellular as well as matrix alterations are detectable by electron microscopy in tendon samples from quinolone-treated rats. Note the vacuoles and large vesicles in the cytoplasm of tenocytes (arrows) resulting from swellings and dilatations of cell organelles (mitochondria, endoplasmic reticulum). Cells are detached from the matrix, and the fibril diameter is decreased in the ciprofloxacin-treated rats. Similar changes were observed in Achilles tendons after treatment with ofloxacin or garenoxacin. Reprinted from reference 33a with permission.

significant reduction of all proteins isolated from the tendons with a buffer that extracted a soluble protein fraction. Results were similar for the ciprofloxacin-treated dogs as well as the magnesium-deficient dogs. These findings support our hypothesis that quinolone-induced toxic effects on connective tissue structures are caused by the magnesium-antagonistic effects of these antibacterial agents. They also indicate that patients with a latent magnesium deficiency could be at an increased risk of quinolone-induced tendon disorders (35).

Effects on Other Structures

Diminished healing during the early stages of femoral fracture repair was described in adult rats after exposure to therapeutic concentrations of ciprofloxacin in serum for 3 weeks. Radiographic, histological, and biomechanical methods were used to evaluate fracture healing. Radiographs revealed significantly more advanced healing of the control fractures than the fractures in the ciprofloxacin-treated group. Fracture calluses in the animals treated with ciprofloxacin showed abnormalities in cartilage morphology and endochondral bone formation and a significant decrease in the number of chondrocytes compared with the controls (12).

CLINICAL DATA

Arthropathy

A clear-cut relationship between quinolones and arthropathia has only been established in animal experiments (see "Experimental Data" above). If there is a risk for acute chondrotoxicity for humans under therapeutic conditions, it is apparently small. The most extensive experience with quinolone therapy in children comes from patients with cystic fibrosis who were treated with ciprofloxacin (28). Overall, arthralgia occurred in 1.5% of the treatment courses ($n = 2,030$ courses in 1,795 children) and resolved without intervention; there was no unequivocal documentation of quinolone-induced arthropathy in any case. The interpretation of these data with respect to the causal relationship is complicated by the fact that the disease cystic fibrosis itself is associated with arthropathy, but there was no evidence that treatment with ciprofloxacin was associated with an increased rate of musculoskeletal adverse events (10).

Because the risk for arthropathy may be higher for other fluoroquinolones (e.g., pefloxacin) and because cartilage lesions are not always associated with clinical symptoms, these studies with ciprofloxacin cannot prove the complete lack of chondrotoxic effects of any quinolone treatment. Furthermore, it cannot be completely excluded that irreversible cartilage alterations arise that may lead to clinical symptoms only after many years.

Several case reports of severe acute arthralgia during therapy with older quinolones, as well as during treatment with fluoroquinolones, are available. Soon after the marketing of nalidixic acid, patients who developed severe arthralgia with painful joint swelling were described (1, 21). The highest incidence of arthropathy in humans reported to date was observed after treatment with pefloxacin. Arthropathies were observed in 8 of 63 (14%) patients with cystic fibrosis during treatment with pefloxacin, but in a similar group of patients treated with ofloxacin no joint complications were observed. These data were not generated from a prospective or direct comparative study, but all patients were suffering from cystic fibrosis and two different quinolones were utilized in the same hospital, in some instances even to the same patients. Five patients who did develop arthralgia under treatment with pefloxacin did not show any joint complications during treatment with ofloxacin (22).

In summary, human experience with ciprofloxacin seems to indicate that no or minimal risks for quinolone-induced arthropathy exist. Animal experiments, on the other hand, have clearly shown that the immature joint cartilage during rapid postnatal growth represents a sensitive target for the toxic effects of quinolones. The effects (i) are dose- and phase-dependent, (ii) probably depend on the duration of treatment, and (iii) are different among the individual quinolones, although all drugs of this class known so far have the *potential* to induce joint cartilage defects. It is still difficult to estimate the relevance of the toxicological data for humans, and it has been argued that the rapid postnatal growth of animals used for toxicological studies provides an explanation for their relative sensitivity to the chondrotoxic effects of quinolones. Certainly, human data must be analyzed for each individual drug, and it is completely unacceptable to generalize, as for example, the favorable experience with ciprofloxacin for the whole group of quinolones. It must be considered that our experience with "quinolones in children" does not equally concern all drugs of that class. Ciprofloxacin and norfloxacin, which are often cited as examples for the fact that "quinolones are safe in children," have in common a rather low bioavailability, with areas under the curve significantly lower than those of other quinolones. This pharmacokinetic feature might explain why the clinical experience is favorable. For other quinolones with a higher "internal exposure" due to better absorption characteristics and/or longer elimination half-life, the risks might be totally different. Available, limited clinical data underline these assumptions, at least in pefloxacin. With the given uncertainties most pediatricians and toxicologists agree in the recommendation that quinolones "should never be used in pediatrics for routine treatment when alternative safe and effective antimicrobials are known" (29).

Tendinopathy

Another toxic reaction of a connective tissue structure is tendinopathy. With regard to the clinical manifestations of this adverse reaction, several phases can be distinguished. Congestive and/or inflammatory edema is the earliest sign and can mimic venous thrombosis. The tendon then becomes painful and swollen, and in half of the cases the symptoms are bilateral. Failure to take appropriate therapeutic measures at this stage may lead to tendon rupture. The manifestations persist for several weeks or months and result in significant functional impairment (15).

Two decades ago Bailey and coworkers first described two patients after renal transplantation who developed tendinitis during treatment with norfloxacin (2). In 1991, the first cases of fluoroquinolone-associated tendon ruptures were reported; nearly 1,000 cases of fluoroquinolone-induced tendinitis had been reported to the French surveillance agency by 1997. Fewer cases have been reported in other countries. Pefloxacin is the fluoroquinolone that is most often associated with cases of tendinitis; the fact that this drug is mainly marketed in France could explain some of the geographic disparities, but underreporting seems to be a more important aspect. In a compilation of more than 400 cases, treatment with ofloxacin, norfloxacin, and ciprofloxacin as well as pefloxacin was associated with tendinitis and tendon ruptures. Of major concern is the fact that Achilles tendon ruptures have been described to occur for as long as 120 days after start of treatment and can occur even several months after withdrawal of the drug (23).

Reports from The Netherlands, Switzerland, and other countries are similar to the French experience. The first extensive retrospective study in approximately 11,000 patients treated with antibiotics identified four cases of tendinitis in 418 patients treated with ofloxacin, indicating that the risk for tendon disorders might be higher than had been assumed. Achilles tendinitis had a relative risk of 10.1 (95% confidence interval (CI), 2.2 to 46.0) for ofloxacin but no significant association was found for ciprofloxacin (relative risk, 2.8; 95% CI, 0.3 to 25.2) or norfloxacin (Table 2). Among 1,030 patients who had received prescriptions for norfloxacin, no case of Achilles tendinitis was identified (52). The authors also provided detailed information on 42 spontaneous reports of fluoroquinolone-associated tendon disorders, including ten patients with tendon rupture. Sixteen cases were attributed to ofloxacin, 13 to ciprofloxacin, 8 to norfloxacin, and 5 to pefloxacin. There was a male predominance, and the median age of the patients was 68 years. In most reports the Achilles tendon was affected, and 57% of the patients had bilateral tendonitis. The latency period between the start of treatment and the appearance of the first symptoms ranged from 1 to 150 days with a median of 6 days. Again, ofloxacin was implicated most frequently, relative to the number of filled prescriptions in The Netherlands (53).

An analysis from the Naval Medical Center San Diego revealed that among 2,122 patients who had received a prescription for ciprofloxacin, no case of Achilles tendon rupture was noticed. Unfortunately, data are only published as a brief letter to the editor and no details, e.g., on the doses of ciprofloxacin, the age of the patients, or underlying diseases, are given (37).

Table 2. Risk for Achilles tendinitis by fluoroquinolones compared with other antibacterial agents[a]

Drug (no. of patients)	No. of patients with tendinitis (total)/ Achilles tendinitis	Risk period[b] (days)	ID /100,000 days[c]	Relative risk (crude) (95% CI)	Relative risk (adjusted)[d] (95% CI)
Reference drugs[e] (9,406)	15/4	458,237	0.87	1.0	1.0
Ofloxacin (418)	4/3	18,929	15.85	18.2 (4.1–81.1)	10.1 (2.2–46.0)
Ciprofloxacin (456)	2/1	20,461	4.89	5.6 (0.63–50.1)	2.8 (0.3–25.2)
Norfloxacin (1,030)	1/0	50,981			

[a] Modified from van der Linden et al. (52) with permission from Blackwell Publishing, Ltd.
[b] Defined as the exposed period plus 1 month.
[c] Incidence density (ID) was calculated by dividing the number of events occurring in the risk windows by the total risk period; expressed as number of events per 100,000 days at risk.
[d] Adjusted for age, gender, GP visits, and concomitant corticosteroid use.
[e] Amoxicillin, trimethoprim, cotrimoxazole, and nitrofurantoin; a fluoroquinolone may have been prescribed to the same patient outside the risk period.

Isolated case reports point out that besides the Achilles tendon other tendons can be regarded as a target of quinolone toxicity. As an example, the case of a spontaneous rupture of the patellar ligament in a 37-year-old man participating in leisure sports can be mentioned. The event occurred one month after a 3-week course of ciprofloxacin (27). The subscapularis tendon was affected in a 54-year-old patient after a 10-week course of ciprofloxacin for recurrent prostatitis (500 mg twice daily). He developed marked anterior shoulder pain associated with mild stretching exercises; magnetic resonance imaging showed a partial tear of the subscapularis tendon (3).

One of the most important aspects connected with quinolone-induced tendinopathies is the question of additional risk factors that render patients susceptible to this rare and unusual adverse effect of a group of antibacterial agents. Uncertainties exist, because although the phenomenon has been known for several decades, the data are still poor. The main sources of information are case reports, compilations from administrative authorities, or isolated retrospective studies that cover only the older compounds. A need clearly exists for a prospective study, especially if valid statements on the incidences of the effects are to be made. A well-conducted case control study would be helpful to clarify the question of additional risk factors. So far, it seems that the risk is increased in older patients (>60 years), patients who are on long-term glucocorticoid treatment, and patients with chronic renal diseases, but it must be stressed that cases have been described in patients without any of these conditions. On the other hand, clinical evidence indicates that spontaneous tendon ruptures can also occur without quinolone treatment, for example in patients on chronic dialysis, and might be associated with poorly controlled hyperparathyroidism (14). These confounding factors emphasize the need for further studies on this topic to better define the role of quinolone treatment in cases of patients with renal diseases. Without any doubt, however, quinolones do have the potential to cause adverse effects on tendons, and these effects are only one of several clinical manifestations of the potential toxic effects of quinolones on connective tissue structures.

REFERENCES

1. Bailey, R. R., R. Natale, and A. L. Linton. 1972. Nalidixic acid arthralgia. *Can. Med. Assoc. J.* **107:**604–607.
2. Bailey, R. R., J. A. Kirk, and B. A. Peddie. 1983. Norfloxacin-induced rheumatic disease. *N. Z. Med. J.* **96:**590.
3. Casparian, J. M., M. Luchi, R. E. Moffat, and D. Hinthorn. 2000. Quinolones and tendon ruptures. *South. Med. J.* **93:**488–491.
4. Christ, W., T. Lehnert, and B. Ulbrich. 1988. Specific toxicologic aspects of the quinolones. *Rev. Infect. Dis.* **10**(Suppl. 1):S141–S146.
5. Fassheber, S., E.-M. Kappel, K. Riecke, U. Rahm, M. Shakibaei, and R. Stahlmann. 2001. Chondrotoxicity of ofloxacin compared with BMS-284756 in juvenile rats, abstr. no. 2207. *In Program and Abstracts of the 41st Interscience Conference on Antimicrobial Agents and Chemotherapy.* American Society for Microbiology, Washington, D.C.
6. Förster, C., K. Kociok, M. Shakibaei, H.-J. Merker, and R. Stahlmann. 1996. Quinolone-induced cartilage lesions are not reversible in rats. *Arch. Toxicol.* **70:**474–481.
7. Förster, C., K. Kociok, M. Shakibaei, H.-J. Merker, J. Vormann, T. Günther, and R. Stahlmann. 1996. Integrins on joint cartilage chondrocytes and alterations by ofloxacin or magnesium deficiency in immature rats. *Arch. Toxicol.* **70:**261–270.
8. Förster, C., R. Schwabe, E. Lozo, U. Zippel, J. Vormann, T. Günther, H.-J. Merker, and R. Stahlmann. 1997. Quinolone-induced arthropathy: Exposure of magnesium-deficient aged rats or immature rats, mineral concentrations in target tissues and pharmacokinetics. *Arch. Toxicol.* **72:**26–32.
9. Gajjar, D. A., D. M. Grasela, A. Bello, Z. Ge, and L. Christopher. 2000. Safety, tolerability, and pharmacokinetics of BMS-284756, a novel des-F(6)-quinolone, following single oral doses in healthy adult subjects, abstr. 2259. *In Progress and Abstracts of the 40th Interscience Conference on Antimicrobial Agents and Chemotherapy.* American Society for Microbiology, Washington, D.C.
10. Hampel, B., R. Hullmann, and H. Schmidt. 1997. Ciprofloxacin in pediatrics: worldwide clinical experience based on compassionate use: safety report. *Pediatr. Infect. Dis.* **16:**127–129.
11. Hayem, G., P. X. Petit, M. Levacher, C. Gaudin, M. E. Kahn, and J. J. Pocidalo. 1994. Cytofluorometric analysis of chondrotoxicity of fluoroquinolone antimicrobial agents. *Antimicrob. Agents Chemother.* **38:**243–247.
12. Huddleston, P.M., J. M. Steckelberg, A. D. Hanssen, M. S. Rouse, M. E. Bolander, and R. Patel. 2000. Ciprofloxacin inhibition of experimental fracture healing. *J. Bone Joint Surg. Am.* **82:**161–173.
13. Ingham, B., D. W. Brentnall, E. A. Dale, and J. A. McFadzean. 1977. Arthropathy induced by antibacterial fused N-alkyl-4-pyridone-3-carboxylic acids. *Toxicol. Lett.* **1:**21–26.
14. Jones, N., and C. M. Kjellstrand. 1996. Spontaneous tendon ruptures in patients on chronic dialysis. *Am. J. Kidney Dis.* **28:**861–866.
15. Kahn, M.-F., and G. Hayem. 1997. Tendons and fluoroquinolones. Unresolved issues. *Rev. Rhum.* (English Edition) **64:**437–439.
16. Kashida, Y., and M. Kato. 1997. Characterization of fluoroquinolone-induced Achilles tendon toxicity in rats: comparison of toxicities of 10 fluoroquinolones and effects of antiinflammatory compounds. *Antimicrob. Agents Chemother.* **41:**2389–2393.
17. Kato, M., and T. Onodera. 1988. Morphological investigation of cavity formation in articular cartilage induced by ofloxacin in rats. *Fund. Appl. Toxicol.* **11:**110–119.
18. Kato, M., S. Takada, Y. Kashida, and M. Nomura. 1995. Histological examination on Achilles tendon lesions induced by quinolone antibacterial agents in juvenile rats. *Toxicol. Pathol.* **23:**385–392.
19. Kawamura, Y., A. Nagai, M. Miyazaki, T. Sanzen, H. Fukumoto, H. Hayakawa, Y. Todo, N. Terashima, Y. Watanabe, and H. Narita. 2000. Articular toxicity of BMS-284756 (T-3811ME) administered orally to juvenile dogs,

poster 277. *In Program and Abstracts of the 40th Interscience Conference on Antimicrobial Agents and Chemotherapy.* American Society for Microbiology, Washington, D.C.

20. **Lawrence, L.E., P. Wu, L. Fran, K. Gouveia, A. Card, K. Denbleyker, and J. F. Barrett.** 2000. The structure-activity relationship of BMS-284756, a novel des-F(6)-quinolone, poster No. 751. *In Program and Abstracts of the 40th Interscience Conference on Antimicrobial Agents and Chemotherapy.* American Society for Microbiology, Washington, D.C.

21. **McDonald, D. F., H. B. Short.** 1964. Usefulnes of nalidixic acid in treatment of urinary infection. *Antimicrob. Agents Chemother.* **4:**628–631.

22. **Pertuiset, E., G. Lenoir, M. Jehanne, F. Douchan, M. Guillot, and C. J. Menkes.** 1989. Tolerance articulaire de la pefloxacine et de l'ofloxacine chez les enfants et adolescents atteints de mucoviscidose. *Rev. Rhum.* **56:**735–740.

23. **Pierfitte, C., and R. J. Royer.** 1996. Tendon disorders with fluoroquinolones. *Therapie* **51:**419–420.

24. **Pfizer.** 1996. *Trovafloxacin Investigator's Brochure.* Pfizer, Groton, Conn.

25. **Riecke, K., E. Lozo, M. Shakibaei, I. Baumann-Wilschke, and R. Stahlmann.** 2000. Fluoroquinolone-induced lesions in the epiphyseal growth plates of immature rats, abstr. 276. *In Program and Abstracts of the 40th Interscience Conference on Antimicrobial Agents and Chemotherapy.* American Society for Microbiology, Washington, D.C.

26. **Rock. E., C. Astier, C. Lab, C. Malpuech, W. Nowacki, E. Gueux, A. Mazur, and Y. Rayssiguier.** 1995. Magnesium deficiency in rats induces a rise in plasma nitric oxide. *Magnes. Res.* **8:**37–242.

27. **Saint, F., G. Gueguen, J. Biserte, C. Fontaine, and E. Mazeman.** 2000. Rupture of the patellar ligament one month after treatment with fluoroquinolone. *Rev. Chir. Orthop. Reparatrice Appar. Mot.* **86:**495–497.

28. **Schaad. U., J. Wedgwood, A. Ruedeberg, R. Kraemer, and B. Hampel.** 1997. Ciprofloxacin as antipseudomonal treatment in patients with cystic fibrosis. *Pediatr. Infect. Dis. J.* **16:**106–111.

29. **Schaad, U. B.** 2000. Use of the quinolones in pediatrics, p. 455–475. *In* V. T. Andriole (ed.), *The Quinolones,* 3rd ed. Academic Press, San Diego, Calif.

30. **Schwabe, R., E. Lozo, I. Baumann-Wilschke, and R. Stahlmann.** 1999. Chondrotoxicity and target tissue kinetics of ofloxacin in immature rats after multiple doses. *Drugs* **58**(Suppl. 2):385–387.

31. **Shakibaei, M., K. Kociok, C. Förster, J. Vormann, T. Günther, R. Stahlmann, and H.-J. Merker.** 1996. Comparative evaluation of ultrastructural changes in articular cartilage of juvenile rats after treatment with ofloxacin and in magnesium-deficient rats. *Toxicol. Pathol.* **24:**580–587.

32. **Shakibaei, M., K. Pfister, R. Schwabe, J. Vormann, and R. Stahlmann.** 2000. Ultrastructure of Achilles tendons of rats treated with ofloxacin and fed a normal or magnesium-deficient diet. *Antimicrob. Agents Chemother.* **44:**261–266.

33. **Shakibaei, M., and R. Stahlmann.** 2001. Ultrastructure of Achilles tendon from rats after treatment with fleroxacin. *Arch. Toxicol.* **75:**97–102.

33a.**Shakibaei, M., and R. Stahlmann.** Ultrastructural changes induced by the des-F(6)-quinolone garenoxacin (BMS-284756) and two fluoroquinolones in Achilles tendon from immature rats. *Arch. Toxicol.,* in press.

34. **Shakibaei, M., I. Baumann-Wilschke, R. Stahlmann.** 2001. Quinolone-induced changes in Achilles tendons from rats persist for several months. *J. Antimicrob. Chemother.* **47**(Suppl. S1):49. (Poster P130.)

35. **Shakibaei, M., P. de Souza, D. van Sickle, and R. Stahlmann.** 2001. Biochemical changes in Achilles tendon from juvenile dogs after treatment with ciprofloxacin or feeding a magnesium-deficient diet. *Arch. Toxicol.* **75:**369–374.

36. **Shakibaei, M., E.-M. Kappel, I. Baumann-Wilschke, and R. Stahlmann.** 2001. Effects of BMS-284756, ofloxacin and ciprofloxacin on the ultrastructure of Achilles tendon in juvenile rats, abstr. 1662. *In Program and Abstracts of the 41st Interscience Conference on Antimicrobial Agents and Chemotherapy.* American Society for Microbiology, Washington, D.C.

37. **Shinohara, Y. T., S. A. Tasker, M. R. Wallace, K. E. Couch, and P. E. Olson.** 1997. What is the risk of Achilles tendon rupture with ciprofloxacin? *J. Rheumatol.* **24:**238–239.

38. **Simonin, M. A., P. Gegout-Pottie, A. Minn, P. Gillet, P. Netter, and B. Terlain.** 1999. Proteoglycan and collagen biochemical variations during fluoroquinolone-induced chondrotoxicity in mice. *Antimicrob. Agents Chemother.* **43:**2915–2921.

39. **Simonin, M. A., P. Gegout-Pottie, A. Minn, P. Gillet, P. Netter, and B. Terlain.** 2000. Pefloxacin-induced Achilles tendon toxicity in rodents: biochemical changes in proteoglycan synthesis and oxidative damage to collagen. *Antimicrob. Agents Chemother.* **44:**867–872.

40. **Stahlmann, R., H.-J. Merker, N. Hinz, J. Webb, W. Heger, and D. Neubert.** 1990. Ofloxacin in juvenile non-human primates and rats. Arthropathia and drug plasma concentrations. *Arch. Toxicol.* **64:**193–204.

41. **Stahlmann, R., C. Förster, M. Shakibaei, J. Vormann, T. Günther, and H.-J. Merker.** 1995. Magnesium deficiency induces joint cartilage lesions in juvenile rats which are identical with quinolone-induced arthropathy. *Antimicrob. Agents Chemother.* **39:**2013–2018.

42. **Stahlmann, R., J. Vormann, T. Günther, C. Förster, U. Zippel, E. Lozo, R. Schwabe, K. Kociok, M. Shakibaei, and H.-J. Merker.** 1997. Effects of quinolones, magnesium deficiency or zinc deficiency on joint cartilage in rats. *Magnes. Bull.* **19:**7–22.

43. **Stahlmann, R., U. Zippel, C. Förster, M. Shakibaei, H.-J. Merker, K. and Borner.** 1998. Chondrotoxicity and toxicokinetics of sparfloxacin in juvenile rats. *Antimicrob. Agents Chemother.* **42:**1470–1475.

44. **Stahlmann, R., R. Schwabe, K. Pfister, E. Lozo, M. Shakibaei, and J. Vormann.** 1999. Supplementation with magnesium and tocopherol diminishes quinolone-induced chondrotoxicity in immature rats. *Drugs* **58**(Suppl. 2):393–394.

45. **Stahlmann, R., S. Kühner, M. Shakibaei, R. Schwabe, J. Flores, S. A. Evander, and D. C. van Sickle.** 2000. Chondrotoxicity of ciprofloxacin in immature Beagle dogs; immunohistochemistry, electron microscopy and drug plasma concentrations. *Arch. Toxicol.* **73:**564–572.

46. **Stahlmann, R., S. Kühner, M. Shakibaei, J. Flores, J. Vormann, and D. C. van Sickle.** 2000. Effects of magnesium deficiency on joint cartilage in immature Beagle dogs: immunohistochemistry, electron microscopy and mineral concentrations. *Arch. Toxicol.* **73:**573–580.

47. **Stahlmann, R.** 2001. Clinical toxicological aspects of fluoroquinolones. EUROTOX 2001, Istanbul. *Toxicol. Lett.,* in press.

48. **Syllm-Rapoport, I., I. Strassburger, D. Grüneberg, and C. Zirbel.** 1958. Über den experimentellen Magnesium-Mangel beim Hund. *Acta Biol. Med. Germ.* **1:**141–163.

49. **Tatsumi, H., H. Senda, S. Yatera, Y. Takemoto, M. Yamayoshi, and K. Ohnishi.** 1978. Toxicological studies on pipemidic acid. V. Effect on diarthrodial joints of experimental animals. *J. Toxicol. Sci.* **3:**357–367.

50. **Takizawa, T., K. Hasimoto, T. Minami, S. Yamashita, K.**

Owen. 1999. The comparative arthropathy of fluoro-quinolones in dogs. *Hum. Exp. Toxicol.* **18**:392–399.

51. Takizawa, T., K. Hasimoto, N. Itoh, S. Yamashita, and K. Owen. 1999. A comparative study of the repeat dose toxicity of grepafloxacin and a number of other fluoroquinolones in rats. *Hum. Exp. Toxicol.* **18**:38–45.

52. Van der Linden. P. D., J. van de Lei, H. W. Nab, A. Knol, and B. H. Ch. Stricker 1999. Achilles tendinitis associated with fluoroquinolones. *Br. J. Clin. Pharmacol.* **48**:433–437.

53. Van der Linden, P. D., E. P. van Puijenbroek, J. Feenstra, B. A. Veld, M. C. Sturkenboom, R. M. Herings, H. G. Leufkens, and B. H. Stricker. 2001. Tendon disorders attributed to flu-oroquinolones: a study on 42 spontaneous reports in the period 1988 to 1998. *Arthritis Rheum.* **45**:235–239.

54. von Keutz, E., and G. Schlüter. 1999. Preclinical safety evalu-ation of moxifloxacin, a novel fluoroquinolone. *J. Antimicrob. Chemother.* **43**(Suppl. B):91–100.

55. Vormann, J., C. Förster, U. Zippel, E. Lozo, T. Günther, H.-J. Merker, and R. Stahlmann. 1997. Effects of magnesium deficiency on magnesium and calcium content in bone and cartilage in developing rats in correlation to chondrotoxicity. *Calcif. Tissue Int.* **61**:230–238.

Quinolone Antimicrobial Agents, 3rd ed.
Edited by David C. Hooper and Ethan Rubinstein
© 2003 ASM Press, Washington, D.C.

Chapter 28

Phototoxicity Due to Fluoroquinolones

JAMES FERGUSON

Abnormal skin responses to sunlight and artificial light sources are common. Within a wide differential diagnosis, the clinician should always remember the possibility of drug-induced photosensitivity, a preventable disorder that should not be missed (29).

Photosensitization is a process in which reactions to normally ineffective UV and visible radiation are induced in a system by the introduction of a specific, radiation-absorbing substance (the photosensitizer) resulting in a change in a substrate, usually the skin. The radiation component, which is often, but not always, UVA (315 to 400 nm), can extend to the shorter wavelengths, UVB (295 to 315 nm), and/or visible wavelengths (400 to 700 nm). The wavelength and dose of irradiation required to produce the effect are of clinical importance. Mild photosensitivity in the UVA region may produce minimal skin damage of which the patient is hardly aware. At the other extreme, marked photosensitivity due to UVA and visible wavelengths can produce severe reactions after minor sunlight or artificial light exposure, even on cloudy days in the winter months.

Drugs, whether applied topically or, more commonly, taken systemically, are the major exogenous source of photosensitized skin reactions. Particular culprits seen commonly in dermatology practice are the sulfonamide-based diuretics, antimalarials, amiodarone, major tranquillizers, the newer parenterally administered photodynamic therapy agents, and fluoroquinolone antimicrobials (FQs).

The drug-induced photosensitivity process generally follows drug or metabolite excitation within the skin, producing a triplet state, with subcellular substrate damage commonly requiring the presence of oxygen. The effect may be direct or via photoproducts that may induce systemic toxicity in mice (2). Local skin effects are drug specific, resulting in acute inflammatory skin damage and occasionally, if the episodes are frequent, a chronic photomutagenic effect, resulting in skin malignancy as seen with psoralen photosensitization (photo-

chemotherapy), a treatment for psoriasis (53, 54). The eye may also be affected with cataracts and retinal damage, both possibilities in humans. The mechanisms whereby drugs induce photosensitization have been reviewed elsewhere (14) Of drug-induced phototoxicity, photoallergy, lupus erythematosus, and pellagra, phototoxicity is the most common. With this mechanism, providing there is enough drug or photoactive metabolite and appropriate irradiation, the skin reaction will arise in any individual. If the drug is a mild photosensitizer, more irradiation is required to produce the effect and vice versa. At the cellular level, some phototoxic agents have an effect directed against cell and subcellular membrane structures, while others, more worrying from a photomutagenic point of view, have DNA targets.

The clinical presentation of phototoxicity is subdivided into five types: (i) a burning, painful, immediate skin reaction as seen with chlorpromazine and amiodarone; (ii) exaggerated sunburn response maximal at 24 h with thiazide diuretics; (iii) 72 to 96-hour delayed erythema and blistering seen with psoralens; (iv) telangiectatic response due to calcium channel antagonists; and (v) a pseudoporphyria response with skin fragility, pigmentation, and blistering induced by numerous agents (14).

Abnormal skin pigmentation is a consequence of several phototoxic drugs; both amiodarone and chlorpromazine are capable in some individuals of the induction of either slate grey or brown pigment which may persist for many years. This pigmentation occurs at sun-exposed skin sites and may be caused by melanin, melanin drug/metabolite complex, or lipofuscin. With psoralens the pigmentation is of a "golden" melanin type, which can also persist for years following photochemotherapy.

An as yet unexplained phenomenon is idiosyncratic phototoxicity, in which an individual experiences phototoxicity after taking a commonly prescribed agent such as a thiazide or quinine, yet in the majority taking

James Ferguson • Photobiology Unit, Ninewells Hospital and Medical School, Dundee DD1 9SY, Scotland.

the agent, it has no such effect. With nonidiosyncratic phototoxic drugs, a range of degree of phototoxicity is seen between individuals taking the same daily dose, despite having an identical racial skin prototype and even similar plasma drug levels.

When considering the origin of an inflammatory skin state, drug photosensitivity should come to mind when the disorder is confined to light-exposed areas such as face, neck, and hands with sparing of the shadow sites of eyelids, beneath the chin, and hair-bearing areas. Involvement of the back of the hands with normal skin over the distal phalanges and a cut off at the start of clothing usually will leave little doubt as to a role for light. In cases in which the disorder is due to UVA or visible wavelengths, which are present in sunlight throughout the year, the ability of these wavelengths to penetrate windowglass and cloud may result in denial by the patient of a sunlight role. Also to be remembered is the phototoxic potential of artificial light sources such as fluorescent or metal halide lamps.

FLUOROQUINOLONE PHOTOSENSITIVITY

FQs are of particular photobiological interest. In the 1960s, the chemical progenitor of the group (nalidixic acid) was known to be capable of photoinduced skin responses (6,45), which ranged from an erythema to a skin fragility/blistering response mimicking porphyria (pseudoporphyria) (3).

With the introduction of a fluorine at position 6 in the quinolone ring, the first generation of FQs was produced. Subsequent chemical substitutions have resulted in a large family of compounds that show various degrees of antibacterial activity across a broad spectrum of organisms. FQs appear to have photosensitizing effects similar to those of nalidixic acid. Early clinical case reports showed a wide range of photosensitizing potential at typical therapeutic dosages. Enoxacin (a naphthyridine, like nalidixic acid) induced photosensitivity in Japanese patients, and pefloxacin, another early fluoroquinolone, appeared to have a phototoxic capacity (8).

Later marketed FQs (ciprofloxacin, ofloxacin, and norfloxacin) have also been reported to be associated with photosensitivity, the severity of which appears mild and the incidence low (<2.4%) (13). Initially, it was felt that members of the group, in general, were weak photosensitizers capable only of mild erythema skin reactions, in particular at elevated daily doses and high levels of UVA exposure. A clinical phototest study of 12 ciprofloxacin-taking subjects (15) clearly demonstrated a mild UVA-dependent phenomenon that was maximal at 24 h

with normalization of phototesting within 2 weeks of stopping the drug. Subsequently, it has been found that some patients with cystic fibrosis receiving high-dose ciprofloxacin (5) seem particularly susceptible and may even be capable of producing skin reactions with indoor fluorescent lighting (28).

The initial impression of a mild phototoxic group effect has required revision. Lomefloxacin, approved in the United States in 1992, was the subject of a U.S. Food and Drug Administration (FDA) Advisory Committee after 182 cases of photosensitivity were reported, the largest number of spontaneous photosensitivity reports for a drug over a 12-month period after initial marketing. Seven of these cases were classed as serious events. The FDA expressed concern, in particular, as in July 1992 a Swedish study of 703 patients who received lomefloxacin reported a 10% incidence of photosensitivity. As a result of the Advisory Committee, the FDA requested a bold-type photosensitivity data section, which included a comment regarding the finding of photocarcinogenicity in mice (12). Subsequently, published clinical cases showed severe blistering skin phototoxic reactions (9, 10). As a result of the phototoxicity and other problems, the future development of lomefloxacin was significantly restricted. Not surprisingly, a further consequence of this event was a heightened awareness of the FDA of about FQ phototoxicity. Guidelines for future submissions for approval of a new FQ drug highlight the need for human phototoxic data (21).

Fleroxacin, first used in 1992, has also been associated with high levels of photosensitivity (~10% [4] to 16% [23]) and was therefore withdrawn later on during the development process. Reported reactions ranged from sunlight-exposed site erythema to blistering, particularly occurring in outdoor workers. In one photosensitive Japanese patient (32) taking long-term fleroxacin, phototesting with a UVA source revealed an abnormally low minimal erythema dose (MED), which normalized on repeat phototesting 4 weeks after stopping the drug. The mechanism was considered phototoxic with a drug dose-related increase in episodes.

Sparfloxacin, initially marketed in Japan in 1993, apparently without photosensitivity problems, has since gained a reputation for photosensitivity; the problem has been recorded in 10% of patients (35, 36) treated with the drug (56). Following launch in France in September 1994, the number of spontaneous reports of phototoxicity was higher than expected; accordingly, an inquiry was set up by the French Medicines Agency. Results (44) revealed 371 cases of severe phototoxicity in the first 9 months of marketing, approximately four to five times that reported for other FQs used in that country. In addition, the date of photo-toxic episodes was linked positively to sunny environmental weather conditions. Interestingly, after severe restrictions were placed on the drug, the reporting per 100,000 prescriptions stayed constant, suggesting that the light avoidance measures that had been put in place had little impact on the numbers of reported cases. Clinical reports (57) pointed to an erythema and blistering, sunburn-like reaction with, in one subject, lichenoid features (25). The phenomenon appeared to be dose-related and the mechanism phototoxic rather than photoallergic. As with lomefloxacin in the United States, sparfloxacin had entered the French marketplace with a significant and, in retrospect, a predictable problem. Considering the effect on patients and the cost to the pharmaceutical industry, the lesson was clear—establish the phototoxic potential of any new FQ during drug development. In fact, FQs now routinely undergo phototoxicity testing during phase 1 of their developmental program.

Moxifloxacin, a more recently developed FQ, had no evidence of phototoxicity when studied in a controlled phototest trial of healthy volunteers taking 200 or 400 mg/day (39). This freedom from phototoxicity is believed due to the methoxy group at position 8 in the quinolone ring (Fig. 1).

PHOTOTOXICITY AND FQ STRUCTURE

Although the relationship between phototoxicity and FQ structure is complex, it does seem (42) that halogenation of position 8 of the quinolone ring structure results in increased phototoxicity (Fig. 1). It also appears that phototoxicity can be enhanced by such other factors as a long biological half-life and high skin penetration, which are both enhanced by the presence of large side chains or a methyl group at the C5 position (40). Conversely, the introduction of a methoxy group at position 8 (43) results in a reduced phototoxic potential.

The mechanism of FQ phototoxicity is unknown; reactive O_2 species such as hydroxyl or peroxide radicals (41) may play a role targeted at DNA in both mitochondria and within the cell nucleus.

FQs are also known to be photoclastogenic (7), photogenotoxic (47, 50), photomutagenic (7) inducers of cyclobutane dimers (48) and are photocarcinogenic in albino nude mice (30, 33, 38). Although there are no clinical reports of FQs implicated in skin cancer in humans, it seems reasonable, when possible, to avoid the use of highly photogenotoxic FQs. In this context, it is often reassuringly stated that FQs are only used in short courses; in fact, some patients

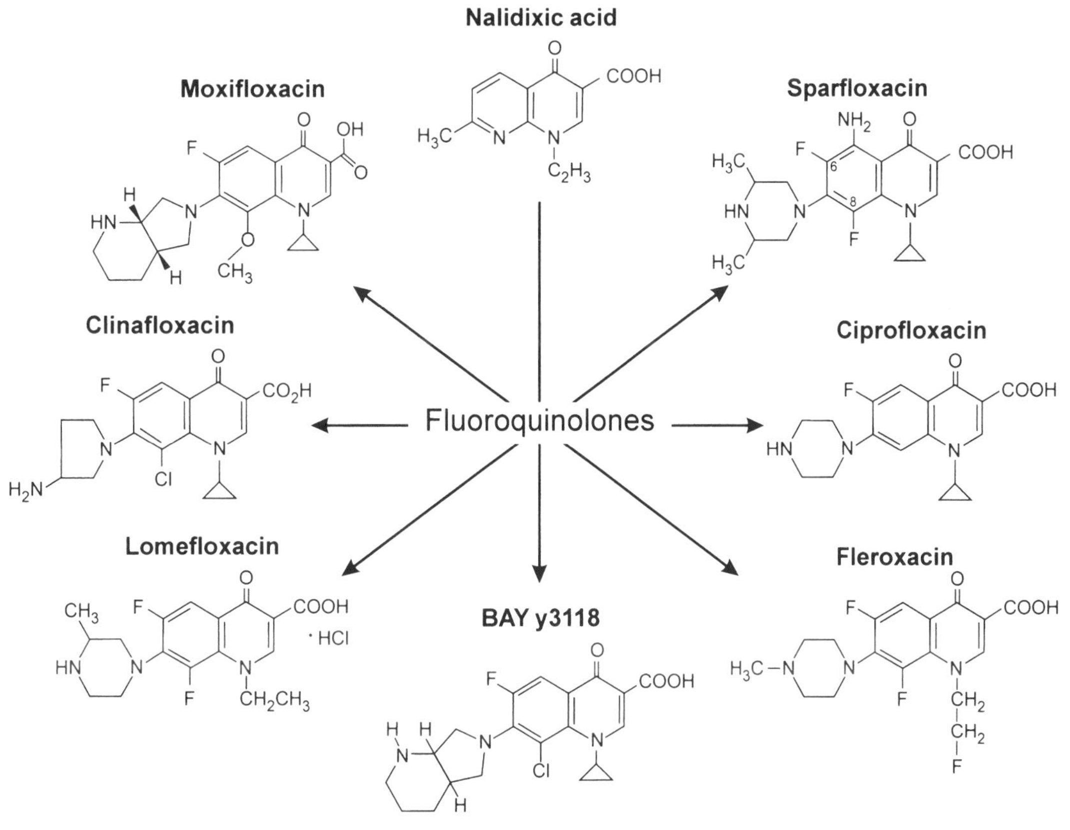

Figure 1. Some members of the quinolone group.

with chronic infections do take this group of drugs repeatedly and for prolonged periods.

Although for some time it has been thought likely that the degree of phototoxicity correlates with the photoclastogenic potential, until recently this has not been proved. In recent work comparing the two effects, a good association has been shown. In particular, FQs with a methoxy group at position 8 had low phototoxicity and photoclastogenicity, whereas those with a halogen at that position had high levels of both (27)—yet another factor that discourages the development of highly phototoxic FQs.

FLUOROQUINOLONE PHOTOALLERGY

Because photoallergic skin reactions to FQs have rarely been reported (31, 34), the doubt must exist as to whether they represent a significant clinical problem. This doubt is not surprising because most photoallergic drug reactions are believed due to topical exposure and not systemic use. In addition, photoallergy is an idiosyncratic process that requires a sensitized immune system suggesting that in susceptible individuals repeated application/exposure to the drug is required. Although topical FQ skin use has been described (24), such use is uncommon.

FQ-ASSOCIATED PHOTOTOXIC EYE EFFECTS

Although reports of FQ-associated mild eye symptoms, such as blurred vision, photophobia, and retroocular pain, are in the literature, no serious ophthalmological effects have been recorded. In albino mice, retinal phototoxicity (vacuolation of photoreceptors) (46, 55) has been detected with sparfloxacin and enoxacin (49). Whether such lesions could occur in humans is doubtful, particularly because UVA wavelengths do not penetrate to the human retina. However, should phototoxicity to a FQ be shown due to visible wavelengths, the potential should be considered.

LABORATORY PHOTOTOXIC STUDIES

Photo-safety testing guidance for industry (21) lays out a sequence of appropriate investigations for the study of a new compound. Absorption spectroscopy of the drug and, as appropriate, metabolites, followed by in vitro mammalian cell line phototoxic (1, 51, 52) test systems do provide useful data, which have been shown to correlate with in vivo information (58).

Murine phototoxic studies confirm the phototoxic effect seen with in vitro studies, yet different models produce different rank orders of phototoxic effect. Albino mouse swelling phototest technique studies indicated that fluoroquinolone ranking of phototoxicity was lomefloxacin > enoxacin > ciprofloxacin but less than ofloxacin (60, 61). With guinea pigs, the order was enoxacin < lomefloxacin < ofloxacin < tosufloxacin < norfloxacin = ciprofloxacin (26).

In recent years there has been a movement away from the use of animal models. The human relevance of the data is often questionable, and whereas some useful controlled-study results can suggest the presence or absence of phototoxicity, detailed information of clinical relevance requires human phototest study.

HUMAN STUDIES

Photosensitivity data reports from preregistration clinical trials are variable and difficult to evaluate. A rough signal highlighting a problem can emerge, particularly when the analysis includes comparator drugs. In a similar way, postmarketing surveillance adverse reporting can be helpful, as seen with lomefloxacin and sparfloxacin, yet by then it could be said to be too late.

Better is the detection of significant phototoxicity during phase 1 study drug development work, initially with in vitro models and, most importantly, human volunteer phototest study. Early controlled work designed to identify drug-induced phototoxicity used groups of volunteers who were sunlight-exposed on a 6-h boat trip off California (22). Following unblinding, the erythema and discomfort scores provided an indication of photoactivity. Since then, an improved artificial-light test system has evolved that uses a randomized controlled blinded technique in volunteers to generate "predrug" artificial-light-source phototest data which, when compared with "on-drug" values, reveals the photosensitizing potential, likely mechanism, clinical features, responsible wavelengths, severity, long-term skin pigmentation effects, and duration of photosensitivity following drug cessation. Such a study should be performed under Good Clinical and Laboratory Practice. The current technique involves healthy volunteers of defined photoskin type (20). Baseline MED values are determined on mid-upper-back skin before taking the drug in question, placebo, or photoactive fluoroquinolone control (usually lomefloxacin), using a monochromator with discrete and overlapping wavebands representing the terrestrial solar spectrum, spanning UVB and UVA into the visible region (290 to 430 ± 30 nm), with additional testing in the most recent studies also using a solar simulator light source. The solar simulator has a broad mix of wavelengths approximating midsummer equatorial sunlight and is used to assess for multiple wavelength dependency phototoxicity, seen with psoralens but not previously detected with fluoroquinolones. On-drug/placebo phototesting is conducted at a time of stable pharmacokinetics (usually days 5 to 6 for FQs) with irradiation at the time of peak plasma level (t_{max}) which for the FQs is usually between 1½ to 2 h after dosing. Phototesting after stopping the drug/placebo is repeated every 24 to 48 h until each subject has returned to within the level of experimental error (40%) of their baseline value.

Presentation of phototoxicity data is best achieved by the calculation of a photosensitivity factor known as the phototoxic index (PI) (median or individual values), which is derived by division of predrug MED by the on-drug MED value at each waveband tested. The degree of phototoxicity can then be categorized within a range of severity (Table 1). The details of such study techniques, which have been refined during the past decade, are described in detail elsewhere (15, 17–19, 37, 39, 59, 62). By such study, FQ phototoxicity has been shown to be predominantly a UVA-dependent phenomenon maximal at 24 h after irradiation, the severity of which is dose related. Recently, sparfloxacin has shown a wavelength dependence that extends into the blue-light region of the visible spectrum, which is unusual for a fluoroquinolone and does raise the possibility of retinal damage in humans (11). Improvement of phototoxic susceptibility after stopping the drug is within 2 weeks and, in general, within 48 h, reflecting the FQ group short elimination half-life.

For the purposes of this chapter, an abridged methodology and results illustrate previously unpublished BAY y 3118 data generated in 1993. This drug has been chosen because it induced unusually high levels of phototoxicity.

A PROSPECTIVE RANDOMIZED DOUBLE-BLIND PLACEBO- AND LOMEFLOXACIN-CONTROLLED PHOTOTEST STUDY IN HEALTHY MALE VOLUNTEERS

BAY y 3118, which was developed in 1992, was noted to have a considerably expanded in vitro antibacterial activity when compared with existing FQs; in particular, it was potent against methicillin- and quinolone-resistant gram-positive bacteria. At the time of phototest study, 120 human volunteers had received the drug. Significant photosensitivity had been noted in six subjects, characterized by severe blistering on exposed sites that took up to 3 weeks to heal (Fig. 2). On the basis of an apparent photosensitizing potential, laboratory in vitro and animal work was conducted by Bayer that confirmed a significant phototoxic potential. UVA-irradiated drug, when injected into guinea pigs, was lethal whereas nonirradiated drug was not, suggesting a toxic photoproduct effect.

Methodology

Thirty-two healthy male volunteers (range, 19 to 45 years, mean 28 years) were enrolled. All were Caucasian residing in Tayside, Scotland, with no significant past illness, abnormal photosensitivity, or concomitant medication. Exclusion criteria included abnormal plasma porphyrins or positive lupus serology. All volunteers were housed for the duration of the investigation within a UV-protected area in an independent part of our hospital (DDS Medicines Research Limited). All volunteers were treated as though they were abnormally photosensitive throughout the period. If they wished to go out of doors they were provided with a broad-spectrum UVB/A protecting sunblock (Sun E45, SPF25).

Medication

BAY y 3118 100- and 200-mg tablets, lomefloxacin (400 mg/day), and placebo were supplied by Bayer United Kingdom. Drugs and placebo were encapsulated in an identical manner. Half-life studies

Table 1. Fluoroquinolone phototoxic index severity grading

Phototoxicity	Phototoxic index	Known example	Reference(s)
Absent	<1.4	Moxifloxacin	39
Mild	1.4–3.0	Ciprofloxacin	15
Moderate	>3.0–6.0	Lomefloxacin	19, 39
Severe	>6.0	Bay y 3118,[a] clinafloxacin[a]	

[a] Drug development abandoned; data on file.

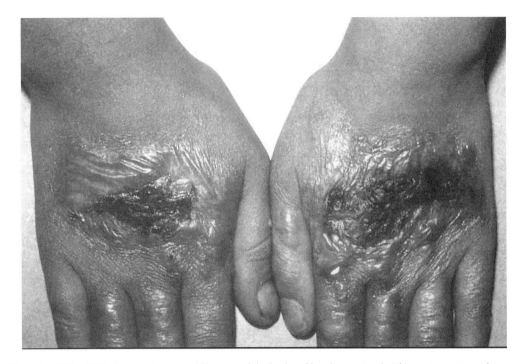

Figure 2. BAY y 3118. Severe phototoxic blistering of the backs of hands in a South African Caucasian volunteer.

for both drugs confirmed that steady-state pharmacokinetics were reached by day 4.

Study Design

The subjects were randomly assigned to one of the four different treatment schedules. If abnormal photosensitivity was detected "on drug," phototesting was repeated every 2 days until the volunteers came within 40% of their baseline MED value.

Compliance

Each identical capsule was administered by nursing staff and the oral cavity checked to ensure ingestion. Plasma sample at the time of phototesting was taken for BAY y 3118 assay to ensure compliance.

Phototesting

Using standard monochromator testing as described previously (16), baseline values were identified during the week prior to study and days 5 and 6 "on drug." The procedure took place 2 h after ingestion (i.e., T_{max}). Immediate and delayed phototest readings were conducted. Repeat testing was conducted on day 9 and, if necessary, day 11 in those with abnormal photosensitivity.

Statistical Methods

The sample-size calculation relied on several assumptions. The standard deviation of $\log_{10}$ MED was taken as a basis for calculation to be 0.3 and was designed to detect a threefold decrease in MED between the placebo and BAY y 3118 groups. A two-sided test at the 5% significance level was considered to have a 90% power to detect this difference. Eight subjects were allocated to each treatment group. The MED determinations were tabulated for each waveband at each stage of the study. The Kruskal-Wallis test was made using on-treatment results to make an overall comparison.

Results

During the trial, history and examination failed to reveal evidence of acute exposed-site phototoxicity in the study volunteers. Plasma scan for porphyrins, antinuclear antibody, anti-Ro and anti-La were normal before and after taking the drug in all subjects (thus excluding drug-induced lupus or porphyria). Good compliance was shown by drug levels in serum at the time of phototesting. With respect to BAY y 3118, 100- and 200-mg doses, respectively, the mean area under the curve values were 5.8 and 12.6 mg/h/liter, which confirmed correct ingestion of the intended medication. All volunteers completed the study.

Table 2. Median PI estimations for BAY y 3118 (100 and 200 mg/day) and
lomefloxacin (400 mg/day)

Drug, dose	Median PI at the following wavelength (nm ± 30)[a]				
	305 ± 5	335	365	400	430
BAY y 3118, 100 mg/day	1.5*	3.8*	7.4*	3.4*	1
BAY y 3118, 200 mg/day	1.4	7.4*	29.3*	7.5*	1
Lomefloxacin	1.2	3.3*	6.7*	1	1
Placebo	1	1	1.1	1	1

[a]The PI is considered to be outside experimental error when >1.4. Asterisks indicate that the
value is statistically significant when compared with placebo ($P \leq 0.05$).

Results indicated statistically significant abnormal phototest results for both BAY y 3118 dosages and lomefloxacin at 335 to 400 ± 30 nm (Table 2). Placebo failed to show evidence of phototoxicity. The phototoxicity for the three active limbs was predominantly UVA in origin (335 to 400 ± 30 nm) and was maximal at 24 h; the susceptibility cleared within 4 days of cessation of the drug. BAY y 3118 extended into the UVB region with abnormal results at 305 ± 5 nm. Abnormal phototest results were obtained in all volunteers in the active limbs. Postphototoxic skin pigmentation (Fig. 3) was seen in both BAY y 3118 groups at "on drug" but not baseline UVA phototest sites. Skin biopsy indicated that abnormal pigmentation was melanin in origin. The phototest site pigmentation was still present although was much faded 1 year after phototesting.

Conclusion

This study revealed BAY y 3118 at 100 and 200 mg/day capable of a phototoxic index in the severe range as defined previously (Table 1). Lomefloxacin in this study showed a PI value also in the severe range (previous work has recorded lomefloxacin to be in the moderate group [PI >3 to 6]), but not

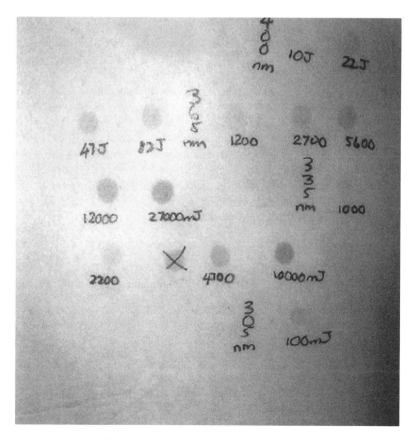

Figure 3. Persistent abnormal pigmentation noted at monochromator phototest sites in a volunteer 3 months after phototesting on BAY y 3118, 200 mg/day.

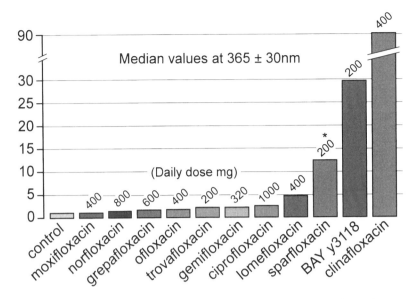

Figure 4. PI values for a range of FQs. * Sparfloxacin maximal phototoxicity was detected at 400 ± 30 nm.

approaching the drug dose-dependent PI values for BAY y 3118 200 mg/day, which had a median PI of 29.3 at 365 ± 30 nm. Because a PI of 30 indicates that an individual's skin will respond to 1/30th of the amount of UVA required to produce erythema before taking the drug, it does provide an indication of the degree of environmental restriction induced. Instead of taking approximately 60 min of midday, midsummer sunlight at 57°N to induce a red-skin reaction, 2 min is all that is required. In addition, the fact that cloud- or windowglass-transmitted light is capable of the effect does provide some idea of the impact of this degree of phototoxicity.

Fortunately, FQs are cleared from the body relatively quickly, so normalization within 4 days is a favourable situation when compared with amiodarone, in which the phototoxicity normalization process may take 12 months. Clearly, at the BAY y 3118 dosages used, phototoxicity was a significant problem that contributed to the halt of its development.

FLUOROQUINOLONE PI VALUES COMPARED

With the described controlled phototest technique, a number of FQs have been studied (15–19, 39). Although most are in the mild PI group (Fig. 4), three drugs stand out with unusually high levels of photosensitization (clinafloxacin, BAY y3118, and sparfloxacin). All have a halogen at position 8 of the quinolone ring. All have been associated with high levels of clinical phototoxicity, and all have either had their development abandoned or are now rarely used.

SUMMARY

Clinical photosensitivity associated with FQs is dose related and phototoxic in origin, predominantly UVA dependent, and rapidly reversible after drug cessation. Although as a group FQs were initially thought to be mildly phototoxic, it is clear from controlled clinical trial data that some FQs are associated with levels of clinical photosensitivity that would be extremely difficult to prevent either in the hospital or the home environment. Because the degree of phototoxicity, postphototoxic pigmentation, and photogenotoxicity appear linked, the development of highly phototoxic FQs should be discouraged. Identification of the phototoxic potential using in vitro and in vivo techniques in phase 1 of new FQ development is required.

REFERENCES

1. **Arlett, C., L. Earl, J. Ferguson, N. Gibbs, J. Hawk, L. Henderson, B. Johnson, W. Lovell, H. D. Menage, and S. Navaratnam.** 1995. Predictive *in vitro* methods for identifying photosensitising drugs. *Br. J. Dermatol.* **132:**271–274.
2. **Bakri, A., G. M. J. Beijersbergen van Henegouwen, and J. L. Chanal.** 1983. Photopharmacology of the tranquillizer chlordiazepoxide in relation to its phototoxicity. *Photochem. Photobiol.* **38:**177–183.
3. **Bilsland, D., and W. S. Douglas.** 1990. Sunbed pseudoporphyria induced by nalidixic acid. *Br. J. Dermatol.* **123:**547.
4. **Bowie, W. R., V. Willetts, and P. J. Jewesson.** 1989. Adverse reactions in a dose-ranging study with a new long-acting fluoroquinolone, fleroxacin. *Antimicrob. Agents Chemother.* **33:**1778–1782.
5. **Burdge, D. R., E. M. Nakielna, and H. R. Rabin.** 1995. Photosensitivity associated with ciprofloxacin use in adult

patients with cystic fibrosis. *Antimicrob. Agents Chemother.* **39**:793.

6. **Burry, J. N., and R. W. L. Crosby.**. 1966. A case of photo-toxicity to nalidixic acid. *Med. J. Australia* **2**:698.

7. **Chetelat, A.-A., S. Albertini, and E. Gocke.** 1996. The photo-mutagenicity of fluoroquinolones in tests for gene mutation, chromosomal aberration, gene conversion and DNA break-age (Comet assay). *Mutagenesis* **11**:497–504.

8. **Christ, W., and T. Lehnent.** 1990. Toxicity of the quinolones, p. 65–185. *In* C. Siporin, C. L. Heifez, and I. M. Domagala (ed.), *The New Generation of Quinolones.* Marcel Dekker, New York, N.Y.

9. **Cohen, J. B., and P. R. Bergstresser.** 1994. Inadvertent pho-totoxicity from home tanning equipment. *Arch. Dermatol.* **130**:804–806.

10. **Correia, O., L. Delgado, and M. A. Barros.** 1994. Bullous pho-todermatosis after lomefloxacin. *Arch. Dermatol.* **130**:808–809.

11. **Dawe, R. S., S. H. Ibbotson, J. B. Sanderson, E. M. Thomson, and J. Ferguson.** A randomised controlled volunteer study of sitafloxacin, enoxacin, levofloxacin, and sparfloxacin photo-toxicity. *Br. J. Dermatol.*, in press.

12. **F-D-C Reports.** 1993. "The Pink Sheet". Searle Maxaquin "Dear Prescriber" letter on phototoxicity should be sent, FDA Advisory Committee urges; group is split on "black box" warning, p. 16–17.

13. **Ferguson, J.** 1995. Fluoroquinolone photosensitization: a review of clinical and laboratory studies. *Photochem. Photobiol.* **62**:954–958.

14. **Ferguson, J.** 2002. Photosensitivity due to drugs. *Photodermatol. Photoimmunol. Photomed.* **18**:262–269.

15. **Ferguson, J., and B. E. Johnson.** 1990. Ciprofloxacin-induced photosensitivity: *in vitro* and *in vivo* studies. *Br. J. Dermatol.* **123**:9–20.

16. **Ferguson, J., and B. E. Johnson.** 1993. Clinical and laborato-ry studies of the photosensitizing potential of norfloxacin, a 4-quinolone broad spectrum antibiotic. *Br. J. Dermatol.* **128**:285–295.

17. **Ferguson, J., and R. Dawe.** 1997. Phototoxity in quinolones: comparison of ciprofloxacin and grepafloxacin. *J. Antimicrob. Chemother.* **40**(Suppl. A):93–98.

18. **Ferguson, J., J. McEwen, K. Gohler, A. Mignot, and D. Watson.** 1999. Phototoxic potential of gatifloxacin, a new fluoroquinolone antimicrobial. *Drugs* **58**(Suppl.):397–399.

19. **Ferguson, J., J. McEwen, H. Al-Ajmi, L. Purkins, P. J. Colman, and S. A. Willavize.** 2000. A comparison of the photosensitizing potential of trovafloxacin with that of other quinolones in healthy subjects. *J. Antimicrob. Chemother.* **45**:503–509.

20. **Fitzpatrick., T. B., A. Z. Eisen, K. Wolff, I. M. Freedberg, and K. F. Austen.** 1993. *Dermatology in General Medicine*, 4th ed., vol. 1. McGraw-Hill Book Co., New York, N.Y.

21. **Food and Drug Administration Center for Drug Evaluation and Research.** Guidance for industry: photosafety testing (recom-mendations). http://www.fda.gov/cder/guidance/index.htm.

22. **Frost, P., G. D. Weinstein, and E. C. Gomez.** 1971. Methacycline and demeclocycline in relation to sunlight. *JAMA* **216**:326–329.

23. **Geddes, A. M.** 1993. Safety of fleroxacin in clinical trials. *Am. J. Med.* **94**(Suppl. 3A):201S–203S.

24. **Ghosh, S., A. Panarese, A. J. Parker, and P. D. Bull.** 2000. Quinolone ear drops for chronic otitis media. *Br. Med. J.* **321**:126–127.

25. **Hamanaka, H., H. Mizutani, and M. Shimizu.** 1998. Sparfloxacin-induced photosensitivity and the occurrence of a lichenoid tissue reaction after prolonged exposure. *J. Am. Acad. Dermatol.* **38**:945–949.

26. **Horio, T., H. Miyauchi, Y. Asada, Y. Aoki, and M. Harada.** 1994. Phototoxicity and photoallergenicity of quinolones in guinea pigs. *J. Dermatol. Sci.* **7**:130–135.

27. **Itoh, S., S. Nakayama, and H. Shimada.** 2002. *In vitro* pho-tochemical clastogenicity of quinolone antibacterial agents studied by a chromosomal aberration test with light irradia-tion. *Mutat. Res.* **517**:113–121.

28. **Jaffe, A., and A. Bush.** 1999. If you can't stand the rash, get out of the kitchen: an unusual adverse reaction to ciprofloxacin. *Pediat. Pulmonol.* **28**:449–450.

29. **Johnson, B. E., and J. Ferguson.** 1990. Drug and chemical photosensitivity. *Semin. Dermatol.* **9**:39–46.

30. **Johnson, B. E., N. K. Gibbs, and J. Ferguson.** 1997. Quinolone antibiotic with potential to photosensitize skin tumorigenesis. *J. Photochem. Photobiol. B Biol.* **37**: 171–173.

31. **Kawabe, Y., N. Mizuno, and S. Sakakibara.** 1989. Photoallergic reaction caused by enoxacin. *Photodermatology* **6**:58–60.

32. **Kimura, M., A. Kawada, T. Kobayashi, M. Hiruma, and A. Ishibashi.** 1996. Photosensitivity induced by fleroxacin. *Clin. Exp. Dermatol.* **21**:46–47.

33. **Klecak, F., F. Urbach, and H. Urwyler.** 1997. Fluoroquinolone antibacterials enhance UVA-induced skin tumours. *J. Photochem. Photobiol. B Biol.* **37**:174–181.

34. **Kurumaji, Y., and M. Shona.** 1992. Scarified photopatch testing in lomefloxacin photosensitivity. *Contact Dermatitis* **26**:5–10.

35. **Lipsky, B. A., and C. A. Baker.** 1999. Fluoroquinolone toxi-city profiles: a review focusing on newer agents. *Clin. Infect. Dis.* **28**:352–364.

36. **Lipsky, B. A., M. B. Dorr, D. J. Magner, and G. H. Talbot.** 1999. Safety profile of sparfloxacin, a new fluoroquinolone antibiotic. *Clin. Ther.* **21**:148–159.

37. **Lowe, N. J., T. D. Fakouhi, R. S. Stern, T. Bourge, B. Roniker, and E. A. Swabb.** 1994. Photoreactions with a fluo-roquinolone antimicrobial: evening versus morning dosing. *Clin. Pharmacol. Ther.* **56**:587–591.

38. **Makinen, M., P. D. Forbes, and D. Stenback.** 1997. Quinolone antibacterials: a new class of photochemical car-cinogens. *J. Photochem. Photobiol. B Biol.* **37**:182–187.

39. **Man, I., J. Murphy, and J. Ferguson.** 1999. Fluoroquinolone phototoxicity: a comparison of moxifloxacin and lome-floxacin in normal volunteers. *J. Antimicrob. Chemother.* **43**(Suppl. B):77–82.

40. **Martinez, L. J., and C. F. Chignell.** 1998. Photocleavage of DNA by the fluoroquinolone antibacterials. *J. Photochem. Photobiol. B Biol.* **45**:51–59.

41. **Martinez, L. J., R. H. Sik, and C. F. Chignell.** 1998. Fluoroquinolone antimicrobials: singlet oxygen, superoxide and phototoxicity. *Photochem. Photobiol.* **67**:399–403.

42. **Marutani, K., M. Matsumoto, Y. Otabe, M. Nagamuta, K. Tanaka, A. Miyoshi, T. Hasegawa, H. Nagano, S. Matsubara, and R. Kamide.** 1993. Reduced phototoxicity of a fluoroquinolone antibacterial agent with a methoxy group at the 8 position in mice irradiated with long-wavelength UV light. *Antimicrob. Agents Chemother.* **37**:2217–2223.

43. **Matsumoto, M., K. Kojima, H. Nagano, S. Matsubara, and T. Yokota.** 1992. Photostability and biological activity of fluoroquinolones substituted at the 8 position after UV irradiation. *Antimicrob. Agents Chemother.* **36**: 1715–1719.

44. **Pierfitte, C., R. J. Royer, N. Moore, and B. Begaud.** 2000. The link between sunshine and phototoxicity of sparfloxacin. *Br. J. Clin. Pharmacol.* **49**:609–612.

45. **Ramsay, C. A., and E. Obreshkova.** 1974. Photosensitivity from nalidixic acid. *Br. J. Dermatol.* **91**:523–528.

46. **Rapp, L. M., B. L. Tolman, and H. S. Dhindsa.** 1990. Separate

mechanisms for retinal damage by ultraviolet-A and mid-visible light. *Investig. Ophthalmol. Vis. Sci.* **31:**1186–1190.

47. **Reavy, H. J., N. J. Traynor, and N. K. Gibbs.** 1997. Photogenotoxicity of skin phototumorigenic fluoroquinolone antibiotics detected using the Comet assay. *Photochem. Photobiol.* **66:**368–373.

48. **Sarvaigo, S., T. Douki, F. Odin, S. Caillat, J.-L. Ravanat, and J. Cadet.** 2001. Analysis of fluoroquinolone-mediated photosensitization of 2′-deoxyguanosine, calf thymus and cellular DNA: determination of type-I, type II and triplet-triplet energy transfer mechanism contribution. *Photochem. Photobiol.* **73:**230–237.

49. **Shimoda, K., M. Yoshida, N. Wagai, S. Takayama, and M. Kato.** 1993. Phototoxic lesions induced by quinolone antibacterial agents in auricular skin and retina of albino mice. *Toxicol. Pathol.* **21:**554–561.

50. **Snyder, R. D., and C. S. Cooper.** 1999. Photogenotoxicity of fluoroquinolones in Chinese hamster V79 cells: dependency on active topoisomerase II. *Photochem. Photobiol.* **69:**288–293.

51. **Spielmann, H., W. W. Lovell, E. Holzle, B. E. Johnson, T. Maurer, M. A. Miranda, W. J. W. Pape, O. Sapora, and D. Sladowski.** 1994. *In vitro* phototoxicity testing (report and recommendations of the ECVAM workshop). *ATLA Abstr.* **22:**314–348.

52. **Spielmann, H., M. Balls, J. Dupuis, W. J. W. Pape, O. De Silva, H. G. Holzhutter, F. Gerberick, M. Liebsch, W. W. Lovell, and U. Pfanenbecker.** 1998. A study on UV filter chemicals from Annex VII of European Union Directive 76 768 EEC, in the in vitro 3T3 NRU phototoxicity text. *ATLA Abstr.* **26:**679–708.

53. **Stern, R. S.** 2001. The risk of melanoma in association with long-term exposure to PUVA. *J. Am. Acad. Dermatol.* **44:**755–761.

54. **Stern, R. S., and N. Laird.** 1994. The carcinogenic risk of treatments for severe psoriasis. *Cancer* **73:**2759–2764.

55. **Takayama, S., M. Hirohashi, M. Kato, and H. Shimada.** 1995. Toxicity of quinolone antimicrobial agents. *J. Toxicol. Environ. Health* **45:**1–45.

56. **Tokura, Y., Y. Iwamoto, K. Mizutani, and M. Takigawa.** 1996. Sparfloxacin phototoxicity: potential photoaugmentation by ultraviolet A and B sources. *Arch. Dermatol. Res.* **288:**45–50.

57. **Tokura, Y., T. Nishijima, H. Yagi, F. Furukawa, and M. Takigawa.** 1996. Photohaptenic properties of fluoroquinolones. *Photochem. Photobiol.* **64:**838–844.

58. **Traynor, N. J., M. D. Barratt, W. W. Lovel, J. Ferguson, and N. K. Gibbs.** 2000. Comparison of an *in vitro* cellular phototoxicity model against controlled clinical trials of fluoroquinolone skin phototoxicity. *Toxicol. In Vitro* **14:**275–283.

59. **Vousden, M., J. Ferguson, J. Richards, N. Bird, and A. Allen.** 1999. Evaluation of phototoxic potential of gemifloxacin in healthy volunteers compared with ciprofloxacin. *Chemotherapy* **45:**512–520.

60. **Wagai, N., and K. Tawara.** 1992. Possible direct role of reactive oxygens in the cause of cutaneous phototoxicity induced by five quinolones in mice. *Arch. Toxicol.* **66:**392–397.

61. **Wagai, N., F. Yamaguchi, M. Sekiguchi, and K. Tawara.** 1990. Phototoxic potentials of quinolone antibacterial agents in Balb/c mice. *Toxicol. Lett.* **54:**299–308.

62. **Young, A. R., T. D. Fakouhi, G. I. Harrison, B. Roniker, E. A. Swabb, and J. L. M. Hawk.** 1996. The UVR wavelength dependence for lomefloxacin photosensitization of human skin. *J. Photochem. Photobiol. B Biol.* **32:**165–170.

Quinolone Antimicrobial Agents, 3rd ed.
Edited by David C. Hooper and Ethan Rubinstein
© 2003 ASM Press, Washington, D.C.

Chapter 29

Central Nervous System Toxicity

S. RAGNAR NORRBY

The first quinolone antibiotic, nalidixic acid, was described in 1962. In the years after its introduction for clinical use in 1965, several reports describing central nervous system (CNS) adverse reactions were published. Cahal (9) reported headache, giddiness, drowsiness, syncope, sensory changes, and grand mal seizures. Reversible psychosis following large nalidixic acid doses was reported by Finegold et al. (15). Islam and Sreedharan (21) described convulsions, hyperglycemia, and glycosuria in a 14-year-old girl after an overdose of 6.5 g of nalidixic acid (normal dose, 500 mg). Kucers and Bennett (25) reported a similar case in a 2-year-old girl who received 500 mg of nalidixic acid. Pediatric use of nalidixic acid has also been related to development of intracranial hypertension (4, 7, 17, 24), a condition that should be considered when quinolone antibacterials are developed for use in children, as is now the case with at least one of the 6-desfluoroquinolones.

CNS reactions have been well known to occur sporadically with all nonfluorinated and fluorinated quinolone antibacterial agents (10, 27). However, as discussed below, considerable differences exist among various derivatives. The frequency of CNS side effects seems to be dose dependent and sometimes also dose limiting. It is therefore of particular interest that animal studies recently published indicate that newly developed quinolones like gemifloxacin and moxifloxacin may have some future use in the treatment of pneumococcal meningitis caused by β-lactam-resistant strains, a condition for which very large β-lactam doses are traditionally given, and which itself has a high risk of convulsions (35, 38, 43).

PHARMACOKINETIC ASPECTS OF CNS EFFECTS OF QUINOLONE ANTIBIOTICS

It is reasonable to assume that the CNS toxicity of quinolones is dependent on the antibiotic concentrations achieved in brain tissue and/or cerebrospinal fluid (CSF). Relatively limited information is available on the penetration of these drugs into brain tissue and the CSF. Available information indicates that the CNS penetration seems not to be related to the lipophilicity of the quinolones (13, 27). Studies using positron emission tomography have shown that fleroxacin is rapidly and equally distributed to the various parts of the brain and that lomefloxacin or ciprofloxacin do not affect cerebral blood flow or oxygen or glucose metabolism (6, 16). Using conventional techniques, Davey et al. (11) studied ciprofloxacin and sparfloxacin kinetics in humans and found concentrations in brain tissue to be similar to those in serum but very much lower than those in CSF. Similar results have been reported with pefloxacin (18). The low concentrations in CSF may be due to an active transport of quinolones out of CSF. Ooie et al. (37) showed that fleroxacin was transported across rat choroid plexus by a saturable pump mechanism, which has previously been described for the elimination of benzylpenicillin from CSF. With an experimental quinolone antibiotic, HSR-903, Murata et al. (33) showed that, in rats, low concentrations in brain tissue were achieved and that the low concentration might be due to several efflux pump mechanisms, of which one seemed to be located in the brain capillary endothelial cells, which constitute the true blood–brain barrier (as opposed to plexus chorioideus, which constitutes the blood–CSF barrier).

Impaired excretory organ function, resulting in slower elimination of quinolones, may result in increased risks of accumulation of the drugs and subsequent CNS toxicity. In animal studies, both acute renal failure and bile duct ligation have been shown to increase drug concentrations in the brain and also the neurotoxicity of ciprofloxacin, levofloxacin, and enoxacin (3, 23, 32, 34).

S. Ragnar Norrby • Swedish Institute for Infectious Disease Control, Nobel's Vg 18, SE17182 Solna, Sweden.

QUINOLONE INTERACTIONS WITH THE GAMMA-AMINOBUTYRIC ACID (GABA) AND THE N-METHYL-D-ASPARTATE (NMDA) RECEPTORS

It has been proposed that the main mechanism behind the CNS toxicity of quinolone antibacterials is a displacement of GABA from the GABA A receptor resulting in CNS stimulation (1, 10, 36, 47, 48). As reviewed by Domagala (13), the C7 side chain seems to be of importance for the degree of binding to the GABA A receptor; the bulkier this side chain, the less efficiently it binds to the receptor. Thus, quinolones with unsubstituted piperazine rings at C7, e.g., ciprofloxacin and norfloxacin, have a high-binding capacity. Quinolones with a pyrrolidinyl side chain, like tosufloxacin and clinafloxacin, have intermediate binding, and those with alkylated side chains, such as temafloxacin and sparfloxacin, have low affinity. Results in agreement with the hypothesis that the C7 substitution is of importance for the GABA A binding have been published also for the new 6-desfluoroquinolone derivatives (12). Other factors also must be of importance, however, because levofloxacin has significantly less binding to the GABA A receptor than ofloxacin, despite the fact that levofloxacin is the l-isomer ofloxacin (2, 49).

It is unlikely that the GABA A receptor interaction is the only mechanism by which quinolones are neurotoxic (44). A possible explanation for why the various quinolones have different types of CNS toxicity and why drugs with very similar binding to the GABA A receptor show considerable variability of their CNS toxicity would be that more than one neurotransmittor receptor is involved. One such receptor is the NMDA receptor, which has been shown to be of importance in the pathophysiology of seizures and also for quinolone CNS side effects (5, 27, 39, 41, 49). One quinolone that interacts strongly with the NMDA receptor is trovafloxacin, which also has a higher degree of neurotoxicity than one would expect from its interaction with the GABA A receptor (41).

DRUG–DRUG INTERACTIONS THAT POTENTIATE QUINOLONE CNS TOXICITY

At an early stage it became apparent that nonsteroidal anti-inflammatory drugs (NSAIDs) could potentiate the neurotoxicity of quinolones. As shown in Table 1, the binding to mouse synaptic GABA A receptors in vitro varies among quinolones and also among NSAIDs (20). A high degree of potentiation of neurotoxicity in animals by biphenyl acetic acid, the active metabolite of the NSAID fenbufen, has been seen with trovafloxacin (27). Other animal studies have verified this variation as shown in Table 2 (2).

Although there is extensive and convincing in vitro and in vivo documentation of the interactions between quinolone antibacterials and NSAIDs, there is minimal documentation in the literature of patients in whom there has been a clear correlation between CNS toxicity and simultaneous administration of the two classes of drugs. In fact, only two such reports were found in a literature search (20, 34). This low frequency of clinically documented quinolone–NSAID interactions could be due to underreporting; most case reports on CNS reactions to quinolones do not mention, nor negate, concurrent NSAID medications. The low reporting could also be due to a lower risk than indicated by preclinical studies. Notably and surprisingly, this type of potentially very serious interaction is not mentioned in the package inserts of any of the marketed quinolones.

Interactions between ciprofloxacin and theophylline and clinafloxacin and theophylline leading to seizures have been reported (22, 30, 40, 42, 46). Most of these patients were elderly. The neurotoxic reactions are most likely caused by increased theophylline concentrations resulting from blockage by

Table 1. In vitro binding of quinolones to GABA A receptors with or without anti-inflammatory drugs (10^{-4} M)[a]

Anti-inflammatory drug	Binding (IC$_{50}$ [M]) by specified quinolone			
	Norfloxacin	Ofloxacin	Ciprofloxacin	Fleroxacin
None	1.4×10^{-5}	1.0×10^{-3}	7.6×10^{-5}	7.6×10^{-4}
Aspirin	1.4×10^{-5}	1.0×10^{-4}	1.0×10^{-4}	7.6×10^{-4}
Fenbufen	1.2×10^{-7}	3.6×10^{-5}	1.3×10^{-6}	5.8×10^{-4}
Indomethacin	1.9×10^{-7}	1.2×10^{-4}	1.0×10^{-4}	5.8×10^{-4}
Flubiprofen	1.4×10^{-8}	3.0×10^{-4}	1.0×10^{-6}	1.0×10^{-6}
Biphenylacetate	$<10^{-8}$	8.3×10^{-7}	3.0×10^{-8}	1.0×10^{-4}

[a] Modified from Hori et al. (20) with permission of the University of Chicago Press.

Table 2. Potentiation of the CNS toxicity
of quinolone antibiotics[a]

Treatment (dose in μg)	Incidence of (no. of affected mice/total)	
	Clonic convulsions	Death
Norfloxacin (5)	9/10[b]	2/10
Ofloxacin (5)	0/10	0/10
Levofloxacin (5)	0/10	0/10
Norfloxacin (50)	10/10	10/10
Ofloxacin (50)	10/10	7/10
Levofloxacin (50)	8/10	2/10
BPAA (50)	0/10	0/10
Norfloxacin (5) + BPAA (50)	10/10[c]	10/10
Ofloxacin (5) + BPAA (50)	3/10	2/10
Levofloxacin (5) + BPAA (50)	1/10	1/10

[a] Antibiotics were administered intracisternally to mice with or without coadministration with biphenylacetic acid (BPAA), the active metabolite of fenbufen. Each treatment was given to a group of 10 mice. Reproduced from Akahane et al. (2) with permission from S. Karger AG, Basel, Switzerland.
[b] Mean time to onset 366 ± 72 s.
[c] Mean time to onset 40 ± 5 s.

the quinolone of the CYP 1A2 isoenzyme of the cytochrome P450 system. With quinolones, which are not metabolized by cytochrome P450 (e.g., ofloxacin and levofloxacin), this interaction will not occur.

Reports have appeared on seizures in patients concomitantly treated with quinolones and the antiviral compound foscarnet (14, 28). An animal study by Matsuo et al. (29) suggested that this occurrence might have been due to a potentiation by foscarnet of the quinolone-induced inhibition of the GABA A receptor.

Interaction between ciprofloxacin and methadone has been described in one patient who developed confusion, sedation, and respiratory depression (19). This interaction was ascribed to inhibition of cytochrome P450 enzymes CYP 1A2 and/or CYP 3A4 involved in the metabolism of methadone.

CNS ADVERSE EVENTS REPORTED IN CLINICAL TRIALS OF QUINOLONES

As reviewed by Stahlmann and Lode (44), CNS adverse reactions to quinolones are often dose dependent. In a trial of fleroxacin, severe insomnia was reported by 8% of patients receiving 400 mg once daily, while 16 of 26 patients (60%) on 800 mg once daily reported this reaction (8). With trovafloxacin, the frequency of dizziness in healthy volunteers increased markedly at oral doses exceeding 300 mg (45). These finding make it important to

reduce doses in patients with the diseases or other conditions which may decrease the rate of elimination of quinolones with the subsequent risks of accumulation. With trovafloxacin, dizziness and light-headedness have been reported most frequently in young women and also when the drug was taken without food (26). That association is contrary to what has been reported with most other quinolones, for which advanced age was a primary risk factor for CNS adverse reactions.

As mentioned above, the frequency of CNS adverse reactions seems to vary considerably between different quinolone antibiotics. Lipsky and Baker (26) graded the quinolones as fleroxacin > trovafloxacin > grepafloxacin > norfloxacin > sparfloxacin > ciprofloxacin > enoxacin > ofloxacin > pefloxacin > levofloxacin. In U.S. post-marketing surveillances, adverse CNS effects were reported in 26 of 100,000 patients treated with trovafloxacin as compared with 4 in 100,000 patients receiving levofloxacin (5). For dizziness, the corresponding frequencies for the two drugs were 12.5 per 100,000 patients and 0.5 per 100,000 patients, respectively. More exact comparisons are not possible since most clinical trials of quinolones have used other classes of antibiotics as comparators. Only in relatively few trials has one quinolone been compared with another. Also, one should be aware of the fact that tendencies by patients and investigators to report adverse events vary considerably between countries, being highest in North America and Northern Europe.

Serious CNS reactions, such as seizures, psychosis, and delirium, are usually not observed in clinical trials but are reported in the literature as cases. Such reactions have been reported with alatrofloxacin, ciprofloxacin, enoxacin, norfloxacin, ofloxacin, and pefloxacin (26, 31).

Variations in the dominating type of CNS reactions to different quinolones are sometimes obvious. With trovafloxacin dizziness and light-headedness dominate ("it is like taking two gin and tonics on a fasting stomach"), while insomnia has been by far the most frequent CNS reaction to fleroxacin. Mechanistic explanations for this variability are lacking.

CONCLUSIONS

Despite the fact that the first quinolone antimicrobial was introduced in the early 1960s and that early on it became obvious that some members of the class have relatively frequent adverse CNS effects, we do not know the exact mechanism(s) behind these reactions. Although serious reactions, seizures, and mental alterations occur, they are very rare. Risk factors for such reactions are high doses (including overdosing as a result of altered excretion, e.g., due to renal or hepatic failure or advanced age), previous epilepsy, and, probably, interactions with NSAIDs or theophylline. Notably, the probability of interactions with NSAIDs is not mentioned in the insert package of any quinolone.

Although serious reactions are uncommon, mild or moderate adverse CNS reactions such as insomnia, dizziness, and headache are relatively common and clearly dose dependent and dose limiting with some quinolones, e.g., trovafloxacin and fleroxacin. With ofloxacin and levofloxacin also these reactions are uncommon. Overall, with most fluoroquinolone antibacterial agents, CNS adverse reactions do not constitute a major clinical problem.

REFERENCES

1. **Akahane, K., M. Sekiguchi, T. Une, and Y. Usada.** 1989. Structure-epileptogenicity relationship of quinolones with special reference to their interaction with gamma-amino butyric acid receptor sites. *Antimicrob. Agents Chemother.* 33:1704–1708.

2. **Akahane, K., Y. Tsutomi, Y. Kimura, and Y. Kitano.** 1994. Levofloxacin, an optical isomer of ofloxacin, has attenuated epileptogenic activity in mice and inhibitory potency in GABA receptor binding capacity. *Chemotherapy* 40:412–417.

3. **Akahane, K., S. Ohkawara, M. Nomura, and M. Kato.** 1996. Effects of bile duct ligation and unilateral nephrectomy on brain concentrations and convulsant potential of the quinolone antibacterial agent levofloxacin in rats. *Fund. Appl. Toxicol.* 29:280–286.

4. **Anderson, E. E., B. Anderson, Jr., and B. S. Nashold.** 1971. Childhood complications of nalidixic acid. *JAMA* 216:1023–1024.

5. **Ball, P., L. Mandell, Y. Niki, and G. Tillotson.** 1999. Comparative tolerability of the newer fluoroquinolone antibacterials. *Drug Safety* 21:407–421.

6. **Bednarczyk, E. M., J. A. Green, A. D. Nelson, G. P. Leisure, D. Little, L. P. Adler, M. S. Berridge, E. A. Panacek, and F. D. Miraldi.** 1992. Comparative assessment of the effect of lomefloxacin, ciprofloxacin, and placebo on cerebral blood flow, and glucose and oxygen metabolism in healthy subjects by positron emission tomography. *Pharmacotherapy* 12:370–375.

7. **Borus, L. O., and B. Sundström.** 1967. Intracranial hypertension in a child during treatment with nalidixic acid. *Br. Med. J.* 2:744–745.

8. **Bowie, W. R., V. Willetts, and P. J. Jeweson.** 1989. Adverse reactions in a dose-ranging study with a new long-acting fluoroquinolone, fleroxacin. *Antimicrob. Agents Chemother.* 33:1778–1782.

9. **Cahal, D. A.** 1965. Reactions to nalidixic acid. *Br. Med. J.* 2:590.

10. **Christ, W.** 1990. Central nervous system toxicity of quinolones: human and animal findings. *J. Antimicrob. Chemother.* 26(Suppl. B):219–225.

11. **Davey, P. G., M. Charter, S. Kelly, T. R. K, Varma, I Jacobson, A. Freeman, E. Precious, and J. Lambert.** 1994.

Ciprofloxacin and sparfloxacin penetration into human brain tissue and their activity as antagonists of GABAA receptor of rat vagus nerve. *Antimicrob. Agents Chemother.* 38:356–1362.

12. **De Sarro, A., V. Cecchetti, V. Fravolini, F. Naccari, O. Tabarini, and G. De Sarro.** 1999. Effects of novel 6-desfluoroquinolones and classic quinolones on pentyleneterazole-induced seizures in mice. *Antimicrob. Agents Chemother.* 43:1729–1736.

13. **Domagala, J. M.** 1994. Structure-activity and structure-side-effects relationships for the quinolone antibacterials. *J. Antimicrob. Chemother.* 33:685–706.

14. **Fan-Harvard, P., V. Sanchorawala, J. Oh, E. M. Moser, and S. P. Smith.** 1994. Concurrent use of foscarnet and ciprofloxacin may increase the propensity for seizures. *Ann. Pharmacother.* 28:869–872.

15. **Finegold, S. M., L. G. Miller, D. Psnick, D. K. Patterson, and A. Davis.** 1967. Nalidixic acid: clinical and laboratory studies. *Antimicrob. Agents. Chemother.* 1966:189–197.

16. **Fischman, A. J., E. Livni, J. Babich, N. M. Alpert, Y-Y Liu, E. Thom, R. Cleeland, B. L. Prosser, J. A. Correia, H. W. Strauss, and R. H. Rubin.** 1993. Pharmacokinetics of [18F] fleroxacin in healthy human subjects studied by using positron emission tomography. *Antimicrob. Agents Chemother.* 37:2144–2152.

17. **Fisher, O. D.** 1967. Nalidixic acid and intracranial hypertension. *Br. Med. J.* 2:744–745.

18. **Gonzales, J. P., and I. M. Henwood.** Pefloxacin: a review of its antibacterial activity, pharmacokinetic properties and therapeutic use. *Drugs* 37:6628–668.

19. **Herrlin, K., M. Segerdahl, L. L. Gustafsson, and L. Kalso.** 2000. Methadone, ciprofloxacin, and adverse drug reactions. *Lancet* 356:2069–2070.

20. **Hori, S., J. Shimada, A. Saito, M. Matsuda, and T. Miyahara.** 1989. Comparison of the inhibitory effects of new quinolones on γ-aminobutyric acid receptor binding in the presence of antiinflammatory drugs. *Rev. Infect. Dis.* 11(Suppl. 5):S1397–S1398.

21. **Islam, M. A., and P. A. Davis.** 1965. Convulsion, hyperglycaemia, and glycosuria from overdose of nalidixic acid. *JAMA* 192:1100–1101.

22. **Karki, S. D., D. W. Bentley, and M. Raghavan.** 1990. Seizure with ciprofloxacin and theophylline combined therapy. *DICP* 24:595–596.

23. **Kawakami, J., K. Ohashi, K. Tamamoto, Y. Sawada, and T. Iga.** 1997. Effect of acute renal failure on neurotoxicity of enoxacin in rats. *Biol. Pharm. Bull.* 20:931–934.

24. **Kremer, L., M. Walton, and E. N. Wardle.** 1967. Nalidixic acid and intracranial hypertension. *Br. Med. J.* 4:488.

25. **Kucers, A., and N. McK. Bennett.** 1975. Nalidixic and oxolinic acids, p. 479–489. *In* A. Kucers, and N. M. Bennett (ed.), *The Use of Antibiotics*, 2nd ed. Wlliam Heinemann Medical Books Ltd., London, United Kingdom.

26. **Lipsky, B. A., and C. A. Baker.** 1999. Fluoroquinolone toxicity profiles: a review focusing on newer agents. *Clin. Infect. Dis.* 28:352–364.

27. **Lode, H.** 1999. Potential interactions of the extended-spectrum fluoroquinolones with the CNS. *Drug Safety* 21:123–135.

28. **Lor, E., and Y. Q. Liu.** 1994. Neurologic sequelae associated with foscarnet therapy. *Ann. Pharmacother.* 28:1035–1037.

29. **Matsuo, H., M. Ryu, A. Nagata, T. Uchida, J.-I. Kawakami, K. Yamamoto, T. Iga, and Y. Sawada.** 1998. Neurotoxicodynamics of the interaction between ciprofloxacin and foscarnet in mice. *Antimicrob. Agents Chemother.* 42:691–694.

30. Matuschka, P. R., and R. S. Vissing. 1995. Clinafloxacin-theophylline drug interactions. *Ann. Pharmacother.* **29:** 378–380.

31. Melvani, S., and B. R. Speed. 2000. Alatrofloxacin-induced seizures during slow intravenous infusion. *Ann. Pharmacother.* **34:**1017–1019.

32. Mizuno, J., S. Dugimoto, A. Kaneko, T. Tsutsui, N. Zushi, and K. Machida. 2001. Convulsions following the combination of single preoperative oral administration of enoxacin and single postoperative intravenous administration of flurbiprofen axetil. *Masui* **50:**425–428.

33. Murata, M., I. Tamai, H. Kato, O. Nagata, H. Kato, and A. Tsuji. 1999. Efflux transport of a new quinolone antibacterial agent, HSR-903, across the blood-brain barrier. *J. Pharmacol. Exp. Ther.* **290:**51–57.

34. Naora, K., N. Ichikawa, H. Hirano, and K. Iwamoto. 1999. Distribution of ciprofloxacin into the central nervous system in rats with acute renal or hepatic failure. *J. Pharm. Pharmacol.* **51:**609–616.

35. Nau, R, T. Schmidt, K. Kaye, J. L. Froula, and M. G. Tauber. 1995. Quinolone antibiotics in therapy of experimental pneumococcal meningitis in rabbits. *Antimicrob. Agents Chemother.* **39:**593–597.

36. Olsen, R. W. 1981. GABA-benzodiazepine-barbiturate receptor interactions. *J. Neurochem.* **37:**1–13.

37. Ooie, T., H. Suzuki, T. Terasaki, and Y. Sugiayma. 1996. Characterization of the transport properties of a quinolone antibiotic, fleroxacin, in rat choroid plexus. *Pharm. Res.* **13:**523–527.

38. Ostergaard, C., T. K. Sorensen, J.D. Knudsen, and N. Frimodt-Müller. 1998. Evaluation of moxifloxacin, a new 8-methoxyquinolone, for treatment of meningitis caused by a penicillin-resistant pneumococcus in rabbits. *Antimicrob. Agents Chemother.* **42:**1706–1712.

39. Sanchez, R. M., C. Wang, G. Gardner, L. Orlando, D. L. Tauck, P. A. Rosenber, E. Aizenman, and F. E. Jensen. 2000. Novel role for the NMDA receptor redox modulatory site in the pathophysiology of seizures. *J. Neurosci.* **20:**2409–2417.

40. Schlienger, R. G., C. Wyser, R. Ritz, and W. E. Haefeli. 1996. Clinico-pharmacological case (4). Epileptic seizure as an unwanted drug effect on theophylline poisoning. *Schweiz. Rundsch. Med. Prax.* **85:**1407–1412.

41. Schmuck, G., A. Schurmann, and G. Schlüter. 1998. Determination of the excitatory potencies of fluoroquinolones in the central nervous system by and in vitro model. *Antimicrob. Agents Chemother.* **42:**1831–1836.

42. Semel, J. D., and N. Allen. 1991. Seizures in patients simultaneously receiving theophylline and imipenem or ciprofloxacin or metronidazole. *South. Med. J.* **84:**465–468.

43. Smirnov, A., A. Wellmer, J. Gerber, K. Maier, S. Henne, and R. Nau. 2000. Gemifloxacin is effective in experimental pneumococcal meningitis. *Antimicrob. Agents Chemother.* **44:**767–770.

44. Stahlmann, R., and H. Lode. 1999. Toxicity of quinolones. *Drugs* **58**(Suppl. 2):37–42.

45. Teng, R., S. C. Harris, D. E. Nix, J. J. Schentag, G. Foulds, and T. E. Liston. 1995. Pharmacokinetics and safety of trovafloxacin (CP-99,219), a new quinolone antibiotic, following administration of single oral doses to healthy male volunteers. *J. Antimicrob. Chemother.* **36:**385–394.

46. Thomson, A. H., G. D. Thomson, M. Hepburn, and B. Whiting. 1987. A clinically significant interaction between ciprofloxacin and theophylline. *Eur. J. Clin. Pharmacol.* **33:**435–436.

47. Tsuji, A., H. Sato, Y. Kume, J. Tamai, E. Okezaki, O. Nagata, and H. Kato. 1988. Inhibitory effects of quinolone antibacterial agents on gamma-aminobutyric acid binding to receptor sites in rat brain membranes. *Antimicrob. Agents Chemother.* **32:**190–194.

48. Tsutomi, Y., K. Matsubayashi, and K, Akahane. 1994. Quantitation of GABAA receptor inhibition required for quinolone-induced convulsions in mice. *J. Antimicrob. Chemother.* **34:**737–746.

49. Williams, P. D., and D. R. Helton. 1991.The proconvulsive activity of quinolone antibiotics in an animal model. *Toxicol. Lett.* **52:**23–28.

Quinolone Antimicrobial Agents, 3rd ed.
Edited by David C. Hooper and Ethan Rubinstein
© 2003 ASM Press, Washington, D.C.

Chapter 30

Effects of Quinolones on the Immune System

LOWELL S. YOUNG

The immune system consists of a complex network of innate and adaptive host responses that defend the host against microbial invaders and the development of neoplastic processes. The cellular components of the innate immune system include neutrophils, macrophages, natural killer cells, and the cell types involved in the adaptive system including antibody-producing B cells and killer or activated T cells. Further investigative knowledge of immune responses at the molecular level reveals a highly evolved but often redundant network of inflammatory responses mediated by messenger molecules such as the cytokines and chemokines.

For several decades there has been considerable interest mounting in the effects of antimicrobial agents on components of the immune system. Some of the extensive review articles that have covered the subject during the past two decades are summarized in Table 1. In these reviews, quinolone agents have been evaluated both in vitro and in vivo. Because quinolone agents are rapidly bactericidal and bacteriolytic, one of the challenges of experimental systems, whether they be purely in vitro or involve animal and human testing, is segregating the effects of the direct antimicrobial effects of an agent versus the more subtle or complex effects on the immune system, which might manifest themselves over many hours or days and exert a global influence on the outcome of an infectious process. Other variables that must be noted are the range of dose responses of the agents evaluated (whether they are at therapeutic levels or at levels not realistically achieved during infection in vivo), and the measures of outcome of the infectious processes (e.g., host survival, in vivo hemodynamic changes, or levels of a microbe-derived antigen). Clearly, different experimental test systems and the variations in drug doses, timing of challenge, selection of challenge organisms (which can differ in virulence), inoculum size, and/or timing of a specific intervention will all influence outcomes. Thus, pin-pointing a specific nonantimicrobial effect of an agent like a quinolone that has clinical significance is challenging.

MECHANISM OF THE ANTIMICROBIAL EFFECT ON IMMUNE MECHANISMS

There are at least five mechanisms by which antimicrobial agents can affect the host–pathogen relationship besides a direct bacteriostatic/bactericidal effect on the microbe (Table 2) (4, 8, 15, 16, 26, 35). First, the agent can block adherence of the microbe to eukaryotic cells and thus limit colonization. Second, the agent can alter components of the innate and acquired immune systems. These include, for the former, phagocytosis by neutrophils and monocytes and, for the latter, production of humoral antibodies or triggered activation of the T-cell response. A third mechanism, and by far one of the most focused of recent research, is that the antimicrobial agent can influence the cytokine network and, specifically, its effector molecules. The fourth potential mode of action is by affecting elaboration of virulence factors by the microbial pathogen. This effect has been reported for agents that inhibit protein synthesis and specifically protein exotoxins (31). Finally, the fifth property is that the antimicrobial agent can affect immune mechanisms by virtue of some pharmacologic property that influences tissue delivery. This property per se might not be considered a direct effect on the immune system but since some antimicrobial agents achieve very high concentrations at localized sites within and outside of cells (monocyte/macrophage phagolysosomes for macrolide derivatives, and in the renal collecting system for other agents excreted primarily by the kidneys) and at these very high concentrations there may be immune effects not usually observed when tests are conducted at "physiologic" or serum concentrations.

Lowell S. Young • Kuzell Institute for Arthritis & Infectious Diseases, California Pacific Medical Center, San Francisco, CA 94115.

Table 1. General reviews of the effects of antimicrobial agents on immune responses

Year	Author(s)	Title	Reference
1982	Hauser and Remington	Effects of antibiotics on the immune response.	8
1989	Korzeniowski	Effects of antibiotics on the mammalian immune system.	15
1993	Rubinstein and Shalit	Effects of the quinolones on the immune system.	26
1996	Van Vlem et al.	Immunomodulating effects of antibiotics: literature review.	35
1998	Dalhoff	Interaction of quinolones with host parasite relationship.	4
2000	Labro	Interference of antibacterial agents with phagocyte functions: immunomodulation or "immuno-fairy tales"?	16

POTENTIAL MECHANISM: AN EFFECT ON ADHERENCE/COLONIZATION

Dalhoff has written a detailed review that includes a comprehensive summary of the reported effects of antimicrobial agents on eukaryotic cells (4). For quinolone agents the great majority of reports cited show a decreased binding of bacteria to eukaryotic cells with simultaneous exposure, although it must be acknowledged that a few exceptions to the usual observations were noted in Dalhoff's review. Cited in detail was a report (summarized in Table 3) that a quinolone, namely sparfloxacin, blocked binding of *Mycobacterium avium* complex organisms to cultured HT-29 intestinal mucosal cells. In this study reported by Bermudez and colleagues, sparfloxacin at dose-ranging concentrations of 0.5 to 7 μg/ml was used in concentrations easily achieved in the intralumenal fluid of the gastrointestinal tract (1). The MIC of the challenge organism for sparfloxacin was 8 μg/ml, and thus the concentrations used in this study were subinhibitory. Over a varying period of bacterial exposure to sparfloxacin, a significant decrease in binding or adherence ranging up to an excess of 90% was observed at the highest test concentration. At the time that this study was reported there was great interest in the potential application of quinolones such as sparfloxacin either to treat *M. avium* complex disease or prevent it in high-risk human populations with advanced AIDS. Not published in this report was a subsequent series of studies in which sparfloxacin was used in the beige mouse model of *M. avium* disease. It was successful in significantly preventing systemic or bacteremic *M. avium* infection, thus validating the *in vitro* observations published. Nonetheless, a small human pilot study using sparfloxacin was inconclusive with respect to a therapeutic benefit in proven *M. avium* complex bacteremia (37). The conclusions from this limited experimental (murine) and human trial was that a quinolone such as sparfloxacin was not sufficiently promising to initiate further studies of the treatment of established *M. avium* disease in humans but was worthy of further clinical investigation as a prophylactic agent for *M. avium* disease that might develop via the gastrointestinal route.

QUINOLONE IMPACT ON COMPONENTS OF INNATE AND ACQUIRED IMMUNITY

Table 4 summarizes some of the published studies of Roszkowski et al. (25) and Riesbeck et al. (24). Comparator agents such as clindamycin had no effect on humoral or cellular responses, and cefotaxime, mezlocillin, and amikacin had modest suppressive effects. In contrast, ciprofloxacin and ofloxacin had modest effects in boosting both humoral and cellular immunity. There was no clear-cut impact of these agents on phagocytosis: the effect with regard to phagocytic cell–microbe interactions was in modifying the bacterial cell surface and thus facilitating uptake by the phagocyte (2, 5). The Roszkowski work included studies performed in BALB/c mice and thus had in vivo experimental support. Because of the large doses of drug used for the experimental animals, the results had uncertain clinical relevance.

A quinolone such as ciprofloxacin did appear to modulate cytokine gene expression, as reported by Riesbeck et al. (24). Hyperinduction of interleukin-2 (IL-2) might be expected to expand the pool of lym-

Table 2. Five mechanisms by which antibiotics affect host–parasite relationships besides bactericidal/static properties

1. Reduce adherence/colonization to eukaryotic cells.
2. Affect components of innate and acquired immunity (e.g., phagocytosis, humoral antibodies).
3. Modulate the cytokine network and its effector molecules.
4. Affect virulence-factor elaboration by microbes.
5. Influence tissue delivery by pharmacologic properties.

Table 3. A quinolone, sparfloxacin, blocks binding of *M. avium* complex organisms to HT-19 intestinal mucosal cells[a]

Sparfloxacin concn (µg/ml)	Time to exposure to antibiotic	% Decrease[b]
0.5	30 min	0
	1 h	16.2
	2 h	51.3*
1	30 min	13.5
	1 h	76.7*
	2 h	86.6*
	30 min	62.1*
	1 h	81.3*
	2 h	93.8*

[a] Adapted from Bermudez et al. (1).
[b] Asterisk indicates $P = 0.05$. Sparfloxacin MIC, 8 µg/ml.

phoid cells, as IL-2 was initially described as T-cell growth factor. Some investigators have shown some effect of quinolones on myelopoiesis, but other studies have not shown a long-term effect on maturation of murine bone marrow (29).

With regard to delayed hypersensitivity or cell-mediated immune mechanisms, various quinolones at concentrations exceeding 50 µg/ml inhibited thymidine uptake by stimulated thymocytes (26). Lymphocyte growth and cell cycle progression from resting phase to DNA synthesis appear to be inhibited by quinolones at concentrations exceeding 20 µg/ml (6, 7). At therapeutic concentrations, however, quinolones have either no effect or a minor inhibitory effect on lymphocyte proliferation in vitro, whereas the higher concentrations are inhibitory for lymphocyte growth in vitro. The clinical relevance of such work is unclear, although one study in mice showed suppressive effects of some quinolones on cell-mediated immunity (11)

All of the results noted above should be interpreted with major reservations, because no comparisons with healthy subjects receiving ofloxacin or ciprofloxacin with infected patients given control antimicrobial compounds have been undertaken and reported. In that light, very few studies have prospectively evaluated the impact of new quinolones on

Table 4. Effect of components of innate and acquired immunity[a]

Drug	Humoral	Cellular
Ciprofloxacin	++	+
Ofloxacin	++	+
Clindamycin	NE	NE
Cefotaxime	−	−
Mezlocillin	−	−
Amikacin	−	−

[a] Adapted from references 24 and 25. Symbols: +, degree of stimulation on a scale of 4; −, degree of suppression on a scale of 4; NE, no effect.

immunoglobulin production or function. Some studies have reported that ciprofloxacin and ofloxacin at clinically achievable concentrations have little or no impact on production of immunoglobulins G and M (26). Given the long half-lives of these immunoglobulins in the circulation, to observe an effect in humans it may be postulated that the duration of exposure would have to be in the order of weeks.

IMPACT OF QUINOLONES ON THE CYTOKINE NETWORK AND ITS EFFECTOR MOLECULES

The explosion in knowledge about immune responses is related, in part, to a better understanding of the complex molecular signals generated when secretory cells of the reticuloendothelial system, particularly monocytes and macrophages, have been studied for cytokine generation. In order of their discovery, the interferons and in particular gamma interferon (IFN-γ), tumor necrosis factor alpha (TNF-α), and the major interleukins have been evaluated in vitro and to a lesser extent in vivo. In particular, IFN-γ and TNF-α have critical roles in immune responses with an impact on activation of macrophages, T cells, natural killer cells, and γδ T cells. The cytokine network clearly influences humoral immune response such as the triggering of immunoglobulin production. It has been known for some time that therapeutic concentrations of quinolones suppress hematopoietic stem cells in the presence of low doses of TNF-α (26). At high doses of ofloxacin, ciprofloxacin, and pefloxacin (25 to 100 µg/ml) increased TNF-α elaboration from cultured cells was observed. Similarly, quinolones have been reported to trigger increased elaboration of IL-2 (24). In contrast, other studies have shown a decrease in cytokine-induced effects when mononuclear cells are exposed to bacteria or bacterial products in the presence of quinolone (14, 22, 32). Using extremely large doses of triggering agents for TNF-α release, a series of studies has been reported by Remington and colleagues. The experimental test system is a murine challenge model in which death induced by administration of large doses of lipopolysaccharide (LPS) can be prevented by simultaneous administration of various quinolone agents (13, 14). Table 5 summarizes the results reported using a challenge of 1 mg of *Escherichia coli* 0111:B4 LPS, an LD100 in mice for the challenge toxin. As indicated, animals were pretreated 47, 17, and 1 h prior to the lethal endotoxin challenge by the fluoroquinolone administered orally at very large doses shown in milligrams per kilogram of body weight (adapted from reference 13). Survival varied from between 67 and 75% and was significant even when the quinolone was administered 1 h prior to endotoxin challenge (a time which in the murine subject should be sufficient for adequate absorption of very high concentrations of quinolone orally). In the studies summarized in Table 5, the investigators demonstrated that a quinolone significantly reduced levels of IL-6 and TNF-α in the serum of these LPS-challenged mice. In vitro studies with trovafloxacin showed suppressed in vitro synthesis of IL-1α, IL-1β, IL-6, IL-10, and granulocyte-macrophage colony-stimulating factor in addition to TNF-α (14). A less detailed study in vitro, but concordant with the preceding results was reported for grepafloxacin (21). The mechanism of grepafloxacin's effect on TNF-α production, as well as IL-1α, IL-1β, IL-6, and IL-8, was felt to be inhibition of gene transcription.

Interpretation of the preceding in vivo studies is difficult because of the extremely large concentrations of challenge endotoxin (a dose that would be clearly lethal for human subjects) and the administration of the "protective" antibiotic or quinolone 1 to 47 h before the endotoxin challenge. Nonetheless, numerous experimental studies of modern interventions for sepsis, including one that has been approved by the U.S. Food and Drug Administration, have used challenge models that involve pretreatment or simultaneous administration of the protective agent and the lethal challenge. Identifying the underlying mechanism of the protection is more complex. If quinolones indeed impair the generation of large concentrations of shock- and death-inducing cytokines, what are the "true" effector molecules that might be triggered? LPS clearly has effects on the cardiovascular system triggering shock and death. A study of patients with cirrhosis suggested that nitric oxide is an effector molecule for the cytokine-mediated vasodilatory effects (36). Nitric oxide (NO) appears to drive the immune system in many ways, so its suppression by quinolones may be synergistic with antibacterial activities. Nitric oxide is a vasodilator in cirrhotic humans (consistent with a cytokine-triggered NO-mediated effect on cardiovascular function as "endothelial relaxing factor").

Thus, the ability of a quinolone to protect against shock and death in an animal test system may be due to the quinolone's ability to antagonize NO-mediated effects on the cardiovascular system. No data, however, are yet available to support this hypothesis.

FURTHER SUGGESTIVE STUDIES WITH INTRA-ABDOMINAL INFECTION AND THE IMPACT OF QUINOLONES ON CARDIOVASCULAR HEMODYNAMIC RESPONSES

Nitsche et al. (20) evaluated the impact of ciprofloxacin in comparison with cefotaxime, imipenem, gentamicin, control animals, and sham-operated animals in an intra-abdominal model of antimicrobial and endotoxin activity. In this test system, Wistar rats were inoculated with 10^7 CFU of E. coli per kg and then treated with the antimicrobial. Plasma endotoxin levels, quantitative bacteremia counts, and mean arterial pressures were subsequently measured for 5 h. The highest endotoxin levels were measured after cefotaxime treatment, whereas the lowest endotoxin levels, as determined by the limulus gelation assay, were in plasma of animals given high-dose ciprofloxacin. The lowest quantitative blood counts of bacteria were measured following treatment with the two bactericidal agents, imipenem and ciprofloxacin. At almost the same time, Prins and colleagues (22) examined different antimicrobial agents for endotoxin-releasing properties. One of the hypotheses tested was that specific antimicrobial structures can influence the speed of defervescence following the initiation of therapy. The conclusion of such studies was that indeed different antimicrobial agents have different effects on such host responses. Furthermore, in one of the relatively few human studies reported to date, imipenem and ceftazidime, with 15 patients treated each who had the clinical diagnosis of Gram-negative bacillary urosepsis were randomized to receive either imipenem or ceftazidime (23). Following the initiation of treatment, 3 of the 15 given imipenem had measurable decreases in LPS levels (as demonstrated by limulus gelation). In contrast, two of four patients given ceftazidime had an increase in LPS levels. The remaining subjects in each group had no measurable endotoxin levels by the technique used. The number of patients studied in this human trial was clearly inadequate, and no conclusions can be drawn until a similar, statistically valid human trial is undertaken. Of interest, however, is another study of LPS release using the limulus assay following ceftazidime or imipenem therapy of meliodosis (28). In the 64 subjects studied, endotoxin levels were 10-fold greater in those treated with ceftazidime than in those

Table 5. *E. coli* 0111:B4 challenge of 1 mg LPS (LD$_{100}$)[a]

P.O. Pre-Rx (× 47, 17, 1 h (before) with:	Survival (%)
Ciprofloxacin (250 mg/kg)	25–30+
Trovafloxacin (100–200 mg/kg)	67–75+
Tosufloxacin (100–200 mg/kg)	30–50

[a] Adapted from reference 13. Sign significance: ↑, survival with even 1 h prechallenge administration of quinolone; +, survival of 25 to 30% even if the fluoroquinolone is administered postchallenge.

given imipenem ($P = 0.008$). An explanation for the differences observed between ceftazidime and imipenem is that they target different penicillin-binding proteins: PBP III for ceftazidime and for PBP IIa imipenem (10). Broad-spectrum cephalosporins appear to cause filimentation and lysis of bacteremia, whereas imipenem results in spheroplast formation. Quinolones also cause filimentation, but their lethal effects are exerted with less LPS release.

QUINOLONES AND GRAM-POSITIVE INFECTIONS

The intriguing data on fluoroquinolone impact on endotoxin-mediated gram-negative bacillary infections has been extended, in principle, to gram-positive infectious processes. With gram-positive organisms the important cell wall components are not LPS but lipoteichoic acid (LTA) peptidoglycan, and teichoic acid (33). Several studies have reported that components of gram-positive coccal cell walls, comparable with the effects of LPS, induce inflammation and the release of TNF-α, IL-1β, and IL-6 (32, 34). Peptidoglycan, teichoic acid, and LTA stimulate human monocytes to release cytokines. The parallels with LPS induction are obvious and, in the treatment of infection, it is clear that limiting the growth or actual lysis and death of bacteria are a critical goal. How it may be accomplished by different antimicrobial agents could affect the disease process or its sequelae. In studies in which *Streptococcus pneumoniae* was exposed to ceftriaxone, meropenem, rifampin, quinupristin, and trovafloxacin, rapid release of LTA and teichoic acid occurred after exposure to β-lactam compounds such as ceftriaxone and meropenem. Trovafloxacin, in contrast, triggered slow release of these two moieties (32). In the well-known rabbit pneumococcal meningitis model (27), LTA release was significantly different between treatment with ceftriaxone and moxifloxacin (27). At 1 and 3 h, respectively, there was a 5-to 6-fold difference in LTA concentrations measured in the cerebral spinal fluid, but by 12 h, no significant difference was noted. It appears that similar quantities of LTA are ultimately released, but the rate of release is significantly slower with moxifloxacin, during an interval when it is exerting a potent bactericidal effect. Similarly, trovafloxacin delayed the antibiotic-induced inflammatory response in experimental pneumococcal meningitis (19). If bacterial product release is directly related to the sequelae of infections (i.e., complications of the disease process such as meningeal scarring, deafness, loss of neurologic function), then the impairment of microbial product release could well have clinical importance.

Overall, the studies of cytokine generation by bacterial products and their influence by the class of antimicrobial agents (quinolone versus β-lactam) has several themes. Many, but not necessarily all, β-lactam agents kill via a lytic process that has been strikingly illustrated. High levels of microbial product release in comparison with levels measured after quinolone treatment are observed. Bacterial products will affect the cytokine response, and excessive quantities of these cytokines may be deleterious to the host. An argument in favor of quinolone usage may be that, initially at least, the cytokine response network in gram-positive and gram-negative bacterial infections may be dampened and less damage to the host may ensue.

AN IMPACT BUT MECHANISM UNKNOWN

A plethora of quinolone effects on specific components of the immune response have been reviewed. Nonetheless, some investigators have been sufficiently candid to note that overall in vivo responses can be measured, but specific mechanisms cannot pinpointed. Perhaps these studies were done at a time when newer technologies for dissecting immune responses and their triggers were not fully elucidated or at least were less well explained in comparison with more contemporary research. As reviewed by Stevens, the quinolone, rufloxacin, increased microbicidal activity against *Klebsiella pneumoniae* in both in vitro and ex vivo test systems (30). Nonetheless, a major methodologic problem exists when the antibacterial agent kills the invading bacterium and at the same time enhances host defense; segregating these properties has proved challenging. Thus, in the study cited (3) a further series of experiments included murine challenge using *Candida albicans*. Rufloxacin markedly improved survival from 5.5% in the placebo-treated animals to 87.5% in the treated group, a dramatic and significant difference. A challenge consisted of 10^9 CFU of the *Candida* organism that clearly was resistant to rufloxacin. While the overall differences were impressive, no specific mechanism for this protection was demonstrated, and one conclusion is that this particular quinolone agent augmented nonspecific host defense mechanisms irrespective of direct antimicrobial effect (3, 30).

THE NEED FOR HYPOTHESIS-TESTING EXPERIMENTS AND HUMAN TRIALS

Despite the plethora of studies cited in Table 1 and reviewed in this chapter, the impact of quinolone agents on the immune response and thus on the outcome of human disease states remains unclear. Rather than pointing out the deficiencies of published studies, one might focus on how best to evaluate the intriguing information that has already been published and improve the design of future studies.

In animal challenge models, one can easily test the concept that a bacterial product release (cytokine modulation) is favorably affected by antimicrobial agents such as a quinolone. An appropriate challenge should include a potentially lethal gram-negative or gram-positive pathogen. Quinolone-susceptible and high-level quinolone-resistant challenge organisms could be compared. Additionally, high and low doses of quinolone drug- and treatment-appropriate controls (other sham treatment and antibacterial agents) would clearly have to be used. The outcomes to be measured would include animal survival, measurement of blood pressure, circulating bacterial products, and cytokine levels in the animal host. A quinolone dose response and appropriate antibiotic controls or comparators would clearly be necessary and these studies assume that quinolone-susceptible and quinolone-resistant bacteria are equally virulent. Doses of drug used for animal challenge should result in body fluid and tissue comparable with those observed in humans.

To test the hypothesis that quinolone "nonantimicrobial" effects on humans make a difference, an empiric therapy setting would have to be selected realistically. These situations would include individuals prone to febrile neutropenia or a similarly defined group at high risk for bacterial disease with postsurgical complications or severe trauma. An intravenous quinolone such as levofloxacin, gatifloxacin, or moxifloxacin could be compared with a β-lactam agent such as cefotaxime, ceftriaxone, or ceftazidime since the latter group have usually been associated usually with the higher levels of LPS or LTA release. The spectrum of the quinolones or of the β-lactams might be sufficiently inadequate to prompt inclusion of a common component of the initial regimen such as an aminoglycoside, at least for the first 3 days. In the human studies, outcomes such as blood pressure, the development of disseminated intravascular coagulation, acute respiratory distress syndrome, renal failure—common "organ failure" outcomes—would be measured, and survival plus rapidity of treatment response could be quantitated. Clearly, all-intravenous therapy regimens would be desirable in this setting. Other adjunctive therapies such as shock-modulating interventions (activated protein C) would have to be "normalized" or controlled for in such a large human trial.

CONCLUSIONS

It remains to be demonstrated that endotoxin- or LTA-iberating activities and marked endotoxin-neutralizing abilities due to dampening of cytokine effects of agents like quinolones contribute to a positive clinical outcome. Downregulation of cytokine responses has also been noted for other antimicrobial agents, including macrolides (9, 12, 17, 18). However, it does appear that quinolones can decrease adherence to various epithelial cells and may interfere with the early phase of infection. Quinolones block the amount or inhibit synthesis of endotoxin and exoproducts, thus reducing their deleterious effects in experimental infection. They are potently bactericidal against susceptible bacteria in all phases of growth. Thus, the effects on the immune system appear to be generally positive and the significance of these effects can be established by appropriately designed animal and human studies.

REFERENCES

1. Bermudez, L. E., L. S. Young, and C. B. Inderlied. 1994. Rifabutin and sparfloxacin but not azithromycin inhibit binding of *Mycobacterium avium* complex to HT-29 intestinal mucosal cells. Antimicrob. Agents Chemother. 38:1200–1202.
2. Boogaerts, M. A., S. Malbrain, W. Scheers, and R. L. Verwilghen. 1986. Effects of quinolones on granulocyte function *in vitro*. Infection 4:258–262.
3. Cuffini, A. M., V. Tullio, A. Allocco, G. Paizis, C. De Leo, and N. A. Carlone. 1994. Effect of rufloxacin upon non-specific immune defences: in-vitro, ex- vivo and in-vivo results. *J. Antimicrob. Chemother.* 34:545–553.
4. Dalhoff, A. 1998. Interaction of quinolones with host-parasite relationship, p. 233–257. *In* J. Kuhlmann, A. Dalhoff, and H.-J. Zeiler (ed.), *Handbook of Experimental Pharmacology*, vol. 127. Springer-Verlag, Berlin, Germany.
5. Forsgren, A., and P. I. Bergkvist. 1985. Effect of ciprofloxacin on phagocytosis. *Eur. J. Clin. Microbiol.* 4:575–578.
6. Forsgren, A., S. F. Schlossman, and T. F. Tedder. 1987. 4-Quinolone drugs affect cell cycle progression and function of human lymphocytes in vitro. *Antimicrob. Agents Chemother.* 31:768–773.
7. Gollapudi, S. V., R. H. Prabhala, and H. Thadepalli. 1986. Effect of ciprofloxacin on mitogen-stimulated lymphocyte proliferation. *Antimicrob. Agents Chemother.* 29:337–338.
8. Hauser, W. E., Jr., and J. S. Remington. 1982. Effect of antibiotics on the immune response. *Am. J. Med.* 72:711–716.
9. Ichiyama, T., M. Nishikawa, T. Yoshitomi, S. Hasegawa, T. Matsubara, T. Hayashi, and S. Furukawa. 2001. Clarithromycin inhibits NF-kappaB activation in human peripheral blood mononuclear cells and pulmonary epithelial cells. *Antimicrob. Agents Chemother.* 45:44–47.
10. Jackson, J. J., and H. Kropp. 1992. beta-Lactam antibiotic-induced release of free endotoxin: *in vitro* comparison of penicillin-binding protein (PBP) 2-specific imipenem and PBP 3-specific ceftazidime. *J. Infect. Dis.* 165:1033–1041.

11. Jimenez-Valera, M., A. Sampedro, E. Moreno, and A. Ruiz-Bravo. 1995. Modification of immune response in mice by ciprofloxacin. *Antimicrob. Agents Chemother.* **39:**150–154.

12. Khan, A. A., T. R. Slifer, F. G. Araujo, and J. S. Remington. 1999. Effect of clarithromycin and azithromycin on production of cytokines by human monocytes. *Int. J. Antimicrob. Agents* **11:**121–132.

13. Khan, A. A., T. R. Slifer, F. G. Araujo, Y. Suzuki, and J. S. Remington. 2000. Protection against lipopolysaccharide-induced death by fluoroquinolones. *Antimicrob. Agents Chemother.* **44:**3169–3173.

14. Khan, A. A., T. R. Slifer, and J. S. Remington. 1998. Effect of trovafloxacin on production of cytokines by human monocytes. *Antimicrob. Agents Chemother.* **42:**1713–1717.

15. Korzeniowski, O. M. 1989. Effects of antibiotics on the mammalian immune system. *Infect. Dis. Clin. N. Am.* **3:**469–478.

16. Labro, M. T. 2000. Interference of antibacterial agents with phagocyte functions: immunomodulation or "immuno-fairy tales"? *Clin. Microbiol. Rev.* **13:**615–650.

17. Morikawa, K., F. Oseko, S. Morikawa, and K. Iwamoto. 1994. Immunomodulatory effects of three macrolides, midecamycin acetate, josamycin, and clarithromycin, on human T-lymphocyte function in vitro. *Antimicrob. Agents Chemother.* **38:**2643–2647.

18. Morikawa, K., H. Watabe, M. Araake, and S. Morikawa. 1996. Modulatory effect of antibiotics on cytokine production by human monocytes *in vitro*. *Antimicrob. Agents Chemother.* **40:**1366–1370.

19. Nau, R., G. Zysk, H. Schmidt, F. R. Fischer, A. K. Stringaris, K. Stuertz, and W. Bruck. 1997. Trovafloxacin delays the antibiotic-induced inflammatory response in experimental pneumococcal meningitis. *J. Antimicrob. Chemother.* **39:**781–788.

20. Nitsche, D., C. Schulze, S. Oesser, A. Dalhoff, and M. Sack. 1996. Impact of different classes antimicrobial agents on plasma endotoxin activity. *Arch. Surg.* **131:**192–199.

21. Ono, Y., Y. Ohmoto, K. Ono, Y. Sakata, and K. Murata. 2000. Effect of grepafloxacin on cytokine production in vitro. *J. Antimicrob. Chemother.* **46:**91–94.

22. Prins, J. M., E. J. Kuijper, M. L. Mevissen, P. Speelman, and S. J. van Deventer. 1995. Release of tumor necrosis factor alpha and interleukin 6 during antibiotic killing of Escherichia coli in whole blood: influence of antibiotic class, antibiotic concentration, and presence of septic serum. *Infect. Immun.* **63:**2236–2242.

23. Prins, J. M., M. A. van Agtmael, E. J. Kuijper, S. J. van Deventer, and P. Speelman. 1995. Antibiotic-induced endotoxin release in patients with gram-negative urosepsis: a double-blind study comparing imipenem and ceftazidime. *J. Infect. Dis.* **172:**886–891.

24. Riesbeck, K., J. Andersson, M. Gullberg, and A. Forsgren. 1989. Fluorinated 4-quinolones induce hyperproduction of interleukin 2. *Proc. Natl. Acad. Sci. USA.* **86:**2809–2813.

25. Roszkowski, W., H. L. Ko, K. Roszkowski, P. Ciborowski, J. Jeljaszewicz, and G. Pulverer. 1986. Effects of ciprofloxacin on the humoral and cellular immune responses in Balb/c-mice. *Zentbl. Bakteriol. Mikrobiol. Hyg. Ser. A* **262:**396–402.

26. Rubinstein, E., and I. Shalit. 1993. Effects of the quinolones on the immune system, p. 519–526. *In* D. C. Hooper and J. S. Wolfson (ed.), *Quinolone Antimicrobial Agents*, 2nd ed. American Society for Microbiology, Washington, D.C.

27. Schmidt, H., A. Dalhoff, K. Stuertz, F. Trostdorf, V. Chen, O. Schneider, C. Kohlsdorfer, W. Bruck, and R. Nau. 1998. Moxifloxacin in the therapy of experimental pneumococcal meningitis. *Antimicrob. Agents Chemother.* **42:**1397–1407.

28. Simpson, A. J., S. M. Opal, B. J. Angus, J. M. Prins, J. E. Palardy, N. A. Parejo, W. Chaowagul, and N. J. White. 2000. Differential antibiotic-induced endotoxin release in severe melioidosis. *J. Infect. Dis.* **181:**1014–1019.

29. Somekh, E., S. West, A. Barzilai, and E. Rubinstein. 1989. The lack of long-term suppressive effect of ciprofloxacin on murine bone marrow. *J. Antimicrob. Chemother.* **24:**209–213.

30. Stevens, D. L. 1996. Immune modulatory effects of antibiotics. *Curr. Opin. Infect. Dis.* **9:**165–169.

31. Stevens, D. L., A. E. Bryant, and S. P. Hackett. 1995. Antibiotic effects on bacterial viability, toxin production, and host response. *Clin. Infect. Dis.* **20**(Suppl. 2):S154–S157.

32. Stuertz, K., H. Schmidt, H. Eiffert, P. Schwartz, M. Mader, and R. Nau. 1998. Differential release of lipoteichoic and teichoic acids from *Streptococcus pneumoniae* as a result of exposure to beta-lactam antibiotics, rifamycins, trovafloxacin, and quinupristin-dalfopristin. *Antimicrob. Agents Chemother.* **42:**277–281.

33. Tuomanen, E., H. Liu, B. Hengstler, O. Zak, and A. Tomasz. 1985. The induction of meningeal inflammation by components of the pneumococcal cell wall. *J. Infect. Dis.* **151:**859–868.

34. van Langevelde, P., J. T. van Dissel, E. Ravensbergen, B. J. Appelmelk, I. A. Schrijver, and P. H. Groeneveld. 1998. Antibiotic-induced release of lipoteichoic acid and peptidoglycan from *Staphylococcus aureus*: quantitative measurements and biological reactivities. *Antimicrob. Agents Chemother.* **42:**3073–3078.

35. Van Vlem, B., R. Vanholder, P. De Paepe, D. Vogelaers, and S. Ringoir. 1996. Immunomodulating effects of antibiotics: literature review. *Infection* **24:**275–291.

36. Yokokawa, K., R. Mankus, M. G. Saklayen, M. Kohno, K. Yasunari, M. Minami, H. Kano, T. Horio, T. Takeda, and A. K. Mandel. 1995. Increased nitric oxide production in patients with hypotension during hemodialysis. *Ann. Intern. Med.* **123:**35–37.

37. Young, L. S., M. Wu, and J. Bender. 1992. Pilot study of sparfloxacin for *M. avium* complex bacteremia complicating AIDS. *In Program and Abstracts of the 37th Interscience Conference on Antimicrobial Agents and Chemotherpy.* American Society for Microbiology, Washington, D.C.

INDEX